FOURTH EDITION

PHYSICAL MEDICINE AND REHABILITATION

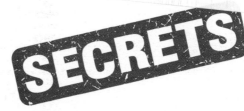

SECRETS

BRYAN J. O'YOUNG, MD, CAc, FAAPMR
Professor and Vice Chair of Education, Department of
    Physical Medicine and Rehabilitation, Lewis Katz
    School of Medicine at Temple University, Philadelphia,
    Pennsylvania, United States
Chief of Outpatient Service, Department of Physical
    Medicine and Rehabilitation, Temple University Health
    System, Philadelphia, Pennsylvania, United States
Clinical Professor, Department of Rehabilitation Medicine,
    New York University Grossman School of Medicine,
    Rusk Rehab at NYU Langone Health, New York, New
    York, United States
Adjunct Clinical Professor, Department of Rehabilitation
    Medicine, Weill Medical College of Cornell University,
    NY Presbyterian Hospital, Weill Cornell Medical Center,
    New York, New York, United States
Adjunct Professor of Rehabilitation Medicine, University of
    the Philippines College of Medicine, Manila, Philippines
Visiting Professor, Department of Rehabilitation Medicine,
    Peking University First Hospital, Peking University
    School of Medicine, Beijing, China
Visiting Professor, Department of Rehabilitation Medicine,
    Sun-Yat Sen University First Hospital, Sun-Yat
    Sen University College of Medicine, Guangzhou,
    Guangdong, China

MARK A. YOUNG, MD, MBA, FACP, FAAPMR, DABPMR
Chair, Department of Physical Medicine & Rehabilitation,
    The Workforce & Technology Center (WTC), The
    Maryland Vocational Rehabilitation Center, State of
    Maryland, Division of Rehabilitation Services (DORS),
    Maryland State Department of Education (MSDE),
    Baltimore, Maryland, United States
Faculty, The Johns Hopkins School of Medicine, Department
    of PM&R, Baltimore, Maryland, United States
Site Director, WTC Vocational Rehabilitation Rotation, Sinai
    Hospital/University of Maryland School of Medicine PM&R
    Residency Program, Baltimore, Maryland, United States
Adjunct Clinical Associate Professor, Department of
    Rehabilitation Medicine, New York University Grossman
    School of Medicine, New York, New York, United States
Professor, Department of Orthopedic Sciences, New York
    College of Podiatric Medicine, New York, New York,
    United States

STEVEN A. STIENS, MD, MS
Curator of Education, Innovated Solutions, Stiens'
    Designs: Personal Enablement, Seattle, Washington,
    United States
Adjunct Clinical Professor, Department of Physical Medicine
    and Rehabilitation, Geisinger Commonwealth School of
    Medicine, Scranton, Pennsylvania, United States

SAM S. H. WU, MD, MA, MPH, MBA
Professor of Clinical Physical Medicine and Rehabilitation,
    Lewis Katz School of Medicine, Temple University,
    Philadelphia, Pennsylvania, United States
Chair of Department of Physical Medicine and
    Rehabilitation, Lewis Katz School of Medicine, Temple
    University, Philadelphia, Pennsylvania, United States
Chief of Service, Department of Physical Medicine and
    Rehabilitation, Temple University Health System,
    Philadelphia, Pennsylvania, United States
Clinical Associate Professor, Department of Physical
    Medicine and Rehabilitation, Rutgers- New Jersey
    Medical School, Newark, New Jersey, United States
Editor-In-Chief, Physiatry Forward, Association of Academic
    Physiatrists, Owings Mills, Maryland, United States
Editor, PM&R Knowledge NOW, American Academy of
    Physical Medicine and Rehabilitation, Rosemont, Illinois,
    United States
Member, Guidelines Development Group, WHO Wheelchair
    Service Guidelines, World Health Organization, Geneva,
    Switzerland

ELSEVIER

Elsevier
1600 John F. Kennedy Blvd.
Ste 1800
Philadelphia, PA 19103-2899

Notice

Practitioners and researchers must always rely on their own experience and knowledge in evaluating
and using any information, methods, compounds, or experiments described herein. Because of rapid
advances in the medical sciences, in particular, independent verification of diagnoses and drug dosages
should be made. To the fullest extent of the law, no responsibility is assumed by Elsevier, authors,
editors, or contributors for any injury and/or damage to persons or property as a matter of products
liability, negligence or otherwise, or from any use or operation of any methods, products, instructions,
or ideas contained in the material herein.

Previous editions copyrighted 2008, 2002, 1997

Senior Content Strategist: Marybeth Thiel
Senior Content Development Specialist: Priyadarshini Pandey
Senior Project Manager: Umarani Natarajan
Publishing Services Manager: Deepthi Unni
Design Direction: Bridget Hoette

Printed in India

Last digit is the print number: 9 8 7 6 5 4 3 2 1

Working together
to grow libraries in
developing countries

www.elsevier.com • www.bookaid.org

To my beloved parents, Sutuan and Merla, for their lifelong love and inspiration.
To my loving and nurturing wife, Fangfang, for her commitment and unwavering support to our family.
To my young children, Aaron, Serena, and Lucas, for their unbridled energy, boundless affection, unceasing curiosity, and wholesome innocence that invigorates my spirit to embrace the moment.
To my siblings, Andrew, Crosby, Dorene, and Eldred, for their support and encouragement.
To my patients, for teaching me that purposeful living is an effective form of healing.
To my medical students, residents, and fellows, who allow me to participate in their educational journey and professional development.
To my teachers and mentors, particularly Dr. Joel DeLisa, Dr. Andrew Fischer, and Dr. Mathew Lee, whose wisdom guided my career.
To my colleagues at Temple University Health System and Lewis Katz School of Medicine for their steadfast commitment to education.
To my fellow editors, Dr. Mark A. Young, Dr. Steven A. Stiens, and Dr. Sam S. H. Wu, who taught me the values of enduring friendship.

Bryan J. O'Young, MD, CAc, FAAPMR

With much love and admiration, I dedicate this book to:
My dearly departed parents, Michael Z"L (a Polish/Ukrainian Holocaust survivor) and Rowena Z"L (a Great Depression survivor), whose shining example of hard work, sincerity and perseverance continue to inspire an unwavering commitment to diligence compassion and professionalism.
My wife, Marlene Malka, whose kindness, courageousness, and forbearance have supported my career and have nurtured our flourishing family, B"H.
To my gifted kids and their spouses, Michelle Shira and Dr. Yehuda Mond; Jennifer Yael and Chad Shapiro; Dr. Michael and Elyse (neé Vilinsky) Young.
My grandchildren: Azriel, Yehoshua, Yisroel, Shoshi Mond, and M'ayan Shapiro.
My brother Evan and sister-in-law Deborah, and my wonderful niece and nephews.
Those who have inspired my career and have led the path to clinical excellence and leadership in medicine: Dr. Jeff Palmer, Dr. Steve Kirshblum, Dr. Jerry Insel, Dr. Ben Carson, Dr. Ronald Rodriguez, Howard Rusk Jr. ("Rusty"), Ms. Jean Jackson, Dr. Maya Desai, Dr. Rhodora Tumanon, and Mr. Louis Levine.
The amazing folks who have provided spiritual sustenance and friendship throughout the years: R. Moshe Hauer, R. Uri Feldman, Mr. Ari Sigal, Dr. David Cassius, and Mr. Abe Rice.
My dearly departed mentors and friends: Dr. Stanley Kornhauser, Dr. Arthur Siebens, Professor Haim Ring, Dr. Andrew Fisher, Dr. Mathew Lee, Dr. Martin Grabois, Mr. Shmuel Chernitzky, Mr. Reggie Honeyblue, and Pr. Tom and Annie Otto.
All my treasured academic and clinical colleagues, including Dr. Bryan J. O' Young, Dr. Steve A. Stiens, Dr. Sam S. H. Wu, Dr. Eli Ehrenpreis, and Dr. Sam Kelman.
Above all, to my patients, residents, and staff, without whose inspiration this book could never have been written.

Mark. A. Young, MD, MBA, FACP, FAAPMR, DABPMR

"The bond that links your true family is not one of blood but of respect and joy in each other's life."
–Richard Bach

For my loving wife Beth (the preschool and special educator) and my children Hanna (the film writer), her husband Jesse McIntosh (the actor), Duffy (the building engineer), and our twins Olivia (the social work scholar) and Luke (the "sparking" Information technology engineer), all making life better for others!
To my parents, who continually develop me with their love, understanding, and direction. Jean (the psychiatrist, 1937–2005) and Bill (the designer and builder, 1927–2015) for their devotion to discovering and actualizing the self in service to others. To my two brothers, Scott (the world developer at the U.S. State Department) and Doug (the interior designer and apartment restorationist), for their vision, insights, implementation, and humor.
To James W. Little, MD, PhD (always have a hypothesis) for his generosity, instruction, and guidance here at University of Washington. To my home state of Ohio mentors: Randal Braddom, MD, MS (successfully adapt!), Earnie Johnson, MD (leadership begins with self-direction), Cart Rogers, PhD (make the client the center), George Engle, MD (the systems around the patient as well as those within responding to treatment), and Gustav Eckstein, MD (the body does have a head).

"In every conceivable manner, the family is a link to our past, bridge to our future."
–Alex Haley

Steven A. Stiens, MD, MS

To my father, Hsueh-Cheng Wu, and my mother, Hsing-Chu Wu, who have both passed on. Their resilience and sacrifices have carried our family across the vast ocean to America, where we have the opportunity to pursue the American Dream.

To my mother-in-law, Rose Tsang, who is always willing to lend a hand.

To my brothers, George Wu, Jen-Hua Wu, and Jan-Haur Wu, for their steadfast support, which enabled me to start the journey of an academic career.

To my patients who showed me how to be a better healer. To my students, residents, and fellows for allowing me to participate in their professional growth. To all my mentors and teachers, especially Dr. Joel DeLisa, Dr. John Melvin, Dr. Richard Salcido, Dr. Stanley Wainapel, Dr. Amy Goldberg, and Dr. Mathew Lee, whose wisdom has shaped my career. I have learned so much from all of them.

To my colleagues at Temple University Health System and the Lewis Katz School of Medicine at Temple University for their inspiration to achieve excellence.

To my fellow editors of this book, Dr. Bryan J. O'Young, Dr. Mark A. Young, and Dr. Steven A. Steins, for their friendship that transcends academia.

To my friends, Leroy Jenkins and Maurice Barnes, for grounding me in what is truly important.

To my children, Samantha Wu and Keefer Wu, who are the pride and joy of my life.

Most importantly, to my wife, Dr. Patricia Tsang, who is always there to help me get back up and who gives meaning to my life.

Sam S. H. Wu, MD, MA, MPH, MBA

A portion of the proceeds from this textbook is donated to Whirlwind Wheelchair International, which works to make it possible for every person in the developing world who needs a wheelchair to obtain one that will lead to maximum personal independence and integration into society. Go to www. whirlwindwheelchair.org

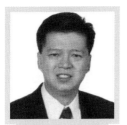

Dr. Bryan J. O'Young

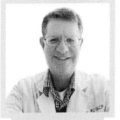

Dr. Mark A. Young

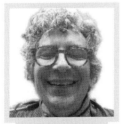

Dr. Steven A. Stiens

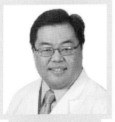

Dr. Sam S. H. Wu

The editors of PM&R Secrets (**Bryan, Mark, Steve, & Sam**) proudly dedicate this fourth edition of our book to People with Disabilities throughout the world and the United Nations.

The heartfelt essence of this dedication is proudly represented by the invocation of Akiko Ito, Chief of the United Nations Secretariat for the Convention on the Rights of Persons with Disabilities.

"We are deeply committed to the inclusion of persons with disabilities in all aspects of our society and development— We are losing out so much when we exclude more than 15% of the world's population. We recognize that persons with disabilities face challenges every single day, and their inclusion in society is taking place at a very slow pace—but it is finally making changes on the ground. Our mission is to accelerate this speed with our medical knowledge as a tool for empowerment.

Let us embrace human diversity to create an inclusive, accessible, and sustainable world for everyone."

The editors are particularly inspired by the passion and spirit displayed by Jean D' Amour (see accompanying photo).

Jean was born with congenital lower extremity deformities and received pediatric rehabilitation at the Gatagara Rehabilitation Center in Rwanda.

Through diligent work of the PM&R team, and the support of the Lilane Foundation, Jean learned to walk again and play soccer, enabling him to enjoy his childhood.

Photo Credit: Monique Velzeboer

LIST OF CONTRIBUTORS

Christopher S. Ahmad, MD
Head Team Physician New York Yankees, Center for
Shoulder, Elbow and Sports Medicine, New York
Presbyterian/Columbia University Medical Center,
New York, United States
Chief, Sports Medicine Service, Center for Shoulder,
Elbow and Sports Medicine, New York Presbyterian/
Columbia University Medical Center, New York,
New York
Vice Chair of Clinical Research, Center for Shoulder,
Elbow and Sports Medicine, New York Presbyterian/
Columbia University Medical Center, New York,
United States
Professor of Orthopedic Surgery, Center for Shoulder,
Elbow and Sports Medicine, New York Presbyterian/
Columbia University Medical Center, New York,
United States

Mindy Aisen, MD
Clinical Professor–Neurology, University of Southern
California, Los Angeles, California, United States

Jason Allen, ND, MPH
Adjunct Professor, Bastyr University, Private Practice,
Seattle, Washington, United States

Gad Alon, PhD, PT
Associate Professor, Emeritus, Physical Therapy and
Rehabilitation Service, University of Maryland, School
of Medicine, Baltimore, Maryland, United States

Ronit Aloni, PhD
Faculty of Medicine, ISHI Clinic, Tel-Aviv University,
Tel-Avi, Israel

Mayur Jayant Amin, MD
Associate, Wound Care/Physical Medicine &
Rehabilitation, Geisinger Medical Center, Danville,
Pennsylvania, United States

Cynthia D. Ang-Muñoz, MD, MSc, FPARM
Associate Professor, Department of Rehabilitation Medicine,
College of Medicine and Philippine General Hospital,
University of the Philippines Manila Manila, Philippines
Chairman, Department of Rehabilitation Medicine,
Chinese General Hospital and Medical Center Manila,
Philippines

Charles E. Argoff, MD
Professor, Department of Neurology, Albany Medical
College, Albany, New York, United States
Director, Comprehensive Pain Center, Albany Medical
Center, New York, New York, United States

Levi (Levan) Atanelov, MD, MS
Adjunct Assistant Professor, Department of Physical
Medicine and Rehabilitation, Johns Hopkins School of
Medicine, Steady Strides: Fall Prevention and Stroke
Rehabilitation Medical Institute, Baltimore, Maryland,
United States

Rita Ayyangar, MD
Clinical Professor, Physical Medicine and Rehabilitation,
University of Michigan, Ann Arbor, Michigan,
United States

John R. Bach, MD
Professor of PM&R, Professor of Neurology, Physical
Medicine and Rehabilitation, Rutgers University NJMS,
Newark, New Jersey, United States

Miroslav "Misha" Bačkonja, MD
Acting Clinical Director, Division of Intramural Research
Supervisory Physician, Clinical Investigations Branch,
National Center for Complementary and Integrative
Health (NCCIH), Bethesda, Maryland, United States
Department of Anesthesiology and Pain Medicine,
University of Washington, Seattle, Washington,
United States

Leela Baggett, JD
Associate, Powers Pyles Sutter & Verville, PC, N/A,
Washington, District of Columbia, United States

Karen P. Barr, MD
Associate Professor, Department of Physical Medicine
and Rehabilitation, University of Pittsburgh, Pittsburgh,
Pennsylvania, United States

J. Christian Barrett, BSEng
Lewis Katz School of Medicine, Temple University,
Philadelphia, Pennsylvania, United States

Matthew Bartels, MD, MPH
Professor and Chairman, Department of Physical
Medicine and Rehabilitation, Albert Einstein College of
Medicine/Montefiore Medical Center, Bronx, New York,
United States

Jeffrey R. Basford, MD, PhD
Professor, Physical Medicine and Rehabilitation,
Mayo Clinic, Rochester, Minnesota, United States

Serap Bastepe-Gray, MD, MScOT
Director, Peabody Occupational Health and Injury
Prevention Program, Peabody Conservatory, Baltimore,
Maryland, United States
Johns Hopkins University School of Medicine,
Department of Neurology, Baltimore, Maryland, United
States

Mahya Beheshti, MD
Research Scientist, Rehabilitation Medicine, NYU
    Langone Health, New York, New York, United States

Scott E. Benjamin, MD, FABPMR, PRM
Section Chief, Pediatric Rehabilitation Medicine
Associate Professor, MUSC Pediatrics, Charleston, South
    Carolina, United States

William A. Bergin, DO
Medical Director, Crichton Inpatient Rehabilitation Unit,
    Memorial Medical Center, Johnstown, Pennsylvania,
    United States

Omar Maurice Bhatti, MD
Clinical Associate Professor, Rehabilitation Medicine,
    University of Washington, Seattle, Washington, United
    States

Ravneet Bhullar, MD
Department of Anesthesiology, Albany Medical Center,
    Albany, New York, United States

Amy Bialek, MS, PT
Advanced Clinician in Physical Therapy and Study
    Coordinator, Wellness Program, Burke Neurological
    Institute, White Plains, New York, United States

Michael L. Boninger, MD
Professor, Physical Medicine & Rehabilitation, University
    of Pittsburgh, Pittsburgh, Pennsylvania, United States

Joanne Borg-Stein, MD
Associate Professor, Physical Medicine and
    Rehabilitation, Harvard Medical School, Boston,
    Massachusetts, United States

Susan Brady, DHEd, MS, CCC-SLP, BCS-S
Vice President, Operations, Northwestern Medicine
    Marianjoy Rehabilitation Hospital, Wheaton, Illinois,
    United States

Marvin McClatchey Brooke, MD, MS
Clinical Associate Professor, Rehabilitation Medicine,
    University of Washington, Seattle, Washington,
    United States

Scott E. Brown, MD, MA
Medical Director, Sinai Rehabilitation Center, Sinai
    Hospital of Baltimore, Chairman, Department of
    Physical Medicine and Rehabilitation, LifeBridge
    Health, Baltimore, Maryland, United States

Steven E. Brown, PhD
Co-Founder, Institute on Disability Culture, NA, Surprise,
    Arizona, United States
Professor (Retired), Center on Disability Studies,
    University of Hawaii, Honolulu, Hawaii, United States

Brandon Bukovitz, MD
Aurora Health Care, Department of Internal Medicine
Milwaukee, Wisconsin, United States

Philippines G. Cabahug, MD, FAAPMR
Assistant Professor, Director, SCI Medicine Fellowship,
    Department of Physical Medicine and Rehabilitation
Johns Hopkins School of Medicine/Kennedy Krieger
    Institute, Baltimore, Maryland, United States

Benjamin S. Carson Sr., MD
Emeritus Professor of Neurosurgery, Johns Hopkins
    Medicine
17th Secretary of the United States Department of
    Housing and Urban Development, Washington DC,
    United States
Founder and Chairman, American Cornerstone Institute
    Washington DC, United States

David A. Cassius, MD
President, Doris Medical Technologies, Seattle,
    Washington, United States

Leighton Chan, MD, MPH
Chief, Rehabilitation Medicine Department, National
    Institutes of Health (NIH), Bethesda, Maryland,
    United States

Stephanie Chan, MD
Chief Resident Physician, Physical Medicine and
    Rehabilitation, Rutgers Robert Wood Johnson Medical
    School, HMH, JFK Johnson Rehabilitation Institute,
    Edison, New Jersey, United States

Caitlin M. Cicone, DO
Interventional Spine/PM&R, OSS Health, Ann Arbor,
    Michigan, United States

Jeffrey Cohen, MD
Clinical Professor of Rehabilitation Medicine, Department
    of Rehabilitation Medicine, Rusk Rehabililitation,
    NYU Langone Medical Center, New York, New York,
    United States

Rory A. Cooper, PhD
Director, Human Engineering Research Laboratories, VA
    Pittsburgh Healthcare System/University of Pittsburgh,
    Pittsburgh, Pennsylvania, United States

Alberto G. Corrales, MD, MS
Clinical Assistant Professor, Physical Medicine and
    Rehabilitation, Geisinger Commonwealth School of
    Medicine, Scranton, Pennsylvania, United States
Associate, Physical Medicine and Rehabilitation,
    Geisinger Musculoskeletal Institute, Danville,
    Pennsylvania, United States

Matthew Cowling, DO
Integrative Rehab Consultants, Chattanooga, Tennessee,
    United States

Sara Cuccurullo, MD
Chair, Professor, Residency Program Director, Physical
    Medicine and Rehabilitation, Rutgers-Robert Wood
    Johnson Medical School, Piscataway, New Jersey,
    United States
Medical Director, VP—Physical Medicine and
    Rehabilitation, JFK Johnson Rehabilitation Institute,
    Edison, New Jersey, United States

Tyler C. Cymet, DO
Vice President for Institutional Effectiveness, Maryland
    College of Osteopathic Medicine (proposed) at Morgan
    State University, Baltimore, Maryland

Kate E. Delaney, MD
Assistant Professor, University of Washington, Department of Rehabilitation Medicine, Seattle, Washington, United States

Laurent Delavaux, MD, MS
Attending Physician, Physical Medicine and Rehabilitation, JFK Johnson Rehab Institute, Edison, New Jersey, United States

Giampaolo de Sena, MD
Spine Clinic, Villa Germana, Clinica Ruesch, Napoli, Italy

Lisa DeStefano, DO
Professor, Osteopathic Manipulative Medicine, College of Osteopathic Medicine, Michigan State University, East Lansing, Michigan, United States

Rubin I. Devon, MD
Professor, Neurology, Mayo Clinic, Jacksonville, Florida, United States, Directory, EMG Laboratory–Neurology, Mayo Clinic, Jacksonville, Florida, United States

Timothy R. Dillingham, MD, MS
Professor and Chairman, Department of Physical Medicine and Rehabilitation, The University of Pennsylvania, Philadelphia, Pennsylvania, United States

Peter Daniel Donofrio, MD
Professor, Neurology, Vanderbilt University Medical Center, Nashville, Tennessee, United States

Freda Dreher, MD
Immediate Past President, American Academy of Medical Acupuncture
Clinical Preceptor, Helms Medical Institute
Owner, Physiatry & Medical Acupuncture, Private Practice, Lebanon, New Hampshire, United States

Andrew J. Duarte, MD
NYU Langone Health, Rusk Rehabilitation, NYU Langone, New York, New York, United States

Rochelle Coleen Tan Dy, MD
Associate Professor, Physical Medicine and Rehabilitation, Baylor College of Medicine, Houston, Texas, United States

Maury Ruben Ellenberg, MD
Clinical Professor-PMR, Wayne State University, Detroit, Michigan, United States

Frank J.E. Falco, MD, FAAPMR
Former Adjunct Associate Professor, Department of Physical Medicine and Rehabilitation, Lewis Katz School of Medicine at Temple University, Philadelphia, Pennsylvania, United States
Founder, Mid-Atlantic Spine and Pain Physicians, Newark, Delaware, United States

Sergey Filatov, MD
Clinical Assistant Professor, Physical Medicine and Rehabilitation, Geisinger Commonwealth School of Medicine, Scranton, Pennsylvania, United States
Associate, Physical Medicine and Rehabilitation, Geisinger Musculoskeletal Institute, Danville, Pennsylvania, United States

Thomas Findley, MD, PhD (Deceased)
Professor, Department of Physical Medicine and Rehabilitation, UMDNJ-New Jersey Medical School, New Jersey, United Sates

Mark Finnegan, RN, MSN
Wound care Nurse–Spinal Cord Unit, Charlile Norwood VAMC, Augusta, Georgia, United States

Michael Flamm, DO
Department of Pain Management, New York Harbor Veteran's Administration Medical Center, New York, New York, United States

Steven Flanagan, MD
Howard A. Rusk Professor and Chair of Rehabilitation Medicine, Rehabilitation Medicine, New York University Langone Health, New York, New York, United States

Michael B. Furman, MD, MS, FAAPMR
Fellowship Director, Interventional Spine and Sports Medicine, OSS Health, York, Pennsylvania, United States
Adjunct Clinical Assistant Professor, Department of Physical Medicine and Rehabilitation, Lewis Katz School of Medicine at Temple University, Philadelphia, Pennsylvania, United States

Vincent Gabriel, MD, FRCPC
Medical Director, Calgary Firefighters Burn Treatment Centre
Assistant Professor, Clinical Neurosciences, Pediatrics and Surgery, University of Calgary, Calgary, Alberta, Canada

Filipinas G. Ganchoon, MD, DPBRM, FPARM
Chair, Department of Physical and Rehabilitation Medicine, The Doctors Hospital, Negros Island, Philippines
Professor, Department of Neurology
University of St. La Salle, College of Medicine, Negros Island, Philippines

Alfred C. Gellhorn, MD
Associate Professor of Clinical Rehabilitation Medicine, Rehabilitation Medicine, Weill Cornell Medicine, New York, New York, United States

Christopher Gharibo, MD
Medical Director of Pain Medicine, Associate Professor of Anesthesiology & Orthopedics, NYU Langone Health, New York, New York, United States

Theresa A. Gillis, MD
Chief, Rehabilitation Service and Associate Attending, Neurology, Memorial Sloan Kettering Cancer Center, New York, United States
Associate Professor of Clinical Rehabilitation Medicine-Division of Rehabilitation Medicine, Weill Cornell Medical College, New York, United States

Francesca Gimigliano, MD, PhD
Professor of Physical and Rehabilitation Medicine, Department of Mental and Physical Health and Preventive Medicine, University of Campania "Luigi Vanvitelli," Naples, Italy, Italy

Lance L. Goetz, MD
Staff Physician, Spinal Cord Injury and Disorders (128),
Department of Veterans Affairs, Central Virginia Health
Care System, Virginia, United States
Associate Professor, Dept. of Physical Medicine and
Rehabilitation, Virginia Commonwealth University,
Richmond, Virginia, United States

Gary Goldberg, MD
Clinical Adjunct Professor–Physical Medicine and
Rehabilitation, Medical College of Virginia/Virginia
Commonwealth University Health System, Richmond,
Virginia, United States

Stephen Goldberg, MD
Professor Emeritus, University of Miami Miller School of
Medicine, Miami, Florida, United States

Marlis Gonzalez-Fernandez, MD, PhD
Associate Professor, Physical Medicine and
Rehabilitation, Johns Hopkins University School of
Medicine, Baltimore, Maryland, United States
Managing Director Outpatient Rehabilitation Services,
Physical Medicine and Rehabilitation, Johns Hopkins
University School of Medicine, Baltimore, Maryland,
United States
Vice-chair for Clinical Operations, Physical Medicine and
Rehabilitation, Johns Hopkins, University School of
Medicine, Baltimore, Maryland, United States

Ryan A. Grant, MD, MS
Associate Neurosurgeon, Department of Neurosurgery,
Geisinger Medical Center, Danville, Pennsylvania,
United States

Behnum Habibi, MD
Assistant Professor, Department of Physical Medicine
and Rehabilitation, Lewis Katz School of Medicine
at Temple University, Philadelphia, Pennsylvania,
United States

Kevin Hakimi, MD
Associate Professor, Rehabilitation Medicine, University of
Washington, Seattle, Washington, United States
Director, Rehabilitation Care Services, VA Puget Sound
Health Care System, Seattle, Washington, United States

Richard L. Harvey, MD
Clinical Chair, Brain Innovation Center and the Wesley
and Suzanne Dixon Stroke Chair of Stroke
Rehabilitation Research, Shirley Ryan AbilityLab,
Chicago, Illinois, United States
Professor of Physical Medicine and Rehabilitation,
Northwestern University Feinberg School of Medicine,
Chicago, Illinois, United States

Jeffrey T. Heckman, DO
Associate Professor, Physical Medicine and
Rehabilitation, University of South Florida, Morsani
College of Medicine Tampa, Florida, United States
Medical Director, Regional Amputation Center–Tampa,
James A. Haley Veterans' Hospital & Clinics, Tampa,
Florida, United States
Fellowship Director, Amputation Rehabilitation, VA Office
of Academic Affiliations, Tampa, Florida, United States

Edward W. Heinle III, MD, MA
Chair, Department of Physical Medicine and
Rehabilitation
Associate Program Director, Physical Medicine and
Rehabilitation Residency, Geisinger, Danville,
Pennsylvania, United States
Clinical Assistant Professor in Physical Medicine and
Rehabilitation, Medical Education, Geisinger
Commonwealth School of Medicine, Scranton,
Pennsylvania, United States

Joseph M. Helms, MD
Director, Helms Medical Institute and Acus Foundation,
Berkeley, California, United States

Rafi J. Heruti, MD
Professor, Director, Rehabilitation Division, Reuth
Rehabilitation Hospital, Tel Aviv, Israel
Head, Sexual Rehabilitation & Therapy Clinic, Reuth
Rehabilitation Hospital, Tel Aviv, Israel
Professor, Sackler School of Medicine Tel Aviv University,
Tel Aviv, Israel

Steven R. Hinderer, MD, MS, PT
Associate Professor Emeritus and Residency Program
Director, Physical Medicine & Rehabilitation, Wayne
State University School of Medicine, Detroit, Michigan,
United States

Chun Ho, MD
Clinical Assistant Professor, Physical Medicine and
Rehabilitation, Geisinger Commonwealth School of
Medicine, Scranton, Pennsylvania, United States
Associate, Physical Medicine and Rehabilitation,
Geisinger Musculoskeletal Institute, Danville,
Pennsylvania, United States

Bethany Honce, MD
Clinical Assistant Professor, Departmet of Orthopaedics,
West Virginia University, Morgantown, West Virginia,
United States

Ileana Michelle Howard, MD
Outpatient Medical Director, Rehabilitation Care Service,
VA Puget Sound Health Care System, Seattle,
Washington, United States
Associate Professor, Rehabilitation Medicine, University of
Washington, Seattle, Washington, United States

DongFeng Huang, MD
Professor and Chair, Faculty of Rehabilitation Sciences,
Sun Yat-Sen University Zhongshan Medical School,
Guangzhou, Guangdong, China
Professor and Chair, Department of Rehabilitation
Medicine, Sun Yat-Sen University Seventh Affiliated
Hospital, Shenzhen, Guangdong, China
Director, World Health Organization Collaborating Centre
for Rehabilitation (CHN-50) Shenzhen, Guangdong,
China
Vice President, Chinese Association of Rehabilitation
Doctors, Beijing, China

Edward A. Hurvitz, MD
Professor and Chair, Department of Physical Medicine
and Rehabilitation, University of Michigan/Michigan
Medicine, Ann Arbor, Michigan, United States

Julia Louisa Iafrate, DO, CAQSM, FAAPMR
Assistant Professor of Orthopedic Surgery and Sports Medicine, Department of Orthopedic Surgery, New York University Grossman School of Medicine, NYU Langone Health, New York, New York, United States

Katarzyna Ibanez, MD
Assistant Attending, Department of Neurology, Rehabilitation Service, Memorial Sloan Kettering Cancer Center, New York, New York, United States

Marta Imamura, MD, PhD
Associate Professor. Departamento de Medicina Legal, Bioética, Medicina do Trabalho e Medicina Física e Reabilitação, The Faculdade de Medicina da Universidade de São Paulo, São Paulo, Brazil.
Coordinator, Pain Laboratory at the Clinical Research Center. Instituto de Medicina Física e Reabilitação, HCFMUSP, São Paulo, Brazil

Akiko Ito, LLM, LLB, MA
Chief, United Nations Secretariat for the Conference on the Convention on the Rights of Persons with Disabilities (CRPD), United Nations, New York, New York, United States
Chief, United Nations Programme on Disability, United Nations, New York, New York, United States
United Nations Focal Point for Gender Equality and Empowerment of Women, Department of Economic and Social Affairs, United Nations, New York, New York, United States

Kristen Jackson, PhD
Assistant Professor, Clinical, Rehabilitation Psychology, The Ohio State University, Columbus, Ohio, United States

Paul Steven Jones, DO
Staff Physiatrist, Physical Medicine and Rehabilitation, Harry S Truman Memorial Veterans Hospital, Columbia, Missouri, United States
Professor of Clinical PM&R, Physical Medicine and Rehabilitation, University of Missouri, Columbia, Columbia, Missouri, United States

Nanette Cunningham Joyce, DO, MS
Associate Clinical Professor, Physical Medicine and Rehabilitation, University of California, Davis School of Medicine, Sacramento, California, United States

Shailaja Kalva, MD
Clinical Associate Professor, Rehabilitation Medicine, New York University Grossman School of Medicine, New York, New York, United States

Chelsea Kane, PsyD
Assistant Professor, Clinical, Physical Medicine & Rehabilitation, The Ohio State University, Columbus, Ohio, United States

Richard T. Katz, MD
Professor–Clinical Neurology (PM&R), Washington University School of Medicine, St. Louis, Missouri, United States

Deidre Casey Kerrigan, MD
Co-Founder, OESH Shoes/JKM Technologies, LLC, Charlottesville, Virginia, United States

Ehtesham Khalid, MD, MRCP, FCPS
Senior Consultant–Neurology, Mukhtar A Shaikh Hospital, Multan, Punjab, Pakistan
Adjunct Clinical Instructor–Neurology, Vanderbilt University Medical Center, Nashville, Tennessee, United States

Fary Khan, MD, MBBS, FAFRM (RACP)
Director, Department of Rehabilitation, Royal Melbourne Hospital, Parkville, Victoria, Australia
Clinical Professor, Department of Medicine, University of Melbourne, Parkville, Victoria, Australia
Adjunct Professor, Disability Inclusive Unit, Nossal Institute of Global Health, Parkville, Victoria, Australia
Adjunct Professor, School of Public Health and Preventative Medicine, Monash University, Clayton, Victoria, Australia

Seema Khurana, DO
Integrated Rehabilitation Adult and Pediatrics, Miami, Florida, United States

Carlotte Kiekens, MD
Dr. Physical and Rehabilitation Medicine, Gruppo MultiMedica, IRCCS MultiMedica, Milan, Italy

Charles Kim, MD, CAc
Assistant Professor, Rehabilitation Medicine and Anesthesiology, NYU Grossman School of Medicine, Director of Clinical Operations, Rusk Spine Service, NYU Langone Orthopedic Center, New York, New York, United States

Kiril Kiprovski, MD
Associate Clinical Professor–Neurology, NYU Langone Medical Center, New York, New York, United States

R. Lee Kirby, MD, FRCPC
Professor, Physical Medicine and Rehabilitation, Dalhousie University, Halifax, Nova Scotia, Canada

Michael L. Knudsen, MD
Assistant, Professor of Orthopedic Surgery, Center for Shoulder, Elbow and Sports Medicine, Department of Orthopedic Surgery, Columbia University Medical Center/New York-Presbyterian Hospital, New York, New York, United States

David J. Kolessar, MD
Chief of Adult Reconstruction, Northeast Division, Department of Orthopaedics, Geisinger Healthcare System, Wilkes Barre, Pennsylvania, United States
Associate Clinical Professor, Geisinger Commonwealth School of Medicine, Scranton, Pennsylvania, United States
Adult Hip and Knee Reconstructive Surgeon, Geisinger Musculoskeletal Institute, Wilkes Barre, Pennsylvania, United States

Franchesca König, MD
Assistant Attending
Medical Director of Cancer Rehabilitation
University of Colorado School of Medicine
Department of Physical Medicine & Rehabilitation
Denver, Colorado, United States

Sarah A. Korth, MD
Director Keelty Center for Spina Bifida & Related
Conditions, Department of Neurorehabilitation,
Kennedy Krieger Institute, Baltimore, Maryland,
United States
Assistant Professor, Department of Physical Medicine and
Rehabilitation, The Johns Hopkins University School of
Medicine, Baltimore, Maryland, United States

Evangeline P. Koutalianos, MD
Assistant Professor, PM&R/Interventional Pain
Management, Department of Physical Medicine &
Rehabilitation, SUNY Upstate Medical University,
Syracuse, New York, United States

Karen J. Kowalske, MD
Professor, Physical Medicine and Rehabilitation,
University of Texas, Southwestern Medical Center,
Dallas, Texas, United States

Jorge Lains, MD
Professor (invited), Faculty of Medicine, Coimbra
University, Coimbra, Portugal
Head of the Physical and Rehabilitation Medicine
Department, Research and Innovation Department,
Continuum of Care Unit–CMRRC-RP, Medical Education
Department, Rovisco Pais, Portugal

David H. Ledbetter, PhD, FACMG
Adjunct Professor, Department of Psychiatry, University of
Florida, College of Medicine, Gainesville, Florida,
United States

Jeffrey Lehman, MD
Head-Rehabilitation, Dorot Geriatric Medical Center,
Netanya, Israel

Yehoshua J. Lehman, MD
Director of Rehabilitation, Dorot Netanya Geriatric
Medical Center, Netanya, Israel

James W. Leonard, DO, PT
Associate Professor of Rehabilitation Medicine,
Department of Orthopedics and Rehabilitation,
University of Wisconsin School of Medicine and Public
Health, University of Wisconsin Hospital and Clinics,
Madison, Wisconsin, United States

Charles Edward Levy, MD
Research Scholar, Center for Arts in Medicine, College of
the Arts, University of Florida, Gainesville, Florida,
United States
Associate Professor (Courtesy), Department of
Occupational Therapy, College of Public Health and
Health Professions, University of Florida, Gainesville,
Florida, United States

Karen Lew, PharmD
Dr., Pharmacy Service, VA Puget Sound, Seattle,
Washington, United States

Leonard S.W. Li, MBBS, FRCP (Lon), FAFRM (RACP)
Honorary Clinical Professor, Medicine, University of Hong
Kong, Hong Kong, Hong Kong

Director, Neurological Rehabilitation Center, Virtus
Medical Center, Hong Kong, Hong Kong
Adjunct Professor, Rehabilitation Sciences, Hong Kong
Polytechnic University, Kowloon, Hong Kong

Janet C. Limke, MD
Spine Center Medical Director, Physical Medicine and
Rehabilitation, South Shore Health, Weymouth,
Massachusetts, United States

Kyle Littell, MD
Assistant Professor, Physical Medicine and Rehabilitation,
Indiana University School of Medicine, Indianapolis,
Indiana, United States
Medical Director of Complex Medical Services,
Rehabilitation Hospital of Indiana, Indianapolis,
Indiana, United States

Francis Lopez, MD, MPH
Assistant Professor, Physical Medicine and Rehabilitation,
New York University, New York, New York, United
States

Samantha Mastanduno, DO
Rothman Orthopedics, New York, New York, United States

Thomas McGunigal, MD
Rehabilitation Hospital of Rhode Island, North Smithfield,
Rhode Island, United States

Jeffrey Saul Meyers, MD, L Ac
Attending Physician, Musculoskeletal Medicine &
Pain Management, Delaware Back Pain & Sports
Rehabilitation Centers, Wilmington, Delaware,
United States

Matthew Mitchkash, MD
Sports Medicine Physician, Department of Physical
Medicine and Rehabilitation, Department of
Orthopedic Surgery, Cleveland Clinic, Cleveland, Ohio,
United States

Jose Alvin Mojica, MD, MHPEd
Clinical Professor, Rehabilitation Medicine, University of
the Philippines Manila, Manila, Philippines

Alex Moroz, MD, MHPE
Professor and Vice Chair for Education, Director of
Physical Medicine and Rehabilitation, Residency
Program, Department of Rehabilitation Medicine,
New York University Grossman School of Medicine,
New York, New York, United States

Stanley J. Myers, MD
A David Gurewitsch Professor Emeritus, Department of
Rehabilitation and Regenerative Medicine, Columbia
University Vagelos College of Physicians and Surgeons,
Columbia University Irving Medical Center,
New York Presbyterian Hospital, New York, New York,
United States

Emma Nally, MD
Assistant Professor of Rehabilitation Medicine
Georgetown University Hospital— Rehabilitation
Medicine, MedStar National Rehabilitation Hospital,
Washington, District of Columbia, United States

Fabreena E. Napier, MD
Assistant Professor, Department of Neurology, Albert Einstein College of Medicine, Bronx, New York, United States
Co-Director, Muscular Dystrophy Association Care Center, Montefiore Medical Center, Bronx, New York, United States
Director, Neuromuscular Medicine, Jacobi Medical Center, Bronx, New York, United States

Noel Rao, MD
Northwestern Medicine, Marianjoy Rehabilitation Hospital, Wheaton, Illinois, United States

Margaret A. Nosek, PhD
Professor, PM&R, Baylor College of Medicine, Houston, Texas, United States

Ib R. Odderson, MD, PhD
Medical Director, Rehabilitation Medicine, University of Washington, Seattle, Washington, United States
Adjunct Associate Professor, Radiology, University of Washington, Seattle, United States

Bryan J. O'Young, MD, CAc, FAAPMR
Professor and Vice Chair of Education, Department of Physical Medicine and Rehabilitation, Lewis Katz School of Medicine at Temple University, Philadelphia, Pennsylvania, United States
Chief of Outpatient Service, Department of Physical Medicine and Rehabilitation, Temple University Health System, Philadelphia, Pennsylvania, United States
Clinical Professor, Department of Rehabilitation Medicine, New York University Grossman School of Medicine, Rusk Rehab at NYU Langone Health, New York, New York, United States
Adjunct Clinical Professor, Department of Rehabilitation Medicine, Weill Medical College of Cornell University, NY Presbyterian Hospital, Weill Cornell Medical Center, New York, New York, United States
Adjunct Professor of Rehabilitation Medicine, University of the Philippines College of Medicine, Manila, Philippines
Visiting Professor, Department of Rehabilitation Medicine, Peking University First Hospital, Peking University School of Medicine, Beijing, China
Visiting Professor, Department of Rehabilitation Medicine, Sun-Yat Sen University First Hospital, Sun-Yat Sen University College of Medicine, Guangzhou, Guangdong, China

Sagar Parikh, MD
Interventional Pain Physician/Fellowship Director, Rehabilitation Medicine, JFK Johnson Rehabilitation Institute, Edison, New Jersey, United States
Director, Center for Sports and Spine Medicine, JFK Johnson Rehabilitation Institute, Edison, New Jersey, United States

Theresa J. C. Pazionis, MD, MA, FRCSC
Assistant Professor of Surgery, Orthopaedic Surgery and Sports Medicine, Lewis Katz School of Medicine at Temple University, Philadelphia, Pennsylvania, United States
Orthopaedic Oncologist, Orthopaedic Surgery and Sports Medicine, Spine Surgeon, Temple University Hospital, Philadelphia, Pennsylvania, United States

Inder Perkash, MD, FACS, FRCS
Emeritus Professor, Stanford University, Stanford, California, United States

Robert Pignolo, MD, PhD
Robert and Arlene Kogod Professor of Geriatric, Department of Medicine, Mayo Clinic School of Medicine, Rochester, Minnesota, United States

Michelle A. Poliak-Tunis, MD
Assistant Professor, Department of Orthopedics and Rehabilitation, University of Wisconsin, Madison, Wisconsin, United States

Joel M. Press, MD
Physiatrist-in-Chief, Physiatry, Hospital for Special Surgery, New York City, New York, United States
Professor of Rehabilitation Medicine, Weill Cornell Medical College, New York, New York, United States

Michael Priebe, MD, MPH
Chief-Spinal Cord Injury Service, Charlie Norwood VA Medical Center, Augusta, Georgia, United States

Jessica Pruente, MD
Assistant Professor, Physical Medicine and Rehabilitation, University of Michigan, Ann Arbor, Michigan, United States

April D. Pruski, MD
Assistant Professor of Physical Medicine and Rehabilitation, Assistant Professor of Neurology, Johns Hopkins University School of Medicine, Baltimore, Maryland, United States

Preeti Raghavan, MD
Sheikh Khalifa Professor, Director Center of Excellence for Treatment, Recovery and Rehabilitation, Sheikh Khalifa Stroke Institute
Vice-Chair Research, Department of Physical Medicine and Rehabilitation Director, Motor Recovery Research Lab
Associate Professor of Physical Medicine and Rehabilitation and Neurology Johns Hopkins University School of Medicine, Baltimore, Maryland, United States

Ira G. Rashbaum, MD
Clinical Professor, Physical Medicine and Rehabilitation, Rusk Rehabilitation/NYU Langone Health, New York, United States

Rajiv R. Ratan, MD, PhD
Chief Operating Officer, Burke Neurological Institute, White Plains, New York, United States
Professor, Neurology and Neuroscience, Weill Cornell Medical College, New York, United States
Associate Dean (Affiliate), Weill Cornell Medical College, New York, United States

Albert Recio, MD, PT
Assistant Professor, Department of Physical Medicine and Rehabilitation
Medical Director Aquatic Program, International Center for Spinal Cord Injury, Kennedy Krieger Institute, Johns Hopkins University School of Medicine, Baltimore, Maryland, United States

James P. Richardson, MD, MPH
Chief, Geriatric and Palliative Medicine, St. Agnes Hospital, Baltimore, Maryland, United States

John-Ross Rizzo, MD, MSCI
Associate Professor, Rehabilitation Medicine, New York University Langone Health, New York, New York, United States
Associate Professor, Neurology, New York University Langone Health, New York, New York, United States

Lawrence R. Robinson, MD
Professor and Division Director, Physical Medicine and Rehabilitation, Rehabilitation Sciences Institute, University of Toronto
Chief of Rehabilitation, St. John's Rehabilitation Hospital, Toronto, Ontario, Canada

Gianna Maria Rodriguez, MD
Associate Professor, Physical Medicine and Rehabilitation, University of Michigan, Ann Arbor, Michigan, United States

Rosa Rodriguez, MD, MS
Physical Medicine & Rehabilitation, Pain Medicine, Miami, Florida, United States

Robert Rondinelli, MD, PhD, MS, MA
CEO & Owner, Pinnacle IME Services, Foxboro, Iowa, United States

Roger P. Rossi, DO
Professor of Physical Medicine and Rehabilitation, Physical Medicine and Rehabilitation, Rutgers—Robert Wood Johnson/Johnson Rehabilitation Institute, Edison, New Jersey, United States

Jacob Rowan, DO
Associate Professor, Osteopathic Manipulative Medicine, Michigan State University, East Lansing, Michigan, United States

Nathan J. Rudin, MD, MA, FAAPMR
Professor of Rehabilitation Medicine, Orthopedics and Rehabilitation Medicine, University of Wisconsin School of Medicine and Public Health, Madison, Wisconsin, United States

Robert Rundorff, MD, PC
Johnstown Medical Director PM&R, Crichton Rehabilitation Services, DLP Conemaugh Memorial Medical Center, Johnstown, Pennsylvania, United States

Ryan J. Roza, MD, CAQSM, R-MSK
Program Director Physical Medicine and Rehabilitation Residency, Core Faculty Sports Medicine Fellowship, Physician of Sports Medicine, Department of Orthopaedics Sports Medicine, Department of Physical Medicine and Rehabilitation, Musculoskeletal Institute, Geisinger Health System, Danville, Pennsylvania, United States

Emily Ryan-Michailidis, DO
National Health Rehabilitation, Atlanta, Georgia, United States

Michael Frederick Saulle, DO, FAAPMR, CAQSM
Assistant Professor Interventional Spine & Sports Medicine, Medical Director of Sports Medicine – Westchester Division, Department of Rehabilitation and Regenerative Medicine, Columbia University Medical Center, New York, New York, United States

Carson D. Schneck, MD, PhD
Professor of Anatomy and Diagnostic Imaging, Department of Anatomy and Cell Biology, Temple University School of Medicine, Philadephia, Pennsylvania, United States

Jeffrey C. Schneider, MD
Medical Director, Trauma, Burn and Orthopedic Program, Physical Medicine and Rehabilitation, Spaulding Rehabilitation Hospital, Boston, Massachusetts, United States
Associate Professor, Physical Medicine and Rehabilitation, Harvard Medical School, Boston, Massachusetts, United States

Shannon L. Schultz, MD, MPH, FAAPMR
Interventional Spine and Sports Medicine, OSS Health, New York, Pennsylvania, United States

Robert G. Schwartz, MD
Executive Director, PMR, Piedmont Physical Medicine & Rehabilitation, PA, Greenville, South Carolina, United States
Chairman of the Board, American Academy of Thermology, Greenville, South Carolina, United States

Jad Georges Sfeir, MD, MS
Assistant Professor of Medicine, Department of Medicine, Mayo Clinic, Rochester, Minnesota, United States

Tarek Shafshak, MB, ChB, ECFMG, Master PMR, PhD, PMR
Professor, Physical Medicine, Rheumatology & Rehabilitation, Faculty of Medicine, Alexandria University, Alexandria, Egypt

Jay P. Shah, MD
Senior Staff Physiatrist and Clinical Investigator, Rehabilitation Medicine Department, Clinical Center, National Institutes of Health, Bethesda, Maryland, United States

Shoshana Shamberg, OTR/L, MS, FOATA
Accessibility Consultant, President/Owner, Abilities OT & Irlen Diagnostic Center, Baltimore, Maryland, United States

Jennifer Shapiro, RDN, LD
Registered Dietitian–Nutrition, Jennifer Shapiro Nutrition, Teaneck, New Jersey, United States
Member of the Academy of Nutrition and Dietetics
Founder of Jennifer Shapiro Nutrition

Shashank Dave, DO, FAAPMR
Associate Clinical Professor, Physical Medicine and Rehabilitation, Indiana University School of Medicine, Indianapolis, Indiana, United States
Associate Clinical Professor, Neurology, Indiana University School of Medicine, Indianapolis, Indiana, United States
Associate Clinical Professor, Marian University, Indianapolis, Indiana, United States

Asad Riaz Siddiqi, DO
Assistant Professor, Rehabilitation and Regenerative Medicine, Columbia University Vagelos College of Physicians & Surgeons, New York, New York, United States

Kenneth H. Silver, MD
Associate Professor, Dept. of Physical Medicine and Rehabilitation, Johns Hopkins School of Medicine, Baltimore, Maryland, United States

Jonathan R. Slotkin, MD, FAANS
Director of Spinal Surgery, Department of Neurosurgery, Geisinger Health System, Danville, Pennsylvania, United States

Cher Smith, OT, MSc
Seating and Mobility Coordinator, Assistive Technology, Nova Scotia Health Authority, Halifax, Nova Scotia, Canada
Adjunct Professor, Occupational Therapy, Dalhousie University, Halifax, Nova Scotia, Canada

Bosco Francisco Soares, MD
Rehabilitation Care Services, VA Puget Sound Health Care Services, Seattle, Washington, United States

Nachum Soroker, MD
Head, Experimental Brain Rehab Lab, Department of Neurological Rehabilitation, Loewenstein Rehabilitation Hospital, Ra'anana, Israel

Rebecca A. Speckman, MD, PhD
Acting Assistant Professor, Rehabilitation Medicine, University of Washington, Seattle, Washington, United States
Medical Director, Regional Amputation Center, VA Puget Sound Health Care System, Seattle, Washington, United States
Fellowship Director, Amputation Rehabilitation, VA Puget Sound and University of Washington, Seattle, Washington, United States

Antonio Stecco, MD, PhD
Assistant Professor, Rusk Rehabilitation, New York University School of Medicine, New York City, United States

Carla Stecco, MD
Associate Professor, Molecular Medicine, University of Padua, Padua, Italy

Joel Stein, MD
Simon Baruch Professor and Chair, Rehabilitation and Regenerative Medicine, Columbia University Vagelos College of Physicians and Surgeons, New York, New York, United States
Professor and Chair, Rehabilitation Medicine, Weill Cornell Medicine, New York, New York, United States
Physiatrist-in-Chief, Rehabilitation Medicine, New York-Presbyterian Hospital, New York, New York, United States

Michelle Stern, MD
Associate Professor Albert Einstein College of Medicine, Department of Physical Medicine and Rehabilitation, H&H Jacobi/North Central Bronx, Bronx, New York, United States

John A. Sturgeon, PhD
Assistant Professor, Department of Anesthesiology and Pain Medicine, Center of Pain Relief, University of Washington, Seattle, Washington, United States

Ninad Durganand Sthalekar, MD
Director, Interventional Pain Management, Bucks County Orthopedic Specialists, Doylestown, Pennsylvania, United States

Beth Stiens, MEd
Educator, St. Luke School, Shoreline, Washington, United States

Steven A. Stiens, MD, MS
Curator of Education, Innovated Solutions, Stiens' Designs: Personal Enablement, Seattle, Washington, United States
Adjunct Clinical Professor, Department of Physical Medicine and Rehabilitation, Geisinger Commonwealth School of Medicine, Scranton, Pennsylvania, United States

Elizabeth A. Stiens, MEd
Educator, St. Luke School, Shoreline, Washington, United States

Margaret Grace Stineman, MD
Professor Emeritus, Department of Physical Medicine and Rehabilitation, Perelman School of Medicine, University of Pennsylvania, Philadelphia, Pennsylvania, United States

Gary Stover Jr., MD
Springfield Clinic, Physical Medicine and Rehabilitation, Springfield, Illinois, United States

Constance L. Strauss, BSN, RN, CWOCN, CFCN, CDE
Spinal Cord Injury, Charlie Norwood VAMC, Augusta, Georgia, United States

Nancy Strauss, MD
John A. Downey Professor and Executive Vice Chair, Rehabilitation and Regenerative Medicine, Columbia University Medical Center, New York, United States

Jonathan Strayer, MD, MS
Medical Director, SCI&D Service, Rehabilitation Medicine, Dayton VA Medical Center, Dayton, Ohio, United States
Volunteer Assoc Prof-Division of PM&R, University of Cincinnati, Cincinnati, Ohio, United States

Areerat Suputtitada, MD
Professor, Rehabilitation Medicine, Faculty of Medicine, Chulalongkorn University, Bangkok, Thailand

Mitchell S. Tepper, PhD, MPH
CEO-drmitchelltepper.com, The Sexual Health Network, Atlanta, Georgia, United States

Matthew Terzella, MD
Medical Director, PM&R, Piedmont Physical Medicine & Rehabilitation, PA, Greenville, South Carolina, United States

Carmen M. Terzic, MD, PhD
Professor, Physical Medicine and Rehabilitation, Mayo Clinic, Rochester, Minnesota, United States
Director Cardiac Rehabilitation, Cardiovascular Diseases, Mayo Clinic, Rochester, Minnesota, United States
Co-Director Rehabilitation Medicine Research Center, Physical Medicine and Rehabilitation, Mayo Clinic, Rochester, Minnesota, United States

Aakash Thakral, MD
Resident, Physical Medicine & Rehabilitation, JFK Johnson Rehabilitation Institute, Edison, New Jersey, United States

Lokendra Thakur, MD
Assistant Professor, Critical Care Medicine, Geisinger Medical Center, Danville, Pennsylvania, United States

Peter Thomas, JD
Principal, Powers Pyles Sutter & Verville, PC, Washington, District of Columbia, United States

Donna C. Tippett, MA, MPH, CCC-SLP
Departments of Neurology, Otolaryngology—Head and Neck Surgery, and Physical Medicine and Rehabilitation, Johns Hopkins University School of Medicine, Baltimore, Maryland, United States

Robert G. Trasolini, DO
Assistant Professor of Orthopedic Surgery, Northwell/Zucker School of Medicine, Huntington, New York, United States

Melissa Trovato, MD
Faculty, Pediatric Rehabilitation Medicine, Kennedy Krieger Institute, Baltimore, Maryland, United States
Assistant Professor, Physical Medicine and Rehabilitation, Johns Hopkins School of Medicine, Baltimore, Maryland, United States

Justin G. Tunis, MD, RMSK, CAQSM
Program Director, Geisinger Northeast Primary Care Sports Medicine Fellowship, Geisinger Health System, Scranton, Pennsylvania, United States
Assistant Clinical Professor, Geisinger Commonwealth School of Medicine, Scranton, Pennsylvania, United States
Sports Medicine Physician, Geisinger Musculoskeletal Institute, Scranton, Pennsylvania, United States

Heikki Uustal, MD
Attending Physiatrist, Rehabilitation Medicine, JFK Johnson Rehab Institute, Edison, New Jersey, United States
Associate Professor, Physical Medicine and Rehabilitation, Rutgers Robert Wood Johnson Medical School, Piscataway, New Jersey, United States
Associate Professor, Physical Medicine and Rehabilitation, Seton Hall Medical School, Nutley, New Jersey, United States

Naheed Asad-Van de Walle MD
Assistant Professor, University of Connecticut, Department of Medicine, Division of PM&R
Attending Physician, Division of PM&R, Hartford Healthcare Rehabilitation Network

Craig Van Dien, MD, FAAPMR, CAQSM
Attending Physician, PM&R and Sports Medicine, Department of Physical Medicine and Rehabilitation, Hackensack Meridian JFK Johnson Rehabilitation Institute, Edison, NJ, New Jersey, United States

Gerard P. Varlotta, DO, FACSM
Attending Physician, Orthopaedics & Rehabilitation, White Plains Hospital, White Plains, New York, United States
Associate Professor, NYIT College Osteopathic Medicine, Old Westbury, New York, United States

Christopher J. Visco, MD
Ursula Corning Associate Professor, Rehabilitation and Regenerative Medicine, Columbia, University, New York, New York, United States

Sheela Vivekanandan, MD
DR., Neurosurgery, Geisinger Health System, Danville, Pennsylvania, United States

Stanley F. Wainapel, MD, MPH
Professor of Clinical Physical Medicine and Rehabilitation, Physical Medicine and Rehabilitation, Albert Einstein College of Medicine, Bronx, New York, United States
Clinical Director, Physical Medicine and Rehabilitation, Montefiore Medical Center, Bronx, New York, United States

Ninghua Wang, MD, PhD
Professor, Rehabilitation Science, Peking University First Hospital, Beijing, Beijing, China

Ruth Westheimer, EdD
Professor, Psychosexual Therapist, Author, Lecturer, New York, New York, United States
Former Adjunct Professor at: Teachers College, Columbia University, New York, New York, United States; Princeton University, Princeton, New Jersey, United States; Yale University, New Haven, Connecticut, United States; and Hunter College, City University of New York, New York, New York, United States

Jonathan H. Whiteson, MBBS
Associate Professor, Rehabilitation Medicine, and Medicine, Rusk Rehabilitation, NYU School of Medicine, New York, New York, United States
Vice Chair Clinical Operations, Rusk Rehabilitation, NYU Langone Health, New York, New York, United States

Medical Director, Cardiac and Pulmonary Rehabilitation, Rusk Rehabilitation, NYU Langone Health, New York, New York, United States

Marc S. Williams, MD
Professor and Director Emeritus, Department of Genomic Health, Geisinger, Medical Center, Danville, Pennsylvania, United States

Olajide Williams, MD, MS
Professor of Neurology, Chief of Staff, Department of Neurology, Associate Dean of Community Research and Engagement, Co-Director, Columbia Wellness Center, Columbia University Irving Medical Center, New York, New York, United States

Susan Wortman-Jutt, MS, CCC-SLP
Research Associate-Center for Speech and Language Recovery, Burke Neurological Institute, White Plains, New York, United States
Speech-Language Pathologist, Advanced Clinician, Outpatient Speech Department, Burke Rehabilitation Hospital, White Plains, New York, United States

Sam S. H. Wu, MD, MA, MPH, MBA
Professor of Clinical Physical Medicine and Rehabilitation, Lewis Katz School of Medicine, Temple University, Philadelphia, Pennsylvania, United States
Chair of Department of Physical Medicine and Rehabilitation, Lewis Katz School of Medicine, Temple University, Philadelphia, Pennsylvania, United States
Chief of Service, Department of Physical Medicine and Rehabilitation, Temple University Health System, Philadelphia, Pennsylvania, United States
Clinical Associate Professor, Department of Physical Medicine and Rehabilitation, Rutgers- New Jersey Medical School, Newark, New Jersey, United States
Editor-In-Chief, Physiatry Forward, Association of Academic Physiatrists, Owings Mills, Maryland, United States
Editor, PM&R Knowledge NOW, American Academy of Physical Medicine and Rehabilitation, Rosemont, Illinois, United States
Member, Guidelines Development Group, WHO Wheelchair Service Guidelines, World Health Organization, Geneva, Switzerland

Henry S. York, MD
Health Sciences Assistant Clinical Professor, UC San Diego Department of Neurosciences, Chief, Spinal Cord Injury Service, VA San Diego Healthcare System, San Diego, California, United States

Mark A. Young, MD, MBA, FACP, FAAPMR, DABPMR
Chair, Department of Physical Medicine & Rehabilitation, The Workforce & Technology Center (WTC), The Maryland Vocational Rehabilitation Center, State of Maryland, Division of Rehabilitation Services (DORS), Maryland State Department of Education (MSDE), Baltimore, Maryland, United States
Faculty, The Johns Hopkins School of Medicine, Department of PM&R, Baltimore, Maryland, United States
Site Director, WTC Vocational Rehabilitation Rotation, Sinai Hospital, University of Maryland School of Medicine PM&R Residency Program, Baltimore, Maryland, United States
Faculty, The Rusk Institute of Rehabilitation Medicine, The New York University Grossman School of Medicine, New York, New York, United States
Adjunct Clinical Associate Professor, Department of Rehabilitation Medicine, New York University School of Medicine, New York, New York, United States
Professor, Department of Orthopedic Sciences, New York College of Podiatric Medicine, New York, New York, United States

Marlene Young, MS, CNS, LD
Licensed Nutritionist, Board Certified, Professional Member, American College of Nutrition, American Diabetes Association, White Marsh, Maryland, United States

Michael J. Young, MD, MPhil
Associate Director, MGH NeuroRecovery Clinic, Center for Neurotechnology and NeuroRecovery (CNTR), Division of Neurocritical Care, Department of Neurology, Massachusetts General Hospital and Harvard Medical School, Boston, Massachusetts, United States

Xiaoning (Jenny) Yuan, MD, PhD
Assistant Professor, Physical Medicine and Rehabilitation, Uniformed Services University of the Health Sciences, Bethesda, Maryland, United States

Jason L. Zaremski, MD, CAQSM, FACSM, FAAPMR
Associate Professor of PM&R and Sports Medicine, Physical Medicine and Rehabilitation, University of Florida, Gainesville, Florida, United States

Richard D. Zorowitz, MD
Chief Medical Informatics Officer, Physical Medicine and Rehabilitation, MedStar National, Rehabilitation Network, Washington, District of Columbia, United States
Professor of Clinical Rehabilitation Medicine, Rehabilitation Medicine, Georgetown University School of Medicine, Washington, District of Columbia, United States

ACKNOWLEDGMENTS

Don't let the sun go down without saying thank you to someone, and without admitting to yourself that absolutely no one gets this far alone.

–Stephen King

A legendary African proverb declares, "*It takes a village to raise a child.*" Just as this proclamation acknowledges the supreme importance of an entire community to nurture a child's growth and development, writing a textbook, no less a medical volume like *PM&R Secrets,* similarly necessitates a coalition of people to cultivate a new edition. This fourth edition of *PM&R Secrets* masterfully combines the skills, talents, and knowledge of so many in our medical and educational village. The editors of this book would like to graciously acknowledge the "citizens" of this literary coterie.

Those who have played an instrumental role in nourishing this volume include academic editors, chapter authors, copy editors, design and graphic associates, academic staff support, administrative help, and the publisher, Elsevier. In true team fashion, these vital "community members" have enabled this new edition to achieve a multitude of impactful "developmental milestones," including revamped content, new diagrams, refreshed and updated references and citations, online and digital content, clickable virtual learning resources, and other benefits that accrue to a mature work.

Ever since the "birth" of the first edition of our book in 1998, we have relished the ongoing dialogue with readers, colleagues, fellow faculty, academics, scholars, residents, and many others on ways we can collaborate to continue to grow our educational book. *You*, the reader, have made all the difference in sustaining the village and encouraging its prosperity. Your observations, suggestions, and pointers have helped us refine and update each edition of *PM&R Secrets*.

We offer applause to the following villagers, without whose help this book would never have become a reality: Ms. Casey Christensen (administrative coordinator, "spreadsheet keeper", and first year medical student); Mr. Ari Sigal (technical & copy editor); Dr. Sweta Thakur, Dr. Nasima Akhter, Mary Lou May, RN, Mia Hannula, and Jason Oleston (librarians at the Seattle VA); Alisa Holcomb; and Christopher Pachero. Critical staff support has been provided by: Savannah Kane, Eunyeong Joo, Seeun Judy Jeong, Alyssa Stuckrath, Bianca Sevidal RN, Beyonce Carrington, Alexis Cyr, Grace Fillmore, Amy Tien, Lauren Ambill, Bryanna Billings, Michael Young, MD, Howard Rusk, Jr., Christopher Radlcz, MD, Dr. Daniel Soloman, Ambreona Thomas, MD, Jeremy Staiman (graphic artist), Sarah Marizan, and Monique Velzebor.

A special thank you to our treasured author faculty. The dedicated and altruistic faculty of international authors embodying the fine academic spirit of teaching, research, and scholarship collaborated to create this newest edition. They have lived Helen Keller's hallowed philosophy, "Alone we can do so little, together so much!"

The editors of *PM&R Secrets* continue to prosper as clinicians, teachers, and scientists through our relationships and friendships with fellow faculty at our home institutions. These connections enabled us to significantly enhance content and style in this fourth edition. Gratitude is extended to our colleagues and residents at Temple University, Johns Hopkins University, Geisinger Commonwealth College of Medicine, the University of Washington, the University of Maryland, the Veterans Administration, and the Maryland Rehabilitation Center & The Workforce & Technology Center. A word of appreciation is due to cherished colleagues associated with the New York College of Podiatric Medicine, especially Louis Levine and Dean Michael J. Trepal.

The highest form of acknowledgment is bestowing thanks and paying homage to people who are no longer with us. Although this is a poignant challenge, we honor colleagues who have perished since the 3rd edition and four (Thomas Findley, Margaret Nosek, Carson Schneck, and Margaret Stineman) who died while working on this edition. The editors offer our heartfelt memorial and kindest remembrance to our beloved colleagues who are dearly departed but whose spirit lovingly remains with us. These include Rene Calliet, MD, Thomas Findley, MD, PhD, Andrew Fischer, MD, PhD, Harlan Hahn, PhD, Stanley Kornhauser, PhD, Mathew Lee, MD, MPH, Martin Grabois, MD, Veronica Fialka Moser, MD, Margaret Nosek, PhD, John B. Redford, MD, Haim Ring, MD, Carson Schneck, Margaret Stineman, MD, and Walter Stolov, MD.

We will particularly miss Thomas Findley, MD, PhD, owing to his lifelong dedication to PM&R research and heartfelt commitment to those that practice PM&R, as well as founding the Fascia Research Congress.

We salute the exemplary administrative, research and clinical leadership of several contemporary academic chairs who have superbly contributed to our lives and our specialty including: Dr. Steven Flanagan (New York University), Dr. Pablo Celnik (Johns Hopkins University), Dr. Joel Stein (Columbia University and Cornell University), Dr. Sam Wu (Temple University) and Dr. Ross Zafonte (Harvard).

Special thanks are due to the industrious and focused publishing staff at Elsevier, including Marybeth Theil, Priyadarshini Pandey, Radjan Selvanadin, Umarani Natarajan, and Saravanan Murugan.

PREFACE

Bryan J. O'Young, MD, CAc, FAAPMR, Mark A. Young, MD, MBA, FACP, FAAPMR, DABPMR,
Steven A. Stiens, MD, MS, Sam S. H. Wu, MD, MA, MPH, MBA

The more that you read, the more things you will know. The more that you learn, the more places you'll go.
—Theodore Seuss Geisel ("Dr. Seuss," 1904–1991)
When it comes to the design of effective learning experiences, one provocative question is worth a hundred proclamations.
—Bernard Bull (1971-)

1. What makes *PM&R Secrets 4th edition* and its online virtual digital companion a unique and indispensable learning tool?

    While there are many helpful physiatric learning resources, including books, videos, podcasts, and online virtual educational material, *PM&R Secrets* has earned a time-honored reputation for excellence because of its distinctive question-and-answer (Q&A) format. As this resource has been crafted in an accessible, entertaining, engaging, and user-friendly format, it has gained academic recognition internationally. Artfully designed to promote better learning through simple and fundamental Socratic dialogue, which skillfully targets essential concepts and basic principles of PM&R ("Just the Facts"), the book has become required reading among learners and teachers of rehabilitation sciences. More than just another text filled with questions and answers, *PM&R Secrets* contains vital content on PM&R philosophy, rehabilitation ideology, disability awareness, and other subjects critical to physiatrist practice. Versions of this book (in multiple languages) have been successfully utilized for nearly three decades by medical students, interns, residents, PM&R examinees, PM&R faculty, and multispecialty medical and allied rehabilitation professionals to maximize their rehabilitation learning and pedagogics.

2. How does the 4th edition of *PM&R Secrets* differ from earlier versions?

    The physician-editors have taken a great product and improved it by adding an abundance of new content in recognition of "keeping current". This edition's refreshed content, revamped contemporary resources, and interactive virtual learning links add 21st-century modernization to this classic. The book's learning value and didactic impact have been significantly enhanced by masterfully leveraging educational technology that includes a unique online digital repository and learning center containing expanded book content. Clickable links, diagrams, photos, schematics, and other important e-learning content are readily and freely accessible to complement the text.

3. What new topics are addressed in this volume?

    The editors have thoroughly and comprehensively revised all content and references to keep readers updated. Although the backbone of *PM&R Secrets* continues to be traditional, fundamental topics, several new chapters address cutting-edge, actionable topics and advances in PM&R. These are, among many others, regenerative medicine, genomics, longitudinal learning, interventional pain physiatry, musculoskeletal ultrasound, and fascia. To help rehabilitations achieve cultural competence, valuable materials relating to PM&R ideology, ethos, and disability sensitivity awareness have been generously covered. With abundant digital and e-learning content, this book and its companion online space assure the reader complete accessibility with the convenience of portability.

4. Why do physiatrists consider *PM&R Secrets* a "Legacy Book"?

    PM&R Secrets has earned the confidence and admiration of readers and educators worldwide. Now in its fourth edition, this volume follows a tradition dedicated to simple, straightforward learning. This commitment to fundamental, accessible learning has resonated with readers at every level of medical education (interns, residents, faculty, and senior clinicians). Available in multiple languages, the book is cited widely in PubMed, journal articles, and other impact-factor resources. On the lighter side, the book has been widely used as a research tool by the media and entertainment industries (e.g., recent episodes of *ER* and Netflix) and has been utilized by governmental and legal consultants. Owing to its reputation for distinction and honor among PM&R learning tools, this 4th edition once again features chapter contributors from many countries.

5. What is the "Secret Sauce" to PM&R education?

    Just as the specialty of PM&R is diverse and includes many subspecialties, learning is best achieved by exposure to various experiences and educational resources. *PM&R Secrets* skillfully fulfills this role by serving as a "bridge-text." The book and its virtual online resources strategically link (bridge) vital information from medical and scientific literature, textbooks, research, and online domains. Clinically relevant and thought-provoking questions are followed by comprehensible answers for every carefully selected topic. Written by prominent, authoritative thought leaders in PM&R, the chapters have been thoroughly updated to include new content, new contributors, and new references. Links to social media, virtual learning resources, videos, diagrams, and educational schematics have enhanced this edition.

6. **Is there any "Magic" to a Q&A approach to PM&R education?**
A famous educator commented, "A good question is seductive; like a work of art, the response it generates is for enjoyment, not analysis" (Morgan N, Saxton J. *Asking Better Questions*. 2nd ed. Pembroke, 2006, p. 14). Similarly, the Q&A's in *PM&R Secrets* have been skillfully designed to spark curiosity and problem-based learning. A review of questions and answers offers a unique and compelling opportunity to serve as a springboard for individual or group learning. Q&A's are an interactive, fun, and convenient way of learning PM&R.

7. **Can Q&A-based learning help across the PM&R educational continuum?**
The customized and curated Q&As included in this book, and its digital counterpart, offer readers essential clinical information suited to all stages of practice development. From the student new to rehabilitation who requires clear definitions of basic physiatric terminology and concepts to the PM&R resident who needs clinical pearls and pointers, and on to the more advanced PM&R clinician and educator who relish sharing rehabilitation knowledge, the Q&A approach embraced by this book is extremely helpful. This book is also well suited for health care providers from other specialties who regularly address PM&R issues in their practices.

8. **Is there scientific evidence supporting the use of Q&A in promoting PM&R education?**
A time-honored tradition in medical education, the Socratic style of teaching skillfully deploys questions and answers to promote dynamic learning. Acquiring knowledge through this interactive, dynamic method has proven to be an engaging and enduring method of teaching compared to "passive learning techniques" (Bruner JS. The act of discovery. *Harv Educ Rev*. 1961;31:21–32). Once again, in this new edition of *PM&R Secrets*, the editors offer a spirited and unpretentious journey through the specialty via a Q&A Socratic approach.

9. **What is the mission and vision of *PM&R Secrets*, 4th ed.?**
As in earlier editions of this legendary book, the newest edition continues its celebrated mission of offering an attractive, portable offline and online educational resource for students, interns, residents, attendings, faculty physicians, and rehabilitation colleagues (PT, OT, SLP, Psychologist, RN). *PM&R Secrets* is a beacon of light to rehabilitation learners by imparting concise clinical knowledge delivered engagingly and interactively. *PM&R Secrets*, supported by expert editors, authors, and faculty, continues to be hailed as an authoritative, straightforward, and powerful educational tool for rehab professionals in clinical and academic environments. Balancing factual details about PM&R with philosophical and ideological concepts, the book provides a well-rounded overview of the specialty. Owing to its unique format and distinctive teaching style, *PM&R Secrets* pays homage to the roots and traditions of physiatry by striving to enhance the quality of care and lives of persons with disabilities.

10. **What is the history of *PM&R Secrets*?**
In 1993, three innovative physiatry clinician-educators (Bryan, Mark, and Steve) had a moment of inspiration that was truly a vision of empowerment and educational action. The trio sought to maximize the learning experience of their students, residents, colleagues, and rehab team members by creating a book with core concepts in a question-and-answer format. For many evenings, the threesome sat around a table in the rehab unit with a few residents, munched on peanuts, and taught PM&R using questions and answers. These sessions were interactive, focused, and quite animated. More PM&R residents attended over time, as well as allied rehabilitation professionals. What began as a casual meet-up to share PM&R knowledge morphed into a written product. A comprehensive book of Q&As focused on all dimensions of the PM&R landscape. The troika was later joined by Sam, a PM&R thought leader with an extensive background in PM&R international leadership and academic education, to enhance the new edition. The book has now gained international acclaim and entered the world of e-learning.

11. **How does the 4th edition of *PM&R Secrets* take the drudgery out of studying?**
Designed to provide brief questions and on-point answers conveniently organized according to a topic in individual chapters, this book is *fun to read, portable, user-friendly*, and a *one-of-a-kind* learning resource.

12. **How have the editors and contributors to *PM&R Secrets* made a positive impact on humanity?**
Just as the famous African proverb goes, "It takes a village to raise a child," the publishing and nurturing of a book require a community of dedicated people. By being true to the roots and traditions of PM&R, every contributor to this book has not only demonstrated their dedication to quality, compassionate care for their patients but has also balanced this commitment by "giving back" by being an author. *PM&R Secrets* would not be possible without the teamwork, altruism, and volunteerism demonstrated. This unique and selfless approach is truly emblematic of the PM&R spirit and is a genuine expression of the physiatrist's call for caring and impassioned advocacy for persons with disability.
As expressed in the pages of *JAMA* by one physiatrist,

> "As practitioners of the healing art, we are often swept away by the mundane minutiae of providing expert technical care to our patients. Often overlooked is the human side of the caring and transcendent sense of seeing life through the eyes of our patients."

Young, MA. Still lives: Narratives of spinal cord injury (Review). *JAMA*. 2005;293(4):497. doi:10.1001/jama.293.4.497-a.

13. What role do "Online Chapters" serve?

    Enhancing PM&R learning through traditional methods (printed books) and online strategies (dedicated online portal) is an integral part of the core mission and vision of PM&R Secrets 4th Edition. This hybrid didactic strategy makes the book unique and truly is the "Secret Sauce" of our academic product. Online content offers the convenience of universal access. (As one resident put it: "Wherever the internet is, PM&R Secrets is.") This makes it easier for busy residents and clinicians "on the run" to access study material across various locations (call rooms, bedrooms, clinics, and airplanes) and from their iPhones, iPad, cell phones, and desktop and laptop computers over the world. ALL print content of the book is easily accessible online.

14. What are "BONUS QUESTIONS & ANSWERS" (Q&A's)?"

    For certain chapters of the PRINTED book, the readers are encouraged to access the online edition of PM&R Secrets for "bonus Q&A'S." Available ONLY virtually, these bonus Q&A's are **included selectively for particular chapters. They are truly a** value-added and enticing web-based feature of this 4th edition".

    To further enhance learning, six additional online-only chapters have been generously included to provide additional valuable content.

PREAMBLE TO THE FOURTH EDITION OF *PM&R SECRETS*: "Answering the Call"

Joel A. DeLisa, MD, MS
Professor Emeritus, Department of PM&R
Rutgers, New Jersey Medical School
Clinical Professor, Department of Orthopedics & Rehabilitation
University of New Mexico
Former Chairman of the Board of the American Board of Medical Specialties

"Answering the Call" is a critical and defining responsibility of every physiatrist. Every day, throughout the world, despite the most adverse of circumstances, the PM&R doctor skillfully and compassionately responds to the needs of his/her patients. The notorious COVID-19 pandemic tested the endurance and resilience of the physiatrist in bold and unprecedented new ways. There, the PM&R team stood passionately and proudly in the ICU—establishing ROM and preventive procedures; at the bedside—maintaining patient recovery and improving function; in the gym—supervising functional restoration and AOL recovery of our patients; and in the continuity clinics—working with persons with disabilities to forge a bold new beginning.

It is no secret that amid the tumultuous COVID-19 era, the altruistic editors of *PM&R Secrets, 4th Edition* and their dedicated faculty of contributing authors have forged ahead to "Answer the Call." Despite a heavy clinical load, challenging family responsibilities, and formidable administrative duties, they have dedicated themselves to producing a new and unique edition of their now legendary volume. The book's uniqueness lies in its simplicity, portability, and distinctive "question and answer" dialogue. It serves as an innovative review style, complementary to other more expansive texts such as my own pioneering work, *Delisa's Physical Medicine and Rehabilitation, Principles and Practice*.

Having dedicated my professional career to "Answering the Call" as the inaugural PM&R Chairman at UMDNJ-New Jersey Medical School, Founding President & CEO of Kessler Medical Rehabilitation, Research, and Education Corporation, Chairman of ABMS, President of ISPRM, and other vital professional roles, I am deeply inspired by the enduring reality that modern medicine adds years to life. At the same time, physiatry contributes to the quality of life during these years. The importance of the specialty is unquestionably reflected by the impressive growth in positions of formal postgraduate educational allopathic and osteopathic training programs. The quality of academic residency training programs and the number of trainees have flourished over the past three decades. This has created an ever-present need for new literature and alternative approaches to didactics and learning.

The specialty of PM&R, long applauded as the "quality of life" medical specialty, powerfully comes alive in this review textbook. The target audience of medical students, residents, faculty, and physiatrists, well entrenched in their careers, are taken on an enlightening educational journey beginning with the fundamental chapter of "What is a Physiatrist" to chapters dedicated to neurorehabilitation, musculoskeletal diagnosis, and procedural intervention through the last chapter, "Future of Physiatry."

Throughout the pages of this volume, the editors and their talented faculty of chapter authors have once again "Answered the Call." They have paid invaluable tribute to the field of PM&R and the education of tomorrow's generation of physiatrists.

INTRODUCTION: PM&R EDUCATION IN THE SOCIAL MEDIA AGE

Mark A. Young, MD, MBA, FACP, FAAPMR, DABPMR, Steven A. Stiens, MD, MS, Bryan J. O'Young, MD, CAc, FAAPMR, Sam S. H. Wu, MD, MA, MPH, MBA

The function of education is to teach one to think intensively and to think critically; intelligence plus character-that is the goal of true education.

—Martin Luther King (1929–1968)

1. **Are there "Best Practices" in PM&R education that guide the attainment of education, knowledge, skills, and aptitude?**

   A "Best Practice" in medical education refers to "a technique or methodology that, through experience and research, has proven to reliably lead to a desired result." In the context of medical education, they generally require *a commitment to utilizing available knowledge, methodology, and technology to achieve success in medical training.* Since its launch in 1997, *PM&R Secrets* has consistently promoted the best practice of PM&R education by combining the pedagogic prowess of the Socratic method with contextual-based learning. Learning tools such as *PM&R Secrets* employ question-and-answer techniques to strengthen problem-solving ability and bolster RQ ("Rehabilitation Quotient"). In the age of social media, this teaching style has grown in importance due to the addition of clickable links and online references. Many of the questions in this book are designed to simulate real-world clinical scenarios that you, the reader, will encounter at the bedside, on clinical rounds, on exams, in evaluations, and throughout your practice.

2. **What is the best way to prepare for board certification, fellowship, and a successful career in physiatry?**

   There are many effective means of learning PM&R, including lectures, grand rounds, journal clubs, bedside rounds, gym rounds, outpatient clinics, Zoom programs, and other online and offline forms of participation. Although there is no perfect formula for studying PM&R, the editors of this book, bolstered by our decades of teaching experience, passionately believe that combining these strategies has the most significant impact. We believe that *PM&R Secrets* (now available digitally) is a valuable adjunctive resource in this process because of its user-friendly Q&A format and contextual-based learning approach. Learning in context is a powerful form of education that places "students" of rehabilitation in an actual or hypothetical clinical context that sparks curiosity and stimulates further learning.

3. **What are the benefits of using the Socratic method to learn medicine and rehabilitation principles?**

   An ancient Greek philosopher, Socrates promoted knowledge through "knowing" and "learning" via critical thinking rather than rote memorization. Accordingly, he emphasized the necessity of dynamic discussion and engaging dialogue between student and teacher to impart wisdom (i.e., educational content). Central to this method is the Q&A approach. *PM&R Secrets*, throughout its time-honored four decades of existence, has enchanted readers with thought-provoking Q&A that stimulates thinking and enhances problem-solving skills. The online edition (e-edition) of the 4th Edition contains an electronic version of all the material in the book, as well as added Q&A content to inform the reader and bolster proficiency in emerging areas of PM&R. This engaging method of teaching has proven a didactic delight to readers at all stages, from medical student to tenured senior attending/faculty.

Katsara O, De Witte K. How to use Socratic questioning in order to promote adults' self-directed learning. *Stud Educ Adults.* 2018;51:109–129. Available at https://cris.maastrichtuniversity.nl/ws/portalfiles/portal/75771302/Wite_2019_how_to_use_Socratic_questioning.pdf.

Pekarsky D. Socratic teaching: A critical assessment. *J Moral Educ.* 1994;23:112–134.

4. How is learning to walk similar to learning rehabilitation?

When we learn to walk, we do so "step by step." Each step we take is a milestone and leads to more advanced functionality later in the developmental stages. When we learn PM&R, we must begin with the basics. A vital prerequisite for rehabilitation students is to understand anatomy, physiology, kinesiology, and the social sciences. These topics are addressed in the beginning pages of *PM&R Secrets* and enable the reader to advance to more complex topics in the field. The questions and answers in *PM&R Secrets* are arranged logically, and an advancing hierarchy enables readers to develop and deploy their clinical skills. For example, manual muscle testing methodology might be presented in a question, followed by a question assessing SCI level, and followed by a question predicting medical complications anticipated by that level. The final question in that chain is functional outcomes (transfer, wheelchair propulsion, and self-care ability). Just as learning to ambulate requires a "step-by-step" approach, learning to maintain balance and stability is an essential characteristic of mobility training. The "balance" of rehabilitation education relates to the ethos of physiatry practice. Learners of rehabilitation must also have a reflective awareness of their personal development and empathic regard for others.

One physiatrist aptly remarked, "As practitioners of the healing art, we are often swept away by the mundane minutiae of providing expert technical care to our patients. Often overlooked is the human side of the caring and transcendent sense of seeing life through the eyes of our patients." The practice of PM&R clearly extends far beyond general diagnosis and treatment to improve the function and quality of life.

Young MA. Still lives: Narratives of spinal cord injury (Review). *JAMA*. 2005;293(4):497. doi:10.1001/jama.293.4.497-a.

Kulkarni VT, Salgado SM, Pelletier SR, Shields HM. Teaching methods used by internal medicine residents on rounds: what works? *Adv Med Educ Pract*. 2019;10:15–21. Available at: https://www.ncbi.nlm.nih.gov/pmc/articles/PMC6345188/pdf/amep-10-015.pdf.

5. What is medical "Show-and-Tell"? Do PM&R physicians use it?

As children, we would often participate in "Show & Tell," a playful practice of showing an object (such as a toy) to an audience and describing it. As academic physicians, we play this game when we participate in Hospital (or Gym) Rounds. Broadly defined as "bedside visitation by a physician and other team members for evaluation, treatment, and documentation," rounds are a daily, time-honored ritual of medicine. The term "rounds" was coined by Sir William Osler, Physician-in-Chief at the Johns Hopkins Hospital. He passionately believed that the patient is at the center of all medical knowledge, and the team of health care providers and doctors gather around. Osler and his clinical entourage would circumnavigate (round) the legendary octagonal hospital ward each morning. In PM&R, rounding has transitioned from the bedside to the therapy gym, where patients can be observed making functional gains while participating in therapy.

Kulkarni VT, Salgado SM, Pelletier SR, Shields HM. Teaching methods used by internal medicine residents on rounds: what works? *Adv Med Educ Pract*. 2019;10:15–21. Available at: https://www.ncbi.nlm.nih.gov/pmc/articles/PMC6345188/pdf/amep-10-015.pdf.

6. How are bedside and gym side rounds fertile grounds for teaching?

Inspired by the clinical environment, Dr. William Osler was acclaimed for his masterful bedside teaching skills, in which he used difficult and obscure questions at the bedside. He was said to have fired these questions at his students and residents like a machine gun. This time-honored academic game came to be known as "pimping," but the term has been replaced by a more acceptable word ("pumping") in more recent years. The tradition of pumping is celebrated each day in rehabilitation education. The physician editors do this every day. The arena for this activity is the bedside, therapy gym, or outpatient clinic. Trainees are asked by supervisors (Attending or Chief Resident) to provide many details of medical background, physical findings, impairments, limitations to barriers, activities, and characteristics of the environment.

When questions about background rehabilitation concepts are asked, the knowledge shared in books such as *PM&R Secrets* can serve as useful preparatory academic "artillery." This academic game of pumping is engaging, animated, and potentially humorous if carried out sensitively and received without pretension or hubris. The bedside and gym are excellent locations.

Ezeoke OM. A guide to pimping in medical education; 2020. Walterskluwer.com Available at: https://www.wolterskluwer.com/en/expert-insights/a-guide-to-pimping-in-medical-education.

Tofade T, Elsner J, Haines ST. Best practice strategies for effective use of questions as a teaching tool. *Am J Pharm Ed*. 2013;77(7):155. https://www.ncbi.nlm.nih.gov/pmc/articles/PMC3776909/.

7. How has "Digital Health" revolutionized the clinical and learning landscape of rehabilitation?

Generally defined as electronic tools and technology that support physicians' clinical decision-making and education, "Digital Health" has had a revolutionary impact on physiatry. According to the FDA, the digital health spectrum includes a variety of categories, including mobile health (mHealth), health information technology (IT), wearable devices, telehealth, telemedicine, and personalized medicine. Examples of educational tools include mobile medical apps and software that inform clinical decision-making, machine learning, and artificial intelligence. Digital medicine can reduce inefficiencies, improve access, reduce costs, increase quality, and make medicine more personalized. Areas of digital health.

Topic Area	Description
Mobile medical applications	"Medical devices that are mobile apps meet the definition of a medical device and are an accessory to a regulated medical device or transform a mobile platform into a regulated medical device."
Digital therapeutics	Regulated, evidence-based software intervention that can be independent or complementary to other therapies.
Telehealth	"Delivery and facilitation of health and health-related services including medical care, provider and patient education, health information services, and self-care via telecommunications and digital communication technologies."
Wearable devices and sensors	"Wearable electronics are devices that can be worn or mated with human skin to continuously and closely monitor an individual's activities without interrupting or limiting the user's motion."
Digital biomarkers	Hardware software-based measurement of physiological data in real-time for prognostic or diagnostic measurements.

Adapted from Aungst TD, Patel R. Integrating digital health into the curriculum—Considerations on the current landscape and future developments. J Med Educ Curric Dev. 2020;7:2382120519901275. doi:10.1177/2382120519901275. Available at https://www.ncbi.nlm.nih.gov/pmc/ articles/PMC6971961/.

8. How has PM&R communication entered the current tech era?

Recently, there has been an enormous growth in the use of the electronic medical record and the adoption of telemedicine-based PM&R evaluations and electronic prescriptions. Although this trend began about 10 years ago, its use was dramatically accelerated by the COVID-19 pandemic. Physician and Physiatry IOS and Android-based communication platforms such as Doximity (LinkedIn for doctors) and Zoom have allowed real-time, user-friendly, HIPPA-compliant clinical and audio and video communication between physicians and patients. Academic educational programming, as well as CME programming, have fostered learning objectives. The "privatization" of physician-patient cell phone communication has been optimized with free HIPPA-compliant apps such as *Doximity Dialer*, which allows the physician to call the patient using their cell phone while displaying the clinic or hospital phone number on caller ID.

Cartledge P, Miller M, Phillips B. The use of social networking sites in medical education, *Med Teach*. 2013;35(10):847–857. doi: 10.3109/0142159X.2013.804909.

9. How can clinicians use social media and electronic communication to facilitate learning?

Digital communication apps have the potential to extend the "reach" and expand the learning potential of physiatrists and members of the PM&R team internationally. Examples include sharing patient vignettes, exchanging radiological and ultrasound images, conducting case discussions and conferences across miles, and fostering participation in grand rounds and journal clubs. Posts on well-known social media apps like WhatsApp, Instagram, Facebook, and Twitter can serve as a valuable platform to facilitate discussion and promote learning. Theme-based content from social media group sites such as @Neuroradiology on Instagram is a unique and indispensable learning resource helpful to physiatrists and neurologists that features high-resolution brain and spine images. A typical post on @Neuroradiology might include questions such as, "What's the diagnosis?" and "How would you manage?" These posts promote independent thinking and enhance learning. Often, digital apps serve a secondary role by building collegiality and developing a community of colleagues who can participate in educational and career cross-talk.

Saha S. *Revised Basic Workshop in Medical Education Networking.* Calcutta National Medical College, August 21–23, 2017. Available at: https://www.slideshare.net/satyajitsaha8/networking-in-medical-education.

10. **How have video-chatting services (VCS) for computers and smartphones revolutionized PM&R education?**

    Wildly popular services (e.g., Zoom, Microsoft Teams, Skype, WebEx, Google Meet, WhatsApp, Doximity, Facetime, and others) have enabled face-to-face, cloud-based, virtual connections among residents, attending faculty, patients, and other educational and clinical stakeholders. The editors and authors of *PM&R Secrets* were able to coordinate the compilation and organization of this book through weekly video-chat meetings conducted across geographic boundaries and time zones. VCS is now liberally used by many academic departments to conduct grand rounds, journal clubs, resident lectures, and teaching rounds. The advantages of VCS in resident education include:

    - Accessibility of speakers across the miles
    - Access to residents across campus or in different 'parts of town'
    - Polling function
    - Recording function

    The added benefit of the "share screen" function of many VCS programs is that they enable joint viewing of videos, articles, pictures, and other content.

Galiatsatos P, Porto-Carreiro F, Hayashi J, Zakaria S, Christmas C. The use of social media to supplement resident medical education—The SMART-ME initiative. *Med Educ Online.* 2016;21(1):29332. Available at https://www.tandfonline.com/doi/pdf/10.3402/meo.v21.29332?needAccess=true&.

11. **How can preparation for the AAPM&R boards (parts 1 and 2) benefit from VCS?**

    In the experience of the editors of *PM&R Secrets*, our residents have successfully leveraged VCS technology to conduct board study sessions, topic reviews, and oral exam one-on-one sessions. The share screen function of many VCS programs enables joint viewing of videos, articles, pictures, and other important board exam-related content.

12. **How does the traditional "Rehabilitation Problem List" guide learning?**

    The demonstrated benefit of the problem list reflects the patient and their unique set of diagnostic findings and social and functional circumstances. Like a fingerprint, the problem list is unique to the patient and helps educate the physician to optimize care. The problem list is organized with the primary diagnosis at the top, followed by secondary conditions and concerns. Next, all impairments, such as pain contracture, are given, followed by activity limitations, including mobility and ADL deficits. Lastly, problems relating to barriers to participation are listed, including psychological adaptation, social role function, community reintegration barriers, architectural accessibility impediments, education, spirituality, and vocation.

13. **How can *PM&R Secrets* in print and online formats help guide my studies and enhance my physiatry practice?**

    Just as thousands of readers of earlier editions of this book have benefited over the past 30 years from the treasure chest of knowledge and wisdom in this work, you too will learn a lot. The chapters are sequentially organized by the development of PM&R knowledge. Although the book need not be read in order, you will appreciate the logical progression of concepts and principles developed from start to finish. Chapters can be read individually in context when the need arises for clinical topics encountered in practice to require closer study. The book and its digital counterpart were designed to be kept close at hand, on the wards, in the call room, clinic, or gym. Clickable links and references generously interspersed throughout the chapters will help illuminate the text. Reviewing questions and answers provides a springboard for group discussions.

Jones RW. Learning and teaching in small groups: Characteristics, benefits, problems, and approaches. *Anaesth Intensive Care.* 2007;35(4):587–592. doi: 10.1177/0310057X0703500420, Available at: https://journals.sagepub.com/doi/pdf/10.1177/0310057X0703500420.

14. **What words of inspiration will help the reader of *PM&R Secrets* thrive as a physiatrist?**

    The knowledge that your patients are your books and that educational tools like *PM&R Secrets* can help promote a vibrant and comprehensive appreciation of the specialty. No matter what you end up doing in your career (e.g., interventional pain or stroke rehab), remain true to the roots and traditions of PM&R. Read on to learn more!

BIBLIOGRAPHY

Chan TM, Stehman C, Gottlieb M, Thoma B. A short history of free open access medical education. The past, present, and future. *ATS Sch*. 2020;1(2):87–100. doi:10.34197/ats-scholar.2020-0014PS. Available at: https://www.ncbi.nlm.nih.gov/pmc/articles/PMC8043296/.

Disabled World. Models of disability: types and definitions. *Disabled World*, 2010. Available at: https://www.disabled-world.com/definitions/disability-models.php.

Gibbons AS, III. *Model-Centered Instruction, the Design, and the Designer*. Faculty Publication 4656, 2008. Available at: https://scholarsarchive.byu.edu/facpub/4656.

Haegele JA, Hodge S. Disability discourse: overview and critiques of the medical and social models. *Quest*. 2016;68(2):193–206. Available at: https://www.researchgate.net/publication/297722476_Disability_Discourse_Overview_and_Critiques_of_the_Medical_and_Social_Models.

Kushner DS, Peters KM, Johnson-Greene D. Evaluating the Siebens model in geriatric-stroke inpatient rehabilitation to reduce institutionalization and acute-care readmissions. *J Stroke Cerebrovasc Dis*. 2016;25(2):317–326. doi: 0.1016/j/jstrokecerebrovasdis.2015.09/036.

Rogers CR, Frieberg HJ. *Freedom to Learn*. 3rd ed. New York: Merrill/Macmillan; 1994.

Smith MK. *Learning Theory*. In *Encyclopedia of Pedagogy and Informal Education, 1999–2020*. Available at: https://infed.org/mobi/learning-theory-models-product-and-process.

Acknowledgments

The editors thank Brandon Brandt, DO, cofounder of PM&R Scholars, for his suggestions and comments on this chapter and its formulation.

FOREWORD

Stanley F. Wainapel MD, MPH
Professor of Clinical Rehabilitation Medicine
Albert Einstein College of Medicine
Bronx, NY, USA

He explained to me with great insistence that every question possessed a power that did not lie in the answer.

Elie Wiesel (1928–2016)

This book has an ironically appropriate title because physical medicine and rehabilitation (PM&R) was something of a secret itself when it was first recognized as a distinct medical specialty three-quarters of a century ago. Lacking the drama of surgical interventions or the specificity of a dedicated organ such as the heart, lungs, or brain to highlight its identity, our specialty introduced a revolutionary paradigm of interdisciplinary, patient-centered care with function and quality of life as its primary focus. Dr. Howard Rusk used to describe our specialty as the third phase of medicine (following preventive and acute care), which can also be likened to the lower motor neuron, which is the final common pathway of the nervous system. PM&R serves as the final common pathway of the health care system, bridging the transition from institution to community. Over the years, our specialty has expanded to encompass a wide range of diseases that results in our interactions with most medical/surgical specialties. In the not-so-distant past, the presence of a distinct academic PM&R Department within a large medical center was far from routine, but such departments are now the rule rather than the exception.

PM&R Secrets is a uniquely invaluable compendium of clinical and educational information for professionals who treat patients with all types of physical disabilities. Its format is a Socratic dialogue between the reader and dozens of leaders in their fields of expertise from around the world. Each new edition has updated its table of contents to reflect recent developments. The range of topics covered in this new edition is breathtaking, including chapters on cutting-edge subjects such as rehabilitation following transplantation, regenerative medicine, and genomics. The expansion from 84 to 92 chapters between the 3rd and 4th Editions attests to the tireless efforts of the editors to stay abreast of the latest state of the art in physiatry. This is the secret to why *PM&R Secrets* will remain an essential textbook that belongs in the library of any clinician devoted to rehabilitation care.

CONTENTS

THE TOP SECRETS: PM&R'S 100 FUNDAMENTAL PRINCIPLES

Bryan J. O'Young, MD, CAc, FAAPMR, Mark A.Young, MD, MBA, FACP, FAAPMR, DABPMR, Steven A. Stiens, MD, MS, and Sam S. H. Wu, MD, MA, MPH, MBA

An investment in knowledge always pays the best interest.

Benjamin Franklin (1706-1790)

This synopsis contains carefully selected rehabilitation concepts, principles, and educational pearls. Designed for multiple audiences, including the PM&R learner, educator, and clinician, this distilled, didactic dialogue promotes mastery of PM&R using the Socratic method. Presented in a unique question-and-answer format, this guide contains crafted contributions by preeminent, internationally-respected academic physiatric expert authors. An indispensable complement to the fourth edition of *PM&R Secrets*, these "Top Secrets" serve as an 'appetizer' for the educational banquet that follows. Within the pages of this book, a treasure chest of knowledge and valuable educational material awaits the reader.

1. ### What is PM&R?
   Physical Medicine and Rehabilitation (PM&R), also known as Physiatry, is the specialty that primarily cares for persons with disability because of its devotion to multisystem medical care for persons with life-long conditions. Preserving and enhancing function is physiatry's ardent call to action. Physiatrists artfully utilize modalities, medications, assistive devices, procedures, and exercise in interdisciplinary rehabilitative formats to deliver functional outcomes.

2. ### How many people worldwide are there with disabilities, and what percent experience significant functional deficits?
   There are more than one billion people with disabilities worldwide, and nearly 200 million experience significant functional deficits.

3. ### What terms are used to describe various aspects of disability?
   The *International Classification of Disability Function and Health* has defined a few related terms.
   Impairment is an abnormality of structure, appearance, and/or function at the end organ level (e.g., a herniated disc with nerve root compression). *Activity limitation* is the inability of a person to perform an activity due to impairment in the normal fashion (e.g., inability to walk or carry groceries). *Participation restriction* is a disadvantage resulting from a disability (and impairment) that limits an individual's ability to fulfill a societal role (e.g., employment).

4. ### Should the words "disability" and "handicap" be used interchangeably?
   No. Simply because a person has a disability does NOT mean they are handicapped. Consider the example of famed singer/composer, Stevie Wonder. Because he is blind, he is a person with a disability. However, his blindness does not hinder him from fulfilling his role as a singer. Therefore, he does not have a handicap. Often, people with disabilities can thrive in various roles with the help of needed personal assistance, adaptations, or modifications.

5. ### How does proper nutrition play an essential role in the restorative and rehabilitative processes?
   Nutrition provides substrates that are the building blocks of rehabilitation outcomes. An individualized and balanced diet that includes whole foods and essential nutrients can help optimize neurological outcomes, pain management, and recovery.

6. ### Name the types of skeletal muscle contractions and their significance?
   A *muscle contraction* activates muscle fibers and force generation, promoting body movement and postural control. Ordinarily, force generation in muscles is produced either by a change in fiber length or by increasing fiber tension. The two main types of muscle contraction are *isometric*, in which muscle tension increases while the muscle length remains the same; and *isotonic*, in which fiber length changes while tension remains uniform. Isotonic contractions have two subtypes: *eccentric* (muscle length increases) and *concentric* (muscle length shortens)

7. ### What is an "eccentric contraction," and how is it unique?
   An eccentric or lengthening contraction occurs when muscle force is *less* than the load. Eccentric contractions are stronger and utilize less energy than concentric contractions ("higher force at lower cost"). Typically, this occurs when gravity is the prime mover (e.g., Tibialis anterior and quadriceps muscle in the gait cycle).

8. Name two neurorehabilitation therapies proven to help facilitate movement and functional restoration?
   Constraint-induced movement therapy (CIMT) involves restraining the unaffected opposite extremity to promote purposeful use of the involved limb. **Locomotor training** utilizes a bodyweight support system over a treadmill with manual gait movement assistance from trainers.

9. What is a physical agent?
   A physical agent is a modality used to achieve a therapeutic effect in tissues. The five categories of physical agents are thermal, electrical, sound, light, and mechanical.

10. Provide three examples of the application of electrotherapy.
    FES (functional electric stimulation) depolarizes nerves or muscles to produce useful movement and exercise. **TENS** (transcutaneous electrical nerve stimulation) temporarily diminishes perceived acute and chronic pain. Invasive **neuromodulation** devices such as deep brain stimulators or spinal cord stimulators minimize chronic pain perception that does not respond to other treatments.

11. What is regenerative rehabilitation?
    Regenerative medicine seeks to repair and replace cells, tissues, and organs to restore function lost due to age, disease, injury, or congenital defects. Regenerative strategies under investigation include prolotherapy, platelet-rich plasma, and stem cell-based therapies to treat musculoskeletal disorders. Research is ongoing to expand these technologies to treat neurological, cardiopulmonary, pediatric, burn, post-amputation, and other medically complex disorders.

12. How are axonal neuropathies unique?
    Axonal neuropathies typically affect the distal territories of the longest nerves and therefore impact the feet first. Proximal nerve conduction is faster because of warmth, thicker myelination, and greater distances between the nodes of Ranvier.

13. How can standard evidence-based medicine be complemented by natural and/or alternative treatments to improve overall outcomes?
    Integrative medicine is the active, patient-centered practice of including the best evidence-based care and a variety of compatible, complementary, and alternative (CAM) treatments that are expected to achieve the fullest adherence, maximal health, and participative function of each patient.

14. Following a burn trauma, which joints are most commonly affected by heterotopic ossification (HO)?
    Following burn injury, HO most commonly presents at the elbow, followed by the shoulder (adult) or hip (pediatric).

15. What are the eight phases of the gait cycle? Are there measurable units?
    The gait cycle is divided into four swing and four stance phases: pre-swing, initial swing, mid-swing, terminal swing, initial contact, loading response, midstance, and terminal stance. Units include stride length, step width, step angle, and cadence (steps per time unit).

16. Is there a difference between a strain and a sprain?
    Yes! A *sprain* affects the ligaments that connect two bones, while a *strain* affects the musculotendinous region.

17. Is Spurling's Test highly specific?
    Yes. If the test is negative, cervical radiculopathy is unlikely to be present.

18. Why is screening for hearing loss in the elderly and in infants important?
    Hearing loss screening is essential in the elderly as hearing loss can mimic dementia and/or aphasia and in infants (as it can contribute to language delay.)

19. What are the classic exacerbating and alleviating factors of disc-related lumbosacral radiculopathy?
    Classic disc-related lumbosacral radicular pain is often exacerbated by sitting and forward-bending and is alleviated by walking, standing, or lying supine.

20. What symptoms and diagnostics aid in the diagnosis of radiculopathy?
    Clinical findings of *weakness* and/or *atrophy*, *sensory impairment*, and *depressed* or *absent* reflexes. Any or all of these can help support the diagnosis. *MRI* may assist with localization and diagnosis, although it alone cannot establish a diagnosis. The electrodiagnostic exam may reveal motor denervation involving the specific nerve root and must be viewed as an extension of the physical exam.

21. What is the classic position that minimizes low back pain associated with neurogenic claudication?
    Patients with neurogenic claudication feel better when walking uphill (spinal flexion) or sitting.

22. Which nerve roots are impinged in an extraforaminal disc herniation versus a central lumbar disc herniation?
    In an extraforaminal (far lateral) lumbar disc herniation, the superior spinal nerve will be affected (e.g., extraforaminal herniation of L4-5 disc will affect the L4 spinal nerve). In a central lumbar disc herniation, the inferior spinal nerve root will be affected (e.g., central herniation of L4-5 disc will affect the L5 spinal nerve).

23. What are the innervation level(s) of the facet joints? And how many nerves are to be injected in a facet joint nerve block?
    For C6-7 facet joint and above, the cervical facet joints are innervated by two nerve branches, both of which are at the same segmental levels. For example, the C5-6 facet joint is innervated by medial branches of the C5 and C6 posterior ramus.
    The C7-T1 facet joint is innervated by medial branches of the C7 and C8 posterior ramus and the T1-T2 facet joint is innervated by the medial branches of the C8 and T1 posterior ramus.
    Facet joints (T2-3 and below) are innervated by two nerve branches: one from the medial branches of the posterior ramus above and one at the same segmental level (e.g., the L2-3 facet joint is innervated by medial branches of the L1 and L2 posterior ramus). The only exception is the L5-S1 facet joint. It is innervated by the L4 medial branch and the L5 posterior ramus, not the medial branch of L5. The L5 posterior ramus is unique in that it runs a longer course, passing the facet joint before giving rise to a medial branch.
    For "n" consecutive, ipsilateral facet joints, n + 1 nerves should be blocked.

24. What is the major risk associated with cervical transforaminal epidural steroid injections?
    Inadvertent steroid injection of the vertebral artery.

25. How are peripheral neuropathies classified?
    Peripheral polyneuropathies may be classified according to the number and distribution of nerves affected: (mononeuropathy, mononeuropathy multiplex, or polyneuropathy), the pathological process (axon loss, demyelinating, or combined), type of fiber involvement (motor, sensory, autonomic, or combined), or process affecting the nerves (inflammation, compression, chemotherapy).

26. What are the two primary birth-related traumatic brachial plexus injuries? Which is the more common?
    Erb's palsy (from shoulder depression) affects the upper brachial plexus (C5,6, and sometimes 7), and **Klempke's palsy** (from arm elevation) affects the lower brachial plexus (C8, T1). Erb's palsy is more common.

27. Which muscles play an important role in standing?
    During standing, the *soleus* muscle and the *gastrocnemius* muscle are the most active lower limb muscles and oppose the line of center of gravity to plantarflex the ankle and extend the knee.

28. What is myasthenia gravis?
    Myasthenia gravis is a postsynaptic autoimmune channelopathy that causes muscle weakness due to antibodies against the acetylcholine (Ach) receptors in the neuromuscular junction.

29. What is Lambert-Eaton Myasthenia Syndrome (LEMS)?
    LEMS is a presynaptic autoimmune channelopathy that causes neuromuscular weakness due to antibodies against voltage-gated calcium channels. LEMS is often associated with small-cell lung carcinoma (SCLC).

30. Is acupuncture effective?
    Studies, including controlled trials, have supported the effectiveness of acupuncture in degenerative joint disease, low back pain, headache, substance abuse, postoperative pain, extremity pain, and many other conditions. Factors impacting treatment efficacy include meridian and point selection, needle retention time, and practitioner skill. Recent research has validated the role of musculoskeletal ultrasound in localizing acupuncture placement points.

Allen D (2014). Precision of acupuncture placement using diagnostic ultrasound. *Intl Musculoskelet Med, 36*(2), 64–74. doi:10.1179/1753615414Y.0000000028.

31. How are myofascial trigger points best managed?
    Treatment of myofascial trigger points is most effective when both the peripheral and central segmental sensitization components are addressed.

32. What is the differential diagnosis of dancing-related groin pain?
    Groin pain in dancers can be caused by acetabular labral tears, femoral neck stress fractures, adductor sprain, rectus femoris tendonitis, and myofascial pain.

33. What are the phases of a well-designed cardiac rehabilitation program?
    Cardiac rehabilitation is a three-phase process consisting of Phase I (Hospital), Phase II (Outpatient monitored) and Phase III (Independent maintenance). Cardiac rehabilitation is designed to assess risk, monitor for complications, treat risk factors, gradually regain mobility, and promote cardiovascular fitness. The long-term goal is to optimize life span, minimize cardiac complications, and promote maximal function.

34. What are the physiological components of voiding?
    a) Detrusor muscle activity (classified as normal, underactive, or non-contractile).
    b) Sphincter activity (classified as normal, detrusor sphincter dyssynergia, or non-relaxing sphincter).
    c) Sensation (classified as normal, overactive/increased, underactive/reduced, or absent, or non-specific).

35. What are the hallmarks of motor neuron disease?
    Atrophy, weakness, spasticity, brisk reflexes, and fasciculations are common. Motor neuron diseases do not affect sensation.

36. What is Henneman's size principle?
    Henneman's size principle states that motor units are recruited starting with smaller motor units first, followed by advancing to progressively larger motor units. This enables initial fine motor control followed by progressive gross motor control.

37. Which are the most commonly injured ligaments in an ankle sprain, medial or lateral ligaments? Of the lateral ligaments, which is the most commonly injured?
    The lateral ligaments, i.e., anterior talofibular ligament (ATFL), calcaneofibular ligament (CFL), and posterior talofibular ligament (PTFL). Of the lateral ligaments, the ATFL is the most commonly injured.

38. What is the most common cause of knee pain in children?
    Osgood-Schlatter disease is characterized by activity-related pain occurring at the tibial insertion of the patellar tendon.

39. When is surgery indicated in a meniscal injury?
    The following symptoms are indicative: persistent knee locking, restriction of knee ROM despite therapy, instability, persistent Baker's cyst resulting from a meniscal injury, and persistent pain despite PT.

40. Can multisystem rehabilitation help improve the quality of life for those with spinal cord injury (SCI)?
    Rehabilitation can improve function and increase patients' quality of life (QOL) with irreversible conditions like SCI. Patient-reported quality of life is unrelated to calculated impairments quantified by motor and sensory examinations (e.g., ASIA Impairment Scores, AIS).

41. What are the differences between "bowel care" and the "bowel program"?
    Bowel care is the procedure for assisted defecation. A bowel program is a comprehensive plan for rehabilitative care that includes multiple components: diet, fluid intake, physical activity, medications, and scheduled bowel care. Refinements and compliance in the bowel program prevent complications and surgical interventions, maximally enrich relationships, and permit full participation throughout life.

42. What physiological changes are observed in autonomic dysreflexia (AD)?
    Changes in AD are a sudden paroxysmal rise in systemic and diastolic BP with compensatory pulse rate slowing. AD typically occurs in persons with SCI lesions above T-5 and T-6 and is frequently triggered by painful stimuli such as a full bladder or rectum.

43. Name five important preventable causes of death for adults with spina bifida.
    The most commonly reported causes of death in adult patients include infections, respiratory failure, renal failure, shunt malfunction, and metastatic cancer.

44. What are the most common presenting complaints of cerebral palsy?
    The usual presenting complaints are developmental delay (e.g., not sitting by 9 months), hand preference before 1 year, trouble feeding, drooling, and arms and/or legs feeling stiff with the legs often crossing over each other (scissoring). In less severe cases, developmental delays and manifestations of spasticity may not be present for up to a year.

45. How can cerebral palsy be differentiated from other diagnoses?
    The most important thing to determine is that there is *no loss of milestones*, which would indicate a neurodegenerative disorder, hydrocephalus, or even a tumor. Metabolic testing to rule out other diagnoses is often indicated. A brain MRI or CT may show lesions that correlate with deficits.

46. What interventions improve the rate of healing of pressure sores?
    Eliminate pressure and shear, debride nonviable tissue, reduce a moist ambient environment, minimize bacterial overgrowth (reduce bioburden), and provide a nutritional plan replete with protein, vitamin C, vitamin A, folate, and zinc, all of which support healing.

47. What are neuromuscular junction disorders, and what are their primary characteristics?
    Neuromuscular junction disorders involve a transmission defect of acetylcholine across the neuromuscular junction. The most common neuromuscular disorder is myasthenia gravis. This group of autoimmune postsynaptic disorders is typically characterized by proximal and oculobulbar weakness.

48. **What are the main pathophysiologic features of multiple sclerosis? What are some of the predictors of reduced survival?**
Multiple sclerosis (MS) is a chronic inflammatory disease of the central nervous system that leads to the formation of demyelinating lesions disseminated in space and time, which result in multifocal damage and neurodegeneration in the brain and spinal cord. Survival is shorter in males and those with progressive MS, cerebellar features, and older age.

49. **What is the difference between apraxia and ataxia?**
Apraxia is a cerebral motor planning disorder characterized by the inability to carry out familiar, purposeful activities despite carrying out skilled movements and gestures and having the desire and the knowledge to perform them. Alternatively, ataxia is a cerebellar disorder characterized by carrying out activities with poor coordination.

50. **What rehabilitation strategies should be used to improve unstable posture in Parkinson's Disease?**
Therapy strategies to offset the tendency toward trunk flexion, improve postural alignment and balance, improve axial range of motion, and address deconditioning. Strategies to enhance coordination and gait, such as Frenkel's exercises, stationary bicycles, arm ergometers, treadmills, etc., and Lee Silverman's BIG and LOUD Voice Training programs are recommended.

51. **Why is it urgent to recognize and treat cerebrovascular disease?**
Rapid identification and early treatment of stroke improve survival and recovery. Early rehabilitation therapy optimizes the likelihood of maximally restoring motor skills, language, and cognitive function by 3 months post-stroke.

52. **What is the most common cause of TBI in the US?**
Falls.

53. **What are the primary reasons for the increasing incidence of TBI in the US?**
The reported incidence is increasing due to the aging population and increased awareness of concussions.

54. **Name several factors that increase the risk for aspiration pneumonia?**
These are altered mental status, recumbent position, neurological disorder, ventilatory dysfunction, or vital signs. Aspiration pneumonia risks include poor oral hygiene, saliva reduction, folate and dopamine deficiencies, and proton pump inhibitors.

55. **What swallowing abnormalities are prevalent among Parkinson's patients?**
Hypokinetic dysarthria, dysphagia problems with oral bolus formation, and loss of coordination between oral and pharyngeal stages of swallowing.

56. **What is fascia?**
Fascia consists primarily of connective tissue layers. Each fascial layer has its orientation and composition of collagen fibers. It surrounds, interweaves, and interpenetrates all organs, muscles, bones, and nerve fibers. It gives the body a web of functional infrastructure.

57. **Does rehabilitation play a crucial role in managing myopathies? What are the basic principles of the exercise prescription?**
Rehabilitation interventions play a vital role in improving the quality of life for patients with myopathies. An exercise program for the myopathic patient should be submaximal in intensity, avoid overfatigue, and be closely supervised.

58. **What are the absolute contraindications to botulinum toxin treatment?**
Firm contraindications to botulinum toxin use include those with known hypersensitivity to any of its ingredients, myasthenia gravis, and infection at the injection site.

59. **What is a fragility fracture? Where are the most vulnerable injury sites?**
A fragility fracture is any fracture that occurs following a fall from standing height or less, indicating poor bone strength, and can be the basis for a diagnosis of osteoporosis. The most common injury sites are the hips, spine, distal forearms, or wrists.

60. **Does exercise reduce the risk of fracture?**
Exercise and physical activity positively affect bone density, spinal alignment, the impact of falls, and reduce the risk of fractures. Moderate- or high-intensity multimodal, progressive resistance training in older women and men for 12-18 months has been shown to be especially beneficial.

61. **What primary tumors should be suspected when bone pain is confirmed to be a metastasis?**
The common tumors that metastasize to bone can be remembered with the mnemonic "lead (Pb) kettle" (PBKTL) and are prostate, breast, kidney, thyroid, and lung. The most common site of skeletal metastases is the thoracic spine.

62. **What is myokymia?**
Myokymia on electromyography is pathognomonic for radiation-induced injury due to the previous radiotherapy.

63. **How is juvenile idiopathic arthritis (JIA) diagnosed?**
JIA is multifactored, classified into six subtypes, with onset $<$ age 16 and the presence of arthritis for $>$ 6 weeks.

64. **How do the coracoclavicular (CC) joint and the acromioclavicular (AC) joint "protect" the shoulder?**
At normal physiologic loads, the CC joint resists axial and superior forces, while the AC joint mainly resists anterior-posterior forces. However, excessive axial or superior forces may tear both joints by placing a greater load on the AC joint.

65. **When is surgical repair indicated for the acromioclavicular (AC) or coracoclavicular (CC) joints?**
Generally, surgery is indicated for AC or CC joint separations only when the clavicle is displaced; most cases of sprains and tears are managed conservatively.

66. **What are the basic principles for managing elbow surgeries due to overuse? When is surgical intervention indicated?**
Elbow injuries from overuse are initially managed conservatively with rest, activity modification, and therapeutic exercise. Surgery is indicated in cases where elbow stability is grossly compromised.

67. **Identify the most sensitive and most specific examination techniques for diagnosing a torn anterior cruciate ligament (ACL)**
The Lachman's test is the most sensitive, while the pivot shift test is the most specific physical test for determining an ACL tear.

68. **Plantar fasciitis is most commonly seen in which two groups?**
Plantar fasciitis is typically seen in two distinct populations, sedentary patients with high BMI and runners who have increased their training.

69. **Identify the classic signs of trigger fingers, mallet fingers, and jersey fingers.**
Trigger fingers lock due to tendon thickening. *Mallet fingers* cannot extend due to extensor tendon avulsion. *Jersey fingers* cannot flex due to flexor tendon tear.

70. **What is iliotibial band syndrome?**
Iliotibial band syndrome is lateral knee pain caused by overuse from repetitive knee flexion activities and commonly occurs in running and cycling.

71. **What are the indications for knee, ankle, or foot orthosis (KAFO)?**
A KAFO should be prescribed when there is instability of the knee and ankle, knee extension strength less than antigravity, and risk for deformity. The knee joint can be free or locked, and the axis is usually situated behind the body's center of gravity to facilitate support in the stance phase. A rigid ankle joint raises the center of gravity in the terminal stance phase of gait and prevents foot drop in the swing phase.

72. **What are some considerations before prescribing and fitting an upper extremity orthosis?**
The conditions include increased tone or spasticity of the upper limb. Treating for controlling the spasticity should be considered before an upper limb orthosis is prescribed. Upper limb orthoses can often be fabricated from low-temperature thermoplastic materials or prefabricated kits available from suppliers.

73. **How is proper use of spinal orthosis for a productive outcome ensured?**
Spinal bracing reduces pain, immobilizes to support healing, aligns to guide growth, and provides a stimulus to correct posture.

74. **What are the benefits of using a rigid removable cast dressing after transtibial amputation?**
Using a rigid dressing such as a cast or off-the-shelf rigid removable dressing after transtibial amputation limits edema, shortens healing time, and permits early standing and ambulation with an attached pylon.

75. **Which rehabilitation device uses simple parts, achieves dramatic improvement in mobility and quality of life, yet requires collaborative expertise and a unique prescription to get the best outcome, regardless of culture and geography?**
The World Health Organization's *International Classification of Function* has validated the critical importance of wheelchairs, which can have a positive impact on *health* by preventing falls while walking, *activity* by improving mobility), and *participation* through a return to work. Although the wheelchair is arguably the most important therapeutic tool in rehabilitation, acute and chronic wheelchair-related injuries may occur, and many wheelchair users do not achieve the level of community mobility they could.

76. The ability to use power mobility is based on what two skills?
Being able to utilize power mobility is not based on age as much as cognitive and perceptual skills.

77. Why should clinicians suspect peripheral vascular disease despite the usual musculoskeletal origins of limb pain?
Early detection of peripheral vascular disease (PVD) can decrease myocardial infarction and stroke risk. Risk factors for PVD include smoking, hypertension, diabetes, hyperlipidemia, homocysteinemia, elevated fibrinogen, and symptoms of ischemia. As claudication pain often mimics musculoskeletal pain, physiatrists must screen for PVD.

78. What are the significant pathophysiological differences between obstructive and restrictive pulmonary dysfunction? What are the therapeutic implications?
Intrinsic or obstructive pulmonary disease results in oxygenation impairment and often manifests as eucapnia or hypocapnia. Patients with mechanical dysfunction of respiratory muscles, lungs, and chest wall restriction have ventilatory pump dysfunction that initially causes retention of CO_2 and later hypoxia secondary to worsening hypoventilation. A cardinal rule in managing patients with restrictive dysfunction is to clear mucus plugs with expectoration, suctioning, and ventilation support rather than supplementing oxygen or initiating intubation.

79. Is sleep apnea common after central nervous system insults?
Yes. TBI is frequently complicated by sleep-disordered breathing caused by obstructive sleep apnea (OSA) and central sleep apnea (CSA). OSA is also common in the first 3 months after a stroke. With SCI, the prevalence is nearly 50%. Prevalence increases with ascending cervical levels and abdominal girth. Fatigue during the day and morning headaches are cardinal symptoms. OSA may also be associated with cognitive and mood dysfunction.
Sleep apnea testing with monitoring of oronasal airflow, thoracic and abdominal effort, oxyhemoglobin saturation, electrocardiogram, and sleep position is effective for home and in-hospital screening. Proper utilization of night positive airway pressure increases energy, prevents complications, and extends life span.

80. What are the most common causes of central pain?
The most commonly cited causes of central pain syndromes are SCI and central post-stroke pain (CPSP). Most cases of CPSP follow ischemic strokes. Thalamic and lateral medullary strokes have the highest incidence of CPSP.

81. What is the role of infrared imaging in identifying the source of chronic pain?
Vasomotor maps generated by infrared skin imaging during cold pressor testing can assist the physiatrist in determining which structure(s) within a dermatome, myotome, or sclerotome may be generating the chronic pain.

82. What is spinal segmental sensitization (SSS)?
SSS is characterized by hyperactivity, facilitation, and hyperexcitability of a spinal segment that develops in reaction to an irritative focus that constantly bombards the sensory ganglion with nociceptive stimuli.

83. What is the role of sensitization in managing chronic pain?
To properly treat chronic pain, it must be understood that pain develops due to peripheral sensitization leading to central sensitization and that only by reducing both peripheral and central sensitization can optimal recovery occur.

84. Besides releasing trigger points, what is another essential principle to manage them?
Myofascial trigger point therapy gives only short-term improvement unless the underlying cause is properly identified and treated.

85. What is the primary mechanism of fibromyalgia (FM)?
FM is a complex clinical syndrome attributed to central neuromodulatory dysregulation with amplified sensory impulses due to central sensitization.

86. What are the primary principles for managing complex regional pain syndrome (CRPS)?
Primary principles in managing CRPS include initiating aggressive treatment as soon as possible by using a combination of pain control (with medications and interventional procedures), rehabilitation, and behavioral therapy for optimal results.

87. What diagnosis affects more Americans than diabetes, heart disease, and cancer combined?
Chronic pain.

88. What are the stages of burn injury?
Burns are classified as superficial (damaging only the epidermis), superficial partial-thickness (injuring the dermis, blistering), deep partial-thickness (destroying deep levels of the dermis), and full-thickness (destroying entire skin through the dermis).

89. How can vocational rehabilitation (VR) help those with a disability rating?
VR recognizes a person with disabilities by identifying their career pathway, passions, strengths, weaknesses, and newly acquired deficits. A VR rehabilitation program seeks to achieve "vocational resuscitation."

90. What are the two major "crutch walking" muscles of the shoulder?
The pectoralis major and latissimus dorsi muscles act on the humerus to resist the upward vector force of crutches on the shoulder.

91. Why are there no sensory abnormalities over the palm in carpal tunnel syndrome?
This is because the palmar cutaneous branch of the median nerve passes superficially to the flexor retinaculum.

92. Name the major ligaments of the spine.
They are the anterior longitudinal ligament, posterior longitudinal ligament, ligamenta flava, interspinous ligament, and supraspinous ligament.

93. What structure gives the strongest support for the acromioclavicular joint?
The coracoclavicular ligament.

94. What are the main types of scapular winging and their mechanisms?
Medial winging occurs when the serratus anterior is paralyzed, the medial border wings away from the chest wall, and is displaced medially by the unopposed retraction of the trapezius. *Lateral winging* happens when the trapezius is paralyzed and the medial border wings are displaced laterally by the unopposed protraction of the serratus anterior.

95. What is longitudinal learning (LL), and how does it relate to PM&R?
LL is a model of education that promotes better development of essential skills among medical trainees and clinicians by observing the same group of patients over a period of time to understand their natural course and adaptions to their conditions. Didactic value is optimized by mimicking the practice of medicine using student-resident-clinician-patient interactions in a clinic setting. In contrast to the traditional classroom, lecture-based learning, LL combines elements of textbook learning, classroom knowledge, and clinical training. It offers many links, diagrams, textual topic discussions, visuals, and other multimedia resources (e.g., books such as *PM&R Secrets*) to promote LL.

96. How does PM&R address the sexuality of patients?
The interdisciplinary, team-focused, problem-based model of rehabilitation helps persons with disabilities compensate for impairments and assists in overcoming barriers to sexuality. As sexuality includes many dimensions, including sexual activity, sexual orientation, cultural identity, gender roles, eroticism, pleasure, intimacy, and reproduction, the interdisciplinary approach used by PM&R is often required.

97. Is genetics relevant to PM&R?
Yes. The genome, defined as the *complete set of genetic material present in an organism*, mediates adaptive inducible changes in response to many rehabilitative therapies. One example is the influence of genetic factors on neural plasticity and recovery after CNS injury. Genes coding for neurotrophic factor and apolipoprotein have been studied in stroke recovery. Other genetic factors have been found to be associated with SCI recovery and other neurologic conditions.

98. What is the rehabilitation approach to the "aging" patient?
With the "graying" of the population, physiatry has come to play a leading role as a quality-of-life specialty for geriatric individuals because of its unique focus on functional restoration. Rehabilitation combines exercise, conditioning, adaptive techniques, behavioral strategies, pharmacotherapy, and procedural interventions to address the aging process.

99. Are all robots in PM&R one-of-a-kind?
Not all robots are alike in PM&R. There are two basic types: *assistive* and *therapeutic*. Each has different objectives. Assistive robots help to compensate for lost skills. Therapeutic robots are designed to train motor function (e.g., improving gait after stroke). Therapeutic robots can be divided into *end-effector* types (attach onto the limb) and *exoskeleton* (worn and provides weight support powered mobility in which neuroplastic improvement occurs by repeating the desired pattern).

100. How is rehabilitation like "surgery from the skin out"?
PM&R strives to improve the quality of life for those with disabilities when environmental demands exceed a person's functional ability. Just as a surgeon treats disease, injury, or deformity using internal operative or manual methods to physically impact body tissues, the physiatrist intervenes externally to mitigate impairment, activity limitations and participation barriers to help people achieve their vital goals.

Look for the light; then, there shall be no darkness.

Bryan J. O'Young

WHAT IS PHYSIATRY?

Mark A. Young, MD, MBA, FACP, FAAPMR, DABPMR, Bryan J. O'Young, MD, CAc, FAAPMR, Steven A. Stiens, MD, MS, Sam S.H. Wu, MD, MA, MPH, MBA, and Stanley F. Wainapel, MD, MPH

The marvelous richness of human experience would lose rewarding joy if there were no limitations to overcome. The hilltop hour would not be half so wonderful if there were not dark valleys to traverse.
                                                                                              —Helen Keller (1880-1968)

KEY POINTS

1. Physiatry, also known as Physical Medicine and Rehabilitation (PM&R) in the United States, and Physical and Rehabilitation Medicine (PRM) internationally, is a dynamic medical specialty highlighting prevention, diagnosis, and treatment of patients with limitations in function from diseases, injuries, or symptoms.
2. The physiatrist's essential call to action is helping patients achieve joy in overcoming physical limitations caused by illness and injury. The physiatrist provides invaluable leadership to the PM&R team and renders meaning to Helen Keller's credo by always recognizing the sanctity and resilience of human existence.
3. Physiatrists are uniquely suited to treat conservatively neurologic, pain, and musculoskeletal conditions through a holistic and balanced combination of exercise, medication, nonoperative procedures, physical modalities, and psychosocial support.
4. Physiatrists work collaboratively with patients, transdisciplinary teams, and other specialties to achieve patient-centered goals and clinical outcomes. Like the conductor of a symphonic orchestra, the physiatrist occupies a "maestro" role by masterfully managing and harmoniously directing the team's symbiotic mission.
5. As the team leader, the physiatrist uses a broad and synergistic variety of treatments and interventions, including biomedical, pharmaceutical, modality, exercise, prosthetic, orthotic, assistive technology, procedural, psychological, and educational based therapies.
6. The crowning achievement of every PM&R physician is facilitating a patient's critical transition from handicapped to "handicapable." The physiatrist restores the richness of human experience by altruistically aiding persons with disabilities to traverse, compensate for, and overcome the challenges of disease and incapacity.
7. The emergence of Coronavirus disease 2019 (COVID-19) and its functional sequela have created a new therapeutic domain for physiatrists. Across the health care landscape, PM&R's role in the acute, chronic, and "long-haul" management of novel and evolving disease states is gaining prominence.
8. The advent of PM&R-themed social media (SM) platforms, websites, blogs, and podcasts, in addition to telemedical virtual communication tools, has contributed generously to the growth and development of PM&R. These powerful resources have facilitated communication, networking, acquisition of new knowledge, and awareness of breaking physiatric scientific research and current content.
9. Physiatric knowledge can be gained through a variety of methods, including bedside teaching, seminars, online education, and books. Resources using a "Question & Answer" (Q&A) didactic approach offer a valuable learning advantage.

1. What is Physiatry (Physical Medicine and Rehabilitation [PM&R])?
   Recognized as the "quality of life" medical specialty across the health care spectrum, physiatry (aka physical medicine and rehabilitation) altruistically accentuates the prevention, diagnosis, and nonoperative management of patients with disabilities and limitations in function from any disease process, injury, or condition.

2. How did PM&R begin?
   Although the specialty is relatively young, the fundamentals of the field originated during ancient times. The birth of contemporary rehabilitation and PM&R occurred in the middle of the 20th century, when a significant shift in thinking among health care providers occurred. Holistic, comprehensive, team-oriented care for people with disabilities came to be recognized as an essential societal obligation. This powerful philosophy sparked a burgeoning interest among health care providers to treat persons with disabilities.
   The year 1928 was a banner year for physiatry. Dr. Frank Krusen inaugurated the first inpatient comprehensive rehabilitation unit at Temple University. Dr. Krusen coined the term *physiatrist* and is credited as the author of the

first comprehensive rehabilitation textbook. Years later, he started the first PM&R residency training program at the Mayo Clinic. Dr. Krusen's monumental work has had a lasting imprint on the field. Improvements in acute medical care (e.g., penicillin) during World War II saved the lives of many soldiers with disabilities who returned home in dire need of rehabilitative care.

Pioneering physicians in the field helped plant the seeds for an exciting new specialty that cared for the whole person, not just the disease. Over time, PM&R has gained recognition across the medical spectrum and has earned its stature in major academic medical centers. Physician historians have acknowledged the critical importance of "nurturing leadership producing a blossoming of the specialty in once barren academic soil."

Atanelov L, Stiens S, Young, MA. History of physical medicine and rehabilitation and its ethical dimensions. *AMA J Ethics.* 2015;17(6):568–74. doi: 10.1001/journalofethics.2015. 17.6.mhst1-1506. Available at: mhst1-1506.pdf (ama-assn.org)

Young MA, Siebens HC, Wainapel SF. A tale of two cities: evolution of academic physiatry in Boston and Baltimore. Part 2: From flower shop to full bloom in Baltimore. *PM&R.* 2020;12(2):202–210. doi:10.1002/pmrj.12252. Available at: A Tale of Two Cities: Evolution of Academic Physiatry in Boston and Baltimore. Part 2: From Flower Shop to Full Bloom in Baltimore—Young—2020—PM&R—Wiley Online Library

3. How do practitioners of PM&R derive their inspiration?

The passion and power of physiatry are inspired by the noble philosophical belief that "ability trumps disability" and that ameliorating symptoms will often help to restore functional wellness. Physiatrists use exercise, physical modalities, injections, pharmaceuticals, and education customized to patients' needs. Restoration of function in all dimensions of life, including medical, psychological, behavioral, social, spiritual, and vocational, is the overarching goal of physiatry.

4. What makes physiatry unique?

Physiatry has been appropriately called the "primary care specialty for persons with disability" due to its emphasis on the health and wellness of persons with medical, musculoskeletal, and neurologic disorders. PM&R specialists provide care for patients with painful and incapacitating neuromusculoskeletal disorders and with acute and chronic disabilities requiring rehabilitation services. As physiatry is the "quality of life medical specialty," PM&R has grown in international recognition because of its commitment to addressing quality of life objectives.

5. What impact has COVID-19 had on physiatry?

Historically, war, epidemics, and widespread cataclysmic events (earthquakes, hurricanes, tsunamis, building collapses) have triggered the need for innovation in restoration and rehabilitation management. The emergence of COVID-19 and its destructive residual functional consequences have created an essential therapeutic and recovery role for physiatrists. PM&R physicians and their multidisciplinary teams rose to the challenge by leading the COVID-19 rehabilitation continuum of care. PM&R specialists in many medical centers were deftly deployed to provide the following essential services: pulmonary rehabilitation to mitigate dyspnea, enhancing airway management and breathing exercises management, implementing "proning" protocols, supervising preventive measures to avert complications of inactivity (decubiti, contractures, thromboembolic prophylaxis), nutrition, stretching, airway management, breathing exercises, manual therapy, and optimizing physical and mobility activity. Although the net long-term impact of these interventions has yet to be characterized, it is now clear that they have helped to minimize complications, mitigate disability, and promote the preservation of function, thereby optimizing the quality of life.

PM&R's "pop-role" in COVID-19 emphasizes the increasing importance of physiatry in new and evolving diseases. With an aging worldwide population and many surviving illnesses once deemed incurable, PM&R's importance has grown mightily.

Weinstein S. How Covid-19 informed the future impact of PM&R across the health care continuum. *PM&R.* 2021;13:551–553. Available at: How COVID-19 informed the future impact of the specialty of physical medicine and rehabilitation across the health care continuum (wiley.com)

Wang TJ, Chau B, Lui M, Lam GT, Lin N, Humbert S. Physical medicine and rehabilitation and pulmonary rehabilitation for COVID-19. *Am J Phys Med Rehabil.* 2020;99(9):769–774. doi: 10.1097/PHM.0000000000001505. Available at: phm-publish-ahead-of-print-10.1097.phm.0000000000001505.pdf (nih.gov)

6. What is social media (SM) and telemedicine, and how have they influenced PM&R?

The advent of PM&R-themed SM platforms, websites, blogs, and podcasts, in addition to telemedical virtual communication tools, has contributed generously to the growth and development of PM&R. *SM* is an interactive technology that enables the creation or exchange/sharing of information, ideas, interests, and expression via virtual communities and networks. SM use among physiatrists has increased exponentially since the previous edition of this book. Readily accessible to all with an internet connection, SM is a convenient communication forum and has facilitated communication, networking, acquisition of new knowledge, and awareness of breaking scientific research.

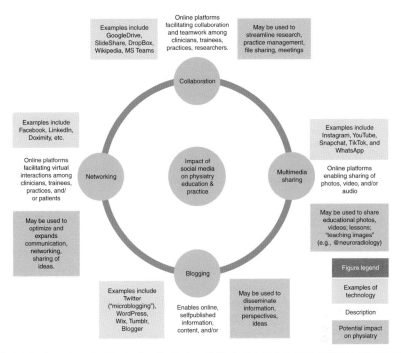

Fig. 1.1 Impact of social media on physiatry education. (Credits: Young MJ [design & content], Thomas A [content], and Radlicz, C [review])

SM is a potent medium for promoting physiatry engagement and awareness. Medical students, interns, residents, academic faculty, and PM&R practitioners increasingly use these tools (Fig. 1.1).

SM platforms and related PM&R Internet resources include Instagram, Twitter, Facebook, Signal, Telegram, LinkedIn, WhatsApp, Doximity, YouTube, and Zoom, and many others have boldly contributed to the growth and development of PM&R. Zoom has created an opportunity for residents and faculty to participate in lectures from the world-renowned rehabilitation leaders. PM&R-oriented blogs and podcasts have fostered additional learning. The online version of PM&R Secrets (4th ed) and connected platforms are examples of dynamic SM resources.

Telemedicine has enabled virtual consults and therapies for rehabilitation patients isolated with COVID-19 and other chronic disabling conditions. In addition, people in rural areas have gained access to health care. The inclusion of telehealth and virtual technology in neurorehabilitation and other PM&R domains has truly transformed traditional physician–patient interactions. The leveraging of virtual online conferencing and communication technology (Zoom, Skype, and Teams) has facilitated the academic collaboration of PM&R scholars and collaborators across the miles, as was the case of the editors and authors contributing to this international volume.

Paganoni S, Frontera WR. Evidence-based physiatry and social media: two new sections. *Am J Phys Med Rehabil.* 2018;97(7): 465–466. doi: 10.1097/PHM.0000000000000952. PMID: 29916901. Available at: Pages from PHM_V98N2_revised-issue-text-proofs_e.pdf (researchgate.net)

Rakesh N. Should we be social in rehab? Social Media 101. Available at: https://www.physiatry.org/general/custom.asp?page=SocialMedia101#.YpUu_Mwiful.link

Young MJ. Neuroethics in the era of teleneurology. *Semin Neurol.* 2022; 42(01):067–076. doi: 10.1055/s-0041-1741496. PMID: 35016251.

7. **How is the important mission of PM&R uniquely carried out?**

    PM&R strives to promote a person's quality of life and functional outcomes through a dynamic team-oriented approach, ideally led by the physiatrist. The physiatrist skillfully balances the fundamentals of traditional medical management ("adding years to life") with the functional model (adding "life to years") in serving the patient's needs. Essential members of the physiatry team include the physical therapist (PT), occupational therapist (OT), speech-language pathologist (SLP), respiratory therapist (RT), nutritionist, psychologists, nursing staff, and others. By blending the best of the traditional medical approach ("adding years to life") with the functional model ("adding life to years"), the PM&R team proudly accomplishes its mission.

8. What is the significance of the name "Physical Medicine and Rehabilitation"?
   PM&R as a specialization encompasses two key areas:
   a. Physical Medicine: Diagnosis, management, and treatment of musculoskeletal and neurologic disorders, using exercise, medications, modalities, biomechanical/kinematic interventions, and procedures.
   b. Rehabilitation: Applying a medical treatment, therapy, adaptive equipment, and environmental adaptation in transforming a patient with disabilities into a person with improved functional skill and performance.

9. Do all medical conditions benefit from PM&R intervention?
   Although many physiatrists view themselves as primary care physicians for people with disabilities (and therefore offer comprehensive care for persons with diverse medical conditions), a growing number of physiatry specialists have elected to focus on specific rehabilitation areas. Common conditions treated by physiatrists include amputations, arthritis, brain injuries, burns, cancer, cardiac disorders, chronic pain, fibromyalgia, industrial injuries, multiple sclerosis (MS), neuromuscular diseases, neuropathies, orthopedic injuries, pain disorders, pediatric disorders, pulmonary disorders, spinal cord injuries (SCIs), stroke, and trauma. Physiatrists are uniquely suited to treat painful neuromusculoskeletal conditions through a holistic and balanced combination of exercise, medication, procedures, and psychosocial support.

10. How is "Working with People with Disabilities" an important physiatric ideal?
    People with disabilities occupy an essential and ever-growing segment of the health care continuum. Physiatrists must always be true to the altruistic roots and traditions of the field and their unique education by being available to manage the individualized needs of persons with disabilities. Whether the task involves readily accepting a consultation on a newly quadriplegic inpatient or assisting a community-based elderly patient who has had a stroke, the physiatrist can truly "make a difference" by virtue of their training. One academic physiatrist wrote in *JAMA*:

    > As practitioners of healing arts, we are often swept away by the mundane minutiae of providing expert technical care to our patients. Often overlooked [however] is the "human side" of caring–that transcendent sense of seeing life through the eyes of our patients.[1]

    Physiatry admirably answers that calling, and because *all* physiatrists have been invested with this training, they must respond unabashedly. No matter which direction your subspecialty takes you, always remember that you are a physiatrist!

[1]Young MA. Review of *Still lives: Narratives of spinal cord injury* by Jonathan Cole. *JAMA* 2005;293(4):497.

11. How does one achieve certification in PM&R?
    It begins with medical school, typically a 4-year journey that ideally includes a rotation in PM&R. Next is an internship, which is either 1 year of a coordinated program of experience in fundamental clinical skills (this is an accredited transitional year) or 6 months or more in accredited training in family practice, internal medicine, obstetrics and gynecology, pediatrics, surgery, or a combination of these patient care experiences. This internship lays the foundation for the aspiring physiatrist to care for complex medical conditions and effectively manage comorbidities. A 3-year residency follows the internship. For some, there is a fellowship (1 to 3 years) in disciplines such as SCI, pediatric rehabilitation, traumatic brain injury, electromyography (EMG), musculoskeletal medicine, interventional spine medicine, neuromuscular medicine, cancer rehabilitation, or pain medicine.
    Like many medical specialization career paths, the road to becoming a PM&R diplomate is exciting and challenging because the field draws from so many sources of knowledge and practice. After the PM&R residency, qualified candidates take a written certification exam (Pt. 1), given by the American Board of Physical and Rehabilitation Medicine (ABPM&R). After residency, another exam (oral, Pt. 2) is administered after the first year of practice. Upon successfully completing both parts, physicians can proudly display a numbered board certification "sheepskin" that recognizes their achievement.

American Board of Physical and Rehabilitation Medicine. Available at: http://www.abpmr.org/

12. What is the best method to prepare for certification?
    - Get to know your patients. Individualize their treatments. Enable their life's passions.
    - Provide comprehensive and compassionate care.
    - Remember that your patients are good teachers.
    - Fashion your practice after caring role models, such as mentors and attending physiatrists.
    - Link your learning to your patients' problems.
    - Throughout the training, supplement your use of textbooks with online learning resources.
    - Make use of validated and reliable web and SM learning resources.
    - Complement your learning and practice knowledge by reading *PM&R Secrets* (4th ed.) *and linking to the online PM&R Secrets site and related SM tools.*

13. How can medical students learn more about PM&R?

Medical schools offering established PM&R rotations are an ideal didactic opportunity. Although many schools offer PM&R exposure as an elective rotation, some have included it as a mandatory component of the medical school curriculum. Students can also learn more about PM&R during the preclinical years by joining their medical school's PM&R student interest group.

A growing number of academic departments have created unique educational opportunities (e.g., lectures, courses, seminars, and symposia) for interested medical students. Some have even developed "shadow experiences" for undergraduates interested in early exposure to physiatry. Part of the physical diagnosis curriculum established in many medical schools involves students spending time in rehabilitation services, where medically stable patients exhibit a broad array of pathologies that allow for an optimal learning environment.

Association of Academic Physiatrists. www.physiatry.org

American Academy of Physical Medicine and Rehabilitation. *Medical Student Resources—A Medical Students Guide to PM&R*. Available at: https://www.aapmr.org/career-support/medical-student-resources/a-medical-students-guide-to-pm-r

Mayer RS, Shah A, DeLateur BJ, et al. Proposal for a required advanced clerkship in chronic disease and disability for medical students. *Am J Phys Med Rehabil.* 2008;87(2):162–7. doi: 10.1097/PHM.0b013e31815b7331.

Perret D, Sunico R, Knowlton T, et al. State of the states: growing physiatry: Association of Academic Physiatrists position statement addressing academic physiatry and physical medicine and rehabilitation growth. *Am J Phys Med Rehabil.* 2018;97(12):921–928. doi: 10.1097/PHM.0000000000001044.

Stiens SA, Berkin DI. A clinical rehabilitation course for college undergraduates provides an introduction to the biopsychosocial interventions that minimize disablement. *Am J Phys Med Rehabil.* 1998;76:462–470.

14. What is there to know about PM&R residency training programs?

With more than 97 accredited residency programs in PM&R in the United States, there are expanding opportunities for postgraduate education. All accredited programs adhere to program requirements written and administered by the Residency Review Committee for PM&R. This ensures uniformity of a high-quality training experience and exposure to the various programs with adequate experience in both inpatient and outpatient rehabilitation. Common procedural exposure includes electromyography (EMG)/nerve conduction velocity (NCV), ultrasound, Botulinum toxin (BOTOX), peripheral joint injections, and interventional procedures. Some programs offer opportunities for advanced degrees (MBA, PhD), specialized electives, and research opportunities as a bonus. A select group of senior residents who become chief residents may have the opportunity to develop additional administrative and leadership skills. Some institutions offer combined programs such as PM&R and neurology, PM&R and pediatrics, and PM&R and internal medicine.

Young MA, Stiens SA, & Hsu P. Chief residency in PM&R. A balance of education and administration. *Am J Phys Med Rehabil.* 1996;75(4):257–262. doi: 10.1097/00002060-199607000-00003. PMID: 8777020. Available at:

Available at: Chief Residency in PM&R: A Balance of Education and Administ...: *American Journal of Physical Medicine & Rehabilitation* (lww.com)

Available at: American Board of Physical Medicine and Rehabilitation. http://www.abpmr.org

15. Is there subspecialty training in physiatry?

Recognized subspecialty fellowship opportunities (both accredited and nonaccredited) exist. ABPMR-certified fellowships are currently available in brain injury medicine, hospice and palliative care medicine, neuromuscular medicine, pain medicine, pediatric rehabilitation medicine, spinal cord injury medicine, and sports medicine. Other fellowships include musculoskeletal (MSK)/spine, stroke, multiple sclerosis (MS), neurorehabilitation, electrodiagnostic medicine, cancer rehabilitation, occupational and environmental medicine, vocational rehabilitation, and research in rehabilitation.

Available at: AAPM&R. Roadmap to a Fellowship. https://www.aapmr.org/docs/default-source/career-center/fellowship/roadmap-to-a-fellowship_2021.pdf

16. How is accreditation of PM&R education achieved?

The Accreditation Council for Graduate Medical Education (ACGME) delegates authority to the Residency Review Committee for PM&R to confer *direct* certification of PM&R residency training programs. Accreditation is a voluntary process and confers approval to a program. The ACGME is the offspring of several important organizations, including the American Board of Medical Specialties (ABMS), Council on Medical Education (CME), American Medical Association (AMA), American Hospital Association (AHA), and Association of American Medical Colleges (AAMC).

17. Which diagnostic modalities are in the physiatrist's "tool kit"?

Aside from standard diagnostic methods routinely used by all physicians, including PM&R (medical history, physical examinations, imaging, functional tests, and laboratory tests), physiatrists use electrodiagnostic techniques, including EMG, nerve conduction studies, and somatosensory and motor evoked potentials. Musculoskeletal ultrasound is also an emerging vital diagnostic tool performed by many physiatrists. Technological developments have enabled miniaturized ultrasound devices, allowing hand-held probes that can be attached to smart devices. This has facilitated portability and increased access to remote diagnostic venues such as sporting events and theaters of war.

Haig A, Stiens SA. *Telerehabilitation: Exercise and Adaptation in Home and Community*. In Moroz A, Flanagan SR, Zaretsky H, eds. *Medical Aspects of Disability*. 5th ed.New York: Springer, 2017:681–696; Introduction available at: Chapter 01.indd (springerpub.com)

18. What treatments do physiatrists offer for pain management?
Treatment options include oral medications, topical analgesics, modalities such as hot packs and cold packs, ultrasound, electrotherapy, laser, assistive devices such as braces and artificial limbs, massage, biofeedback, traction, and therapeutic exercise. Physiatrists, with added training, also perform acupuncture, injections, interventional procedures, including peripheral articular injections (increasingly guided by ultrasound), spinal blocks, and botulinum toxin injections. Increasingly, musculoskeletal ultrasound is used with great success for needle localization and diagnostic applications.

19. Is physiatry a worldwide specialty?
Known in many countries as Physical and Rehabilitation Medicine (PRM), physiatry's importance and utility have been recognized globally. This field continues its popularity among international doctors because of the aging population globally and the need for functional restoration. The International Society of Physical and Rehabilitation Medicine (ISPRM) is a unique global organization that works to assist PRM specialists, doctors, and other health care workers to become more effective practitioners and improve the quality of life for those worldwide with impairments and disabilities.

Efforts to achieve this goal are by convening international congresses and providing rehabilitation medicine input to international health organizations such as the World Health Organization (WHO). Many countries maintain special boards of PM&R analogous to the ABPM&R. Notable examples are the European Board of PM&R, the Australasian Faculty of PRM, and the Israel Society of PM&R (see Chapter 86, "International PM&R"). The Haim Ring International Rehabilitation Summer School offers trainees an annually sponsored residential rehabilitation learning retreat in Italy.

Euro Mediterranean Rehabilitation Summer School. Available at: http://www.emrss.it/ENG/styled/

International Society of Physical and Rehabilitation Medicine. Available at: http://www.isprm.org/

20. What about international learning opportunities in PM&R?
The International Exchange Committee (IEC), a unique international educational project sponsored by the ISPRM, serves as a central clearinghouse for novel educational, humanitarian, and learning opportunities in PM&R in all continents. Inspired by the late Professor Haim Ring of Israel, the then-President of ISPRM, the IEC is composed of an international faculty of physiatrists and committee members. Two of the authors of this book have proudly served as Chair of the IEC: Dr. Mark Young (Inaugural and Founding Chair) and Dr. Bryan O'Young. The goals of the IEC include:
- Serving as a clearinghouse for international learning opportunities in rehabilitation.
- Facilitating placement of medical students, residents, faculty physicians, and allied rehabilitation professionals in global, voluntary didactic rotations.
- Sharing information about global PRM educational opportunities with the membership of the organization.
- Tracking the outcomes, progress, and successes of the committee's educational initiatives
- Interfacing and networking with other rehabilitation educational organizations in pursuit of international education and scholarship in the field
- Tracking individual accomplishments and the endeavors of the committee
- Providing academically based PM&R-related humanitarian assistance. Examples include COVID-19, Hurricane Katrina, and the tsunami in the Indian Ocean.
- Awarding an annual recognition award (the "Professor Haim Ring Memorial Award") to an individual and institution that have distinguished themselves in altruistic international exchange.

21. To review the fundamentals of PM&R in an engaging, concise, and entertaining way, which learning resource is recommended?
Physical Medicine and Rehabilitation Secrets is a veritable "treasure trove" of knowledge-packed questions and answers. Rehabilitation learning is made more accessible using the question-and-answer approach. This volume is all about simple, straightforward education. For every topic, carefully selected, clinically relevant, thought-provoking questions are accompanied by straightforward answers. It is presented in a distinctive Socratic format and is designed to provide readers with a fundamental PM&R education. Many have used it to pass exams. For

the past three decades, students, clinicians, and faculty have successfully used the book to become better physiatrists and educators. Tweet your sentiments! (@PMRSecrets)

Learning is not attained by chance; it must be sought for with ardor and attended to with diligence.
—Abigail Adams (1744–1818)

ACKNOWLEDGMENTS

Thanks to Dr. Michael Young, Dr. Ambreona Thomas, and Chris Radlicz for their assistance.
Content and figure design ©2021 by MJ Young, MD

WEBSITES

American Academy of Physical Medicine and Rehabilitation. Available at: http://www.aapmr.org
American Board of Physical and Rehabilitation Medicine. Available at: http://www.abpmr.org/
American Congress of Rehabilitation Medicine. Available at: http://www.acrm.org/
Association of Academic Physiatrists. Available at: https://www.physiatry.org/
International Society of Physical and Rehabilitation Medicine. Available at: http://www.isprm.org/
Union Européenne des Médecins Specialistes (U.E.M.S., European Union of Medical Specialists). Available at: https://uems-prm.eu/the-specialty/

BIBLIOGRAPHY

Atanelov L, Stiens S, Young, MA. History of physical medicine and rehabilitation and its ethical dimensions. *AMA J Ethics.* 2015;17(6):568–574. doi: 10.1001/journalofethics.2015. 17.6.mhst1-1506.
European Physical and Rehabilitation Medicine Bodies Alliance. *White Book on Physical and Rehabilitation Medicine (PRM) in Europe.* Chapter 3. A primary medical specialty: the fundamentals of PRM. *Eur J Phys Rehabil Med.* 2018;54(2):177–185. doi: 10.23736/S1973-9087.18.05146-8.
Stiens SA, Berkin DI. A clinical rehabilitation course for college undergraduates provides an introduction to the biopsychosocial interventions that minimize disablement. *Am J Phys Med Rehabil.* 1998;76:462–470.
Wang TJ, Chau B, Lui M, et al. Physical medicine and rehabilitation and pulmonary rehabilitation for COVID-19. *Am J Phys Med Rehabil.* 2020;99(9):769–774. doi:10.1097/PHM.0000000000001505
Weinstein SM. How Covid-19 informed the future impact of PM&R across the health care continuum. *PM&R.* 2021;13(6):551–553.
Young MA, Siebens HC, Wainapel SF. A tale of two cities: evolution of academic physiatry in Boston and Baltimore. Part 2: From flower shop to full bloom in Baltimore. *PM&R.* 2020;12(2):202–210. doi:10.1002/pmrj.12252.
Young MA, Stiens SA, Hsu P. The PM&R chief resident: a balance between administration and education. *Am J Phys Med Rehabil.* 1996;75:257–262.
Young MJ. Neuroethics in the era of teleneurology. *Semin Neurol.* In press.

CHAPTER 2

THE PHYSIATRIC CONSULTATION: ACUTE TREATMENT, IMMEDIATE REHABILITATION, FUTURE ENABLEMENT, AND SYSTEM DESIGNS

Steven A. Stiens, MD, MS and Lawrence R. Robinson, MD

Everything that exists in your life does so because of two things: something you did or something you didn't do.
—Albert Einstein (1879–1955)

KEY POINTS: ESSENTIAL COMPONENTS OF THE PHYSIATRIC CONSULTATION

1. Discover the patients' life roles and future aspirations.
2. Confirm current diagnoses and risk factors.
3. Quantify impairments, disabilities, and barriers to participation.
4. Develop a problem list.
5. Formulate a goal-driven treatment plan.
6. Orchestrate interdisciplinary team interventions.
7. Re-evaluate progress toward goals.

1. **What is a physiatric consultation?**
   In the past, a consultation consisted of two physicians evaluating the patient together. Today, this process is asynchronous and requires collaborative coordination. ***Consultation*** provides an expert, situation-specific formula to the patient's attending physician and treatment team. Recommendations are unique because physicians and their appraisals of patients and effectiveness of interventions determine sequenced capability goals that catalyze necessary outcomes. The mediums for interaction include in person, tele-rehabilitation, interdisciplinary meetings, and remote tele-monitoring. The essential tasks include identifying the foci for intervention, tailoring the treatment options for the setting, communicating and agreeing on outcomes, and orchestrating the team to meet identified goals.

Galea MD. Telemedicine in rehabilitation. *Phys Med Rehabil Clin N Am.* 2019;30(2):473–483. doi: 10.1016/j.pmr.2018.12.002.

2. **Why are physical medicine and rehabilitation (PM&R) consultations requested?**
   Typically, patients do not have sufficient capabilities for transiting between care settings or life roles. Ideally, physiatrists are consulted to keep patients maximally capable in order to enable them to meet life demands and aspirations. Consultation patterns and outcomes should be followed in a database that is designed for each medical system of care because PM&R is underutilized, referral sources require directed education, and early intervention improves the outcomes and reduces the cost of care. Consultations are an opportunity to provide education to the treating team, patient, and family. PM&R is underused and should be more pervasive throughout healthcare systems, addressing perioperative, palliative, and intensive care.

Nickerson RB, McDowell SM, Gaters DR. An exploratory examination of an academic PM&R inpatient consultation service. *Disabil Rehabil.* 2003;25(7):354–359. Available at: https://doi.org/10.1080/0963828031000090498

3. **How can physiatric consultation fit into the medical continuum?**
   The medical continuum is actually a cycle including ***prevention***, ***acute treatment***, and ***rehabilitation***. Howard Rusk (1901–1989), considered the founder of rehabilitative medicine, announced rehabilitation was the "third phase of medical care." Alternatively, the interdisciplinary team can intervene throughout the medical continuum

by using multiple mechanisms simultaneously. Physiatric consultation in the future must be timed and implemented as a matrix, addressing each patient's situation, prognosis, goals, and resources. ***Rehabilitation competency frameworks*** need to be designed and implemented to bring, train, and deploy interdisciplinary teams as needed for each patient population.

World Health Organization. *Rehabilitation Competency Framework*. 2019. Available at: https://www.who.int/multi-media/details/rehabilitation-competency-framework

4. Should rehabilitation really be limited to the last phase of medical care?

The interdisciplinary rehabilitation team can intervene throughout the medical continuum. Early intervention with rehabilitation, during or before acute treatment, can shorten the overall time required for rehabilitation and prevent morbidity and mortality (especially in stroke, cardiac, spinal cord, and amputation rehabilitation). Rehabilitation can also address needs to be maximally functional in late life, during palliative care, by adaptively supporting quality of life.

Corcoran JR, Herbsman JM, Bushnik T, et al. Early rehabilitation in the medical and surgical intensive care units for patients with and without mechanical ventilation: An inter-professional performance improvement project. *PMR*. 2017;9(2):113–119. doi:10.1016/j.pmrj.2016.06.015.

5. What skills and knowledge are necessary for the savvy consulting physiatrist and the interdisciplinary team?

Physiatrists are patient-centered function doctors who are knowledgeable about the daily routine and life goals of patients with new impairments and activity limitations. The physiatrist must know people, personalities, coping styles, and be able to estimate patients' tolerances for treatment and equipment (***gadget tolerance***). The consultant should know the hospital or practice setting very well, including diets, supplies stocked, therapies, other ancillary support, and past policies. Finally, it is good to know the "territory" of the communities of the patients. Knowledge of the community, landscape, housing designs, transportation, and access to places of business helps the physiatrist prepare the patient for the fullest participation upon discharge.

6. What are the objectives of a comprehensive physiatric consultation?

Confirm the diagnosis, pathology, and active pathophysiology.

Quantify functional levels and provide a functional prognosis.

Design a rehabilitation problem list (*see* Chapter 14, "Person and Process of Rehabilitation").

Answer the question of the initial consultation and then educate the team about the rehabilitation interventions.

Formulate short-term, intermediate, and long-term ***rehabilitation goals***.

Translate the plans and interventions for the originators of the consult and for the patient and family, and arrive at agreement on treatment plans.

Orchestrate the secondary consultations and direct interventions through the interdisciplinary process to immediately begin to achieve goals on schedule and advance function.

Establish an activity, education, and rest schedule for the patient.

Should a ***transfer to inpatient rehabilitation*** be planned, confirm with the treating team if acute medical interventions have been completed and/or which treatments need to be continued.

Tan X, van Egmond L, Partinen M, et al. A narrative review of interventions for improving sleep and reducing circadian disruption in medical inpatients. *Sleep Med*. 2019;59:42–50. doi: 10.1016/j.sleep.2018.08.007

7. When you go into the room to take the patient's history, how many experts will be present?

At least two: the **patient** and hopefully the ***physiatrist***. Every experience of an injury or disease is unique because the course of injury and recovery always varies, and the person impacted by the bodily changes has a unique development, life experiences, and goals. The patient is an expert on his or her unique ***illness experience*** (a subjective sense of not being well) and the impact of ***disability*** (the sum of impairments, activity limitations, and barriers to participation). Other "experts" in the room may include nurses therapists, family, close friends, attendants, and roommates. Each has a perspective of the challenges the patient faces and may have a vision of what recovery is and their role in it. These expectations need to be elicited and addressed in the design of a cohesive rehabilitation plan that the patient and the interdisciplinary team can adopt. In acute inpatient cases, it is often necessary to conduct ward-based patient, family, and ***team goal-setting meetings*** to explain the rehabilitation process and decide on the facility for future post-acute rehabilitation. Strategic human resources, planning for development of rehabilitation programs, requires recruitment, training, and education, with all competencies considered necessary for quality and efficient progress.

Sanchez-Gomez MD, Novo-Munoz M, Rodriguez-Gomez JA, et al. Methodology proposal for the management of nursing competencies towards a strategic training. A theoretical analysis. *Healthcare* (Basel). 2020;8(2):170. doi:10.3390/healthcare8020170. Available at: https://www.ncbi.nlm.nih.gov/pmc/articles/PMC7349343/

8. How do you elicit information from family, friends, and attendants about the actual/specific help the patient gets at home?

Establishing an *atmosphere of acceptance* permits patients' and families' honest expression of functional solutions and requests for improvement in the system that is in place. Keep the *patients in charge* of their life activity. Ask: "Who do you direct in assisting you with transfers, such as dressing, bathing, and meal preparation?" The role of the clinician is to *frame the interaction as a learning activity*. Each patient then becomes an "anthropologist" reporting on his or her experience in a unique environmental matrix. It is the work of the physiatrist to recognize, define, and *negotiate goals in the context of the patient's life* and to commit to achieving solutions. Indeed, each situation is a perception, activity, psychosocial, and economic equation in itself. The challenge is to understand each patient's specific self-care methods and refine these processes with new techniques and equipment.

Karrer M, Schnelli A, Zeller A., Mayer H. A systematic review of interventions to improve acute hospital care for people with dementia. *Geriatr Nurs.* 2021;42(3):657–673. doi: 10.1016/j.gerinurse.2021.03.006. Available at: https://www.sciencedirect.com/science/article/pii/S0197457221000859?via%3Dihub

Lawler K, Taylor NF, Shields N. Family-assisted therapy empowered families of older people transitioning from hospital to the community: A qualitative study. *J Physiother.* 2019;65(3):166–171. doi: 10.1016/j.jphys.2019.05.009. Available at: https://www.sciencedirect.com/science/article/pii/S1836955319300566?via%3Dihub

9. What options are there for sequencing the history-taking from the patient?

First, an *introduction of the clinician* and their role is presented. An *understanding of the patient* as a whole person is then derived. Next, the *menu of rehabilitation services* is presented as a directory related to patient-centered needs. A medical and functional history is elicited from the patient, detailing the *impact of the illness on life activity*. One method is to record the history chronologically, starting by asking the patient how they noticed their injury, pain, or diagnosis and what worried them most about how it would affect their life. If the patient is newly injured, exploring immediate goals may be a next step. If the patient is being seen in an outpatient setting or has a chronic disability, proceed from the history into a description of the disability as experienced by the patient.

Another approach would be to focus on the patient's function before the injury or illness, then review the changes afterward in a format guided by a problem list or by organ system. Be sure to elicit comments about function as well as symptoms. Identify immediate *barriers* and focus the rehabilitation process. Expand the conversation from current and local challenges to future target disposition requirements.

Laerum E, Indahl A, Skouen JS. What is "The Good Back Consultation"? A combined qualitative and quantitative study of chronic low back pain patients' interaction with and perceptions of consultations with specialists. *J Rehabil Med.* 2006;38(4):255–262. doi: 10.1080/16501970600613461. Available at: https://www.medicaljournals.se/jrm/content/abstract/

10. How can the examination be an education for the patient and provide therapy that could contribute to recovery?

Many patients with pain, paralysis, and on anesthesia are not fully aware of their capabilities and learn much from a *guided examination*. In addition, spouses, attendants, and nurses caring for the patient may have questions about methods for improving the patient's care. Sensory testing allows discussion of the receptive fields of various peripheral nerves and dermatomes. In the patient with myelopathy, sacral sparing can be explained and used as an incentive to be attentive to and attempt to regain control of bowel, bladder, and sexual function. *Range-of-motion (ROM) testing* allows for *instruction in self-stretching* and ROM with assistance. Strength testing permits instruction in *proprioceptive neuromuscular facilitation techniques*. Functional motor and coordination testing can lead to demonstration of exercises prescribed for the patient. At the conclusion of a visit, the patient can be set up with a *written set of exercises and schedule for practice* that can be posted at the bedside or used in the home before therapy visits start.

Table 2.1 Contents of a Consultation

Problem list—Include primary diagnoses, secondary diagnoses, impairments, activity limitations, and barriers to participation. Follow each of the problems with a brief assessment description.

Introduction—Record referring physician and reason for referral.

Current treatment

Patient identity, life roles past and present

History of injury or disease process, life impact

Interventions, medications, treatments,

Past history

Past medical history—diagnoses and impact

Family history—risk for conditions

Social history—past and current life roles, potential support options

Current function

Mobility—assistive devices, transfers, ambulation, setting required

Activities of daily living (ADLs)—eating, hygiene, bowel/bladder management, bathing, dressing

Vocational function—include volunteering, parenting, work from home

Leisure activities—enjoyment, engagement with others, channels for satisfaction

Equipment and home architecture, vehicles

Examination—Focus on diagnosis confirmation, impairment and activity limitation quantification, and areas of rehabilitation. Record functional neuromuscular examination, including mental status, cognition, mobility, and ADLs.

Assessment—Develop a summary statement of diagnosis, medical stability (improving, plateau, declining), preparedness for rehabilitation, and setting for further interventions.

Recommendations—List in the same order as the problem list. Record recommendations for further testing, treatment options, patient's daily schedule, and prognosis. Include short- and long-term goals and prognosis. Describe an immediate plan (i.e., acute rehabilitation), an intermediate plan (i.e., transfer to subacute rehabilitation), and a long-term plan (i.e., discharge to home).

11. What essential components should be included in the consultation report?

Remember, the consultation report may be used not only by the referring provider but also by the patient, rehabilitation therapists, lawyers, and insurance providers (Table 2.1). Indicate who will order necessary studies and medications as well as provide ongoing care for the patient. A copy of the consultation should be sent to the referring physician and to the primary medical care provider, patient, and family.

Keely E, Dojeiji S, Myers K. Writing effective consultation letters: 12 tips for teachers. *Med Teacher.* 2009;24(6):585–589.

12. How is the problem list organized in consultation report notes?

As the chart is reviewed, a problem list is derived that includes ***diagnoses***, ***impairments***, ***activity limitations***, and ***barriers to participation***, arranged in that order. This process might occur at bedside, on the phone with family, or in earshot of the patient's nurse. Specifics of the hospital course need not be recorded. The diagnoses themselves, duration of time under treatment, and recent severity measures are most useful in each problem. Each problem should be a short phrase that describes the unique situation of that patient. ***Potential problem domains*** are primary injury or diagnosis, other diagnoses, spine stability, neurogenic bowel, neurogenic bladder, neurogenic skin, pressure ulcers, mobility, activities of daily living (ADLs), communication, psychological adaptation, sexuality, social role function, architectural accessibility, community reintegration, and discharge management. Patient-centered domains, such as unique roles or vocations, should be included as well.

13. Whose consult is it anyway?

Whose life is it anyway? The patient's, of course. In practicing patient-centered medicine, we must receive confirmation of and engage the patient's interest and willingness to participate in the evaluation process and treatment. Sensitivity and perceptiveness are required as the patient's needs are elicited, and the plan of care is designed. First, physiatric assessments and treatment recommendations should be discussed and communicated to the attending physician or the directly responsible resident for discussion and concurrence. Immediately thereafter, a report should be made to the patient for his or her concurrence with the plan. This allows the patient to know the plan before it is disseminated to other providers, preventing misunderstanding, promoting consistency in information transmitted to the patient, and maximizing cooperation.

14. What is a physiatric prescription?

A **prescription** is a written formula for the preparation and administration of a therapeutic remedy. The physiatrist leads the interdisciplinary rehabilitation team by prescribing specific interventions to meet short- and long-term goals of various patient problem domains. Prescriptions for treatment come in the form of orders for nursing care and consultative referrals for the interdisciplinary rehabilitation team. The physician as team leader must balance specific requests for interventions with the objectives or outcomes that may be achieved through a variety of means. Therefore, therapeutic prescriptions are often an amalgamation of objectives, requests for evaluation, specific requests for treatment, and problem solving to achieve various outcomes. Contemporary innovations, using software and the electronic medical record, allow for consolidating essential information in uniform referrals.

Trauma Audit & Research Network. *Major trauma rehabilitation prescription 2019. TARN data entry guidance document.* 2018. Available at: https://www.c4ts.qmul.ac.uk/downloads/mt-rehabilitation-prescription-2019-guidance.pdf

15. How do you write a prescription for treatment that integrates other members of the interdisciplinary team into the rehabilitation process?

The basic components of the physiatric prescription are:

- Identification of **discipline consulted** (e.g., physical, recreational, occupational therapy)
- Major and significant secondary **diagnoses**
- Pertinent **impairments, activity limitations, and barriers to participation** that may be a focus of therapy
- **Precautions**: cardiac, weight-bearing, pulmonary (O_2 sat monitoring)
- **Short- and long-term goals** and objectives of therapy, including a copy of physiatric consult as needed
- **Specific therapeutic prescription** that includes areas to be treated, modality, intensity, duration, and frequency, as needed
- **Frequency of visits** and over what period
- **Date of physiatric re-evaluation**, request for a summary report detailing response to therapy

16. How would you construct a consultation on a 55-year-old married white man with a new left-middle cerebral artery stroke?

On approach to the ward, **identify the patient's nurse** for a review of current condition and particular needs. Abstract from the chart a **list of problems,** such as cerebrovascular accident (CVA), risk factors, and complications. Use a phrase with each problem to specify severity. For example, identify **location, size, and etiology of stroke**. List the **risk factors** for CVA as separate problems as well. For example, a description of diabetes mellitus might read, "IDDM for 10 years with HgbA1C of 8." Follow with a list of various **complications**, such as deep venous thrombosis, edema, and skin breakdown. Then, list the **impairments** (perception/neglect) and **activity limitations** (mobility, ADLs, communication ability, cognition, leisure activities). Specific functional limitations in self-care can be included in or under the ADL limitation problems.

Thereafter, problems at the **barrier to participation** level can be listed: **psychological adaptation** (depression), **social role function** (e.g., husband, neighbor), and **architectural access** (ramp to door, bathroom access). Recommendations and prioritization of short-term goals should be listed, making sure to include the family in training. **Immediate progress** might be achieved with medication adjustments or by posting a schedule for goal-based activity throughout the day: ROM, sitting time, Foley drainage to leg bag, dressing, supervised meals, prescribed family activities, and identifying one primary nurse. After stabilization, the patient should be **transferred to the least restrictive setting** for continued rehabilitation.

17. How can PM&R consultation contribute to patient care after trauma?

Retrospective studies have demonstrated early PM&R consultation during acute care can improve many outcome parameters, reduce required acute length of stay (LOS), and prevent sedative overmedication. In burn care, a dedicated and trained burn physiatrist can improve efficiency of care delivery, get an early start on the rehabilitation process, and reduce required LOS once patients are transferred to inpatient rehabilitation. Quality improvement projects provide a practical refinement methodology to improve timing, location, nature, and methodology of interventions.

Alizo G, Sciarretta JD, Gibson S, et al. Multidisciplinary team approach to traumatic spinal cord injuries: A single institution's quality improvement project. *Eur J Trauma Emerg Surg.* 2018;44(2):245–250. doi: 10.1007/s00068-017-0776-8. Available at: https://link.springer.com/article/10.1007/s00068-017-0776-8

Robinson LR, Godleski M, Rehou S, Jeschke M. The impact of introducing a physical medicine and rehabilitation trauma consultation service to an academic burn center. *J Burn Care Res.* 2019;40(5):648–651. doi: 10.1093/jbcr/irz079

Robinson LR, Tam AKH, MacDonald SL, et al. The impact of introducing a physical medicine and rehabilitation trauma consultation service to an academic level 1 trauma center. *Am J Phys Med Rehabil.* 2019;98(1):20–25. doi: 10.1097/PHM.0000000000001007

18. What is a clinical pathway or care map?

A *clinical pathway*, or *clinical care map*, is a uniform procedure for coordinating interventions by a variety of medical disciplines in patients within a given diagnostic group. The development of a clinical pathway requires a sufficient number of cases seen per year to justify pathway design. Management of past cases is reviewed by all disciplines that care for patients with the diagnosis. The sequence schedule and details of interventions are designed and revised until unanimous agreement is reached. Then, a form or software for the chart is created that lists the interventions and disciplines. The pathway is typically triggered by one order made by the attending physician. Other referrals and orders are made automatically with clinical pathway implementation. The process is refined with retrospective review, prospective interactive redesign, and ratifications of revisions by the care team.

Albert T, Blanquart F, Le Chapelain L, et al. Physical and rehabilitation medicine (PRM) care pathways: "Spinal cord injury." *Ann Phys Rehabil Med.* 2012;55:440–450. Available at: http://dx.doi.org/10.1016/j.rehab.2012.04.004

Yelnik AP, Schnitzler A, Pradat-Diehl P, et al. Physical and rehabilitation medicine (PRM) care pathways: "Stroke patients." *Ann Phys Rehabil Med.* 2011;54:506–518. doi:10.1016/j.rehab.2011.09.004

19. How can the PM&R consultation be used as a mechanism for teaching?

A PM&R consultation can fulfill many teaching missions. Bringing rehabilitation to other floors of the hospital, to clinics, or to patients' homes showcases rehabilitation in process and demonstrates functional outcomes in patients with many diagnoses. Bringing medical students and pre-medical students on PM&R consultation rounds introduces them to patients with a wide spectrum of disablement experiences who are treated in various settings. The consult service offers an opportunity to provide a broad overview of a number of various medical problems and rehabilitation solutions.

Stiens SA, Berkin DI. A clinical rehabilitation course for college undergraduates provides an introduction to biopsychosocial interventions that minimize disablement. *Am J Phys Med Rehabil.* 1998;76:462–470.

ACKNOWLEDGMENT

The authors acknowledge their indebtedness to Walter C. Stolov, MD (1928–2018), for his PM&R consult format, used for decades at the University of Washington.

BIBLIOGRAPHY

Fredrickson M, Cannon NL. The role of the rehabilitation physician in the postacute continuum. *Arch Phys Med Rehabil.* 1995;76: SC5–SC9.

Groenveld B, Melles M, Vehmeijer S, et al. Developing digital applications for tailored communication in orthopaedics using a Research through Design approach. *Digit Health.* 2019;5:2055207618824919. Available at: https://doi.org/10.1177/2055207618824919; https://journals.sagepub.com/doi/pdf/10.1177/2055207618824919

Lawler K, "aylor NF, Shields N. Family-assisted therapy empowered families of older people transitioning from hospital to the community: A qualitative study. *J Physiother.* 2019; 65(3):166–171. doi:10.1016/j.jphys.2019.05.009 Available at: https://www.sciencedirect.com/science/article/pii/S1836955319300566?via%3Dihub

Marin EL, Colandner AS. *Therapeutic Prescription.* In B O'Young, MA Young, SA Stiens (Eds.). *PM&R Secrets.* Philadelphia: Hanley & Belfus, 1997:509–512.

Robinson LR. *Trauma Rehabilitation.* Philadelphia: Lippincott, William Wilkins; 2006.

Rotter T, Kinsman L, James EL, et al. Clinical pathways: Effects on professional practice, patient outcomes, length of stay and hospital costs (Review). *Cochrane Collaboration.* 2010;7. Available at: https://akademia.nfz.gov.pl/wp-content/uploads/2016/08/CD006632. pdf

Tarrant C, Stokes T, Colman AM. Models of the medical consultation: Opportunities and limitations of a game theory perspective. *Qual Saf Health Care.* 2004;13:461–466. doi: 10.1136/qshc.2003.008417. Available at: https://www.ncbi.nlm.nih.gov/pmc/articles/PMC1743922/pdf/v013p00461.pdf

Tenforde AS, Jaye E, Kodish-Wachs JE, et al. Telehealth in physical medicine and rehabilitation: A narrative review. *PM R.* 2017;9(5S): S51–S58. doi:10.1016/j.pmrj.2017.02.013.

Tolchin DW. Recommendations Relevant to Physiatrists in New Clinical Practice Guidelines for Quality Palliative Care. *Am J Phys Med Rehabil.* 2020;99(5):444–445. doi:10.1097/PHM. 0000000000001381. Available at: https://journals.lww.com/ajpmr/Fulltext/2020/05000/Recommendations_Relevant_to_Physiatrists_in_New.14.aspx

Zimmermann KZ, Brown RD. Rehabilitation technology prescription: Determinations of failure and elements of success in advances in rehabilitation technology. *Phys Med Rehabil State Art Rev.* 1997;11:1–12.

ANATOMY AND KINESIOLOGY OF THE MUSCULOSKELETAL SYSTEM

Carson D. Schneck, MD, PhD

CHAPTER 3

No knowledge can be more satisfactory to a man than that of his own frame, its parts, their functions and actions.

—Thomas Jefferson (1814)

KEY POINTS

1. Key structures comprising the intervertebral disc include the annulus fibrosus and the nucleus pulposus.
2. Most intervertebral disc protrusions occur posterolaterally.
3. Joint motion can be facilitated by agonist, antagonistic, and synergistic muscles.
4. Types of muscle contractions include concentric/isotonic/shortening contractions; isometric/static contractions; eccentric/lengthening contractions.
5. The two major "crutch walking" muscles of the shoulder are: lower pectoralis major, latissimus dorsi.
6. Carpal tunnel syndrome does not typically cause proximal palm sensory abnormalities.

1. Which forces typically act to produce motion at joints?
   Gravity and muscle contraction produce motion at joints. Each serves as the prime mover for approximately 50% of all joint movements.

2. What role do agonist, antagonist, and synergistic muscles play in facilitating joint motion?
   - An **agonist**, or prime mover, is any muscle that can provide the needed force to cause a specific joint motion. For example, the triceps brachii contracts to cause elbow extension.
   - An **antagonist** is any muscle that can provide the needed force to cause a motion opposite to the specific agonist motion. For example, the biceps brachii is an antagonist to elbow extension. Antagonists are typically relaxed during agonist contraction (except near the end of a rapid ballistic motion).
   - A **synergist** typically stabilizes joints around where movement is occurring or contracts to remove unwanted agonist actions.

3. How is muscle strength graded?
   Manual muscle strength assessment is accomplished by proceeding anteriorly downward in the order of innervation from the brachial plexus through the lumbosacral plexus. Examine muscles in the proximal-to-distal order in which they receive their motor branches if specific nerves are in question. The "make and break" technique, which is when the examiner overpowers a patient's fixed mid-muscle length contraction, is the best way to assess resistance. Ordinal-ranked categories used in clinical practice are:

Grade	Description
0	Absent muscle contraction
1	Minimal contraction
2	Active movement with gravity eliminated
3	Active movement against gravity only
4	Active movement against gravity and some resistance
5	Normal muscle strength

Ferri FF. *Ferri's Practical Guide: Fast Facts for Patient Care.* 9th ed. Philadelphia, PA: Mosby/Elsevier; 2014:306–339.

4. Two muscles often perform the same function. How can the examiner eliminate one of the muscles to evaluate the other muscle in relative isolation?

Three muscle isolation procedures are commonly used:

- *Mechanical Disadvantage:* The muscle to be eliminated must be positioned so that it will have no substantial vector component in the direction of the function to be tested.
- *Physiologic or Length Disadvantage:* The muscle to be eliminated must be positioned so that it will be slackened or use up majority of its shortening capability by performing a function other than the one being tested.
- *Reciprocal Inhibition:* If the muscle to be eliminated has several functions, reciprocally inhibit it from participating in the tested function by forcibly performing a function antagonistic to one of its other functions.

5. What are the parts of the intervertebral disc?

The intervertebral disc consists of an outer peripheral, laminated, fibrocartilaginous *anulus fibrosus* and an inner central, gel-like *nucleus pulposus* (Fig. 3.1). The anulus fibrosus contains the nucleus pulposus and lies in between adjacent vertebral bodies. The nucleus pulposus functions as a hydraulic load-dispersing mechanism, ensuring that compressive forces are redistributed over a larger surface area, thereby reducing the overall pressure.

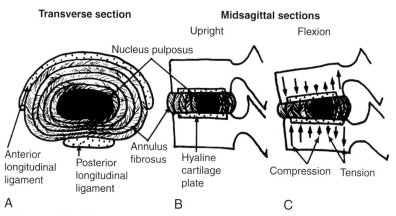

Fig. 3.1 The intervertebral disk. *A,* A transverse section. *B,* A midsagittal section through the intervertebral disk with the spine in an upright neutral position to display its normal structure and relationships. *C,* A midsagittal section of the disk with the spine in flexion to demonstrate the compressile and tensile stresses in this position. (From Schneck CD: Functional and clinical anatomy of the spine. Spine State Art Rev 9:571–604, 1995.)

6. Describe the course of the spinal nerves in relationship to the spine.

The paired *dorsal and ventral roots* of *spinal nerves* are continuous with the spinal cord and enter the intervertebral foramen. The *dorsal root ganglia* are located on each root within the spinal nerves. The spinal nerves terminate by dividing into *dorsal and ventral rami* when exiting the intervertebral foramen. Cervical spinal nerves exit above the vertebra of the same number while the C8 spinal nerve emerges between the C7 and T1 vertebrae, causing all thoracic, lumbar, and sacral nerves to exit below the vertebrae of the same number. Lower spinal nerves typically occupy the upper portion of lumbar intervertebral foramen because they must descend to their intervertebral foramina from their higher point of origin (Fig. 3.2).

7. Why do herniated lumbar intervertebral discs commonly miss the nerve that exits at that level and instead affect the next lower spinal nerve roots?

Posterolateral disc herniations typically affect the roots of the next lower spinal nerve instead of the nerve that exits at that level because the nerves occupy the upper part of the large lumbar intervertebral foramen while the disc is related to the lower part of the foramen. The herniations commonly miss the nerve in the foramen and affect the nerves that occupy the most lateral part of the spinal canal before exiting from the lower intervertebral foramen. For example, a herniated L3–L4 disc will typically miss the L3 nerve and affect the L4 roots.

8. What do dorsal rami of spinal nerves innervate?

The dorsal rami contain nerves that carry visceral motor, somatic motor, and somatic sensory information to and from the skin of the interauricular line to the coccyx (head to tail), deep muscles of the back, posterior ligaments of the spine, and the facet joint capsules.

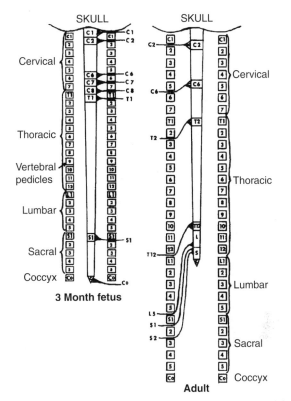

Fig. 3.2 Dorsal view of spinal nerves in relation to vertebral levels and spinal cord segments in the 3-month fetus and adult. (From Schneck CD: Functional and clinical anatomy of the spine. Spine State Art Rev 9:571–604, 1995.)

9. Name the major ligaments of the spine and the spine motions they resist.
   - Posterior longitudinal ligament: flexion
   - Ligamenta flava and facet joint capsule: flexion
   - Interspinous and supraspinous ligaments: flexion
   - Anterior longitudinal ligament: extension

10. Which muscles are responsible for producing the major spine motions?
    The major spine motions include lateral bending, rotation, flexion, and extension. While the deep back muscles are included in all of these motions, some abdominal muscles are also involved in producing spinal motions.
    - *Lateral bending* is initiated by the ipsilateral *deep back, abdominal, psoas major, and quadratus lumborum* muscles. Once started, gravity becomes the prime mover under the control of eccentric contraction of the same muscles on the contralateral side, which also contract concentrically to return the spine to the upright position.
    - **Rotation** of the front of the trunk to one side is produced by the ipsilateral **erector spinae, internal abdominal oblique muscles, the contralateral deeper back muscles, and the external abdominal oblique.** Rotation of the face to one side involves the ipsilateral **splenius, contralateral sternocleidomastoid, and other cervical rotators.**
    - *Flexion* of the spine is initiated by the *anterior abdominal muscles*. As soon as the spine is out of equilibrium, the deep back muscles contract eccentrically, allowing gravity to become the prime mover. A concentric contraction of the *deep back muscles* returns the spine to the upright position.
    - *Extension* of the spine is initiated by the *deep back muscles*. The *anterior abdominal muscles* control gravity with an eccentric contraction and return the spine to an upright position with a concentric contraction.

11. **What are the uncovertebral or Luschka's joints?**

The C3–C7 vertebrae contain lip-like crests called **uncinate processes**. As a result of normal degenerative changes, these processes begin to articulate with the depression in the inferior aspect of the vertebral body to form **Luschka's joints**. Luschka's joints form at this point because this is where the cervical discs are narrowest and susceptible to the greatest tensile stress. Luschka's joints can serve as a buffer to protect surrounding structures from disc herniation due to their posterolateral location relative to the vertebral body.

12. **What are lateral recesses? What is their significance?**

Lateral recesses are narrow bony canals in which the spinal nerves pass through at the L4, L5, and S1 levels before exiting their intervertebral foramen. This narrowing occurs because the pedicles become shorter in the anteroposterior dimension of the lateral portion at this level. The lateral recess is formed by the medial border of the superior facet and medial border of the pedicle.

Hypertrophic degenerative changes within the superior articular process can cause stenosis, or narrowing, of the space between this process and the vertebral body. If the distance becomes less than 3 mm, **lateral stenosis** occurs with the potential for nerve root impingement. Lumbar level L4–L5 is most commonly involved in lateral recess stenosis. Similar hypertrophic changes within the more medially situated inferior articular process will cause a **central stenosis**. Hypertrophy of the superior articular facets can cause **foraminal stenosis** (Fig. 3.3).

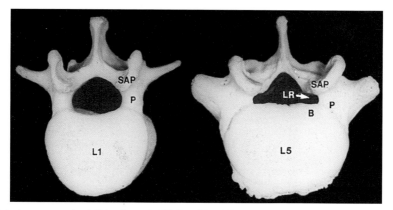

Fig. 3.3 Lateral recesses are absent at L1 and present at L5. (From Schneck CD: Functional and clinical anatomy of the spine. Spine State Art Rev 9:571–604, 1995.)

13. **Why do most intervertebral disc protrusions occur posterolaterally?**

- The intervertebral disc is supported anterolaterally by the anterior longitudinal ligament and posteromedially by the posterior longitudinal ligament. There are no extrinsic supporting ligaments posterolaterally.
- The posterior anulus has the small radial dimension and offers the least support given that the nucleus pulposus is located closer to the posterior aspect of the disc.
- The posterior anulus is thinnest in the superior-inferior dimension at the cervical and lumbar levels, which increases strain. Disc protrusions tend to occur where the anulus fibrosis is thinner, lacking structural support.
- The posterior anulus is under repetitive stress given that flexion is the most predominant spine motion.
- The posterolateral anulus is subject to the highest intralaminar shear stresses, causing intralaminar separations.

14. **What anatomic and mechanical features of the lumbosacral junction predispose L5 to spondylolysis and spondylolisthesis?**

The L5–S1 junction is susceptible to misalignment and injury because the top of the sacrum is typically positioned at a steep angle that shifts under gravitational load. The L5 vertebra tends to shift forward on the S1 vertebra under stress; however, the impingement of the inferior articular processes of L5 against the superior articular processes of the sacrum typically resist this shift. These substantial forces cause stress on the **par interarticularis** (which connects the upper and lower facets) of the L5 lamina and can result in a stress fracture or **spondylolysis**. Spondylolysis can predispose the vertebral body to displacement or **spondylolisthesis** (Fig. 3.4).

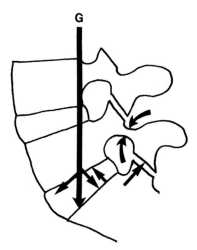

Fig. 3.4 Spondylolysis at L5. (From Schneck CD: Functional and clinical anatomy of the spine. Spine State Art Rev 9:571–604, 1995.)

15. **Are the deep back muscles contracted or relaxed in the upright position?**
    The spine is in relatively good equilibrium when in the upright position because the line of gravity falls through the points of inflection of each of the spinal curves. Therefore, activity in the major deep back muscles (erector spinae, semispinalis, multifidus, and rotators) is insignificant. The ligaments of the spine provide the most resistance to any applied movement.

16. **What structural features cause the shoulder (glenohumeral) joint to be a highly mobile but relatively unstable joint?**
    The relatively poor bony congruence between the glenoid and humeral head and a relatively slack capsule contribute to instability of the shoulder. Much of the stability of the shoulder is provided by the surrounding muscles and soft tissue structures.

17. **What dynamic features help maintain shoulder joint contact through the full range of abduction?**
    The ***rotator cuff muscles,*** which are the supraspinatus, infraspinatus, subscapularis, and teres minor, are responsible for stabilization and movement of the shoulder. The ***deltoid*** tends to sublux the humeral head superiorly in early abduction. The simultaneous contraction of the ***supraspinatus*** and the slightly downward vector pull of the ***subscapularis***, ***infraspinatus***, and ***teres minor*** muscles offset this subluxation. In the middle range of abduction, the subscapularis will turn off to allow the ***infraspinatus*** and ***teres major*** to externally rotate the humerus and bring the greater tubercle posteriorly under the acromion. This prevents impingement against the coracoacromial arch.

Miller MD, Thompson SR. Shoulder Anatomy and Biomechanics. In: *DeLee, Drez, and Miller's Orthopaedic Sports Medicine.* 5th ed. Elsevier; 2019:393–401.

18. **What structure provides the strongest support for the acromioclavicular joint?**
    The coracoclavicular ligament attaches the distal clavicle to the coracoid process of the scapula, hence providing support in a superior-inferior direction.

19. **What are the two major "crutch-walking" muscles of the shoulder?**
    The downward pull of the ***lower pectoralis major*** and ***latissimus dorsi*** muscles acting on the humerus offset the upward vector force of the crutches.

20. **How do medial and lateral winging of the scapula occur?**
    The trapezius and serratus anterior provide the force necessary to keep the medial border of the scapula close to the thoracic wall. However, injuries may occur that cause the medial border to wing away from the thoracic wall

either medially or laterally. ***Medial winging*** is typically due to serratus anterior paralysis. The medial border will wing away from the thoracic wall and be displaced medially by the unopposed retraction of the trapezius. ***Lateral winging*** is typically caused by trapezius paralysis. The medial border wings but is displaced laterally by the unopposed protraction of the serratus anterior.

21. **Why is the elbow a relatively stable joint?**
    The trochlear notch of the ulna, which is formed by the coronoid process and olecranon, firmly grips the humeral trochlea increasing joint stability. Additionally, the surrounding radial and ulnar collateral ligaments are strong and taut.

22. **How are major loads transferred from the radius at the wrist to the ulna at the elbow?**
    Loads are transferred across a fibrous connective sheath called the ***interosseous membrane.*** Loads ascending the radius cause the interosseous membrane fibers to become taut and shift the load from the distal radius to the proximal ulna.

23. **Where is the axis for pronation and supination of the forearm located?**
    The axis passes through the center of the radial head proximally and through the ulnar head distally.

24. **What is the normal digital balance mechanism of the fingers?**
    There is one extensor, the extensor digitorum (although there is an additional extensor of the index and little fingers), at the metacarpophalangeal (MCP) joint balanced against four flexors—the interossei, lumbrical, flexor digitorum profundus, and superficialis. Three extensors—the interossei, lumbrical, and extensor digitorum—at the proximal interphalangeal (PIP) joint are balanced against two flexors, the flexor digitorum profundus and superficialis. There are three extensors (the interossei, lumbrical, and extensor digitorum) at the distal interphalangeal (DIP) joint balancing against one flexor (flexor digitorum profundus). The extensor tendons form an extensor hood mechanism that further splits into lateral and central bands over the PIP joint. The central band inserts into the base of the middle phalanx and the lateral bands insert into the base of the distal phalanx. All three bands are connected by the ***triangular membrane***, which holds the lateral bands in their normal dorsal position, over the PIP joint. The lateral bands are split and tethered ventrally to the proximal phalanx by the ***oblique retinacular ligament of the Landsmeer***.

25. **Which carpal bones are most frequently injured?**
    The most frequently injured carpal bones are the major weight-bearing bones: the scaphoid and the triquetrum. Scaphoid fractures account for 60% of all carpal fractures. About 70% to 80% of scaphoids receive a blood supply via the radial artery to their distal ends while 20% to 30% receive a blood supply only to their distal ends. Hence, 20% to 30% of scaphoid fractures are nonunion, which is a permanent failure to heal.

    Triquetrum fractures account for 15% of all carpal fractures; specifically, the dorsal cortical fracture that accounts for 93% of all triquetral fractures. Extreme palmar flexion and hyperextension with ulnar deviation are the two main mechanisms of injury.

Lee SK. Fracture of the Carpal Bones. In: *Green's Operative Hand Surgery*. 7th ed. Elsevier; 2017:588–652.

Williams DT, Kim HT. Wrist and Forearm. In: *Rosen's Emergency Medicine: Concepts and Clinical Practice*. 9th ed. Elsevier; 2017: 508–529.

26. **Why are the motions of the thumb at right angles to the similar motions of the fingers?**
    The motions of the thumb are at right angles compared to the rest of the fingers because the thumb is internally rotated at 90 degrees relative to the fingers. Flexion and extension of the thumb, for example, occur in a plane parallel to the palm while thumb abduction and adduction occur in a plane perpendicular to the palm.

27. **How can the flexor digitorum profundus be eliminated in order to test the flexor digitorum superficialis tendons in isolation?**
    In order to test the ability of the flexor digitorum superficialis to flex the PIP joint of a finger, press down on the distal phalanges of all other fingers except of that being tested. This causes the other fingers to remain hyperextended, which causes the profundus to be taut and eliminates it as a PIP joint flexor. This is because the tendons of the profundus arise from a common tendon attached to its muscle mass while the tendons of the superficialis each have their own muscle belly.

28. **How can the extensor digitorum be eliminated to isolate and test the extensor indicis as the last muscle innervated by the radial nerve?**
    Extensor indicis is tested by extending the index finger while holding the remaining fingers in tight flexion at their MCP and interphalangeal (IP) joints. This eliminates simultaneous extensor digitorum contraction as the tendons of the extensor digitorum are pulled distally over their MCP and IP joints.

29. Why doesn't carpal tunnel syndrome cause sensory abnormalities over the proximal palm?
Carpal tunnel syndrome causes sensory abnormalities in the median nerve distribution only, which consists of the thumb, index finger, long and radial aspect of the ring finger. The palmar cutaneous branch of the median nerve passes superficial to the flexor retinaculum.

30. What are the unique features of the hip joint capsule and its blood supply? What is their clinical significance?
The femoral head and majority of the femoral neck are intracapsular. This is because the anterior hip joint capsule attaches to the **intertrochanteric line** of the femur enclosing the anterior femoral neck and the posterior capsule encloses the proximal two-thirds of the femoral neck. This capsule requires that most of the blood supply to the femoral head ascend from the femoral neck. Aside from the small branch of the **obturator artery** that enters the head with the ligament of the femoral head, majority of the blood flow to the femoral head is supplied by *the* **medial circumflex femoral artery**, which passes through the layers of the joint capsule. Hence, most of the blood supply to the femoral head is at risk of compromise due to femoral neck fractures.

Additionally, the upper femoral metaphysis is intracapsular because the capsule attaches to the femoral neck so low. In most other joints, the metaphyses, which are the most vascular parts of long bones, are extracapsular; therefore, hematogenously spread infection to the upper femoral metaphysis can easily produce septic arthritis.

31. What structural features make the hip a relatively stable joint?
The femoral head and acetabulum, which form a ball-and-socket joint, contribute to the stability of the hip. The acetabulum has a surrounding fibrocartilaginous lip called a labrum that deepens the socket and provides greater stability. Surrounding the joint are three strong capsular ligaments, two of which, the iliofemoral and ischiofemoral ligaments, are maximally stretched in the usual weight-bearing position.

32. Though the long, obliquely situated femoral neck predisposes the hip to high shearing forces and fracture, are there physiologic advantages to this unique design?
The long, obliquely situated femoral neck has the salutary effect of displacing the greater trochanter farther from the abduction-adduction axis of the femoral head, thereby lengthening the moment arm of the gluteus medius and minimus muscles. In standing on one leg, the gravitational vector acting on the adduction side of the hip joint is on a moment arm approximately three times as long as the gluteus medius and minimus moment arm.

Therefore, these muscles have to produce a force approximately three times as great as the gravitational vector to offset its hip adduction tendency. If the femoral neck were any shorter or more vertically oriented, as in a valgus hip, the gluteus medius and minimus moment arm would be shortened, requiring these muscles to apply more force to offset the gravitational vector. The long moment arm of the normal femoral neck thereby reduces the loads across the hip and helps protect the hip from degenerative arthritis.

Turek SL. *Orthopedics: Principles and Their Application.* 6th ed. Lippincott, Williams, & Wilkins; 2005.

33. When is the iliopsoas most active during the gait cycle? Why?
The iliopsoas is most active during toe-off. The iliopsoas acts posteriorly on the hip and causes hip extension.

34. At what point in the gait cycle is the gluteus maximus most active? Why?
The gluteus maximus is most active at the heel strike of the ipsilateral limb. This causes the trunk to flex the thigh.

35. What is the best way to test the right gluteus medius and minimus muscles?
The best way to test the right gluteus medius and minimus muscles is to perform the Trendelenburg test. The patient is asked to stand on the right leg while the examiner watches the movements of the pelvis. If the pelvis on the left side falls, this test is considered positive as it indicates weakness in the hip abductor muscles, specifically in the gluteus medius, on the right side.

36. Why is the knee joint most stable in extension?
The knee is most stable in extension because the contact between the **femoral and tibial condyles** are greatest in extension, lowering the pressures acting across the knee. The knee is "locked" in extension and is at this point the most stable. The knee is also surrounded by supporting ligaments that provide stability. The **tibial and fibular collateral ligaments** are maximally taut in extension while the **anterior cruciate ligament** is maximally taut only in extension.

37. Why are the gastrocnemius and soleus muscles the most active lower limb muscles in standing?
The center of gravity when standing passes slightly through the back of the hip, anterior to the knee, and slightly anterior to the ankle joint. The iliofemoral (and ischiofemoral) ligaments prevent hyperextension of the hip while the posterior capsule prevents hyperextension of the knee. The gastrocnemius muscle, which primarily provides ankle stability, also helps prevent back-knee. The line of gravity acting anterior to the ankle makes it a strong ankle dorsiflexor. The gastrocnemius and soleus muscles resist this ankle dorsiflexion.

38. When are the ankle dorsiflexor muscles active during gait?
The ankle dorsiflexors must be equally active during the supporting and swinging phases of walking. They help the leg incline forward during the supporting phase and prevent foot-drop during the swinging phase.

39. What is the most osteologically stable position of the ankle? Why?
Dorsiflexion. The talar trochlea and tibiofibular mortise are wedge-shaped with wide anterior surfaces and narrow posterior surfaces. As the foot moves into dorsiflexion, the talar trochlea glides posteriorly and the wider portion becomes wedged into the narrow part of the tibiofibular mortise.

40. Which nerve of the foot is homologous to the median nerve in the hand?
The medial plantar. This nerve is a major sensory nerve in the sole of the foot that innervates the following: skin on the medial two-thirds of the foot and medial three and one-half digits, the intrinsic muscles of the great toe except for the adductor hallucis, the first lumbrical, and the flexor digitorum brevis. The lateral plantar nerve is homologous to the ulnar nerve.

41. At what joint does most of the pronation and supination of the foot occur?
The transverse tarsal (or midtarsal), tarsometatarsal, and subtalar joint all contribute to most of the pronation (eversion) and supination (inversion) of the foot.

BIBLIOGRAPHY

Books
Benzon HT, Rathmell JP, Wu CL, et al. *Practical Management of Pain.* 5th ed. Philadelphia, PA: Mosby; 2013:185–242.
Roberts JR, Custalow CB, Thomsen TW, et al. eds. *Roberts and Hedges' Clinical Procedures in Emergency Medicine and Acute Care.* 7th ed. Elsevier; 2018:980–1026.
Spondylosis—Definition, Causes and Treatment. Available at: https://boneandspine.com/what-is-spondylosis/

CHAPTER 4

NERVOUS SYSTEM ANATOMY: CENTRAL AND PERIPHERAL

Stephen Goldberg, MD

The human brain starts working the moment you are born and never stops until you stand up to speak in public.
George Jessel (1898–1981)

KEY POINTS: RAPID LOCALIZERS OF NEUROLOGIC LESIONS

1. Pain in an extremity or a sensory deficit along a dermatome suggests a lesion outside the spinal cord.
2. A facial deficit on one side and an extremity deficit on the other side suggests a brain stem lesion.
3. A visual deficit that only affects one eye suggests a lesion anterior to the optic chiasm.
4. Paralysis and loss of proprioception—stereognosis on one side of the body combined with pain-temperature loss on the other side—suggests a spinal cord lesion (Brown-Sequard).
5. Paralysis and hyperactive reflexes suggest a central nervous system (CNS) (upper motor neuron) lesion.
6. A cerebellar lesion is characterized by awkwardness of intended movements. A basal ganglia lesion is better characterized as unintended movements while at rest.

CENTRAL NERVOUS SYSTEM

1. What structures comprise the central nervous system (CNS)?
   - Spinal cord (cervical enlargement, lumbar enlargement, conus, cauda equina)
   - Brain stem (medulla, pons, midbrain)
   - or
   - Cerebellum (lateral lobes, central vermis)
   - Cerebrum
   - Diencephalon (everything that contains the name *thalamus*—thalamus, hypothalamus, epithalamus, subthalamus)
   - Basal ganglia (caudate nucleus, globus pallidus, putamen, claustrum, amygdala)

   Meditay, Central Nervous System Anatomy, Available at: https://www.youtube.com/watch?v=Z3fLmpepJfg&list=PLmzZnYRTmRK8BTd1iJtzry0WhOYkpca0g

2. How many nerve structures make up the peripheral nervous system?
   - 12 cranial nerves (although the optic nerve technically is an outgrowth of the CNS)
   - 31 pairs of spinal nerves

   Anatomy and Physiology I: Peripheral Nervous System. Available at: https://www.youtube.com/watch?v=SxMoBeev-2E

3. What is the autonomic nervous system? What role does it play?
   The autonomic nervous system innervates smooth muscle, cardiac muscle, and glands. It includes:
   - **Sympathetic nerves,** from the **intermediolateral column** of spinal cord segments T1–L2
   - **Parasympathetic nerves,** which originate from spinal cord segments S2–S4 (conus)
   - **Four cranial nerves:** CN3 (oculomotor nerve fibers to pupil and ciliary body), CN7 (facial nerve fibers to sublingual, submaxillary, and lacrimal glands), CN9 (glossopharyngeal nerve fibers to parotid glands), and CN10 (vagus nerve fibers to heart, lungs, and gastrointestinal [GI] tract to the splenic flexure of the colon)
   - Autonomic nervous system anatomy

   Available at: https://www.youtube.com/watch?v=Fh9cTO2hmM0

4. What type of nerve fibers are found in anterior (ventral) nerve roots?
   Mainly motor axons

5. What type of nerve fibers are found in posterior (dorsal) nerve roots?
   Mainly sensory axons

6. What structures are located in posterior (dorsal) root ganglia?
   Posterior root ganglia are located outside the central nervous system and contain cell bodies of sensory axons but no synapses. This has important implications for nerve conduction studies. If the lesion is proximal to the dorsal root ganglion, then sensory conduction will be normal in the peripheral nerve, since the cell bodies are spared.

7. Is a peripheral nerve lesion different from a CNS lesion in terms of sensory features?
   Peripheral nerve lesions can be distinguished from CNS lesions by the different kinds of sensory and motor deficits that arise:
   - **Peripheral nerve lesions** result in **dermatome-type** sensory deficits (i.e., there is a strip-like loss of sensation along a particular area of the body, corresponding to the extension of individual peripheral nerves away from the spinal cord). L4–L5 (anterior calf, large toe) radiculopathies are particularly common, as are C6 (thumb), C7 (middle finger), and C8 (small finger) radiculopathies.
   - However, the CNS is not organized by dermatomes. A CNS motor lesion will more likely result in a **general sensory loss** in an extremity, rather than in the strip-like dermatome deficit.

8. Which dermatomes are innervated by which nerves?
   - **C1:** No sensory distribution
   - **C2:** Skull cap
   - **C3:** Collar around the neck
   - **C4:** Cape around the shoulders
   - **C6:** "Thumb suckers suck C6"
   - **T5:** Nipples
   - **T10:** Belly button
   - **L1:** IL (region of inguinal ligament)
   - **L3:** Rhymes with knee
   - **L4**: Knee jerk
   - **L5:** Medial hamstrings
   - **S1:** Ankle jerk

Dermatomes and Cutaneous Fields. Available at: https://www.youtube.com/watch?v=FpdL24OUYMs

9. Is it possible for features to distinguish a peripheral nerve lesion from a CNS lesion?
   Peripheral nerve lesions produce lower motor neuron deficits, whereas CNS lesions produce upper motor neuron deficits (Table 4.1).

10. Which roots comprise the brachial plexus?
    The brachial plexus contains the ventral rami of C5, C6, C7, C8, and T1.

Brachial Plexus—YouTube. Available at: https://www.youtube.com/watch?v=RLJ8aUw468M

Myotomes and Peripheral nerves—YouTube. Available at: https://www.youtube.com/watch?v=4fMgypHEozo

Table 4.1 Upper Versus Lower Motor Neuron Defects

UPPER MN DEFECT	LOWER MN DEFECT
Spastic paralysis	Flaccid paralysis
No significant muscle atrophy	Significant atrophy
No fasciculations or fibrillations	Fasciculations and fibrillations
Hyperreflexia	Hyporeflexia
Babinski reflex may be present	Babinski reflex not present

11. Which nerves arise from the anterior (ventral) rami of the roots, prior to the formation of the brachial plexus?
    - The **dorsal scapular nerve,** from C5 to the **rhomboid and levator scapula muscles**, is responsible for elevating and stabilizing the scapula.
    - The **long thoracic nerve,** from C5, C6, and C7 to the **serratus anterior muscle**, is responsible for abduction of the scapula.

12. Which roots form the trunks of the brachial plexus?
    The superior trunk arises from C5 and C6. The **suprascapular nerve** (C5) comes off the upper trunk and supplies the **supraspinatus** (abduction) and **infraspinatus** (external rotation) muscles of the shoulder. The middle trunk comes from C7. The lower trunk comes from C8 and T1.

13. What is the "Waiter's tip" injury?
    A lesion to the upper trunk of the brachial plexus interrupts the C5–C6 nerve roots, with weakening of the **infraspinatus** and **bicep muscles**. This results in shoulder in-turning, with the hand held in the flexed position, as if the waiter is "asking for a tip," behind his back.

14. What types of injury typically may cause a "Waiter's tip" deficit?
    Stab wounds to the neck, birth injuries (Erb's paralysis), and falls in which the angle between the shoulder and neck is suddenly widened (**stinger** injury).

15. Where in the brachial plexus could an injury cause a "claw hand?"
    An injury to the lower trunk of the brachial plexus affects the C8–T1 nerves, resulting in a combined ulnar and median nerve deficit, paralyzing **wrist flexors, flexor carpi ulnaris, ulnar half of flexor digitorum profundus, and intrinsic hand muscles**.

Claw Hand, Ape Hand, and the Sign of Benediction: Animated Review. Available at: https://www.youtube.com/watch?v=0AAligXLJ1A

16. What types of injury typically may cause a brachial plexus "claw hand?"
    - Extra cervical rib
    - Sudden pulling the arm up (as in trying to grab onto an object to break a fall)
    - Birth injury
    - Compression from lymph node metastases

17. Where in the brachial plexus could an injury result in a wrist drop?
    An injury to the posterior cord affects the extensors of the wrist because this cord gives rise to the radial nerve.

18. What type of brachial nerve injury could give rise to a wrist drop?
    This is commonly the result of pressure from inappropriately applied crutches that press on the axilla. Compression of the radial nerve against the humerus can arise from sleeping on an outstretched arm (**honeymoon palsy**), sleeping with the arm over the back of a chair or park bench (**Saturday night palsy**), or misusing axillary crutches.

19. What nerve is commonly affected in shoulder dislocations or humerus fractures?
    The axillary nerve is commonly affected, resulting in weakness or abduction of the shoulder and anesthesia over the lateral proximal arm.

20. What is the thoracic outlet syndrome?
    This syndrome, usually caused by an extra cervical rib that compresses the medial cord of the brachial plexus and the axillary artery, results in tingling and numbness in the medial aspect of the arm, along with decreased upper extremity pulses.

21. Describe the anatomy of the peripheral nerves to the upper extremity.
    See Fig. 4.1.

22. What motor functions are impaired by peripheral nerve injuries in the upper extremity?
    - **Radial nerve (C5–C8):** elbow and wrist extension (patient has wrist drop); extension of fingers at metacarpophalangeal (MCP) joints; triceps reflex
    - **Median nerve (C8–T1):** wrist, thumb, index, and middle finger flexion; thumb opposition, forearm pronation; ability of wrist to bend toward the radial (thumb) side; atrophy of thenar eminence (ball of thumb)
    - **Ulnar nerve (C8–T1):** flexion of wrist, ring and small fingers (claw hand); opposition of little finger; ability of wrist to bend toward ulnar (small finger) side; adduction and abduction of fingers; atrophy of hypothenar eminence in palm (at base of ring and small fingers)
    - **Musculocutaneous nerve (C5–C6):** elbow flexion (biceps); forearm supination; biceps reflex
    - **Axillary nerve (C5–C6):** ability to move upper arm outward, forward, or backward (deltoid atrophy)
    - **Long thoracic nerve (C5–C7):** ability to elevate arm beyond horizontal (winging of scapula; **serratus anterior atrophy**)

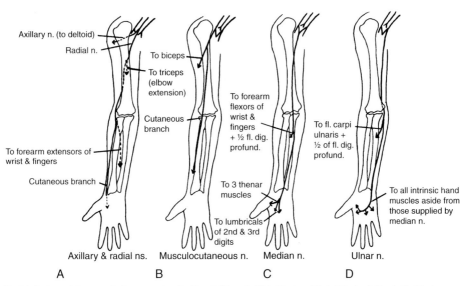

Fig. 4.1 Anatomy of the nerves to the upper extremity. (From Goldberg S. *Clinical Anatomy Made Ridiculously Simple*. MedMaster, 2016. Available at: www.medmaster.net.)

23. Describe the anatomy of the lumbosacral plexus.

The roots of L1–S4 contribute to the lumbosacral plexus, which innervates the skin and skeletal muscles of the lower extremity and perineal area (Fig. 4.2). As in the brachial plexus, its motor nerve fibers are extensions of anterior (ventral) rami. The **inferior gluteal nerve** supplies the gluteus maximus. The **superior gluteal nerve** supplies the gluteus medius and minimus. Injury to the superior gluteal nerve (e.g., direct trauma, polio) results in the "**gluteus medius limp**"; the abductor function of gluteus medius is lost, and the pelvis and trunk tilt to the unaffected side when the unaffected extremity is lifted in walking because the affected side is unable to keep the pelvis level.

Lumbosacral Plexus—Everything You Need to Know—Dr. Nabil Ebraheim. Available at: https://www.youtube.com/watch?v=-OqTl7DihPc

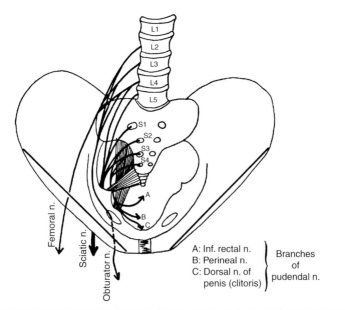

Fig. 4.2 Overview of the lumbosacral plexus. (From Goldberg S. *Clinical Anatomy Made Ridiculously Simple*. MedMaster, 2016. Available at: www.medmaster.net.)

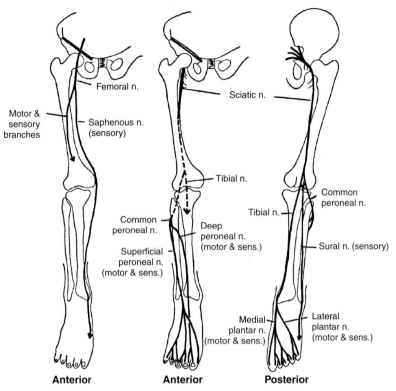

Fig. 4.3 Anatomy of the nerves to the lower extremity. (From Goldberg S. *Clinical Anatomy Made Ridiculously Simple*. MedMaster, 2016. Available at: www.medmaster.net.)

24. Describe the route of the peripheral nerves to the lower extremity.
    See Fig. 4.3.

25. What motor functions are impaired by peripheral nerve injuries in the lower extremity?
    • **Femoral nerve (L2–L4):** hip flexion, knee extension, knee jerk
    • **Obturator nerve (L2–L4):** hip adduction (patient's leg swings outward when walking)
    • **Sciatic nerve (L4–S3):** knee flexion (**hamstrings**) plus other functions along its branches, the tibial, and common peroneal nerves (ankle dorsiflexion)
    • **Tibial nerve (L4–S3):** foot inversion, ankle plantar flexion, ankle jerk reflex
    • **Common peroneal nerve (L4–S2):** foot eversion, ankle and toes dorsiflexion (patient has high-stepping gait due to foot-drop)

26. Name the other branches of the lumbar plexus.
    • **Iliohypogastric nerve (L1):** supplies abdominal muscles and skin over the hypogastric and gluteal areas
    • **Ilioinguinal nerve (L1):** innervates skin over the groin and scrotum/labia
    • **Genitofemoral nerve (L1, L2):** runs in the inguinal canal to reach the skin at the base of the penis and scrotum/clitoris and labia majora

---

Lumbosacral Plexus Drawing and Spinal Segments. Available at: https://www.youtube.com/watch?v=GLJeEVm2aHl

27. What is meralgia paresthetica?
    Commonly found in obese individuals, it is a numbness over the lateral thigh that results from compression of the **lateral femoral cutaneous nerve**, where it runs under the inguinal ligament.

28. Which nerve supplies the perineum?
The **pudendal nerve** (S2, S3, and S4). Parasympathetic branches of S2, S3, and S4 supply the bladder and are critical in bladder emptying. Sympathetic fibers to the bladder (T11–L2) support retention of urine, although severing sympathetic fibers to the bladder does not significantly affect bladder function.

29. Which nerve roots are usually affected by a herniation of the disc between vertebrae L4 and L5?
Although the L4 nerve root exits between vertebrae L4 and L5, it is generally the L5 nerve root that is compromised by a herniation, while L4 is spared. Similarly, a herniation between vertebrae L5 and S1 typically affects S1, even though the L5 root exits between L5 and S1.
    (Recommended Readings show MRI images of a herniated disk and a diagram that demonstrates relationship)

How to Read a Spine MRI—YouTube. Available at: https://www.youtube.com/watch?v=FkxvTsfDQ0Y

30. Name the five major divisions of the spinal cord.
Cervical, thoracic, lumbar, sacral, and coccygeal.

31. Where does the spinal cord end?
The spinal cord ends about at the L1–L2 vertebral level.

32. How many nerves exit the spinal cord?
There are 31 pairs of spinal nerves: 8 cervical, 12 thoracic, 5 lumbar, 5 sacral, and 1 coccygeal. Each spinal nerve is a fusion of the dorsal and ventral nerve roots.

33. What are the coverings (meninges) of the spinal cord?
The meninges surround the entire CNS and consist of the **pia,** which hugs the spinal cord and brain; the **arachnoid membrane;** and the **dura,** which is closely adherent to bone.

34. Where do you find the cauda equina?
The cauda equina ("horse's tail") is the downward extension of spinal cord roots, starting at the inferior end of the spinal cord.

35. A Brown-Sequard lesion that compromises one side of the spinal cord will cause ipsilateral deficits, except for one sensory modality. Which one?
Pain-temperature sensation below the site of the lesion will be lost two dermatomes below on the contralateral side; the pain-temperature pathway crosses over through the **anterior commissure** of the spinal cord soon after the nerve enters the spinal cord. A Brown-Sequard lesion is a spinal cord hemisection, which results in primarily ipsilateral (same side) deficits, except for pain temperature sensation.

Motor and Sensory Pathways. Available at: https://www.youtube.com/watch?v=gMCHVls_2oQ

36. What are the major motor pathways to the extremities?
  • **Corticospinal tract (pyramidal tract):** extends from the motor area of the cerebral frontal cortex (**Brodmann's areas 4, 6**) through the internal capsule, brain stem, and spinal cord, crossing over at the junction between the brain stem and spinal cord at the level of the foramen magnum. Therefore, lesions to the corticospinal tract, above the level of the foramen magnum, result in contralateral weakness, whereas lesions below the level of the foramen magnum result in ipsilateral weakness.
  • **Rubrospinal tract:** This connects the **red nucleus** of the midbrain with the spinal cord.
  • **Tectospinal tract:** This connects the **tectum** of the midbrain with the spinal cord.
  • **Reticulospinal tract:** This connects the **reticular formation** of the brain stem with the spinal cord.
  • **Vestibulospinal tract:** This connects the **vestibular nuclei** of the brain stem with the spinal cord.

Spinal Cord Mnemonics: Memorable Neurology. Available at: https://www.youtube.com/watch?v=JpA1NHDww3s

37. What distinguishes an upper motor neuron lesion from a lower motor neuron lesion?
  • An **upper motor neuron** lesion generally refers to an injury to the corticospinal tract. The corticospinal pathway synapses in the anterior horn of the spinal cord just before leaving the cord.
  • A **lower motor neuron** lesion is an injury to the peripheral motor nerves or their cell bodies in the gray matter of the anterior horn on which the corticospinal tract synapses.
    See Table 4.1.

38. **How do the effects of corticospinal tract injuries differ from those of cerebellar and basal ganglia injuries?**

    All of the injuries produce motor problems:
    - **Corticospinal tract** injuries cause upper motor neuron paralysis (see Table 4.1).
    - **Cerebellar** injuries are characterized by awkwardness of movement **(ataxia)**, not paralysis. The awkwardness is on intention—(i.e., at rest, the patient shows no problem) but ataxia becomes noticeable when the patient attempts a motor action. There may be awkwardness of posture and gait, poor coordination of movement, **dysmetria** (overshoot of intended limb position), **dysdiadochokinesia** (difficulty with quick alternating movements), **scanning speech** (abnormally long pauses between syllables and words), decreased tendon percussion reflexes on the affected side, **asthenia** (abnormal fatigue), tremor, and **nystagmus** (involuntary back and forth eye movements).
    - **Basal ganglia** disorders, like cerebellar disorders, are characterized by awkward movements rather than paralysis. The movement disorder, however, is present at rest, including such problems as **Parkinsonian "pill rolling" tremor, chorea, athetosis,** and **hemiballismus**.

Basal Ganglia Mnemonics: Memorable Neurology. Available at: https://www.youtube.com/watch?v=e9jSeRBJH8U

39. **Name three major sensory pathways in the spinal cord.**
    - **Pain–temperature:** Spinothalamic tract
    - **Proprioception–stereognosis:** posterior columns—(Proprioception is the ability to tell, with the eyes closed, if a joint is flexed or extended. **Stereognosis** is the ability to identify, with the eyes closed, an object placed in one's hand.)
    - **Light–touch:** Spinothalamic tract and posterior columns

40. **Name the three parts of the brain stem.**

    Midbrain (most superior), pons, and medulla (most inferior).

41. **What are the functions of the cranial nerves?**
    - **CN1 (olfactory):** Smell
    - **CN2 (optic):** Sight
    - **CN3 (oculomotor):** Constricts pupils, accommodates, moves eyes
    - **CN4 (trochlear), CN6 (abducens):** Move eyes
    - **CN5 (trigeminal):** Chews, feels front of head
    - **CN7 (facial):** Moves face, taste, salivation, crying
    - **CN8 (vestibulocochlear):** Hearing, regulates balance
    - **CN9 (glossopharyngeal):** Taste, salivation, swallowing, monitors carotid body, and sinus
    - **CN10 (vagus):** Taste, swallowing, lifts palate; communication to and from thoracoabdominal viscera to the splenic flexure of the colon
    - **CN11 (accessory):** Turns head (**sternocleidomastoid** muscle), lifts shoulders (**trapezius** muscle)
    - **CN12 (hypoglossal):** Moves tongue

42. **What is Horner's syndrome?**

    Horner's syndrome is **ptosis** (eyelid dropping), **miosis** (small pupil), and **anhidrosis** (lack of sweating) from a lesion of the sympathetic pathway to the face. The lesion may lie within the sympathetic pathway in the brain stem, the spinal cord, the superior cervical ganglion, or its sympathetic extensions to the head.

43. **Which cranial nerves exit from the three parts of the brain stem?**
    - Midbrain—CN3, CN4
    - Pons—CN5, CN6, CN7, CN8
    - Medulla—part of CN7 and CN8, CN9, CN10, CN12

    CN11 exits from the upper cervical cord, goes through the foramen magnum, touches CNs 9 and 10, and then returns to the neck via the jugular foramen. The optic nerve (CN2) lies superior to the brain stem. The olfactory nerve (CN1) lies in the cribriform plate of the ethmoid bone.

44. **What CNS structures connect with the brain stem?**

    The midbrain connects with the diencephalon above the brain stem. The medulla connects with the spinal cord below it. Each section of the brain stem has two major connections (right and left) with the cerebellum: two superior cerebellar peduncles connect with the midbrain, two middle cerebellar peduncles connect with the pons, and two inferior cerebellar peduncles connect with the medulla.

Neuroanatomy for Dummies. Available at: https://www.youtube.com/watch?v=QL20YcbeZY4

45. What are the two pigmented areas of the brain stem?

The **substantia nigra**, which lies in the midbrain, and the **locus ceruleus**, which lies in the pons.

46. What is the red nucleus?

The red nucleus, involved in motor coordination, lies in the midbrain. It receives major output from the cerebellum via the **superior cerebellar peduncle**. It has major connections to the cerebral cortex, as well as to the spinal cord via the **rubrospinal** tract.

47. What is the medial longitudinal fasciculus (MLF)?

The MLF is a pathway that runs through the brain stem and interconnects the ocular nuclei of CNs 3, 4, and 6 and the vestibular nuclei. It plays an important role in coordinating eye movements with head and truncal posture.

48. What is the Edinger-Westphal nucleus?

It is the **parasympathetic nucleus** of the third cranial nerve (oculomotor nerve) in the midbrain. It supplies motor fibers responsible for pupillary constriction and lens accommodation.

49. What is an Argyll-Robertson pupil?

One of the classic signs of **tertiary syphilis**. The pupil constricts on accommodating but does not constrict to light. The lesion is believed to be in the midbrain.

50. Describe the pathway for vision.

Optic nerve fibers extend from the retina to the **optic nerve**, to the optic chiasm, through the **optic tract**, to the **lateral geniculate body**, and to the visual area of the brain via **optic radiation** fibers. Some fibers extend laterally through the parietal lobe and end up superior to the **calcarine fissure** in the occipital lobe. Optic radiation fibers that extend through the temporal lobe end up inferior to the calcarine fissure in the occipital lobe; these can be damaged with anterior temporal lobe injuries, causing superior field cuts.

51. What causes a left homonymous hemianopsia? Bitemporal hemianopsia? Superior quadrantanopsia?

- **Left homonymous hemianopsia:** A lesion to the right optic tract, right lateral geniculate body, right optic radiation, or right occipital lobe
- **Bitemporal hemianopsia:** A lesion to the optic chiasm, generally from a pituitary tumor
- **Superior quadrantanopsia:** A lesion in the inferior aspect of the optic radiation

---

Visual Pathways Animated. Available at: https://www.youtube.com/watch?v=ETlp8kZPoBw

52. What is most peculiar about the exit point of CN4 from the brain stem?

CN4 (**trochlear nerve**) is the only cranial nerve to exit on the posterior side of the brain stem. In addition, it crosses over the midline before continuing on its course.

53. If a child has a head tilt, how do you know if it is due to a CN4 palsy or a stiff neck?

Cover one eye. If the head straightens out, then the tilt is due to **CN4 palsy**. The child tilts the head in a CN4 palsy to avoid double vision. Covering one eye eliminates double vision, so the head straightens out.

54. Which CRANIAL NERVES exit at the pontomedullary junction?

CN6 (**abducens nerve**) exits by the midline; CNs 7 (**facial nerve**) and 8 (**vestibular/auditory nerve**) exit laterally.

55. Where do the motor and sensory branches of CN5 exit the brain stem?

Both exit the brain stem at the same point, which is in in the lateral aspect of the pons.

56. What are the sensory branches of CN5?

V1: **Ophthalmic**; V2: **Maxillary**; V3: **Mandibular**

57. Which cranial nerve nucleus extends through all sections of the brain stem?

The **trigeminal sensory nucleus**. Its **mesencephalic nucleus** (facial proprioception) lies in the midbrain. Its **main nucleus** (facial light touch) lies in the pons. Its **spinal nucleus** (facial pain/temperature) lies in the medulla and upper spinal cord.

58. What is the function of CN7?

CN7 (the facial nerve) innervates the muscles of facial expression; supplies parasympathetic fibers to the lacrimal, submandibular, and sublingual glands; receives taste information from the anterior two-thirds of the tongue; and receives a minor sensory input from the skin of the external ear.

59. How does the facial weakness that results from a CN7 lesion differ from that caused by a lesion of the facial motor area of the cerebral cortex?

A CN7 lesion (as in **Bell's palsy** of CN7, which occurs in the facial nerve canal) results in ipsilateral facial paralysis, which includes the upper and lower face. A cerebral lesion results in contralateral facial paralysis confined to the lower face because the nucleus sends bilateral innervation to the upper face.

60. What is Möbius syndrome?

A congenital absence of both facial nerve nuclei, resulting in bilateral facial paralysis. The **abducens nuclei** may also be absent.

61. What are the nucleus ambiguus, nucleus solitarius, and salivatory nucleus?

- The **nucleus ambiguus,** which lies in the medulla, is a motor nucleus (CNs 9 and 10) that innervates the deep throat (i.e., the muscles of swallowing [CN 9 and 10] and speech [CN10]).
- The **nucleus solitarius** is a visceral sensory nucleus (CNs 7, 9, 10) that lies in the medulla. It receives input from the viscera, as well as taste information. It is a relay in the gag reflex.
- The **salivatory nucleus,** which contains superior and inferior divisions, innervates the salivary glands (CNs 7 and 9) and lacrimal glands (CN7).

62. What does CN9 do?

CN9, the **glossopharyngeal nerve**, innervates the **stylopharyngeus muscle** of the pharynx and the **parotid gland**. It receives taste information from the posterior one-third of the tongue, sensory tactile input from the posterior one-third of the tongue and the skin around the external ear canal, and sensory oxygen concentration and arterial pressure input from the **carotid body** and **sinus**.

63. To which side does the tongue deviate if CN12 (hypoglossal nerve) is injured?

The tongue deviates to the side of the lesion. Imagine you are riding a bicycle and your left hand becomes paralyzed. When you push on the handlebars, the wheel will turn to the left. The **genioglossus muscle**, which is innervated by CN12 and pushes out the tongue, operates on a similar principle.

64. A patient has a neural deficit involving the extremities on one side but the face on the other side. Where is the lesion?

The combination of a facial neural deficit on one side and an extremities deficit on the other suggests a brain stem lesion. The lesion cannot be below the brain stem because a cranial nerve is involved. The lesion cannot be above the brain stem because those lesions tend to cause strictly contralateral deficits.

CEREBRUM

65. What does the frontal lobe do?

Motor areas of the frontal lobe control **voluntary movement** on the opposite side of the body, including eye movement. The dominant hemisphere, usually the left, contains **Broca's speech area**, which when injured results in **motor aphasia** (motor **language** deficit). Areas of the frontal lobe anterior to the motor areas are involved in complex **behavioral** and **executive** activities. Lesions here result in changes in judgment, abstract thinking, tactfulness, and foresight.

66. What does the parietal lobe do?

It receives contralateral light touch, proprioceptive, and pain sensory input. Lesions to the dominant hemisphere result in tactile and proprioceptive **agnosia** (complex receptive disabilities). There may also be confusion in left-right discrimination, disturbances of body image, and **apraxia** (complex cerebral motor disabilities caused by cutting off impulses to and from association tracts that interconnect with nearby regions).

Bonus questions and answers available online.

WEBSITES

Digital Anatomist Project. Available at: http://da.si.washington.edu/da.html

Neurologic Exam Videos and Descriptions: An Anatomical Approach. Available at: https://neurologicexam.med.utah.edu/adult/html/home_exam.html

Pediatric Neurologic Examination Videos & Descriptions. Available at: https://neurologicexam.med.utah.edu/pediatric/html/home_exam.html

RECOMMENDED READINGS

Carpenter MB, Sutin J. *Human Neuroanatomy*. Baltimore: Williams & Wilkins; 1983.

Goldberg S. *Clinical Neuroanatomy Made Ridiculously Simple*. Miami: MedMaster; 2014. Available at www.medmaster.net

Haines DE. *Neuroanatomy: An Atlas of Structures, Sections and Systems*. Baltimore: Urban & Schwarzenberg; 1991.

Kandel ER, Schwartz JH, Jessell TM. *Essentials of Neural Science and Behavior*. Norwalk, CT: Appleton & Lange; 1995.

Martin JH. *Neuroanatomy: Text and Atlas*. Norwalk, CT: Appleton & Lange; 1996.

CHAPTER 5

NEUROPHYSIOLOGY AND COGNITIVE NEUROSCIENCE: FROM MEMBRANES TO FUNCTIONAL BRAIN NETWORKS

Gary Goldberg, MD, and Nachum Soroker, MD

The human brain, then, is the most complicated organization of matter that we know.
— Isaac Asimov (1920–1992)

1. Explain the significance of neurophysiology and its relevance to rehabilitation
   Rehabilitation is person-centered, function-oriented, and process-based. It is fundamentally relational, in that personal performance depends critically on proper interacting dynamic relationships between multiple peripheral and central nervous system (CNS) components. Rehabilitation clinicians must have a basic working understanding of how these processes operate normally, how activity is coordinated, and how performance degrades due to effects of pathology. To restore rather than compensate for a lost neurologic function, clinicians must recognize the basic principles of neuroplasticity and the novel experimental means to elicit activation of latent neural pathways in an effort to facilitate adaptive remapping and functional recovery. Assuming the basic function of the nervous system is to ensure survival by minimizing free energy and addressing uncertainty, rehabilitation serves to facilitate the mitigation of uncertainty.

2. How do neurons integrate and transmit information?
   Via chemicals released at the **synapses**. These **neurotransmitters** either excite the postsynaptic neuron by depolarizing its membrane, creating an excitatory postsynaptic potential, or inhibit the neuron by hyperpolarizing the membrane, producing an inhibitory postsynaptic potential. The **action potential** subsequently generated is conducted along the neuron's axon to other neurons via synaptic junctions. Neural network processing combines analog summation in the dendritic tree with digital transmission via action potentials.

3. How do voltage-dependent ion channels work to produce an action potential?
   In neuronal and muscle specialized membrane (the **neurolemma** and **sarcolemma**, respectively), **voltage-dependent ion channels**, primarily for sodium and potassium, open up transiently when the intracellular voltage shifts positive toward zero (i.e., the membrane depolarizes). At the threshold voltage, an explosive process is initiated in which **voltage-dependent sodium channels** open in rapidly increasing numbers, and the transmembrane voltage increases sharply as sodium ions rush into the cell, producing a further increase in intracellular voltage and further depolarization of the cell membrane. The voltage levels off as sodium channels inactivate and as **voltage-dependent potassium channels** open, allowing potassium to move out. The transmembrane voltage then reverses. The membrane then becomes hyperpolarized for a short time, called the **refractory period**, during which it is relatively resistant to excitation.

4. What is an ectopic action potential?
   An **ectopic action potential** is an *anomalously produced* action potential. Any problem with the membrane-based ion-exchange pump or the relative permeability of the membrane to any of the major ionic species can result in pathological instability and major fluctuations of the resting membrane potential in nerve and muscle fibers. These fluctuations can lead to a spontaneous depolarization of the membrane to the threshold level, resulting in the production of an aberrant, or ectopic, action potential. This produces manifestations of pathology such as pain, fibrillations, and fasciculations (see later).

5. How do calcium ions participate in neural transmission?
   When the action potential reaches the distal end of the axon at the presynaptic terminal, in a neuromuscular junction, it initiates the flow of calcium ions into the presynaptic terminal through voltage-dependent calcium channels concentrated in the membrane at the presynaptic terminal. This influx of calcium ions facilitates the process through which a neurotransmitter such as acetylcholine is released from vesicles in the presynaptic terminal, leading to excitation (i.e., depolarization) or inhibition (i.e., hyperpolarization) of the postsynaptic cell membrane.

6. What is a motor unit?
   The motor unit is the basic *functional element of voluntary movement* occurring through controlled voluntary activation of somatic muscle. It consists of the anterior horn cell body in the spinal cord, motor axon, terminal branches, neuromuscular junctions, and all the muscle fibers innervated by the anterior horn cell. Descending

pathways originating in cortical and brainstem upper motor neurons (UMNs) activate the anterior horn cell, which in turn activates the muscle fibers in the motor unit to produce movement.

7. **How does the motor unit work?**

The anterior horn cell typically controls several muscle fibers, ranging up to several thousand muscle fibers in a single motor unit. Each time the anterior horn cell fires, the result is a **synchronous** twitch of all the muscle fibers in the motor unit. Tension is graded by recruiting additional motor units and by increasing the firing rate of the activated motor units in the available pool. The rate at which a motor unit starts firing when it is first recruited is called the **onset firing rate**. The rate at which a motor unit is firing when the next motor unit is recruited is called the **recruitment firing rate** or **recruitment frequency**.

KEY POINTS: MEMBRANE PUMPS

1. All cellular membranes have a sodium-potassium ATP-(adenosine triphosphate) dependent ion exchange pump that produces relative electronegativity inside the cell. Its primary purpose is the control of cell volume and osmotic pressures. In excitable tissues, this sustains the "resting membrane potential" at approximately − 100 mV inside the cell relative to the extracellular environment.
2. Only excitable membranes of nerve and muscle cells have voltage-dependent ionic channels to support action potential generation and a directional wave of depolarization.
3. Muscle fibers normally contract only when depolarized by their innervating motor neuron (i.e., the anterior horn cell). Spontaneous, autonomous muscle fiber contraction is called **fibrillation** and is abnormal.

---

8. **What are fibrillations and fasciculations?**

In muscle fibers with defective membranes that cannot maintain stable transmembrane ionic gradients, spontaneous membrane depolarization leads to anomalous generation of muscle fiber action potentials. This autonomous activation of a muscle fiber occurs when pathologic conditions compromise normal neural influence over the electrical stability of the muscle fiber or directly damage the muscle fiber membrane. This autonomous muscle fiber contraction is called a **fibrillation**. Fibrillations can be detected as fibrillation potentials when recording spontaneous electromyographic activity through a needle electrode placed in a relaxed muscle.

Electrical destabilization of the cell membrane of the motor neuron or motor axon leads to spontaneous generation of an **ectopic nerve action potential**, which is conducted to all muscle fibers innervated by the motor neuron. This results in a synchronous, isolated contraction of all the fibers in the motor unit. This can produce a visible spontaneous twitch of the muscle called a **fasciculation**. Fasciculations are detectable as spontaneous firing of a single motor unit potential through a needle electrode placed in a relaxed muscle.

A1 (Kandel et al.) Chapters 4–14; B1 (Brodal) Chapters 1–5

---

9. **Outline the somatic and autonomic parts of the peripheral nervous system (PNS) and their major functions**

- The somatic PNS enables access to the CNS for afferent input originating in organs of somatic sensation. It also transmits CNS control to skeletal muscles acting as effector organs in maintenance of body posture and execution of voluntary movement.
- The autonomic nervous system has two parts, parasympathetic and sympathetic, holding a dynamic balance between them in the control of vegetative functions and the body internal milieu (energy homeostasis), such that growth and preservation of resources ("rest and digest") during periods of energy conservation and acquisition (under parasympathetic direction) can change in stress conditions ("fight or flight") needing high energy expenditure (under sympathetic dominance) (Table 5.1).

Table 5.1 Afferent and Efferent Components of the Peripheral Nervous System	
Somatic	
Afferent (sensory)	Transmits sensory information from periphery (skin, muscles, joints) about the dynamic state of limbs, their articulation in space, and external environment
Efferent (motor)	Conducts voluntary control messages to skeletal muscle
Autonomic	
Afferent	Receives sensory information about internal environment of body
Efferent	Sends control messages to smooth muscle of blood vessels, cardiac muscle, exocrine glands, and internal viscera

10. How are the afferent sensory systems organized?
Several afferent sensory systems convey information to the CNS from the body and the external environment. Afferent stimulation reaching the cerebral cortex is processed in primary cortical regions (e.g., primary visual cortex in Brodmann area 17 of the occipital lobe) for decoding of elementary attributes of stimuli. Afterward, afferent stimulation is processed in unimodal association cortices for more elaborate stimulus identification and localization purposes, enabling conscious manipulation of perceived information (e.g., visual association cortex mainly in Brodmann areas 18 and 19 of temporooccipital and parietooccipital cortical regions). Afferent information terminates also in structures outside the cortical mantle (e.g., in the cerebellum). This information does not reach conscious awareness but plays a crucial role in feedback provision for the purpose of motor control.
- General somatic afferents (GSAs) transmit somatosensory and kinesthetic information originating in receptors located in the skin, skeletal muscles (muscle spindles, Golgi tendon organs), and connective tissue.
- Special somatic afferents (SSAs) transmit visual, auditory, and vestibular information.
- General visceral afferents (GVAs) transmit information from smooth and cardiac muscles.
- Special visceral afferents (SVAs) transmit olfactory and gustatory information.

The GSA system is subdivided into the **lemniscal system**, subserving *epicritic* sensations of light touch, kinesthesis; and vibration sense; and the **spinothalamic system**, subserving the *protocritic* sensations of pain and temperature. The GSAs and SSAs transmit information to specialized modality-specific relay nuclei in the thalamus from which sensory data are transmitted to the corresponding primary sensory cortical regions. The SVAs project directly to specialized regions of the cerebral cortex bypassing the thalamus.

A1 (Kandel et al.) Chapters 21–32; B1 (Brodal) Chapters 12–19.

11. How are the extrathalamic ascending neuromodulatory systems organized?
In addition to the specific GSA, SSA, and SVA projections to the cerebral cortex, a number of widely projecting systems connect to the cerebral cortex directly from nuclei in the reticular core of the brain stem, also known as the **ascending reticular activating system (ARAS)**, and from cell aggregates in the basal forebrain. These ascending neuromodulatory systems are characterized by the major neurotransmitter that each system uses to modulate cortical activity. They are extremely important in controlling neuronal excitability and responsiveness in different parts of the cortical mantle, thus exerting a major impact on the functioning of special-purpose (vector) cortical functions (e.g., language, visual perception, memory). This "state-regulation" function of the neuromodulatory systems is important also in sleep-wake cycle regulation and in the transitions between different phases in sleep. It is also involved in the regulation of mood and emotional states as well as neuroplasticity and learning. Disruption of these systems may lead to widespread malfunctioning of different special-purpose systems, as can be seen, for example, in degeneration of central cholinergic systems in Alzheimer disease. Widespread damage to white matter ascending tracts in cranial trauma with diffuse axonal injury may lead to protracted impairment of consciousness. Many neurotransmitter-based psychoactive medications function by influencing the operation of one or more of these neuromodulatory systems (Table 5.2).

12. Which efferent tracts enable the brain to control lower motor neuron (LMN) activity?
The brain controls the activity of LMNs in the spinal cord directly through the pyramidal (corticospinal) tract and indirectly through a series of descending pathways originating in the brainstem and acting largely on spinal interneurons.
- **The corticospinal (pyramidal) tract (CST)**—originates in the **precentral gyrus** (primary motor cortex), with additional sources in the **premotor cortex**, the primary and secondary sensory cortices, and other parts of the **parietal cortex**. It descends in the **corona radiata**, the posterior limb of the **internal capsule**, the ventral brainstem, and the lateral compartment of the spinal cord (after decussation of its major part in the medulla oblongata). A small uncrossed portion descends in the ventral part of the cord. The CST is of crucial importance for the ability to produce precise, voluntary movements.
- **The rubrospinal tract**—originates in the magnocellular part of the **red nucleus** in the midbrain and descends in the lateral compartment of the spinal cord, next to the lateral CST. Its function and importance to motor

Table 5.2 Major Extrathalamic Neurotransmitter Systems

NEUROTRANSMITTER	MAJOR SOURCE NUCLEUS	TYPICAL MEDICATION
Acetylcholine	Nucleus basalis of Meynert	Donepezil (agonist) Benztropine mesylate (antagonist)
Dopamine	Substantia nigra (pars compacta) Ventral tegmental area	L-dopa, bromocriptine (agonist) Droperidol (antagonist)
Norepinephrine	Nucleus locus coeruleus	Methylphenidate (agonist)
Serotonin	Brainstem raphe nuclei	Selective serotonin reuptake inhibitor (SSRI) (e.g., fluoxetine [agonist])

control in humans is not clear, although it may be crucially involved in the facilitation of antigravity flexor musculature in the upper limb of the bipedal human being (see later).

- **The lateral and medial vestibulospinal tracts**—originate in the **vestibular nuclei**, near the pontomedullary junction. They descend in the ventral compartment of the cord and act mainly on LMNs activating trunk and proximal limb muscles. These tracts (especially the lateral) help to maintain balance and posture.
- **The tectospinal tract**—originates in the **superior colliculus**, descends in the ventral compartment of the cord, up to the cervical level, and is involved in reflex movements of the eyes and head (as in orientation toward a rapidly approaching visual object or in response to a loud sound).
- **The medial (pontine) and lateral (medullary) reticulospinal tracts**—originate in the **reticular formation** (in the pons and medulla, respectively), descend in the ventral compartment of the cord, and participate in posture control and also in execution of crude limb movements under ipsilateral (medial reticulospinal [RS] tract) and bilateral (lateral RS tract) cortical control.

13. **How does each of the different efferent tracts modulate muscle tone in health and disease?**
Each of the motor descending pathways has a different influence on the background tone and dynamic activation of motor neuron pools and interneuronal circuits in the spinal cord.
- The **vestibulospinal** and **reticulospinal** tracts are involved in the postural biasing of axial and truncal muscles and in execution of anticipatory postural adjustments that precede voluntary movements. The vestibulospinal and reticulospinal output neurons are generally excitatory to spinal motor neurons innervating extensor muscles in the arms and legs and are thought to be under inhibitory control from the cortical level. The loss of cortical inhibitory control over these pathways tends to facilitate extensor tone in both arms and legs, resulting in **decerebrate rigidity**.
- The **CST** and **rubrospinal** tracts both tend to balance the extensor drive by facilitating drive to flexor muscles. The rubrospinal tract in humans extends only down to the cervical cord and thus can possibly counterbalance extensor drive in the arms but not the legs. The **decorticate rigidity** in humans with large cerebral hemisphere lesions is primarily one part of a net facilitation of flexors in the arms and extensors in the legs. This is because loss of descending inhibitory control from the cerebral cortex releases excitatory extensor drive from the vestibular and reticular formation areas to the lower limb extensor muscles, whereas flexor facilitation is released from the red nucleus to upper limb flexor muscles. The lateral CSTs control rapid, fractionated, fine motor coordination in the contralateral hands and feet, primarily. The ventral CSTs tend to be less lateralized and are focused on more proximal musculature in the limbs.

14. **What is the upper motor neuron (UMN) syndrome?**
This syndrome is a collection of clinical "negative" (lack) and "positive" (excess) symptoms and signs, arising after damage to the descending motor pathways (UMNs) that regulate the activity of spinal interneurons and LMNs. In the case of unilateral brain damage, the UMN syndrome is reflected in the form of (1) unilateral (contralesional) muscle weakness—hemiparesis or hemiplegia, reflecting diminished recruitment of motor units or/and pathologic co-contraction of agonist and antagonist muscles preventing movement; (2) impaired movement control and loss of dexterity (difficulty producing isolated movement out of synergy); (3) impaired posture control (leading to typical or atypical abnormal resting posture); and (4) impaired reflex activity and spasticity resulting from dysregulated stretch reflex.

15. **What parts of the nervous system are involved in the control of voluntary movement?**
- The **primary motor cortex** is the cortical region involved in the **"execution"** phase of motor control. It resides in the precentral gyrus (Brodmann area 4 and posterior area 6). It is the major location of origin of neurons comprising the pyramidal tract with its corticospinal and corticobulbar components. It is somatotopically organized (the "homunculus"), with internal parcellation reflecting the complexity of control and degree of precision exercised in movement by different muscle groups. The primary motor cortex is involved in the execution of precise, rapid, "fractionated" voluntary movements of the contralateral limbs (notably, distal movements). Damage confined to the primary motor cortex and/or the corticospinal tract results in contralateral hemiparesis.
- **Motor control** is studied in the context of **behavior control** because it is through muscular activity and movement that one acts on his or her environment to satisfy drives and intents and to obtain personal goals. Therefore the cascade of events preceding execution of movements is often described as starting in a phase termed **"intent,"** where intentions and drives are processed in **midline thalamic nuclei**, in the **limbic system** (notably, the **cingulate cortex**), and in the **medial prefrontal cortex (PFC)**.
- Following the "intent" phase comes a phase termed **"idea,"** where different options for the fulfilment of the intent are processed, mainly in **dorsolateral prefrontal cortex**. Here goals are set, relevant data are retrieved, and decisions on what to do are taken; therefore these activities are also termed **"executive functions."**
- Next comes a stage termed **"plan,"** where the **premotor cortex** and regions of the **posterior parietal cortex** are involved in translating the preceding intent-idea processing into more concrete movement planning, relating to movement aspects such as its spatiotemporal organization, sequential linkage of different subroutines, trajectory planning in relationship to external objects in peripersonal and extrapersonal space, and coordination between postural stabilization and distal limb control in the organization of coordinated limb movement.

The **dorsolateral premotor cortex** is more likely to dominate motor planning aimed to answer ongoing environmental challenges in a **"bottom-up,"** responsive fashion, whereas the **medial premotor cortex** (including **supplementary motor cortex**) is more likely to dominate motor planning driven by internal goals (i.e., in a **"top-down,"** predictive manner).

- Next comes a stage termed **"program"** involving the recruitment of appropriate **motor engrams (programs)** formed by **procedural learning** in repeated past events sharing the same action parameters. This stage involves activation of a **cortex-basal ganglia-cortex loop** and a **cortex-cerebellum-cortex loop** (see later).
- The aforementioned intent-idea-plan-program phases precede a phase termed **"execution,"** where movement is finally overtly executed, with participation of the **primary motor cortex** and the medial parts of the cerebellum (**spinocerebellum**), continuing with activation of spinal interneurons and **motor neurons in the anterior horns of the spinal gray matter**, which in turn activate muscles and produce movements.
- The final (sixth) phase in the cascade is termed **"evaluate"** and is comprised by **feedback** information conveyed by spinothalamocortical pathways (**dorsal column—medial lemniscus system** and the **lateral spinothalamic tract**) transmitting information from the effector organs to the sensory cortex, and ascending tracts leading to the cerebellum (**dorsal and ventral spinocerebellar tracts**).
- It should be noted that the aforementioned simplified scheme is far from encompassing all the relevant processing that takes place in preparation for movement. For example, it is clear that selective attention is involved in processing the target stimulus of an action. Two attentional systems—the **dorsal attentional network (DAN)** composed of interconnected dorsal regions of the frontal and parietal cortices in both hemispheres and the **ventral attentional network (VAN)** composed of interconnected more ventral regions of the frontal and parietal cortices, mainly in the right hemisphere [RH]—are both involved in behavior and motor control, with the DAN taking part in goal directed task-relevant exploratory activity, and the VAN being involved in exogenously triggered response to unexpected environmental sensory events.

16. What are the roles of the basal ganglia and the cerebellum in the control of voluntary movement?

As explained earlier, in the stage of motor control termed **"program,"** cortical regions involved in motor planning recruit **motor engrams (programs)** appropriate for the planned act, which have been formed by **procedural learning** in the past, using a reentrant **cortex-basal ganglia-cortex loop** and a reentrant **cortex-cerebellum-cortex loop**.

- The **basal ganglia** consist of the input nuclei of the striatum (**caudate** and **putamen**), the external and internal segments of the **globus pallidus**, the two parts of the **substantia nigra** (**compacta** and **reticulata**), and the **subthalamic nucleus**. The basal ganglia reconnect to the motor and premotor cortex by way of the ventrolateral and ventral anterior thalamic nuclei. Note that the basal ganglia are involved also in nonmotor aspects of behavior and cognition through a series of reentrant loops with different other parts of the cortical mantle. The medial and rostroventral structures of the basal ganglia and adjacent nuclei constitute a **cortico-ventral basal ganglia loop** serving as a "reward circuit" involved in the motivational and drive-related aspects of action selection.
- The **cerebellum** is involved in the control and coordination of precise timing relationships between activity in different muscles firing within a pattern, whereas the basal ganglia are involved in the more global control of the timing of the pattern as a whole (i.e., its relative expansion or compression in time) and are also involved in strategic learning of the general scheme and structure of a sequential sensorimotor coordination task.
- The **striatum** receives widespread input from all over the cerebral cortex, and the output of the globus pallidus goes (via the above thalamic relay nuclei) to a more limited area of the premotor and supplementary motor cortex. The **striatum** appears to be subdivided into segregated modules, each of which receives input from a different subregion of the cerebral cortex, suggesting a highly modularized system of parallel reentrant loops. The basal ganglia may be viewed as a selective filter for the temporal coordination of competing sensorimotor linkages such that at each moment a single particular sensorimotor linkage is facilitated and selected while all other potential linkages are inhibited in a "winner takes all" competitive interaction.

17. What are the three functional subunits of the cerebellum?

The cerebellum consists of three functional units:

1. **cerebrocerebellum** (the main portion of the cerebellar hemispheres). Input—from the contralateral association cortex via the middle cerebellar peduncle following relay in pontine nuclei. Output—to the contralateral motor cortex, premotor, prefrontal, and parietal cortices via the dentate nucleus, superior cerebellar peduncle, ventrolateral nucleus of the thalamus. **Role—motor programming**.
2. **vestibulocerebellum** (the floculonodular lobe). Input—from somatosensory receptors in the neck, labyrinths (via vestibular nuclei), visual information. Output—to vestibular nuclei. **Role—balance and posture control.**
3. **spinocerebellum** (vermis and pars intermedia). Input—from somatosensory receptors in the moving effector organs via the dorsal spinocerebellar tract, along with auditory, visual, and vestibular information. In addition—information originating in the motor cortex providing the cerebellum with an afferent copy of the intended movement via the ventral spinocerebellar tract. Output—to spinal interneurons via fastigial and interposed nuclei, vestibular nuclei, red nucleus and reticular nuclei, and to the motor cortex via the ventrolateral thalamus. **Role—online correction of spinal motor activity during the "execution" phase,** by comparison of the actual ongoing

movement with information on the intended movement, which produces a corrective output with a modulating influence on the executive activity emanating from primary motor cortex.
- The cerebellum enables the refinement and fine-tuning of the temporal details of motor performance through feedback that dynamically modulates outflows from the motor cortex. This is done by correcting relative deviations detected between the sampled outflow from the motor cortex, which conveys the details of the intended movement, and the kinesthetic somatosensory feedback from the periphery, which conveys the details of the actual movement. The cerebellum is also involved in continuous adjustment and recalibration of sensorimotor linkages to maintain optimal function under transformed sensorimotor circumstances (e.g., when a subject wears reversing or inverting prism glasses).

KEY POINTS: CEREBELLUM AND BASAL GANGLIA

1. Both the cerebellum and the basal ganglia operate through cortically reentrant subcortical loops that begin and end at the cerebral cortex.
2. Outflows from the cerebellum and the basal ganglia are relayed to the cortex through specific relay nuclei in the ventral thalamus.
3. Cerebellar circuitry is set up to make fine-grained timing adjustments in corticospinal outflow to motor neuron pools in the spinal segments.
4. The basal ganglia are more involved in the selection and initiation of motor subroutines and sensorimotor linkages as well as in adjustment of the overall time scale of motor performance.
5. Beside their role in the "program" stage of motor control (i.e., in the stage where learned motor engrams are recruited and activated to serve the motor plan), the basal ganglia and the cerebellum are important in different aspects of motor learning and procedural memory (in a way somewhat similar to the role played by the hippocampus in declarative memory). The cerebellum may serve as a general purpose coprocessor involved in timing, prediction, and learning, spanning all intrinsic aspects of cognition, not only voluntary movement.
6. Cerebellar damage leads typically to manual dysmetria (lack of precision in the spatiotemporal parameters of movement and in force regulation, reflecting failed coordination of agonist, antagonist and synergist muscles involved in the movement), hypotonia, and gait ataxia.
7. Basal ganglia damage may lead to muscular rigidity, tremor, bradykinesia, hypokinesia, amimia, impaired postural reactions, and impaired motor learning.

Bonus questions and answers available online.

RECOMMENDED WEBSITES

The Brain from Top to Bottom. Available at: http://thebrain.mcgill.ca/index.php
Neuroscience Educational Animations. Available at: http://www.sumanasinc.com/webcontent/animations/neurobiology.html
The Mind Project. Available at: http://www.mind.ilstu.edu/curriculum/
Neuroanatomy. Available at: http://www.med.harvard.edu/AANLIB/home.html
Functional Neuroanatomy. Available at: http://fn.med.utoronto.ca/
Open Access Neuroscience e-Textbook. Available at: https://nba.uth.tmc.edu/neuroscience/index.htm

BIBLIOGRAPHY

Neuroscience—From Cellular Level to Functional Systems:
Kandel ER, Koester JD, Mack SH, Siegelbaum SA, eds. *Principles of Neural Science*. 6th ed. New York: McGraw-Hill; 2021.
Purves D, Cabeza R, Huettel SA, et al. *Principles of Cognitive Neuroscience*. 2nd ed. Sunderland: Sinauer; 2013.
Structural and Functional Neuroanatomy:
Brodal P. *The Central Nervous System*. 5th ed. Oxford: Oxford University Press; 2016.
Hendelman WJ. *Atlas of Functional Neuroanatomy*. 3rd ed. Boca Raton, FL: CRC; 2016.
Cognitive and Linguistic Neuroscience:
Gazzaniga MS, Ivry RB, Mangum GR. *Cognitive Neuroscience: The Biology of the Mind*. 5th ed. New York: Norton; 2018.
Kemmerer D. *Cognitive Neuroscience of Language*. Hove: Psychology Press; 2015.
Clinical Manifestations of Damage to Functional Systems of the Brain:
Andrewes D. *Neuropsychology—From Theory to Practice*. 2nd ed. Abingdon: Routledge; 2016.
Krakauer JW, Carmichael ST. *Broken Movement—The Neurobiology of Motor Recovery after Stroke*. Cambridge, MA: MIT Press; 2017.

CHAPTER 6

EDUCATING LEARNERS IN PM&R: THE VALUE OF LONGITUDINAL LEARNING

Sam S. H. Wu, MD, MA, MPH, MBA, Bryan J. O'Young, MD, CAc, FAAPMR, Steven A. Stiens, MD, MS, Mark A. Young, MD, MBA, FACP, FAAPMR, DABPMR

Live as if you were to die tomorrow. Learn as if you were to live forever.

Mahatma Gandhi (1869–1948)

KEY POINTS

1. PM&R learning is a lifelong cumulative process focused on knowledge attainment through book study, clinical experience, formal didactics (lectures, podcasts, videos, websites, and internet resources), literature analysis, and other multi-media resources.
2. Longitudinal learning (LL) is a model of education that seeks to promote better development of essential skills among medical trainees. This educational paradigm brings physicians and patients together often in their natural environment-the medical clinic visit. These clinical encounters are often multiple and spaced out over time and offer the trainee a privileged opportunity to learn.
3. Longitudinal clinical observation and monitoring of a disease process and its impact on function, physical and behavioral well-being (through a portion of a patient's lifetime) offers learners a vital educational "lens."
4. An idealized example of LL through the care continuum is a medical student or resident monitoring a person with a cerebrovascular accident (CVA) from the early acute (neuro-intensive acute care stage) throughout the subsequent rehabilitation journey. This process may include multiple phases including acute inpatient rehabilitation, outpatient stage, community integration, vocational rehabilitation, and employment.

1. What is learning?

   Learning is defined as "acquiring knowledge or skills through experience, study or being taught." Within the physical medicine and rehabilitation (PM&R) educational world, learning frequently takes place in a multidisciplinary milieu and often includes a matrix of clinicians, administrators, support staff, students, and patients.

2. Who are learners?

   According to a famous Chinese proverb: *"Learning is a treasure that will follow the owner everywhere."* So too, learners in physiatry are dedicated lifelong students who seek to master a subject or skill over time and in many different settings. Learning of medical and rehabilitation principles is a journey that starts in medical school and advances to internship, residency, and for some, fellowship. Learners transition from "learning to earning" once they take their first job. Once employed, learners never stop learning but continue to participate in continuing medical education (CME) and courses.

3. What is longitudinal learning?

   Longitudinal learning (LL) is a model of education that seeks to promote better development of essential skills among medical trainees. In contrast to the traditional classroom, lecture-based learning, LL strives to combine elements of textbook learning, classroom knowledge, and clinical experiential training. Didactic value is optimized by simulating the actual practice of medicine through student-resident patient interactions in a clinical setting.

Ellaway R, Graves L, Berry S, Myhre D, Cummings B, Konkin J. Twelve tips for designing and running longitudinal integrated clerkships. *Med Teach.* 2013 Dec;35(12):989–995. Available at: https://www.ncbi.nlm.nih.gov/pmc/articles/PMC3836395/

4. Is longitudinal learning impactful?

Medical Students certainly think so and they have reported that LL creates a dynamic integrated environment, provides a broader understanding of all aspects of illness, offers a deeper relationship with patients, transforms student physician's roles, reveals systems-based practice, and inspires commitment, advocacy, and idealism.

Ogur B, Hirsh D. Learning through longitudinal patient care-narratives from the Harvard Medical School-Cambridge Integrated Clerkship. *Acad Med.* 2009;84(7):844–850. doi: 10.1097/ACM.0b013e3181a85793. Available at: https://journals.lww.com/academicmedicine/Fulltext/2009/07000/Learning_Through_Longitudinal_Patient.11.aspx

Hemmer P. Longitudinal, integrated clerkship education: is different better? *Acad Med.* 2009;84(7):822. doi: 10.1097/ACM.0b013e3181a843b1. Available at: https://journals.lww.com/academicmedicine/Fulltext/2009/07000/Longitudinal,_Integrated_Clerkship_Education__Is.6.aspx

5. How is longitudinal learning different from traditional learning methods in clinical settings?

Traditional clinical medical education utilizes a sequential "block rotation" structure that places students in a specific specialty setting. This approach can have significant limitations, including a lack of continuity of care and learning (especially on an inpatient rotation) due to the acuity of patients and the frequent tendency of transfer between care settings. This inevitably impedes students' capacity to longitudinally follow illness episodes and gain exposure to outpatient continuity of care. The limited participatory roles of students and haphazard and random sequence of rotations can lead to incomplete clinical and educational skill development.

Poncelet AN, Hauer KE, O'Brien B. The longitudinal integrated clerkship. *Virtual Mentor: AMA J Ethics.* 2009 November;11(11): 864–869.

In contrast to "block learning," a longitudinal medical education experience emphasizes continuity during the clinical years. LL encourages medical students and other learners to engage in the comprehensive and ongoing management of patients over time. This helps bolster relationships between students and attending clinicians and satisfying key core clinical competencies in multiple disciplines and specialties. Additionally, LL can take place in various educational and clinical settings, including academic centers, community hospitals, primary care practices, specialty care, and rural centers.

Mylopoulos M, Kulasegaram KM, Weyman K, Bernstein S, Martimianakis MAT. Same but different: exploring mechanisms of learning in a longitudinal integrated clerkship. *Acad Med.* 2020;95(3):411–416. doi: 10.1097/ACM.0000000000002960. Available at: https://journals.lww.com/academicmedicine/Fulltext/2020/03000/Same_but_Different__Exploring_Mechanisms_of.32.aspx

6. What simple interventions can make conventional PM&R rotations, services, and clinics more longitudinal in experience for learners and patients?

Trainees may be assigned to **evaluate patients at the point of entry** into the PM&R continuum. Often this initial encounter can be accomplished through phone, clinic, consult or telemedicine visit. Trainees commonly **follow those patients through the process** of care in a variety of settings including: emergency medicine unit, acute medical inpatient unit, acute inpatient rehabilitation unit, home visits and outpatient clinic visits and vocational rehabilitation milieu. Assessment of readiness for discharge and person-centered outpatient care designs can be fashioned based on multiple factors. **Outings with recreation therapy** to accomplish community reintegration and home visits to assess accessibility and the need for adaptations help to optimize outcome. Learners can perform **telemedicine visits after discharge** to reevaluate treatment plans, utilization of resources, medications, equipment, and quality of life. Students can see patients at **outpatient education events** or volunteer with **adaptive recreation** in the community. The advent and maturation of telemedicine and physician-based social media platforms such as Doximity and Doximity-Dialer have streamlined learner-patient telemedicine interactions and physician to physician electronic consultation methodology.

7. What role does the vocational rehabilitation center play in the longitudinal learning process and the education of PM&R students and residents?

The vocational rehabilitation center is an ideal environment for students and residents to observe the culmination of the LL process for many persons with disabilities who have previously participated in the rehabilitation acute process. The personal satisfaction and gratification attained by the trainee in observing a person return to work and achieve career goals after a CVA or SCI can help to complete the rehabilitation. The relationship between vocational rehabilitation and personhood as it relates to the physiatrists' role is explored in a later chapter of this book.

Reference: PM&R SECRETS 4th edition, Chapter 81 *Vocational Rehabilitation and Personhood: A Physiatrist's Vital Calling*

Young MA, Stiens SA, Carson B Ankam NS, Bosques G, Sauter C, Stiens S, Therattil M, Williams FH, Atkins CC, Mayer RS. Competency-based curriculum development to meet the needs of people with disabilities: a call to action. *Acad Med.* 2019 June;94(6):781–788. Available at: https://pubmed.ncbi.nlm.nih.gov/30844926

8. Can longitudinal learning develop and sustain the active competency of PM&R clinicians?
   Evidence-Based Medicine (EBM) can be challenging for PM&R, where there is often a dearth of outcome research data. Learning is facilitated by using the **5 As of EBM**: ask, acquire, appraise, apply, and assess. A longitudinal blended learning EBM curriculum was designed for PM&R residents (R2-4) with a journal club spanned over months. Residents drove the process from patient care generated clinical questions presented using the **PICOTT format** (patient, intervention, comparison, outcome, type of question, type of study). Continuity was accomplished with reports of patient management, and progress and perspectives were provided by senior residents and faculty relating outcomes of similar case examples. Connecting current patient problems with the choice of evidence-based interventions resulted in a prospective increase in residents' diagnoses and interventions using EBM with future patients.

   Recently, the American Board of Physical Medicine and Rehabilitation has replaced the maintenance of certification examination with the longitudinal assessment program for physical medicine and rehabilitation (LA-PM&R). Preliminary evaluation suggests the program leads to better learning and retention of information than the 10-year maintenance of certification examination.

Yoon S, Kim M, Tarver C, Loo LK. "ACEing" the evidence within physical medicine and rehabilitation (PM&R). *J Teach Open Resour.* OPEN ACCESS December 11, 2020. Available at: https://www.mededportal.org/doi/10.15766/mep_2374-8265.11051

Yoon SH, Kim M, Tarver C, Loo LK. "ACEing" the evidence within physical medicine and rehabilitation (PM&R). *MedEdPORTAL.* 2020 Dec 11;16:11051. doi: 10/15766/mep_2374-8265.11051. AAMC, MedPortal

Robinson LR, Raddatz MM, Kinney CL. Evaluation of longitudinal assessment for use in maintenance of certification. *Am J Phys Med Rehabil.* 2020;99(5):420–423.

9. What is a "learning organization?" How can systems of learning and care delivery curate knowledge and experience to provide an enriched environment for pathways through longitudinal learning?
   PM&R is a medical specialty that requires active patient participation throughout the rehabilitation process, creating a variety of learning methods for patients, staff, and trainees. The concepts of the learning organization were founded on the **process of continuous improvement** programs and can be simply described as places where people continuously expand their capacity to create results. To achieve this for everyone requires skilled faculty adept at creating, acquiring, and transferring knowledge. Longitudinal learners must apply variants of the **PDCA Cycle** (Plan, Do Check, Act) to address recognized problems and seek solutions. The environment must therefore be enriched with access to procedures, policies, medical literature, and faculty discourse to catalyze the patient service and learning process. Knowledge management is, therefore, imperative for the learner and institutional leaders that appraise intellectual capital, organizational competencies, and all the concurrent learning pathways. The translated outcome is **knowledge,** a context-specific combination of experience, interpretation, and reflection that contributes to action upon problem recognition.

Basten D, Haamann T. Approaches for organizational learning: a literature review. AGE Open. 2018; July–September:1–20. Available at: https://journals.sagepub.com/doi/pdf/10.1177/2158244018794224

Evans JM, Brown A, Baker RG. Organizational knowledge and capabilities in healthcare: Deconstructing and integrating diverse perspectives. *SAGE Open Med* 5:1–10. Available at: https://journals.sagepub.com/doi/pdf/10.1177/2050312117712655

10. What is the ACGME position on lifelong learning?
    The Accreditation Council for Graduate Medical Education (ACGME) Program Requirements for Graduate Medical Education in PM&R indicates that "Graduate medical education occurs in clinical settings that establish the foundation for practice-based and lifelong learning. The professional development of the physician begins in medical school and continues through faculty modeling of the effacement of self-interest in a humanistic environment that emphasizes joy in curiosity, problem-solving, academic rigor, and discovery. This transformation is often physically, emotionally, and intellectually demanding and occurs in a variety of clinical learning environments committed to graduate medical education and the well-being of patients, residents, fellows, faculty members, students, and all members of the health care team." In addition, "Longitudinal experiences, such as continuity clinic in the context of other clinical responsibilities, must be evaluated at least every 3 months and at completion."

ACGME. Available at: https://www.acgme.org/.

Norris TE, Schaad DC, DeWitt D, Ogur B, Hunt DD; Consortium of Longitudinal Integrated Clerkships. Longitudinal integrated clerkships for medical students: an innovation adopted by medical schools in Australia, Canada, South Africa, and the United States. *Acad Med.* 2009;84(7):902–907.

BIBLIOGRAPHY

Bartlett M, Couper I, Poncelet A, Worley P. The do's, don'ts and don't knows of establishing a sustainable longitudinal integrated clerkship. *Perspect Med Educ.* 2020;9:5–19. Available at: s40037-019-00558-z.pdf (springer.com)

Poncelet A, Hirsh D. *Longitudinal Integrated Clerkships: Principles, Outcomes, Practical Tools, and Future Directions.* Omaha, NE: Alliance for Clinical Education, 2016:326. Available at: https://www.amazon.com/s?i=stripbooks&rh=p_27%3AAlliance+for+Clinical+Education&s=relevancerank&text=Alliance+for+Clinical+Education&ref=dp_byline_sr_book_1

Stiens S, Berkin D. A clinical rehabilitation course for college undergraduates provides an introduction to biopsychosocial interventions that minimize disablement. *Am J Phys Med Rehabil.* 1997;76(6):462–470. doi: 10.1097/00002060-199711000-00006

COMMUNICATION STRATEGIES FOR REHABILITATION PROFESSIONALS: EMPOWERMENT MEDICINE CATALYZES PERSONAL POTENTIAL ACTUALIZATION

Steven A. Stiens, MD, MS, Steven E. Brown, PhD, Margaret A. Nosek, PhD, and Margaret Grace Stineman, MD

We reject the notion that we need "experts" to tell us how to live, especially experts from the able-bodied world. We are not diagnoses in need of a cure or cases to be closed. We are human, with human dreams and ambitions.
—John R Woodward, MSW, A Disabled Manifesto

KEY POINTS: COMMUNICATION STRATEGIES

1. The lived disability experience of each person is a unique resource for that person and a critical perspective to share as a clinician designing a treatment program.
2. Communication is an exercise of the therapeutic encounter process and results in mutually determined and attainable goals.
3. Empowerment medicine is the method for recognizing a patient's personhood and realizing the full expression of their capabilities and life roles as advocates.
4. The independent living movement defined and manifested the rights of all to live in the least restrictive settings possible.
5. Empowerment medicine utilizes the therapeutic relationship to reestablish patients' self-concept, self-determination, self-actualization, life-roles, and unique contributions to society.

1. Imagine yourself recognizing a person with a disability. As you approach, you wonder, "Can disability etiquette help with this conversation?"
   Disability etiquette puts the humanity of the person first and any disabilities second. People with disabilities have the same needs for respect, dignity, and autonomy as anyone else. In the ***patient-clinician encounter***, a variety of emotional reactions may occur based on similarities of the people or situations of the past. ***Transference*** is the unconscious tendency of a patient to assign emotion expectations from prior experiences to a person in their current environment. ***Countertransference*** is the reaction of the treating clinician to the patient based on past experiences and emotional needs. Clinicians must be constantly aware of these inevitable reactions, and recognize situations that can limit or distract from the successful process of rehabilitation.

Tips on Interacting with People with Disabilities. Available at: https://www.nfc.usda.gov/AdditionalResources/Civil_Rights/interaction.php

Cohen J. *Disability Etiquette.* Jackson Heights, NY: Eastern Paralyzed Veterans Association; 1998. Available at: https://www.youtube.com/watch?v=W6c6JLbczC8 (*How to Treat a Person with Disabilities, According to People with Disabilities*)

Ozmen M. Transference and countertransference in medically ill patients. *Turk Psikiyatri Derg.* 2007;18(1):1–7.

Freeman AG. Looking through the mirror of disability: transference and countertransference issues with therapists who are disabled. *Women Ther.* 1994;14(3–4):79–90. doi:10.1300/ J015v14n03_09

2. What is "the shock response"? How can the health professional guard against this normal response to unexpected or unusual pathology?
   The ***shock response*** occurs when the professional is distracted by the most visible or unusual aspects of the patient's history, physical presentation, job, or life-role. This can eclipse recognition of more important symptoms,

signs, and other positive and unique patient attributes in a way that may influence treatment and patient-centered outcomes. If the patient brings up the characteristic in question, frankly ask about the patient's experience, opinions, and methods for management. Then address the characteristic as it relates to achievement of the patient's goals. The best ways to avoid the shock response are to desensitize yourself, and explore and understand all aspects of each person. Evaluate the person's presentation of self and, most importantly, formulate pathways to the potential you can help them achieve.

The power of the patient voice: how health care organizations empower patients and improve care delivery. Available at: https://cssjs.nejm.org/landing-page/cj-ebook-2021/The-Power-of-the-Patient-Voice.pdf

3. **Is it normal to have emotional responses to (or feel uncomfortable around) people with some types of impairments or problems? How can you use humor effectively to relieve stress and build empathy?**
   First, acknowledge that these feelings may exist. Then recognize, specify, and analyze them from your perspective. By confronting and analyzing such feelings directly, rehabilitation professionals will be better able to manage them productively. It is important for all clinicians to have close friendships with a few peers with and without disabilities in order to confidentially review and process such responses. Such review can result in enhanced capacity for observation, empathy, and creative innovation for solutions. The context of the situation dictates the demand for active listening, providing a permissive response to patients' levity.

Bennet HJ. Humor in medicine. *South Med J.* 2003;96(12):1257–1261. doi:10.1097/01. SMJ. 0000066657.70073.14.

Gallows humour by BMJ Talk Medicine (Available at: soundcloud.com)

4. **How do you use person-first and identity-first language?**
   Language and the images it promotes mirror attitudes toward particular groups of people. When communicating with or about people with disabilities, some (but not all) of those with disabilities argue that it is essential to use ***person-first language*** **(PFL)** (Table 7.1), and avoid focusing on the disability before recognizing the person. Saying, "person with a disability" or "person who uses a wheelchair" recontextualizes the relationship rather than defining the person with these characteristics. Also, avoid using "normal" as the opposite of disabled, suggesting a dichotomous separation rather than a spectrum of function. "Normal" implies that people with disabilities are not normal. Use "nondisabled" or "persons without disabilities."

Table 7.1 Person-First Terminology

POOR TERM	BETTER TERM	EXPLANATION
Cerebral-palsied	Has cerebral palsy	Use person-first, non-emotional language that describes the condition.
Cripple, invalid	Has a disability	"Invalid" implies not acceptable
Paralytic, weakling	Has paralysis or is paralyzed	Individual impairments do not determine personal effectiveness.
Hunchback	Person with spinal curvature	Do not identify the person with deformity.
Wheelchair bound/confined	Uses a wheelchair	Wheelchairs are liberating to people with severe walking impairments
Home bound/confined	Is limited by barriers outside the home	People are not tied to the device. Homes should be places of refuge and hopefully comfort
Physically challenged	Has activity limitation	Implies unmet challenge
Afflicted/victim	Simply state that the person has a particular condition.	The terms *disabled* and *handicapped* are still accepted by many but are being replaced by terms that are more neutral.
Normal or healthy	People without disabilities or nondisabled	Avoid "tragic;" but "brave" and "courageous" stereotypes. Emphasize abilities, but do not describe successful people with disabilities as "superhuman" Avoid terms that imply serious misfortune and emotional disability.

An important contingent of people with disabilities prefers to use ***identity first language*** (IFL). An example is "disabled person." They claim disability permeates their entire being and since it is their dominant characteristic and a source of pride, it should be mentioned first.

Young MA, Morgan SB. Strategies for fostering communication between physician and patients with disabilities. *Wis Med J.* 1997;96: 36–37..

Ladau E. *Why Person-First Language Doesn't Always Put the Person First* (blog post). Available at: https://www.thinkinclusive.us/why-person-first-language-doesnt-always-put-the-person-first/

5. **What pitfalls need to be avoided when conceptualizing about and communicating with people with disabilities?**
   Carefully examine your mindset as you analyze situations. ***Ableism*** embraces ability preferences that inaugurate the norm. ***Disablism*** is a set of assumptions (conscious or unconscious) and practices that promote the differential or unequal treatment of people because of actual or presumed disabilities. The difference is that *disablism* discriminates against disabled people while *ableism* does so in favor of nondisabled people. Do not assume anything based on your experience alone. Use active listening techniques to develop an understanding of how each patient experiences disability and how and why they choose to adapt. Pave and celebrate many pathways to individual and community success.

Storey K. Combating ableism in schools: preventing school failure. *Alternative Education for Children and Youth*, 2010;52: 56–58. Combating Ableism in Schools. Available at: http://www.nln.org/docs/default-source/professional-development-programs/ace-series/gettting-started-communication-with-pwd.pdf?sfvrsn58

Smeltzer SC, Mariani B, Meakim C. *Communicating With People With Disabilities.* National League of Nursing; 2017. Available at: http://www.nln.org/docs/default-source/professional-development-programs/ace-series/disability-overview.pdf?sfvrsn=6

6. **Why do some people with disabilities object to being called "patients"? Is there any escape from being a perpetual patient for any of us?**
   For some, the designation of "patient" may imply ongoing sickness requiring perpetual treatment in spite of their stable impairments and overall health. For others, it may indicate a lack of awareness that patients have a life beyond the medical or clinical encounter. For example, despite extreme illness, they may sustain immediate productivity and creative inventions utilizing contemporary platforms and direct communication with collaborators. These persons might object to being addressed solely as a patient when that is not their only life-role.
   In response to these objections, some health care systems have chosen the terms "person served," "consumer," or "client" but still reinforce their participation as the prime beneficiary of services. It is therefore inappropriate to refer to healthy people living with fixed impairments that are not under current treatment as "patients."
   Clinicians need to be particularly receptive to the personal presentation of each person they serve, and avoid emphasizing only the medical aspects of encounters. Contemporary technology permits a variety of creative ways for persons to interface with others that might celebrate otherwise eclipsed attributes. For example, a ***cyborg*** is a hybrid entity that has both biological and robotic components enabling presence, appearance, and voice that reflect intention but transcend the impairments.

Episode 66: *Cyborgs: Disability Visibility Project.* Available at: https://disabilityvisibilityproject.com/2019/12/18/ep-66-cyborgs/

Disabled or cyborg? How bionics affect stereotypes toward people with physical disabilities. Available at: https://www.frontiersin.org/articles/10.3389/fpsyg.2018.02251/full#:,:text=We%20argue%20that%20the%20increasing,and%20popular%20culture%20is%20typically

7. **How can we connect with patients by circumnavigating our various habits and limitations?**
   Mobility impairments make good examples. People who use wheelchairs live well below the eye level of standing adults. Even positioned in full view of others, those with disabilities are commonly ignored. Communication is facilitated by recognizing the person and getting to eye level. **Sitting down** goes a long way in establishing contact. Both the patient and clinicians should feel comfortable and respect each other's personal space. Proximity communicates the alliance for understanding but must be exercised with respect for personal space. People without disabilities need to be conscious of their gait speed while accompanying a person using crutches or a manual wheelchair. When walking with someone using a device for assisting ambulation, allow them space, and let them set the pace. Use eye contact from the side, and invite them to sit with you and talk. For those in a wheelchair or bed, sit or kneel on one knee beside them. If the conversation lasts for longer than a few minutes, find some place to sit so they know you are comfortable.

Iezzoni LI. What should I say? Communication around disability. *Ann Intern Med.* 1998;129:661–665.

8. How do you communicate effectively with people who have severe speech or hearing impairments?

The key is planning and patience. When encountering a patient who has difficulty speaking, the tendency for some physicians is to listen until their patience runs out, then look for help to the person who accompanies the patient, or look away. A better approach would be to repeat what you understand back to the patient for validation. If you have misunderstood, ask them to say it again until you are truly communicating. If you are unable to do this, ask the patient's permission to communicate with the person who accompanies them, or ask one of your staff for assistance. Your primary concern is to maintain the dignity of the patient, and value effective, direct communication. Hearing impairments can be addressed by using the dictation-to-text feature on a smartphone to provide the patient with the option to read.

For patients who prefer to communicate through a certified interpreter, plans should be made in advance. Advise appointment staff or the ward clerk to screen patients for that need. They may bring along an interpreter of their choice, or ask that the physician's office provide one from a local agency.

AAC for ICU. University of Nebraska. *Lincoln Department of Special Education & Communication Disorders.* 2020. Available at: https://cehs.unl.edu/aac/aac-icu-0/

Patak L, Wilson-Stronks A, Costello J, et al. Improving patient-provider communication: a call to action. *J Nurs Adm.* 2009;39(9): 372–376. Available at: https://www.ncbi.nlm.nih.gov/pmc/articles/PMC2904301/

9. What communication methods help in caring for patients with memory and orientation impairments?

The goal is a prosthetic design to supplement function to meet goals of patient awareness of deficits and independent compensation. Collaboration with speech therapy to design a ***memory book*** with ***photos*** documenting significant others and important events in rehabilitation is helpful for remembering and reminiscence. Use of a ***communication log*** where staff, family, and visitors make dated and timed written, drawn, or photographic entries summarizing conversations helps the patient and the interdisciplinary team interact about past, current, and upcoming events.

10. What are inappropriate responses and turn-offs?

The first step in an effective ***therapeutic interaction requires suspension of judgment*** in order to present positive regard and active listening to understand the patient as a person. Creative skill and experience is required to extrapolate their potential with rehabilitation and educational intervention. When the clinician judges (prejudges) the patient through the misuse or misperception of some bit of history or medical information, it can become a barrier that blocks patient self-actualization. Responding with opinions, invalidating statements, or nonspecific medical knowledge used in ways that are insensitive, distorted, or fail to address the full circumstances of the patient's life are inappropriate. The "turn-off" occurs after the physician has alienated or embarrassed the patient in some way. This disengages the process and detracts from patient cooperation and synergistic team collaboration.

Shenk CE, Fruzzetti AE. The impact of validating and invalidating responses on emotional reactivity. *J Soc Clin Psychol.* 2010;30(2):163–183.

11. Give an example of an inappropriate response

Patient "tune out" or "turn off" occurs when the physician fails in openly eliciting the patient's perspective, needs, and intent. It may also occur if a physician misunderstands, discounts, or patronizes patients. These kinds of responses or observations might lead a patient to have nagging and inappropriate self-doubts that are injurious and prevent progress.

Edlund SM, Wurm M, Hollandare F, et al. Pain patients' experiences of validation and invalidation from physicians before and after multimodal pain rehabilitation: Associations with pain, negative affectivity, and treatment outcome. *Scan J Pain.* 2017;17(1): 77–86.

12. How can inappropriate responses be avoided?

Use medical knowledge to positively support and empower the patient. Use an exploratory approach. For example, "I understand you would like to become pregnant. Let's talk about the pros and cons for you, and how your disability might play a role." This requires active listening, self-monitoring, and visionary outcomes. The ability to see beyond the medical aspects to the humanity and potential of the person is derived from experience and essential for advanced rehabilitation program design and direction. It is essential to recognize with sensitivity aspirations as well as defenses constructed by the patient. Avoid conflicts that pit medical knowledge against the patient's knowledge of her- or himself. Again, see the person as more than the processes of his or her diseases and disabilities by projecting developmental imperatives and expressed goals into rehabilitation design. Remember that the experience of disability is not the same as being sick, suffering symptoms, or living through a finite illness.

Linton SJ, Fink IK, Nilsson E, Edlund S. Can training in empathetic validation improve medical students' communication with patients suffering pain? A test of concept. *Pain Rep.* 2017;2(3):1–5.

13. What are masked concerns in communication?

Masked concerns occur when the patient describes one symptom, feeling, or condition that is related to, but does not represent their primary complaint. Sometimes patients raise issues explicitly but have hidden or masked concerns. Discussing difficulty getting out of the house for social occasions or excessive fatigue is an explicit, seemingly clear issue. However, digging deeper, the professional might find that the patient fears falling (because of weakness), is limited in ambulatory endurance by severe arthritis pain, or will not leave for fear of incontinence or another reason that may not be obvious to the physician—and possibly even to the patient. This is why digging deeper is crucial.

Active Listening – National Disability Services. Available at: https://www.nds.org.au/images/resources/person-centred/Active-listening.pdf

14. How does communication accomplish the best outcome?

Speaking directly to the patient rather than through family or companions is an affirmation. It is essential to hear and formulate an understanding of each patient as a person. This evolving person-first approach must be celebrated by the entire rehabilitation team. Establishing an optimal patient-clinician relationship requires interest and sensitivity. Active listening and perceptive questioning lead to positive patient encounters. Each person has a unique perspective and experience of their own disability (disablement); understanding that perspective is essential for collaborative rehabilitation processes. Maximal success is accomplished by designing a rehabilitation plan that leads to functional, psychological, and social recovery in a sequence that empowers the patient to be interdependent in accomplishing broader life goals.

Some unique experiences of life with disability can result in creative solutions that escape the attention of people who are nondisabled. Yet many people have difficulty living independently in a society designed for those with average capacity. Nevertheless, regarding disability as an *experience* rather than a source of pathology can provide a different perspective that is enriching and can lead to innovation. When a physician acknowledges these creative responses, the therapeutic bond is stronger, giving the physician an opportunity to learn and grow with the patient.

Challenging behaviour and learning disabilities: independent living (YouTube) Available at: https://www.youtube.com/watch?v=9YrXmG6qO9E

Cohn KH. Developing effective communication skills. *J Oncol Pract.* 2007;3(6):314–317.doi: 10.1200/JOP.0766501. Available at: https://www.ncbi.nlm.nih.gov/pmc/articles/PMC2793758/

National League for Nursing. *Communicating With People With Disabilities* (Advancing Care Excellence for Persons with Disabilities Professional Development Programs). Available at: http://www.nln.org/ professional-development-programs/teaching-resources/ace-d/additional-resources/communicating-with-people-with-disabilities (for healthcare providers)

University of New Hampshire. Responsive practice: accessible & adaptive communication, Available at: https://unh.az1.qualtrics.com/jfe/form/SV_3I8BLOm7U1COj5z Video Training (0.5 CME credits)

15. What are some special issues with regard to communicating with people with life-long disabilities?

Recognize and respect the lessons of long life experience. People are the experts on their own unique personal histories, goals, and lifestyle. Make them your teachers. Recognize and express your appreciation for and interest in the way they solve problems and how and why they have adapted physically, productively, and interpersonally. Ask them to teach you how they decided on various adaptive equipment and techniques. People with life-long disabilities usually incorporate their disability and functional solutions into their self-concept. They have the benefit of time to accommodate and present themselves as they integrate with society. Yet they remain at a potential disadvantage in communicating with others who have had the experiences that people without disabilities share.

Different and able: Empowering people with differences. A support and resource platform. Available at: https://differentandable.org/

Examining sexuality for people with disabilities (YouTube). Available at: https://youtu.be/FxMjhYo4oKA

16. **What are some special issues in communicating with a person who becomes disabled later in life?**
People with disabilities are a minority that anyone can join at any time. Fortunately, people who become disabled later in life have the benefit of knowing how society works and have had the opportunity to develop their social skillsets as nondisabled people. Yet it can also be a burden to remember what it was like to live without disability. The process of facing and living with the real and often extreme changes in their lives can be overwhelming or depressing. The health professional, through their communications with the individual, has the opportunity to lead them toward self-determination and away from potentially self-destructive feelings. Frame these challenges positively, and facilitate successful adaptation and life-role performance.

17. **You believe a person with physical disabilities may need help getting into your office, undressing, or getting onto your examination table. What should you do?**
Put the individual in charge, assuming their strengths. Never assume that a person needs help just because he or she has some visible physical limitations. ***Ask the patient: "How can I be of assistance."*** Respect the person's answers and thank them for what you learn. Unless the circumstance clearly warrants quick action to avoid injury, do not provide physical assistance unexpectedly to a person who is already walking or standing. The first steps are to provide an accessible environment and the helping resources needed to overcome any barriers. All clinicians have the obligation to offer their services as part of environments that are fully accessible and accommodate the needs of people with disabilities.

Agaronnik N, Campbell EG, Ressalam J, & Iezzoni LI. Accessibility of medical diagnostic equipment for patients with disability: observations from physicians. *Arch Phys Med Rehabil.* 2019;100(11): 2032–2038. doi:10.1016/j.apmr.2019.02.007 Available at: https://www.ncbi.nlm.nih.gov/pmc/articles/PMC6761045/pdf/nihms-1525342.pdf

18. **What are some common Issues and pitfalls examining people with disabilities?**
Doing an examination while a patient remains in a wheelchair can lead to suboptimal pulmonary, abdominal, musculoskeletal, and neurological assessments compared to a person who is disrobed on an examining table. An appropriately equipped office with trained personnel can communicate an accessible invitation to the patient for inclusion in the process of medical care. Determining the degree to which the person is able to stand, walk, and move around on the examination table is an essential part of the functional examination. If the patient has serious mobility difficulties, take appropriate safety precautions. Ask the patient whether they can stand and transfer onto the examination table. Ask patients to explain how difficult it is, how they do it, and how they direct the assistance of others. This communication ahead of time will help plan transfers and avoid unsafe situations. It is also a good way to assess and learn from the patient's insight, safety awareness, and resourcefulness.

19. **What is the "lump syndrome"?**
In hospitals, medical equipment, food or laundry carts, and people sitting in wheelchairs or lying on gurneys are all hauled about and can be left parked in corridors indiscriminately, like "heaps" or "lumps." Patients embody the purpose of the institution and deserve recognition and control. Never begin pushing patients in wheelchairs or on gurneys without greeting them and saying where you propose to take them, and ask if they need assistance. Never leave a patient without an explanation. State where they are, and why you are parking them there. Introduce them to someone in that environment, a receptionist or a nurse, to announce their presence. Thoughtful gestures take little time but are tremendous opportunities to recognize and greet patients as people outside of medical rituals, provide service they direct, and show genuine interest in them through action and conversation. For example, "Would it be okay to leave you here in the waiting room until transportation meets you? This is Wilma, the receptionist. She can call if they need a reminder," or "Would you like a magazine to read?" Remember people with mobility limitations. Effective and thoughtful positioning and communication prevent the lump syndrome.

20. **What are some possible biasing effects of medical training?**
Pathology-focused training tends to encourage clinicians to see cure as success and chronic disease and progressive disability as failure. Practitioners often focus on pathology and are inattentive to the patient's function and strengths. A functional review of systems provides patients with excellent opportunities to discuss concerns about their disabilities and a context for the personal impact, as well as explain their adaptive capabilities and plans. It should include mobility activities of daily living (ADLs), instrumental activities of daily living (IADLs), mobility and environmental barriers, and facilitators.
Another serious bias in medical training is the ***default-to-male tendency***. By omitting known gender differences in presenting symptoms and responses to treatment, educators are setting up their students for potentially lethal errors. Cardiology is a classic case in point: Women die when physicians persist in acknowledging only male characteristic symptoms of myocardial infarction, ignoring female characteristic symptoms, such as jaw, neck, and back pain. Similarly, in rehabilitation medicine, especially when treating disorders that occur more frequently in men (e.g., spinal cord injury, traumatic brain injury), specific concerns of women are underrepresented in curricula. As a result, physicians examining recurrent urinary tract infections almost never ask

women about their pregnancy history. The same is true even when treating disorders that occur more often in women (multiple sclerosis, stroke, arthritis, and other autoimmune diseases). Women with disabilities need to be sought out as part of the curriculum.

Ankam NS, Bosques G, Sauter C, Stiens S, et al. Competency-based curriculum development to meet the needs of people with disabilities: a call to action. *Acad Med.* 2019;94(6):781–788. Available at: https://pubmed.ncbi.nlm.nih.gov/30844926/

21. What is the independent living movement?

The disability rights and independent living movements of the 1960s and 1970s, both worldwide movements, led to major changes in the way people with disabilities were viewed, educated, respected, and appreciated. These movements were the result of those with disabilities wanting access and full participation in society. They challenged (and still challenge) health care providers to reevaluate how they perceive, understand, and serve patients. The dignity of those with disabilities must be honored at all times, and they must be integrated into society as self-determining contributors.

The **Americans with Disabilities Act of 1990** (ADA) recognized that people with disabilities have the right to pursue and participate in socially meaningful activities, including their own medical care. Ideas embodied within the movement declare that people with disabilities have the right to live in the least restrictive setting possible of their choice. For hundreds of years, many individuals with disabilities of all kinds were placed in institutions. These institutions often became notorious for the mistreatment of their residents.

One of the most-publicized cases was Willowbrook in New York, which became national news in the United States in the 1960s and 1970s with the publication of Blatt and Kaplan's *Christmas in Purgatory: A Photographic Essay on Mental Retardation* (1966). This book led to the closing of Willowbrook in 1987. In 1999, the US Supreme Court affirmed in the landmark case of *Olmstead v. L.C.* (now known as the "Olmstead Decision") the position of the independent living movement: Life in a community is preferable to institutionalization. The Court found that the unjustified segregation of people with disabilities is a form of unlawful discrimination under the ADA. The independent living movement and federally funded independent living centers celebrate the dignity and individuality of each person with a disability as a self-determining contributor integrated into society, which includes their being a relevant participant in their own medical care.

Blatt B, Kaplan F. *Christmas in Purgatory: A Photographic Essay on Mental Retardation.* Boston: Allyn and Bacon; 1966.

Health and Human Services. *Serving People With Disabilities in the Integrated Setting: Community Living and Olmstead.* 2018. Available at: https://www.hhs.gov/civil-rights/for-individuals/special-topics/community-living-and-olmstead/index.html

Ratzka A. *What is independent living?* 2005. Available at: https://www.independentliving.org/ indexen.html

22. What terminology is recommended when writing about people with disabilities?

Many people now object to putting person first language first. I think we should not eliminate it but should be aware that it is no longer standard.

Use person-first language in descriptions, and avoid categories such as "autistics." Use "person living with HIV," "person who is blind," or "person who uses a wheelchair." The term "nondisabled" is most appropriate for those without disabilities. Less appropriate are "normal," "able-bodied" and "temporarily able-bodied," "healthy," or "whole." Portrayals of people with disabilities should emphasize their capabilities.

- The Life Span Institute guidelines *Reporting and Writing about People with Disabilities* recommend avoiding terminology that is not person-first:
- Do not focus on disability to the exclusion of the person's capabilities.
- The term "wheelchair-bound" does not portray the mobility-enhancing effect of that adaptive tool.
- Do not portray successful people with disabilities as superheroes or necessarily extraordinary. Do not sensationalize disability by referring to the person as "afflicted with," "crippled with," "victim of," or "suffers from" an illness or diagnosis.
- Do not use euphemisms such as "physically inconvenienced" or "physically challenged."
- Do not use generic labels that generalize about groups such as the deaf.
- The term "retarded" is derogatory and misrepresents the multiple causes for "intellectual disability."
- Do not imply active disease processes when they are not present.
- If persons live with chronic impairments that are not under treatment, the word *patient* is inappropriate.

Ferrigon P. Person-first language vs. identity-first language: An examination of the gains and drawbacks of disability language in society. *J Teaching Disability Studies.* 2019. Available at: https://jtds.commons.gc.cuny.edu/person-first-language-vs-identity-first-language-an-examination-of-the-gains-and-drawbacks-of-disability-language-in-society/

University of Kansas. *Research and Training Center on Independent Living Guidelines: How to Write about People With Disabilities.* 9th ed. Available at: https://www.aucd.org/docs/phe/9%20ed%20guidelines%20pamphlet%207.24.pdf

23. What is intersectionality?

Intersectionality is a qualitative analytical framework that utilizes intersecting sets to illustrate how various identities, characteristics, demographics, capabilities, disabilities, and resources can interact to compound problems or may present solutions for individuals. These subset intersections present an understanding of the patient that summarizes simultaneous relationships with multiple community groups. Presentation and utilization of this patient formulation with the interdisciplinary team can rapidly communicate personal complexity, potential barriers, and options for integration.

One method to view and analyze your own cultural identity(ies) is via a tool called a **bubble map**. These templates facilitate persons envisioning the complexities of their own lives and cultures.

Bubble Map templates for cultural identity. Available at: https://www.google.com/ search?q=Bubble+map+templates&tbm=isch&s ource=univ&sa=X&ved=2ahUKEwjMOf0Jt8PhAhVTFjQlHWhlBcUQsAR6BAgHEAE&biw=1042&bih=498&dpr=1.25

Columbia University School of Law. *Kimberlé Crenshaw on Intersectionality, More Than Two Decades Later*. 2017. Available at: https://www.law.columbia.edu/news/archive/kimberle-crenshaw-intersectionality-more-two-decades-later

Crenshaw K. *Demarginalizing the Intersection of Race and Sex: A Black Feminist Critique of Antidiscrimination Doctrine, Feminist Theory and Antiracist Politics*. 1989. Available at: https://chicagounbound.uchicago.edu/cgi/viewcontent. cgi?article=1052&context=uclf

Erevelles N Minear A. Unspeakable offenses: untangling race and disability in discourses of intersectionality. *J. Lit. Cult. Disabil. Stud.* 2010;4(2):127–145.

Gray K. *Intersectionality & Disability*. 2020. (YouTube). Available at: https://www.youtube.com/ watch?v=p2XNOCQazr0

University of Hawaii. Center on Disability Studies. *Bubble Maps from Teaching All Students, Reaching all Learners, Including Students With Disabilities as Diverse Learners*. 2011. Available at: http://www.ist.hawaii.edu/modules/multiculturalism/

24. What is empowerment medicine?

Empowerment medicine is the process of using available knowledge and resources to guide patients toward establishing a positive self-concept, self-determination, and pursuit of life aspirations. The goal of empowerment medicine is to use medical knowledge to increase the freedom, awareness, and civil rights of those with disabilities. Through a reciprocal patient-clinician exchange, patients explain their goals and values while working with the interdisciplinary team to reduce physical, attitudinal, and societal barriers to achievement. Ultimately, this approach to treatment helps the patient gain maximal control over their life and captures the patient's values. As the acute phase of injury or illness subsides, a return to personal autonomy is sought for the patient through simultaneously rehabilitating and removing environmental barriers. The process includes identifying and extinguishing pathological processes but also synergizes actions on the set of unique rehabilitation problems through catalyzing interdisciplinary team and patient engagement.

Hahn H. An agenda for citizens with disabilities: Pursuing identity and empowerment. *J Voc Rehabil.* 1997;9(1):31–37.

Nosek MA. Women with disabilities and the delivery of empowerment medicine. *Arch Phys Med Rehabil.* 1997;78(12 Suppl 5):S1–S2.

Stineman MG. Medical humanism and empowerment medicine. *Disabil Stud Q.* 2000;20(1):11–16.

25. How did empowerment medicine begin?

One of the fundamental principles of the disability rights movement is to reverse damage done by the medical model. This model dictates that an individual should want a cure for their disability and to that end must comply with all directions given by medical authorities. As a result, many individuals with disabilities have **experienced devaluation** in their interaction with the health care system and health care staff. In addition, they felt they were **viewed as abnormal, pathetic, helpless** victims with **little to no value to society**. This **stigmatization of pathology, dysfunction**, and **disfigurement provoked the independent living** and **disability rights movements** to respond with a call for **empowerment medicine**. This change from traditional approaches focuses on treating **people with disabilities as equal partners** in their health care and **offering them information** about how their disability affects maintenance of good health and functioning within their chosen lifestyle.

Health services researchers have taken up these concepts and coined the terms **patient-centered outcomes, patient-provider communication**, and **patient engagement**. Be aware, however, that although the principles of empowerment underlie these terms, remnants of provider superiority appear when they are put into practice. For example, guidelines for improving patient engagement often only measure the degree to which patients comply with physician orders and not the degree to which patients are involved in coming up with treatment plans.

The challenge for each clinician is to become familiar with problems faced by people with disabilities (as well as other oppressed and disadvantaged segments of the population) and to examine the discriminatory barriers they face. In addition, effective clinicians develop the fullest understanding of individual patient problems by understanding personally successful adaptation techniques from successful people with disabilities. Understanding disability rights movements and **disability studies** and providing exposure of clinical trainees to people with disabilities who live fulfilling lives leads to a more realistic perspective of true person-centered re-habilitation potential.

DeJong G. Health care reform and disability: affirming our commitment to community. *Arch Phys Med Rehabil.* 1993;74:1017–1024.

Ennis-O'Connor M. *What Does It Mean to Be an Empowered Patient?* 2018. Available at: https://powerfulpatients.org/2018/05/22/what-does-it-mean-to-be-an-empowered-patient/

26. How does empowerment medicine relate directly to communication with patients?
    Empowerment medicine leads to a greater depth of communication, providing patients with the optimal medical rehabilitation information necessary for them to make informed choices that will maximize their particular capabilities and quality of life. It is intended to increase trust by sharing information, communication, ideas, and planning for improved health between the patient and clinician. This increased trust can positively affect how patients view themselves and their clinicians, their lives, and their futures, thus positively influencing patient outcomes. The empowerment medicine approach to patient-provider communication requires mutual respect and cooperation. The effort is on the rehabilitation provider, who traditionally assumes the lead role but must now focus instead on establishing a communication style based in equality, trust, and vision.

Nosek MA. Women with disabilities and the delivery of empowerment medicine. *Arch Phys Med Rehabil.* 1997;78(12 Suppl 5):SI–S2.

27. How do you communicate the need for assistive technology in a positive manner?
    Some health professionals and most patients loathe discussing the need for a wheelchair or other types of assistive technology because of the symbolic association with infirmity and loss. Present considerations of the wheelchair as an adaptive tool used to meet their specific life goals. The wheelchair is a potent functional catalyst that enables mobility. Appearance is key. Encourage the patient to select personalized features. The appropriate wheelchair can enhance life, providing new possibilities, giving tremendous relief, and providing wonderful liberation from a restricted circumstance.

Nordgren A. How to respond to resistiveness towards assistive technologies among persons with dementia. *Med Health Care Philos.* 2018;21:411–421. Available at: https://doi.org/10.1007/s11019-017-9816-8

28. Are there any tools for enhancing the depth and meaningfulness of communication with patients?
    Recovery preference exploration (RPE) is an emerging technology based on the Features Resource Trade-Off Game. Patients or family members are first introduced to the Functional Independence Measure (FIM) or other sets of functional status scales to be utilized in therapy. Next, they are asked to imagine complete disability in all items, and choose patterns of optimal recovery, assuming they could control all aspects. The game forces choice of amount of recovery from varied activity limitations based on their own values and life worlds.

    When rehabilitation practitioners played the game, they utilized the three forms of clinical reasoning for problem solving: ***procedural*** (seeking conditions that may respond to treatment), ***conditional reasoning*** (consideration of the patient's past, meaning of the condition, and best possible outcomes), and ***interactive reasoning*** (customize treatment through continual patient dialog). ***Selection drivers*** represented these logic-based strategies applied to integrating recovery preference priorities. As clinicians assign meaning to recovery paths in a simulated lived experience of imagined disability, the patient's context becomes more understandable in the process of treatment planning. The two main selection driver themes of ***building a foundation*** and ***balance of recovery*** are excellent topics for clinician-patient transaction.

Stineman MG, Maislin G, Nosek MA, et al. *Comparing Consumer and Clinician Values for Alternative Functional States: Application of a New Feature Trade-Off Consensus Building Tool.* Available at: https://www.archives-pmr.org/article/S0003-9993(98)90413-0/pdf

Future-Resource Trade-Off Game of Functional Recovery (page 1524).

Kurtz AE, Saint-Louis N, Burke JP, et al. Exploring the personal reality of disability and recovery: a tool for empowering the rehabilitation process. *Qual Health Res.* 2008;18(1): 90–105. Available at: https://www.ncbi.nlm.nih.gov/pmc/articles/PMC2879973/pdf/nihms-162277.pdf

Communicating with people with disabilities. *Advancing Care Excellence for Persons With Disabilities. 2017.* Available at: http://www.nln.org/professional-development-programs/teaching-resources/ace-d/additional-resources/communicating-with-people-with-disabilities (for healthcare providers)

University of New Hampshire. *Responsive Practice: Accessible and Adaptive Communication.* Available at: https://unh.az1.qualtrics.com /jfe/form/SV_3I8BL0m7U1COj5z

Making Health Communication Programs Work. NIH Office of Communications and Public Liaison. 2009. Available at: https://www.cancer.gov/publications/health-communication/pink-book.pdf

29. **What media attempts to celebrate the contemporary perspectives of the lived disability experience?**
To enhance communication, the rehabilitationist needs to be familiar with a basic disability studies bibliography and to remain current with prominent disability issues as reported in magazines such as *New Mobility* and *Paraplegia News*. In addition, knowledge of disability studies will enhance clinical skills, forge a deeper connection with patients, and make it possible for health professionals to recommend media to patients with disabilities, families, and caregivers, providing valuable sources of meaning and purpose for their lives.

Disability Studies Quarterly. Available at: https://dsq-sds.org/

Northern Arizona University. *Disability Experience Module*. Available at: https://nau.edu/ihd/disability-experience/

Disability and Health. Available at: https://www.cdc.gov/ncbddd/disabilityandhealth/stories.html

Disability Visibility Project. Available at: https://disabilityvisibilityproject.com/

New Mobility. A magazine available in print or online at: http://www.newmobility.com/

Journal of Teaching Disability Studies. Available at: https://jtds.commons.gc.cuny.edu/

30. **How can patient and family education make communication more efficient?**
Communication with the patient and his or her family should begin with the first referral. Selectively recommended internet-based videos and focused reading material, and plan a conference to answer their list of questions.

Model Systems Knowledge Translation Center. Available at: https://msktc.org/Knowledge_Translation

31. **How have Health Insurance Portability and Accountability Act (HIPAA) regulations affected communication with patients?**
Physicians can feel constraints on their ability to communicate with and about their patients due to the HIPAA, which prohibits the disclosure of a patient's personal health information for any purpose unless the individual has authorized this disclosure with a signature. Furthermore, a patient has the right to restrict disclosure of his or her health information to individuals, such as family members. These regulations can put limitations on communication between health care providers, patients, and families and compromise care. Nevertheless, techniques for maintaining effective patient communication within these limits are plentiful. Electronic medical records, such as **MyChart**, offer a secure channel for two-way communication. Most medical institutions offer affiliated physicians an email service that includes encryption and secure emailing options. Goals include the correct care at the critical time in the least restrictive place. Contemporary pertinent and understandable information is best available to the patient and all members of the interdisciplinary team simultaneously to focus quality communication and action toward aims and goals with maximal impact.

HIPAA Notice of Privacy Practices. Available at: http://www.hhs.gov/ocr/hipaa/finalreg.html

Meirte J, Hellemans N, Anthonissen M, et al. Benefits and disadvantages of electronic patient-reported outcome measures: systematic review. *JMIR Perioper Med*. 2020;3(1): e15588. doi: 10.2196/15588

JMIR Perioperative Medicine—Benefits and Disadvantages of Electronic Patient-Reported Outcome Measures: Systematic Review.

Webber EC, Brick D, ScibiliaJB, Dehnel P. Electronic communication of the health record and information with pediatric patients and their guardians. *Pediatrics*. 2019;144(1):e20191359. Available at: https://doi.org/10.1542/peds.2019-1359

Electronic communication of the health record and information with pediatric patients and their guardians

32. **How should the physiatrist balance short and long-term goals in facilitating treatment by the interdisciplinary team?**
The realities of practice today may leave insufficient time to personally follow all problems through to their optimal resolution at each clinical encounter or admission. This makes timely interactions between providers essential to linking new capabilities with new activities. A complete and individualized problem list should be maintained but interpreted and addressed with constant awareness of the patient's life context, strengths, passions, and aspirations. Understanding these aspects contributes to a more holistic approach, even in a short problem-focused visit. Sustained conversation about patient life goals and passions drives success with compliance in turning aptitude into action and outcomes.

Craven BC, Alavinia SM, Wiest MJ, et al. Methods for development of structure, process, and outcome indicators for prioritized spinal cord injury rehabilitation domains: SCI-High Project. *J Spinal Cord Med*. 2019;42:(supp 1):51–67. Available at: https://www.ncbi.nlm.nih.gov/pmc/articles/PMC6781197/pdf/YSCM_42_1647386.pdf

BIBLIOGRAPHY

Albrecht C, Seelman K, Bury M. *Handbook of Disability Studies.* Thousand Oaks: Sage; 2003.

Davis, LJ. *The Disability Studies Reader.* 5th ed. New York: Routledge; 2016.

Gill CJ, Mukherjee S, Garland-Thomson R. Disability stigma in rehabilitation. *PM&R.* 2016;8:997–1003. doi: 10.1016/j.pmrj.2016.08.028:

Girma HH. *The Deafblind Woman Who Conquered Harvard Law.* New York: Twelve, Illustrated Edition; 2019.

Heumann J, Joiner K. *Being Heumann: An Unrepentant Memoir of a Disability Rights Activist.* Boston: Beacon; 2020.

Stineman MG, Rist PM, Burke JP. Through the clinician's lens: objective and subjective views of disability. *Qual Health Res.* 2009;*19*(1):17–29. doi: 10.1177/1049732308327853

DEDICATION

This chapter has been an ongoing exercise, of collaboration with, and devotion from two ever-enlightening, invigorating, and always laughing co-authors: Professors **Margaret Grace Stineman, MD** (1952-2020) and **Margaret Ann (Peg) Nosek, PhD** (1952–2020). They contributed to the actualization of many clinicians, patients, communities, and social movements!

CHAPTER 8

ENVIRONMENT AS PERSONAL HABITAT: ECOLOGY OF FUNCTION AND PARTICIPATION FROM INTERIOR BODY TO THE METAVERSE

Steven A. Stiens, MD, MS, and Shoshana Shamberg, OTR/L, MS, FOATA

Rehabilitation is often like surgery from the skin...out

— Steven A. Stiens

KEY POINTS: ENVIRONMENTAL ADAPTATIONS

1. Representations of the environment in the form of body imaging, photography, video recording, and simulation amplify rehabilitation assessment, reveal possibilities, and direct assembly of active solutions.
2. Contemporary concepts of the patient environment include a spectrum of locations for monitoring and intervention from dynamic biochemistry internally through to virtual environments and interface simulations for the purpose of therapy, personal projection, and connection to communities.
3. The attentive clinician visualizes all concentric spaces within and without the patient and imagines and animates these areas for maximal health, function, education, togetherness, and productivity.
4. A functional history combined with a sketch of a home floor plan and community map is an effective method for documenting and enabling life activity.
5. Use of retrospective sociospatial mapping and family scenario mapping can suggest environmental changes and allow for virtual projection of the proposed impact as well as actual outcome assessment.
6. Interdisciplinary connections to multiple environmental foci, common communication mechanisms, and resources for implementation maximize patient performance.

---

1. From a rehabilitation perspective, what aspects of the environment require evaluation and prospective treatment?

    The environment is everything that surrounds and reciprocally interacts with the patient, providing a unique habitat array for each person:

    - The ***physical aspects*** include the object constellation and morphology as well as the energy distribution.
    - The ***social aspects*** are the responses of the living community surrounding the patient: family, neighbors, inter-disciplinary team, and any others who may have contact with the patient.
    - The ***political aspects*** dictate laws and specify characteristics of the built and community environments as well as the rights of persons living with disablement.
    - The ***social capital theory*** integrates and supports integration, inclusion, power, and social cohesion.
        Various models of the environment are described in the current literature: ***The World Health Organization Model*** (2001), the ***Quebec Model*** (1995), the ***Institute of Medicine*** (1997), and the recent ***Craig Hospital Inventory of Environmental Factors (CHIEF) and the Craig Hospital Inventory of Environmental Factors Short Form (CHIEF-SF)***, both designed as questionnaires.

Craig Hospital Inventory of Environmental Factors; 2013. Available at: https://www.sralab.org/ rehabilitation-measures/craig-hospital-inventory-environmental-factors

IDEA—Center for Inclusive Design and Environmental Access. Available at: https://idea.ap.buffalo.edu/

Magasi S, Wong A, Gray DB, et al. Theoretical foundations for the measurement of environmental factors and their impact on participation among people with disabilities. *Arch Phys Med Rehabil.* 96(4):569–77; 2015.

Your Voice Matters—Including People with Disabilities in Research; 2018. Available at: https://www.youtube.com/watch?v= euAj6Me2jos

2. Describe the relationship between personhood and the physical environment.

Human behavior is carried out through interaction with the physical environment. Normal human development requires in-depth perception and manipulation of the environment as well as self-propulsion through the environment. From these interactions, one develops a working knowledge of the environment. Capabilities acquired from these interactions define our freedom to move about and modify the surroundings to our personal preferences. These experiences of mastery are internalized through self-discovery. Mastery then becomes a habit that is successfully executed in relationship to the surrounding world. In addition, it is uniquely human to observe and adapt the environment within and outside ourselves.

Demirkan H, Olguntüürk N. A priority-based "design for all" approach to guide home designers for independent living. *Archit Sci Rev*. 2014;*57*(2);90–104.

3. How does a new injury or illness affect the person-environment relationship?

Immediately after a catastrophic illness or injury, the experience of the body is radically distorted. ***Body image*** may be altered because of new deficits in perception, sensation, motor performance, and loss of body parts. Environmental perception may be altered as a result of sensory deficits or neglect. This situation is compounded by the ***depersonalization*** of hospitalization: patients are separated from the familiar, immediate environment of their clothes and personal items and may be confined to a bed in a horizontal position.

Initially, communication as a means to share personal identity and affect the physical environment frequently dominates the interaction. During this vulnerable period, patients' requests should be encouraged and fulfilled as reassurance that patients can meet their needs in spite of new functional limitations. Effective nursing, adaptive call lights, and access to television and telephone provide critical personal environmental control.

4. Can anticipatory milieu design and receptiveness in the environment dramatically improve outcomes?

A person in a new body interacting with their new environment is like an infant testing the environment of a crib. Testing and modifying the environment through verbal and physical interaction are crucial for beginning the problem-solving process and eliminating potential barriers to independence. Patients carry old memories, impressions, and attitudes into their current experience of disablement. Early experiments of environmental interaction in the new state confirm or refute their expectations and adaptive behaviors.

This ongoing iterative process of adaptation is an ***operant operation*** that is shaped with a variety of perceptual and physical interactions, including multiple spontaneous activities, repetitions, and problem solving. In this context, rehabilitation is a process of acquisition of functional skills, known as ***disability-appropriate behaviors***, and extinction of maladaptive, ***disability-inappropriate behaviors***. The adaptive habits need to be cued, supported, and enabled by the adapted habitats. Many of the limitations experienced by persons with physical, cognitive, and sensory limitations can be attributed to their environment.

Independent Living Institute (Adaptive Environments Center). Available at: https://www.independentliving.org/donet/11_adaptive_environments_center.html

5. Can the physical environment be divided into spaces that guide intervention from a person-centered perspective?

Fig. 8.1 depicts the spaces of the physical environment from a person-centered perspective:
- The ***internal environment*** is inside the body and includes components within spaces occupied by the organ systems.
- Rehabilitation treatment within the ***immediate environment*** (in constant direct contact with the person) includes specialized dressings, orthotics, prosthetics, adaptive clothing, communication devices, adaptive or assistive technology for toileting and feeding, and mobility devices. These aspects can be addressed in any care-giving setting.
- The ***intermediate environment*** (adapted specifically for inhabitants, adapted home or office) includes designs emphasizing function, safety, and personal style.
- The ***community environment*** (surrounds the homes) includes not only the physical structure but also people and institutions governed by a common culture and law.
- The ***political component*** includes dynamic attitudes, opinions expressed, and laws that specify access and the rights of persons with disabilities.
- The ***built environment component*** includes public and private buildings. Many structural changes have been implemented in accordance with the *Americans with Disabilities Act* (ADA), the *Rehabilitation Act* (Section 504), and *Fair Housing Act* (FHA) legislation.

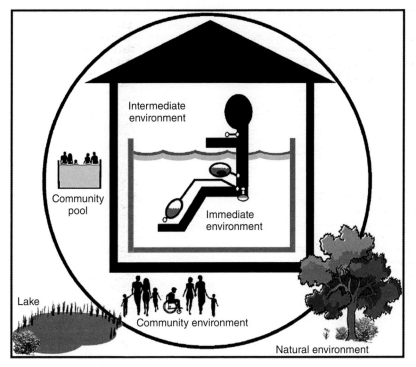

Fig. 8.1 Spaces of the physical environment from a person-centered perspective

- Finally, the ***natural environment*** (surrounds the community-modified space) presents access challenges that can be overcome with specialized skill acquisition, adaptive landscaping, and terrain-specific mobility aids

Environmental Barriers; 2008. Available at: https://www.researchgate.net/publication/301076759

Stiens SA. Personhood disablement and mobility technology: personal control of development. In: Gray DB, Quatrano LA, Liberman M, eds. *Designing and Using Assistive Technology: The Human Perspective.* Towson: Paul Brookes; 1998:29–49.

6. How can the rehabilitation team enhance patient interactions with the environment?
   Environmental spaces are substrates for interdisciplinary renovations. The goal is for the patient to rediscover a healthy, productive interaction with the environment that allows achieving life goals. Clinicians and therapists should explore patient memories of a particular satisfaction, prowess, and access in certain places. By analyzing these interactions, an intervention plan is formulated that makes stepwise changes to the patient's environment, progressing from the immediate environment out. The interdisciplinary team collaborates to link adapted tasks to sequential approximation of patients to the least restrictive environments of choice.

7. What techniques can the interdisciplinary team USE to target environmental barriers and maximize functional independence?
   Patient life behaviors can be elicited with ***retrospective sociobehavioral mapping***, which is a step-by-step review of where patients have gone, who they were with, what they were doing, as well as their intentions in activities. Negative findings are often the most significant intervention foci (where patients do not go, what they are not doing). The information can be diagrammed on floor plans or community maps.
   Intervention in the form of adaptive equipment often evolves as a continuum, starting with the design of the person's immediate environment (e.g., braces, wheelchair) and progressing to the intermediate environment (the patient's home). The community and natural environments are emphasized during the latter phases of the process.

Assessment of the home environment can include drawn floor plans, photographic/video depictions, or home visits. Success in the home and community is achieved with passes, predischarge home visits, and community outings. In essence, the goal is to progressively design an environment that enhances personhood (with objectives of safety and independence) and reflects the characteristics and goals of the patient in concert with others. *Successive approximation* of the home environment is through adaptation of the hospital bed, room, and trial living quarters as informed design experiments.

Easy Architectural Drawing & Rendering 2D &3D. Available at: https://youtu.be/a71D3Ms-sAU

How to draw a room in 2-point perspective. Available at: https://youtu.be/rCanYY7eLeA

Drawing Techniques. Available at: https://www.youtube.com/channel/UCuc81B9rEB2AdfaM8HxEaKA

Keysor J, Jette A, Haley S. Development of the home and community environment (HACE) instrument. *J Rehabil Med.* 2005:37; 37–44.

8. Describe four transitional environments in current use as part of community rehabilitation units.
   Hospital beds and rooms on a series of units are designed for various independence levels: intensive care, step down, telemetry, and rehabilitation unit.
   Independent living trial apartments have real-world, generic, unmodified, and modifiable characteristics to adapt for home simulation and to challenge the patients, caregivers, and family to develop adaptive solutions.
   Simulated community environments are designed for trial life scenarios without leaving the hospital.
   Selected community environments are for activity-specific trials.

9. In planning discharge to home, what other assessments are needed to help change the patient's immediate environment to meet personal needs?
   Role changes may result from functional limitations that prevent the patient from performing various activities or home duties. Preparation is accomplished through *family scenario mapping* (i.e., verbal review of family activities to redefine tasks by interest and aptitude). In addition, transitions can be facilitated by practice with therapy, as needed for bathroom and kitchen activities, housekeeping, gardening, home maintenance, childcare, and marital relations.

Fange A, Iwarsson S. Changes in accessibility and usability in housing: an exploration of the housing adaptation process. *Occup Ther Int.* 2005:12(1);44–59.

10. What adaptive options should be CONSIDERED in a functional home assessment that will enhance a patient's activity and participation?
    The rehabilitation clinician should accompany the patient and other occupants to follow the sequence of movements he or she would take to, and through, the home. The clinician should consider such environmental elements as:
    - **Public transportation access** (stops, shelter safety, barriers on route from home)
    - **Parking** (wide, covered, and level; motion-activated lighting)
    - **Steps** (ramp, 20/1-inch length over rise; ratio, 4 degrees or 12/1 is maximum steepness)
    - **Entrances and doorways** (level porch, flat or ramped threshold, light switch, security system)
    - **Telephones** (cordless, multiple, headset options)
    - **Exterior walkways and driveway** (level, lighted, rails)
    - **Interior stairs** (gates, bilateral rails, lift options)
    - **Bathroom** (door, commode height, grab bars, shower transfer, handheld sprayer, controls, drainpipe insulation)
    - **Kitchen** (reach ability, storage, food preparation, cooking sequences, clean up, and reach for dishes)
    - **Security** (on-person alert system for falls, building wide with intercom, cameras, remote lock control)
    - **Storage** (including closets and dressers)
    - **Laundry facilities** (front loading, reacher)
    - **Interior hallways** (avoid loose rugs)
    - **Access to floors** (outside walks, entrances, stair lifts, elevators)
    - **Living/dining room** (furniture height, serving access)
    - **Breaker/fuse boxes** (location labeling)
    - **Floor surfaces** (durable, nonslip)
    - **Environmental control units (ECUs)** (location, power backups)

- **Interior lighting** (activated by touch, voice, motion, or ECU)
- **Emergency** (lighting, escape pathways, fire extinguisher, smoke alarms)

ADA Barrier Removal Checklist. Available at: www.usdoj.gov/crt/ada/racheck.pdf

Adapted Life (Easy Street). Available at: https://www.youtube.com/watch?v=pQFhgqt2iKM&authuser=0

Cook DJ, Crandall AS, Thomas BL, Krishnan NC, CASAS: a smart home in a box. *Computer.* 2013;*46*(7);62–69. Available at: https://www.ncbi.nlm.nih.gov/pmc/articles/PMC3886862/

Smart home in a box kit. Available at: https://www.ncbi.nlm.nih.gov/pmc/articles/PMC3886862/figure/F2/

McClusky JF. Creating engaging experiences for rehabilitation. *Top Stroke Rehabil.* 2008;*15*(2):80–86. doi:10.1310/tsr1502-80. PMID: 18430671.

Wilson, L. What non-home health providers & clinicians should know about patients' homes: a home health occupational therapist perspective. VA home based primary care: Available at: https://medschool.cuanschutz.edu/docs/librariesprovider82/default-document-library/what-non-home-health-providers-and-clinicians-should-know-about-patients-homes-l-wilson.pdf?sfvrsn=a0d06bb9_2

11. How is accessibility defined in the community environment?

In the United States, the **Federal Access Board** does extensive accessibility research with a variety of experts in design, architecture, medicine, and technology. Guidelines are generated for the federal level, but state and local guidelines vary. The access board in Washington, D.C. has extensive information, publications, and technical assistance available to address the government regulations for compliance with the ADA, the *Rehabilitation Act*, and the *Architectural Barriers Act.* A hard copy of accessibility guidelines is available by calling 202-272-5434.

Access Board. Available at: https://www.access-board.gov/guidelines-and-standards

ADA Standards. Available at: https://www.ada.gov/2010ADAstandards_index.htm

12. What are the rights of a tenant with disability?

The **Fair Housing Act of 1988** mandates accessibility compliance and civil rights protection in advertised rental properties. Persons with disabilities are provided equal access. The resident cannot be denied the opportunity to modify the rented home to meet individual accessibility needs (documented by a licensed medical professional). The cost of modification is paid by the renter. In addition, the landlord may require that the work be done by an approved professional, and an escrow account may be established in which the tenant must place funds for returning the residence to its original state. Modifications that are easily used by future renters (universal design) can be left intact. If approved by the landlord, a physician's prescription for modifications as medically necessary permits a tax deduction for expense. Section 504 of the **Rehabilitation Act of 1973** mandates that public housing and housing subsidized with federal funds be accessible and adaptable to meet the needs of tenants with disabilities.

Fair Housing Act Design Manual. Available at: https://www.huduser.gov/portal/publications/PDF/FAIRHOUSING/fairfull.pdf

Fair Housing Tool Kit. Available at: www.knowledgeplex.org/

Universal Design Accessibility article. Available at: https://www.resna.org/Portals/0/Documents/ Position%20Papers/Rehabilitation%20Engineering%20Professionals%20-%20White%20Paper%20-%20RESNA%202017%20-%20Final%20-%20Approved.pdf

13. What are environmental adaptations for bathrooms?

Bathroom accidents are one of the leading causes of death and disability in the older population. Shower and tub falls rank as the third leading cause of accidental death in the 50-plus age group. More than half of all accidents could be prevented with some sort of environmental modification.

The following list gives ways to increase safety:

- Multilevel or **adjustable sink heights** and countertops provide accessibility from standing and seated positions.
- Plumbing should be installed toward the back wall with **hot water pipes insulated** and water temperature set to prevent burns.
- **Single-levered faucet** handles are universal.
- Automatic faucets, wall-mounted electric toothbrushes, soap/shampoo dispensers, and hair dryers may be installed for a person with limited hand function and upper body strength.
- **Toilet height of 17 to 19 inches** allows horizontal transfers from wheelchairs and eases standing and sitting. However, child access with a stool and/or exclusion with lid-lock may be needed for safety.
- An **ideal grab bar system** is customized for tub and toilet access that enables greatest efficiency and safety.
- A **handheld showerhead** on an adjustable-height track can be used for bathing from a seated or standing position.
- **Padded shower chairs** with back support are safe and practical.

- *Tub lifts*, which lower a person into a tub, can be controlled by hydraulic, battery, or manual mechanisms.
- A *rubberized mat* and tub strips provide a nonslip surface.
- An *angled mirror* and a side-mounted medicine cabinet can be used from a standing or seated position.
- Adequate *lighting is nonglare*, preferably with sconces and multiple bulbs or adjustable intensity.
- A *ground fault intercept (GFI)* outlet prevents electrocution from the use of electrical appliances near a sink or other source of water.
- *Contrasting the color of surfaces*, especially background and foreground, enables people with visual or cognitive impairments to see and define surfaces.

Adaptable Bathrooms Manual (2005–2006). Available at: https://www.fairhousingfirst.org/documents/BATHROOM_FINAL_BOOK.pdf; www.abilitycenter.org/webtools/links/adaresources/AdaptableBath.pdf

Wheelchair Mobility Standards. Available at: https://www.huduser.gov/portal/publications/pdf/fairhousing/fairch7.pdf

Adaptable Bathrooms Manual. Available at: https://www.huduser.gov/portal/publications/pdf/fairhousing/fairch7.pdf

14. **List design possibilities and features for mobility-challenged adaptations for kitchens.**
    Access-friendly kitchens should have cabinets with high, deep kick plates for toe space, a U- or L-shaped floor plan for traffic flow, an appliance and storage sequence for recipe completion to service and clean up, and a stove in lowered countertop with side or front controls and angled mirror overhead. For ease of mobility, a side-swinging oven door, pullout shelves, and Lazy Susans are helpful. In addition, continuous countertops for sliding heavy vessels, pullout or lap cutting boards, shallow sinks, long, retractable sprayer hoses, task lighting, reachable fire extinguishers, and strip outlets with on/off switches are popular innovations.

15. **A single woman with mild dementia had to be discharged home. Suggest possible environmental solutions for challenges she may face.**
    - Provide *environmental* cues to address safety, memory, and communication deficits.
    - Personal *emergency response system*, with medication management and training in the use of the devices, with monitoring of her ability to learn.
    - *Automatic medication management* system set up weekly by a caregiver or home care nurse.
    - *Burglar alarm* and posted fire escape plan that has been learned, practiced, and monitored regularly.
    - *Smoke alarms* hot-wired with battery backup.
    - *Emergency lighting* in case of power failure.
    - *Daily calls* to monitor her ability to care for herself.
    - "Meals on Wheels" and use of *microwave* with *electric hot-water pot*.
    - *Electric range* or microwave oven. Avoid using a gas stove. *Automatic turn-off controls* to address memory deficits.
    - Posted instructions on the step-by-step use of all appliances and their safety issues.
    - Preprogramming frequently used telephone numbers for *one-button speed calling*.
    - Using a digital voice recorder to record daily instructions or for message taking.
    - Providing opportunities for patient to *access as many community resources* as needed to maintain her independence, health, and safety and to promote socialization (e.g., support groups, religious associations, social service agencies, and transportation).

ADA Documents Center. Available at: https://askjan.org/articles/What-to-Include-in-Your-ADA-Accommodation-Toolkit.cfm?csSearch=2737809_1

ADA Accessibility Guidelines on Recreational Facilities. Available at: https://adata.org/ada-document-portal/results

16. **What is visitability? Why is this movement important?**
    Visitability is a design concept for residential households that promotes the creation of communities in which people of all abilities and disabilities, especially mobility impairments, can get into the door and use at least one bathroom when visiting neighbors. This concept provides a bridge from the intermediate to the surrounding community environment and fosters social interdependence (neighbor role) and relationships that can offer natural supports for persons with disabilities.

Accessible Housing by Design; 20018. Available at: https://fpg.unc.edu/sites/fpg.unc.edu/files/resource-files/NCODH_RemovingBarriersToHealthCare.pdf

Center For an Accessible Society. Available at: www.accessiblesociety.org

Housing Design Standards for Accessibility and Inclusion. The Kelsey. 2022. Available at: https://thekelsey.org/learn-center/design-standards/

Center for Universal Design; 2006. Available at: https://projects.ncsu.edu/ncsu/design/cud/pubs_p/docs/UDinHousing.pdf

17. **What interior home and community features enhance success for persons with visual impairments?**

Home interior:

- Increase lighting intensity and spectrum but *reduce glare* to increase acuity.
- Contrast solid colors to *define surfaces and edges*.
- Post *large print* with raised letters or use *voice output on signage* and controls.
- Vary *textures to define edges* and boundaries.
- *Illuminate switches*
- Install *nonskid*, matte-finish floor surfaces.

Exterior public spaces:

- Use *auditory signals* for crosswalks, transmit guidance signal to phones and smartcanes.
- Record short verbal messages about opportunities or barriers in the area.

Iwamiya S, Yamauchi K, Takada M. Design specifications of audio-guidance systems for the blind in public spaces. *J Physiol Anthropol Appl Human Sci.* 2004:23;267–271.

Introduction to smart homes for people who are blind or visually impaired; 2018. Available at: https://youtu.be/jPO9zrMn78E

18. **What might aid persons with hearing impairments?**

Facing furniture arrangements with good lighting and wall-mounted mirrors to present faces for interpretation. Communication technology such as *telecommunications device for the deaf (TDD)* telephone, fax machine, and telephone relay system. Vibrating or light cues for clocks, telephones, doorbells, and baby monitors.

Johnson CA. Articulation of deaf and hearing spaces using deaf space design guidelines: a community based participatory research with the Albuquerque Sign Language Academy; 2010. Available at: http://digitalrespository.umn.edu/arch_etds/18

19. **What does the phrase "aging in place" mean?**

Over the past decade, older persons have overwhelmingly reported that they would prefer to remain in their homes as long as possible. Single-level homes with wide floor plans and attached separate apartments on bus lines, near shopping, and potential attendant help are most ideal.

AARP Home Modifications Guide. Available at: https://www.aarp.org/home-family/your-home/?migration=rdrct

Administration on Aging—Remodeling resources. Available at: https://acl.gov/news-and-events/news/contributor-discusses-process-finding-aging-place-specialist

CASPAR Extended Home Living Services—home mods assessment tool. Available at: https://homemods.org/wp-content/uploads/2019/06/Assessments_3.20.19_Professionals.pdf

Universal Home Design Guide. Available at: http://www.mnhousing.gov/get/MHFA_002502

20. **Describe a series of steps that might identify safety risks, functional barriers, and an economical response to identified needs.**

- Client activities of daily living (ADLs): *home safety screening survey* by mail or telephone visit.
- Home environment: *On-site home safety assessment* in cases defined by survey thresholds.
- Functional and environmental assessment with *individualized modification* and patient rehabilitation on program operated by specially trained occupational and physical therapists
- Occupational and physical therapy with *trial of interventions* and specified planning for modifications and installations
- Product installation and home modification

Client/caregiver training to help maximize the client's independence, wellness, and quality of life, as well as increasing the efficiency and safety of caregiver assistance

RECOMMENDED READINGS

National Organization on Disability (NOD)—Access to Worship Checklist; 2020. Available at: www.nod.org/index.cfm?fuseaction=page.
viewPage&pageID=1430&nodeID=1&FeatureID=399&redirected=1&C FID=5162137&CFTOKEN=16611784
Practical Guide to Universal Home Design. Available at: http://www.universaldesign.com/
Removing Barriers to Health Care Guide; 2020. Available at:
United Spinal Association publications. Available at: www.unitedspinal.org/pages.php?catid=7

21. **What should be considered when formulating solutions to functional and environmental barriers to maximize independence and safety?**
    - Emphasize the goals of the client to achieve the maximum level of independence and safety for daily activities at home to the jobsite/school environment/community.
    - Integrate the caregivers and others living in the home.
    - Identify strengths and weakness in sensorimotor, cognitive, and psychosocial functions.
    - Adapt to the progressive nature of the client's illness/disability by articulating future needs.
    - Target environmental barriers along a route from parking to building entrances and throughout the interior space, considering safety, maximum independence, and adaptability of the environment.
    - Assess the need for specialized equipment and training in its use. Internet product research is now a very effective way to find products, evaluations of those products, and distributors.
    - Prioritize all suggestions (client/caregiver in consult with the team) according to the immediate requirements needed for functioning/caregiving, including getting in and out of the home, training in transfers, ADLs, mobility, compensation techniques, stress management, and safety issues according to the financial resources available to the client.
    - Provide resources to the client and caregivers, including specially trained professionals, support services, and funding options.
    - Provide ongoing consultation to designers, building contractors, and client during the design and construction phase.
    - Consider financial constraints and potential resources from medical insurance, community resources, and loans/grants.

    Consideration of all these factors will ensure greater levels of success in carryover of the rehabilitation process and community integration once discharged from inpatient, intermediate care, and home-care therapy. In addition, ***periodically monitor progress and challenges*** once environmental modifications and assistive technology are in place and in use. Address issues of the person when functioning in his or her environment, as well as issues of the caregiver. Adjust elements as needed to promote success, maximum safety, function, and independence.

    National Resource Center on Supportive Housing and Home Modification. Available at: www.homemods.org

22. **Can virtual presence in a synthetic environment meet socialization goals, accomplish tasks, and improve performance in the actual physical environment? How can the risk of "cybersickness" be diminished?**
    Social presence can start with the telephone and advance to videoconferencing, self-presentation controlling a robot, and shared "virtual spaces" as animated avatars or holograms. These virtual definitions include ***cyberspace*** (interconnected digital technology), ***mirrorworld*** (reality overlaid with digital augmented reality), and ***metaverse*** (a collective, persistent virtual shared space that converges with reality). Transformation of physical presence into a virtual space is accomplished using ***cybermetric*** approaches of simultaneous presentation of synchronized sensory stimuli via specialized headset, presenting stereoscopic views and surround sound, kinetic vibratory seating, and manipulation of handsets and devices in a wind- and temperature-controlled space.

    Presence, or "being there," is enhanced by approaching and establishing "context" and immersing in the "illusion" with navigation control and sensory feedback. ***Engrossment*** or ***immersion*** occurs with focus or attendance to task. These are digital mechanisms with potential to therapeutically unite patients with family, community, work, therapy, and play. ***Cybersickness*** is a constellation of malaise similar to motion sickness and associated with asynchronous, dissonant sensory stimuli having aberrant sensory presentation from the virtualization system. Symptoms improve with immersion, accommodation, and improvement in the quality or the synchrony of the simulation.

    ADA and IT; 2010. Available at: https://www.ada.gov/regs2010/2010ADAStandards/2010ADAstandards.htm

    Weech S, Kenny S, Barnett-Crown M. Presence and cybersickness in virtual reality are negatively related: a review. *Front Psychol.* 2019;10:158. 10.3389/fpsyg.2019.00158.

    Full text. Available at: https://www.researchgate.net/publication/330849499_Presence_and_Cybersickness_in_Virtual_Reality_Are_Negatively_Related_A_Review

23. **How does the "paradox of overcoming barriers" imperceptibly determine life trajectories?**
    Environmental factors have profound roles in shaping activity as a "scene setter" for life by expanding or constraining the task choices and determining available options. Examples include: segregated "accessible" seating in public venues, wheelchair spaces "in front of the bus," and adaptive technologies that do not achieve equal opportunity for all users. Paradoxically, this self-selection process provides some but not all opportunities, limiting the sphere of being. Universal design opens more pathways and reaps greater rewards for and from each person.

24. Can the rehabilitation clinic be "transported" to the patient's home?
    Clearly, patient's function in their homes and communities is the objective of the interdisciplinary team, but access to specialized services has kept patients at tertiary care institutions. Contemporary solutions are emerging in the form of home-based rehabilitative care and **_telerehabilitation_** with robotics to bring physical treatment to patients guided by therapists in real time and computer monitored for compliance, progress, and complications between visits. Repetitive robotic exercise allows patients to achieve performance refinements, and caregivers can immediately translate functional gains into productive person-centered activities, reinforcing and augmenting their achievements.

Haig A, Stiens SA. Telerehabilitation: Exercise and adaptation in home and community. In: Moroz A, Flanagan SR, Zaretsky H, eds., _Medical Aspects of Disability_. 5th ed. New York: Springer; 2017:681–696.

WEBSITES

ABLEDATA, database of information (Available at: https://abledata.acl.gov/) on assistive technology and rehabilitation equipment designed to serve persons with disabilities and rehabilitation professionals. Contact: 800-227-0216.
ADAPT (Advocacy for Independent Living); 2020. Available at: www.adapt.org

RAMPS

Adaptive Environments Center (AEC); 1994. Available at: https://www.ada.gov/checkweb.htm
Andrus Center. At-home modification publications and information/directory of consultants. Available at: www.homemods.org
Center for Universal Design; 1994. Available at: https://projects.ncsu.edu/ncsu/design/cud/

ACCESSIBLE HOUSE DESIGN AND UNIVERSAL DESIGN

American Occupational Therapy Association (AOTA). Available at: https://www.aota.org//media/Corporate/Files/Practice/Researcher/Complex_Environmental_Modifications_review_draft.pdf
Occupational Therapy and Home Modifications: Breaking New Ground With Rebuilding Together. Available at: https://www.aota.org/About-Occupational-Therapy/Professionals/PA/Facts/Home-Modifications.aspx
Accessible housing by design. Available at: https://www.cmhc-schl.gc.ca/en/developing-and-renovating/accessible-adaptable-housing/accessible-housing-by-design
Accessible and adaptable housing. Available at: https://www.cmhc-schl.gc.ca/en/developing-and-renovating/accessible-adaptable-housing
Universal design and adaptable housing models. Available at: https://www.cmhc-schl.gc.ca/en/developing-and-renovating/accessible-adaptable-housing/universal-design-adaptable-housing-models
The Principles of Universal Design. Available at: https://projects.ncsu.edu/ncsu/design/cud/pubs_p/docs/poster.pdf
The Center for Universal Design Available at: https://projects.ncsu.edu/ncsu/design/cud/pubs_p/docs/stockHouse-Plans.pdf

BATHROOMS

Essential Guide to Accessible Bathroom Design. Live in Place Designs. Available at: https://liveinplacedesigns.com/guide-to-remodeling-a-handicap-bathroom/

KITCHENS

Canada Mortgage and Housing Corporation (CMHC). Available at: https://www.cmhc-schl.gc.ca/en/search#q=accessable&sort=relevancy
Accessible Kitchen Design. Available at: https://www.youtube.com/watch?v=EJKu6gh5TOk
73 Wheelchair Acessible Kitchen Ideas. Available at: https://www.pinterest.com/modica03/wheelchair-accessible-kitchens/

HOME AUTOMATION

Setz B, Graef S, Ivanova D, Tiessen A, Aiello M. "A Comparison of Open-Source Home Automation Systems", _IEEE Access_. 2021;9:167332-167352. Available at: https://ieeexplore.ieee.org/stamp/stamp.jsp?tp=&arnumber=9652536
Lazazzara A, Ricciard F, Za S. Exploring Digital Ecosystems: Organizational and Human Challenges, Springer, Switzerland. 2020. Available at: https://doi.org/10.1007/978-3-030-23665-6

CEILING LIFTS AND ELEVATORS

Baird C. Types of Home Accessibility Lifts: Choosing What is Best for You. Available at: https://liftandaccessibilitysolutions.com/types-home-accessibility-lifts-choosing-whats-best/

ASSESSMENT TOOLS

Home Assessments for Falls Prevention. Available at: https://homemods.org/wp-content/uploads/2019/06/Assessments_3.20.19_Professionals.pdf

BIBLIOGRAPHY

Abilities OT Services and Seminars: See www.aotss.com for a complete listing of organizations and publications (3309 W. Strathmore Ave., Baltimore, MD 21215; Phone: 410-358-7269; Fax: 410-358-6454). Technical assistance, publications, and Internet and on-site training programs for medical and design/build professionals on home modifications, job-site modifications, disability legislation compliance, and assistive technology.

Compendium of home modification and assistive technology policy and practice across the states: state policy and practice, 2006. Available at: https://aspe.hhs.gov/basic-report/compendium-home-modification-and-assistive-technology-policy-and-practice-across-states-state-profiles

Designing a More Usable World; 1994. Available at: https://trace.umd.edu/

Easter Seals: Available at: www.easterseals.com/site/PageServer?pagename=ntl_resource_room &s_esLocation=res (230 W. Monroe St., Suite 1800, Chicago, IL 60606; Phone: 800-221-6827; 312-726-6200; 312-726-4258 (TTY)).

Hamraie A. *Building Access: Universal Design and the Politics of Disability.* 3rd ed. Minneapolis: University of Minnesota Press; 2017.

Sabata DV, Shamberg S, Williams M. Optimizing access to home, community, and work environments In: Trombley CA, Radomski MV, eds. *Occupational Therapy for Physical Dysfunction.* 5th ed. Philadelphia: Kluwer; 2008:952–973.

Shamberg S. Occupational therapy practitioner: role in the implementation of worksite modifications. *IOS 24*: 2005;185–197.

Stark S, Landsbaum A, Palmer JL, et al. Client-centred home modifications improve daily activity performance of older adults. *Can J Occup Ther.* 2009;*76*(1 suppl):235–245. Available at: https://pubmed.ncbi.nlm.nih.gov/19757729/ doi:10.1177/000841740907600s09

Stiens DW, Stiens SA. Environmental modifications and role functions: Redesign of a house for a family with a paraplegic father. *J Am Parapleg Soc.*1993;16:278–279.

Wylde M, Baron-Robbins A, S Clark. Building for a lifetime: the design and construction of fully accessible homes. Newtown: Taunton; 1994.

CHAPTER 9

PSYCHOLOGICAL METHODS THROUGH REHABILITATION: THEORY, ASSESSMENT, AND INTERVENTION

Kristen Jackson, PhD, Chelsea Kane, PsyD, and Steven A. Stiens, MD, MS

…disability is only one aspect, and often a very minor aspect, of a person. We should always attend primarily to the person.
— Harold E. Yuker (1924–1997)

KEY POINTS

1. The clinician must assess the entire patient situation beyond mere diagnosis.
2. Multiple psychological interventions are essential to the rehabilitation process.
3. Emotions, cognitions, and behaviors are discrete yet mutually interdependent. Patient attitudes, beliefs, and engagement are decisive and essential targets for exploration and intervention.
4. Successful life through and beyond rehabilitation is a process of acquiring adaptive behaviors to support health and wellbeing while also reducing unhelpful behaviors.
5. Understanding the patient as related to the environment and society contextualizes treatment and demands a continual redesign of rehabilitation systems.
6. The patient is the most important part of his or her own recovery.
7. Rehabilitation is a dynamic interdisciplinary process requiring committed collaboration between multiple disciplines, providers, and the patient and family with thoughtfulness to the ever-changing conditions.

1. What is psychology?

   Psychology is the study of mind and behavior. Humans have always sought to understand human experience. Historically, psychology started within philosophy and became a scientific discipline with primary areas in perception, cognition, development, personality, and social interaction. The American Psychological Association (APA) defines the **practice of psychology** as "the use of psychological knowledge for any of several purposes: to understand and treat mental, emotional, physical, and social dysfunction; to understand and enhance behavior in various settings of human activity (e.g., school, workplace, courtroom, sports arena, battlefield); and to improve machine and building design for human use."

   APA Dictionary of Psychology. Available at: https://dictionary.apa.org/psychology

2. Are there specialists within the rehabilitation setting for psychological, behavioral, and cognitive patient needs?

   Yes, several subspecialty domains within psychology, including **rehabilitation psychology,** concentrate theory and methods to facilitate the rehabilitation process. **Rehabilitation psychologists** focus on maximizing patients' independence, choice, agency, and participation and, as a result, support improved functional status and wellbeing. Naturally, patients have reactions to changing health and functional status, and these reactions can impact their adaptation to disability. Successful **transdisciplinary team function** demands universal reporting of psychological functioning and collaboration on mutual goals that support patient mood and behavior.

   Rehabilitation Psychology from Division 22. Available at: https://www.ncbi.nlm.nih.gov/pmc/articles/PMC3410123/

   Wahass SH. The role of psychologists in health care delivery. *J Family Community Med.* 2005;12(2):63–70.

3. Why should psychological assessment and intervention be included as a part of rehabilitation? Why is it important to consider a patient's mood and social factors when providing health care?

   Psychiatrist Dr. Lean Eisenberg famously wrote, "Biomedical knowledge is essential for providing sound medical care, but it is not sufficient. The nature of dysfunctions and the physicians' transaction with the patient must also be informed by the psychosocial understanding." George Engel developed the biopsychosocial model of health, illustrating the links between interacting body and community systems. Disability is a lived experience, one which is pervasive and maintained through these interdependent systems. The World Health Organization (WHO) defines **disability** as "a complex phenomenon, reflecting the interaction between features of a person's body and features of the society in which he or she lives." **Self-efficacy** is constantly redefined through dynamic appraisal, choice, and action.

WHO. *Disability.* Available at: https://www.who.int/topics/disabilities/en/

Heinemann AW, Wilson CS, Huston T, et al. Relationship of psychology inpatient rehabilitation services and patient characteristics to outcomes following spinal cord injury: the SCIRehab project. *J Spinal Cord Med.* 2012;35(6):578–592. Available at: https://doi.org/10.1179/2045772312Y.0000000059

Strasser DC, Falconer JA, Stevens AB, et al. Team training and stroke rehabilitation outcomes: a cluster randomized trial. *Arch Phys Med Rehabil.* 2008;89(1):10–15. Available at: https://doi.org/10.1016/j.apmr.2007.08.127.

4. **How can including psychological theory and methods make a treatment team more effective?**
   Multidisciplinary treatment has proven to be superior to isolated physician visits. Integration of psychological theory and interventions has been critical to advancing health quality. For example, trauma-informed care and motivational interviewing (MI) are two examples of psychological theory and practice which have been promoted in health care to enhance outcomes and relationships between health care providers and patients. New systems of interdisciplinary care with simultaneous multisystem interventions (a la the **Biopsychosocial Model**) continue evolving. Team members must prioritize interventions to meet team consensus on sequential goal attainment.

Integrated Care Research and Practice. Available at: https://www.scie.org.uk/integrated-care/research-practice/activities/multidisciplinary-teams

Rusk HA. The growth and development of rehabilitation medicine. *Arch Phys Med Rehabil.* 1969;50:463–466.

Altmaier EM, Lehmann TR, Russell DW, et al. The effectiveness of psychological interventions for the rehabilitation of low back pain: a randomized controlled trial evaluation. *Pain.* 1992;49(3):329–335. Available at: https://doi.org/10.1016/0304-3959(92)90240-C

https://www.brighamandwomens.org/assets/BWH/womens-health/connors-center/pdfs/tic-in-medicine-raja-2015.pdf

5. **How have psychologists shaped the ethical foundations of rehabilitation as a field?**
   Beatrice Wright's (1983) **20 value-laden beliefs and principles** have notably guided the field of rehabilitation psychology and rehabilitation generally. These universal psychosocial guidelines should be printed and posted for regular review. The **themes of these principles** are: everyone is worthy of encouragement, the physical and social environment profoundly impacts coping and adjustment, all individuals possess unique assets that aid rehabilitation, clients benefit the process and the team as comanagers, and psychological issues change but are constants throughout rehabilitation. These principles have been central to disability ethics, disability advocacy and justice issues, and how we respond to the real-world issues of people with disability.

Dunn DS, Elliott TR. Revisiting a constructive classic: Wright's physical disability: a psychosocial approach. *Rehabil Psychol.* 2005;50(2):183–189. Available at: https://psycnet.apa.org/fulltext/2005-05481-013.pdf

Value Laden Beliefs & Principles for Rehabilitation. Available at: https://abpp.org/BlankSite/media/Rehabilitation-Psychology-Documents/ABRP-Value-Laden-Beliefs-Principles.pdf

6. **What is "contextualization," and why is it important within rehabilitation treatment?**
   Contextualization is the dynamic process of assessment of all the pertinent relational, historical, and environmental factors that may impact patients as well as their perceptions and reactions. The psychosocial team often works in a transdisciplinary way to translate the voices of the patient and family, integrating and prioritizing information about the patient's medical status, background (culture, race, ethnicity, and religion), level of medical literacy/understanding, cognition, values, education, personality style, and psychological and psychiatric background and current conditions. This allows the team to hold a more holistic conceptualization of the individual patient: immediate coping reactions, resources for adaptation, passions, and pathways to achieve their unique goals.

Bogner J, Dijkers M, Hade EM, et al. Contextualized treatment in traumatic brain injury inpatient rehabilitation: effects on outcomes during the first year after discharge. *Arch Phys Med Rehabil.* 2019;100(10):1810–1817. Available at: https://doi.org/10.1016/j.apmr.2018.12.037

7. **What other factors, in addition to known biological aspects, should the team think about when conceptualizing health and rehabilitation progress?**
A patient's presentation during rehabilitation can be impacted by multiple factors, many of which can impact health and recovery. Additional considerations that the treatment team may benefit from incorporating into their understanding of their patients include many known **determinants of health** which include a wide range of factors: biological aspects (e.g., genetic predispositions or risks), behavioral factors (e.g., stress, health beliefs, lifestyle habits), and social conditions (e.g., social support, socioeconomic status, family relationships, environment, larger cultural influences and impact). How patients think (**mindset**) determines their response to life events, with adaptive healthy behaviors or habits that can suppress progress.

Hosseini SM, Oyster ML, Kirby RL, et al. Manual wheelchair skills capacity predicts quality of life and community integration in persons with spinal cord injury. *Arch Phys Med Rehabil.* 2012;93(12):2237–2243. Available at: https://doi.org/10.1016/j.apmr.2012.05.021

Saunders LL, Krause JS, Acuna J. Association of race, socioeconomic status, and health care access with pressure ulcers after spinal cord injury. *Arch Phys Med Rehabil.* 2012;93(6):972–977. Available at: https://doi.org/10.1016/j.apmr.2012.02.004

Frier A, Barnett F, Devine S. The relationship between social determinants of health, and rehabilitation of neurological conditions: a systematic literature review. *Disabil Rehabil.* 2017;39(10):941–948. DOI: 10.3109/09638288.2016.1172672

8. **Do patients without a mental health diagnosis benefit from psychosocial assessment and intervention?**
Certainly. All patients can benefit from attention to their psychological reactions and adjustment to changes in their health, functioning, and body status. Health improvement requires active engagement to make changes and in rehabilitation; it requires physical participation. Many times, patients are aware of what they need to do to promote health and/or healing but are unsure of how to structure their efforts, how to start, and, importantly, how to maintain their behaviors over time. For example, patients may say something to the effect of, "My doctor told me to quit smoking, but he didn't tell me how." There are also times when patients do not feel engaged nor motivated to make changes to their behavior or functioning and may appear disconnected from the rehabilitation process. Occasionally, there are times when patients are flatly resistant to engagement and may not wish to participate in rehabilitation efforts for one reason or another. Implementation and maintenance of health-related behavior change often requires psychological intervention.

Wilding S, Conner M, Prestwich A, et al. Using the question-behavior effect to change multiple health behaviors: an exploratory randomized controlled trial. *J Exp Soc Psychol.* 2019;81:53–60. Available at: https://doi.org/10.1016/j.jesp.2018.07.008

Knecht S, Kenning P. Changing health behavior motivation from I-must to I-want. *Prog Brain Res.* 2016;229:427–438. Available at: https://doi.org/10.1016/bs.pbr.2016.06.013

Johnson SK, von Sternberg K, Velasquez MM. Changing multiple health risk behaviors in CHOICES. *Prev Med Rep.* 2018;11:69–73. Available at: https://doi.org/10.1016/j.pmedr.2018.05.006

9. **What are the major steps for implementing self-management approaches for people with chronic health concerns?**
Patients must:
   1. **accept responsibility** for their health and for seeking solutions
   2. **acquire specific health knowledge** regarding the causes and treatments for health conditions
   3. **implement solutions in partnership** with the treatment team and family
   4. Sustain success by establishing **habits**

Hart T, Dijkers MP, Whyte J, et al. A theory-driven system for the specification of rehabilitation treatments. *Arch Phys Med Rehabil.* 2019;100(1):172–180.

10. **I have explained the new injury or illness, but the patient does not appear to understand the need for adaptive methods. How should the rehabilitation team approach this concern?**
During rehabilitation, patients are confronted with multiple simultaneous changes that can overwhelm and disorient. Sudden dysfunction threatens sense of self, identity, life roles, relationships, and capacity to engage in desired activities. For example, patients with new spinal cord injury (SCI) may reject the use of wheelchairs in spite of the functional benefits; it is important to try to elicit a better understanding of the patients' perceptions rather than forcing new demands. The adjustment process is fraught with **conflicts between stereotypic views of disability and distorted views of self**. These include worry about how others will view and react to their new status. Individuals with disabilities regularly must navigate often inhospitable/inaccessible public spaces, manage transportation challenges, and confront issues of prejudice and discrimination related to disability status, even

within the health care system. Patients often ruminate rather than explore how disability will impact their valued roles and activities. Assistance with **cognitive "reframing"** and open-minded **active trial of adaptive methods** in chosen environments often catalyzes success.

Villarosa-Hurlocker MC, O'Sickey AJ, Houck JM. Examining the influence of active ingredients of motivational interviewing on client change talk. *J Subst Abuse Treat.* 2019;96:39–45. Available at: https://doi.org/10.1016/j.jsat.2018.10.001

11. How do we therapeutically support patients' emotional reactions to illness, injury, or disability?

Many people have heard of the five stages of grief model, or the **Kübler-Ross Model** of grief, which proposes that one goes through a series of five emotional stages including denial, anger, bargaining, depression, and then finally reaches acceptance. While this theory is widely known within popular culture and referenced frequently, studies have not empirically demonstrated the sequential progression of these stages.

For those experiencing injury and confronting the possibility of long-term disability, ranges of emotions including sadness, anger, and fear are situationally congruent. These intense and strong emotions do not necessarily require a diagnosis, and the absence of these emotions or the presence of happiness, hope, and indicators of **resilience** do not necessarily indicate a pathological state of denial. However, it is important to distinguish between normative emotional reactions versus those that may interfere with the person's rehabilitation performance and would benefit from intervention. Research demonstrates mental health symptoms can negatively impact various health outcomes; thus it is important to assess and treat these symptoms early in the rehabilitation process.

Morin R, Galatzer-Levy I, Bonanno G. Experiencing multiple major health events does not reduce resilience: a comparison of depression and mortality following single and multiple events. *Arch Phys Med Rehabil.* 2016;97(10):E126–E127. Available at: https://doi.org/10.1016/j.apmr.2016.08.394

Hewson D. Coping with loss of ability: "Good grief" or episodic stress responses? *Soc Sci Med.* 1997;44(8):1129–1139. Available at: https://doi.org/10.1016/S0277-9536(96)00244-4.

Elliott TR, Frank RG. Depression following spinal cord injury. *Arch Phys Med Rehabil.* 1996;77(8):816–823. Available at: https://doi.org/10.1016/S0003-9993(96)90263-4

12. My patient says, "I don't want to live like this!" What should I do?

Acute functional loss, coping with complications and consequences, as well as the new, challenging, and **painful processes of adaptation** commonly contribute to existential **expressions of suffering**. These expressions may be related to suicidal thoughts and intent; however, they can also be expressed in the absence of intent for self-harm or intent to die. Sometimes, patients are simply unable to envision a future in their new state and feel hopeless about their ability to endure and adapt. If can often be helpful for patients to explore their worries with a supportive and knowledgeable team member who can then assist them with gathering additional information to either educate them on realistic challenges or contradict their preillness/injury assumptions about disability. In all cases, it is important to discuss with the patient what he or she is experiencing and when it began, to consider how to intervene and support. **Open communication, nonjudgment,** and **acceptance of authentic expressions of mood are critical for the success of these conversations.**

Whenever a health care provider is confronted with a suicidal or death-focused statements (e.g., thoughts of hopelessness, death, and overt suicidality), it is important to immediately **assess for risk of suicide attempt** and to triage to additional evaluation and care if needed. Desire to die without plans or intent for suicide is often referred to as **passive thoughts of suicide**. Providers need to communicate to patients that an assessment of risk is a direct response to our concern for them as individuals. While this process can be distressing for patients, frequently the patient can also recognize **the genuine caring of the team**, which can be therapeutic in itself.

Anyone making these types of comments needs to be followed closely including consideration of psychological intervention and/or suicide precautions. Both passive and active suicidal statements indicate a **dynamic mix of ambivalent thoughts and feelings** about death. While this may be along a continuum of severity, it **can fluctuate quickly** depending on a number of risk factors.

Dazzi T, Gribble R, Wessely S, et al. Does asking about suicide and related behaviours induce suicidal ideation? What is the evidence? *Psychol Med.* 2014;44(16):3361–3363.

13. Suicidal ideation seems like an uncomfortable topic to bring up. Is there guidance on how to specifically talk with and assess patients?

The Suicide Assessment Five-step Evaluation and Triage (SAFE-T) provides a sequential procedure:
- Identification of **risk factors**
- Identification of **protective factors**
- Direct inquiry about **suicidal thoughts**, **plan(s)**, **behavior(s)**, and **intent**

- **Risk determination** and **intervention selection**
- **Documentation** and **follow-up**

  The Chronological Assessment of Suicidal Events (CASE) approach is also a helpful.

  Asking about "giving up or hurting yourself" can in many ways be therapeutic; asking about suicide and self-harm is shown to reduce suicidal ideation and provides an opportunity for help and treatment.

  A psychological expert should be available to every treatment team. It is appropriate to consult an expert in cases of suicidal ideation to assist with evaluation and treatment planning. However, if risk is high, getting the patient to emergency services (i.e., emergency department [ED], psychiatric intake/triage for hospitalization) should be the highest priority.

Betz ME, Boudreaux ED. Managing suicidal patients in the Emergency Department. *Ann Emerg Med*. 2016;67(2):276–282. Available at: https://doi.org/10.1016/j.annemergmed.2015.09.001.

Shea SC. The chronological assessment of suicide events: a practical interviewing strategy for the elicitation of suicidal ideation. *J Clin Psychiatry*. 1998;59(Suppl 20):58–72.

14. What psychological interventions are commonly used to address mood, coping, and participation?

    Interventional modalities are selected based on the diagnostic and symptom presentation, taking into consideration the specific needs, personality, thoughts, and communication style of each patient.

    - **Cognitive behavioral therapy (CBT)** first codeveloped by Dr. Aaron Beck in the 1960s is now framed in the **Mediational Model**, which recognizes **emotions, cognitions, and behaviors are interlinked and mutually dependent**. Thus a change in one will affect the other two. For example, an intervention designed to change the patient's perception of a situation impacts mood and willful acts. CBT has been scientifically demonstrated as an evidence-based intervention for a number of different chronic conditions.

Butler AC, Chapman JE, Forman EM, et al. The empirical status of cognitive-behavioral therapy: a review of meta-analyses. *Clin Psychol Rev*. 2006;26(1):17–31. Available at: https://doi.org/10.1016/j.cpr.2005.07.003

Hoffman JM, Ehde DM, Dikmen S, et al. Telephone-delivered cognitive behavioral therapy for veterans with chronic pain following traumatic brain injury: rationale and study protocol for a randomized controlled trial study. *Contemp Clin Trials*. 2019;76:112–119. Available at: https://doi.org/10.1016/j.cct.2018.12.004

Cohen JN, Gopal A, Roberts KJ, et al. Ventilator-dependent patients successfully weaned with cognitive-behavioral therapy: a case series. *Psychosomatics*. 2019;60(6):612–619. Available at: https://doi.org/10.1016/j.psym.2019.02.003

Hofmann SG, Asmundson GJG. *The Science of Cognitive Behavioral Therapy*. Available at: https://www.sciencedirect.com/book/9780128034576/the-science-of-cognitive-behavioral-therapy

15. What is MI?

    How can the care team improve culture to refine family centered care?

    1. The **Rehabilitation Engagement Collaborative** (REC) is a collaboration between Johns Hopkins University School of Medicine's Department of Physical Medicine & Rehabilitation and Craig Rehabilitation Hospital. REC aims to assist rehabilitation professionals in delivering patient- and family-centered care and promote a collaborative rehabilitation culture. Their website includes a variety of resources for rehabilitation clinicians and teams/institutions; they have videos focusing on how to handle treatment impasses, managing social avoidance, balancing reality and hope, patient hopes, and provider expertise, and promoting independence in self-care.
       a. REC
    - **MI**: MI is a patient-centered intervention designed to assist the individual in eliciting motivation and advancing to establishing a plan for specific behavior change. MI works by resolving ambivalence through directed conversation and questioning to drive patient-centered decision-making. Specific methods include asking permission, evoking change talk, exploring confidence and importance, use of open-ended questions, use of reflective listening, and assessing readiness to change.

Rollnick S, Miller W. What is motivational interviewing? *Behav Cogn Psychoth*. 1995;23(4):325–334. Available at: https://doi.org/10.1017/S135246580001643X

BOOKS

Atul G. *Being Mortal: Medicine and What Matters in the End*. New York, NY: Metropolitan Books, Henry Holt and Company; 2014.

Brenner LA, Reid-Arndt SA, Elliot TR, et al. *Handbook of Rehabilitation Psychology*. 3rd ed. Washington, D.C. American Psychological Association; 2019:559.

Engel G. The need for a new medical model: a challenge for biomedicine. *Science*. 1977;196:129–136.

Kabat-Zinn J. *Full Catastrophe Living: Using the Wisdom of Your Body and Mind to Face Stress, Pain, and Illness.* New York, NY: Dell Publishing; 1991.

Mackinnon RA, Michaels R, Buckley PJ. *The Psychiatric Interview in Clinical Practice.* 3rd ed. Washington, DC: American Psychiatric Association Publishing; 2016:704.

Miller WR, Rollnick S. *Motivational Interviewing: Helping People Change.* 3rd ed. New York, NY: Guilford Press; 2013.

Paul K, ed. *Psychological Management of Physical Disabilities: A Practitioner's Guide.* London Rootledge/Taylor & Francis Group; 2007.

Posner K, Oquendo MA, Gould M, et al. Columbia classification algorithm of suicide assessment (C-CASA): classification of suicidal events in the FDA's pediatric suicidal risk analysis of antidepressants. *Am J Psychiatry.* 2007;164(7):1035–1043.

Wright BA. *Physical Disability: A Psychosocial Approach.* 2nd ed. New York, NY: Harper & Row; 1983.

Yuker HE, ed. *Attitudes Toward Persons With Disabilities.* New York, NY: Springer; 1998.

BIBLIOGRAPHY

Betz ME, Boudreaux ED. Managing suicidal patients in the Emergency Department. *Ann Emerg Med.* 2016;67(2):276–282. Available at: https://doi.org/10.1016/j.annemergmed.2015.09.001. http://www.sciencedirect.com/science/article/pii/S0196064415012640

Emmons KM, Rollnick S. Motivational interviewing in health care settings: opportunities and limitations. *Am J Preventive Med.* 2001;20(1):68–74. Available at: https://www.sciencedirect.com/science/article/pii/S0749379700002543?via%3Dihub

Grzesiak RC, Hicok DA. A brief history of psychotherapy and physical disability. *Am J Psychother.* 1994;48(2):240–250. Available at: https://doi.org/10.1176/appi.psychotherapy.1994.48.2.240

Hewson D. Coping with loss of ability: "Good grief" or episodic stress responses?. *Soc Sci Med.* 1997;44(8):1129–1139. Available at: http://www.sciencedirect.com/science/article/pii/S0277953696002444

Huffman JC, Feig EH, Rachel A. Usefulness of a positive psychology-motivational interviewing intervention to promote positive affect and physical activity after an acute coronary syndrome. *Am J Cardiol.* 2019;123(12):1906–1914. Available at: https://www.science-direct.com/science/article/pii/S0002914919303212?via%3Dihub

NEUROMUSCULOSKELETAL EVALUATION OF THE REHABILITATION PATIENT: INTEGRATING DIFFERENT PIECES OF THE PUZZLE TO LOCALIZE LESION, ASSESS FUNCTION, AND PLAN THERAPY

Albert Recio, MD, PT, Susan Wortman-Jutt, MS, CCC-SLP, Amy Bialek, MS, PT, and Rajiv R. Ratan, MD, PhD

CHAPTER 10

You may not control all the events that happen to you, but you can decide not to be reduced by them
— Maya Angelou (1928–2014)

KEY POINTS

1. Delirium affects a person's attention, whereas dementia affects memory.
2. Although the distribution of weakness is similar in myasthenia gravis and neuromuscular junction disorders, neuromuscular junction disorders are characterized by **fatigability,** worsen with use, and recover with rest.
3. **Apraxia** is a cerebral motor planning disorder of purposeful movements, whereas **ataxia** is a cerebellar disorder of motor coordination.

1. What are the objectives of the neuromusculoskeletal examination in physical medicine and rehabilitation (PM&R)?
   - Confirm the diagnosis
   - Quantify impairment
   - Identify functional capabilities for compensation
   - Record a baseline for future comparisons
   - Screen for complications, deterioration, and additional neuromusculoskeletal disorders

2. Identify the key components of the neurological examination.
   The neurologic evaluation of the rehabilitation patient includes:
   - Mental status
   - Cranial nerves
   - Motor function (tone, reflexes, strength, adventitial movements)
   - Sensory function (touch, pain, temperature, proprioception, vibration, stereognosis, two-point discrimination)
   - Cerebellar function
   - Functional motor activity (screening for apraxia, dressing, and gait)
   - Speech, language, swallowing function

Neuroexam.com: www.neuroexam.com

Manji H, Connolly S, Kitchen N, et al. *Oxford Handbook of Neurology.* 2nd ed. Oxford: Oxford University Press. 2014

3. What is the Mini-Mental State Exam (MMSE)?
   The **MMSE** is a short (5 to 10 minutes) 30-point questionnaire used to detect cognitive impairment. It quantifies and estimates the severity of cognitive changes over time. It assesses functions including **registration** (repeating named prompts), **attention** and **calculation**, **recall, language**, ability to follow simple **commands, and orientation**.

Folstein M, Folstein S. *Mini-Mental State Examination.* 2nd ed™. Available at: https://www.parinc.com/Products/Pkey/238

4. How does one differentiate between delirium and dementia?

Delirium affects a person's attention, whereas **dementia** affects memory. Often, delirium is caused by an illness or drug toxicity and is most often a reversible condition. Dementia is caused by anatomic changes in a person's brain and is irreversible. See Table 10.1 for additional comparison between delirium and dementia.

Marshall K , Hale D. Delirium , dementia, and depression. *Home Healthc Now*. 2017 Oct;35(9):515–516.

5. How does one differentiate between dementia and aphasia?

Dementia is a clinical state characterized by the significant loss of function in multiple cognitive domains and interferes with activities of daily living (ADLs). Unlike patients with dementia who may experience concomitant language deficits, patients with aphasia do well during nonverbal memory tasks.

Medscape. Articles on Neurology. Available at: www.emedicine.com/neuro/index.shtml

6. How does one determine the difference between aphasia and agnosia?

Aphasia is a language disorder that may be accompanied by motor speech deficits and is generally described as either "fluent" or "nonfluent." Difficulty with naming, grammar, and comprehension is common in aphasia. **Agnosia** is a deficit in perceiving or recognizing people or objects. In visual agnosia, the patient may not recognize that two objects are identical. Other forms of agnosia include auditory agnosia or **prosopagnosia** (inability to recognize faces).

National Aphasia Association. Agnosia. Available at: https://www.aphasia.org/aphasia-resources/agnosia

7. Define unilateral neglect.

Unilateral neglect is a lack of orienting responses to stimuli presented unilaterally. Neglect cannot be diagnosed unless the primary sensory or motor modalities required to sense or orient the particular stimulus are intact. Neglect can be unimodal (i.e., visual neglect) or multimodal (i.e., performing complex tasks, such as dressing, in which the patient fails to cover the neglected side). **Hemineglect** is most commonly associated with right hemisphere damage but can be caused by strokes or tumors affecting either hemisphere. Neglect is prognostic of poor functional recovery but can improve with targeted therapies and challenging positioning.

Azouvi P , Jacquin-Courtois S , Luauté J. Rehabilitation of unilateral neglect: evidence-based medicine. *Ann Phys Rehabil Med* . 2017 Jun;60(3):191–197.

8. After excluding visual field defects and disorders of eye movements, how does one evaluate neglect at the bedside?

- Line bisection: Have the patient mark the center of five horizontal lines, each presented separately on a sheet of paper.
- Line cancelation: Present the patient with a single sheet of paper on which 20 lines in varying orientations are drawn on each half of the page.
- Letter cancelation: Instruct the patient to mark all the As on a sheet of paper. There should be eight As on the sheet, four on each side, with 70 distractor letters (e.g., D, L, F, R).
- Clock construction: Have the patient place numbers as they would appear on a clock face, with a circle outline on a piece of paper.

With the aforementioned test, performance on the left side can be compared with performance on the right side.

Azouvi P. The ecological assessment of unilateral neglect. *Ann Phys Rehabil Med* . 2017 Jun;60(3):186–190

CRANIAL NERVE EVALUATION

9. How should one evaluate the integrity of the patient's visual fields?

Stand approximately 3 feet in front of the patient, and ask him or her to focus on your nose. Hold your hands to either side of your face, midway between your eyes and the patient. Briefly present one or two fingers from each hand, and ask the patient to indicate the number of fingers on each hand. Give the patient one or two trials to make sure that the nature of the trial is understood. The hands should be moved so that all four quadrants of the visual field are tested. These tests will enable detection of a field defect or neglect.

During testing, encourage the patient to maintain fixation on your nose. If the patient is uncooperative, bedside confrontation of the visual fields can provide diagnostic information. In the patient who is uncooperative or lethargic, a visual threat may cause an asymmetric blink response if there is field deficit or neglect.

10. What is the first question to ask a patient who complains of diplopia (double vision)?

"Does the diplopia go away when you cover one eye?" **Monocular diplopia** (double vision that persists with only one eye viewing) is usually caused by a problem with the lens or cornea. **Binocular diplopia** (double vision that disappears with only one eye viewing) is usually a result of paralysis of extraocular muscles.

11. How does one evaluate the seventh cranial nerve?

Paying particular attention to the nasolabial folds and palpebral fissures, look for facial asymmetry at rest and during spontaneous facial movements. Then systematically test the **frontalis muscle** ("raise your eyebrows"), **orbicularis oculi** ("close your eyelids, and don't let me open them"), **buccinator** ("blow out your cheeks"), elevators of the lips ("show me your teeth; smile"), **orbicularis oris** ("purse your lips, and don't let me open them").

Upper motor lesions generally cause lower facial weakness with a slight asymmetry of the palpebral fissures and little or no weakness of the orbicularis oculi or frontalis muscles. Lower motor neuron lesions result in weakness of the upper and lower parts of the face and can involve **taste (chorda tympani)** and **tearing (greater superior petrosal nerve)**.

MOTOR EXAMINATION

12. How do you distinguish between upper motor neuron (UMN) and lower motor neuron (LMN) deficits?

UMN deficit leads to hypertonicity, hyperreflexia, spasticity with a positive Babinski sign, and/or muscle atrophy due to disuse. LMN injury results in hypotonicity, hyporeflexia, flaccidity, and/or muscle atrophy due to denervation. The function of the **hypoglossal nerve, CN XII,** can be observed by asking the patient to protrude the tongue at the midline. A tongue that deviates opposite the side of the lesion indicates UMN damage. A tongue deviating toward the side of the lesion indicates an LMN lesion. LMN lesions may also be characterized by tongue fasciculation and atrophy.

13. What is the Hoffman sign?

The **Hoffman sign** or reflex is a test to examine for hyperactive reflexes of the upper extremities and can discriminate between central and peripheral lesions. Flexion of the index finger and thumb indicates a positive Hoffman sign. Hoffman reflex is elicited by first supporting the patient's relaxed suspended hand by holding at the wrist. The examiner then triggers a quick brisk stretch of the patient's finger flexors by slipping his or her thumbnail down off the edge of the patient's middle fingernail, causing a quick extension as it slips off the edge. A positive abnormal reflex demonstrates **spreading** of finger flexion onto all fingers and the thumb.

14. What is the Babinski sign?

The **Babinski sign** is dorsiflexion of the great toe in response to a plantar stimulus. It indicates an interruption of UMN tracts to the lumbosacral spinal reflex centers, as seen in spinal cord injury, stroke, and multiple sclerosis.

15. Describe one grading system for reflexes.

- Grade 0 = absent reflex
- Grade 1 = hypoactive reflex, or normal reflex that can be elicited only with reinforcement
- Grade 2 = normal reflex
- Grade 3 = hyperactive reflex
- Grade 4 = clonus

16. What can one do if one cannot obtain a response when eliciting a reflex? What is the Jendrassik maneuver?

Make sure to bounce the hammer on the taught tendon to produce a quick stretch. Reflexes can be "tuned" to maximum by varying tension of the musculotendinous unit voluntarily or passively. Reinforcement can be achieved by having the patient perform a strong voluntary contraction of a muscle the examiner is not testing. The **Jendrassik maneuver** is a reinforcement for muscle stretch reflexes below the arms. The patient hooks hands together by the flexed fingers and isometrically pulls apart as hard as possible.

Gregory JE, Wood SA, Proske U. An investigation into mechanisms of reflex reinforcement by the Jendrassik's manoeuvre. *Exp Brain Res.* 2001;1383:366–374.

17. What does the presence of clonus indicate?

Hyperreflexia caused by a central nervous system (CNS) lesion although nonsustained clonus can also be elicited in patients with acute anxiety.

18. **How is clonus at the ankle elicited?**
Quick dorsiflexion of the foot is the stimulus followed by continuous light supportive pressure under the ball of the foot. The brisk dorsiflexion triggers reflex plantarflexion that reoccurs felt in "beats."

19. **Define spasticity versus rigidity, and how is it assessed?**
Spasticity is velocity-dependent resistance to passive joint movement. Spasticity usually involves some specific groups of muscles more than others. For instance, after a cerebral lesion, a patient may become hemiplegic and have greater spasticity in flexor muscles of the upper extremity and extensor muscles of the lower extremity (**decorticate pattern**). **The Modified Ashworth Scale and Tardieu Scale provide guidelines for quantifying severity of spasticity.**
   Rigidity is defined as consistent resistance appreciated by the examiner throughout the range of joint movement. The **cogwheel sign** corresponds to an intermittent but rachety opposition to passive motion. The resistance affects flexor and extensor muscles in the involved limb equally.
   "Lead pipe" rigidity suggests damage or dysfunction of the **extrapyramidal system (basal ganglia)** such as idiopathic Parkinson disease or drug-induced parkinsonism (e.g., metoclopramide, haloperidol, reserpine).

Bohannon RW, Smith MB. Interrater reliability of a modified Ashworth scale of muscle spasticity. *Phys Ther.* 1987;67:206–207.

20. **What are the clinical manifestations of proximal versus distal muscle weakness?**
Lower Extremity:
   • Proximal weakness: Inability to get up from a chair or toilet without using one's hands; Inability to get out of a car
   • Distal weakness: Frequent tripping or unusual wear on the toes of the shoes
Upper Extremity:
Proximal weakness: Inability to lift arm up to touch head or face during grooming tasks; inability to carry grocery bags or young children
   • Distal Weakness: Inability to fasten buttons, open jars, or hold onto things

21. **What are the common causes and clinical features of myopathy?**
Common causes of myopathy may include steroids, alcohol, zidovudine (azidothymidine [AZT]), hypothyroidism, Duchenne muscular dystrophy, polymyositis, acquired immunodeficiency syndrome (AIDS), and mitochondrial diseases.
   Nearly asymmetric proximal muscle weakness without muscle wasting, with normal sensory examination, and with intact or slightly decreased reflexes.

22. **What is the critical clinical difference between myopathies and disorders of the neuromuscular junction (e.g., myasthenia gravis)?**
Although the distribution of weakness is similar in these disorders, neuromuscular diseases are characterized by **fatigability.** They worsen with use and recover with rest.

RANGE OF MOTION

23. **Define active range of motion (AROM) and passive range of motion (PROM).**
AROM is the ROM through which the patient can move the joint. PROM is the ROM through which the examiner can move the joint.

24. **Can PROM be less than AROM?**
Never. PROM must be greater than or equal to AROM.

25. **Are there other forms of ROM besides PROM and AROM?**
Yes.
   • Active-assisted ROM: Patient assisted by the therapist
   • Progress-resistive exercises (PREs): Progressively heavier weights are used while applying a formula based on the subject's maximum strength at onset

Gallo FP. *Energy Diagnostic and Treatment Methods.* New York, NY: W W Norton & Co; 2000.

26. **What joints do the ROM of shoulder abduction measure?**
Glenohumeral and scapulothoracic. There are approximately 2 degrees of a glenohumeral joint motion for every degree of scapulothoracic joint motion, termed **scapulohumeral rhythm.**

27. **In shoulder abduction ROM, how does the glenohumeral joint move as the scapulothoracic joint moves?**
There are approximately 2 degrees of a glenohumeral joint motion for every degree of scapulohumeral joint motion.

28. **Which shoulder ROM is usually limited by early inflammatory arthritis?**
    Internal rotation.

29. **Describe the Schroeber test.**
    It measures the patient's ability to flex their lower back. The posterior spinous processes do not spread apart as the patient bends forward, and flexion occurs predominantly from hip motion.

30. **What does the Spurling test detect?**
    Cervical spine radiculopathy suggested by simultaneous cervical lateral flexion and cervical spine extension to narrow the neural foramina and generate symptoms that radiate in a dermatomal pattern.

31. **What does the Thomas test evaluate?**
    The presence of a hip flexion contracture. It is measured when the patient is lying supine on a firm surface, and the hip opposite the side measured is flexed, holding the thigh to the chest to eliminate lumbar lordosis.

32. **Does the straight-leg-raising test measure full ROM (FROM) of hip flexion?**
    No. The knee must be flexed to eliminate hamstring resistance and measure the full extent of hip joint flexion.

MANUAL MUSCLE TESTING (MMT)

33. **Why is MMT performed, and what do results indicate?**
    Results help to define impairment and focus a program to improve function. Results indicate the one-repetition maximal concentric contraction of the muscle. Be aware of abnormal muscle tone because this is not an indicator of strength. Assessors should ensure appropriate and consistent positioning for accurate results.

34. **How are muscles graded in MMT?**
    - 0/5 = No palpable contraction or motion
    - 1/5 = Trace motion observed
    - 2/5 = FROM when not against gravity only
    - 3/5 = FROM against gravity, but not against additional resistance
    - 4/5 = FROM against gravity and minimal to moderate resistance
    - 5/5 = Normal strength; FROM against gravity and normal resistance for age and size

Hislop HJ, Montgomery J. *Daniels and Worthington's Muscle Testing: Techniques of Manual Examination.* 7th ed. Philadelphia: W.B. Saunders; 2002.

Peterson Kendall F, Kendall McCreary E, Geise Provance P, McIntyre Rodgers M, Romani WA. *Muscles: Testing and Function, with Posture and Pain (Kendall, Muscles).* Fifth, North American Edition; 2005

35. **Does deconditioning cause focal muscle weakness?**
    No. Deconditioning leads to decreased endurance in all muscles.

36. **What can cause focal muscle weakness?**
    Focal neuropathies, nerve entrapment, mononeuritis, injuries, trauma, or myopathies.

37. **What does a hand-held dynamometer measure?**
    It measures force in pounds or kilograms of the contracting muscle at midrange using the "make and break" technique.

Andrews AW, Thomas MW, Bohannon RW. Normative values for isometric muscle force measurements obtained with hand-held dyna-mometers. *Phys Ther.* 1996;76:248–259.

SENSORY EVALUATION

38. **Define the primary and secondary sensory modalities.**
    Primary sensory modalities include pain, temperature, light touch, proprioception, and vibratory sensation. Primary sensory loss can be caused by a lesion in the periphery, spinal cord, brain stem, or thalamus. **Stereognosis** (form sense, as in identifying a nickel or penny placed in the hand) and **topognosia** (ability to localize skin stimuli) are **secondary sensory** or cortical sensory modalities.

39. **What is a proper way to test pain sensation?**
    With a clean safety pin. The advantage of a safety pin is that it has a blunt end and a sharp end, thus allowing the reliability of the patient to be tested.

40. What is an optimal way to test position sense?
Position sense should be tested in the hands or feet. The distal end of the third or fourth digit or toe should be used because these have the least cortical innervation and are thus the most sensitive to a loss in position sense. The digit should be grasped laterally and moved up or down or maintained in a neutral position. It is helpful to perform the test a few times with the patient's eyes open to be sure communication is established. With the eyes closed, the patient should make no mistakes on five trials. If abnormalities are found in one digit or two, other digits or toes should be tested.

41. What frequency tuning fork should be used for vibration testing?
256 Hz.

SENSORY AND MOTOR ANATOMIC LANDMARK

42. Name the anatomic landmarks that delineate different dermatomes and myotomes.

Dermatomes	Myotomes
• C2—angle of the jaw	Neck flexion
• C3—supraclavicular fossa	Neck side flexion
• C4—acromioclavicular joint	Shoulder elevation
• C5—proximal forearm	Biceps (elbow flexion)
• C6—thumb	Extensor carpi radialis (wrist extension)
• C7—middle finger (third digit)	Triceps (elbow extension)
• C8—little finger (fifth digit) Finger Flexors (flexor carpi ulnaris)	
• T1— medial antecubital fossa	Small finger Abduction (abductor digiti minimi)
• T4—nipple	
• T10—umbilicus	
• L2—anterior medial thigh	Hip Flexion
• L3—medial femoral	Knee Extension
• L4—knee cap	Knee Extension and Quadriceps
• L5—big toe	Tibialis Anterior
• S1—lateral foot	Gastrocnemius Muscle
• S4, S5—perianal area	External Anal Sphincter

CEREBELLAR ASSESSMENT

43. What are the clinical features of cerebellar disease?
The main features of cerebellar dysfunction can be remembered by the mnemonic
HANDS Tremor:
- H = Hypotonia
- A = Asynergy (lack of coordination)
- N = Nystagmus (ocular oscillation)
- D = Dysarthria (speech abnormalities/scanning speech)
- S = Station and gait (ataxia)
- Tremor = Coarse intention tremor

44. Distinguish cerebellar ataxia from sensory ataxia.
- Cerebellar ataxia
  - Nystagmus
  - Hypotonia
  - Coarse intention tremor
  - Dysarthria
- Sensory ataxia
  - Loss of vibration and position sense
  - Loss of reflexes
  - Ataxia worse with eyes closed (positive Romberg sign)

45. What is the best way to describe someone with cerebellar dysfunction?
They look intoxicated with a broad-based gait.

46. Identify some common causes of cerebellar dysfunction seen in the rehabilitation setting.
Strokes, multiple sclerosis, and anticonvulsants (phenytoin, phenobarbital, carbamazepine).

47. How can coordination of the arms be tested?

Have the patient perform a finger-to-chin test. Instruct the patient to touch the examiner's finger, then touch his or her own chin. Repeat this sequence several times while altering the position of your finger with each trial. The chin is used instead of the nose because many patients with cerebellar dysfunction have such poor coordination that they are in danger of poking their own eye. If the patient undershoots or overshoots the examiner's fingers (**past pointing**), the test is considered indicative of cerebellar dysfunction.

Detailed neurologic exam of the adult. Available at: www.uptodate.com

Powers DW. Assessment of the stroke patient using the NIH stroke scale. *Emerg Med Serv.* 2001;30(6):52–56.

48. Describe the heel-to-shin test.

This is another test evocative of leg ataxia. While lying down or sitting, the patient is instructed to place the heel of one leg on the opposing knee and to run the heel straight down to the shin to the ankle.

Bonus questions and answers available online.

CHAPTER 11

GAIT: A CLINICAL AND BIOMECHANICAL OVERVIEW

Deidre Casey Kerrigan, MD, MS

And he do the walk, do the walk of life. Yeah, he do the walk of life.

— Dire Straits (1985)

KEY POINTS: GAIT

1. Walking and running are distinguished by the presence or absence of a "double limb support" phase of gait.
2. Double limb support typically comprises 20%–25% of a normal walking gait cycle.
3. Key factors that determine gait include heel rise, pelvic rotation, pelvic tilt, knee flexion, foot and knee motion, and lateral displacement of the pelvis.
4. At a normal walking speed, generally 60% of a gait cycle is spent in stance and 40% in swing. The time in stance decreases as walking speed increases.
5. An ankle-foot orthosis (AFO) lowers energy utilization by simulating push-off and raising the center of gravity (COG) in terminal stance.

1. **Describe the gait cycle and associated terminology.**
   - **Gait cycle**: Fundamental unit of gait. Defined as one foot strike* to a repeat of same foot strike.
   - **Stride length**: Distance between sequential points of contact of the same foot.
   - **Step length**: Distance between corresponding contact points of opposite foot.
   - **Cadence**: Number of steps per unit time (e.g., steps/min).
   - **Speed**: Calculated as cadence × step length.

Biomechanics of Foot Strikes & Applications to Running Barefoot or in Minimal Footwear. Available at: http://barefootrunning.fas.harvard.edu/4BiomechanicsofFootStrike.html. (Accessed 2019).

   See Fig. 11.1.

2. **What is the terminology of gait analysis?**
   Older terms used to describe gait, such as heel strike, heel-off, and toe-off, are dated because they often do not apply to the range of gait types (e.g., walking, running, and other gait patterns) observed in clinical practice and across varying disabilities. Fig. 11.2 illustrates the components differentiated according to function: weight acceptance, single limb support, and limb advancement. The first two terms constitute the stance period, and the last is the swing period. Stance is further subdivided into four phases: initial contact, loading response, midstance, terminal stance, and preswing. Swing is composed of three phases: initial swing, midswing, and terminal swing.

3. **Discuss the classical determinants of gait.**
   Factors that determine gait were originally described (Saunders, Inman, & Eberhart) as natural mechanisms in human motion used to reduce movement and create a smooth path for the body's center of mass (COM). More recently, three of the factors originally described (pelvic rotation, pelvic tilt, and knee flexion) were shown to affect the vertical displacement of the COM by only a small amount. The heel rise of the trailing limb in double limb support is now considered the major element minimizing vertical displacement of the COM.

4. **Does the COM matter? Does COM shift during ambulation?**
   Although the exact location of the COM varies with body type and limb position, it is usually 5 cm anterior to the second sacral vertebra. The average total displacement of the COM is generally 5 cm along the vertical axis and 5 cm on the horizontal axis for a typical adult male step. The displacement of the COM changes depending on

---

*Foot strike: Portion of the gait cycle where the foot (heel or forefoot) hits the ground.

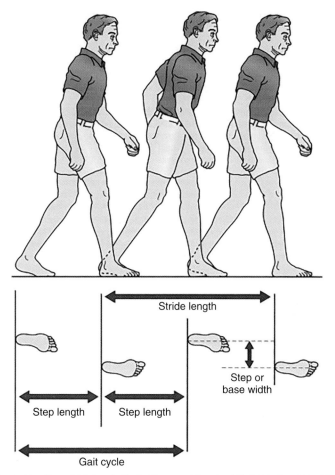

Fig. 11.1 Gait cycle. (From Magee DJ. Orthopedic Physical Assessment. Saunders: Philadelphia; 2014:981–1016 [Chapter 14].)

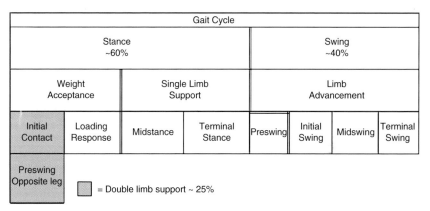

Fig. 11.2 Gait cycle and its phases.

one's height and step length but is close to half of what it would be except for the determinants of gait listed as follows.

Key factors that determine gait and their impact:

- **Heel rise**: Reduces the COM's overall displacement by usually 6 to 8 mm. This is the main factor reducing COM displacement.
- **Pelvic rotation**: Generally raises the COM's predicted lowest point by 2.0 to 2.5 mm.
- **Pelvic tilt (also called "list" or "obliquity")**: Happens at midstance, increases effective leg length, and lowers the COM's predicted highest point by 2 to 3 mm.
- **Knee flexion**: Takes place at midstance and lowers the COM's predicted highest point by 2 mm.
- **Foot and knee motion**: The ankle pivots on the posterior heel during initial contact. The pivot point progresses to the forefoot by terminal stance, and knee and foot motions serve to smooth motion into a sinusoidal curve.
- **Lateral displacement of the pelvis**: Valgus alignment at the knees, along with hip adduction, place the feet closer together and create less movement of the center of gravity (COG) in the horizontal plane.

5. Distinguish walking and running.
   Double limb support is typically 20% to 25% of a normal walking gait cycle. As walking speed increases, the time spent in double support decreases. Walking then becomes running when there is no period of double support.

6. During walking and running, when is COG highest and lowest?
   While walking, COG is the highest in midstance during single-limb support and lowest at first contact during double support. However, during running, it is at its highest point in the "flight" portion and its lowest in midstance of single limb support.

7. Explain why walking and running require more energy than wheelchair mobility.
   While walking and running, the body's COM must rise and fall with each step. However, in wheelchair ambulation, the COM stays horizontal. The work done in walking a certain distance can be determined by the vertical displacement of the COM $\times$ body weight $\times$ number of steps.

8. What is a comfortable walking speed?
   A comfortable walking speed occurs when the energy expended per unit distance is at a minimum (i.e., comfort equals efficiency). In an able-bodied adult, this rate is usually 80 m/min, or 3 mph. The energy used is 0.15 mL O_2/kg/m. When biomechanical function is not normal, an increased energy cost results and often lowers the walking speed.

9. During a typical walking cycle, how much time is allocated to stance versus swing phases?
   At a normal walking speed, generally 60% of a gait cycle is spent in stance and 40% in swing. The time in stance decreases as walking speed increases.

10. What is the difference between kinematics and kinetics?
    Kinematics studies the motions of joint and limb segments. Kinetics focuses on the forces and torques causing joint and limb motion. Gait laboratories currently use a three-dimensional (3D) multicamera system to gather kinematic data in all three planes of motion (sagittal, coronal, and transverse) and a computer to combine ground reaction forces from forceplates to create a 3D picture of torques and joint forces.

11. Is a gait laboratory analysis really necessary? If so, when?
    An analysis is useful for cases of upper motor neuron pathology in which static evaluation of strength and tone may be inaccurate. For example, spasticity that is evident during static examination may not be seen during ambulation. Gait analysis measures the requirement and the effect of therapeutic intervention. It can also aid in selecting a correct orthosis, a program of therapy, or surgery. In addition, the results sometimes are able to suggest a different treatment plan for a patient whose performance has leveled.

12. What is antalgic gait?
    When a person with lower extremity pain walks, gait is modified to reduce weight bearing on the involved side. The normal limb rapidly advances to shorten stance on the affected side. Gait is often slow and steps are short, to limit the weight-bearing period.

13. Define steppage gait.
    A compensatory gait that uses excessive hip and knee flexion to assist a "functionally long" lower leg and foot to clear the ground. This is seen with equinus deformity (excessive plantar flexion) during swing caused by weak dorsiflexors, heel cord contracture, or gastrocsoleus spasticity.

14. What is gluteus medius (Trendelenburg) gait and its etiology?
    This gait results from either weak hip adductors (gluteus medius) or hip pain from osteoarthritis and is recognized by increased pelvic tilt opposite the affected side. To compensate for this tilt, the trunk bends toward the affected side so the COG directly above the hip during the stance phase remains unchanged. This bend lessens the large adductor moment, avoids the need for hip abductors, and reduces the forces across the hip joint. A useful treatment is a cane used contralaterally during the stance period of the affected side. With increasing speed and less time in the stance phase, the gait deviation is less noticeable.

15. Which gait pattern can be identified by its sound?
The foot-slap of a patient with a partial foot-drop can be heard as the foot moves quickly from initial contact to loading response. This is caused by moderately weak (grades 3 or 4) dorsiflexors. During the time from initial contact to loading response, the dorsiflexors must eccentrically contract to slow the forward fall of the body. If they are very weak (grade 2 or less), a steppage gait appears because there is not enough strength to lift the forefoot from the ground. This gait is silent.

16. Which gait pattern relates to weak hip extensors?
The person walks with an extensor lurch. The trunk is hyperextended at the hip to prevent a rapid forward fall at initial contact ("jackknifing").

17. How do changes in gait and assistive devices impact energy use?
The amount of energy expenditure is related to the type of gait abnormality and the assistive device used. See *Data Set 11.1*.

18. How does an elderly person's gait differ from that of someone younger?
There are numerous differences in lower extremity joint parameters in older adults compared with younger ones. However, the only persistent difference when older adults walk at an increased speed, compared with younger subjects, is a decreased peak hip extension. This extension is reduced further in older adults who have a history of falls, compared with older adults without such a history.

19. During quiet standing, which muscles maintain the body in an upright (erect) position?
The ground reaction force for erect posture acts along the line of gravity through the COM and passes in front of the ankle and knee and behind the hip. The hip is then supported by the iliofemoral ligament and the knee by the posterior popliteal capsule without muscle involvement. Ankle stability is achieved by continuous contraction of the gastrocsoleus to produce a stabilizing ankle joint moment (i.e., a torque).

20. Give possible causes of genu recurvatum during the stance.
   • Plantarflexion contracture (which causes a knee extension moment through a closed kinetic chain);
   • Quadriceps weakness;
   • Plantar flexor spasticity;
   • Quadriceps spasticity.

21. At what point does knee flexion contracture significantly affect gait?
Any knee flexion contracture compromises gait function. However, a contracture of 30 degrees or more affects all aspects of the gait cycle. Contractures of this severity (or greater) often produce a leg-length discrepancy.

22. Does varus or valgus knee alignment affect the progress of knee osteoarthritis during walking?
Yes. Ambulating with greater than 5 degrees of varus alignment increases the risk that medial compartment knee osteoarthritis will worsen. Similar results happen for valgus alignment and lateral compartment knee osteoarthritis. An increase in varus knee torques has been correlated with worsening medial compartment knee osteoarthritis.

Data Set 11.1 Energy Cost of Lower Extremity Impairments: Impairment Increase in Energy Use by Percentage[a]

Ankle fusion: 13
Bilateral TF/TF: 120
Bilateral TT/TT: 33
Crutches NWB: 41–78
Crutches PWB: 18–36
Hemiparesis: 88
Hip fusion: 47
Knee flexed, 15 degrees: 13
Knee flexed, 30 degrees: 27
Knee immobilized: 33
Traumatic TF: 33
Traumatic TT: 7
Vascular TF: 87
Vascular TT: 13

NWB, Non–weight-bearing; *PWB*, partial weight-bearing; *TF*, transfemoral amputation; *TT*, transtibial amputation.
[a]Energy expenditure is usually measured at comfortable walking speed with prosthesis in place and without an upper extremity assistive device, except for crutches.

23. **Can a shoe insole modify joint biomechanics in patients with knee osteoarthritis?**
Quantitative gait analysis of a 5-degree lateral-wedge insole has shown a significant reduction (6%) of peak knee varus torques. Although a 10-degree lateral-wedge insole reduces the same torques by 8%, study subjects did not tolerate it as well.

24. **Do high-heeled shoes increase the risk of osteoarthritis of the knees?**
Gait analysis of women who wear high-heeled shoes ($\geq$2.5 in.) has revealed increased force across the patellofemoral joint and a 23% greater compressive force on the medial compartment of the knee while walking in high heels compared with walking barefoot. As bilateral osteoarthritis of the knee is twice as common in women as in men, it is likely that high heels are a predisposing risk factor.

25. **Are moderately high–heeled shoes also a risk factor?**
Gait analysis has also shown that women's shoes with a moderate heel elevation (1.5 in.) increase knee varus torque by 14% and knee flexor torque by 19%. This is considered a risk factor in developing knee osteoarthritis and its progression.

26. **What effects do traditional athletic shoes having a slight heel elevation and arch support cause?**
An athletic shoe with a somewhat elevated heel and arch support significantly increases knee varus torque by almost 10% during walking. Increases in both knee varus and knee flexion torques (38% and 36%, respectively) have been recorded. An arch support alone significantly increases peak knee varus torque by 6% while walking and 4% while running.

27 **How does plastic or metal ankle-foot orthosis (AFO) reduce the energy used in hemiparetic movement?**
AFO lowers energy utilization by simulating push-off, and raising the COG in terminal stance. This is its most important feature. Walking speed increases, and foot-drop is prevented in the swing phase. In patients with hemiparesis that affects their gait, energy expenditure per unit distance is often 74% greater than normal with an AFO but 88% higher without one. There is no significant difference in energy expenditure between various AFOs.

28. **Are children small adults in their gait?**
No!

29. **List mobility milestones in infants.**
- Walks with support by 1 year;
- Walks unsupported by 15 months;
- Runs by 18 months, on average;
- Mature gait by 3 years.

30. **How does a toddler's gait differ from an adult's?**
- Wider base of support;
- Reduced stride length with a higher cadence;
- No heel strike;
- Only slight knee flexion during standing;
- Reciprocal arm swing not present;
- External rotation of the entire leg during the swing phase, periods, tasks, and phases of the gait cycle.

WEBSITES

American Society of Biomechanics. Available at: www.asb-biomech.org
Clinical Gait Analysis. Available at: http://espace.curtin.edu.au/handle/20.500.11937/51997
Gait and Clinical Movement Analysis Society. Available at: www.gcmas.net/index.html
International Society of Biomechanics. Available at: www.isbweb.org
University of Virginia Physical Medicine and Rehabilitation Gait Lab. Available at: www.healthsystem.virginia.edu/internet/pmr/Biomechanics.cfm

BIBLIOGRAPHY

Fisher SV, Gullickson G Jr. Energy cost of ambulation in health and disability: a literature review. *Arch Phys Med Rehabil.* 1978;59(3):124–133.
Franz JR, Dicharry J, Riley PO, et al. The influence of arch supports on knee torques relevant to knee osteoarthritis. *Med Sci Sports Exerc.* 2008;40(5):913–917.
Gard SA, Childress DS. The effect of pelvic list on the vertical displacement of the trunk during normal walking. *Gait Posture.* 1997;5:233–238.
Gard SA, Childress DS. The influence of stance-phase knee flexion on the vertical displacement of the trunk during normal walking. *Arch Phys Med Rehabil.* 1999;80:26–32.
Gonzalez E, Corcoran PJ. Energy expenditure during ambulation. In: Downey JA, ed. *Physiological Basis of Rehabilitation Medicine.* 2nd ed. Boston, MA: Butterworth-Heinemann; 1994:413–446.

Harris GF, Wertsch JJ. Procedures for gait analysis. *Arch Phys Med Rehabil.*1994;75:216–225.

Keenan GS, Franz JR, Dicharry J, et al. Lower limb joint kinetics in walking: the role of industry recommended footwear. *Gait Posture.* 2011;33(3):350–355.

Kerrigan DC, Della Croce U, Marciello M, et al. A refined view of the determinants of gait: significance of heel rise. *Arch Phys Med Rehabil.* 2000;81:1077–1080.

Kerrigan DC, Franz JR, Keenan GS, et al. The effect of running shoes on lower extremity joint torques. *PM R.* 2009;1:1058–1063.

Kerrigan DC, Johansson JL, Bryant MG, et al. Moderate-heeled shoes and knee joint torques relevant to the development and progression of knee osteoarthritis. *Arch Phys Med Rehabil.* 2005;86:871–875.

Kerrigan DC, Lee LW, Collins JJ, et al. Reduced hip extension during walking: healthy elderly and fallers versus young adults. *Arch Phys Med Rehabil.* 2001;82:26–30.

Kerrigan DC, Lelas JL, Goggins J, et al. Effectiveness of a lateral-wedge insole on knee varus torque in patients with knee osteoarthritis. *Arch Phys Med Rehabil.* 2002;83:889–893.

Kerrigan DC, Riley PO, Lelas JL, et al. Quantification of pelvic rotation as a determinant of gait. *Arch Phys Med Rehabil.* 2001;82:217–220.

Pease WS, Bowyer BL, Kadyan V. Human walking. In: Delisa JA, Gans BM, eds. *Physical Medicine and Rehabilitation Medicine Principles and Practice.* 4th ed. Philadelphia, PA: Lippincott Williams and Wilkins; 2005:155–167.

Saunders JB, Inman VT, Eberhart HD. The major determinants in normal and pathological gait. *J Bone Joint Surg Am.* 1953;35-A:543–558.

Sharma L, Song J, Felson DT, et al. The role of knee alignment in disease progression and functional decline in knee osteoarthritis. *JAMA.* 2001;286:188–195.

Waters RL, Mulroy S. The energy expenditure of normal and pathologic gait. *Gait Posture.* 1999;9:207–231.

5 ELECTRODIAGNOSTIC EVALUATION OF NEUROMUSCULAR CONDITIONS

BASIC ELECTRODIAGNOSIS: INTERPRETATION OF ELECTRICAL MANIFESTATIONS OF NEUROMUSCULAR DISORDERS

Marvin McClatchey Brooke, MD, Rubin I. Devon, MD, Janet C. Limke, MD, Steven A. Stiens, MD, MS, and Lawrence R. Robinson, MD

Genius hath electric power which earth can never tame.

— Lydia M. Child (1802–1880)

KEY POINTS

1. Nerve conduction studies (NCSs) and electromyography are the most frequent electrodiagnostic studies. They give objective measurements of electrical activity in peripheral nerves, nerve roots, and muscles.
2. NCSs allow you to electrically stimulate at multiple locations along a nerve and record the conducted depolarization waveforms. These waveform responses can be normal or abnormal in shape. The nerve conduction velocity (NCV) is calculated as measured distance/divided by the recorded response latency time.
3. Electromyography records the muscle's electrical activity to reveal the electrophysiological function of muscle fibers, anterior horn cells, axons, myoneural junctions, and terminal axon branches.
4. The location and type of abnormalities also help indicate a diagnosis, a more exact process location, timing since onset, stage, how extensive, and recovery progress.
5. Electrodiagnostic findings correlate closely with electrophysiology and diagnosis and should be combined with the history and physical examination and other evidence to confirm, suggest, or rule out diagnoses and aid in the monitoring of disease, treatment, and prognosis.

1. What is electrodiagnosis?
   Electrodiagnosis uses electrodiagnostic studies that record evolved and spontaneous electrical potentials that are volume conducted through the body to detect normal and pathologic patterns that are helpful in diagnosis and prognosis. Nerve conduction studies (NCSs) and electromyography are most frequently done.
   Other central nervous system electrodiagnostic studies such as electroencephalography, evoked potentials, operative monitoring, and neuromuscular stimulation and research topics are not discussed here.

Electromyography and Nerve Conduction Studies: Background, Indications, Contraindications. Available at: https://emedicine.medscape.com/article/2094544-overview#a6

Interpreting Neurophysiology (EMG & NCS)—YouTube. Available at: https://www.youtube.com/watch?v=k8OX8j3Dqn4

2. What is the role of electrodiagnosis in the evaluation of a patient?
   General electrodiagnostic testing (i.e., NCSs, needle electromyography) is used as an extension of the neurologic examination to evaluate patients with neuromuscular conditions.
   An NCS is done by first stimulating the **distal** nerve with a superficial electrode. The response, a **compound motor action potential** (CMAP), is recorded from an active electrode over the muscle. This **response** will appear on screen after the stimulus artifact and further to the right at the time in millisecond called the **latency**. The nerve conduction velocity (NCV) of a nerve from a proximal to a distal stimulation site produces recorded proximal and "distal latency" times from stimulation artifact to response action potentials. The measured **distance** over the nerve segment divided by the **time** difference of latencies gives a NCV. Distal latencies and conduction velocities can be compared to other nerve segments and the lab or published normal values (see Fig. 12.1).

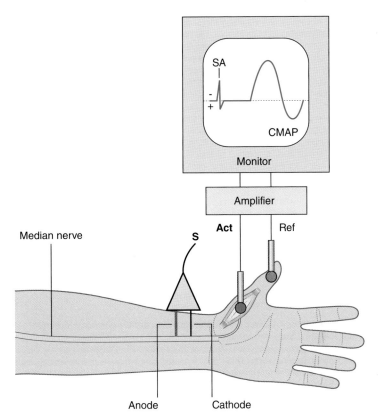

Fig. 12.1 Basic setup for recording a compound motor unit action potential (MUAP) and a distal latency for a median motor nerve conduction study.
1. The active electrode (A) is placed over the abductor pollicis brevis (APB) muscle belly at the midpoint between the distal wrist crease and the metacarpolphalangeal (MCP) joint of the thumb.
2. The reference electrode (R) is placed over the APB tendon at the first MCP joint.
3. The ground electrode (G) is placed on the palm or dorsum of the hand. The median nerve is stimulated at the wrist between the tendons of Flexor Carpi Radialis (FCR) and Palmaris Longus, 8 cm proximal to the Active electrode (A).
4. The distance is measured in a hockey-stick-shaped line from the A electrode to the midpoint of the distal wrist crease and then to the point of stimulation following the anatomic course of median nerve.
Permission Reproduced with permission Mtui E, Gruener G, Declory P. *Fitzgerald's Clinical Neuroanatomy and Neuroscience.* 8th ed. Elsevier; 2021. Chapter 12 electrodiagnostic examination. (Fig. 12.1 basic set up for recording a compound motor unit action potential. Fig. 12.4 NCV motor nerve conduction velocity and Fig. 12.16 reinnervation of motor end plates. Motor unit action potential.) Fitzgerald Fig. 12.1.

The **goals** of an electrodiagnostic examination are to: (1) confirm a suspected clinical diagnosis, (2) exclude alternative diagnoses, (3) localize a lesion, (4) identify subclinical involvement in other regions, (5) determine underlying pathophysiology, (6) determine chronicity, and (7) determine severity. The common NCSs and needle examination can also be used as an objective measure to follow over time, such as in patients with inflammatory myopathy, autoimmune neuropathies, or myasthenia gravis. **Urgent acute nerve injury studies** can help determine if a nerve decompression, reanastomosis (or graft) is needed. Other less common electrodiagnostic studies (e.g., somatosensory evoked potentials, motor evoked potentials) are used to assess the integrity of the central somatosensory and motor pathways and can be used to assist in the diagnose of central nervous system disorders. These techniques are also used in the intraoperative setting to monitor for central and peripheral nervous system injuries during surgery.

3. What nervous system anatomic pathways are assessed by electrodiagnostic studies?
    Electromyography and NCSs test for disorders of the peripheral nervous system, including the levels of the spinal cord, reflex pathways, motor and sensory nerves, and motor unit (MU). The basic electrodiagnostic tests of electromyography and NCSs stimulate and measure the **anatomic structures and physiology** of the: (A) MU, including the anterior horn cell and axons coursing through ventral nerve root and nerve and the innervated muscle fibers, and (B) **sensory nerve** axons extending up to the cell body in the dorsal nerve root ganglion, from which some projections and interneurons modulate the firing of anterior horn cells.

The higher central nervous system **voluntary motor pathway anatomy and physiology** is not directly tested during routine NCSs and needle electromyography. The **contralateral** motor cortex has 90% of cortex axonal **pyramidal track** output descend, cross in the lower medulla to the opposite side, descend into the **lateral cortical spinal tract**, and terminate primarily on spinal cord **interneurons** or directly on the **anterior horn cells**, which discharge and activate the MU. Muscle tone is not directly studied in electrodiagnosis but can be affected by the sensory nerve stretch and pain receptors, including spindle reflexes (e.g., deep tendon reflexes) and gamma motor neurons affecting intra-fusil muscle fibers with their own stretch receptors.

The multiple **other cortical and spinal pathways** include multiple intra-cortical and crossing contralateral cortical and descending pathways that are not usually assessed with electrodiagnostic testing and are not as accessible because of their central location. The 10% of primary motor cortex output that does not descend to the pyramidal track includes descending motor pathways to the basal ganglia and contralateral cerebellum. They impact motor control, coordination, associated movements (e.g., trunk and balance) and muscle tone much more than isolated movements. They may impact patient function and examination procedure. These other pathways are correlated with other diseases and other parts of functional motor control. Future research, diagnosis, and therapy may make them more pertinent to electrodiagnosis. One example is increasing evidence, and use of electromyographic EMG triggered functional neuromuscular electrical stimulation of movement. Another future example is research on the cerebellar nucleus interpositus, which is contralateral to the primary motor cortex and stimulates primate C56 shoulder abduction and flexion and then wrist and hand extension before grasp.

Thanawalla AR, Chen AI, Azim E. The cerebellar nuclei and dexterous limb movements. *Neuroscience.* 2020;450:168–183. doi: 10.1016/j.neuroscience.2020.06.046.

Daube JR, Rubin DI. Needle electromyography. *Muscle Nerve.* 2009;39:244–270.

Course 1—EMG and NCV Principles—YouTube. Available at: https://www.youtube.com/watch?v=PURNQ15oUnU&t=57s

4. What are the limitations of nerve conduction and electromyographic studies?
NCSs are performed by electrically stimulating a nerve and recording either: (A) **axonal depolarization** over the nerve (during a sensory or mixed nerve study [MNS]); or (B) a **motor action potential** over the muscle innervated by the nerve (during a motor nerve study). NCSs study the integrity of the nerve, neuromuscular junction, and muscle. Several parameters are recorded including amplitude, conduction velocity, and distal latency. The findings are compared to reference values.
The following are several limitations of these tests:
- **NCSs** only test large, myelinated nerves. In neuropathies that affect small, unmyelinated fibers (e.g., **small fiber neuropathies**), routine NCSs are normal.
- NCSs may only demonstrate an **amplitude reduction** when there is a significant loss of axons or muscle fibers. Therefore, in mild neurogenic disorders (e.g., mild radiculopathies) or myopathies, NCSs are commonly normal and may not identify the underlying problem. Furthermore, even though the amplitudes of the NCSs responses may correlate to some degree with functional deficits, the NCSs amplitudes can be maintained with reinnervation. This means that, even with a loss of MUs, this correlation is not always precise.
- Routine NCSs test **distal** segments of the limbs. While proximal NCSs can be performed, they are technically more difficult.
- Sensory NCSs are abnormal in disorders involving the **sensory axons at or distal to the dorsal root ganglion** (DRG). In nerve root diseases that affect the dorsal rami, before the DRG for the cell body, sensory NCSs will not demonstrate an abnormality, even in the context of clinical sensory loss or pain.
  All NCSs are prone to a multitude of **technical problems** (e.g., cold temperature, improper filter or gain settings, electronic noise) that can result in false-negative or false-positive findings. **Operator-dependent factors**, such as inappropriate nerve or muscle selection, measurement error, or under stimulation, can also result in erroneous findings. Careful attention to the details of the technique and identification of the technical problems is critical to obtaining reliable results.
Electromyography is the recording of electrical activity that occurs from muscle fibers at rest, and during voluntary activation, in order to detect electrophysiological abnormalities.
Routine intramuscular needle EMG primarily evaluates the small type 1 MUs and does **not assess sensory fibers**.
The needle electrode only detects signals a **few millimeters from** the tip of the needle and **does not determine the size of the entire MU.**
Needle EMG provides only **pathophysiologic** information and does **not** translate directly to an **etiology** in most cases.

A Basic Intro to NCS/EMG for Neurologists—YouTube. Available at: https://www.youtube.com/watch?v=HZH95nMsVKM

5. What are the contraindications of nerve conduction study and needle examination?
NCS and needle examination are safe procedures when performed by experienced personnel. However, some contraindications and possible risks may be present, so patients should be informed of the risks and side effects.

The main risk of NCS is transient discomfort from the electrical stimuli. There is a relative contraindication of stimulation near a **pacemaker, cardiac defibrillator, or other implanted electrical device**. Routine NCS in limb nerves, including repetitive nerve stimulation, can be safely performed in most cases.

One potential risk of needle EMG is hematoma formation. Consideration for whether to perform needle EMG in patients with **bleeding disorders** such as hemophilia or severe thrombocytopenia should be carefully made. Anticoagulation is a relative risk for bleeding, bruising, and pain. Needle examination should not be performed in an area of skin infection due to the risk of introducing infectious organisms when penetrating the skin. Needle examination near peri-plural muscles, such as serratus anterior or diaphragm, poses a potential risk of pneumothorax.

6. How do you plan and carry out the electrodiagnostic examination?
   The goals of the electrodiagnostic examination, which is also an electrodiagnostic **consultation,** are to provide sufficient diagnostic **confirmation** and **elimination** of other possible **differential diagnoses** within a reasonable timeframe and with the least patient discomfort. The electrodiagnostician puts the patient at ease and obtains the history and physical examination.

   Based on the referral question, history, and examination, a list of differential diagnoses to rule in or out can be developed and the appropriate anatomic structures and locations to test strategically selected. Nerve conduction and needle electromyography studies can be planned. For example, if one diagnosis to confirm is right L5 spinal level radiculopathy in a patient with a history of back pain for 6 weeks, weak extensor hallucis longus and ankle dorsiflexion weakness (i.e., a "footdrop, slapping or skipping" gait); the first test planned might be motor NCSs and needle EMG of distal and proximal right L5-S1 muscles, including the tibialis anterior and posterior muscles, gluteus medius and maximus muscles, and paraspinals. Other non-L5-S1 muscles would also be checked (expecting them to be normal) to help localize the appropriate root.

7. How are the electrodiagnostic parameters affected by the frequency of the filters?
   All waveforms recorded during electrodiagnostic studies are composed of various frequencies. To eliminate non-physiologic noise, high- and low-frequency filters (LFF) are used in EMG machines. Alteration of low and high-frequency filters can affect NCS and needle EMG waveforms. Raising the LFF has more effect on the CMAP than sensory nerve action potential (SNAP) since the CMAP contains more lower frequencies. On the other hand, CMAP is not significantly affected by slightly lowering the high-frequency filter. Raising the LFF will filter lower frequency components of the motor unit potential (**MUP**) or motor unit action potential (**MUAP**) during needle EMG, resulting in a shorter MUP duration (*see* Table 12.1).

Table 12.1 Effect of Filter Frequency on SNAP Parameters

PARAMETERS OF SNAP	ELEVATED LOW-FREQUENCY FILTER	LOWERED HIGH-FREQUENCY FILTER
Onset latency	No change	Increased
Peak latency	Decreased	Increased
Amplitude	Decreased	Decreased

SNAP, Sensory nerve action potential.

8. What is the impact of temperature on electrodiagnostic measurements?
   Temperature changes have an impact on NCS and, less so, on needle EMG. Cool limb temperature slows the kinetics of channels along the membrane, thereby slowing depolarization and repolarization and slowing conduction time.

   Nerve conduction velocities: Cooling results in a longer time for the action potential to propagate and a net slowing of conduction. For each $1\,^{\circ}C$ drop in temperature, there is an approximately 5% decrease in NCV.

   SNAP and CMAP amplitude: When cool, the duration of an action potential gets longer, and the amplitude gets larger. Because of prolonged opening times of the sodium channels, larger action potentials are seen from individual axons and the nerve as a whole.

   Conduction block: With low temperature, slow opening and even slower closing of ion channels lead to prolonged ion channel opening time and increased influx of Na^+, resulting in prolonged action potential duration. This extra duration may be long enough to excite or skip a short, demyelinated segment. Therefore, the conduction block can be overcome by cooling.

   Spontaneous and voluntary EMG potentials: Cooling leads to desynchronization, which results in an increase in the duration of the **MUAP** and increased polyphasia. The amplitude of the MUAP may or may not increase depending on the pattern of cooling. Fibrillations and positive waves decrease in frequency with cooling, whereas fasciculations may increase.

Rutkov SB. Effects of temperature in neuromuscular electrophysiology. *Muscle Nerve.* 2001;24:867–882.

Neurophysiology for Neurologists—YouTube. Available at: https://www.youtube.com/watch?v=WmmV3xiYAdE

9. How does age impact electrodiagnostic testing?

NCV slows with age, and different normal ranges of conduction velocity can be used, for example, over the age of 80. It is best if each laboratory has its own normal values to determine if the results are normal or abnormal, and the normal range is included in the report itself. Extremity length is controlled for by measuring a standard length of the nerve segment between two stimulation points to calculate the velocity. Muscle mass as well as strength decrease with age separately from the impact on NCV. NCS amplitudes and conduction velocities vary with age groups in the pediatric population, and reference tables for age should be used in the interpretation of studies in children.

Punga AR, Jabe JF, Amandusson Å. Facing the challenges of electrodiagnostic studies in the very elderly (>80 years) population. *Clin Neurophysiol.* 2019; 130:1091–1097.

10. Describe the difference between a monopolar and concentric needle electrode used during needle EMG?

Needle EMG is performed by inserting a thin recording needle electrode into a muscle to record the muscle fiber action potentials. Two types of electrodes are used routinely: **monopolar** and concentric. A monopolar electrode is a fine Teflon-coated needle with a conical recording tip. A separate surface electrode is applied to the skin as a reference electrode. A **concentric** needle electrode is a single needle with a hollow shaft and a fine recording needle in the center. The central wire is referenced to the shaft of the electrode (*see* Figs. 12.2–12.5).

(Basic Overview of Electromyography David C. Preston MD, Shapiro BE. Electromyography and neuromuscular disorders: clinical-electrophysiologic-ultrasound correlations, fourth edition. *J Clin Neurophysiol.* 2021;38(4):e19. Figs. 12.1–12.4.) Note figures may be from 3rd ed adjust citation and link as needed to bring up the same images.)

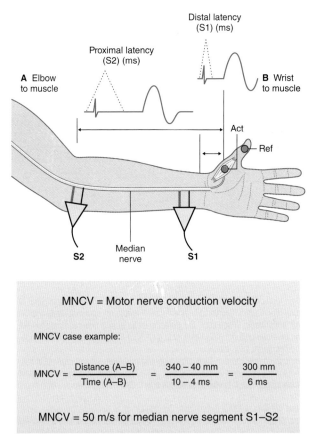

MNCV = Motor nerve conduction velocity

MNCV case example:

$$\text{MNCV} = \frac{\text{Distance (A–B)}}{\text{Time (A–B)}} = \frac{340 - 40 \text{ mm}}{10 - 4 \text{ ms}} = \frac{300 \text{ mm}}{6 \text{ ms}}$$

MNCV = 50 m/s for median nerve segment S1–S2

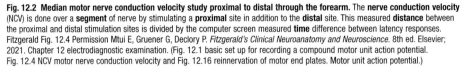

Fig. 12.2 Median motor nerve conduction velocity study proximal to distal through the forearm. The **nerve conduction velocity** (NCV) is done over a **segment** of nerve by stimulating a **proximal** site in addition to the **distal** site. This measured **distance** between the proximal and distal stimulation sites is divided by the computer screen measured **time** difference between latency responses. Fitzgerald Fig. 12.4 Permission Mtui E, Gruener G, Declory P. *Fitzgerald's Clinical Neuroanatomy and Neuroscience.* 8th ed. Elsevier; 2021. Chapter 12 electrodiagnostic examination. (Fig. 12.1 basic set up for recording a compound motor unit action potential. Fig. 12.4 NCV motor nerve conduction velocity and Fig. 12.16 reinnervation of motor end plates. Motor unit action potential.)

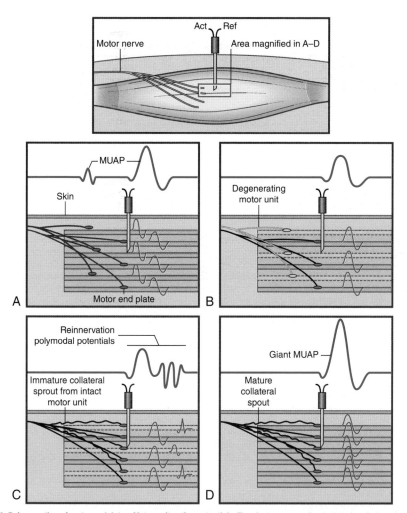

Fig. 12.3 Reinnervation of motor endplates. Motor unit action potentials. The **electromyography** study is done by inserting a needle into the muscle to record the electrical **motor unit action potential** (MUAP) responses. There is some **insertional** activity caused by moving the needle through muscle fibers. **Resting** activity while the muscle is resting is usually absent or minimal but may show abnormal potentials after insertion of the needle. When the patient is asked to **contract** the muscle slightly, a single motor unit (MU) **axon** depolarizes through **terminal axons** to **motor end plates** on multiple muscle **fibers**. (A) A single compact **MUAP** is generated by the motor fibers near the needle depolarizing at the same time. (B) If the axon is abnormal, the potential may be **smaller** and may be more spread out. (C) If terminal axons or slowed or reinnervation is occurring, the potential may be spread out and be **polyphasic**. (D) Later, the **"mature"** axon may be depolarizing many more fibers at one time and appear as a **giant** MUAP. Fitzgerald Fig. 12.16. Permission Mtui E, Gruener G, Declory P. Fitzgerald's Clinical Neuroanatomy and Neuroscience. 8th ed. Elsevier; 2021. Chapter 12 electrodiagnostic examination. (Fig. 12.1 basic set up for recording a compound motor unit action potential. Fig. 12.4 NCV motor nerve conduction velocity and Fig. 12.16 reinnervation of motor end plates. Motor unit action potential.)

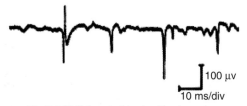

Fig. 12.4 Fibrillation potential and positive sharp waves.

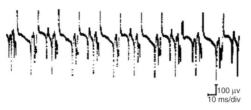

Fig. 12.5 Complex repetitive discharge.

Monopolar electrodes are less expensive than concentric needles. They have a larger recording area than concentric needles, and because they are referenced to a distant surface electrode, they record more baseline noise than concentric needles. MU potentials are slightly larger when recorded with monopolar electrodes than with concentric needles.

11. **What is insertion activity?**
Insertion activity refers to myoelectric **depolarization potentials triggered by a needle** moving through a resting muscle. When a needle electrode is inserted into a resting muscle, it causes brief depolarization of a few muscle fibers that are irritated by the electrode, producing a burst of spikes. Usually, the spikes only fire briefly during the needle movement, and no continuous activity occurs following the cessation of needle movement. However, conditions associated with denervation or dysfunction of muscle membranes may cause insertion activity to be **increased** with repeated spikes after cessation of needle movement. Conditions associated with muscle fiber atrophy or replacement by connective tissue may cause **decreased** electrical activity during needle movement and decreased insertion activity. After insertion of an EMG needle into the normal muscle **at rest, no electrical activity** is usually seen after the initial burst of insertional activity unless the needle is near an end-plate zone.

Neuropathy EMG Changes explained—YouTube. Available at: https://youtu.be/3i1xc9ddr4k

12. **Describe the sounds, waveforms, and firing patterns of common spontaneous potentials recorded inside of muscles**
Spontaneous activity refers to involuntary electrical potentials recorded in muscle at rest. There are several types of spontaneous waveforms, which can be distinguished by their firing patterns (defined by the change in the interpotential intervals) and sounds. These include:
- **Fibrillation potentials**: Regular firing pattern (often with gradual slowing of rate). They sound like a "ticking" clock.
- **Positive sharp waves (PSWs)**: Regular firing pattern, often with gradual slowing of rate (e.g., the sound of a "tocking" clock).
- **End-plate spikes (EPSs)**: Irregular firing pattern (e.g., the sound of fat frying in a pan).
- **Fasciculation potentials**: Irregular firing pattern (e.g., the sound of first few kernels of corn beginning to pop).
- **Complex repetitive discharges (CRDs)**: Regular firing rate; start, stop, or change abruptly (e.g., the sound of a motorboat or jackhammer).
- **Myokymic discharges**: Regular or semi-rhythmic firing pattern of bursts of potentials (e.g., the sound of soldiers marching in formation).
- **Myotonic discharges**: Exponentially changing firing pattern (e.g., the sound of dive-bombers attacking a target).
- **Neuromyotonic discharges**: Exponentially changing firing pattern at rates greater than 150Hz (e.g., the sound of a high-pitched "ping"; a racecar traveling at very high RPMs).

Daube JR, Rubin DI. Needle electromyography. *Muscle Nerve*. 2009;39:244–270.

EMG Waveform Trainer. Available at: http://www.aanem.org/Education/All-Education-Products/Product-Details?productid={8CEC405D-500C-E411-B3BF-00155D0A6803}

American Association of Neuromuscular & Electrodiagnostic Medicine. Improving the Lives of Patients with Neuromuscular Diseases. Available at: www.aanem.org

13. Define a motor unit and motor unit action potential
The **motor unit** is defined as a single anterior horn cell, the axon and its branches, and all the muscle fibers (10 to 1500 fibers) innervated by that motor neuron. A MU territory is 5 to 10 mm in diameter. Normally, each muscle fiber produces an action potential with a duration of approximately 1 to 3 ms. A motor unit action

potential (**MUAP**), seen and heard on an EMG machine, video display, and speaker, is the machine-processed representation of the summation of electrical potentials recorded from muscle fibers of a MU close to the needle and discharging when the anterior horn cell "fires." A MUAP is usually composed of 5 to 20 muscle fibers. The morphology of the MUAP can be extrapolated to determine the overall size and function of the MU and determine the type of neuromuscular disease.

Quantitative EMG 3—YouTube. Available at: https://youtu.be/rARqGYKiNMI

14. What are the EMG characteristics of fibrillation potentials?

Fibrillation potentials are the spontaneous firing single muscle fiber action potentials generated from fibers that have lost their innervation. The precise mechanism for the generation of fibrillation potentials is not known, although they may be due to acetylcholine hypersensitivity, the regulation of receptors, and fluctuating muscle membrane resting potential in a denervated fiber. This reduces the threshold for depolarization. Fibrillation potentials are recognized by their regular firing pattern, often with a gradual slowing of rate. Fibrillations are non-specific and found in many different neurogenic and myopathic disorders. They are seen in neurogenic disorders in which there has been a loss of axons (e.g., radiculopathies, axonal polyneuropathies, mononeuropathies, motor neuron disorders) and are also found in myopathies characterized by muscle fiber necrosis, splitting, or vacuolar changes (e.g., inflammatory myopathies, muscular dystrophies). They are rarely seen in severe neuromuscular transmission disorders.

Fibrillation potentials have amplitudes from 20 to 1000 μv that vary with the proximity of the needle electrode to the muscle fiber generating the action potential and the diameter of the muscle fiber. The morphology of a fibrillation potential varies and may be biphasic or triphasic.

Positive Waves and Fibrillation Potentials—YouTube. Available at: https://youtu.be/jjUZMf8_B1k

EMG Waveform Trainer. Available at: http://www.aanem.org/Education/All-Education-Products/Product-Details?productid={8CEC405D-500C-E411-B3BF-00155D0A6803}

15. What are positive sharp waves and their EMG characteristics?

Positive sharp waves (PSWs) are a form of fibrillation (spontaneous depolarization of a single muscle fiber), which is seen as a biphasic morphology consisting of a sharp initial positive (downward) deflection followed by a return to baseline. Amplitudes range from 10 μv to 3 mv.

The PSWs' morphology occurs when the action potential is generated at a distance from the tip of the recording needle electrode but cannot propagate past the electrode due to damage to the muscle fiber by the needle electrode or disease. PSWs often appear with spike form fibrillation potentials but may be seen earlier than spike form fibrillation potentials after a nerve injury. PSWs are seen in the same types of disorders as spike form fibrillation potentials.

Gatens PF, Saeed MA. Electromyographic findings in the intrinsic muscles of normal feet. *Arch Phys Med Rehabil.* 1982;63:317–318.

Kimura & Kohara: F17 Fibrillation Potentials and Positive Sharp Waves—YouTube. Available at: https://www.youtube.com/watch?v=k1RIQv6rdWQ

16. Describe the EMG characteristics of end-plate spikes and miniature end-plate potentials

End-plate spikes (EPSs) are single muscle fiber local depolarizations originating from the end-plate zone, triggered by the needle electrode. They usually have an initial negative muscle fiber action potential, although they can be initially positive if recorded just outside the end-plate zone. EPSs are irregular in rhythm and, unlike fibrillations, are only recorded at the end-plate zone. Miniature end-plate potentials (MEPPs) are also known as **end-plate noise** and have been compared to the noise heard when holding a seashell to one's ear. MEPPs are non-propagating potentials recorded from the end-plate zone and result from the spontaneous release of acetylcholine vesicles during the resting state.

17. What are complex repetitive discharges?

Complex repetitive discharges (CRDs) are continuous "**trains**" of complex action potential discharges that may begin spontaneously or after needle movement (*see* Fig. 12.2). They have a regular firing pattern with constant frequency, shape, and amplitude. They may sound like very regular and moderately fast train wheels hitting steel rail bumps. However, there may be abrupt changes in configuration or firing rates. Firing rates are typically 20 to 150 Hz. They probably originate from **ephaptic activation** (i.e., direct activation by local electrical currents) of groups of adjacent muscle fibers and are seen in chronic neuropathic and myopathic disorders.

Complex Repetitive Discharges Explained—YouTube. Available at: https://youtu.be/EFJsxseTjJE

18. What are fasciculation potentials?

Fasciculation potentials are the spontaneous discharge of either an entire MU (all innervated muscle fibers connected to their **anterior horn cell**) or a portion of fibers in the same MU. Fasciculations are often visible or palpable in the superficial muscles but may not be visible in the deep muscles. The source is usually instability of the motor neuron cell body, its axon, or the distal nerve terminals. The waveforms of fasciculation potentials reflect the morphology and distribution of the underlying motor fiber potential—they may be normal morphology or large in neurogenic disorders. Fasciculation potentials fire in an irregular, random pattern. Fasciculations may be seen in normal individuals. Benign and pathologic forms of fasciculations can look similar and are best distinguished by looking for associated abnormalities such as fibrillation potentials or abnormal MU morphology.

Kimura & Kohara: F32 Typical Fasciculation Potentials—YouTube. Available at: https://youtu.be/6-3PP_S-Q8I

19. What are the EMG characteristics of myokymic discharges? Neuromyotonic discharges?

Myokymic discharges are rhythmic, spontaneous bursts of an MU potential (i.e., grouped fasciculations) probably resulting from **ephaptic transmission** between the motor axons along demyelinated segments of the nerve. There are variable numbers of potentials in each group or burst. Interburst frequency is 0.1 to 10 Hz along the demyelinated segments of nerves, whereas the intraburst potentials fire at 20 to 150 Hz. Myokymic discharges have been reported in a variety of focal and generalized neuromuscular disorders, including radiation-induced nerve damage and Isaacs' syndrome.

Neuromyotonic discharges are continuous "trains" or shorter bursts of MUAPs that originate in motor axons and fire at high rates (150 to 300 Hz). These discharges can be seen in many conditions, including neuropathies, tetany, spinal muscular atrophy, and Isaacs' syndrome.

Daube JR, Rubin DI. Needle electromyography. *Muscle Nerve.* 2009;39:244–270.

Myokymia on EMG—YouTube. Available at: https://youtu.be/f0eM_M5IpM4

20. What changes occur in the motor unit and motor unit potentials in neuromuscular diseases?

In neurogenic disorders due to loss of axons or anterior horn cells, there are multiple changes in adjacent surviving cells, neurotransmitters, and other substances. This is in essence a form of neuroplasticity early after cell loss. Adjacent surviving anterior horn cell terminal axons sprout out to and innervate adjacent denervated muscle fibers. This may occur in the post-acute phase of **acute flaccid paralysis** similar to acute poliomyelitis, acute flaccid myelitis post COVID-19, or ongoing ALS. The MUP will change in morphology with reinnervation, as there is an increase in fiber density and distribution of fibers within the recording area, thereby increasing the size of the recorded MUP. In **myopathies**, a loss or destruction of muscle fibers within MUs occurs, resulting in a decrease in the overall size of MUPs.

21. Describe the EMG characteristics of a motor unit action potential

A variety of MUAP parameters are evaluated during clinical electromyography, each reflecting the function, timing, and distribution of fibers within the MU. Changes in each of the parameters can help determine the underlying disease and temporal course of the condition.

The most important parameters of a MUAP are duration, firing rate (recruitment), stability, different waveform phases, and amplitude.

- **Duration** reflects the area and distribution of the fibers of the MU near the recording electrode. (Normal MUAP durations vary according to muscle but are typically 6 to 15 ms). The duration of a MUAP is longer with monopolar needle recording than with concentric needle and increases with lower temperature and advanced age. MU durations increase in chronic neurogenic disorders and typically decrease in myopathies.
- **Firing rate** is used to determine MUP recruitment, which represents the orderly addition of MUPs and increased firing rates of MUPs with increasing force.
- **Stability** represents the moment-to-moment changes of a repetitively firing MUP. Normal MUPs are stable and have the same morphology each time they fire. Unstable MUPs indicate a defect of neuromuscular transmission, as can be seen in neuromuscular junction disorders or reinnervating neurogenic disorders.
- **Phases** are determined by counting the deflections of the waveform away from and back to the baseline. The number of phases increases with greater differences in the transmission along the terminal axon and myoneural junction, causing greater differences in the timing of discharge of bundles of MU muscle fibers within the area adjacent to the needle and supplied by one anterior horn cell.
- **Amplitude** is determined by fiber density (the number of muscle fibers in the same MU near the recording electrode) and not by the total number of muscle fibers in that MU (size), because only several fibers close to the needle determine the amplitude.

22. What are "myopathic" MUAPs?

MUAPs with short duration and small amplitude are sometimes referred to as "**myopathic MUAPs.**" The amplitude and duration of these potentials are smaller than normal due to fewer single muscle fibers contributing to the potential. While short duration, low amplitude MUAPs are characteristic of myopathies, they can also be seen in other conditions involving decreased number of contributing muscle fiber action potentials (i.e., neuromuscular transmission diseases, early regeneration of nerve fibers after injury, neuropathies affecting the terminal branches of the nerve fiber and myopathies). Therefore, the term "myopathic MUAP" should be avoided and the MUAPs described (e.g., **small amplitude, short duration MUAP**).

Larry Robinson: ICU Weakness—YouTube. Available at: https://www.youtube.com/watch?v=w5W9X5VWvLU

23. Explain Henneman's "size principle" of motor unit recruitment. What is the recruitment rate and ratio?

The primary mechanism for increasing muscle shortening/contracting force is the additional activation of more MUs (**spatial recruitment**) rather than an increased firing rate of MUs (**temporal recruitment**). MUs are recruited in size order from small to large, because larger units require greater central facilitation for depolarization than smaller MUs (**Henneman's size principle**). The recruitment is a function of the central nervous system, not a function of the peripheral nervous system, but can be altered in diseases of the peripheral nervous system.

- **Recruitment rate** is defined as the firing rate of the first MU when the second is recruited (usually 10 to 12 Hz, <15 Hz in a normal individual). A single MU firing rate can be as rapid as 50 Hz in pathologic conditions.
- **Recruitment ratio** is calculated by the highest firing rate of MU among all on the screen, divided by the number of MUs recruited. Recruitment ratio is normally less than 5.

Henneman E, Somjen G, Carpenter DO. Functional significance of cell size in spinal motor neurons. *J Neurophysiol.* 1965;28:560–589.

Motor Unit Recruitment.avi—YouTube. Available at: https://www.youtube.com/watch?v=pC3NJZ1cjuM

24. Describe the significance of both decreased and increased MUAP recruitment rates

In the early phase of proximal motor axon, lesions including diseases of anterior horn cell, nerves or roots (i.e., early radiculopathy), the only electrodiagnostic finding may be **decreased recruitment,** characterized by a high firing rate of MUs. Early or **rapid recruitment** signifies that too many MUAPs are recruited in proportion to the level of muscle force upon initiating contraction. This can be observed in myopathies.

25. What information can be obtained with a nerve conduction study?

An NCS induces and detects the waves of depolarization along the nerve axons and muscle depolarization. The types of nerves tested are sensory, motor, or mixed. NCS can provide information about the integrity of the axons, myelin, and, indirectly, muscle fibers. NCV represents the velocity of the fastest fibers depending on axon diameter, quality/thickness of the myelin sheath, internodal distance, and temperature. NCV is decreased in demyelinating disease with relatively preserved amplitude unless significant conduction block coexists. NCV may remain normal with reduced amplitude in diseases with axonal degeneration. Some slowing of the NCV occurs with the loss of fast, large-diameter fibers during the progression of axonal neuropathy. The amplitude of the recorded responses reflects the number of axons and functioning muscle fibers (in motor NCSs). In axonal neuropathies, a loss of functioning axons may result in lower CMAP or SNAP amplitudes.

Nerve Conduction Studies (NCV) Fundamentals—YouTube. Available at: https://www.youtube.com/watch?v=Dom18f9l7BY

26. What is the "mixed" nerve study? When is it useful?

A **mixed** nerve study (MNS) is a NCS that stimulates and records **sensory and motor** axons. Examples of mixed NCS include **orthodromic** (from distal towards proximal) **palmar studies** when a median or ulnar nerve is stimulated in the palm and recorded at the wrist. In contrast, an **antidromic** (from proximal to distal) **median or ulnar** study is where only sensory fiber action potentials are recorded from the digits. **Mixed nerve recordings** include action potentials of both motor and sensory fibers. Some advantages of mixed nerve studies include the avoidance of volume conducted compound muscle action potentials. Median and ulnar MNS across the wrist is useful for diagnosing carpal tunnel syndrome. Medial and lateral plantar MNS across the ankle is useful for diagnosing tarsal tunnel syndrome because a SNAP is technically difficult to obtain from toe stimulation.

The electrodiagnostic instrument should be set for the sensory conduction study mode because it only records compound nerve action potentials. The initial deflection of the compound mixed nerve potential probably represents the larger myelinated sensory fibers due to salutatory, rapid conduction, and greater axon diameter, providing increased capacitance.

Alanazy MH. Clinical and electrophysiological evaluation of carpal tunnel syndrome: approach and pitfalls. *Neurosciences.* 2017;23:169–180.

27. How does the F-wave differ from the H-reflex?

The **F-wave** response is a small action potential elicited by antidromic supramaximal stimulation upward in a proximal direction of motor nerve fibers, causing depolarization and repolarization backfiring. This test assesses spinal cord and proximal motor nerve conduction. It causes "backfiring" of 3% to 5% of the motor neuron pool and occurs later than other waves because of the distance traveled. The F-wave latency is approximately 30 ms in the upper limb (side-to-side difference <2 ms) and 50 to 60 ms in the lower limb (side-to-side difference of <4 ms).

- **Hoffman (H) reflexes** are the electrical equivalent of the muscle stretch reflex and are usually only recorded in the soleus and flexor carpi radialis at rest in healthy adults. H reflexes are elicited by selectively stimulating different fibers using a low stimulus amperage with long stimulus duration. The afferent sensory action potentials synapse in the spinal cord and the orthodromically motor action potentials are recorded. H reflexes assess proximal segments of sensory and motor nerves. H-reflexes may be recorded in a variety of muscles in infants, in some types of central neuropathology, and in healthy adults during an isometric contraction.

  F-wave and H-reflex are most useful for suspected proximal-segment pathologies when the other electrodiagnostic parameters are normal, especially in the early stage of disease (*see* Table 12.2).

Bodofsky EB. Contraction-induced upper extremity H reflexes: normative values. *Arch Phys Med Rehabil.* 1999;80(5):562–565.

Table 12.2 F-Wave Versus H-Reflex		
	F-WAVE (NOT A REFLEX)	**H-REFLEX**
Afferent arc	Alpha motor neuron	I-A fiber
Efferent arc	Alpha motor neuron	Alpha motor neuron
Stimulation intensity	Supramaximal	Submaximal
Stimulation duration	Same as motor conduction study	Long duration (>500 ms for I-A fibers)
Muscles recorded	All distal muscles	Soleus, flexor carpi radialis
Consistency	Variable latency and configuration	Consistent latency and configuration
Amplitude	3%–5% of M-response	
Side-to-side difference (upper extremity)	<2 ms	<2 ms in soleus
Side-to-side difference (lower extremity)	<4 ms	

28. Describe the types of nerve injury according to the Seddon classification system

- **Neurapraxia:** Failure of impulse conduction across the affected nerve segment combined with normal conduction above and below the affected segment; carries a good prognosis for recovery; no Wallerian degeneration involved.
- **Axonotmesis:** Disruption of axonal continuity with Wallerian degeneration.
- **Neurotmesis:** Severance of entire nerve; carries a poor prognosis, and surgical repair is needed for functional recovery.

  These studies may be more critical now that early peripheral nerve surgery is possible in this optimum time of early regeneration.

29. What is the purpose of electrodiagnosis soon after nerve injury (10 days after injury)?

The goal of EMG early after injury is to distinguish **neurapraxia from axonotmesis** or **neurotmesis**. Axonotmesis and neurotmesis are not easily distinguished because the difference is primarily the integrity of supporting structures with no electrophysiologic function.

The best way to distinguish neurapraxia from axonotmesis or neurotmesis is by examining the amplitude of the distal CMAP. In neurapraxia, the distal CMAP (stimulating and recording distal to the lesion) is maintained, whereas in axonotmesis or neurotmesis, the distal CMAP disappears after 10 days as a result of Wallerian degeneration. The larger the distal CMAP, the better the prognosis.

Robinson LR. Traumatic injury to peripheral nerves. *Muscle Nerve.* 2000;23(6):863–873.

30. **What is the meaning of a lesion proximal to the dorsal root ganglion?**
   In most, but not all, cases for radiculopathy, the pathology is proximal to the **DRG**. Despite sensory loss, routine sensory conduction studies in the limb show no abnormalities. This is because the distal sensory fibers continue to be supplied by axoplasmic flow from the DRG. An abnormal SNAP occurs infrequently in discogenic radiculopathy, such as when a far lateral disc causes damage to the DRG. The DRG can also be damaged in diseases such as diabetes mellitus and herpes zoster (ganglionopathy).

31. **List common reasons for an unstable baseline during electrodiagnostic studies**
   - Poor contact between ground electrode and patient.
   - Broken recording electrode wire (G1 or G2).
   - Placing stimulating cathode near the recording electrode and stimulating anode away from the nerve trunk minimizes anodal block.
   - Excessive stimulus duration and intensity.
   - Crossing of stimulation wire leads with the other leads and cables.
   - Recording electrodes contacting parts of body other than recording site.

Gitter AJ, Stolov WC. AAEM minimonograph #16: instrumentation and measurement in electrodiagnostic medicine—part I. *Muscle Nerve*. 1995;18:799–811.

Dr. Stolov Reflects on His Presidency—YouTube. Available at: https://www.youtube.com/watch?v=aXyyP9wuJRl

32. **List five common pitfalls in reporting electrodiagnostic results**
   The use of vague terminology and the inclusion of too many findings and differential diagnoses can confuse the referring physicians.
   Diagnoses should not be outlined in a random order without explanation. Organize diagnoses from the most likely to least likely.
   Absence of explanation of the limitations of electrodiagnosis to the referring physician.
   The lesion should be described in terms of neuromuscular localization rather than musculoskeletal localization. For example, a radial nerve lesion should be described as: "distal to innervation of the triceps, proximal to innervation of brachioradialis"; instead of lesion in spiral groove, because the specific fascicular lesion at proximal site can mimic the lesion at a distal location.

Johnson EW. Why and how to request an electrodiagnostic examination and what to expect in return. *Phys Med Rehabil Clin North Am*. 1990;1:149–158.

WEBSITES

American Association of Neuromuscular & Electrodiagnostic Medicine. Available at: https://www.aanem.org/Home
Test questions, go to each issue of *Positives Waves,* a publication of the AANEM. Available at: LMS (aanem.org)
Order electronic media for waveform identification. Interactive Product: Rapid WaveformTester. Available at: https://education.aanem.org/Public/Catalog/Home.aspx
https://www.nandedkarproductions.com/shop
Patient resource information. Available at: https://www.aanem.org/Patients
Preston DG, Shapiro BE. *Electromyography and Neuromuscular Disorders: Clinical-Electrophysiologic-Ultrasound Correlations.* 4th ed. Elsevier; 2020. Available at: https://teleemg.com/

BIBLIOGRAPHY

Alanazy MH. Clinical and electrophysiological evaluation of carpal tunnel syndrome: approach and pitfalls. *Neurosciences.* 2017;23:169–180.
Berne and Levy Physiology. 7th ed. Philadelphia, PA: Elsevier; 2018.
Bodofsky EB. Contraction-induced upper extremity H reflexes: normative values. *Arch Phys Med Rehabil.* 1999;80(5):562–565.
Dumitru D. *Electrodiagnostic Medicine.* 2nd ed. Philadelphia, PA: Hanley & Belfus; 2002.
EMG Waveform Trainer. Available at: http://www.aanem.org/Education/All-Education-Products/Product-Details?productid={8CEC405D-500C-E411-B3BF-00155D0A6803}
Gatens MA, Saeed PF. Electromyographic findings in the intrinsic muscles of normal feet. *Arch Phys Med Rehabil.* 1982;63:317–318.
Gitter AJ, Stolov WC. AAEM minimonograph #16: instrumentation and measurement in electrodiagnostic medicine–part II. *Muscle Nerve.* 1995;18(8):812–824.
Henneman E, Somjen G, Carpenter DO. Functional significance of cell size in spinal motor neurons. *J Neurophysiol.* 1965;28:560–589.
Johnson EW. Why and how to request an electrodiagnostic examination and what to expect in return. *Phys Med Rehabil Clin North Am.* 1990;1:149–158.
Katirji B, Kaminski HJ, Preston DC, et al. *Neuromuscular Disorders in Clinical Practice.* Boston, MA: Butterworth-Heinemann; 2002.
Learn EMG. Available at: https://education.aanem.org/Public/Catalog/Home.aspx
McPhedran AM, Wuerker RB, Henneman E. Properties of motor units in a homogeneous red muscle (soleus) of the cat. *J Neurophysiol.* 1965;28:71–84. Available at: http://jn.physiology.org/cgi/reprint/28/1/71
Preston BE, Shapiro DC. (1998). *Electromyography and Neuromuscular Disorders.* Boston, MA: Butterworth-Heinemann; 1998.

Preston D, Shapiro B. *Electromyography and Neuromuscular Disorders: Clinical-Electrophysiologic-Ultrasound Correlations.* 4th ed. Elsevier; 2021: 275.

Preston DC. *Electromyography and Neuromuscular Disorders.* Philadelphia, PA: Elsevier; 2021.

Punga AR, Jabe JF, Amandusson A. Facing the challenges of electrodiagnostic studies in the very elderly (>80 years) population. *Clin Neurophys.* 2019;130:1091–1097.

Robinson LR. Traumatic injury to peripheral nerves. *Muscle Nerve.* 2000;23(6):863–873.

Rubin DI, Daube JR, eds. *Clinical Neurophysiology.* 4th ed. New York, NY: Oxford University Press; 2016.

Rutkov SB. Effects of temperature in neuromuscular electrophysiology. *Muscle Nerve.* 2001;24:867–882.

Srinivasan J. *Netter's Neurology.* Philadelphia, PA: Elsevier; 2020.

Stinear CM, Lang CR, Zeiler WD. Advances and challenges in stroke rehabilitation. *Lancet Neurol.* 2020;19:4348–4360.

Tan FC, ed. *EMG Secrets.* Philadelphia, PA: Hanley & Belfus; 2004.

Thanawalla AR, Chen AI, Azim E. The cerebellar nuclei and dexterous limb movements. *Neuroscience.* 2020;450:168–183. doi:10.1016/j.neuroscience.2020.06.046

Weiss J, Weiss L, Silver J. *Easy EMG.* Philadelphia, PA: Elsevier; 2016.

CHAPTER 13

RADICULOPATHIES: CLINICAL MANIFESTATIONS, DIFFERENTIAL DIAGNOSES, ELECTRODIAGNOSTIC APPROACH, AND MANAGEMENT

Timothy R. Dillingham, MD

Pain is inevitable. Suffering is optional.

— Buddhist proverb

1. **What are radiculopathies?**
   Radiculopathies are conditions resulting from pathologic processes affecting the spinal nerve root. Common pathologies may include herniated nucleus pulposus, spinal stenosis, degenerative spondylosis, spondylolisthesis, and inflammatory radiculitis.

   Dawson E. *Herniated Discs: Definition, Progression, and Diagnosis.* Available at: www.spineuniverse.com/displayarticle.php/article1431.html

KEY POINTS: COMMON CAUSES OF RADICULOPATHY

1. Herniated nucleus pulposus
2. Spinal stenosis
3. Degenerative spondylosis
4. Spondylolisthesis
5. Inflammatory radiculitis

2. **What are the nondiscogenic/nonspondylitic causes of radiculopathies?**
   - Tumors
     - Primary: meningiomas, neurofibromas, lipomas (cauda equina and conus medullaris)
     - Secondary: breast, prostate, lung, colorectal, thyroid, etc.
   - Leptomeningeal metastasis (leukemias, lymphoproliferative diseases)
   - Abscess, hemorrhage, cysts
   - Infection: herpes zoster, tuberculosis, Lyme disease, syphilis, human immunodeficiency virus (HIV) infection
   - Arachnoiditis: myelogram, surgery, anesthetics, steroid injections
   - Sarcoidosis, Guillain-Barré syndrome, diabetes

3. **Describe the relationship of the exiting spinal nerve to the numbered vertebral segment**
   In the cervical region, there are eight cervical nerve roots and only seven vertebrae. The first seven cervical roots (C1 to C7) exit above the same numbered vertebrae. C8 exits above T1.
   In the thoracolumbar spine the nerve roots exit the spinal canal by passing below the pedicle of their named vertebrae.

   American Association of Orthopaedic Surgeons: Available at: www.aaos.org

   www.spineuniverse.com/displayarticle.php/article265.html

4. **What symptoms are associated with radiculopathies?**
   - Radiating limb pain greater than axial pain; aggravated by sneezing, coughing, or Valsalva maneuver
   - Numbness or tingling extending into the limb
   - Weakness in a myotomal distribution
   - Rarely, bowel and/or bladder retention, urgency, or incontinence

KEY POINTS: AGGRAVATING AND ALLEVIATING FACTORS

1. Classic disc-related lumbosacral radicular pain is often aggravated by sitting and forward-bending and is alleviated by walking, standing, or lying supine.
2. Lumbar stenosis–related radicular pain is often exacerbated by walking and relieved by sitting or lumbar flexion.
3. Cervical radicular pain may be aggravated by neck extension, which causes narrowing of the intervertebral foramen.

5. **Discuss the most important elements of the examination in patients with potential radiculopathies**
A focused neuromuscular examination to determine the presence or absence of a neurologic deficit is mandatory. For each nerve root, assessment of strength, sensation, and, when appropriate, reflex testing should be completed. Patients with radiculopathy may demonstrate subtle weakness, a reduced reflex, or sensory loss. A positive straight-leg raising test (pain radiating below the knee) can be seen despite normal strength, sensation, and reflex findings. Central nerve system (CNS) disorders (e.g., stroke or spinal myelopathy) may result in sensory loss and weakness similar to that found in radiculopathy; however, reflexes are usually increased in these CNS conditions.

6. **Describe the classic patterns of pain radiation and the corresponding physical exam findings seen in common cervical and lumbar radiculopathies**
See Table 13.1.

KEY POINTS: PHYSICAL EXAM PEARLS

1. Upon hearing a heavy foot slap as your patient enters the room, think L5 radiculopathy (ankle dorsiflexor weakness).
2. If your patient cannot walk on his or her toes, think S1 radiculopathy.
3. If your patient cannot extend the elbow, think C7 radiculopathy.

7. **What conditions can mimic cervical radiculopathy?**
For a list of musculoskeletal conditions that commonly mimic cervical radiculopathy, see Table 13.2. Common entrapment neuropathies, plexopathies, and idiopathic brachial neuritis can present similarly. Brachial neuritis usually begins with severe proximal shoulder girdle pain, and then weakness develops. The weakness is characteristically in a focal nerve distribution such as the suprascapular or long thoracic nerve.

8. **What conditions may mimic lumbosacral radiculopathy?**
For a list of musculoskeletal conditions that commonly mimic lumbosacral radiculopathy, see Table 13.3. Neuralgic amyotrophy (caused by nerve ischemia) from diabetes often presents with thigh pain and proximal

Table 13.1 Classic Patterns of Pain Radiation and Physical Exam Findings in Common Cervical and Lumbar Radiculopathies

ROOT	PAIN RADIATION	REFLEX	SENSATION	MOTOR WEAKNESS
C5	Shoulder blade and lateral arm	Biceps	Lateral arm	Shoulder flexion and abduction, elbow flexion
C6	Shoulder blade, radial arm, and forearm	Brachioradialis and biceps	Radial distal arm and forearm, thumb	Elbow flexion, forearm pronation, wrist extension
C7	Posterior arm and forearm	Triceps	Posterior arm and dorsal forearm, middle finger	Elbow extension, wrist flexion
C8	Medial arm and forearm	Triceps	Medial forearm, fourth and fifth fingers	Finger flexion and abduction
L4	Anterior thigh and knee, medial calf	Patellar	Anterior thigh, medial calf/foot	Knee extension, ankle dorsiflexion
L5	Buttocks, lateral thigh and calf, dorsal foot and great toe	Medial hamstring	Lateral leg and dorsum of foot	Ankle dorsiflexion, great toe extension
S1	Posterior thigh and calf, lateral/plantar foot	Achilles	Posterior calf, lateral foot	Ankle plantar flexion

Table 13.2 Musculoskeletal Conditions That Commonly Mimic Cervical Radiculopathy

CONDITION	CLINICAL SYMPTOMS/SIGNS
Fibromyalgia syndrome	Pain all over, female predominance, sleep problems, tender to palpation in multiple areas
Regional myofascial pain	Trigger point reproducing localized or radiating pain syndrome
Polymyalgia rheumatica	Age >50 years; pain and stiffness in neck, shoulders, and hips; high ESR
Sternoclavicular joint arthropathy	Pain in anterior chest, pain with shoulder movement, pain on direct palpation
Acromioclavicular joint arthropathy	Pain in anterior chest, pain with shoulder movement, pain on direct palpation, pain with crossed adduction of shoulder
Shoulder bursitis, impingement syndrome, bicipital tendonitis	Pain with palpation, positive impingement signs, pain in C5 distribution
Lateral epicondylitis, "tennis elbow"	Pain in lateral forearm, pain with palpation and resisted wrist extension
de Quervain tenosynovitis	Lateral wrist and forearm pain, tender at abductor pollicis longus or extensor pollicis brevis tendons; positive Finkelstein test
Trigger finger, stenosing, tenosynovitis of finger flexor tendons	Intermittent pain and locking of digit in flexion

ESR, Erythrocyte sedimentation rate.

Table 13.3 Common Musculoskeletal Disorders Mimicking Lumbosacral Radiculopathy Condition Clinical Symptoms/Signs.

Fibromyalgia, myofascial pain syndrome, polymyalgia rheumatica	See Table 14.2
Hip arthritis	Pain in groin and anterior thigh, pain with weight bearing, positive Patrick test
Trochanteric bursitis	Lateral hip pain, pain with palpation over lateral and posterior hip
Iliotibial band syndrome	Pain along outer thigh, pain with palpation, tight iliotibial band (positive Ober test)
Knee arthritis	Pain with weight-bearing
Patellofemoral pain	Anterior knee pain, worse with prolonged sitting, positive patellar compression test
Pes anserinus bursitis	Medial proximal tibia pain, tender to palpation
Hamstring tendinitis, chronic strain	Posterior knee and thigh pain, can mimic positive straight-leg raise, common in runners
Baker cyst	Posterior knee pain and swelling
Plantar fasciitis	Pain in sole of foot, worse with weight-bearing activities, tender to palpation
Gastrocnemius-soleus tendonitis, chronic strain	Calf pain, worse with sports activities, usually limited range of motion compared with asymptomatic limb

weakness. On electromyography (EMG), it appears more like proximal lumbosacral plexopathy with frequent involvement of the femoral nerve. Distal mononeuropathies such as common peroneal neuropathy can present with similar symptoms.

9. **Which diagnostic tools are useful for further evaluating patients with suspected cervical or lumbosacral radiculopathy?**
   When a person reports in their history certain "red flags" (fever, trauma, weight loss, loss of bladder or bowel control, night pain, or history of malignancy), diagnostic studies that include spinal magnetic resonance imaging (MRI)

are needed to exclude malignancy, infections, fractures, spinal compression, or cauda equine syndrome from a herniated lumbar disc or spinal stenosis. Any signs of myelopathy from the cervical or thoracic spine region on physical exam should be evaluated with spinal MRI. **Plain radiographs** reveal bony alignment, disc space narrowing, and bony trauma but are insensitive for radiculopathy.

- Dynamic flexion/extension views can reveal instability such as spondylolisthesis.
- MRI provides the best resolution of water, colloidal tissue, and spinal structures. Gadolinium enhancement should be considered if tumor is suspected. Clinical correlation with imaging findings is essential for optimal patient care as there are frequently identified findings on spinal imaging that are irrelevant to the patient's symptoms.
- Computed tomography (CT) is especially valuable in assessing bony encroachment. Use of intrathecal contrast can enhance visualization of soft tissues and neural structures.
- Electrodiagnostic testing consists primarily of EMG and nerve conduction studies (NCSs). EMG/NCSs provide an assessment as to whether motor axonal damage is occurring, help localize the lesion to a specific root level, and complement spinal imaging, particularly when the imaging findings are subtle or can be attributed to age-related changes. EMG/NCSs are useful to assess a coexistent peripheral polyneuropathy, focal entrapment neuropathy, or myopathy, especially when presenting symptoms and signs are vague, diffuse, or nonlocalizing.
- Laboratory testing: Complete blood count (CBC), erythrocyte sedimentation rate (ESR), and serum electrophoresis (SPEP) may be indicated if infection, tumor, or metabolic disease is suspected.

American Association of Neuromuscular and Electrodiagnostic Medicine: Available at: www.aanem.org

Mobic MT, Obuchowski NA, Ross JS, et al. Acute low back pain and radiculopathy: MR imaging findings and their prognostic role and effect on outcome. *Radiology.* 2005;237:597–604.

Bonus questions and answers available online.

11. **What is the most important and useful electrodiagnostic test for radiculopathy?**

    EMG using concentric or monopolar needles to examine muscles for signs of denervation in a myotomal distribution is the single most useful electrodiagnostic test to assess for radiculopathy. By examining muscles in the limb and the paraspinal muscles, the examiner can elucidate signs of root level axonal loss and determine the most likely root level involved.

12. **Are NCSs helpful in assessing for radiculopathy?**

    The motor and sensory NCSs are usually normal with single-level radiculopathies. The sensory nerve action potential (SNAP) should be unaffected with a typical compressive radiculopathy given that the lesion is proximal to the dorsal root ganglion. Motor latencies and conduction velocities are normal in persons with radiculopathy.

    Guidelines published by American Association of Neuromuscular and Electrodiagnostic Medicine (AANEM) suggest techniques and reference values for motor and sensory nerve testing in the upper and lower limb when performing NCSs. These reference values are derived from rigorously conducted normative studies that assessed the influences of age, gender, body mass index, and height on NCS parameters for commonly tested upper and lower limb nerves (chen, Dillingham refs).

    For identifying or confirming radiculopathy, H reflexes may help in the setting of a suspected S1 radiculopathy yet have only modest sensitivities. F waves are late responses involving the motor axons and axon pool at the spinal cord level; they have low sensitivities for radiculopathy and are not very useful (cho ref).

Chen S, Andary M, Buschbacher R, Del Toro D, Smith B, So Y, Zimmermann K, Dillingham TR. Electrodiagnostic reference values for upper and lower limb nerve conduction studies in adult populations. *Muscle Nerve*. 2016;54(3):371–377.

Cho C, Ferrante MA, Levin KH, Harmon RL, So YT. AANEM Practice topic: utility of electrodiagnostic testing in evaluating patients with lumbosacral radiculopathy: an evidence-based review. *Muscle Nerve*. 2010;42:276–282.

Dillingham T, Chen S, Andary M, Buschbacher R, Del Toro D, Smith B, Zimmermann K, So Y. Establishing high quality reference values for nerve conduction studies: a report from the Normative Data Task Force of the American Association of Neuromuscular & Electrodiagnostic Medicine. *Muscle Nerve*. 2016;54(3):366–370.

Bonus questions and answers available online.

14. **Why is the EMG normal for many people with radiculopathies?**

The needle EMG assesses only the motor axons. Motor axonal loss is necessary for creating denervated muscle fibers within a muscle. An EMG examination of that muscle with denervated muscle fibers will demonstrate fibrillation potentials that are derived from these fibrillating (denervated) muscle fibers. A radiculopathy that involves only the sensory nerve roots and causes radicular pain and numbness will demonstrate a normal EMG. Radiculopathies that cause only motor neurapraxia at the nerve root level (not axonal loss) will not show spontaneous activity (fibrillations and positive sharp waves) on EMG. Radiculopathies that result in chronic, slow axonal loss that is balanced with reinnervation may not show spontaneous activity but rather may show more subtle findings, such as polyphasic motor units or large motor units firing in a reduced recruitment pattern.

KEY POINTS: NONOPERATIVE TREATMENT FOR RADICULOPATHIES

1. Control pain with over-the-counter analgesics or prescription nonsteroidal antiinflammatory medications.
2. Encourage positional pain relief techniques, avoiding prolonged bed rest.
3. Incorporate cervical or lumbar stabilization exercises and continue walking for exercise
4. Consider epidural steroid injections for intractable radicular pain unresponsive to the aforementioned measures.

15. **Outline the initial treatment plan for a patient with an active radiculopathy.**

The initial goals of treatment are to control pain and reduce inflammation. Treatment strategies include over-the-counter analgesics or nonsteroidal antiinflammatory medications, prescription analgesic medications for acute intractable pain, intermittent localized icing, and positional pain relief techniques. Opiate medications are generally not needed except for severe pain and then for a short period.

Prolonged bed rest is not recommended. Activity modification is recommended, avoiding bending, lifting, and twisting, which tend to increase lumbar intradiscal pressure. Patients should continue daily walking for exercise.

Malanga GA. The diagnosis and treatment of cervical radiculopathy. *Med Sci Sports Exerc*. 1997;29(7)Suppl:S236–S245.

Brat GA, Agniel D, Beam A, Yorkgitis B, Bicket M, Homer M, Fox KP, Knecht DB, McMahill-Walraven CN, Palmer N, Kohane I. Postsurgical prescriptions for opioid naive patients and association with overdose and misuse: retrospective cohort study. *BMJ*. 2018;360:j5790.

Bonus questions and answers available online.

19. Can EMG findings predict clinical outcomes and response to treatment?

A positive EMG of the lower limb and spine showing unequivocal lumbosacral radiculopathy is a strong predictor of a good outcome with conservative management. Furthermore, a positive EMG means that the patient is more likely to respond better to epidural steroid injections if these are felt to be necessary to control pain symptoms. This all means that a positive EMG should be viewed as reflective of a clear underlying pathophysiology and indicative of a better clinical course.

Annaswamy TM, Bierner SM, Chouteau W, Elliott AC. Needle electromyography predicts outcome after lumbar epidural steroid injection. *Muscle Nerve*. 2012;45(3):346–355.

Savage NJ, Fritz JM, Kircher JC, Thackeray A. The prognostic value of electrodiagnostic testing in patients with sciatica receiving physical therapy. *Eur Spine J*. 2015;24:434–443.

20. Describe a rehabilitation plan of care for a patient with an acute lumbosacral radiculopathy.

Goals of physical therapy include centralization of peripheral radicular pain, improvement in basic and advanced activities of daily living, and restoration of function. Treatment includes pain management, education in proper back protection techniques, initiation and progression of core strengthening through lumbosacral stabilization exercises, and correction of lower extremity musculoligamentous imbalances. Aerobic exercise such as a walking program should be encouraged.

21. What are the long-term outcomes for persons with a herniated cervical disc managed nonoperatively?

Saal, Saal, and Yurth demonstrated that persons with cervical disc herniations have a very favorable clinical course. Their cohort of patients was managed with pain management strategies that incorporated medications, rehabilitation with cervical traction and exercises, and epidural or selective nerve root injections if medications failed to control pain. In this series the majority (24 of 26) of patients with herniated cervical discs achieved successful outcomes without surgery. Overall, 83% of the nonoperative group had a good or excellent outcome. A total of 89% of patients with disc extrusions treated nonoperatively achieved a good or excellent outcome, compared with 80% of patients with contained disc herniations. No patients had progressive neurologic loss or new-onset myelopathy.

Saal JS, Saal JA, Yurth EF. Nonoperative management of herniated cervical intervertebral disc with radiculopathy. *Spine*. 1996;21:1877–1883.

22. What are the long-term outcomes for persons with a herniated lumbar disc managed nonoperatively?

They are quite good. A classic investigation by Henrik Weber, a randomized, prospective study of surgery versus conservative care for herniated nucleus pulposus, demonstrated that surgery was somewhat more effective at pain control during the first year. However, beyond 1 year, conservative treatment had equal results compared with the surgically managed group. Even for persons with motor weakness, a good outcome with conservative treatment was the norm, and surgery did not improve motor return. Other investigators in cohort outcomes studies have demonstrated that the majority of persons suffering lumbosacral radiculopathy can resolve their symptoms. In fact, on follow-up MRI studies, lumbosacral disc herniations and disc fragments resolve in 76% of patients.

Atlas S, Keller RB, Wu YA, et al. Long-term outcomes of surgical and nonsurgical management of sciatica secondary to a lumbar disc herniation: 10-year results from the Maine Lumbar Spine Study. *Spine*. 2005;30(8):927–935.

Lipetz JS, Misra N, Silber JS. Resolution of pronounced painless weakness arising from radiculopathy and disk extrusion. *Am J Phys Med Rehabil*. 2005;84:528–537.

Saal JA, Saal JS. Nonoperative treatment of herniated lumbar intervertebral disc with radiculopathy. An outcome study. *Spine (Phila PA 1976)*. 1989;14(4):431–437.

Saal JA. Dynamic muscular stabilization in the nonoperative treatment of lumbar spine pain syndormes. *Orthop Rev*. 1990;19(8):691–700.

Weber H. Lumbar disc herniation: a controlled, prospective study with ten years of observation. *Spine*. 1983;8:131–140.

KEY POINTS: INDICATIONS FOR SURGICAL REFERRAL

1. Progressive neuromotor deficits
2. Cauda equina syndrome
3. Cervical or thoracic myelopathy
4. Intractable pain, unresponsive to comprehensive nonoperative treatment
5. Spinal tumors causing radiculopathy symptoms
6. Spinal infections causing radiculopathy symptoms
7. Fractures of the spine
8. Pronounced spondylolisthesis with neurological symptoms and signs

23. What are the indications for referral of a patient with radiculopathy to a spine surgeon?
    The indications for more urgent referral of a patients with lumbosacral radiculopathy to a spine surgeon include cauda equina syndrome with bowel or bladder dysfunction, saddle paresthesias, and/or severe and progressive lower extremity weakness. For cervical radiculopathy or thoracic myelopathy, surgical consultation should be considered when gait disturbance, pronounced or progressive upper extremity weakness, and bowel and bladder dysfunction are present.
    Surgical referral should be considered for
    • Intractable pain despite aggressive nonoperative care
    • Severe or progressive motor weakness
    • Bowel or bladder dysfunction and evidence of cauda equine syndrome.
    • Infections of the spine
    • Spinal malignancies
    • Spinal fractures
    • Severe spondylolisthesis with pain or weakness

BIBLIOGRAPHY

American Association of Electrodiagnostic & Neuromuscular Medicine. AANEM's top five choosing wisely recommendations. *Muscle Nerve.* 2015;51(4):617–619.
Bush K, Cowan N, Katz DE, Gishen P. The natural history of sciatica associated with disc pathology: a prospective study with clinical and independent radiological follow-up. *Spine.* 1992;1:1205–1212.
Dowell D, Haegerich TM, Chou R. CDC Guideline for Prescribing Opioids for Chronic Pain—United States, 2016. *MMWR.* 2016, March 15;65:617–619
Dumitru D, ed.. *Electrodiagnostic Medicine.* 2nd ed. Philadelphia: Hanley & Belfus; 2002.
Jensen MC, Brant-Zawadzki MN, Obuchowski N, et al. Magnetic resonance imaging of the lumbar spine in people without back pain. *N Engl J Med.* 1994;331:69–73.
Krebs EE, Gravely A, Nugent S, Jensen AC, DeRonne B, Goldsmith ES, Kroenke K, Bair MJ, Noorbaloochi S. Effect of opioid vs nonopioid medications on pain-related function in patients with chronic back pain or hip or knee osteoarthritis pain: The SPACE Randomized Clinical Trial. *JAMA.* 2018;319(9):872–882.
Qaseem A, Wilt TJ, McLean RM, Forciea MA; Clinical Guidelines Committee of the American College of Physicians. Noninvasive treatments for acute, subacute, and chronic low back pain: a clinical practice guideline from the American College of Physicians. *Ann Intern Med.* 2017;166(7):514–530.

CHAPTER 14

PERIPHERAL NEUROPATHY: DIAGNOSIS, PREVENTION, AND REHABILITATION

Ehtesham Khalid, MD, MRCP, FCPS, Peter Daniel Donofrio, MD, and Steven A. Stiens, MD, MS

Sensation is not the conduction of a quality or state of external bodies to consciousness, but the conduction of a quality or state of our nerves to consciousness, excited by an external cause.
— Johannes Peter Muller (1801–1858) (Law of Specific Nerve Energies 1835)

1. **How are diffuse polyneuropathies categorized by their underlying pathologic mechanisms?**
   Most polyneuropathies can be subdivided into those that are **motor, sensory, or both** and into those that are **axon loss, demyelinating, or combined**. The demyelinating neuropathies can be further grouped as **multifocal acquired** or **uniformly demyelinating**. The acute inflammatory demyelinating polyradiculoneuropathy (AIDP) presentation of Guillain-Barre syndrome is a good example of a motor greater than sensory acquired multifocal demyelinating polyneuropathy. Whereas most toxic neuropathies, such as alcohol overuse, or medication-induced neuropathies, affect the sensory axons more than motor fibers. Inherited neuropathies often cause uniform demyelination of a nerve. Charcot-Marie-Tooth (CMT) Type 1-A is a good example of uniformly demyelinating polyneuropathy (Fig. 14.1).

   Reilly MM. Classification and diagnosis of the inherited neuropathies. *Ann Indian Acad Neurol.* 2009;12(2):80–88.

2. **Which drugs cause peripheral neuropathy?**
   Peripheral sensory and motor fibers react to toxins (in this case, medications) in a limited manner. Schaumburg and Spencer theorized that toxins cause disease at one of four regions of the peripheral nerve:

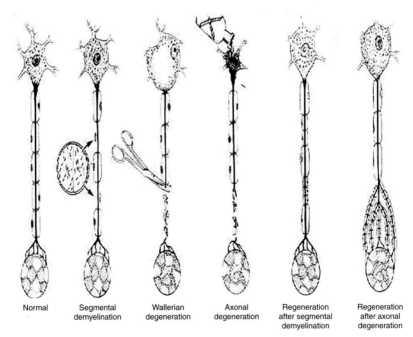

| Normal | Segmental demyelination | Wallerian degeneration | Axonal degeneration | Regeneration after segmental demyelination | Regeneration after axonal degeneration |

Fig. 14.1 Schematic representation of nerve degenerations.

- Distal sensory and motor axon (axonopathy)
- Schwann cell
- Dorsal root ganglion (ganglionopathy or neuropathy)
- Anterior horn cell or motor neuron
  Many of the medications that cause neuropathy belong to chemotherapy, immunosuppresants, and anti-microbial classes peripheral nerves at different locations. Rarely, anti-seizure and anti-arrhythmic medications can induce neuropathy.

Schaumburg HH, Spencer PS. Toxic neuropathies. *Neurology.* 1979;29:429–431.

Donofrio PD. Electrophysiologic evaluations. *Neurol Clin Neurobehav Toxicol.* 2000;18:601–613.

Chan CW, Cheng H, Au SK, et al. Living with chemotherapy-induced peripheral neuropathy: uncovering the symptom experience and self-management of neuropathic symptoms among cancer survivors. *European J Oncol Nurs.* 2018;36:135–141.

3. What tests are pertinent to identify the cause of diffuse polyneuropathy?
   History and examination are paramount in guiding further testing but have poor diagnostic utility. The initial testing includes complete blood count, fasting blood sugar or hemoglobin A1c, serum **B12 level**, **serum protein electrophoresis**, **erythrocyte sedimentation rate**, **metabolic panel,** and **ANA survey with reflex**. Thyroid function testing is rarely helpful as hypothyroidism or hyperthyroidism are rare causes of neuropathy. If the above studies are negative, additional evaluation can be performed including HIV testing, vitamin E, B6, and B1 levels, 24-hour urine screen for heavy metals, and lumbar puncture. Other studies that can be ordered include anti-SSA and SSB, anti-gliadin, and ACE levels.

Barrell K, Smith GA. Peripheral neuropathy. *Med Clin N Am.* 2019;103:383–397.

4. What is the role of nerve conduction study (NCS)/electromyography (EMG) in assessing polyneuropathy?
   Nerve conduction studies are useful to demonstrate the presence of neuropathy and to determine if the neuropathy is sensory and/or motor, axon loss, or demyelinating and can give clues to the chronicity of the neuropathy. They can also decipher if another neuromuscular condition co-exists, such as a plexopathy, polyradiculopathy, anterior horn cell disorder, or mononeuritis multiplex.

5. How are inherited neuropathies classified?
   More than 70 distinct genes have been identified which have been associated with neuropathy. Any length-dependent polyneuropathy should be addressed as a potential genetic neuropathy. Inherited neuropathies may be isolated neurological manifestations or part of a multisystemic genetic disorder with other organs involved. Current investigations are exploring the role of genetic mutation in the classification of CMT disease (Table 14.1).

6. What are the genetic defects in CMT?
   Most patients with CMT disease have mutations in the following genes, but the types of genetic mutations vary from deletions and duplications to point mutations. The four most common genetic mutations (listed below) account for less than 30% of the patients with CMT, implying that the other 70% are due to many other mutations, some of which are undiscovered.

Table 14.1 Classification of the Genetic Neuropathies

Neuropathies in which the neuropathy is the sole or primary part of the disorder

Charcot-Marie-Tooth disease (CMT)
Hereditary neuropathy with liability to pressure palsies (HNPP)
Hereditary sensory and autonomic neuropathies/hereditary sensory neuropathies (HSAN/HSN)
Distal hereditary motor neuropathies (dHMN)
Hereditary neuralgic amyotrophy (HNA)

Neuropathies in which the neuropathy is part of a movie widespread neurological or multisystem disorder

Familial amyloid polyneuropathy (FAP)
Disturbances of lipid metabolism (e.g., adrenoleukodystrophy)
Porphyrias
Disorders with defective developmental diseases of the nervous system (DNS) (e.g., ataxia telangiectasia)
Neuropathies associated with mitochondrial diseases
Neuropathies associated with hereditary ataxias

- PMP-22—19.6%
- Connexin 32—4.8%
- MPZ—1.1%
- MFN—3.2%

Braathen GJ. Genetic epidemiology of Charcot–Marie–Tooth disease. *Acta Neurol Scand Suppl.* 2012;(193):iv-2 2.

KEY POINTS: POLYNEUROPATHIES

1. Polyneuropathies can be classified in many ways, including the primary pathological process as axon loss, demyelinating, or combined, or type of fiber involvement as motor, sensory or combined.
2. Axonal neuropathies primarily manifest in a length-dependent manner, starting distally with progressive proximal involvement.

7. List the common sites of nerve entrapment in the upper and lower limbs.
   See Table 14.2

8. How does carpal tunnel syndrome present?
   Carpal tunnel syndrome (CTS) is the most common focal nerve entrapment syndrome. The presentation includes pain and paresthesia (tingling, burning, and numbness) in the median nerve distribution, and sometimes radiation of those symptoms into the forearm (often worse at night). In moderate to severe cases, weakness of the median-innervated hand muscles is present. Minor, nonspecific symptoms include clumsiness, tightness, and complaints of dropping objects. Symptoms are often induced by overuse of the hand, especially forceful gripping or repetitive hand/wrist motion. CTS can be bilateral in about 25% of patients. Bilateral CTS can be a manifestation of amyloidosis, hypothyroidism, acromegaly, rheumatoid arthritis, and diabetes.

Padua L, Coraci D, Erra C, et al. Carpal tunnel syndrome: clinical features, diagnosis, and management. *Lancet Neurol.* 2016;15: 1273–1284.

9. How is the Phalen wrist flexion test carried out?
   The patient places his or her flexed elbows on a table and allows the wrists to fall freely into maximum flexion (no forced flexion by the patient or examiner). This positioning should elicit numbness and tingling in a median distribution in 75% of patients with CTS symptoms after 2 minutes. The reverse Phalen can be performed, but tests should be reproducible to be helpful for diagnosis.

10. How is the Tinel's test performed at the wrist?
    Percussion over the median nerve at the wrist with a reflex hammer produces a tingling sensation in the distribution of the median nerve. False positives range from 6% to 45%. Tinel's sign is not specific to the median nerve and can be elicited at other sites where nerves are superficial (ulnar, peroneal, radial, sural, plantars).

11. What are the ergonomic risk factors for CTS?
    High force, high repetition, vibration, awkward posture, and temperature extremes have been implicated as ergonomic risk factors for occupational hand and wrist disorders, including CTS. Although not ergonomic, obesity and pregnancy are also independent risk factors.

Table 14.2 The Common Sites of Nerve Entrapment in the Upper and Lower Limbs

NERVE	SITE OF ENTRAPMENT	CLINICAL PATTERN
Median nerve	Wrist	Carpal Tunnel syndrome
	Forearm	Anterior interosseous syndrome
Ulnar nerve	Elbow	Cubital tunnel syndrome
	Wrist	Guyon's canal syndrome
Peroneal nerve	Knee or fibular head	Cross leg syndrome
Lateral femoral cutaneous nerve of thigh	Medial to anterior superior iliac spine (ASIS)	Meralgia paresthetica
Tibial nerve	Under flexor retinaculum	Tarsal tunnel syndrome

12. **How is the diagnosis of CTS made?**

Median nerve impingement at the wrist (CTS) can be verified using NCSs, nerve ultrasound, magnetic resonance imaging (MRI), or open surgical exploration. Some clinicians make the diagnosis solely on the clinical history and physical exam and recommend surgery after conservative measures have failed. However, many conditions can be confused with CTS, including C6 radiculopathy, upper and middle trunk plexopathy, a proximal median neuropathy above the wrist, or arterial disease of the upper limb. In studies in which patients were surgically treated for symptoms of CTS without NCS, a significant number did not improve and were eventually found to have other conditions.

Limke JC, Stiens SA. Carpal tunnel syndrome and/or median neuropathy at the wrist. In: O'Young B, Young M, Stiens SA, eds. *Physical Medicine and Rehabilitation Secrets*. 2nd ed. Philadelphia: Hanley and Belfus; 2002:137–144.

13. **List the differential diagnosis of CTS.**

See Table 14.3

If median neuropathy of the wrist is suspected, what is a common electrodiagnostic approach?
- Sensory NCS of the median nerve across the wrist, and if latency is abnormal, comparison to another sensory study in the symptomatic limb.
- If the initial median sensory NCS across the wrist has a conduction distance greater than 8 cm and the results are normal, additional studies should be pursued: a) median sensory NCS across the wrist over a short (7 to 8 cm) conduction distance and comparison of median sensory NCS across the wrist to the radial or ulnar sensory conduction across the wrist in the same limb. The American Association of Neuromuscular and Electrodiagnostic Medicine practice parameter recommends motor NCS of the median nerve compared to one other motor nerve in the symptomatic limb.

14. **What factors are associated with false-positive nerve conduction velocity results in CTS?**

Cold temperature, increasing age and height, and finger circumference.

15. **Which technical problems can result in inaccurate results?**

A cold hand will slow conduction velocities and increase latencies and amplitudes. This phenomenon would apply to other nerves studied in the cold hand (ulnar and radial). Submaximal stimulus intensity may elicit an erroneously small-amplitude response and a longer latency because the fastest fibers may not be depolarized. Sensory studies performed with less than a 4 cm electrode separation between active and reference electrodes may result in a smaller amplitude and shorter peak latency. For motor studies, the recording electrode must be centered over the belly of the muscle, or the amplitude of the motor response will be low, and the onset of the waveform may be distorted.

16. **Describe anomalous innervation affecting interpretation of the NCSs in CTS?**

The **Martin-Gruber anastomosis**, a median to ulnar connection in the forearm of motor fibers from the median or anterior interosseous nerve, occurs in 15% of individuals and affects both median and ulnar recordings. In an individual without median neuropathy at the wrist, this anomaly will result in a larger compound muscle action potential (CMAP) amplitude when stimulating the median nerve at the elbow than at the wrist. In the presence of median neuropathy, the anastomosis causes an initial positive deflection of the CMAP when stimulating at the elbow, despite proper centering of the recording electrode over the belly of the thenar muscle. The same deflection is not noted on distal wrist stimulation. This appearance is explained by stimulation of the unaffected ulnar innervated

Table 14.3 List the Differential Diagnosis of Carpal Tunnel Syndrome
Neurologic Disorders
• Cervical radiculopathy (roots C6, 7, 8) • Brachial plexus lesions, including thoracic outlet syndrome • Ulnar, radial, or proximal median nerve lesions • Syringomyelia • Cervical cord lesions
Musculoskeletal Disorders
• Tenosynovitis, including de Quervain's (inflammation of synovial tendon sheaths) • Osteoarthritis of the metacarpal-trapezial joint (thumb carpometacarpal arthritis) • Kienbock's disease (avascular lunate necrosis) • Scaphoidal-trapezial arthritis • Digital neuritis
Vascular Disorders
• Raynaud's phenomenon • Radial artery thrombosis

muscles in the hand (from the anastomosis) before those stimulated by the median nerve (slowed by the median neuropathy) reach the (abductor pollicis brevis) muscle.

17. **What are the clinical and electrodiagnostic features of anterior interosseous nerve entrapment?**
Typically, the patient complains of vague aching pain in the forearm and weakness in the muscles supplied by the anterior interosseous nerve (i.e., flexor pollicis longus, flexor digitorum profundus (lateral head), and pronator quadratus). These muscles work together to make the **"okay" sign** with the hand. There is no sensory deficit. The anterior interosseus mononeuropathy is commonly caused by the anterior interosseous nerve being entrapped in the forearm by a fibrous band.

18. **What does the needle EMG exam contribute to the differential diagnosis of CTS?**
Results of the needle exam of the thenar muscles assess for evidence of acute and/or chronic motor axon injury. It confirms motor axon loss in severe CTS and may help to determine chronicity and the need for surgery. It is necessary to rule out separate or concomitant pathology, such as proximal median neuropathy, cervical or thoracic radiculopathy, or plexopathy.

19. **What are the non-operative therapies for CTS?**
Nonoperative therapy includes **wrist splinting** in a neutral position, **passive stretching** of the transverse carpal ligament, **range of motion** (ROM) exercises, **diuretics**, and **nonsteroidal anti-inflammatory drugs** (NSAIDs), ergonomic modifications, and oral or **injectable steroids** into the wrist. Modest oral doses of pyridoxine (**vitamin B6**) have been advocated, although controlled trials have not demonstrated its efficacy, and pyridoxine excess can cause a polyneuropathy.

20. **What surgical treatments can be performed for CTS?**
The most traditional technique for CTS release is an open decompression using a curved, longitudinal incision that provides good exposure of the transverse carpal ligament. Endoscopic techniques have been developed. A recent analysis of published series describes comparable rates of complications between open and closed techniques. Still, the endoscopic release is associated with less tissue trauma, pain at the surgical site and higher level of functioning, a better patient satisfaction rate, and fewer days of convalescence. Some case reports have described a heightened risk of complications from endoscopic release, such as the transection of the median nerve. Overall, the success rate for surgical treatment of CTS approaches 90%.

American Academy of Orthopedic Surgeons. *Management of Carpal Tunnel Syndrome: Evidence Based Clinical Practice Guideline.* 2016. Available at: http://www.orthoguidelines.org/topic?id=1020.

21. **What is Saturday night palsy? Honeymoon palsy?**
Saturday night palsy is one of the "sleep palsies" that results from compression of the radial nerve at the brachium (spiral groove) as it pierces the lateral intermuscular septum in the upper part of the arm. Compression often occurs in patients who fall asleep with the arm resting against the firm edge of a chair or couch.
Honeymoon palsy results from compression of the radial nerve more distally in the arm when the spouse's head injures the nerve resting in the crook of the patient's arm.

22. **Describe the three distinct compressive ulnar neuropathies at the wrist and two at the elbow.**
   • Compression of the superficial and deep branches within **Guyon's canal.**
   • Compression of the ulnar nerve after it exits Guyon's canal.
   • Compression of superficial branch of the ulnar nerve in Guyon's canal.
   • Elbow ulnar compression under the **humeroulnar aponeurotic** arcade.
   • External compression of ulnar at the **retroepicondylar groove** of the non-dominant arm of administrative desk workers.

Doughty CT, Bowley MP. Entrapment neuropathies of the upper extremity. *Med Clin North Am.* 2019;103:357–370.

23. **What is double crush syndrome?**
The double crush nerve entrapment syndrome was described in 1973 by **Upton and McComas**. In this syndrome, the sensory or motor fibers emanating from a particular root, if compressed proximally, are more susceptible to compression distally. A good example is a patient with a C6 or C7 radiculopathy and entrapment of the median nerve at the wrist. The two crushes would be the radiculopathy of C6 and/or C7 and the distal compression of the median nerve.

24. **Describe the clinical features of meralgia paresthetica. How is it treated?**
Meralgia paresthetica results from compression of the **lateral femoral cutaneous nerve** of the thigh (a pure sensory nerve), as it passes beneath or through the **inguinal ligament**, medial to the anterior superior iliac spine (ASIS). This condition is often associated with pregnancy, obesity, diabetes, and the use of tight belts, corsets, and

underwear. The patient usually complains of paresthesia and pain over the anterolateral aspect of the thigh. There may be point tenderness, a positive **Tinel's sign**, or a positive compression test, medial to ASIS. Treatment includes eliminating the causative factor (weight loss, better control of diabetes, wearing looser clothing, and delivery of the baby), a temporary block with a local anesthetic and steroid, and surgical release of the nerve.

25. What are the common sites of entrapment in the sciatic nerve?

The **sciatic nerve** can be injured at several sites along the nerve as a result of neoplasia, pelvic fractures, pelvic infection, penetrating injuries, surgical trauma, aneurysm, intramuscular injections, a thick billfold, prolonged sitting on the edge of a hard surface, or entrapment by the **piriformis muscle**. The exact site depends on the location of the pathology.

Bowley MP, Doughty CT. Entrapment neuropathies of the lower extremity. *Med Clin North Am.* 2019;103:371–382.

26. Where does the entrapment of the tibial nerve commonly occur?

The tibial nerve can be entrapped under the **foot flexor retinaculum** or just posterior to the medial malleolus. This is popularly known as **tarsal tunnel syndrome** and may occur due to tenosynovitis, venous stasis, edema, trauma, **pronated foot (pes planovalgus)**, arthritis of the subtalar joint, or a ganglia arising in the area of the medial aspect of the ankle. Lesions distal to the flexor retinaculum can compress the medial or lateral plantar branches of the tibial nerve. An uncommon entrapment is in the popliteal fossa by a **Baker's cyst**.

27. Describe the clinical presentation of tarsal tunnel syndrome.

- Painful dysesthesias of the soles and toes, associated with a sensory deficit on the plantar aspect of the foot and toes and weakness in the intrinsic muscles of the feet. Symptoms depend on whether the medial or lateral plantar nerves or both are affected.
- Pain occurs at rest while the patient is sitting or in bed.
- Positive Tinel's sign (paresthesia in the nerve distribution) after percussion over the nerve at the entrapment site posterior to the medial malleolus.

28. What is Morton's neuroma?

Entrapment of the **interdigital nerve** between the second and third or the third and fourth metatarsal heads. The symptoms include shooting pain and burning of the second, third, or fourth toes. Examination reveals the tenderness of the sole and affected web spaces. Conservative treatment of **Morton's neuroma** includes positioning of a pad just proximal to the metatarsal heads and/or an injection of Bupivacaine and corticosteroid. Surgery is advised if conservative treatments fail.

29. Outline the approach to the prevention and treatment of entrapment neuropathies.

Prevention:
- Avoid sustained pressure or tethering at the entrapment sites.
- Optimized control of diabetes. (Diabetics are more vulnerable to developing not only a polyneuropathy but also entrapment neuropathies.)

Treatment:
- Non-operative
  - Splint the limb in a neutral position; this maximizes space for the entrapped nerve.
  - Modify activity and avoid positions that can be a source of nerve trauma.
  - Consider using ice, NSAIDs, and corticosteroids injections in structures surrounding the nerves.
- Operative
  - Surgical decompression—open or endoscopic

KEY POINTS: ENTRAPMENT NEUROPATHIES

1. Median nerve compression can be at multiple points along the course of the nerve: at the wrist, anterior interosseous branch, between the two heads of the pronator teres, and at the supracondylar ligament of Struthers.
2. Entrapment neuropathies are common at the distal locations and are exacerbated by proximal entrapment.

Bonus questions and answers available online.

CHAPTER 15

NEUROMUSCULAR JUNCTION DISORDERS: PHYSIOLOGY, CLINICAL MANIFESTATIONS, AND ELECTRODIAGNOSIS

Michelle Stern, MD, Thomas McGunigal, MD, Olajide Williams, MD, and Fabreena Napier, MD

Let the young know they will never find a more interesting, more instructive book than the patient himself.
— Giorgio Baglivi (1668–1707)

KEY POINTS

1. The neuromuscular junction is a specialized synapse between a motor nerve and a muscle fiber, consisting of a presynaptic nerve terminal, synaptic cleft, and postsynaptic end plate of the muscle fiber. Acetylcholine is the active neurotransmitter at this synapse.
2. Neuromuscular junction disorders involve a transmission defect of acetylcholine across the neuromuscular junction.
3. Repetitive nerve stimulation and single-fiber electromyography (EMG) are used in evaluating neuromuscular junction disorders. Antibody testing may be of additional value in immune-mediated neuromuscular junction disorders.
4. Myasthenia gravis is an immune-mediated, postsynaptic neuromuscular junction disorder, most commonly caused by antibodies to the acetylcholine receptor.
5. Lambert-Eaton myasthenic syndrome is an immune-mediated, presynaptic neuromuscular junction disorder caused by antibodies to the P/Q voltage-gated calcium channels. The clinical trial in Lambert-Eaton is proximal weakness, dysautonomia, and areflexia.

1. **Describe the neuromuscular junction (NMJ) and function.**
   The NMJ is the synapse between a motor nerve and a muscle fiber, consisting of a presynaptic nerve terminal, synaptic cleft, and postsynaptic end plate of the muscle fiber. Acetylcholine (Ach), the neurotransmitter released from the presynaptic nerve terminal at the NMJ, allows for depolarization of the muscle fiber by binding to the nicotinic Ach receptor (AChR) on the postsynaptic plate. Acetylcholinesterase is in the synaptic cleft and recycles Ach by breaking it into choline and acetate. Choline reuptake occurs by the presynaptic terminal. The primary physiologic functions at the NMJ leading to muscle depolarization include (1) presynaptic storage, synthesis, and release of Ach; (2) synaptic transmission and degradation of Ach; and (3) postsynaptic coupling with receptors (Fig. 15.1).

2. **Describe NMJ transmission and quantal release.**
   Ach is stored in the presynaptic terminal in vesicles called quanta. Ach storage occurs in three interrelated compartments, the primary, secondary, and tertiary stores. The primary (or immediate-release) store, which contains approximately 1000 quanta, is immediately available for release upon depolarization. The secondary (or mobilization) store, containing about 10,000 quanta, resupplies the primary source when depleted. The tertiary store is the reserve, which contains more than 100,000 quanta. When an action potential reaches the presynaptic nerve terminal, it causes a voltage-sensitive influx of calcium ions, which signals the vesicles to release Ach into the synaptic cleft. Binding of Ach to the postsynaptic cleft on the muscle fiber leads to depolarization, referred to as the end plate potential (EPP).

3. **What is the relationship between calcium and ach release?**
   Depolarization of the motor nerve terminal causes calcium ion influx into the presynaptic terminal via voltage-gated calcium channels. Specialized proteins on the vesicles and presynaptic membrane activate in response to calcium concentrations in the nerve terminal. This group of proteins are termed SNARE proteins (soluble N-ethylmaleimide-sensitive factor attachment receptor). Through a series of interactions of these proteins in response to calcium influx, the vesicles are guided to the postsynaptic membrane for export into the NMJ. Calcium accumulation with

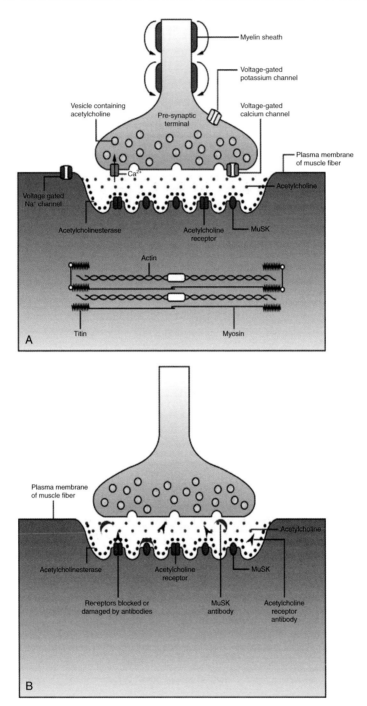

Fig. 15.1 Schematic diagrams of (A) a normal neuromuscular junction illustrating locations of the presynaptic vesicles, acetylcholine within the synapse, and the postsynaptic acetylcholine receptors, as well as (B) a neuromuscular junction affected by myasthenia gravis with antibodies that interfere with the binding and/or structure of the acetylcholine receptors and muscle-specific kinase (MuSK) (note that antibodies to both proteins are not typically present in the same individual, although this phenomenon has been reported on occasion). (From Kang PB, Liew WKM, Oskoui M, et al. In: Darras BT, Jones HR Jr, Ryan MM, et al., eds. *Neuromuscular Disorders of Infancy, Childhood, and Adolescence: A Clinician's Approach.* 2nd ed. San Diego: Academic Press; 2015:482–496 [Chapter 27].)

each depolarization requires 100 to 200 ms to diffuse away from the nerve terminal. Therefore stimulation that arrives at rates greater than 5 to 10/s (5 to 10 Hz) causes calcium to accumulate, leading to the release of vesicles.

4. **Is there a safeguard for transmission at the NMJ?**

Yes. The release of more Ach from the presynaptic terminal than what is needed to produce an EPP is referred to as the *safety factor*. This ensures that in normal NMJ transmission, every above-threshold stimulus results in depolarization of the muscle fiber. In disease states, such as myasthenia gravis (MG), the NMJ transmission is much more tenuous. With fewer functioning receptors, a slight drop in Ach concentration may block transmission.

5. **Describe repetitive nerve stimulation (RNS)?**

RNS is an electrophysiologic study whereby a motor nerve is stimulated repetitively while recording compound muscle action potentials (CMAPs) from an appropriate muscle. Trains of supramaximal stimuli are delivered to a peripheral nerve at rates of less than 5 Hz (usually 2 to 3 Hz). RNS at this rate serves to stress dysfunctional NMJs by depleting the primary store of Ach, which causes failure of neuromuscular transmission in a portion of motor end plates, resulting in fewer muscle fibers contributing to the CMAP. This failure of transmission leads to lower amplitude CMAPs over successive stimulations, termed a decremental response. The decremental response is defined as the percentage of change between the amplitude and area of the first potential to the lowest potential (usually the fourth or fifth in a train of ten). A decrement of 10% or greater is abnormal, which can be seen in presynaptic or postsynaptic disorders.

6. **How can one distinguish between presynaptic and postsynaptic dysfunction electrophysiologically?**

If the initial CMAP is small due to a presynaptic disorder, brief activation (10 to 15 seconds) can produce a marked increase in the CMAP amplitude. The physiologic effect of such activation results from the accumulation of calcium in the nerve terminal, which enhances the release of Ach. This phenomenon is termed *postactivation facilitation*. An increase in the amplitude of more than 100% is most definitive for a presynaptic disorder.

In postsynaptic disorders, a more sustained activation ($\geq$30 seconds) depletes the readily releasable stores of Ach, which overrides the effects of calcium accumulation in the nerve terminal and also depresses endplate excitability. This effect is most marked 2 to 4 minutes after activation and is referred to as *postactivation exhaustion*. The electrodiagnostic manifestation of this phenomenon is an exaggeration of the decremental response at low-frequency RNS compared with the pre-exercise values (Fig. 15.2).

7. **Describe jitter and block in single-fiber EMG (SFEMG)?**

SFEMG uses a specialized needle electrode that allows recording of two individual muscle fiber action potentials within a motor unit. When a motor nerve is depolarized, all of the muscle fibers within one motor unit are activated at about the same time in a normally functioning NMJ. The slight difference in time of activation of individual muscle fibers in one motor unit is called *jitter* and is determined by the time it takes for the EPP to reach the threshold. An increase in jitter is the most sensitive electrophysiologic evidence of a defect in neuromuscular transmission. When the defect is more severe, some nerve impulses fail to elicit muscle fiber action potentials, and SFEMG recordings demonstrate an intermittent absence of one or more single muscle-fiber action potentials on consecutive firings. This is called *impulse blocking* and represents neuromuscular transmission failure at the involved end plate.

Cherian A, Baheti NN, Iype T. Electrophysiological study in neuromuscular junction disorders. *Ann Indian Acad Neurol*. 2013;16(1): 34–41. Available at: https://www.ncbi.nlm.nih.gov/pmc/articles/PMC3644779/.

8. **Classify the main categories of NMJ disorders.**

See Table 15.1.

9. **What are the clinical manifestations of MG?**

MG is an immune-mediated, postsynaptic NMJ disorder. There is a bimodal incidence of MG, with peaks in the third decade in females, and after age 50 in males. MG has a female-to-male ratio of 1.5:1. Ocular symptoms, including ptosis and diplopia, are the most common complaint in MG, occurring in 90% of cases, and is the presenting complaint in two-thirds of patients. While a subset of patients can remain purely ocular, symptoms can become generalized in about 75% of patients involving facial, bulbar, trunk, limb, respiratory, and masticatory muscles. The hallmark of this syndrome is muscle weakness, which fluctuates, worsening as the day progresses or with repetitive use. Thymomas can occur in 10% to 15% of patients with generalized MG.

Hehir MK, Silvestri NJ. Generalized myasthenia gravis: classification, clinical presentation, natural history, and epidemiology. *Neurol Clin*. 2018;36(2):253–260. Available at: https://doi.org/10.1016/j.ncl.2018.01.002.

10. **Describe ancillary testing and management of MG.**

Antibodies to various targets on the postsynaptic membrane of the NMJ, mediated by complement, cause MG. The most common antibody involved in MG is the AChR antibody, which is present in about 80% of cases. The remainder of

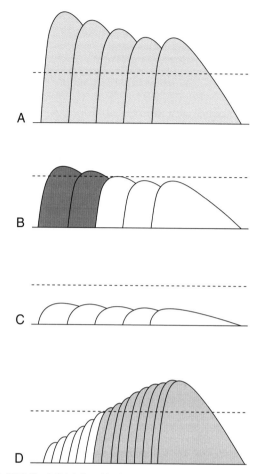

Fig. 15.2 End plate potentials (EPPs). Threshold is indicated by the dashed line. Shaded EPPs are those that rise above the threshold and generate a muscle fiber action potential. (A) Three-Hertz repetitive nerve stimulation (RNS), normal neuromuscular junction (NMJ). Note that all potentials remain well above the threshold despite the normal decline in EPP amplitude (safety factor). (B) Three-Hertz RNS, postsynaptic NMJ disorder. Note the lower EPP amplitudes. With further acetylcholine depletion, the last three potentials are below the threshold, and a muscle fiber action potential is not generated. (C) Three-Hertz RNS, presynaptic NMJ disorder. Note that all EPPs are less than the threshold, and no muscle fiber action potentials are generated. The EPP declines in amplitude, but the decrement is not as marked in normal subjects or patients with postsynaptic NMJ disorders. (D) Fifty-Hertz RNS, presynaptic NMJ disorder. Note the progressive increment in the EPP amplitude to the above threshold and the subsequent generation of muscle fiber action potentials. (From: Preston D, Shapiro B. *Electromyography and NM Disorders.* 2nd ed. Boston: Butterworth-Heinemann; 2005:65–75 & 553–564.)

Table 15.1 Common Disorders of Neuromuscular Transmission

IMMUNE-MEDIATED DISORDERS	TOXIC/METABOLIC DISORDERS	CONGENITAL MYASTHENIC SYNDROME
Lambert-Eaton myasthenic syndrome Myasthenia gravis	Arthropod venom poisoning (e.g., black widow spider) Botulism Hypermagnesemia Medication side effects (e.g., aminoglycosides, procainamide, penicillamine) Organophosphate insecticide poisoning Snake venom poisoning Tick paralysis	Defective synthesis or packaging of acetylcholine (Ach) Deficiency of acetylcholinesterase Deficiency of Ach receptors

cases can have antibodies to muscle-specific tyrosine kinase (MUSK) or low-density lipoprotein receptor-related protein 4 (LRP4) or are antibody negative. Antibody testing is key in confirming a diagnosis of MG. In patients with objective weakness, the Tensilon (edrophonium) test or ice-bag test may be used to support a clinical suspicion. RNS and SFEMG are especially useful in antibody-negative cases. Treatment includes acetylcholinesterase inhibitors and immunosuppression (steroids, steroid-sparing agents, Intravenous Immunoglobulin (IVIG), and complement inhibitors). Computed tomography (CT) of the chest is recommended to exclude thymoma. However, studies show that thymectomy of even healthy thymus tissue may be therapeutic in patients who are AChR antibody positive *and* have generalized symptoms.

Cetin H, Vincent A. Pathogenic mechanisms and clinical correlations in autoimmune myasthenic syndromes. *Semin Neurol.* 2018; 38(3):344–354.

Gilhus NE, Verschuuren JJ. Myasthenia gravis: subgroup classification and therapeutic strategies. *Lancet Neurol.* 2015;14:1023–1036.

Benatar M. A systematic review of diagnostic studies in myasthenia gravis. *Neuromuscul Disord.* 2006;16(7):459–467. Available at: https://www.ncbi.nlm.nih.gov/books/NBK73346/. Of note edrophonium had been discontinued in the US as of 2018.

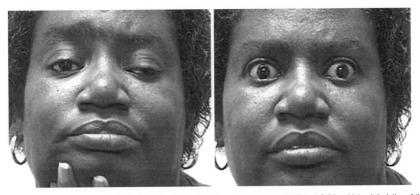

Fig. 15.3 Edrophonium test in myasthenia gravis. Before testing *(left)*, there is marked ptosis of the left lid and lateral deviation of the left eye, and the jaw must be supported. Within 5 seconds after injection of 0.1 mg edrophonium *(right)*, the function of both lids and left medial rectus are improved. (From: Sanders DB, Massey JM. Clinical features of myasthenia gravis. *Handb Clin Neurol.* 2008;91:229–252.)

11. **What is the electrophysiology seen in MG?**
    In MG, the CMAP amplitudes are usually normal. With 2 to 3 Hz of repetitive stimulation, a decremental response of 10% or greater in CMAP amplitude is diagnostic. Diagnostic RNS occurs in approximately 75% of patients with generalized MG and in less than 50% of patients with ocular MG. SFEMG is the most sensitive test for assessing the NMJ and is abnormal in more than 90% of patients with MG.

12. **What is Lambert-Eaton myasthenic syndrome (LEMS)?**
    LEMS is due to a presynaptic abnormality of Ach release at the NMJ secondary to an autoimmune attack against the P/Q voltage-gated calcium channel on the presynaptic motor nerve terminal. The clinical triad of LEMS is proximal weakness, dysautonomia, and areflexia. Weakness of the proximal lower extremities occurs early in the course, although it progresses to involve the shoulder girdle and oculobulbar muscles. Dysautonomia most frequently involves dry mouth but may also include erectile dysfunction, orthostasis, and constipation. LEMS patients may experience an increase in muscle power with exercise. LEMS may be secondary to a paraneoplastic syndrome in 50% to 60% of cases; the most common cancer association is small cell lung cancer (SCLCA). The remainder of LEMS cases (non-paraneoplastic) is related to idiopathic autoimmune dysregulation.

Kesner VG, Oh SJ, Dimachkie MM, et al. Lambert-Eaton myasthenic syndrome. *Neurol Clin.* 2018;36:379–394. Available at: https:// doi.org/10.1016/j.ncl.2018.01.008.

13. **Describe ancillary testing and management of LEMS.**
    In LEMS, autoantibodies against the presynaptic P/Q calcium channels are detectable in 85% to 90% of patients. CT chest, abdomen, and pelvis or positron emission tomography (PET) is recommended to exclude malignancy. SOX1 antibodies may be seen in approximately 60% of patients with SCLCA. RNS and postexercise CMAPs are useful in diagnosis. Treating the malignancy, if present, can help to improve motor symptoms. Immunosuppression (steroids, steroid-sparing agents, IVIG) is also very effective. Amifampridine (3,4 diaminopyridine) is a US Food and Drug Administration (FDA)-approved oral medication specifically for LEMS patients, which increases Ach release in nerve terminals by potassium channel blockade.

14. What is the electrophysiology in LEMS?

In LEMS, the baseline CMAP amplitudes are usually low. With 2 to 3 Hz of stimulation, there may be a decremental response. With 30 to 50 Hz stimulation or a 10-second contraction (which approximates a 50-Hz stimulation), there is an increase in the CMAP amplitude that is usually greater than 100%.

15. Describe adult and infantile botulism.

Botulism is caused by an NMJ toxin, which is produced by *Clostridium botulinum*. Botulinum toxin affects the presynaptic nerve terminal by targeting SNARE proteins, preventing release of Ach. This results in an acute, generalized, descending paralysis.

Symptoms of adult botulism may occur after ingestion of toxin-tainted food, spore inhalation, or spore-colonized wounds. The syndrome includes acute onset of blurred vision and diplopia, which may be accompanied by anorexia, nausea, and vomiting. Pupillary dysfunction, dysarthria, and dysphagia follow rapidly and are soon joined by respiratory insufficiency and quadriparesis. Treatment is with botulism antitoxin.

Infantile botulism is a result of *C. botulinum* colonizing the immature gut. The typical food exposure is honey. Symptoms include early constipation and weak cry and suck, followed by a quadriparesis and poorly reactive pupils. Most patients require intubation for respiratory support. Treatment is with intravenous (IV) botulism immunoglobulin.

In both forms of the disease, RNS shows facilitation of the motor response at high rates of stimulation (30 to 50 Hz) and with brief exercise.

Rosow LK, Strober JB. Infant botulism: review and clinical update. *Pediatr Neurol*. 2015;52(5):487–492.

16. Summarize nerve conduction study (NCS) findings in NMJ transmission defects.

See Table 15.2.

Cherian A, Baheti NN, Iype T. Electrophysiological study in neuromuscular junction disorders. *Ann Indian Acad Neurol*. 2013;16(1):34–41. Available at: https://www.ncbi.nlm.nih.gov/pmc/articles/PMC3644779/.

17. Identify key rehabilitation principles in managing MG patients.

Weakness in MG will increase with exercise and heat. Energy conservation techniques are useful, with afternoon rest periods and avoidance of warm environments. Strength training has not been extensively studied; therefore maximal stress exercise cannot be recommended. A few small trials have been performed examining exercise (aerobic, resistance, balance, respiratory muscle training) in mildly affected patients with MG; however, larger studies are needed to determine practice parameters.

Table 15.2 Nerve Conduction Study Findings in Neuromuscular Junction Transmission Defects

NMJ DEFECT	HZ	FINDING IN NCS	WITH EXERCISE	POSTEXERCISE FINDINGS OF NCS
Postsynaptic	2–5 Hz	>10% decrement Normal CMAP amplitude	10 s	Repair of decrement postexercise
			30–60 s	Postactivation exhaustion 2–4 min
Presynaptic	2–5 Hz	>10% decrement, low CMAP amplitude	10 s	Postactivation facilitation postexercise
	20–50 Hz	>100% increase CMAP amplitude		

CMAP, Compound muscle action potential; *NCS*, nerve conduction study.

BIBLIOGRAPHY

Preston D, Shapiro B. *Electromyography and NM Disorders*. 2nd ed. Boston: Butterworth-Heinemann; 2005:65–75 & 553–564.

WEBSITES

Myasthenia Gravis Foundation of America. Available at: www.myasthenia.org.
Neuromuscular Disease Center. Available at: https://neuromuscular.wustl.edu.
Sanders D, Wolfe G, et al. International consensus guidance for management of myasthenia Gravis. Neurology 2016;87:419–425.
Available at: https://n.neurology.org/content/87/4/419.long.

PERSON-CENTERED REHABILITATION: INTERDISCIPLINARY CONTEXT-SPECIFIC TREATMENT REQUIRES COMPONENT CUSTOMIZATION

CHAPTER 16

Steven A. Stiens, MD, MS, Bryan J. O'Young, MD, CAc, FAAPMR, Sam S. H. Wu, MD, MA, MPH, MBA, and Mark A. Young, MD, MBA, FACP, FAAPMR, DABPMR

The mainspring of creativity appears to be the same tendency we discover so deeply as the curative force in psychotherapy, man's tendency to actualize himself, to become his potentialities. By this, I mean the organic and human life, the urge to expand, extend, develop, mature—the tendency to express and activate all the capacities of the organism, or the self.
— Carl Rogers, PhD (1902–1987)

KEY POINTS

1. ***Impairment*** is any loss or abnormality of anatomic structure, physiologic, or psychological function of an organ or system.
2. ***Activity limitation*** is any deficit in a person's ability to complete a task that would otherwise be within the range considered normal for a person of a particular age.
3. ***Participation*** is performance in all the areas of life, including societal opportunities in which an individual is actively involved in meeting life goals and fulfilling roles
4. ***Rehabilitation*** is the collaborative process of development of a person to his or her fullest physical, psychological, social, educational, and vocational potential by eliminating or compensating for any biochemical pathophysiology, anatomic impairments, activity limitations, participation restrictions, and environment barriers.
5. The ***rehabilitation problem list*** is a sequence of diagnoses, impairments, activity limitations, and participation barriers that guide goal setting. It is organized as a spectrum starting from active injuries and diagnoses through the domains of disability (disablement).

1. How are the person and personhood relevant to rehabilitation?
   The ***person*** is a living human being with characteristic unique genetic, physical, mental, social, and spiritual dimensions. Each is guided by experiences and developmental changes and has the free will to make life decisions. Therefore the person is the current "real self" subject of rehabilitation intervention. As such, ***personhood*** is the dynamic process of being and becoming the self; ***function is the catalyst***. Awareness of the patient's self-understanding is critical to enabling efficacy. The person has the right to solve his or her problems and plays an essential role in health goal setting. As Carl Rogers explained, "The hypothesis is that the patient has within him or herself the capacity latent, if not evident, to understand those aspects of life and the capacity to organize a relationship to live in the direction of self-actualization and maturity with resulting inner comfort."[a] People are in constant dynamic development and require reserve capabilities to meet health challenges. Anticipatory ***prehabilitation*** and continued community interventions are contemporary innovations.

Bean JF, Brown L, DeAngelis TR, et al. The rehabilitation enhancing aging through connected health prehabilitation trial. *Arch Phys Med Rehabil.* 2019;100(11):1999–2005.

Kirschenbaum H. Carl Rogers's life and work: an assessment on the 100th anniversary of his birth. *J Counsel Devel.* 2004;82: 116–124.

Ziegelstein RC. Personomics and precision medicine. *Trans Am Clin Climatol Assoc.* 2017;128:160–168. Available at: https://www.ncbi.nlm.nih.gov/pmc/articles/PMC5525386/.

[a]Rogers C. A current formulation of client-centered therapy. *Soc Serv Rev.* 1950;24(4):442–450.

2. How can person-centered rehabilitation be defined and related to the new concepts of precision and personalized medicine?

   Person-centeredness is a philosophy for organizing, designing, and delivering a plan of care directed by the patient's individual needs, preferences, capabilities, resources, and goals. As such, aspects of the person as an individual related to family, employment, leisure, personal passions, culture, and community transcend the biological reality. The unique **personal context-driven** plan complements evidence-based biomedical care with an intent to achieve optimum outcomes. **Precision medicine**, **personalized medicine**, and **theranostics** use predictive models to guide biomedicine derived from population studies of molecular and genetic profiles compared with the patient's unique **genotype** and **proteome**.

Gareth T, Kayes N. Person centered care in neurorehabilitation: a secondary analysis. *Disabil Rehabil.* 2020;42(16):2334–2343. Available at: https://doi.org/10.1080/09638288.2018.1561952.

Sacristán JA. Patient-centered medicine and patient-oriented research: improving health outcomes for individual patients. *BMC Med Inform Decis Mak.* 2013;13:6. Available at: https://doi.org/10.1186/1472-6947-13-6.

3. What are the five responsibilities of the clinician in the clinician-patient relationship?
   a. Suspension of judgment—Use empathy.
   b. Evaluation for health risks—Recognition of assets, resources, potential.
   c. Diagnosis by problem, identify pathophysiologic processes. Identify intervention mechanisms.
   d. Reporting, analysis—Interpreting in context of disability experience and environment of choice.
   e. Treatment Cooperative agreement—Interdisciplinary formulation, informed consent, prescription, consultation, and plan.

Emanuel EJ, Emanuel LL. Four models of the physician-patient relationship. *JAMA.* 1992;267:2221–2226.

Personalized Medicine Coalition. www.personalizedmedicinecoalition.org

Pinto RZ, Ferreira ML, Oliveira VC, et al. Patient-centred communication is associated with positive therapeutic alliance: a systematic review. *J Physiother.* 2012;58(2):77–87. Available at: https://www.sciencedirect.com/science/article/pii/S1836955312700875?via%3Dihub. doi: 10.1016/S1836-9553(12)70087-5.

4. Define health, illness, and disease.
   - **Health** is an optimum condition of a person's physical, mental, and social well-being **in action**. Health is not merely the absence of disease or infirmity; it is the **dynamic situation of self-action** through functional activity.
   - **Illness** is the patient's unique subjective lived experience of "unwellness" distress or threat of failed function. Illness is not only a biologic state but can also be an existential transformation that affects trust in the body and reliance on the future. The illness experience contributes to the psychological state, which influences the perception of the body's ability to function in the present and future.
   - **Disease** is a medical construct that diagnoses a disorder characterized by a set of symptoms, signs, and pathology and is attributable to infection, diet, heredity, or environment.

5. Define impairment.

   Impairment is any loss or abnormality of anatomic structure, physiologic, or psychological function of an organ or system. Examples include loss of limb, weakness, sensory deficit, facial disfigurement, and being immune-compromised.

6. How can the effects of disease on a person be practically classified?

   The World Health Organization originally published the International Classification of Impairments, Disabilities, and Handicaps (ICIDH) in 1980 and released a revision (ICIDH-2) in 2001. Within the International Classification of Disability Functioning and Health (ICF) **Disability** is the current summary term for the collective consequences of the disease on the person. Consequences are considered within three interrelated **domains**: (1) the **organ** or system, (2) the whole **person**, and (3) **society**. In ICF/ICIDH-2 terminology, limitations or barriers within these domains are named **impairments** (organ domain), **activity limitations** (person domain), and **barriers to participation** (societal domain).

Gray DB, Hendershot GE. The ICIDH-2: developments for a new era of outcomes research. *Arch Phys Med Rehabil.* 2000;81(suppl 2): S10–S14. Available at: https://pubmed.ncbi.nlm.nih.gov/11128899/.

World Health Organization. Available at: www3.who.int/icf (http://www.who.int/).

7. How do impairments and activity limitations interact?

   A **task** is a purposeful activity that requires the engagement of the whole person. Examples are an ability to perform activities of daily living, such as dressing, driving, shopping, or cooking. **Impairments** are the organ domain, and **activity limitations** are deficits in personal performance. Therefore **activities**, according to the ICF and the ICIDH-2, are the performance of personal-level tasks or human endeavors.

8. What is the relationship between handicap and participation?

The relationship is **reciprocal**. **Participation** is defined as a person's involvement in life situations. **Involvement** means inclusion and contributions to life activities in the context of the person's community. As participation increases, handicap decreases. The restriction of participation or involvement in life activities by external factors (social roles) is termed **participation limitation/restriction** or **barrier to participation**.

Dijkers MP. Issues in the conceptualization and measurement of participation: an overview. *Arch Phys Med Rehab.* 2010;91(9 Suppl 1): S5–16. Available at: https://www.archives-pmr.org/article/S0003-9993(10)00095-X/fulltext.

9. What are contextual factors?

Contextual factors are the "situations" within and around the person. ICF/ICIDH-2 describe environmental and personal contextual factors as follows:

- **Environmental factors** include many categories, such as natural environments; human-made changes to the environment; products and technology; support and relationships; attitudes, values, beliefs, services, and systems and policies.
- **Personal factors** refer to patient characteristics that may contribute to or limit adaptation. They include genome, proteome, age, gender, diagnoses, fitness, lifestyle, upbringing, coping styles, social background, education, profession, past experiences, character style, and physical and psychological assets.

Stucki G, Ewert T, Cieza A. Value and application of the ICF in rehabilitation medicine. *Disabil Rehabil.* 2003;25(11–12):628–634 Available at: https://efisiopediatric.com/wp-content/uploads/ 2017/06/ Value-and-application-of-the-ICF-in-rehabilitation-medicine.pdf.

10. What are the influences on environmental characteristics on the rehabilitation decision-making process?

Function in the ICFDH "is defined as an interaction of a person with a health condition and the material and social environment." The rehabilitation leader integrates this information with interdisciplinary team conversation. The patient's pertinent environment includes the **micro** (immediate interventions, adaptations), **meso** (health care system, service organization), and **macro** (community resources, social systems, payors).

The progressive clinician maintains anticipatory surveillance for all potential opportunities that patients can utilize. Team leaders innovate, certify, and proactively evolve the immediate rehabilitation program, informing and adapting the health care system and building bridges to community support for patients' benefit.

Commission on Accreditation of Rehabilitation Facilities. Available at: http://www.carf.org/.

Gutenbrunner C, Nugraha B. Decision-making in evidence-based practice in rehabilitation medicine: proposing a fourth factor. *Am J Phys Med Rehabil.* 2020;99:436–440. doi: 10.1097/PHM.0000000000001394.

11. What is rehabilitation? Does it optimize function and improve lives?

Rehabilitation is the collaborative process of development of a person to his or her fullest physical, psychological, social, educational, and vocational potential by eliminating or compensating for any biochemical pathophysiology, anatomic impairments, activity limitations, participation restrictions, and environment barriers. In contrast to classic reductionist medical therapeutics, which emphasize diagnosis and focused treatment directed against the pathologic process alone, rehabilitation directs treatment against the pathologic process. However, it also applies multiple simultaneous interventions addressing both the cause and secondary effects of injury and illness at multiple system levels *(biopsychosocial model)*.

Traditionally, medical science has directed treatment at the cause of the disease *(biomedical model)*, neglecting the secondary effects of illness. The very nature of rehabilitation includes assessment and achievement of the patient's personal capacities, role performance, and life aspirations.

Comprehensive rehabilitation requires five necessary and sufficient subcomponents:

a. Unique, patient-centered plan
b. Goals derived and prioritized through an interdisciplinary process
c. Patient, family, and community participation required to achieve the goals
d. Results in improvement in the patient's personal potential and spontaneous activity
e. Outcomes demonstrate enablement (i.e., improved organ system function, activity, and participation)

Imrie R. Rethinking the relationships between disability, rehabilitation, and society. *Disabil Rehabil.* 1997;19:263–271.

Jesus TS, Bright F, Kayes N, et al. Person-centered rehabilitation: what exactly does it mean? Protocol for a scoping review with thematic analysis towards framing the concept and practice of person-centred rehabilitation. *BMJ Open.* 2016;6(7):e011959. Available at: https://bmjopen.bmj.com/ content/6/7/e011959.

Terry G, Kayes N. Person centered care in neurorehabilitation: a secondary analysis. *Disabil Rehabil.* 2020;42(16):2334–2343. doi: 10.1080/09638288.2018.1561952. Available at: https://doi.org/10.1080/09638288.2018.1561952.

12. **What components mutually support patient-centered rehabilitation medicine practice?**
The process that maximizes all of the patient's capabilities and animates potential has the following seven inter-active components:
    a. *Understanding of the whole person*: Identity, occupation, lifestyles, ideology, and aspirations
    b. *Exploration of the illness experience and compensation*: Pathologic process, disability, capabilities, and resources
    c. *Formulate a comprehensive problem list* with patient contributions
    d. *Deriving short- and long-term goals*: Prioritizing sequential steps to least restrictive settings of choice
    e. *Incorporating prevention, health promotion, patient education, and adaptation*
    f. *Enhancing the treatment relationships* among the interdisciplinary team and the patient, family, friends, and volunteers
    g. Establishing *home- and community-based habits*, *a routine of self-care*, and scheduled treatment visits, and advancing goals.

Cott CA. Client-centred rehabilitation: client perspectives. *Disabil Rehabil.* 2004;26:1411–1422.

Schut HA, Stam HJ. Goals in rehabilitation teamwork. *Disabil Rehabil.* 1994;16(4):223–226. Available at: https://pubmed.ncbi.nlm.nih.gov/7812023/.

Martin D. Martin's Map: a conceptual framework for teaching and learning the medical interview using a patient-centered approach. *Med Educ.* 2003;37:1145–1153. Available at: https://www.researchgate.net/publication/6354901_Martin%27s_Map_A_conceptual_framework_for_teaching_and_learning_the_medical_interview_using_a_patient-centred_approach.

13. **What is the multidisciplinary practice of patient care? How do contemporary opportunities enable interdisciplinary and transdisciplinary practice?**
Multidisciplinary teams consist of various professionals treating the patient separately, with discipline-specific goals. The patient's progress with each discipline is communicated primarily through various documents.
    In the *interdisciplinary* collaborative practice model, each profession evaluates the patient separately, simultaneously shaping documentation, and interact together at team meetings, where they collaborate on short- and long-term goals. The team collectively develops a synchronized vision for patient outcomes, as informed by their assessments and patient aspirations. The goals of each discipline are combined into a *unified*, *coordinated plan* through the synergistic interaction of the team, patient, and family. Photographs of successful adaptive events can be used to share achievements.
    In addition, the team collaboratively participates in problem solving and decision-making as the plan unfolds. Evidence for decision-making includes measurements of various disability domains and task performances. Patients with intellectual disabilities and achievements "in the field" can contribute to the process with photographs and videos of successful life activities that can be assessed by the team for incremental goal setting. The *whole outcome* is synergistic! Life performance is more than the sum of specific interventions or discrete patient achievements.

Whyte J, Barrett AM. Advancing the evidence base of rehabilitation treatments: a developmental approach. *Arch Phys Med Rehabil.* 2012;93(8 Suppl 2):S101–10. Available at: https://www.ncbi.nlm.nih.gov/pmc/articles/PMC3732479/.

14. **How can rehabilitation treatments be specified, dosed, and monitored?**
Keith and Lipsey define *treatment theory* as "propositions that explain the actual nature of the process that transforms received therapy into improved health." The customized rehabilitation is delivered in a schedule by a network of providers directed at various targets. *Targets* are specific, measurable aspects of patient functioning responsive to individual *treatment components*. Three *treatment characteristics* are considered: aspects of functioning intended to change, ingredients administered, and mechanisms of action. *Aims* are outcomes that require changes in multiple targets and typically relate to the independent performance of various task functions. Treatments can be grouped based on their direct targets: *organ functions*, *skills and habits*, and *representations* (knowledge, attitudes, motivation, volition). Experience with treatment effectiveness, dosing, required duration, and intermediate outcomes required for the advancement of care settings toward the community is essential for leadership in simultaneously executing interventions.

Van Stan JH, Dijkers MP, Whyte J, et al. The rehabilitation treatment specification system: implications for improvements in research design, reporting, replication, and synthesis. *Arch Phys Med Rehabil.* 2019;100:146–155, 2019. doi: 10.1016/j.apmr.2018.09.112 Available at: https://www.ncbi.nlm.nih.gov/ pmc/articles/PMC6452635/.

MossRehab/Einstein Healthcare Network. *Manual for Rehabilitation Treatment Specification.* Elkins Park, Pennsylvania; 2019. Available at: https://mrri.org/innovations/manual-for-rehabilitation-treatment-specification/.

15. **What nine conditions maximize the success of interdisciplinary rehabilitation teams?**
    • Adherence to a *mission statement* (i.e., person-centered rehabilitation in the least restrictive setting)
    • *Delineated roles* for each discipline

- *Balance of participation* by each professional
- Agreement on, and implementation of, ground *rules for interaction*
- Clear and effective *communication* and *documentation*
- *Scientific approach* to patient problems, and development of strengths
- Clearly defined, *measurable goals*
- Working *knowledge of group process*
- *Expedient procedures* for coming to consensus and decision-making

Sinclair LB, Lingard LA, Mohabeer RN. What's so great about rehabilitation teams? An ethnographic study of interprofessional collaboration in a rehabilitation unit. *Arch Phys Med Rehabil.* 2009;90:1196–1201. Available at: https://www.archives-pmr.org/article/S0003-9993(09)00219-6/fulltext.

16. Describe the phases of the rehabilitation process.

Rehabilitation intervention is best orchestrated to meet goals in a sequence that advances the patient efficiently to the fullest function in the least restrictive setting. These phases are guidelines for simultaneous overlapping interventions. Efficiently achieving life-enhancing outcomes reinforces effort. A comprehensive problem list guides monitoring of index measures of pathophysiology, and success in functional capabilities within domains of disability: impairment, activity, and participation.

- *Phase I (evaluation).* Prehabilitation through initiation, recognition of priorities.
- *Phase II (initial treatment).* Arrest the pathophysiologic processes, prevent complications, provide substrate for regeneration, establish psychological support, and assess response. Utilize and order definitive adaptive equipment.
- *Phase III (therapeutic exercise).* Remobilization on healing, enhancement of organ performance, and maximization of all capabilities.
- *Phase IV (task reacquisition).* Educate and confirm personal knowledge, adaptive techniques, and spontaneous disability-appropriate adaptive behavior.
- *Phase V (patient-family adaptation and environmental modification).* Organizing, synchronizing, a scheduled network for sustained progress, environmental enhancement (physical, psychological, social, and political) to eliminate barriers and establish participation.

These phases approximate the emphasis of the team's interventions during daily and through a community reintegration continuum. The *rehabilitation problem list* (Box 16.1) is a spectrum of diagnoses, impairments, activity limitations, and participation barriers that guide goal setting priorities and periods. The patient drives the process by demonstrating his or her particular predicament with disability and treatment priorities. Adaptation is achieved by *enhancing the patient's personal characteristics* that mediate or limit disability. The overall goal is the fullest personal enablement and action toward fulfillment of life roles that are actively played out.

de Kleijn-de Vrankrijker M, Seidel C, Tscherner U. The International Classification of Impairments, Disabilities, and Handicaps (ICIDH): its use in rehabilitation. *World Health Stat Q.* 1999;42:151–156.

17. How does a transdisciplinary team interact to facilitate progress?

Transdisciplinary teams are designed through cross-training of members and procedure development to allow an *overlap of responsibilities* between disciplines (Fig. 16.1). This overlap enables collaboration in problem solving and increases interdependence. Disciplines with extensive direct involvement with the patient during particular phases may rotate into leadership *case managers* and coordinate team efforts. Establishing and achieving goals

Box 16.1 Rehabilitation Problem List: Ordered Categories

Impairments (e.g., neurogenic, bladder, bowel, sexual function)
Activity limitations (e.g., mobility, activities of daily living, communication)
Education
Participation barriers
Psychological adaptation
Social role function
Architectural accessibility
Community reintegration
Vocational adaptation
Spiritual practice

The rehabilitation problem list is organized as a spectrum of areas for intervention, starting from active injuries and diagnoses through the dimensions of disability (disablement). It is individualized for each patient and organizes short- and long-term goals.

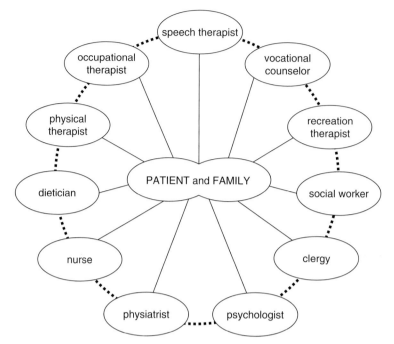

Fig. 16.1 Interdisciplinary team interaction. (From: Mumma CM, Nelson A. Models for theory-based practice of rehabilitation nursing. In: Hoeman SD, ed. *Rehabilitation Nursing: Process and Application.* St. Louis: Mosby; 1995:32–53.)

starts with unconditional positive regard but may require a more direct approach, such as **motivational interviewing**, in patient interactions at times during rehabilitation. This requires empathy, identification of discrepancies between patient behaviors and personal goals, development of self-efficacy, and reconfirmation of commitment.

Wagner CC, McMahon BT. Motivational interviewing and rehabilitation counseling practice. *Rehabil Counsel Bull.* 2004;47:152–161.

WEBSITE

World Health Organization. Available at: www.who.org.

BIBLIOGRAPHY

Cristian A, Batmangelich S. *Physical Medicine and Rehabilitation Patient-Centered Care: Mastering the Competencies.* New York: Demos Medical; 2014.

Dunn DS, Elliott TR. The place and promise of theory in rehabilitation psychology. *Rehabil Psychol.* 2008;53(3):254–267. doi:10.1037/a0012962.

Granger CV, Gresham CE. International Classification of Impairments, Disabilities, and Handicaps (ICIDH) as a conceptual basis for stroke outcome research. A tribute to Philip H.N. Wood. *Stroke.* 1999;21(Suppl II):1166–1167.

Haig A, Stiens SA. Telerehabilitation: exercise and adaptation in home and community. In: Moroz A, Flanagan SR, Zaretsky H, eds. *Medical Aspects of a Disability.* 5th ed. New York, NY: Springer; 2017:681–696.

Jacob ME, Ni P, Driver J, et al. Burden and patterns of multimorbidity: impact on disablement in older adults. *Am J Phys Med Rehabil.* 2020;99:359–365. doi: 10.1097/PHM.0000000000001388.

Jesus TS, Landry MD, Hoening H. Global need for physical rehabilitation: systematic analysis from the Global Burden of Disease study 2017. *Int J Environ Res Public Health.* 2019;16:E980.

Lundgren C, Molander C. *Teamwork in Medical Rehabilitation.* New York: Routledge; 2017.

Morrison C, Dearden A. Beyond tokenistic participation: using representational artefacts to enable meaningful public participation in health service design. *Health Policy.* 2013;112:179–186. Available at: https://doi.org/10.1016/j.healthpol.2013.05.008.

Ozer MN, Payton OD, Nelson CE. *Treatment Planning for Rehabilitation: A Patient-Centered Approach.* New York: McGraw-Hill; 2000.

Pere D. Building physician competency in lifestyle medicine: a model for health improvement. *Am J Prev Med.* 2017;52(2):260–61. Available at: http://dx.doi.org/10.1016/j.amepre.2016.11.001.

Stiens SA, Haselkorn JK, Peters DJ, et al. Rehabilitation intervention for patients with upper extremity dysfunction: challenges of outcome evaluation. *Am J Ind Med.* 1996;29: 590–601.

World Health Organization (WHO). *ICIDH-2: International Classification System of Functioning and Disability—Beta-2 Draft, Short Version.* Geneva: WHO; 1999.

MANUAL MEDICINE: PHILOSOPHY, ASSESSMENT, AND MANIPULATIVE TECHNIQUES

Lisa DeStefano, DO, Jacob Rowan, DO, Jeffrey Meyers, DO, and Tyler Cymet, DO

Healing is a matter of time, but it is sometimes also a matter of opportunity…

— Hippocrates

KEY POINTS

1. A joint is not a passive structure. Each joint needs to be conceptualized as an actively stabilized dynamic center of the kinetic energy transition, proprioceptively monitoring total body position and contributing to segmental function.
2. Stabilization of any joint requires flawless interdependent active, passive, and neural subsystem activity.
3. The mechanisms that contribute to manipulative techniques' effectiveness are inherent in optimizing the tissues within the joints' role in transferring kinetic energy, proprioception, mechanoreception, and segmental function.
4. The scope of the manual medicine practice is much greater than cracking a joint. It requires the knowledge of understanding the musculoskeletal system's normal function and the skill in optimizing that function to achieve pain-free motion of the musculoskeletal system to enhance whole-person wellbeing.
5. Manual medicine is undervalued and underused in health care. Chronic musculoskeletal pain and arthritic conditions are effectively and efficiently addressed by optimizing function and improving joint function and stability.

1. **What is the manual medicine perspective of patient health, assessment, intervention, and outcomes?**
   A joint is not only a mechanical structure that functions as a hinge or guides motion between two bones. **Joint systems** involve a sophisticated interplay between active (muscle), passive (joint capsule, ligament, tendon), and neural subsystems. **Joint dysfunction** or reduced range of motion of a joint causes an imbalance in these subsystems' function. This imbalance has negative local and distal implications in musculoskeletal function and general health. The goal of manual medicine is to restore pain-free motion of the musculoskeletal system to enhance whole-person well-being.

2. **What is spinal stability? Name the stabilizing subsystems?**
   The normal function of the **spinal stabilizing system** is to provide enough support to the spine to match the instantaneously varying stability demands due to changes in spinal posture and static and dynamic loads. Three subsystems work together to achieve these goals: **passive (ligamentous), active (musculotendinous),** and **neural control systems** (Fig. 17.1).

   Active, passive, and neural subsystem integration for stability of the spine, emphasizing that the local and global musculature provide feedback and feedforward information into the peripheral nervous system for spinal stability.

Panjabi MM. The stabilizing system of the spine. Part II. Neutral zone and instability hypothesis. *J Spinal Disord*. 1992;5(4):390–396; discussion 397. doi: 10.1097/00002517-199212000-00002.

Bergmark A. Stability of the lumbar spine. A study in mechanical engineering. *Acta Ortho Scand*. 1989;230(suppl):20–24.

3. **What is arthrokinetic reflex activation or inhibition?**
   Coined by medical researchers at the University of Pittsburgh's Medical School, Department of Physiology, in 1956 to refer to how joint movement can reflexively cause muscle activation or inhibition. The prefix "arthro-" means joint, "kinetic" signifies motion. A **reflex** in humans refers to an involuntary movement in response to a given

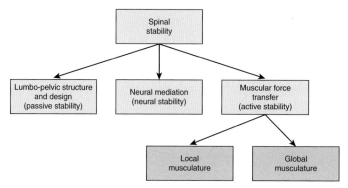

Fig. 17.1 Spine Stabilizing Subsystems.

stimulus. Thus the **arthrokinetic reflex** refers to the involuntary response when a joint is moved, namely that relevant muscles fire reflexively.

Wyke BD. Temporomandibular arthrokinetic reflex control of the mandibular musculature. *Br J Oral Surg.* 1975;13(2):196–202.

Ramcharan JE, Wyke B. Articular reflexes at the knee joint: an electromyographic study. *Am J Physiol.* 1972;223(6):1276–1280. doi:10.1152/ajplegacy.1972.223.6.1276

Cohen LA, Cohen ML. Arthrokinetic reflex of the knee. *Am J Physiol.* 1956;184(2):433–437. doi:10.1152/ajplegacy.1956.184.2.433.

4. How vital are alignment and functional range of motion?

The joint's range of motion is essential because the **mechanoreceptors** within the ligamentous system signal muscles to provide instantaneous stabilizing demands. The musculotendinous system is dependent on alignment for dynamic posture to optimize the lever arms and inertial loads of different masses and external loads. Properly maintained alignment in posture resists progressive deformity and requires resisted functional range in daily activity, preserving the "muscle memory." The act of committing a specific motor task into memory through repetition develops dynamic balance and resilience, thus preventing injury.

5. How does the joint affect muscle function?

Each joint capsule is monitored by a constellation of mechanoreceptors (neural control system), which signal where the joint is in three-dimensional space. The peripheral nervous system perceives deficiencies in the joint range of motion and central circuits attempt to compensate by redistributing tensions through the insertion arrays of local muscle groups.

6. Don't all muscles work the same way? How is dysfunction detected?

It is useful to consider the classification of muscles in relation to function when considering **dynamic stabilization**. Functionally, the **stabilizer muscles** tend to have a postural holding role associated with eccentrically decelerating or resisting momentum. They control the neutral range of motion and monosynaptically take their cues from mechanoreceptors of the joint they stabilize.

In contrast, the **mobilizer muscles** (e.g., rectus femoris and latissimus dorsi) tend to have a movement production role associated with concentric muscle acceleration. **Mobilizer muscles** tend to cross many segments, but they do not have attachments at all segments between origin and insertion (e.g., sternocleidomastoid, rectus abdominis). **Mobilizer muscles** tend to become facilitated in the presence of joint dysfunction. Due to the loss in stimulus of mechanoreceptors within a joint, joint dysfunction leads to deafferentation of the **stabilizer muscles** (Table 17.1).

Goff B. The application of recent advances in neurophysiology to Miss R. Rood's concept of neuromuscular facilitation. *Physiotherapy.* 1972;58(2):409–415.

Janda V. On the concept of postural muscles and posture in man. *Aust J Physiother.* 1983;29(3):83–84.

Comerford MJ, Mottram SL. Movement and stability dysfunction–contemporary developments. *Man Ther.* 2001;6(1):15–26.

Strengthminded. *Muscle Roles: Synergist, Agonist, Antagonist, Stabilizer & Fixator.* Available at: https://www.strengthminded.com/muscle-roles-synergist-agonist-antagonist-stabilizer-fixator/.

7. What knowledge is necessary to better understand the etiology of common musculoskeletal pain syndromes?

The incidence of musculoskeletal pain syndromes emanating from the facet joints or spinal nerve roots is minor compared with muscles. The etiology is often overuse or microtrauma due to aberrant muscle behavior and suggestive of

Table 17.1 Muscle Classification

LOCAL STABILIZER	GLOBAL STABILIZER	GLOBAL MOBILIZER
• Muscle stiffness to control segmental motion • Controls the neutral joint position • Contraction = no/min. length change 4 does not produce range of motion (ROM). • Activity is often anticipatory (or at the same instant) to functional load or movement to provide protective stiffness prior to motion stress • Activity is independent of direction of movement • Continuous activity throughout movement • Proprioceptive input re: joint position, range, and rate of movement	• Generates force to control ROM • Contraction = eccentric length change 4 control throughout range especially inner range "muscle active = joint passive") and hyper-mobile outer range • Low load deceleration of momentum (especially axial plane: rotation) • Activity is direction-dependent	• Generates torque to produce a range of movement • Contraction = concentric length change 4 concentric production of movement (rather than eccentric control) • Concentric acceleration of movement (especially sagittal plane: flexion/extension) • Shock absorption of load • Activity is direction-dependent • Noncontinuous activity (on/off phasic pattern)

Stability and movement dysfunction related to the forearm and elbow
Gibbons SGT, Mottram SL, Comerford MJ. https://www.researchgate.net/publication/262912716_Stability_and_movement_dysfunction_
related_to_the_forearm_and_elbow. September/October 2001—Orthopaedic Division Review 17.

joint dysfunction. Joint dysfunction (decreased range of motion, altered stress on the joint capsule) causes incomplete mechanoreceptive afferent communication with the spinal cord, which leads to poor efferent communication (inhibition) to the local stabilizer muscles. Most pain syndromes arise from overuse of a global mobilizer muscle, which compensates for joint dysfunction inhibition of the local stabilizer muscle function.

8. What questions and interview techniques are most effective in guiding the examination?
   A keen sense of clinical experience and curiosity is critical when questioning patients about their pain. Not only the timing and frequency but the **events that proceed** the aberrant muscle behavior (i.e., dental procedure or new abdominal strengthening exercise) must be considered. One must also clearly understand **muscle referral patterns** associated with the global muscle system, guiding the clinician to the associated **local muscle inhibition** and corresponding joint dysfunction.

9. What is a "structural examination"? Is there a sequence that makes it most informative and revealing?
   Physical examination of the musculoskeletal system tends to focus on the location of pain and regional gross range of motion. The **structural examination** is a more detailed examination of the neuromusculoskeletal system through observation, inspection, palpation, and motion testing to identify somatic dysfunction areas within each body quadrant. Pelvic and trunk stabilization are critical to the lower quarter examination. Trunk and scapular stabilization is critical to upper quarter examination.

10. What is the "body framework," and how does this relate to somatic dysfunction?
    The **body framework** is composed of skeletal, arthrodial, and myofascial structures. Somatic dysfunction is the impaired or altered function of related components of the somatic (skeletal, arthrodial, myofascial) system and the related vascular, lymphatic, and neural elements.

Anatomy Slings and Their Relationship to Low Back Pain. Available at: www.physio-pedia.com/Anatomy_Slings_and_Their_Relationship_to_Low_Back_Pain.

11. How are the structural examination results documented to consider in diagnosis, gauge severity of involvement, and recognize treatment success prospectively?
    The structural exam evaluates the neuromusculoskeletal system through inspection, palpation, and motion testing. Results are documented in terms of asymmetry, range-of-motion restrictions, or tissue texture abnormalities (e.g., the first cervical vertebrae, C1, resists rotation right). The severity is sometimes noted as none, mild, moderate, or severe.

12. How does the structural examination reveal the subcomponents of somatic dysfunction?
    The subcomponents of somatic dysfunction, *vascular, lymphatic*, and *neural changes*, can be noted through history and/or physical examination.

13. Besides musculoskeletal pain, what other symptoms might suggest the need for a manual medicine approach?

Relevant examples of the varied inpatient conditions that may benefit include constipation, ileus, atelectasis, and vertigo. Weakness, paresthesias, and edema are signs that the patient may have impaired or altered function due to somatic connections, which could benefit from a manual medicine approach.

14. What is a viscerosomatic reflex dysfunction? How does a somatovisceral reflex dysfunction differ?

A localized visceral stimulus is producing patterns of reflex response in segmentally related somatic structures. A viscerosomatic example would be the classic chest pain from myocardial infarction.

A localized nociceptive somatic stimulation produces patterns of reflex response in segmentally related visceral structures. Somatic afferent nerve stimulation can regulate various visceral functions via reflex reactions. The effects of somatic afferent stimulation are dependent on the particular organ and on the spinal afferent segments. For example, gastrointestinal motility is strongly inhibited by nociceptive stimulation of the abdominal skin (sympathetic-gastric) yet is increased with the noxious stimulus of the lower extremity (vagal-gastric). The types of manipulative techniques utilized to treat somatovisceral dysfunctions will depend on the type and location of the nociceptive stimulus.

Sato A, Schmidt RF. The modulation of visceral functions by somatic afferent activity. *Jpn J Physiol.* 1987;37(1):1–17. doi:10.2170/J Physiol.37.1.

Reflex Activity. Available at: www.hal.bim.msu.edu/CMEonLine/Autonomic/Sympathetic/ReflexActivity.html.

15. Describe range assessment and "end feel." Is "joint play" a game?

Typically, evaluation of a joint's motion is described in terms of quality, which encompasses **range, symmetry, and "end feel." Range** of motion refers to the distance or quantity a joint can move. **Symmetry** is defined in terms of motion compared to the contralateral side or two halves of a plain of motion (i.e., sagittal). Symmetry can also be evaluated at the joint's **midrange** or the location within the joint with the least amount of tension. **"End feel"** is a characteristic sensation perceived by the examiner when the *end of joint range of motion is reached.* The **six joint "end types"** most often described are **bone to bone (hard or abrupt), soft tissue (elastic)** approximation, **spasm** end feel, **empty** end feel, **capsular** end feel, and **springy block**.

John Mennell defined **"joint play"** as small and critical joint movements independent of voluntary muscle contraction. Typically, one would assess each joint by moving it through its full range, assessing midrange symmetry and "end-feel" at each end of the range.

Physiopedia. *End-Feel.* Available at: https://physio-pedia.com/End-Feel.

Boston Body Worker. *What is the "End Feel"?* Available at: https://bostonbodyworker.com/blog/what-is-the-end-feel/.

Dalton Myoskeletal. *Joint Play the Mennell Way.* Available at: https://erikdalton.com/blog/joint-play-the-mennell-way/.

16. What is the difference between direct and indirect manipulative methods?

Often manipulation is described by the *structure (joint), manner (direct), intensity (high velocity), and direction of the force applied.* A *"direct technique"* is a manipulative force applied in the direction of the most significant resistance to overcome motion restriction. An *"indirect technique"* involves applying force in a direction opposite to where the musculoskeletal restriction exists (Table 17.2).

Giusti R. *Glossary of Osteopathic Terminology.* Available at: https://www.aacom.org/docs/default-source/insideome/got2011ed.pdf.

Osteopathic Manipulative Treatment (OMT). Available at: www.spine-health.com/treatment/spine-specialists/osteopathic-manipulative-treatment-omt.

17. What is the "CRACK" you hear during a manipulation? Does the "impulse" create an explosion?

The noise heard when a joint is manipulated is the result of cavitation and is the breaking of the surface tension of the synovial fluid and releases gases into the fluid from vacuum pressure changes within the joint capsule. Generally referred to as an "audible release," it often occurs when the manipulation is a high-velocity, low-amplitude technique and is not required for a therapeutically successful manipulation. Most successful manipulative techniques are not necessarily associated with an audible "crack."

Real-Time Visualization of Joint Cavitation—YouTube. Available at: https://www.youtube.com/watch?v=aJLU-4M-hdE.

Physiological Mechanism of Popping ("Cracking") Joints—YouTube. Available at: https://www.youtube.com/watch?v=1gsjS4ZKmpo.

Table 17.2 List of Manipulative Medicine Techniques

OSTEOPATHIC MANIPULATIVE TECHNIQUES

Osteopathic Cranial Manipulative Medicine	Myofascial release of the osseous cranium and its sutures to optimize cranial and cerebrospinal fluid (CSF) hemodynamics
Counterstrain	Spontaneous release by positioning
High velocity–low amplitude (HVLA)	The classic "thrust" technique.
Muscle energy	Passive positioning with active counterforce.
Myofascial release	Application of gentle sustained pressure to myofascial connective tissue restrictions to eliminate pain and restore function.
Ligamentous release	Disengagement, exaggeration and balancing of opposing ligaments.
Lymphatic Technique	Remove impediments to lymphatic drainage.
Soft tissue techniques	Separation of origin and insertion
Visceral techniques	Treatment directed to the viscera to improve function.

18. What are the theories for mechanisms of manipulation?

Joint dysfunction may result from entrapment of synovial material, lack of congruence in the point-to-point contact of opposing joint surfaces, alteration in the biomechanical and biochemical properties of the myofascial elements, alteration in the physical and chemical properties of the synovial fluid and synovial surfaces, or restriction of motion because of altered length and tone of muscle. Optimizing joint arthrokinematics via manipulation ensures associated neuroreflexive responses (e.g., mechanoreceptor and proprioceptor), improving joint stability and function. For example, when addressing spine pain, manipulation allows for increased tolerance for a sustained muscle contraction to maintain proper posture and enables active stabilizer muscle function throughout the normal range of motion, allowing for pain-free motion.

Lascurain-Aguirrebeña I, Newham D, Critchley DJ. Mechanism of action of spinal mobilizations: a systematic review. *Spine (Phila Pa 1976)*. 2016;41(2):159–172. doi:10.1097/BRS.0000000000001151.

19. What are the absolute contraindications to mobilization and manipulation?

None, if there is an accurate diagnosis of somatic dysfunction that requires treatment to affect the patient's overall management and the manual medicine procedure is appropriate for that diagnosis and the patient's physical condition. However, several conditions require clinician recognition and special precautions requiring restraint in situations of excessive risk-benefit analysis. These conditions may include vertebral malignancy, active inflammatory arthropathy, acute spondyloarthropathy, ligamentous instability (Marfan's, Ehlers-Danlos), tumor or metastasis, active spinal infection or osteomyelitis, acute fracture or dislocation, severe osteoporosis, acute myelopathy, cauda equina syndrome, poor outcome to prior manipulation, ankylosing spondylitis or spondyloarthropathy, symptoms of vertebrobasilar insufficiency, or severe spondylosis.

Although reports of cervical spine manipulation complications have gained attention, literature reviews have noted the incidence to be rare.

Powell FC, Hanigan WC, Olivero WC. A risk/benefit analysis of spinal manipulation therapy for relief of lumbar or cervical pain. *Neurosurgery*. 1993;33(1):73–79. doi:10.1227/00006123-199307000-00011.

WHO Guidelines—Contraindications to SMT. Available at: http://wikichiro.org/en/index.php/WHO_Guidelines_-_Contraindications_to_ SMT#:,:text=Contraindications%20to%20joint%20manipulation%20by%20category%20of%20disorder,4%20Neurological%20disorders.%20…%205%20Psychological%20factors.%20.

20. What treatment modalities can complement or be synergistic with manipulative treatment?

Although manipulation alone is often used as a procedure, therapeutic exercises and other manual techniques (e.g., massage) and physical modalities (e.g., acupuncture, trigger point injections) can be synergistic. Research suggests the efficacy of combining manipulation with other modalities, including general anesthesia, epidural steroid injection, epidural and joint anesthesia, and manipulation included with injectants such as steroids and proliferative agents.

Ongley MJ, Klein RG, Dorman TA, et al. A new approach to the treatment of chronic low back pain. *Lancet*. 1987;2(8551):143–146. doi:10.1016/s0140-6736(87)92340-3.

21. Can manipulation lower the cost of patient care?

Yes, an example is low back pain, which has no cure and is fraught with frequent acute exacerbations throughout the patient's lifetime. Low back pain is the leading cause of activity limitation and work absence throughout much of the world. Exacerbations lead to an increase in the use of medications, including opioids, added radiographic studies, physical therapy visits, or injections, all of which are costly. The goal of spinal manipulative treatment is to increase neuromusculoskeletal function in persons struggling with chronic back pain, which markedly reduces acute exacerbations and thus cost.

Tsertsvadze A, Clar C, Court R, et al. Cost-effectiveness of manual therapy for the management of musculoskeletal conditions: a systematic review and narrative synthesis of evidence from randomized controlled trials. *J Manipulative Physiol Ther*. 2014;37(6): 343–362. doi:10.1016/j.jmpt.2014.05.001.

Korthals-de Bos IB, Hoving JL, van Tulder MW, et al. Cost-effectiveness of physiotherapy, manual therapy, and general practitioner care for neck pain: economic evaluation alongside a randomized controlled trial. *BMJ*. 2003;326(7395):911. doi:10.1136/bmj.326.7395.911.

22. What mechanistic processes and system targets guide clinicians and patients?

Models of Manipulation

Respiratory-circulatory	Decongest and improve cellular respiration
Biomechanical-structural	Optimize the musculoskeletal system function
Metabolic-nutritional	Optimize metabolic exchange/detoxification
Neurologic	Optimize neural mechanisms
Behavior-biopsychosocial	Improve function and wellbeing

When using manipulation in patient-care, five models are considered; respiratory-circulatory, biomechanical-structural, metabolic-nutritional, neurological, and behavior-biopsychosocial.

Manipulation helps neuromusculoskeletal conditions such as low back pain and neck pain that can be chronic with frequent acute exacerbations and thus should be managed as a chronic condition. Using manipulation in the comprehensive care of these chronic conditions is extremely helpful and highly valued by patients. In patients with multiple comorbidities who may not be good candidates for interventions such as surgery, opioids, or injections, gentle manipulation is valuable to safely and effectively manage their condition.

Spinal Manipulation: What You Need to Know. Available at: https://nccih.nih.gov/health/pain/spinemanipulation.htm.

Pickar JG. Neurophysiological effects of spinal manipulation. *Spine J*. 2002;2(5):357–371. doi:10.1016/s1529-9430(02)00400-x.

Rist PM, Hernandez A, Bernstein C, et al. The impact of spinal manipulation on migraine pain and disability: a systematic review and meta-analysis. *Headache*. 2019;59(4):532–542. doi:10.1111/head.13501.

Rubinstein SM, de Zoete A, van Middelkoop M, et al. Benefits and harms of spinal manipulative therapy for the treatment of chronic low back pain: systematic review and meta-analysis of randomised controlled trials. *BMJ*. 2019;364:l689. doi:10.1136/bmj.l689.

23. What is the expected frequency and duration of manipulation treatment?

Three main factors influence manual medicine patient care: the **setting/place/location** of the patient (outpatient clinic, hospital, athletic field, home), the patient's **condition** and **chronicity** of the problem, and the patient and practitioner **preference**. It would not be uncommon to see an inpatient daily for manual medicine treatment. Outpatient treatment varies considerably. Commonly patients are treated once or twice weekly for a couple of months, then monthly for several visits, then every 6 to 12 weeks for an undetermined period.

It is not unusual for a patient to want manipulation regularly to achieve their overall well-being and health goals. In these instances, a home maintenance program of stretching and postural control, tailored for each individual combined with manipulation every 6 to 12 weeks, is best practice. Self-manipulation or self-adjustment can be a beneficial consequence of a home stretching program. Used to maintain mobility of the thoracic spine, lumbar spine, and rib cage, many people habitually self-adjust. Self-manipulation of the cervical spine can put a patient at risk for vertebral artery injuries and must be discouraged.

Physiopedia. *Spinal Manipulation*. Available at: https://www.physio-pedia.com/Spinal_Manipulation.

Spine-health. *Chiropractic Treatment Program Guidelines*. Available at: https://www.spine-health.com/treatment/chiropractic/chiropractic-treatment-program-guidelines.

Local Coverage Determination (LCD): Osteopathic Manipulative Treatment (L33616). Available at: https://osteopathic.org/wp-content/uploads/Local-Coverage-Determination-for-Osteopathic-Manipulative-Treatment-L33616.pdf.

Thoracic Spine Mobility | Self Adjust Mid Back. Available at: https://www.youtube.com/watch?v=7sZcCcV9UTo.

Biller J, Sacco RL, Albuquerque FC, et al. Cervical arterial dissections and association with cervical manipulative therapy: a statement for healthcare professionals from the American Heart Association/American Stroke Association. *Stroke*. 2014;45(10):3155–3174. Available at: https://www.ahajournals.org/doi/full/10.1161/STR.0000000000000016.

BIBLIOGRAPHY

DeStefano L. *Greenman's Principles of Manual Medicine*. 4th ed. Philadelphia, PA: Lippincott Williams & Wilkins; 2011.

DiGiovanna E, Amen C, Burns D, eds. *An Osteopathic Approach to Diagnosis and Treatment*. 4th ed. Philadelphia, PA: Wolters Kluwer; 2021.

Isaacs ER, Bookhout MR. *Bourdillon's Spinal Manipulation*. Boston: Butterworth-Heinemann; 2002.

Janda VL. Pain in the locomotor system. A broad approach. In: Glasgow EF, ed. *Aspects of Manipulative Therapy*. Melbourne: Churchill Livingstone; 1985:148–151.

Mennell JM. *The Musculoskeletal System: Differential Diagnosis from Symptoms and Physical Signs*. United States: Aspen Publishers; 1992.

Nicholas A, Nicholas E. *Atlas of Osteopathic Techniques*. 3rd ed. Philadelphia, PA: LWW; 2021.

Sahrmann SA. *Diagnosis & Treatment of Movement Impairment Syndromes*. USA: St. Louis Missouri: Mosby; 2002.

Savarese R, Adesina A, Capobianco J, et al. *OMT Review*. 4th ed. Wolters Kluwer: Philadelphia; 2018.

Seffinger M. *Foundations of Osteopathic Medicine: Philosophy, Science, Clinical Applications, and Research*. 4th ed. Philadelphia, PA: Wolters Klower; 2019.

Vleeming A, Mooney V, Stoeckart R. *Movement, Stability & Lumbopelvic Pain*. Philadelphia, PA: Churchill Livingstone Elsevier; 2007. doi: 10.1016/B978-0-443-10178-6.X5001-4.

White A, Panjabi M. *Clinical Biomechanics of the Spine*. Philadelphia PA: J. B. Lippincott, cop; 1990.

CHAPTER 18

TRACTION, MANIPULATION, AND MASSAGE: SELECTION APPLICATION AND OUTCOME

Steven R. Hinderer, MD, MS, PT; William A. Bergin, DO; and Steven A. Stiens, MD, MS

If you put yourself in a position where you have to strengthen outside your comfort zone, then you are forced to expand your consciousness

Les Brown (1945–)

KEY POINTS: FUNDAMENTALS OF MANUAL TECHNIQUES

1. Manual Medicine uses hands in palpation to detect segmental dysfunction, deficits in movement and limited range.
2. The goals of manipulation are to optimize motion, relieve pain, promote symmetry, and enhance physical function.
3. Traction—translates forces across tissues to therapeutically distract structures to relieve an impingement and reestablish normal alignment.
4. Massage—tactual appraisal of segmental temperature, tone, and range guides therapeutic application of pressure, friction, tension, and distraction to promote relaxation, circulation, range of motion, and pain relief.

1. **What is anisotropism? How can it guide my palpation and mobilization skills?**
   Anisotrophy is the property of being directionally dependent, which implies different properties in different directions. All tissues and organs have a molecular structure and shape that adapts to their purpose. They all respond differently to forces from various directions applied to their surfaces or translated with tension. The role of the clinician is to apply the anatomy, kinesiology, and clinical assessment to the prescription for intervention with forces properly directed in the proper impulse. Massage, manipulation, and traction are potent interventions in the hands of the trained experienced clinician.

Manual Medicine. Available at: https://www.aaomed.org/Manual-medicine

Smith MS, Olivas J, Smith K. Manipulative therapies: what works. *Am Fam Phys.* 2019;99(4):248–252

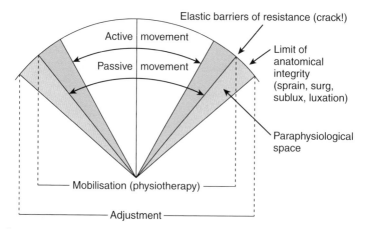

Fig. 18.1 The diagram represents an arch of joint movement in two directions in one plane. The ranges of active movement by the patient, passive movement with assisted stretch, and adjustment movement into the paraphysiological space by a manual medicine clinician. (Adapted from: Normal Joint Movement, Module 7, Understanding Manipulation. Available at: http://www.chiro-online.com/lc/principles/module7/module7_8.html)

2. What techniques are available for applying traction?

   Manual—applied after palpation of passive and active range and monitored with patient tolerance, **tension**, **give**, and **end feel**.

   Mechanical—administered using a pulley and gradually loading a free weight system

   Motorized—mechanical traction applied by a motorized system, administered in continuous or intermittent intervals.

   Gravity—securing limbs and using inversion or inclined lean using body weight as a force

   Autotraction—Patients are instructed to use their own strength and self-monitoring to distract various joints, sometimes using adaptive devices.

3. What are the physiologic effects of traction?

   While many studies have shown that elongation of the cervical spine by 2 to 20 mm can be achieved with 25 lb or more of traction force, 10 lb is needed to counterbalance the weight of the head (less in some persons, more in others). Prolonged pull on the cervical spine with adequate force may lead to cervical paraspinal muscle fatigue, which may alleviate the muscle spasm.

4. What advantages does home mechanical traction have over a clinic-based traction program?

   Mechanical traction is often prescribed early on in the treatment course and later continued with home traction. Administration of **continuous or intermittent (timed on-and-off periods) mechanical traction** applied with a motorized device is commonly limited to physical therapy clinics because of the need for close monitoring of position and its effect on symptoms. Most patients tolerate greater forces of pull with intermittent administration.

   Transition to home for cervical traction for neck or radicular pain requires therapist instruction. Typical devices include a pulley that mounts on the top of a door and a water-filled weight.

Fritz JM, Thackeray A, Brennan GP, Childs JD. Exercise only, exercise with mechanical traction, or exercise with over-door traction for patients with cervical radiculopathy, with or without consideration of status on a previously described subgrouping rule: a randomized clinical trial. *J Orthop Sports Phys Ther*. 2014 Feb;44(2):45–57. doi: 10.2519/jospt.2014.5065. Epub 2014 Jan 9.

5. Is there a role for gravity traction?

   Gravity (inversion) traction attempts to distract the lumbar spine with body weight, by hanging upside down. Numerous side effects such as persistent headaches, blurred vision, petechiae, and numerous musculoskeletal complaints have prevented effective clinical use.

Gianakopoulos G, Waylonis GW, Grant PA, et al. Inversion devices: their role in producing lumbar distraction. *Arch Phys Med Rehabil*. 1985;66 100–102.

6. When prescribing traction, what parameters should be specified?

   - Positioning: specific patient position and angle of alignment to pull
   - Administration: intermittent or continuous
   - Force of traction: increased gradually, demonstrate tolerability
   - Frequency: guided by symptoms
   - Duration- twenty minutes of full effectiveness
     Helpful adjunctive modalities include heat, TENS, ice, cold spray, and trigger point procedures.

7. Discuss positioning.

   Positioning is a key element of a traction prescription. For **cervical traction,** specification of sitting or supine position should be based on patient comfort and maximal muscle relaxation. If cervical traction is being administered to relieve symptoms of nerve root compression, 25 to 35 degrees of forwarding neck flexion will optimally open the intervertebral foramina. Less flexion is required for the treatment of muscle spasms in the absence of radicular symptoms.

   The supine position with 90 degrees of hip and knee flexion is the most common position for **lumbar traction**. In this position, the lumbar lordosis is maximally reduced with the lower back well supported on the traction table. The spine is distracted into a relatively flexed position to facilitate optimal vertebral separation.

Onel D, Tukzlaci M, Sari H, Demir K. Computed tomographic investigation of the effect of traction on lumbar disc herniations. *Spine*. 1989;14:82–90.

8. What is the difference between intermittent and continuous traction?

   In practice, a greater force of pull can be tolerated with incremental increases. Utilized to achieve vertebral distraction. Continuous prolonged stretch is effective for muscle relaxation.

9. How much pull is usually used and for how long?

For **cervical spine distraction**, forces greater than 25 lb need to be achieved but forces greater than 50 lb probably do not provide any additional advantage. However, with lumber traction forces greater than 50 lb are required to achieve posterior vertebral separation and forces greater than 100 lb are required for anterior separation. Unfortunately, the countertraction over 100 lb to stabilize the chest and shoulders is often poorly tolerated. Therapeutic effects are maximized with durations of 20 minutes.

10. What are the contraindications to traction?

The potential for **cervical ligamentous instability**, as might occur with rheumatoid arthritis, Down's syndrome, achondroplastic dwarfism, Marfan syndrome, or previous trauma, are absolute contraindications. **Cervical extension** during **traction** should be avoided, especially in the presence of vertebrobasilar insufficiency. Documented or suspected **tumors** in the region of the spine, **osteopenia**, infectious process of the spine or surrounding soft tissue, and **pregnancy** are also absolute contraindications. The geriatric population is a relative contraindication secondary to the expected spondylosis with osteoarthritic spine changes (stenosis, spicules, osteophytes).

Massage Therapy: What You Need to Know National Center for complementary and integrative health. Available at: https://nccih.nih.gov/health/massage/massageintroduction.htm

11. What is manipulation? Is it practiced in paraphysiological space?

Manual Medicine is the use of palpation and operator directed techniques to aid in the diagnosis and treatment of musculoskeletal disorders. Manual medicine is based on the self-regulating process of the body. A normal structural relationship makes the person maximally capable of self-healing with defense against disease. The goal of manipulation is to restore maximal pain-free movement of the musculoskeletal system in postural balance. The International Federation of Manual Medicine defines **manipulation** as the use of the hands and the patient management process using instructions and maneuvers to maintain maximal painless movement of the musculoskeletal system and postural balance. Manipulation as a treatment has been demonstrated to be effective in reducing acute low back pain but is less effective in chronic.

Bialosky JE, Beneciuk JM, Bishop MD, Coronado RA, Penza CW, Simon CB, George SZ. Unraveling the mechanisms of manual therapy: modeling an approach. *J Orthop Sports Phys Ther.* 2020;48(1):8–18.

12. What are the goals of manipulation?

The goal of **manipulation or manual medicine** is to help maintain optimal body mechanics and improve motion in restricted areas. Enhancing maximal pain-free movement in a balanced posture and optimizing function are major goals. The ultimate goal of manipulation is to improve the function and well-being of patients. This can include pain reduction, improved biomechanical performance, gait enhancement and achievements in ADLS.

Smith MS, Olivas J, Smith K. Manipulative therapy: what works. *Am Fam Physician.* 2019;99(4):248–252.

13. When do you use manipulation?

Manipulation is used to remedy **somatic dysfunction,** which is defined as an impaired or altered function of the radicular nerve root and autonomic innervated components of the musculoskeletal, visceral system, and integumentary systems. These connections are established via embryologic development and persist throughout life. Segmentally, neural, skeletal, muscular, ligamentous, myofascial, vascular, and lymphatic elements are related. **Somatic dysfunction** can be detected on physical exam, as summarized by the acronym

TART:
- T = Tenderness, skin, facial
- A = Asymmetric structure
- R = Range of motion abnormalities
- T = Tissue texture changes, piloerection, flushing

Brantingham JW, Cassa TK, Bonnefin D, Jensen M, Globe G, Hicks M, Korporaal C. Manipulative therapy for shoulder pain and disorders: expansion of a systematic review. *J Manipulative Physiol Ther.* 2011;34:314–346.

Licciardone J, Gatchel R, Aryal S. Recovery from chronic low back pain after osteopathic manipulative treatment: a randomized controlled trial. *J Am Osteopath Assoc.* 2016;116(3):144–155. DOI: 10.7556/jaoa.2016.031.

14. In which conditions might manipulation prove helpful?

Manipulation can be helpful, when appropriate, in the following conditions:
- Acute or chronic back and neck pain
- Rib pain including intercostal pain
- Radiculopathies Neck/back radicular pain secondary to herniation or impingement
- Facet syndrome for localized neck or back pain
- Piriformis syndrome
- Sciatica
- Headaches cervicogenic, migraine, sinus, TMJ related
- Sacroiliac syndrome including pelvic and innominate disparities improving leg length discrepancies
   There is fair evidence for the success of manipulative therapy of upper and lower extremity joints for pain and limited range. Combination with modalities and exercise improves outcomes.

Mirtz TA, Morgan L, Wyatt LH, Greene L. An epidemiological examination of the subluxation construct using Hill's criteria of causation. *Chiropr Osteopat.* 2009;17:13. doi:10.1186/1746-1340-17-13

Brantingham JW, Cassa TK, Bonnefin D, Pribicevic M, Robb A, Pollard H, Tong V, Korporaal C. Manipulative and multimodal therapy for upper extremity and temporomandibular disorders: a systematic review. *J Manipulative Physiol Ther.* 2013;36:143–201.

15. What are commonly used techniques of therapeutic massage?

Classical massage involves **stroking and gliding movements (effleurage), kneading (pétrissage)**, and **percussion (tapotement)**. Stroking, gliding, and friction movements are helpful for locating areas of muscle spasm or focal pain. Stroking can help produce muscle relaxation in locations where spasm exists. Kneading techniques are performed on muscle and subcutaneous tissue for the purposes of muscle relaxation, improving circulation, and reducing edema. Percussion is primarily used for chest therapy in conjunction with postural drainage.

Field T. Massage therapy research review. *Complement Ther Clin Pract.* 2014;20:224–229.

Brantingham JW, Globe G, Pollard H, Hicks M, Korporaal C, Hoskins W. Manipulation of lower extremity conditions. *J Manipulative Physiol Ther.* 2009;32:53–71.

16. When is a massage medium required?

A **massage medium** is used topically to reduce friction over the skin. Examples include mineral oil, glycerin, coconut oil, cocoa butter, and other moisturizing creams. Such media are used when the massage is intended for edema reduction, relaxation/sedation, or relief of muscle spasm/tightness. In contrast, when the massage is used to loosen or stretch scar tissue, fascia, or subcutaneous tissue, no medium is used, allowing the therapist to gain control by grasping and moving appropriate tissue structures.

17. What physical parameters of massage can be altered to achieve the desired therapeutic effect?
- Myofascial release has been defined as a hands-on technique that applies prolonged light pressure in specific directions into the fascia system. It is applied in conjunction with a passive range of motion with the purpose of identifying and removing tissue restrictions in combination with other modalities such as those listed below.
- Deep friction massage is used to prevent adhesions in acute muscle injuries and to break up adhesions in subacute and chronic injuries. Deep friction is applied transversely across the muscle fiber, tendon, or ligament.
- Soft-tissue mobilization is a forceful massage and resistance of the muscle-fascial system element and differs from most massages in that it is done with fascia and muscle in a stretched position rather than relaxed or shortened. It is particularly effective as an adjunct to passive stretching for the reduction of contractures.
- Acupressure is the application of sustained deep pressure over trigger points, as defined by Travell. Acupressure is often done in conjunction with the application of other therapeutic modalities (e.g., ice, ultrasound, electrical stimulation) to the trigger points.

Denneny D, Frawley HC, Petersen K, McLoughlin R, Brook S, Hassan S, Williams AC. Trigger point manual therapy for the treatment of chronic noncancer pain in adults: a systematic review and meta-analysis. *Arch Phys Med Rehabil.* 2019;100:562–577.

18. Are there any contraindications to massage?

Yes—there can be potential harm from **massage**. It is contraindicated over malignancies, open wounds, thrombophlebitis/deep vein thrombosis, infected tissues, areas of lymphangitis, or areas of recent trauma or bleeding. Peripheral nerve compression from hematoma formation has been reported when acupressure was applied too vigorously.

WEBSITES

1. Available at: https://aapmr.org/
2. American Association of Orthopedic Medicine. Available at: HTTPS://WWW.AAOMED.ORG/
3. Massage Therapy: What You Need To Know. Available at: https://www.nccih.nih.gov/health/massage-therapy-what-you-need-to-know
4. Wieting J. Massage, Traction, and Manipulation. Available at: https://emedicine.medscape.com/article/324694-overview#a16
5. Wieting J. Massage, Traction, and Manipulation. Available at: http://www.emedicine.com/pmr/topic200.htm

BOOKS

Cyriax JH. Textbook of Orthopaedic Medicine: Treatment by Manipulation, Massage and Injection, 10th ed. London: Bailliere-Tindall; 1982.

DiGiovanna E. Somatic dysfunction. In DiGiovanna E, Schiowitz S, Dowling D, eds. An Osteopathic Approach to Diagnosis and Treatment. 3rd ed. Lippincott Williams and Wilkins Philadelphia; 2005:16–23.

Greenman PE. Principles of Manual Medicine. 2nd edn. Baltimore: Williams & Wilkins; 1996.

Travell J. Myofascial Pain and Dysfunction. 2nd edn. Baltimore: Williams & Wilkins; 1999.

Schiotz EH, Cyriax J. Manipulation: Past and Present. London, UK: William Heinemann Medical Books; 1974.

BIBLIOGRAPHY

Bagheripour B, Kamyab M, Azadinia F, Amiri A, Akbari M. The efficacy of a home-mechanical traction unit for patients with mild to moderate cervical osteoarthrosis: a pilot study. *Med J Islam Repub Iran.* 2016;30:386. Published online 2016, Jun 12.

Bridger RS, Ossey S, Gourie G. Effect of lumbar traction on stature. *Spine* 1989;14:82–90.

Cameron M. Traction, physical agents and rehabilitation from research to practice. 3rd ed. St. Louis: Saunders Elsevier; 2009:287–316. PMCID: PMC4972072 PMID: 27493930.

Prinsen J, Hensel KL, Snow R. Osteopathic manipulative therapy associated with reduced analgesic prescribing and fewer missed work days in patients with low back pain: an observational study. *Am Osteopath Assoc.* 2014;114(2):90–98. doi:10.7556/jaoa.2014.022.

Slattengren A, Nissly T, Blustin J, Bader A, Westfall E. Best uses of osteopathic manipulation, *J Fam Pract.* 2017;66(12):743–747

CHAPTER 19

EXERCISE

Shashank J. Davé, DO, FAAPMR; Kyle Littell, MD, FAAPMR; Gary Stover, MD; and Albert Recio, MD, RPT, PTRP

Take care of your body. It's the only place you have to live.

—Jim Rohn

If I knew I was going to live this long, I'd have taken better care of myself.

—Eubie Blake

KEY POINTS

1. In the first few weeks of a training program, there is an increase in strength not related to hypertrophy. An increase in integrated electromyographic (EMG) activity during this time period implies that there are *neural factors leading to increased strength*. This may be caused by increased synchronization and coordination of muscle firing. Only later does hypertrophy take effect.
2. Aging reduces isometric and concentric muscle strength because of atrophy, deterioration of mechanical properties, and motor unit breakdown. Maximal physical capacity is typically between ages 20 and 30 with pronounced physiological changes occurring after age 50.
3. VO_{2max} decreases with increasing age in concordance with a decrease in maximum heart rate, cardiac output, and lean body mass. Maximum heart rate declines with age and is not influenced by exercise training. However, the decline of lean body mass can be slowed with exercise training with the potential for slowing the decline of VO_{2max}.
4. According to the Henneman size principle, motor units are recruited in order of increasing size, increasing contraction strength, and diminishing fatigue resistance.
5. VO_{2max} is the maximum rate of oxygen consumption and is a measure of the maximum intensity of exercise that can be sustained.
6. Women have lower levels of testosterone and thereby experience less hypertrophy of the muscles and have less of an increase in VO_{2max} with exercise.
7. Early mobilization with progression from passive to active exercises has been effective even with those on continued mechanical ventilation to help combat intensive care unit (ICU)-acquired weakness.

1. What is exercise?
   a. **Exercise** is sustained exertion using neuromuscular function carried out on a schedule to induce performance-enhancing physiological improvements in systems, function, physical fitness, and wellness.
   b. **Exercise** is a subcomponent of daily physical activity that contributes to increased capacity for peak and endurance performance. Improvements are mediated primarily via neuroplastic muscular and cardiovascular effects.
   c. **Everyone** should exercise at a moderate-intensity level of aerobic exercise at least 150 minutes/week or 75 minutes of high-intensity AND perform muscle-strengthening activities at least 2 days/week.
   d. **Evidence** demonstrates a greater increase in the upper and lower body one repetition, maximum with 3 sessions per week compared with 1 week/year.
   e. **Resistance** training with free weights has demonstrated no significant difference in strength gains versus using exercise machines with the same weights.
   f. **The challenge** of the rehabilitation clinician is to understand each patient as an individual and help them be more active by "doing what moves them!"

McLester JR, Bishop E, Guilliams ME. Comparison of 1 day and 3 days per week of equal-volume resistance training in experienced subjects. *J Strength Cond Res.* 2000;14:273–281.

Silvester LJ, Stiggins C, McGown C, Bryce GR. The effect of variable resistance and free-weight training programs on strength and vertical jump. *Natl Strength Cond Assoc J.* 1981;3:30–33.

Table 19.1 Muscle Fiber Types and Their Characteristics

CHARACTERISTIC	TYPE I: SLOW OXIDATIVE	TYPE IIA: FAST OXIDATIVE GLYCOLYTIC	TYPE IIX: FAST GLYCOLYTIC
Histology and biochemistry	Numerous mitochondria	Increased electrochemical transmission of action potentials; increased calcium release and uptake by sarcoplasmic reticulum and cross-bridge turnover	
Activity level of myosin ATPase	Low	High	High
Speed of contraction	Slow	Fast	Fast
Glycolytic/anaerobic potential	Low	Moderate	High
Oxidative potential	High	Moderate	Low
Resistance to fatigue	High	Moderate	Low
Uses	Posture/endurance muscles	Quick force contractions	

2. What are the three types of muscle fibers? Can you help clear the F.O.G?
   a. See Table 19.1 to clear the "F.O.G." (Fast [and slow] Oxidative, Glycolytic)

The Khan Academy. Available at: https://www.khanacademy.org/science/health-and-medicine/human-anatomy-and-physiology/introduction-to-muscles/v/type-1-and-2-muscle-fibers

3. What determines the fiber type of a given muscle cell?
   a. The **fiber type** is determined by the **nerve fiber** that innervates it. All fibers innervated by a given motor neuron have the same physiologic and histochemical properties. The type of motor neuron and pattern of nerve impulses transmitted play the main roles in determining the mechanical and histochemical properties of the muscle fibers. After denervation, if nerve regrowth and sprouting occur, the muscle fiber will take on the characteristics determined by the new nerve fiber. Animal modeling has suggested the role of gene marker expression during development may also play a part in embryologic cell differentiation of muscle type that is additionally altered by the innervation process.

Bacou F, Rouanet P, Barjot CP, et al A. Expression of myosin isoforms in denervated, cross-reinnervated and electrically stimulated rabbit muscles. *Eur J Biochem.* 1996;236:539–547.

Berti F, Nogueira JM, Wöhrle S, et al. Time course and side-by-side analysis of mesodermal, pre-myogenic, myogenic and differentiated cell markers in the chicken model for skeletal muscle formation. *J Anat.* 2015;227(3):361–382.

Qiu X, Chen D, Liu F, et al. Transition of myosin heavy chain isoforms in human laryngeal abductors following denervation. *Eur Arch Otorhinolaryngol.* 2015;272(10):2915–2923.

Li J, Liu S, Cheng Q, et al. Changes in electrical response function and myosin heavy chain isoforms following denervation and reinnervation of bilateral posterior cricoarytenoid muscles in dogs. *Acta Otolaryngol.* 2014;134(3):318–325.

4. What is the Henneman size principle?
   a. **Motor units** are recruited in order of increasing size, increasing contraction strength, and diminishing fatigue resistance. Therefore, the smaller, less powerful, fatigue-resistant fibers are recruited before the larger, more powerful, fatigable fibers, regardless of the speed of contraction. This makes sense because these fibers are weaker. When initially moving a muscle, not much strength is needed, and activating the weaker fibers (motor units) gives finer motor control. When more strength is needed, increasingly larger fibers are recruited to

generate more gross muscle strength. To reduce fatigue, the firing rate of earlier recruited motor units is greater than that of later recruited motor units.

Thomas GT, Munson CK, Stein RB. The resilience of the size principle in the organization of motor unit properties in normal and reinnervated adult skeletal muscles. *Can J Physiol Pharmacol.* 2004;82(8–9):645–661.

De Luca CJ, Contessa P. Hierarchical control of motor units in voluntary contractions. *J Neurophysiol.* 2012;107:178–195.

5. **What two-dimensional measurements of muscle correlate best with strength?**
   a. Simply put, it's mostly the muscle's cross-sectional area. Other factors are listed in Fig. 19.1.

Edstrom L, Grimby L. Effect of exercise on the motor unit. *Muscle Nerve.* 1986;9:104–126.

6. **Describe different types of muscle shapes.**
   a. **Parallel** muscle fibers travel longitudinally along the entire length of the muscle. The majority of the muscles in the body have this shape. A muscle fiber ordinarily contracts by approximately 50% of its resting length (length if removed from the body). Thus, parallel muscle fibers can generate a large amount of shortening but have lesser strength (see Fig. 20.1). Example: biceps brachii.
   b. **Pennate** (penne = "feathers") muscles have fibers that insert onto a tendon that runs centrally throughout the muscle length at an angle, which allows a greater number of muscle fibers. Although the total size of the muscle may be the same as in a parallel arrangement, the total effective cross-sectional area is greater and thus provides greater strength. Because the muscle fibers shorten by approximately 50% of their resting length and the fibers attach at an angle onto the tendon, the total movement is less than in parallel muscle fibers. Example: rectus femoris (Fig. 19.2).
   c. **Circular** muscles typically called **sphincters** are concentrically arranged bundles of muscle around an opening. When they contract, they will make the opening smaller. Example: orbicularis oculi.

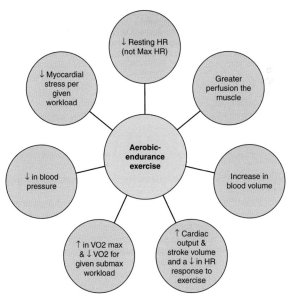

Fig. 19.1 Effects of aerobic endurance exercise.

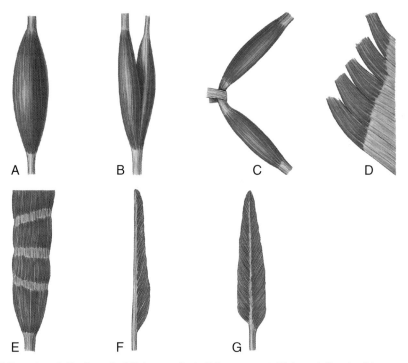

Fig. 19.2 Types of muscle. Muscles can be divided up according to (1) the arrangement of their muscle fibers (parallel course to the pull direction of the tendon with substantial movements using low force, or pennate = diagonal course of muscle fibers at a particularly acute angle [pennation angle] with long, wide tendons using high muscle force); (2) the number of muscle heads (1, 2 or more); (3) differences in joint involvement (depending on whether a muscle is involved in movements in one or two joints or has no relationship to a joint: single-joint muscles, two-joint muscles, mimic muscles without joint involvement); (4) or form. Under the microscope skeletal muscles have a transverse stripe and can be divided according to their shape into (A) single-headed, parallel fibrous muscles (Musculus fusiformis); (B) two-headed, parallel fibrous muscles (Musculus biceps); (C) two-lobed, parallel fibrous muscles (Musculus biventer); (D) multi-lobed, flat muscles (Musculus planus); (E) multi-lobed muscles divided by intermediate tendons (Musculus intersectus); (F) semipennate muscles (Musculus semipennatus); (G) multipennate muscles (Musculus pennatus). (Paulsen, Waschke, Sobotta Atlas of Human Anatomy, 16th Edition 2018 © Elsevier GmbH, Urban & Fischer, Munich.)

Biga LM, Dawson S, Harwell A, et al. *Explain the organization of muscle fascicles and their role in generating force.* In *Anatomy & Physiology.* Corvallis: Open Oregon State. 2019. Oregon State University; 701–703. Available at: https://open.oregonstate.education/aandp/chapter/11-2-explain-the-organization-of-muscle-fascicles-and-their-role-in-generating-force/

7. Can training programs improve the muscle strength of unexercised limbs or muscles without hypertrophy?
   a. Moritani and deVries showed in the first few weeks of training that there is an increase in strength without hypertrophy. An increase in integrated electromyographic (EMG) activity during this time period implies that there are neural factors leading to increased strength. This may be achieved with increased synchronization and coordination of muscle firing. Only later does hypertrophy take effect. They also showed that neural training effects are transferred to some extent to the opposite (untrained) limb. However, a regimented resistive exercise routine will promote marked increases in muscle strength and hypertrophy, with improvements seen irrespective of age and gender.

Moritani T, deVries HA. Neural factors versus hypertrophy in the time course of muscle strength gain. *Am J Phys Med.* 1979;58: 115–130.

Schoenfeld BJ, Peterson MD, Ogborn D, Contrares B, Sonmez GT. Effect of low vs high-load resistance training on muscle strength and hypertrophy in well trained men. *J Strength Cond Res.* 2015;9(10):2954–2963.

Miller MS, Callahan DM, Tourville TW, Slauterbeck JR, Kaplan A, Fiske BR, Savage PD, Ades PA, Beynnon BD, Toth MJ. Moderate-intensity resistance exercise alters skeletal muscle molecular and cellular structure and function in inactive older adults with knee osteoarthritis. *J Appl Physiol*. 2017;122:775–787.

8. Can a muscle fiber's type be changed by exercise?

a. There can be a training-induced fiber-type transformation with sport-specific training and possibly with short-term training. However, most commonly the changes are in muscle groups that are considered hybrids. Type IIA/IIB fibers with high intensity resistive or sprint training can cause a shift of these fibers toward a pure type IIA. Similar changes can be seen with endurance training hybrid muscles tend to shift toward a pure type I. Strength training causes muscle hypertrophy of both type I and II muscles. Endurance training increases the mitochondrial content and respiratory capacity making them less fatigable.

Bogdanis GC. Effects of physical activity and inactivity on muscle fatigue. *Front Physiol*. 2012, May 18;3:142.. doi:10.3389/fphys.2012.00142

Qaisar R, Bhaskaran S, Van Remmen H. Muscle fiber type diversification during exercise and regeneration. *Free Radic Biol Med*. 2016;98:56–67.

Available at: https://sandcresearch.medium.com/explaining-how-hypertrophy-works-using-only-basic-principles-of-muscle-physiology-48beda5fbf1b

Kazior Z, Willis SJ, Moberg M, et al. Endurance exercise enhances the effect of strength training on muscle fiber size and protein expression of Akt and mTOR. *PLoS One*. 2016;11:e0149082.

Hawley JA. Adaptations of skeletal muscle to prolonged, intense endurance training. *Clin Exp Pharmacol Physiol*. 2002;29:218–222.

9. Describe three types of resistance training techniques.

a. See Table 19.2.

Lieberman, J. Resistance training, Therapeutic Exercise. Medscape. 2018. Available at: https://emedicine.medscape.com/article/324583-overview#a5

10. What is the difference between concentric and eccentric muscle contraction?

a. See Table 19.3.

Padulo J, Laffaye G, Chamari K, Concu A. Concentric and eccentric: muscle contraction or exercise? *Sports Health*. 2013;5(4):306.

Table 19.2 Types of Resistance Training Techniques

	ISOMETRIC	ISOTONIC	ISOKINETIC
Definition	Equal distance	Equal tone	Equal speed
Joint movement	No	Yes	Yes
Example	Pushing on a wall	Weight-lifting	Cybex machine
Important principles	Muscle has some internal shortening, but no gross movement of the joint	Constant resistance throughout the joint motion. See question 15.	Speed of movement remains constant no matter how hard the subject pushes against the machine

Table 19.3 Concentric versus Eccentric Contraction

	CONCENTRIC	ECCENTRIC
Muscle action	Shortening	Lengthening
Example:	Biceps brachii: lifting a weight in a curl	lowering the weight back through elbow extension
Characteristics	Less muscle tension	Greater muscle tension; hence more potential for tissue injury, but also more potential for hypertrophy

Table 19.4 Open versus Closed Kinetic Chain Exercises		
	OPEN KINETIC CHAIN	**CLOSED KINETIC CHAIN**
Definition	Distal end not fixed	Distal end fixed
Example	Extending leg with free weight	Squatting
Comments	More shear stress	Less shear stress

11. Why choose open or closed kinetic chain exercises? Can they affect muscle shear?
    a. See Table 19.4.
    b. Excessive **muscle shear** (tearing of myofibers and the connective tissue) during exercise can predispose the muscle-tendon unit to damage. Comparative EMG analysis has shown that closed kinetic chain exercise produces less shear force compared to open kinetic chain exercise.

Lutz GE, Palmitier RA, An KN, Chao, EY. Comparison of tibiofemoral joint forces during open-kinetic-chain and closed-kinetic-chain exercises. *J Bone Joint Surg.* 1993;75(5):732–739

Kwon YJ, Park SJ, Jefferson J, Kim K. The effect of open and closed kinetic chain exercises on dynamic balance ability of normal healthy adults. *J Phys Ther Sci.* 2013;25(6):671–674.

Closed vs Open Kinematic Chain—YouTube. Available at: https://www.youtube.com/watch?v=TV2CyvmMhRE Accessed April 7, 2019

12. What is the DeLorme technique?
    a. The DeLorme technique, used to strengthen muscles, is also called **progressive resistance exercise**. Classically, the subject is tested to determine the maximum weight that she or he can lift 10 times using good form and technique—this is called the **10-repetition maximum (10 RM).** DeLorme would have the person train lifting various percentages of their maximum in sets of 10, starting at 10%, 20%, 30%, etc., up to 100%. Later it was adapted to only 3 sets with 50% 10RM, 75% 10RM, then 100% 10RM.

deLateur BJ, Lehmann JF, Fordyce WE. A test of the DeLorme axiom. *Arch Phys Med Rehabil.* 1968;49:245–248.

13. What is the DeLorme axiom?
    a. The **DeLorme axiom** states that high-intensity, low-repetition exercise builds strength, and low-intensity, high-repetition exercise builds endurance and that each of these two types of exercise is incapable of producing the results obtained by the other type. This is too extreme. There is some crossover effect from one exercise type to the other.

Todd JS, Shurley JP, Todd TC, Thomas L. DeLorme and the science of progressive resistance exercise. *J Strength Cond Res.* 2012;26:2913–2923. doi:10.1519/JSC.0b013e31825adcb4.

14. What is the Oxford technique?
    a. The Oxford technique basically turned the DeLorme method on its head by doing the exercises at 100% 10 RM, then 75% 10 RM, then 50% 10 RM. Thus far both the DeLorme and the Oxford protocols improve strength with equivalent efficacy.

Zinovieff AN. Heavy resistance exercises: the Oxford technique. *Br J Phys Med.* 1957;14:129–132.

Fish DE, Krabak BJ, Johnson-Greene D, et al Optimal resistance training: comparison of DeLorme with Oxford techniques. *Am J Phys Med Rehabil.* 2003;82:903–909.

15. How do the effects of free weights, pulleys, and cam-varied resistance differ during the range of motion (ROM)?
    a. **Free-weight** lifting is usually considered a type of isotonic exercise. However, the actual muscle tension is *not equal* throughout the ROM because of gravity and joint position, which is a limitation of using free weights. You can only lift as much as the weakest part of the motion.
    b. **Circular Pulleys** *even out* the tension and create the same amount of resistance throughout the entire ROM of the muscle. Nevertheless, this still does not match the curve of muscle contraction, because muscle generates near maximum force at optimum actin and myosin overlap.

c. **Cam-varied resistance** utilizes an ovoid-shaped pully and *varies* the torque throughout the ROM of the muscle. By attempting to match the torque curvature of the muscle. This provides maximal tolerable resistance and maximal stimulus for hypertrophy to the muscle throughout the contraction.

16. What is plyometric exercise?
    a. **Plyometric exercises** are functional types of exercise, which apply the principle of a brief stretch followed by contraction. A brief stretch (such as during a muscle stretch reflex) will elicit a contraction, and by briefly preloading (stretching) the muscle, facilitates the subsequent contraction. Exercises using this principle include jumping up and down or jumping over boxes. Plyometric exercise is useful because many sports involve plyometric-type maneuvers. Although, it is also more likely to cause injury. However, in children, these fun exercises improve bone mineral content, density and structural properties (Fig. 19.3).

Gómez-bruton A, Matute-llorente Á, González-agüero A, Casajús JA, Vicente-Rodríguez G. Plyometric exercise and bone health in children and adolescents: a systematic review. *World J Pediatr.* 2017;13(2):112–121.

17. Ouch! Why do muscles become sore after a workout?
    a. Heavily loaded lengthening **(eccentric) contractions** are probably responsible for **delayed-onset muscle soreness (DOMS)** by causing structural damage yet are probably better at generating muscle hypertrophy than concentric contractions. This soreness usually starts a day or two after exercise and lasts a few days. Metabolically the efflux of cytokines and reactive oxygen species can lead to muscle damage and in severe cases rhabdomyolysis. For temporary relief of DOMS active exercise of the muscles is the best way to clear inflammation. NSAIDs may provide some benefits by preventing and reducing soreness.

Clarkson PM, Hubal MJ. Exercise-induced muscle damage in humans. *Am J Phys Med Rehabil.* 2002 Nov;81(11 Suppl):S52–S69.

Qaisar R, Bhaskaran S, Van Remmen H. Muscle fiber type diversification during exercise and regeneration. *Free Radic Biol Med.* 2016;98:56–67.

Kedlaya D. Postexercise Muscle Soreness. Available at: https://emedicine.medscape.com/article/313267-overview

Pyne DB. Exercise-induced muscle damage and inflammation: a review. *Aust J Sci Med Sport.* 1994;26:49.

Hotfiel T, Freiwald J, Hoppe MW, et al. Advances in delayed-onset muscle soreness (DOMS): part I: pathogenesis and diagnostics. *Sportverletz Sportschaden.* 2018;32(4):243–250.

Heiss R, Lutter C, Freiwald J, et al. Advances in delayed-onset muscle soreness (DOMS) - part II: treatment and prevention. *Sportverletz Sportschaden.* 2019;33(1):21–29.

Cheung K, Hume P, Maxwell L. Delayed onset muscle soreness: treatment strategies and performance factors. *Sports Med.* 2003;33(2):145–164.

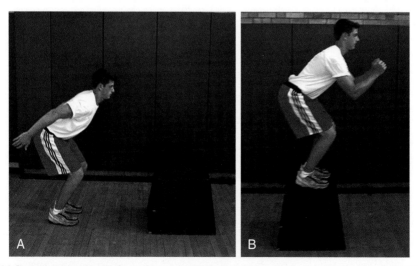

Fig. 19.3 Plyometric training and drills. (Source: Cuoco, Anthony, DPT, MS, CSCS; Tyler, Timothy F., PT, MS, ATC. Published January 1, 2012. Pages 571–595. © 2012. Physical Rehabilitation of the Injured Athlete. Fourth Edition.)

18. **What is endurance exercise? Endurance fitness?**
    a. **Endurance exercise** is the prolonged reciprocal use of large muscle groups. It is differentiated from **muscle endurance**, which refers to the length of time that a muscle can contract at a given tension (isometric).
    b. The terms *stamina, endurance fitness, cardiovascular fitness,* and *aerobic fitness* refer to the body's ability to generate adenosine triphosphate (ATP) aerobically. Aerobic energy, or the long-term energy system, is primarily measured by an individual's VO_{2max}. VO_{2max} is considered the fundamental measurement of aerobic capability in exercise physiology.

19. **Define VO_2 and VO_{2max}.**
    a. In VO_{2max} the V refers to the **rate**, and the O_2 refers to the **oxygen** being consumed. Put together, this is the **rate of oxygen consumption**. VO_{2max} is the **maximum rate of oxygen consumption** and is a measure of the maximum intensity of exercise that can be sustained. VO_{2max} is limited by the oxygen-carrying and utilization capacity of the body. Exceeding the VO_{2max} for brief periods can be accomplished by reverting to glycolytic energy production; however, this creates a buildup of lactic acid and cannot be sustained.

Lundby C, Montero D, Joyner M. Biology of VO_{2max}: looking under the physiology lamp. *Acta Physiol (Oxf)*. 2017;220(2):218–228.

Sousa A, Rodríguez F, Machado L, Vilas-Boas J, Fernandes R. Exercise modality effect on oxygen uptake off-transient kinetics at maximal oxygen uptake intensity. *Exp Physiol*. 2015;100(6):719–729.

Faude O, Kindermann W, Meyer T. Lactate threshold concepts. *Sports Med*. 2009;39(6):469–490.

20. **What are the different techniques for flexibility exercises?**
    a. **Passive stretching:** Also known as relaxed stretching or static-passive stretching, in this form of stretching exercise the person stretching assumes a position and holds it with another part of the body or with assistance from a partner or some apparatus such as a machine. For example, when standing with the ball of the foot on a step and the heels hanging down, bodyweight will stretch the gastrocsoleus complex (Fig. 19.4).
    b. **Static stretching:** Static stretches involve stretching the muscle and staying in that position for some time period. Generally, at least 15 to 20 seconds is required to provide any benefit. Static stretching is relatively safe.
    c. **Ballistic stretching:** Ballistic stretching involves bouncing-type maneuvers. This exercise was popular several decades ago, but it is now out of favor because muscle stretch reflex is activated similar to plyometric exercise triggering partial muscle contraction and which can hinder stretching.
    d. **Dynamic stretching:** Dynamic stretching is different from ballistic stretching in that ballistic stretching forces a limb or part of the body beyond its usual ROM. Dynamic stretching involves moving parts of the body in a controlled manner (e.g., dance or martial arts) and gradually increasing the reach and speed of movement.
    e. **Proprioceptive neuromuscular facilitation (PNF):** This is a form of pre-contraction stretching and is similar to osteopathic muscle energy techniques. For this type of stretching, the muscle is contracted and then stretched to its fullest extent. Although the joint position does not change, this is felt to cause internal shortening of the connective tissues of the muscle, and after a few seconds of contraction, the muscle is relaxed and again stretched a bit more. This is generally done three times in any given position and can sometimes be done with a partner. Subtypes of PNF stretching include:
        i. **Contract relax** (contraction of the muscle through its spiral-diagonal PNF pattern followed by stretching).
        ii. **Hold relax** (contraction of the muscle through the rotational component of the PNF pattern followed by stretching).

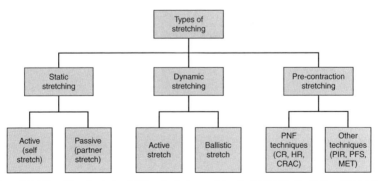

Fig. 19.4 Types of stretching. *CR,* contract relax; *CRAC,* contract relax, agonist contract; *HR,* hold relax; *MET,* medical exercise therapy; *PIR,* post-isometric relaxation; *PNF,* Proprioceptive neuromuscular facilitation; *PFS,* post-facilitation stretching.

iii. **Contract-relax agonist contract** (contraction of the muscle through its spiral-diagonal PNF pattern followed by contraction of the opposite muscle to stretch target muscle).

iv. These stretches are typically performed at 75% to 100% of maximal contraction, holding for 10 sections, then relaxing.

f. Additional pre-contraction stretching techniques

i. **Post-isometric relaxation** uses a less intense 25% muscle contraction followed by stretching the target muscle.

ii. **Post-facilitation stretch** utilizes maximal contraction of a muscle at mid-range of motion, rapid stretch to maximal length, then a held static stretch.

g. While the benefits of stretching are known, controversy remains about the best type to perform.

Behm DG. Blazevich AJ, Kay AD, McHugh M. Acute effects of muscle stretching on physical performance, range of motion, and injury incidence in healthy active individuals: a systematic review. *Appl Physiol Nutr Metab.* 2016;41:1–11.

Lieberman J. *Therapeutic Exercise.* Available at: https://emedicine.medscape.com/article/324583-overview

Page P. Current concepts in muscle stretching for exercise and rehabilitation. *Int J Sports Phys Ther.* 2012;7(1):109–119.

KEY POINTS: TYPES OF FLEXIBILITY EXERCISES

1. **Static stretching**: a gradual stretch over 15 seconds
2. **Ballistic stretching**: repeated rapid stretching such as bouncing
3. **PNF**: stretching followed by muscle contraction, then further stretching
4. **Passive stretching**: a partner applying a stretch to a relaxed muscle
5. **Dynamic stretching**: controlled movement of body parts gradually increasing reach and range of motion (such as martial arts)

21. How do I measure flexibility?

a. Although there are various methods to measure flexibility, the **goniometer** is the most commonly used tool to determine the joint range of motion. Measuring 0 to 180 degrees, values are then compared to standardized values of normal joint ROM. When measuring spine ROM, a goniometer is less reliable. An **inclinometer** is a device placed on the spine used to assess gross ROM, where sagittal plane (*not* coronal or transverse) measurements are taken. However, it has been shown that, at least in the lumbar spine, flexion measurement is more reliable than extension measurement. There are now apps for your phone to help with these measurements.

Saur PM, Ensink FB, Frese K, et al. Lumbar range of motion: reliability and validity of the inclinometer technique in the clinical measurement of trunk flexibility. *Spine.* 1996;21(11):1332–1338.

Hancock GE, Hepworth T, Wembridge K. Accuracy and reliability of knee goniometry methods. *J Exp Orthop.* 2018;5(1):46. doi: 10.1186/s40634-018-0161-5.

22. Do I have to warm up?

a. Individuals may complete a brief session of less intense exercise to "warm up" the muscles prior to the initiation of more intense exercise. **Warming up** is generally accepted as a valid procedure before vigorous exercise. Subjects can utilize both passive and active warm-up techniques that affect temperature, metabolic, neural, and psychology-related effects with the benefit of improved performance and decreased risk of injury. A 1°C increase in muscle temperature can increase exercise performance by 2% to 5%. A typical warm-up should be less than 15 minutes of an active warm-up with 1 to 5 minutes of race pace exercise. **Passive warm up** techniques such as heated garments can be helpful to prolong the active warm-up benefits with prolonged wait times until the activity begins.

McGowan CJ, Pyne DB, Thompson KG, Rattray B. Warm-up strategies for sport and exercise: mechanisms and applications. *Sports Med.* 2015;45:1523–1546.

23. What is the difference between upper-extremity and lower-extremity exercise?

a. Blood pressure (both systolic and diastolic) rises more with upper-body exercise versus lower-body exercise. This is most likely a result of the smaller muscle mass and vasculature of the upper extremities, which offer greater resistance to blood flow than the larger muscle mass and vasculature of the lower body and legs. Upper extremity exercises also increase perceived exertion over lower body exercise even at the same heart rate, thus making perceived exertion an important part of exercise training along with heart rate and blood pressure responses.

Di Blasio A, Sablone A, Civino P, et al. Arm vs. combined leg and arm exercise: blood pressure responses and ratings of perceived exertion at the same indirectly determined heart rate. *J Sports Sci Med.* 2009;8:401–409.

24. How does aging affect muscle strength?
    a. Aging reduces isometric and concentric muscle strength due to the reduced quantity and size of muscle fibers. If the fibers shrink to a critical minimal size, they begin to undergo apoptosis. As aging occurs muscle fibers are more susceptible to damage with decreased muscle metabolism and reduced capability to repair. Maximal physical capacity is typically between ages 20 and 30 with pronounced physiological changes occurring after age 50. Factors for intervention include nutritional inadequacies, hormonal changes, effects of disease, and a sedentary lifestyle. It has been shown that conventional resistance training is possible, even for very old adults, and can reverse some of the effects of aging on muscular strength.

Fiatarone MA, Marks EC, Ryan ND, et al. High-intensity strength training in nonagenarians. Effects on skeletal muscle. *JAMA.* 1990;263:3029–3034.

Keller K, Engelhardt M. Strength and muscle mass loss with aging process. Age and strength loss. *Muscles Ligaments Tendons J.* 2013;3(4):346–350.

Lopez P, Pinto RS, Radaelli R, RechA, Grazioli R, Izquierdo M, Cadore EL. Benefits of resistance training in physically frail elderly: a systematic review. *Aging Clin Exp Res.* 2018 ;30:889–899.

25. How does gender affect muscle strength and response to exercise?
    a. Women have lower levels of testosterone therefore they experience less hypertrophy of the muscles and have less of an increase in VO_{2max} with exercise. Women tend to have a greater amount of body fat and less lean muscle mass as a percentage of total body mass. However, some studies suggest with endurance exercises women's lower extremity muscles may be less susceptible to fatigue.

Daskalopoulou C, Stubbs B, Krali C, et al. Physical activity and healthy aging; a systemic review and meta-analysis of longitudinal cohort studies. *Ageing Res Rev.* 2017;38:6–17.

Shepard RJ. Exercise and training in women. I. Influence of gender on exercise and training responses. *Can J Appl Physiol.* 2000;25(1):19–34.

Hunter SK. The relevance of sex differences in performance fatigability. *Med Sci Sports Exerc.* 2016;48(11):2247–2256.

26. How does the cardiovascular system adapt (or not) to aerobic, endurance-type exercise?
    a. See Fig. 20.2.

Hellsten Y, Nyberg M. Cardiovascular adaptations to exercise training. *Compr Physiol.* 2015;6(1):1–32.

27. How does regular aerobic exercise affect diabetics?
    a. For **non–insulin-dependent** diabetic persons, aerobic exercises increase end-organ cell receptor sensitivity to insulin reducing circulating blood glucose levels. Glucose-lowering treatments may provide a correct insulin level at rest but may become unsafe during exercise by preventing a normal physiological decrease of circulating insulin that allows a shift from energy storage to energy utilization. Exercise will also decrease obesity, which will help in blood sugar control. Be careful to watch for the **Somogyi effect** (epinephrine release with low blood glucose, causing hyperglycemia) when exercising, especially late in the day.
    b. In **insulin-dependent** diabetic persons, exercise does not change the nature of the disease but certainly will change insulin requirements. Moderate-intensity and aerobic exercise can cause hypoglycemia. Meanwhile, high-intensity training and anaerobic exercise may induce hyperglycemia due to a significant rise in catecholamines causing stimulation of muscle glycogenolysis and inhibition of glucose uptake.
    Silent cardiac ischemia is a risk and requires electrocardiographic or perfusion studies for detection.

Lumb A. Diabetes and exercise. *Clin Med (Lond).* 2014;14(6):673–676.

Younk L, Mikeladze M, Tate D, Davis S. Exercise-related hypoglycemia in diabetes mellitus. *Expert Rev Endocrinol Metab.* 2011;6(1):93–108.

28. How to write an exercise prescription?
    a. A handy mnemonic is **TOIL:**
        i. **T** = **T**ype: remember to include components of question 9 as well as exercises the patient will most likely stick with.
        ii. **O** = How **O**ften: per day/week/month, etc.
        iii. **I** = **I**ntensity
        iv. **L** = **L**ength of time

29. How does being in the intensive care unit (ICU) affect your muscles?
    a. **ICU-acquired weakness (ICUAW)** can cause a daily loss of muscle mass averaging 2% to 3% over the first 10 days. This is due to atrophy, muscle fiber necrosis and denervation. ICUAW can occur in up to 80% of patients admitted to the ICU. ICUAW can be manifested in **three forms: muscle atrophy, polyneuropathy, and myopathy**. Early mobilization with progression from passive to active exercises starting while on continued mechanical ventilation reduces ICUAW.

Puthucheary, Z. An update on muscle wasting in the ICU. *Signa Vitae.* 2017;13(Suppl 3):30–31

Jolley SE, Bunnell AE, Hough CL. ICU-acquired weakness. *Chest.* 2016;150(5):1129–1140.

Arias-Fernández P, Romero-Martin M, Gómez-Salgado J, et al. Rehabilitation and early mobilization in the critical patient: systematic review. *J Phys Ther Sci.* 2018;30(9):1193–1201.

30. What is Aquatic Exercise?
    a. Water is an essential ingredient for life and is the medium that transmits pneumatic forces within the internal environment of the body. As a solvent for nutrients and a conveyance for propulsion and an outward sign for sacraments water has been an ancient and remains a contemporary link to physical and spiritual health.
       Creative utilization of water in nutrition activities of daily living, regular exercise, recreation and social togetherness is an essential mission in rehabilitation. There are a myriad of hospital, home, community, and nature-based options to utilize.

Palamara G, Gotti F, Maestri R, et al. Land plus aquatic therapy versus land-based rehabilitation alone for the treatment of balance dysfunction in Parkinson disease: a randomized controlled study with 6-month follow-up. *Arch Phys Medi Rehabil.* 2017;98(6) 1077–1085.

Recio, A, Stiens S, Kubrova E. Aquatic-based therapy in spinal cord injury rehabilitation: effective yet underutilitzed. *Curr Phys Med Rehabil Rep.* 2017;5(3):108–112.

31. What properties make water so effective as a therapeutic medium?
    a. **Buoyancy:** aids in creating resistance and diminishes effects of gravitational pull creating partial body weight support.
    b. **Resistance:** aids in strength and balance.
    c. **Hydrostatic pressure**: depth gradient increases venous and lymphatic return.
    d. **Temperature**: convection currents maintain a constant temperature. The optimal aquatic therapy environment is between 91 and 95 degrees Fahrenheit.

32. What are the indications for Aquatic Therapy?
    a. **Weakness**: many times patients can move further with buoyant limb support and maintenance of upright position and decreased fear of falling.
    b. **Pain**: in water pain is decreased, or gone due to skin stimulation, buoyancy, warmth, and facilitated movement.
    c. **Swelling**: hydrostatic pressure helps mobilize tissue fluid.
    d. **Gait dysfunction**: the entire body (including lower extremities) is off lifted versus harness systems over land where only the trunk is off lifted.
    e. **Shortened muscles**: warmth of water assists in stretching and tissue length changes.
    f. **Tone/Spasticity**: warmth and rotational movements facilitate gradual and sustained stretches to decrease tone/spasticity.
    g. **Balance impairments**: The decreased fear of falling enables patients to work harder and challenge themselves more than on land.
    h. **Impaired functional mobility**: if the floor to stand on is a goal breaking it into parts and being successful in water can translate to land.
    i. **Decreased independence**: water offers an environment where adults and kids who cannot normally interact and move or keep up with their peers can—once they learn water safety.

Becker B. Aquatic therapy: scientific foundations and clinical rehabilitation applications. *PM&R.* 2009;1(9):859–872.

33. Is aquatic therapy safe for patients with invasive devices (pressures ulcer dressing, supra-pubic catheters, indwelling catheters, colostomy bags, and tracheostomy tubes)?
    a. YES! Aquatic therapy, with correct procedures, policies, and protocols is proven efficacious and safe for patients even with invasive devices.
    b. Note: aquatics should always be performed with the ultimate goal of transition back to land. We don't live in the water.

Recio AC, Kubrova E, Stiens SA, Exercise in aquatic environments for patients with chronic spinal cord injury and invasive appliances: successful integration and therapeutic interventions. *Am J Phys Med Rehabil.* 2020; 99:109–115

34. What is activity-based restorative therapy? Who coined the term *ABRT*?
    a. The phrase **activity-based restorative therapy or ABRT**, was originally coined by Drs. Cristina L Sadowsky and John W. McDonald. ABRT is a life-long intervention to achieve activity-dependent neural plasticity driven by repetitive activation of the neuromuscular system above and below the injury level. ABRT is intended to optimize neuromuscular function and offset the rapid aging, physical deterioration, and secondary complications associated with neurological deficits. ABRT is guided by the principle of neuroplasticity and the evidence that even those with chronic SCI can benefit from repeated activation of the spinal cord pathways located both above and below the level of injury.

Dolbow D, Gorgey A, Recio A, McDonald J, Curry A, Martin R, Sadowsky C, Gater D, Stiens SA. Activity-based restorative therapies after spinal cord injury: inter-institutional conceptions and perceptions. *Aging Dis.* 2015;6(4):254–261.

35. What Are the Principles Behind ABRT?
    a. The guiding principles of ABRT are: high-intensity practice, task-specific and functionally patterned activity **above and below** the level of the neurologic lesion, normalizing kinematics and coordination, and aimed at recovery of motor and sensory function.

Sadowsky CL, McDonald JW. Activity-based restorative therapies: concepts and applications in spinal cord injury-related neurorehabilitation. *Dev Disabil Res Rev.* 2009;15(2):112–116.

36. Although different, how can ABRT and traditional therapies be integrated as treatment designs to achieve the best outcomes?
    a. ABRT overcomes the barriers of gravity and exertion to achieve the repetition necessary to functionalize latent pathways and establish new neural connections. ABRT supports new functional utilization of robotic kinematics, functional electrical stimulation, and electronic neural stimulation under permissive biological conditions. Contemporary biological and tissue supportive therapies that include stem cell transplant, growth factors, and supportive nutrients establish a bioenvironment for recovery that is particularly responsive and enabled by ABRT. Traditional supportive brace ambulation adaptive techniques and supportive environments result in better-sustained outcomes with maximal motor recovery.

McDonald J, Sadowsky C, Stampas A. The changing field of rehabilitation: optimizing spontaneous regeneration and functional recovery. *Handb Clin Neurol.* 2012;109:317–336.

Belegu V, Oudega M, Gary D, McDonald JW. Restoring function after spinal cord injury: promoting spontaneous regeneration with stem cells and activity-based therapies. *Neurosurg Clin N Am.* 2007;18(1):143–168.

McDonald JW. Repairing the damaged spinal cord: from stem cells to activity-based restoration therapies. *Clin Neurosurg.* 2004;51:207–27.

BOOKS

• Becker BE, Cole AJ. *Comprehensive Aquatic Therapy.* 3rd ed. Pullman: Washington State University Publishing, 2011.
• Gibson AL, Wagoner DR, Heyood VA. *Advanced Fitness Assessment and Exercise Prescription.* 8th ed. Humankinetics; Human Kinetics Publishers, 2019:560

NEXT STEP REFERENCES

• American Alliance of Health, Physical Education, Recreation, and Dance. Available at: www.aahperd.org/
• American College of Sports Medicine. Available at: www.acsm.org/
• American Council on Exercise. Available at: www.acefitness.org
• American Heart Association. Available at: www.americanheart.org/
• Becker BE, Cole AJ. *Comprehensive Aquatic Therapy.* 3rd ed. Pullman: Washington State University Publishing; 2011.

- President's Council on Physical Fitness and Sports. Available at: www.fitness.gov/
- More on muscle types: Available at: https://www.khanacademy.org/science/health-and-medicine/human-anatomy-and-physiology/introduction-to-muscles/v/type-1-and-2-muscle-fibers
- More on stretching: Available at: www.emedicine.com/pmr/topic199.htm
- More on VO2: 13th Edition, 2016—Guyton and Hall Textbook of Medical Physiology, Chapter 85, 1085–1096. Available at: https://www-clinicalkey-com.proxy.medlib.uits.iu.edu/#!/content/book/3-s2.0-B978145577005200086X
- More on resistance training techniques: Available at: https://emedicine.medscape.com/article/324583-overview#a5
- More on physical activity guidelines: Available at: https://health.gov/paguidelines/second-edition/pdf/Physical_Activity_Guidelines_2nd_edition.pdf

CHAPTER 20

PHYSICAL MODALITIES: THERAPEUTIC AGENTS IN THE CLINIC

Jeffrey R. Basford, MD, PhD

Wade into the water to live again, and reach out for healing hands

—Sir Elton John (1989)

KEY POINTS

1. Physical agents, for the most part, produce only a limited number of effects of which heating, cooling, analgesia, compression, and neuromuscular stimulation are the most common.
2. Tissue temperatures can be altered in only three ways: conduction, convection, or conversion of another form of energy to heat.
3. Major contraindications to therapeutic heat include: acute hemorrhage, inflammation, or trauma, ischemia, insensitivity/inability to respond to pain, bleeding dyscrasias, atrophic or scarred skin, and, while poorly documented, perhaps malignancy.
4. Ultrasound requires a medium for transmission and can be focused, reflected, or refracted. Although frequencies between 0.3 and 3 MHz are used for therapeutic purposes, the 0.8 to 1.0 MHz frequency range may be the best trade-off between focusing properties and tissue penetration.
5. There are two common choices for transcutaneous electrical nerve stimulation (TENS) parameters: high (conventional) TENS with frequencies of 60 to 80 Hz and barely perceptible stimulation intensities and low TENS that uses larger-amplitude, low-frequency (<4 to 8 Hz) signals. Either can be modulated by varying its frequencies and amplitudes.

IMPORTANT FACTS ABOUT PHYSICAL AGENTS

1. What is the role of a physical agent?

   Physical agents are almost always in conjunction with a therapy program that may also involve exercise, stretching, and education. As such, they may be viewed as an adjunct to the program's other components. A possible exception may occur with transcutaneous electrical nerve stimulation (TENS) for chronic pain.

2. What are the limitations of the physical agents?

   Although each agent has unique characteristics, most ultimately rely on heating, cooling, or electromagnetic stimulation to gain their effects. As a result, many are limited by the fact that temperatures above 45°C (100°F) or below 0°C (32°F) may injure tissue. Treatments involving higher intensities or more extreme temperatures are limited to restricted portions of the body.

HEAT AND COLD

3. How do physical agents heat or cool tissue?

   There are only three ways that tissue temperature can be altered:
   - **Conduction: transference of heat** between two bodies in contact at different temperatures. Examples include hot packs and ice massage.
   - **Convection: transference of heat between two objects** at different temperatures in which one, the medium, flows past the other. This flow, with wind chill being an example, facilitates a more rapid and intense heating and cooling than would be otherwise possible.
   - **Conversion** involves the transformation of one form of energy to another. Heat lamps and ultrasound (US), for example, rely on the conversion of infrared (IR) light and sound to heat.

4. How many types of heat therapy are available?

   There are only two ways to heat tissue. Superficial agents such as heat lamps heat the skin and subcutaneous tissues. Deep heating agents, such as US, heat more deeply and can raise temperatures to therapeutic levels at depths of 3.5 to 7 cm.

5. What forms of cold therapy (cryotherapy) are available?

Cold is produced by the reduction of a body's thermal energy. As there is no known way to extract energy at a distance, only superficial agents such as ice can be used.

6. What are the goals of heat and cryotherapy?
   - Analgesia
   - Hyperemia/vasoconstriction
   - Increased collagen extensibility (heat)
   - Acceleration (heat) and slowing (cold) of metabolic processes
   - Muscle spasm relaxation

7. What are the major contraindications to therapeutic heat?
   - Acute hemorrhage, inflammation, or trauma
   - Ischemia
   - Insensitivity/inability to respond to pain
   - Malignancy (which is poorly documented)
   - Bleeding dyscrasias
   - Atrophic or scarred skin

8. What are some common examples of superficial thermal agents?
   - Hot packs
   - Heat lamps
   - Hot-water soaks
   - Whirlpools

9. How are hot packs used?

Hot packs are usually kept immersed in water baths at 70 to 80°C (168 to 175°F). During treatment, they are removed from the bath and excess water is permitted to drain off. They are then placed in an insulated cover and *laid on, not under* the patient. Packs typically hold therapeutically useful temperatures for 20 to 30 minutes.

10. What are some useful facts about heat lamps?
   - Special IR heating elements are probably no more effective than standard incandescent bulbs.
   - Most lamps behave as "point" sources with the intensity of their heating decreasing inversely with the square of their distance from the body ($1/d^2$).
   - Most heat lamps use 60 to 150 W bulbs and are placed 50 to 75 cm from the body.
   - Chronic exposure to superficial heat can produce a permanent skin mottling known as erythema ab igne (erythema from fire).

11. What about paraffin baths?

Paraffin baths have fallen out of favor but once had an established place in the treatment of rheumatoid arthritis, contractures, and scleroderma. They do, however, remain available on the internet and typically consist of 1:7 mixtures of mineral oil and paraffin maintained at about 52°C. Treatment commonly takes one of three forms:
   - Dipping (the most common) involves placing the part to be treated in the bath, removing it, letting the wax harden, and repeating the cycle 10 times. The treated area is then covered with a plastic sheet and an insulating mitt for about 20 minutes.
   - Immersion provides more vigorous heating and involves dipping the treated area into paraffin several times and then keeping it immersed for about 20 minutes.
   - Brushing is used to provide paraffin treatment to parts of the body that cannot be placed in a bath. Paraffin baths are filled with hot molten wax and bath temperatures must be monitored (e.g., with an installed thermometer) carefully to avoid burns.

12. What is a contrast bath? How were they used?

Contrast baths are far less common now but in the past were used primarily for their purported desensitization and vasogenic reflex effects in patients with rheumatoid arthritis and complex regional pain. They consist of two reservoirs with one filled with warm water (43°C) and the other cool (16°C). Treatment was usually limited to the hands or feet and typically began with a 10-minute soak in the warm bath and then cycling between the two baths. Soaking duration varied but was often about 4 minutes in the warm and 1 to 2 minutes in the cool bath.

13. What are the most common forms of cryotherapy?
   - Ice, whether in the form of ice packs, ice massage, or ice slushes remains the most common form of cryotherapy. Most importantly, it is central to the rest, ice, compression, and elevation (RICE) approach to musculoskeletal injury. Ice massage is frequently used for intense treatment of localized areas of musculoskeletal pain, such as lateral epicondylitis. Ice slushes and whirlpools are less commonly used and tend to be restricted to sport training rooms.

- Chemical ice packs, while convenient, typically do not provide as intense cooling as ice packs. (Many find a bag of frozen peas more convenient and less expensive.)
- Vapocoolant spray and stretch treatments involve spraying a rapidly evaporative skin refrigerant on the skin (i.e., spray and stretch). While now rare in clinics, they remain commercially available.

14. **What are the effects of cryotherapy?**
   Cryotherapy typically results in longer-lasting effects than heat. A desire for analgesia, vasoconstriction, and control of the swelling associated with acute injury are the most obvious indications for longer duration (>3 min) cryotherapy. Prolonged cooling reduces spasticity and slows both nerve conduction and metabolism.

Brosseau L, Yonge KA, Robinson V, et al. Thermotherapy for treatment of osteoarthritis. *Cochrane Database Sys Rev.* 2003;4:CD004522.

15. **When is cryotherapy contraindicated?**
   The most common contraindications for cryotherapy include ischemia, Raynaud's syndrome, insensitivity, cryoglobulinemia, and cold-induced pressor responses. As is true for all physical agents, contraindications are often relative. For example, ice massage of a diabetic with neuropathy and atherosclerotic disease might be appropriate for trochanteric bursitis but not for a foot condition.

16. **What do I need to know about whirlpool baths?**
   - Whirlpools use agitated water to produce convective heating or cooling, massage, and gentle debridement.
   - Tub size, water temperature, agitation intensity, and solvent properties are adjusted to the patient's situation.
   - Water temperature is determined by the amount of the body submerged, the patient's health, and goals of treatment. A limited portion of a limb with intact sensation may tolerate temperatures up to 45°C, but as more of the body is submerged, temperatures should decrease, commonly to 40 to 41°C for immersion to the waist and 38 to 39°C if more of the body is submerged. The condition of the patient is important; an elderly diabetic would be treated more cautiously than a young athlete.

17. **How are wounds treated with hydrotherapy?**
   Wounds treated with hydrotherapy typically have open areas with necrotic debris, adherent dressings, or contamination and can range from hand cuts and abrasions to large and even open abdominal wounds. The latter require careful selection of bath temperature, osmolality, and agitation as well as supervision by an experienced therapist. Patients with large wounds can be reassured as correctly adjusted baths are surprisingly comfortable. Hand held showerheads, sprays, and dental water jets may be used for more forceful debridement.

18. **Can hydrotherapy solvent properties be manipulated? If so, why?**
   Warmed tap water (which is amazingly sterile) is usually used alone. Gentle detergents and antiseptic solutions may be added to improve debridement and wound cleansing. Salt can be dissolved in a bath to produce a normal saline (0.9% NaCl) solution to improve comfort and reduce concerns about hemolysis and water intoxication in patients with large wounds.

19. **What are common indications for hydrotherapy?**
   - Open, contaminated wounds
   - Contractures
   - Muscle spasm
   - Burns
   - Immobile obese patients who cannot be cleansed in another manner

20. **What is diathermy, and what are the diatheric agents?**
   Diathermy (literally "heating through") is available in three forms: US, shortwave, and microwave. All heat tissue by conversion.

21. **What are the characteristics of shortwave diathermy?**
   Shortwave diathermy (SWD) is becoming less common, and microwave diathermy (MWD) is now a rarity in clinics. While three SWD frequencies (40.68, 27.12, and 13.56 MHz) are approved for medical use in the United States, 27.12 MHz is the most common. Treatments aimed at warming tissue generally involve energy outputs of several hundred watts.

22. **How is SWD delivered?**
   Energy is transferred to the body in two ways:
   - Capacitive coupling: the tissue to be treated is placed between two plates, and the body acts as a dielectric in a series circuit. Heating is greatest in high-impedance, water-poor tissues, such as fat.
   - Inductive coupling: the body acts as a receiver, and eddy currents are induced by the SWD machine. Heating is most intense in low-impedance, water-rich tissues, such as muscle. Temperature elevations of 4 to 6°C are seen at depths of 4 to 5 cm.

23. **What are the contraindicated uses of SWD?**
    - Water and metal are electrical conductors and can cause burns if exposed to SWD. Therefore, patients must remove jewelry, and perspiration should be absorbed by toweling.
    - Metal implants and perhaps metallic sutures may produce local areas of heating; treatment with SWD is not recommended.
    - SWD produces wide fields, and precautions include not treating pregnant women, a uterus during menstruation, or patients with implanted metal devices, pacemakers, defibrillators, pumps, or contact lenses.

24. **What is MWD?**
    MWD, like SWD, uses electromagnetic waves to heat tissue. However, the frequencies used are 30 to 100 times higher than those of SWD. MWD was common but now has been replaced by US. Microwave beams are much easier to direct than SWD but, because of their higher frequencies, attenuate more rapidly and often lose much of their energy in subcutaneous tissue. The precautions of SWD apply to MWD. In addition, microwaves produce cataracts and MWD should be avoided in the vicinity of the eyes' fluid-filled cavities and may affect the growth plates of young bones.

25. **What is therapeutic US?**
    US is identical to audible sound but limited to frequencies above the 18 to 20,000 Hz limit of human hearing. As such, it requires a medium for transmission and can be focused, reflected, or refracted. Although therapeutic frequencies (in distinction to the higher frequencies required for diagnostic imaging) range between 0.3 and 3 MHz, the 0.8 to 1.0 MHz region is favored as the best trade-off between focusing and tissue penetration.

26. **What are the effects of US on the body?**
    Heating is the most important effect. Nonthermal effects, such as cavitation, media motion, and standing waves, occur, but their risks and benefits are poorly understood. Cavitation, for example, produces bubbles, which can disrupt tissue by their oscillation and bursting. Small-scale media motion may occur from US exposure. Standing-wave patterns in a stationary US field produce fixed areas of elevated and low pressure.

27. **How far does therapeutic US penetrate?**
    The depth of clinically beneficial heating depends on the power applied, the nature of the tissue, and the direction/frequency of the beam. For example, 50% of a US beam may penetrate 7 to 8 cm of fat but less than 1 mm of bone. Direction can also be important: A US beam may penetrate 7 cm when traveling parallel to the fibers of a muscle but only 2 cm when perpendicular. Frequency also has significant effects as well. Beam penetration in tissue may fall by about 85% as its frequency increases from 0.3 to 3.3 MHz. Therapeutic US treatment with frequencies of 0.8 to 1.0 MHz can produce 4 to 5°C temperature elevations at depths of 8 cm.

28. **Where does heating occur during US treatment?**
    US can heat skin, fat, muscle, and bone with the most pronounced heating occurring at tissue interfaces. Bone-soft tissue discontinuities produce the most intensive areas of heating. Most avoid treatment in the vicinity of metal (e.g., implants) or laminectomies.

29. **How is US applied?**
    Acoustic gels or mineral oil are used to maximize acoustic coupling. Treatment is performed with the applicator being moved in a circular motion. Irregular body parts (e.g., the ankle) may be submerged in degassed water with the applicator slightly offset from the surface. Dosage depends on location and goals, but treatment sessions usually last 7 to 15 minutes and may utilize either pulsed or continuous waveforms. Treatments aimed at warming tissue heating typically involve intensities of 0.5 to 1.5 W/cm^2, while those hoping to emphasize US's nonthermal properties tend to utilize lower intensities.

30. **What is phonophoresis?**
    Phonophoresis is a US technique in which medication is mixed with the acoustic-coupling medium in the expectation that the US beam will drive the pharmacologic agent into the tissue. Penetration depths depend on the nature of the substance involved, and significant amounts of drug are absorbed by the subcutaneous circulation. Studies involving topical anesthetics and corticosteroids have suggested benefits, but more work is needed to establish whether this technique is more effective than medication or even US alone.

31. **When should US be used?**
    Research is limited but often supports treating:
    - Soft tissue wounds
    - Contractures
    - Calcific tendonitis
    - Non-healing fractures (pulsed US only)
    - Musculoskeletal pain

32. When is US contraindicated?
    - All general contraindications for therapeutic heat
    - Fluid filled organs such as a gravid uterus, eyes, and heart
    - Immature or acutely inflamed joints
    - Laminectomy sites
    - Tumors

33. What is TENS?
    TENS is a form of therapy that applies low intensity electrical signals to the body with skin electrodes which may be placed over peripheral nerves, nerve roots, and acupuncture points, as well as proximal to, distal to, over, and (more debatable) contralateral to the areas of pain.

34. How does TENS produce relief?
    The exact mechanism remains unclear. Melzack and Wall's "gate theory of pain" (1965) proposed that stimulation of large myelinated afferent fibers blocks the transmission of pain by small unmyelinated fibers at the level of the spinal cord. Although plausible in many ways, the theory does not explain all aspects of TENS analgesia (i.e., prolonged pain relief following use). Alterations of cerebrospinal endorphin concentrations are also reported but difficult to correlate with therapeutic response.

Melzack R, Wall PD. Pain mechanisms: a new theory. *Science*. 1965;150(3699):971–979.

35. Can electrical stimulation increase muscle strength and function?
    Electrical stimulation has been shown to maintain and increase muscle bulk and strength in immobilized limbs and paretic muscles. In addition, functional electrical stimulation (FES) can provide functional movement of one or more muscles in a coordinated manner. Limitations due to complexity, cost, reliability, and safety have restricted its use. Exercise and training devices for patients with spinal cord injury and stroke are the best-known applications of this approach.

36. Is it safe to use electrical stimulation in patients with cancer?
    This is generally true. Most would avoid treatment near the site of the tumor or a metastasis, but otherwise, electrical stimulation, including FES, appears safe.

Crevenna R. From neuromuscular electrical stimulation and biofeedback-assisted exercise up to triathlon competitions—regular physical activity for cancer patients in Austria. *Eur Rev Aging Phys Act.* 2013;*10*:53–55.

Jones S, Man WD, Gao W, et al. Neuromuscular electrical stimulation for muscle weakness in adults with advanced disease. *Cochrane Database Sys Rev.* 2016;10(10):CD009419.

37. What is interferential current?
    Interferential devices rely on two electromagnetic characteristics: (1) while low frequency stimulation (such as from TENS) of skin can be painful, they are not responsive to higher frequencies and (2) electrical waves differing slightly in frequency can interact (i.e., beat) with each other and produce waveforms with frequencies equal to the sum or difference of the original waves. Interferential current (IFC) devices use these properties and generate waves at different frequencies (e.g., 2000 and 2040 Hz), which can penetrate the skin without discomfort. Treatment involves placing pairs of electrodes so that the waves cross at the site of treatment. In a clinical situation, only the low-frequency difference waves are important. IFC can be used to produce TENS-like effects or stimulate muscle contraction.

38. What is iontophoresis?
    Iontophoresis uses positively and negatively charged electrodes to force electrically charged or polar substances into the skin. Any charged or polar substance can theoretically be phoresed, and medications have included agents such as lidocaine, iodine, salicylates, antibiotics, and silver. Iontophoresis with tap water is an effective treatment of hyperhidrosis. This approach has also been used to deliver antibiotics to poorly vascularized tissue, produce local anesthesia, speed wound healing, and treat musculoskeletal pain. Although iontophoresis can be effective, it can be a cumbersome way to provide treatment that could be more easily accomplished by an injection or a pill.

39. What are graduated compressive garments?
    Graduated compression garments are designed to apply higher pressures distally and lesser pressures proximally in a graduated manner. Garment pressures and style (i.e., calf-high, thigh-high, or leotard) are dictated by edema severity and location as well as the patient's ability to tolerate and don the garment. Lower-extremity stockings

are typically chosen in the 20 to 30 or 30 to 40 mm Hg ranges with choice influenced by the limb's sensation and perfusion and patient compliance. Off-the-shelf garments are usually suitable, although custom-measured garments may be necessary for people who are obese, difficult to fit, or need compression over irregular areas. Compressive garments are used primarily for the prevention of deep venous thrombosis and the control of edema. There is strong evidence of their effectiveness in both of these roles.

Sachdeva A, Dalton M, Lees T. Graduated compression stockings for prevention of deep vein thrombosis. *Cochrane Database Sys Rev.* 2018;11(11):CD001484.

40. ## How should compression wraps be used?
Compressive wrapping is of therapeutic value on its own but may be used to lessen edema or heal venous ulcers prior to the time that a compressive garment can be used. While its use in edema control is well known, there is ample evidence that it is effective in improving the healing of venous ulcers. A number of wraps and techniques are available. Each has its advantages, and often, a number of approaches will be combined. For example, short-stretch as well as more elastic wraps may be used in conjunction with padding when treating leg ulcers and reducing refractory edema.

O'Meara S, Cullum N, Nelson AE, et al. Compression for venous leg ulcers. *Cochrane Database Sys Rev.* 2019;3(1):CD000265.

41. ## What are the risks of compressive garments and wraps?
Compression has risks. Most are commonsensical in nature. For example, shear forces on atrophic or injured skin should be avoided. Use on insensate limbs should also be avoided if possible and monitored carefully if initiated. Arterial insufficiency is a concern with many guidelines recommending that patients with leg ulcers undergo ankle-brachial pressure index screening before treatment.

42. ## What are common uses for compressive garments?
- Edema due to congestive heart failure
- Treated deep venous thrombosis
- Lymphedema treated deep venous thrombosis
- Venous incompetence
- Postmastectomy edema
- Orthostatic hypotension (abdominal compression with a binder may be helpful; lower extremity garments must be thigh-length to be effective)

43. ## What are basic rules for wearing compression garments?
- Garments are less effective and more poorly tolerated by obese people.
- Thigh-length garments slide down the limb without the use of straps or adhesive.
- Use the shortest garment possible.
- Men are resistant to leotards.

44. ## What role do pneumatic pumps have in therapy?
Pneumatic devices are used in various medical settings. While sequential compression devices (SCDs) that are used to reduce the risk of deep venous thrombosis in immobilized patients are outside the scope of this chapter, other pneumatic devices are used in clinics. Intermittent compression with different cycling characteristics has been utilized to treat conditions such as lymphedema, leg ulcers, and arterial perfusion in the distal extremities. The evidence for benefit is mixed and often of poor quality. Regardless, treatment should only be performed by a skilled therapist. Relative and absolute contraindications include acute deep venous thrombosis, cellulitis, impaired perfusion, and insensate limbs.

45. ## What is the role of photobiomodulation (laser therapy) in the clinic?
Photobiomodulation (also known as light, low level, and laser therapy) has been used since the 1960s to promote wound healing, lessen pain, and speed recovery from musculoskeletal injury. Many devices have been used, but most have powers less than 100 mW and utilize red (0.6 μm) and IR (0.82 to 1.06 μm) wavelengths. Irradiation produces striking effects on cellular processes, immune function, and collagen formation in the laboratory. Use is widespread and safety well-established, although proof of efficacy and the choice of optimal clinical parameters remain controversial.

Yousefi-Nooraie R. Low level laser therapy for nonspecific low-back pain. *Cochrane Database of Sys Rev.* 2007;(2):CD005107.

Fleming PS, Strydom H, Katsaros C, et al. Non-pharmacological interventions for alleviating pain during orthodontic treatment. *Cochrane Database Sys Rev.* 2016:12(12):CD010263.

Available at: https://waltpbm.org/documentation-links/recommendations

46. Are there other new physical agents or new applications of older agents?

Laser therapy has had the most attention recently, but other new as well as older agents with new uses exist. For example, US and low-intensity electromagnetic fields accelerate fracture healing. In addition, there are other newer agents with varying proof of effectiveness. Among these are the use of US mist therapy for wound treatment, transcortical electrical/magnetic stimulation to relieve pain or enhance learning and recovery from brain injury, and the use of "micro-electro-magnetic" fields to treat a variety of wounds and painful conditions.

Akyuz G, Kenis O. Physical therapy modalities and rehabilitation techniques in the treatment of neuropathic pain. *Am J Phys Med Rehabil.* 2013:1(4). doi:10.1097/ PHM.0000000000000037

Basford JR. Physical agents. In *DeLisa's Physical Medicine and Rehabilitation: Principles and Practice.* 6th ed. Philadelphia, PA: Lippincott Williams & Wilkins.

Galea MP. Physical modalities in the treatment of neurological dysfunction. *Clin Neurol Neurosurg.* 2012;114(5):483–8. doi:10.1016/j. clineuro.2012.01.009. Available at: https://pubmed.ncbi.nlm.nih.gov/22296649/.

CHAPTER 21

ELECTROTHERAPY: MEDICAL TREATMENTS USING ELECTRICITY

Gad Alon, PhD, PT, Ryan A. Grant, MD, MS, Sheela Vivekanandan, MD, and Jonathan R. Slotkin, MD, FAANS

Listening is a magnetic and strange thing, a creative force. When we really listen to people there is an alternating current, and this recharges us so that we never get tired of each other. We are constantly being recreated.
— Brenda Ueland (1891–1986)
With electricity we extend our central nervous system globally, instantly interrelating every human experience.
— Marshall McLuhan (1911–1980)

KEY POINTS

1. Noninvasive neuromuscular electrical stimulation and functional electrical stimulation (FES) minimize physical impairments by improving muscle strength, peripheral circulation, and joint range of motion.
2. Noninvasive FES enables patients to improve locomotion and upper extremity daily functions abilities.
3. Implanted FES benefits mainly those with a high spinal cord injury.
4. Invasive and noninvasive neuromodulation is used to minimize chronic pain perception that does not respond to other treatments.
5. Transcutaneous electrical nerve stimulation is used to temporarily diminish perceived acute and chronic pain of various origins and causes but has no meaningful post-stimulation lasting effect.
6. Using a specific and sterile protocol, electrical stimulation should be the first-line option to accelerate the healing of slow-to-heal wounds.

1. **What is neuromodulation's role in rehabilitation?**
   Neuromodulation is a broad term describing the application of electrical currents used clinically (invasively or noninvasively) over the spinal cord or head to modulate neural transmission within different levels of neural networks. The intent is to reduce and/or suppress pain and also modulate micro- and macro-circulation. Common to all stimulators is the delivery of electrical pulses of various waveforms, varying durations, pulse frequencies, and parameter control. Waveforms can be unidirectional or bidirectional.

   This form of therapy has become a key intervention option in recent years and can be done using fully or partially implantable stimulators. Neuromodulation by noninvasive conductive stimulation (TENS, NMES) or electromagnetic stimulation (TMS) is an equally available clinical option. Most invasive systems are surgically implanted over regions of the spinal cord or selected internal organs. Other systems are implanted in the brain (deep brain stimulation, or DBS). The clearest indication for spinal cord stimulation is to minimize pain perception in patients suffering from chronic musculoskeletal or peripheral vascular pain who are unresponsive to other interventions.[1] Partially implanted systems (implanted lead-wire with non-implanted stimulator), also termed "percutaneous," have been used to minimize persistent shoulder pain.[2,3]

   Neuromodulation by noninvasive stimulation has been the focus of peer-reviewed research including managing tension and migraine headaches or controlling epileptic seizures.[4] Generally, the trigeminal, occipital, or both nerves are stimulated in conjunction with behavior modification methods.

   Another approach to modulating brain connectivity has been to apply conductive stimulation (transcutaneous direct current [tDCS], pulsed current [tPCS][5,6] or electromagnetic stimulation termed [TMS]).[7] The objectives of these approaches are to enhance the recovery of motor control following damage to the brain or to minimize chronic pain following spinal cord injury (SCI). Although the evidence for its efficacy and effectiveness appears insufficient, both the conductive and electromagnetic approaches are also being used to treat clinical depression or insomnia.

2. **What are TENS, NMES, and FES?**
   a. Transcutaneous electrical nerve stimulation (TENS) reduces and/or suppresses pain from various sources by modulating neural transmission within different levels of the neural networks that control pain perception. By definition, TENS is noninvasive.
   b. Neuromuscular electrical stimulation (NMES) induces contraction of skeletal muscles in order to strengthen weak or sarcopenic muscles and enhance peripheral, arterial, venous, and lymphatic circulation. NMES is generally noninvasive.

c. Functional electrical stimulation (FES) improves the performance of daily living tasks, including locomotion, upper extremity function, and internal organ functions. FES can be noninvasive or invasive (known as Implantable Electrical Stimulation).

3. **What distinguishes TENS, NMES, FES, and neuromodulation?**
Unlike TENS, NMES, and FES have modulations called "on" and "off" times that provide intermittent contraction and relaxation of stimulated muscles. The difference between NMES and FES in clinical practice is arbitrary and not supported by evidence-based research. When an NMES device is used with task-specific or functional training, the term FES should be used. The difference between TENS and neuromodulation is that TENS is applied noninvasively while neuromodulation can be applied noninvasively, partially invasively, or completely invasively. Both neuromodulation and TENS seek to eliminate or lessen pain perception of various origins. Cochlear or DBS are also called invasive neuromodulation.

4. **Do TENS, NMES, FES, or neuromodulation affect the brain?**
Studies show that applying any form of electrical stimulation over the lower or upper extremities, torso, face, or head changes brain activity, as shown by various imaging or mapping techniques.

5. **What are the contraindications for FES, NMES, TENS, and neuromodulation?**
Although there are no absolute contraindications for use of commercially available stimulation systems, caution should be used in the following instances:
   a. Patients with cardiac, bladder, or other electronic pacing devices. Electrical stimulation applied anywhere on the body can disrupt the electronic sensing of these devices.
   b. Patients with cardiac monitoring or congestive heart failure.
   c. Pregnancy.
   d. Sensitivity to the electrode material.
   e. Wounds that are healing. Muscle contraction from NMES may adversely impact tissues that are healing.
   f. Implantable FES devices are generally MRI compatible, but noninvasive FES units are not. However, each device must be considered individually for compatibility before imaging is done.
   g. If any noninvasive stimulators cause skin irritation, stimulating the irritated site must stop until the irritation is resolved.

6. **How is FES used?**
FES systems can be completely or partially implanted (i.e., minimally invasive), or applied noninvasively over the skin. For most patients seeking rehabilitation, implanted FES is not an option because it requires major surgery yet offers limited improvement. In contrast, using non-implanted FES (surface electrodes), regardless of the source of injury, has been supported by numerous evidence-based, peer-reviewed published research.

   FES activates paretic muscles resulting from damage to the brain. Typical examples include multiple sclerosis (MS), trauma (including traumatic brain injury, TBI), surgery, stroke, and cerebral palsy (CP). It can also activate paretic muscles following damage to the spinal cord. Noninvasive FES can be FES-dependent (which lets patients perform specific tasks or functions that they otherwise could not perform), or FES-independent (relearned). In the latter, the patient uses FES for a specified time to minimize impairments and dysfunctions while relearning to eventually perform the tasks and functions without FES.[8] FES-dependent treatment is also called neuro-prosthesis.

7. **Do FES/NMES systems directly stimulate nerves or muscles?**
Motor units are activated electrically by depolarizing sensory and motor nerve fibers of mixed nerves, including median, radial, ulnar, femoral, sciatic, tibial and fibular (common peroneal), or their terminal nerve branches. Unlike normal propagation, in which action potentials of afferent and efferent fibers propagate unidirectionally, electrically depolarized nerves propagate bidirectionally. When the action potentials of a motor nerve reach the muscle, they spread over via the T-tubules and cause contraction.

   A muscle that has lost its innervation can be directly depolarized by electrical current, but the amount of pulse charge (current-time integral) necessary to induce contraction is considerably greater than that needed to depolarize the nerve.[9,10] Therefore, for clinical purposes, FES systems stimulate nerves and not muscles.

8. **What happens to electrically activated muscles over time?**
The following cascade begins at the molecular level[9,10]:
   a. Up-regulation of IGF-1
   b. Modulation of MuRF-1
   c. Up-regulation of relevant markers of differentiating satellite cells
   d. Extracellular matrix remodeling, which maintains satellite cell function and reduces fibrosis.

   Electrically induced contractions significantly increase total RNA content and reduce protein degradation,[11] increase body cell mass, attenuate reduction of intracellular water, alleviate arterial hemodynamic disturbance,[12] reduce tumor necrosis factor (TNF-alpha),[13] and increase β-endorphin levels.

   Enhancing these molecular and cellular metabolic events are all markers supporting long-established clinical data demonstrating that FES/NMES use likely provides significant muscle strength gains, regardless of whether the strength deficits resulted from damage to musculoskeletal, neurological, or cardiovascular-pulmonary systems.[11,14–17] FES/NMES activation of skeletal muscles has been shown to also enhance arterial, venous, and lymphatic flow while concurrently transmitting multimodal afferent signals to multiple sites in regions of interest in the brain.[18]

9. **What is the difference between implanted and non-implanted FES systems?**

Implanted FES systems require complex surgery and have been successfully implanted in patients with cervical or high thoracic SCI and those with foot-drop as a result of a stroke. At the FES Center (Cleveland, OH), advanced FES units are used to help those with SCI move their arms or legs, control their bowels and bladder, treat or prevent pressure sores, and provide male erection and ejaculation. However, only a few survivors of SCI benefit from implanted FES because they are part of research protocols, not clinical practice.

By contrast, non-implanted systems, including wearable or non-wearable FES and motorized cycle FES systems are commercially available and many survivors of SCI, stroke, TBI, MS, and CP, as well as patients in CCU/ICU, appear to benefit from using these systems. The primary limitations of noninvasive FES are its inability to induce contraction in deeply situated muscles (i.e., iliopsoas and muscles "covered" by bone such as subscapularis)[8] and the inconvenience of placing and removing the system.

---

http://fescenter.org
http://www.bionessmobility.com

Restorative Therapies. Available at: https://www.restorative-therapies.com

10. **List pathophysiological changes following SCI.**

Depending on the degree of damage and whether it is complete or incomplete, those with SCI share the following:
- Become more sedentary
- Paralysis is compounded by impaired autonomic nervous system function
- Cardiovascular response to exercise is limited, especially in individuals with lesions at T6 or above
- Muscle mass, strength, and endurance all decrease, and muscle fibers convert to primarily anaerobic metabolism after injury
- Muscles are infiltrated by fibrotic and fatty cells
- Paralysis of intercostal musculature reduces vital capacity and cough efficiency
- Control of bladder and bowel functions are lost or impaired
- Peripheral circulation, lean body mass, and bone density are impaired
- Altered endocrine responses.

11. **How does FES assist in treating SCI?**

In cervical injuries, restoring hand function is the main focus in order to increase independence with personal care. Lower SCI restoration focuses on the ability to stand and step. All the changes following SCI can be partially reversed or improved with FES. Specific benefits include:
- Muscle strengthening
- Increasing lean muscle mass and decreasing adipose tissue
- Decreasing spasticity
- Improving ASIA motor and sensory scores
- Increasing stepping responses
- Recovering lost bone mass
- Improving cardiovascular conditioning, oxygen uptake, and ventilation
- Enhanced venous return from the legs
- Decreased blood glucose and insulin levels
- Better bowel and bladder function
- Psychological benefits
- Electro-ejaculation for fertility.

12. **Does implanted FES improve sitting balance, standing, and walking in those with SCI?**

The Cleveland FES Center found that it is possible to improve balance, standing, and walking in some patients with SCI following implantation and extended training. Several approaches to using FES for lower-extremity standing and walking in paraplegia are being researched. Implantable lower-extremity FES using percutaneous electrodes and implantable stimulator-receivers with epimysial or intramuscular electrodes have also been developed to aid in activating deep musculature. Hybrid approaches, such as reciprocating gait orthosis (RGO), use exoskeletal and mechanical bracing with FES. However, the technique remains controversial, and practitioners are unsure of the added value of this hybrid approach to "activity of daily living," as well as the cost of long-term technical support.

13. **Can implanted FES restore hand-grasp in tetraplegia?**

Tetraplegic hand grasp systems have focused on those with C5 and C6 SCI. Data for people with C4 injury are anecdotal. Those injured at C7 and lower have multiple voluntary active forearm muscles (e.g., brachioradialis, extensor carpi radialis longus and brevis, pronator teres), which can be used in many activities, making tendon transfer and FES somewhat beneficial.

14. **What benefits can patients with SCI receive from training with motorized FES cycle ergometry?**
Cardiac output and muscle oxidative capacity both improve with FES ergometry. Some patients using FES ergometry reach aerobic metabolic rates (as measured by peak VO_2) comparable to those without disabilities. Electrical exercise also increases peripheral venous return and fibrinolysis. In one report, FES combined with heparin therapy was more effective in preventing DVT than heparin alone. There are, however, limits to the cardiovascular benefits of FES ergometry for those with lesions at or above T5. In these patients, there is a loss of supraspinal sympathetic control, which limits the body's ability to increase heart rate, stroke volume, and cardiac output.[17]

15. **What are the benefits of training with motorized FES?**
Advanced, motorized FES systems let patients exercise some or all extremities. Some systems are designed to train the patient in simulated upright walking, cycling, sitting, and can be done while lying in bed. These computerized exercise systems use multiple stimulation channels and surface electrodes to sequentially induce the contraction of muscles at the correct time during cycling or walking. By activating multiple muscles in a coordinated series of specific tasks (e.g., cycling or walking) patients gain muscle strength, joint motion, motor-control, and cardiovascular fitness. One recent study post-stroke also reported gains in walking speed, distance, and balance.[19]

16. **What role does FES have in respiratory assistance?**
In high-level tetraplegic injuries (C1 or C2), the use of the phrenic pacemaker has become a standard alternative to chronic ventilator dependence. Those with spinal cord damage at C3 and C4 often have damaged the anterior horns of those segments, resulting in Wallerian degeneration of the phrenic nerves. Therefore, phrenic nerve conduction testing before FES use is mandatory because intact phrenic nerves are required.

   Diaphragmatic pacing is attractive to patients with high cervical SCI because it makes possible the removal of a tracheostomy in people who require mechanical ventilation while they sleep. Also, for patients who require full-time mechanical ventilation, FES can give them freedom from the ventilator for speech and other activities. Some centers are also using it to wean patients off ventilators faster.

17. **What changes occur following brain injury?**
Unlike SCI, damage to the brain disrupts connectivity among and between numerous brain networks, including motor and sensorimotor networks. Consequently, patients lose varying degrees of motor control over the trunk, and upper and lower limbs. The resulting pathophysiological impairments may include abnormal sympathetic-parasympathetic autonomic nervous responses, causing eutrophic changes in dermal and subdermal tissues.

   Limited mobility also contributes to loss of muscle strength, shortening and adhesions within the myofascial system leading to joints' contracture. Impaired motor control is typically accompanied by flaccid paralysis or paresis, and various degrees of spasticity of the affected muscles. These, in turn, further contribute to myofascial shortening and may impair peripheral blood flow.

18. **Is there a reason to delay FES in cases of stroke or TBI?**
No. A number of clinical trials, including some that are randomized and controlled, have reported that initiating FES within 7 to 20 days post-stroke resulted in benefits, including:
    a. Minimizing shoulder subluxation and shoulder pain.
    b. Improving active range of motion (ROM).
    c. Reducing spasticity.
    d. Regaining hand function.
    e. Regaining the ability to walk.
    f. No report of increased risk of recurrent stroke, TIA, seizures, shoulder-hand syndrome, or edema.

19. **List common outcomes from training with noninvasive FES and NMES?**
In recent years, commercial FES and NMES systems are available as wearable wireless or wired, non-wearable. Traditionally, NMES has been used to manage impairments, while FES has been used to overcome impairments and functional deficits. Typical clinical outcomes include:
    - Strengthening weak, atrophied, sarcopenic skeletal muscles (NMES/FES).
    - Maintaining or improving joint mobility (NMES/FES).
    - Enhancing peripheral arterial, venous, and lymphatic flow (NMES/FES).
    - Improving volitional motor control (NMES/FES), locomotion ability (FES), and upper extremity function (FES).

20. **What is the reason for and common uses of TENS?**
TENS has been used in clinical practice using two settings. One is termed "low intensity, higher frequency" (60 to 150 Hz). The other is called "high intensity, low frequency" (2 to 10 Hz). Animal-derived mechanisms underlying the former setting include release of γ-aminobutyric acid (GABA), decrease in glutamate at the spinal level, activation of δ-opioid and muscarinic receptors in the spinal cord and δ-opioid receptors supra-spinally. The "low-frequency" approach releases serotonin and activates serotonin receptors 5-HT2 and 5HT3, muscarinic and muscarin-opioid receptors in the spine, and muscarin-opioid receptors at the supra-spinal level. Pain relief with TENS is expected during stimulation but typically has a short duration post stimulation (<2 to 3 hours).

Meta-analyses have shown that a strong, subnoxious intensity at a higher frequency is a better choice to significantly reduce analgesic consumption and control postoperative pain.[20] In contrast, a systematic review provided inconclusive evidence of TENS benefit in low back pain patients because the quality of the studies was low and adequate parameters and timing of assessment were not uniformly used or reported.[21–23] In one recent study, it was reported that using TENS units in the hospital emergency department reduced pain in 99% of cases. When surveyed, 83% of patients reported a functional improvement while using the TENS, and all would recommend a TENS unit to a family or friend.[24]

21. How should TENS be used?

The literature supports that TENS might prove beneficial in diminishing acute, subacute, or chronic pain regardless of its source. Combining TENS with active motions is recommended. Equally important, due to its short-lasting effect, good practice implies applying it several times each day (including at home) as long as it is effective. Being aware that not everyone in pain can benefit from TENS, initial screening by a clinician is needed.

22. What evidence supports using ES to accelerate the healing of open wounds and ulcers?

Numerous clinical reports, including randomized, placebo-controlled trials, pre-post comparison trials, and many case reports, support using ES to manage slowly healing pressure ulcers and diabetic neuropathic ulcers. In a recent review, ES was associated with faster wound area reduction and/or a higher proportion of wounds that healed. In most studies, a monophasic waveform was used. Sterile and biocompatible positive (anode) or negative (cathode) electrodes were placed directly onto the wound. Daeschlein et al.,[25] found that the highest reduction factor (RF) for different organisms was done with positive polarity. The maximum RF was measured for *Escherichia coli* and the lowest for *Staphylococcus epidermidis*. There was no significant difference between Gram-positive and Gram-negative organisms. Therefore, infected wounds should be treated with ES to eliminate infection and accelerate healing.

Stimulators using a monophasic waveform, very short (5 to 100 microsecond) pulse durations, and a pulse rate of 100 to 120 per second are typically used. The mechanism of healing may be based on an electrically mediated increase in microcirculation via activation of vasoactive peptides (e.g., calcitonin gene-related peptide or vasoactive intestinal polypeptide). A possible concurrent mechanism is that electrically induced protein synthesis may produce collagen fiber regeneration.

REFERENCES

1. Viswanath O, Urits I, Bouley E, et al. Evolving spinal cord stimulation technologies and clinical implications in chronic pain management. *Curr Pain Headache Rep*. 2019;23(6):39. doi: 10.1007/s11916-019-0778-9.
2. Ilfeld BM, Finneran 4th JJ, Gabriel RA, et al. Ultrasound-guided percutaneous peripheral nerve stimulation: neuromodulation of the suprascapular nerve and brachial plexus for postoperative analgesia following ambulatory rotator cuff repair. A proof-of-concept study. *Reg Anesth Pain Med*. 2019;44(3):310–318. doi: 10.1136/rapm-2018-100121.
3. Wilson RD, Harris MA, Gunzler DD, et al. Percutaneous peripheral nerve stimulation for chronic pain in subacromial impingement syndrome: a case series. *Neuromodulation*. 2014;17(8):771–776. doi: 10.1111/ner.12152.
4. Lauritsen CG, Silberstein SD. Rationale for electrical parameter determination in external trigeminal nerve stimulation (eTNS) for migraine: a narrative review. *Cephalalgia*. 2019;39(6):750–760. doi: 10.1177/0333102418796781.
5. Sours C, Alon G, Roys S, et al. Modulation of resting state functional connectivity of the motor network by transcranial pulsed current stimulation. *Brain Connect*. 2014;4(3):157–165. doi: 10.1089/brain.2013.0196.
6. Alon G, Roys SR, Gullapalli RP, et al. Non-invasive electrical stimulation of the brain (ESB) modifies the resting-state network connectivity of the primary motor cortex: a proof of concept fMRI study. *Brain Res*. 2011;1403:37–44. doi: 10.1016/j.brainres.2011.06.013.
7. Zis P, Shafique F, Hadjivassiliou M, et al. Safety, tolerability, and nocebo phenomena during transcranial magnetic stimulation: a systematic review and meta-analysis of placebo-controlled clinical trials. *Neuromodulation*. 2019;23(3):291–300. doi: 10.1111/ner.12946.
8. Alon G. Functional electrical stimulation (FES): transforming clinical trials to neuro-rehabilitation clinical practice-a forward perspective. *J Novel Physiotherapies*. 2013;3:176–185.
9. Albertin G, Kern H, Hofer C, et al. Two years of functional electrical stimulation by large surface electrodes for denervated muscles improve skin epidermis in SCI. *Eur J Transl Myol*. 2018;28(1):7373. doi:10.4081/ejtm.2018.7373.
10. Kern H, Hofer C, Loefler S, et al. Atrophy, ultra-structural disorders, severe atrophy and degeneration of denervated human muscle in SCI and Aging. Implications for their recovery by Functional Electrical Stimulation, updated 2017. *Neurol Res*. 2017;39(7):660–666. doi: 10.1080/01616412.2017.1314906.
11. Dirks ML, Hansen D, Van Assche A, et al. Neuromuscular electrical stimulation prevents muscle wasting in critically ill comatose patients. *Clin Sci* (Lond). 2015;128(6):357–365. doi: 10.1042/CS20140447.
12. Huang S-C, Wong AM-K, Chuang Y-F, et al. Effects of neuromuscular electrical stimulation on arterial hemodynamic properties and body composition in paretic upper extremities of patients with subacute stroke. *Biomed J*. 2014;37(4):205–210. doi:10.4103/2319-4170.117892.
13. Li G, Li S, Sun L, et al. A comparison study of immune-inflammatory response in electroacupuncture and transcutaneous electrical nerve stimulation for patients undergoing supratentorial craniotomy. *Int J Clin Exp Med*. 2015;8(1):1156–1161.
14. Yue C, Zhang X, Zhu Y, et al. Systematic review of three electrical stimulation techniques for rehabilitation after total knee arthroplasty. *J Arthroplasty*. 2018;33(7):2330–2337. doi: 10.1016/j.arth.2018.01.070.
15. Ploesteanu RL, Nechita AC, Turcu D, et al. Effects of neuromuscular electrical stimulation in patients with heart failure—Review. *J Med Life*. 2018;11(2):107–118.

16. Frost J, Robinson HF, Hibberd J. A comparison of neuromuscular electrical stimulation and traditional therapy, versus traditional therapy in patients with longstanding dysphagia. *Curr Opin Otolaryngol Head Neck Surg*. 2018;26(3):167–173. doi: 10.1097/MOO. 0000000000000454.
17. Bickel CS, Yarar-Fisher C, Mahoney ET, et al. Neuromuscular electrical stimulation-induced resistance training after SCI: a review of the Dudley protocol. *Top Spinal Cord Inj Rehabil*. 2015;21(4):294–302. doi: 10.1310/sci2104-294.
18. Kimberley TJ, Lewis SM, Auerbach EJ, et al. Electrical stimulation driving functional improvements and cortical changes in subjects with stroke. *Exp Brain Res*. 2004;154(4):450–460. doi: 10.1007/s00221-003-1695-y.
19. Aaron SE, Vanderwerker CJ, Embry AE, et al. FES-assisted cycling improves aerobic capacity and locomotor function postcerebro-vascular accident. *Med Sci Sports Exerc*. 2018;50(3):400–406. doi: 10.1249/MSS.0000000000001457.
20. Bjordal JM, Johnson MI, Ljunggreen AE. Transcutaneous electrical nerve stimulation (TENS) can reduce postoperative analgesic consumption. A meta-analysis with assessment of optimal treatment parameters for postoperative pain. *Eur J Pain*. 2003;7(2): 181–188. doi: 10.1016/S1090-3801(02)00098-8.
21. Gladwell PW, Cramp F, Palmer S. Matching the perceived benefits of transcutaneous electrical nerve stimulation (TENS) for chronic musculoskeletal pain against patient reported outcome measures using the International Classification of Functioning, Disability and Health (ICF). *Physiotherapy*. 2020;106:128–135. doi: 10.1016/j.physio.2019.01.017.
22. Jamison RN, Wan L, Edwards RR, et al. Outcome of a high-frequency transcutaneous electrical nerve stimulator (hfTENS) device for low back pain: a randomized controlled trial. *Pain Pract*. 2019;19(5):466–475. doi: 10.1111/papr.12764.
23. Binny J, Wong NL, Garga S, et al. Transcutaneous electric nerve stimulation (TENS) for acute low back pain: Systematic review. *Scand J Pain*. 2019;19(2):225–233. doi:10.1515/sjpain-2018-0124.
24. Grover CA, McKernan MP, & Close RJH. Transcutaneous electrical nerve stimulation (TENS) in the emergency department for pain relief: a preliminary study of feasibility and efficacy. *West J Emerg Med*. 2018;19(5):872–876. doi: 10.5811/westjem.2018.7.38447.
25. Daeschlein G, Assadian O, Kloth LC, et al. Antibacterial activity of positive and negative polarity low-voltage pulsed current (LVPC) on six typical Gram-positive and Gram-negative bacterial pathogens of chronic wounds. *Wound Repair Regen*. 2007;15(3):399–403. doi: 10.1111/j.1524-475X.2007.00242.x.

NUTRITION AND DIET IN REHABILITATION: OPTIMIZING OUTCOMES

Mark A. Young, MD, MBA, FACP, FAAPMR, DABPMR, Marlene Young, MS, CNS, LD, Jennifer Shapiro, RDN, LD, Michael J. Young, MD, MPhil, Bryan J. O'Young, MD, CAc, FAAPMR, and Steven A. Stiens, MD, MS

Let food be thy medicine.

— Hippocrates

KEY POINTS

1. Nutritional screening includes a comprehensive review of medical history, labs, diet history, functional feeding ability, and nutrition-focused physical exams.
2. Important nutrients that are key to neurological health include B vitamins, omega-3 fatty acids, vitamin D, and zinc. The most optimal way to incorporate these nutrients into the diet is through the consumption of whole foods rich in these nutrients, but supplementation should be considered if specific nutrient deficiencies are identified.
3. Consumption of anti-inflammatory, antioxidant-rich foods may reduce chronic pain and inflammation. Anti-inflammatory foods include salmon, leafy green vegetables, avocado, pineapple, berries, nuts, olive oil, ginger, and turmeric.
4. Calorie and protein requirements depend on multiple factors including body weight, nutritional status, metabolic state, and activity levels. Energy requirements can be assessed by measuring height and weight along with calculating a patient's basal metabolic rate.
5. Malnutrition must be identified and treated as early as possible to prevent conditions from worsening. Interventions include increasing calorie and nutrient intake, individualized supplementation, treating underlying medical conditions, and addressing environmental factors that may impact a patient's nutrition intake. Enteral or parenteral nutrition may be indicated for patients who cannot eat or drink orally.

1. **What role does nutrition play in Physical Medicine & Rehabilitation?**
   Optimizing nutritional status is critically important in all aspects of rehabilitation. People with disabilities, including those with pain, neurologic, musculoskeletal, and orthopedic diagnoses, are positively impacted by dietary optimization. Physical Medicine & Rehabilitation (PM&R) recommendations include strengthening, stretching, and aerobic enhancement demand for proper nutrition to maximize outcome. Physiatric application of holistic dietary principles is key and impacts all biopsychosocial levels, thereby reducing impairment and improving outcomes.

   As specific nutritional substrates are essential for cellular, tissue, and organ-based function, proper nutrition is intrinsically linked to functional outcomes in all aspects of rehabilitation. The publication of recent "Food for Thought" guidelines and policy statements by leading rehabilitation organizations have created further awareness. Fundamental knowledge of nutritional principles is critical for all rehabilitation providers.

Philippou E, Polak R, Michunovich A, et al. Food for thought: basic nutrition recommendations for the mature brain. *Arch Phys Med Rehabil.* 2019;100(8):1581–1583. doi: 10.1016/j.apmr.2019.01.006.

2. **Describe functional foods (FF).**
   As defined by the Nutritional Academy of Sciences Food and Nutrition Board, FF are, "any modified food or food ingredient that may provide a health benefit beyond the traditional nutrients it contains." The definition from the Academy of Nutrition & Dietetics builds on this, stating that FF are "'whole fortified, enriched or enhanced' [foods] that should be consumed regularly and at effective amounts in order to derive health benefits." Examples of such foods are enriched flour, vitamin D fortified milk, and iodized salt.

Leveille, GA. Trailblazer lecture: a journey through the past and a perspective on the future of nutrition, food science, and health. *J Acad Nutr Diet.* 2016;116(6):1031–1034. doi:10.1016/j.jand.2016.02.004.

3. **Can food rebuild the brain and improve cognition?**
   The development of "gut hormones" created in the brain (or capable of entering the brain), which can affect cognitive functioning, is often called the "brain-gut axis." There are several known "brain foods" that contribute to brain

function as a whole, including omega-3 fatty acids and vitamin B12, among others. Ingesting these foods can signal metabolic modulators, exerting an influence on synaptic plasticity (e.g., brain-derived neurotrophic factor). Through the addition of these key dietary elements, brain health can be supported, and rehabilitation improved.

Gómez-Pinilla F. Foods: the effects of nutrients on brain function. *Nat Rev Neurosci.* 2008;9(7):568–578. doi:10.1038/Nrn2421.

4. How is ideal body weight (IBW) calculated?

Body mass index (BMI) provides a useful estimate of body fat using height and weight. This eliminates frame size differences to assess body composition differences. The formula is:

$$\frac{weight(kg)}{height(m)}$$

While BMIs for men and women vary, it serves as a useful categorization.
- Underweight = <18.5
- Normal weight = 18.5–24.9
- Overweight = 25–29.9
- Obesity = >30

As BMI increases above 20 kg/m, the risk of morbidity from conditions such as heart disease, stroke, type 2 diabetes, hypertension, cancer, and osteoarthritis increases incrementally. This risk increases dramatically with a BMI over 25 (National Health and Nutrition Examination Survey 3).

The **IBW**—the "normal" weight for a particular age, sex, and body frame—is estimated from comparison tables, most commonly the Metropolitan Life Insurance Tables.

Available at: www.nhlbisupport.com/bmi/bmicalc.htm

5. What process does the physiatrist follow to perform a simple bedside nutritional screen?

1. Medical Record Review
   - History of any systemic diseases (intestinal disease), dietary constraints, or nutritional deficiency
   - Documented weights, heights, and waist measurements from past clinical visits.
2. Complete Nutritional History
   - Alterations in food consumption, body weight, gastrointestinal (GI) symptoms, general mental health, food access, swallowing, and absorption capability (digestion).
3. Careful Clinical Evaluation
   - Anthropometric measurements: height, weight, and waist measurements
   - Physical examination: skin evaluation, muscle strength, and neurologic exam
   - Functional assessment: mobility, self-feeding, chewing, and swallowing.

6. How common is malnutrition?

Malnourishment is common in rehabilitation patients. In the United States, the incidence of malnutrition is between 30% and 50% of hospitalized medical patients and can worsen before rehabilitation starts. The chronic illnesses requiring prolonged hospitalizations that are characteristic of many rehabilitation patients make malnutrition an unfortunate consequence for many. Fortunately, optimal nutritional support in times of critical illness can reduce body protein loss by as much as half.

Tobert, CM, Mott SL, Nepple KG. Malnutrition diagnosis during adult inpatient hospitalizations: analysis of a multi-institutional collaborative database of academic medical centers. *J Acad Nutr Diet.* 2018:118(1). doi.org/10.1016/j.jand.2016.12.019.

7. How many ways can a patient be malnourished?

Malnutrition is a medical condition resulting from an imbalanced diet containing too *little*, too *much*, and/or insufficient food. While malnutrition is frequently diagnosed on the basis of unintentional weight loss or a low BMI, it is becoming imperative to determine the pathophysiological mechanisms. With this approach, malnutrition can be characterized as various, treatable disordered nutritional states. Combinations of improper nutrient balances, inflammation, and other metabolic aberrations lead to changes in body composition, function, and outcome.

Some of the most common forms of malnutrition include:
- **Micronutrient malnutrition**: the inadequate availability of essential nutrients such as vitamins (organic compounds broken down by the body) and trace minerals (inorganic elements that keep their structure) required by the body in small quantities (e.g., vitamin A, iron, iodine) for critical enzyme function and as cofactors in cellular reactions. This is often seen clinically as stunted growth, decreased cognitive ability, and reduced intelligence.

- **Protein-energy malnutrition (PEM)** is the inadequate availability or absorption of proteins and energy substrates in the body, preventing peak and endurance performance.

Soeters P, Bozetti F, et al., Defining malnutrition: a plea to rethink. *Clin Nut.* 2017;36(3):896–901. doi: 10.1016/j.clnu.2016.09.032.

8. What are common risk factors for malnutrition in geriatric patients?
   Geriatric patients most at-risk for malnutrition include those with one or more of the following: insufficient diet, underlying disease, sudden weight change, financial challenges, multiple medications, and dental problems.

9. What common serum markers are diminished in malnourished patients, and are there acute measures for them?
   - Pre-albumin levels: frequently used to assess recent nutritional metabolism, as they are closely associated with fluctuations in protein-energy status. Due to the short half-life of approximately 2 days, pre-albumin levels reflect only a brief period but are valuable to evaluate the success of intensive interventions.
   - Total lymphocyte count
   - Blood urea nitrogen
   - Creatinine
   - Total protein
   - Albumin
   - Triglycerides
   - Cholesterol

10. What aspects of nutritional support should rehabilitation professionals know?
    For patients who cannot ingest nutrients (water, calories, protein, vitamins, minerals) orally, nutritional support serves as an alternate conduit. The most common ways to bypass oral ingestion are through the **parenteral route** (intravenous feeding) or the enteral route (**nasogastric tube**, endoscopically or surgically placed **gastrostomy** or **jejunostomy**).

11. When might total parenteral nutrition (TPN) be needed in rehabilitation patients?
    - Pre- and post-surgery with an expected prolonged course before return to normal bowel function
    - Difficulty eating
    - Malnourished preoperative patients
    - Hypermetabolic conditions involving decreased ability to intake nutrients (i.e., polytrauma, infection)
    - Adjunctive therapy in patients with GI disease or dysfunction (e.g., inflammatory bowel disease)
    - Improperly functioning GI tract
    - Protracted nutrient losses with severe malnutrition

12. Why is it important to treat B12 deficiencies?
    Deficiencies in B12 have become increasingly prevalent and clinically significant, particularly in the spinal cord injury population and the elderly (incidence runs up to 14.5%). Results of these deficiencies include poor memory, decreased cognitive skills, peripheral neuropathy, slow wound healing (B12 is a protein synthesis cofactor), and pernicious anemia. High homocysteine levels can also be an effect, which contributes to coronary artery disease. Common treatment involves monthly intramuscular injections, although oral therapy can be used in lieu of injections, with effective dosing of 1000 μg/day.

Petchkrua W, Burns S, Stiens S, et al: Prevalence of vitamin B12 deficiency in patients with spinal cord injury or disease. *Arch Phys Med Rehabil.* 2003; 84:1675–1679.

13. Can an anti-inflammatory diet be prescribed?
    Chronic pain syndrome is often associated with suboptimal appetite and poor nutrition, underscoring the need for proper hydration and nutrition to aid rehabilitation. Evidence-based practice includes targeted food selection to reduce pain and support recovery. For example, turmeric (the most potent anti-inflammatory spice), and an extract from the pineapple plant, bromelain, can potentially serve as an effective alternative treatment for pain syndromes due to their analgesic and anti-inflammatory properties.

Mandolfo C, Baumgart C, Weiss E, et al. Consuming an anti-inflammatory diet to alleviate chronic pain. *J Acad Nutr Diet.* 2018;118(9):A21.

14. How can rehabilitation synergize with the nutritional counseling process?
    Optimal nutrition via patient choices is but one of many patient-dependent rehabilitative processes. The rehabilitation clinician not only identifies the diagnoses but also recognizes patient strengths and resources that will

make treatment successful. The team leader establishes interdisciplinary collaboration with the dietician to design a strategy that capitalizes on patient personality, style, and strengths. Research supports combinations of exogenous behavioral and endogenous cognitive approaches in a transtheoretical model carried out in stages (pre-contemplation, contemplation, preparation, action, and maintenance). Specific measures (e.g., consumption, weight, and exercise) are recorded and intermediate goals are negotiated. Effective designs include active problem solving, stimulus control, and patient self-monitoring. Over time, the clinician must self-educate, practice, and develop a successful repertoire of interaction styles in response to varied patient needs.

Spahn JM, Reeves RS, Keim KS, et al. State of the evidence regarding behavior change theories and strategies in nutrition counseling to facilitate health and food behavior change. *J Am Diet Assoc*. 2010;110(6):879–891. doi:10.1016/j.jada.2010. 03.021.

15. How can the energy requirements of a rehabilitation patient be assessed by determining the basal metabolic rate (BMR)?
Simple estimation: 30 kcal/kg—25%
Harris-Benedict equation:
Female kcal: 655 + (9.6 × weight [kg]) + (1.8 × height [cm]) − (4.7 × age)
Male kcal: 66 + (13.7 × weight [kg]) + (5 × height [cm]) − (6.8 × age)

16. How is body fat distributed differently in men and women? Does this have clinical implications for drug bioavailability?
While women tend to have a higher percentage of body fat than men across all age groups, men tend to have a greater distribution of excess body fat. Men tend to store body fat in their abdomen, and women store it in their thighs and buttocks, which has significant implications for drug metabolism and bioavailability. This may explain why men and women show different responses to certain medications (e.g., analgesics and other pain medications). A simple way to remember the difference in body shape is apples (men) and pears (women) (Fig. 22.1).

17. Can good nutrition play a role in musculoskeletal ailments and pain management?
Poor nutrition and suboptimal appetite are common concomitants of chronic pain syndrome and also medications used. Bolstering nutrition and proper hydration can significantly improve outcomes for pain patients. Scientific evidence supports the role of targeted food selection in pain reduction and rehabilitation. The following foods

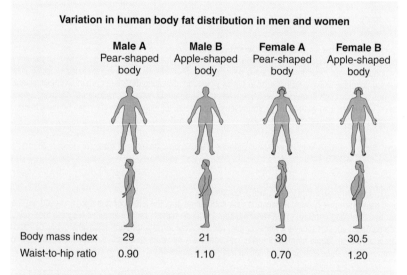

Variation in human body fat distribution in men and women

	Male A Pear-shaped body	Male B Apple-shaped body	Female A Pear-shaped body	Female B Apple-shaped body
Body mass index	29	21	30	30.5
Waist-to-hip ratio	0.90	1.10	0.70	1.20

In each pair of men and pair of women (subjects A and B), the body mass indices are similar. However, the waist circumference and waist-to-hip ratios of subjects B are much higher, indicating a greater distribution of body fat around the abdomen as well as a decreased amount of muscle mass around the hips.

Fig. 22.1 Body shape in men and women. (*Source*: Han TS, Lean MEJ. Metabolic syndrome. *Medicine*. 2015;43(2):80–87. Available at: doi: 10.1016/j.mpmed.2014.11.006.)

have been identified as having anti-inflammatory and analgesic properties, possibly providing nutritionally astute treatment alternatives for pain syndromes.

18. **Discuss the hazards of thiamine (B1) deficiency?**
    B1 deficiency is a common and pernicious deficiency syndrome seen in alcoholics, geriatrics, and in those on chronic diuretics. Frequently it is mistaken for dementia/delirium. Thiamine deficiency can be associated with length-dependent peripheral neuropathy, ophthalmoplegia, ataxia and confabulation (Wernickes), and psychosis (Korsakoff).

19. **Provide examples of other common nutrient-associated neurologic sequela?**
    1. Pyridoxine (B6) excess: sensory neuropathy
    2. Zinc excess: copper deficiency myelopathy
    3. Vitamin D deficiency: cognitive decline

20. **Elaborate on vitamin D's neuroprotective role?**
    Vitamin D targets factors that lead to neurodegeneration, including antioxidant, immunoregulatory, anti-ischemic factors, neurotrophic factors, and acetylcholine neurotransmitters. Also, Vitamin D helps prevent hyperparathyroidism and clear amyloid-β peptide.

What role does vitamin d play in neurologic diseases? *Neurol Rev.* 2012;20 (8):9.

21. **Is celiac disease associated with neuropathology?**
    Celiac disease is an autoimmune intestinal mucosal inflammatory disease treated by limiting gluten consumption. Neuropathy and cerebellar ataxia have been noted in more severe cases.

RECOMMENDED READINGS

Finestone HM, Greene-Finestone LS. Rehabilitation medicine. 2. Diagnosis of dysphagia and its nutritional management for stroke patients. *CMAJ.* 169(10):2003;1041–1044.
Young, MA, Barr K. *Women and Pain: Why It Hurts and What You Can Do.* New York, NY: Hyperion-AOL Time Warner; 2002:18–25.
National Institute on Aging (n.d.).. Healthy Eating. Available at: https://www.nia.nih.gov/healthy-eating
Alzheimer's Association. Food and Eating (italicize page name). 2022. Available at: https://www.alz.org/help-support/caregiving/daily-care/food-eating
Academy of Nutrition and Dietetics. *Eat Right.* 2022. Available at: www.eatright.org/cps/rde/xchg/ada/hs.xsl/index.html
US Department of Agriculture. Available at: www.nutrition.gov/
American Society for Nutrition Available at: www.nutrition.org/
Global Council on Brain Health. Available at: www.aarp.org/health/brain-health/global-council-on-brain-health/

CHAPTER 23

MEDICATION THERAPY MANAGEMENT TO ACHIEVE ENABLEMENT: RECOGNIZING INDICATIONS AND TARGETING OUTCOMES

Edward W. Heinle III, MD, MA, Karen Y. Lew, PharmD, and Steven A. Stiens, MD, MS

It is easy to get a thousand prescriptions, but hard to get one single remedy.

— Chinese proverb

KEY POINTS

1. The ever-increasing number of clinical indications for which pharmacological agents are available require that the physiatrist be attentive to the patient's needs, critical in evaluating the response to newly prescribed agents, and alert to adverse effects and drug interactions.
2. Reviewing a well-designed problem list will prompt a realization of the opportunities for medication use but must also create an appreciation of the risks for adverse effects and potential drug interactions.
3. Including an interdisciplinary team collaboration with a pharmacist trained in physical rehabilitation methods allows for implementing medications directed toward multiple mechanisms, monitoring, and establishing trans-disciplinary independent patient medication management.
4. Establish procedures for monitoring success and complications with sensitive and consistent measures to document improvements or adverse effects.
5. Stepwise decrease dosing or deprescribe medications as dictated by indications, complications, lack of desired effect, or intolerability.
6. Reinforce compliance by utilizing primary nursing practice, patient-centered education, and medication-dispensing technologies.

MEDICATION SAFETY

Optimization is achieved through recognizing indications, drug interactions, adverse effects, and resultant positive outcomes with treatment.

Compliance is improved by patient medication education and simplified medication therapy.

Polypharmacy is reduced by discontinuing, or ***deprescribing***, medications no longer indicated or effective.

1. How should rehabilitation clinicians think about medications as parts of a complex individual interdisciplinary plan?

   Each patient's rehabilitation program has a unique patient-centered design with implementation systems that bring "years to life and life to years." Medications are ingredients for longevity, wellness, comfort, and enablement. Comprehensive pharmacology references are available for use from the physiatric perspective. This chapter is designed to guide the utilization and monitoring of medications that can be successful catalysts of physical medicine and rehabilitation collaborative care.

2. How does pharmacologic management fit into the processes of rehabilitation and continued primary care?

   Patient and family participation in interdisciplinary rehabilitation allows everyone maximum ability to meet individual life goals. Ever-expanding options in medications let the clinician target drug therapy for disease prevention, interrupt pathophysiology, control symptoms, minimize organ dysfunction, enhance functional activity, and promote full social participation. Pharmacologic treatment is applied at the molecular level via the biopsychosocial model, but outcomes are realized on multiple system levels requiring comprehensive goal-directed investigation and anticipation for therapeutic opportunities and monitoring for compliance, complications, and outcomes. Drug therapy should therefore be carefully targeted in concert with other treatment modalities and evaluated by a systematic review of the problem list.

3. Describe the pharmacist's role in rehabilitation medicine.

Pharmacists, as part of the interdisciplinary health care team, optimize pharmacotherapy by performing **medication review** and **reconciliation**. This ensures appropriate indication, fosters appropriate medication de-escalation and deprescribing, minimizes adverse effects and drug-drug interactions, and simplifies medication therapy. In addition, the pharmacist is consulted on drug **serum level monitoring**, such as for vancomycin and warfarin therapy for positive outcomes. Pharmacists also provide education (e.g., how to take and what to expect, oral inhaler technique and care, and **medication management** in a pill organizer), which improves patient **medication compliance** and satisfaction with their health care experience.

Pharmacists' role on the rehabilitation interdisciplinary team was demonstrated in a 38-bed Spinal Cord Injury (SCI) unit. A systematic and comprehensive review of medication profiles and clinical conditions by SCI pharmacists, combined with a weekly conference (**SCI/Pharmacy Rounds**), identified clinically significant changes in patient medication management plans and provided education to SCI physicians and providers.

Lew KY, et al. American Paraplegia Society 53rd Annual Conference Poster Presentation: pharmacist recommendations achieve medication optimization in patients with chronic spinal cord injury. *J Spinal Cord Med.* 2007;30(4):399–412.

Michalets E, Creger J, Shillinglaw WR. Outcomes of expanded use of clinical pharmacist practitioners in addition to team-based care in a community health system intensive care unit. *Am J Health Syst Pharm.* 2015;72(1):47–53. doi:10.2146/ajhp140105

Sjölander M, Lindholm L, Pfister B, et al. Impact of clinical pharmacist engagement in ward teams on the number of drug-related readmissions among older patients with dementia or cognitive impairment: an economic evaluation. *Res Social Admn Pharm.* 2019;15(3):287–291. doi:10.1016/j.sapharm.2018.05.006.

Warrington L, Ayers P, Baldwin AM, et al. Implementation of a pharmacist-led, multidisciplinary diabetes management team. *Am J Health Syst Pharm.* 2012;69(14):1240–5. doi: 10.2146/ajhp110297

4. What principles guide drug therapy for patients with chronic, often permanent, disabilities?

Use medications only when necessary, **dose sparingly**, and **monitor for outcomes**. Provide accessible and **practical schedules** and methods of administration. Use the minimum potency and dosage that will achieve desired outcomes. Recognize that the **body is dynamic** and may not need all medications continually for success. **Reevaluate the necessity** of medications by reducing doses to eliminate those no longer required.

5. Which agents treat agitation in traumatic brain injury (TBI)?

Large-scale, controlled studies are sparse, but enough evidence exists to suggest that benzodiazepines and typical antipsychotics are not optimal first-line agents. As such, consider specific symptoms, desired behavioral outcomes, environmental modifications, and minimizing comorbidities. The only level 1a (randomized, controlled trial) evidence for an agent reducing agitation in acquired brain injury is **amantadine**, which is often used as a neurostimulant in this population, with hypomania as a side effect. Antiepileptics, including **lamotrigine**, **valproic acid,** and **carbamazepine** may be the first choice for patients also experiencing seizures. Agitation in patients with anxiety or depression after TBI often responds to **amitriptyline**, a tricyclic antidepressant, or **sertraline**, an SSRI, with fewer side effects. Beta blockers (**pindolol** and **propranolol**) studied in this population have level 1b evidence supporting their efficacy and may concomitantly treat hypertension and paroxysmal sympathetic hyperactivity.

Antipsychotics have been used to address aggressive behavior in many patient populations. These medications include typical (**droperidol** and **methotrimeprazine**) and atypical (**quetiapine** and **ziprasidone**) antipsychotics. They are effective, but with a strongly sedating side effect that may put this population at risk for falls, aspiration, and decreased participation in therapy. Adverse events with daily use include seizures and neuroleptic malignant syndrome. Short-term use is recommended apart from patients who have a separate indication for an antipsychotic.

Mehta S, McIntyre A, Janzen S, et al. Pharmacological management of agitation among individuals with moderate to severe acquired brain injury: a systematic review. *Brain Inj.* 2018;32(3):287–296. doi: 10.1080/02699052.2017.1419377.

6. What are the advantages and disadvantages of prescribing hypnotics (sleep aids)?

Commonly used agents to complement a program of sleep hygiene

- **Benzodiazepines,** such as **temazepam**, have anxiolytic effects that may benefit certain patients. These are generally safe but should be tapered off if used for more than 2 weeks. However, they may impede or delay next-day cognitive performance, depending on whether a longer-acting form is used or if use has been over an extended period.
- Gamma amino-butyric acid (GABA$_A$) receptor agonists **zolpidem**, **zaleplon**, and **eszopiclone** may disrupt normal sleep architecture (stages 3 and 4, "restorative" sleep) less than benzodiazepines. They are administered just before sleep because of their rapid onset and short duration. **Eszopiclone** may be used for longer-term treatment. Zolpidem has a black box warning, as it is associated with complex sleep behaviors including sleep-driving. Its use should be limited, and discontinued if the patient experiences complex sleep behaviors.

- *Triazolopyridines*, such as *trazodone*, have a positive effect on sleep architecture, but side effects include vivid dreams and enhanced appetite. Longer-term use is helpful for sleep maintenance. It should be administered at least 1 hour before bed.
- *Melatonin*, and analogs *ramelteon* and *tasimelteon*, are well tolerated for longer durations and do not impair next-day cognitive performance.
- *Tricyclic antidepressants* can be given for their sedative side effects (see antidepressant question for details).
- Orexin receptor antagonist, *suvorexant*, a newer agent, is taken right before sleep when the patient can stay in bed for at least 7 hours. Lower dosage for the elderly.
- *Doxepin*,a tricyclic antidepressant and H_1 antagonist, is indicated for sleep maintenance insomnia but may worsen depression.
- *Diphenhydramine* is available over the counter. Often used in "nighttime" formulations and frequently self-administered, it has significant anticholinergic side effects and is therefore not recommended for the elderly.

Nazareth K, Burkhardt K. Hypnotics and anxiolytics practice guide. Available at: http://www.wales.nhs.uk/sites3/Documents/582/Guide_Hypnotics%20%26%20Anxiolytics%20Practice%20Guide_version02.pdf

7. Are there special considerations when using antihypertensives in those with SCI?

First, discriminate essential hypertension from autonomic dysreflexia (AD) and other secondary forms of hypertension.
- For essential hypertension, the dihydropyridine class of calcium channel blockers, which includes *felodipine* and *amlodipine*, is a good choice because of the absence of negative inotropic effects but may cause reflexive tachycardia initially. Angiotensin converting enzyme (*ACE*) *inhibitors* in low doses have been successfully used and enhance renal function as well.
- *Diuretics* and *vasodilators* (*nitrates* and *hydralazine*) may increase orthostatic hypotension in a population that is already prone to this effect. *Clonidine* and *beta blockers may* suppress compensatory tachycardia.
- *Nonselective beta blockers* (*propranolol*, *nadolol*, *labetalol*) may increase bronchospasm. *Cardioselective beta blockers* (*atenolol*, *metoprolol*, *betaxolol*) generally cause less bronchospasm but lose their cardioselectivity at higher doses. Additionally, beta blockers decrease high-density lipoprotein (HDL) and exacerbate insulin resistance.

James PA, Oparil S, Carter BL, et al. 2014 evidence-based guideline for the management of high blood pressure in adults: report from the panel members appointed to the Eighth Joint National Committee (JNC 8). *JAMA*. 2014;311(5) 507–520. doi: 10.1001/jama.2013.284427. Available at: https://jamanetwork.com/journals/ jama/fullarticle/1791497

8. How is hypertension resulting from AD managed?

Acute hypertension in AD is caused by reflex triggered, and sympathetic mediated, constriction of the peripheral vasculature. This is treated first by eliminating the noxious stimuli that triggered the event. Bladder or bowel distension are common causes, but pressure wounds, ingrown toenails, and tight clothing may also be modifiable, instigating factors. If pharmacologic intervention is necessary, *transdermal nitrates* applied above the level of the SCI work quickly and can be wiped off once blood pressure control is achieved. *Hydralazine* or *clonidine* may also be used. Short-acting *nifedipine*, a calcium channel blocker, is less frequently used, as it has a risk for profound hypotension. *Prazosin*, an alpha-1 adrenergic receptor antagonist, is increasingly used long-term to moderate the severity of AD events. It has little effect on cardiac function or resting blood pressure.

Eldahan KC, Rabchevsky AG. Autonomic dysreflexia after spinal cord injury: systemic pathophysiology and methods of management. *Auton Neurosci*. 2018;209:59–70. doi: 10.1016/j.autneu.2017.05.002. Available at: https://www.ncbi.nlm.nih.gov/pmc/ articles/PMC5677594/

9. Which medications attenuate orthostatic hypotension after SCI?

One of the most effective "medications" for the treatment of orthostatic hypotension is *water*! Individuals with neurotrauma may lose the ability to peripherally constrict vasculature. Encouraging adequate fluids, with balanced electrolyte intake, abdominal binders, and lower extremity compression wraps, may adequately treat symptomatic hypotension. Should pharmacologic intervention be necessary, *midodrine*—a sympathomimetic with predominant alpha-receptor binding—dosed 30 minutes before the patient gets out of bed may be helpful. To avoid hypertension, it is recommended that patients wait 4 hours before lying again down after the last dose. *Fludrocortisone*, a mineralocorticosteroid, may be effective but increases fluid retention. *Salt tablets* are effective but also cause fluid retention and are not very palatable.

10. What medications are used to treat neuropathic pain?

All mechanisms of neuropathic pain have yet to be elucidated. Known mechanisms include the dysfunction of serotonergic and norepinephrine systems that modulate pain transmission in the spinal cord.

Pregabalin and *gabapentin* are analogues of the inhibitory neurotransmitter GABA that are effective in treating neuropathic pain and generally well tolerated. Side effects include peripheral edema and constipation. *Duloxetine* is effective and especially useful for patients who have depression. Side effects include constipation and dizziness. *Tricyclic antidepressants* are effective but be aware of anticholinergic side effects and orthostatic hypotension.

Attal N, Mazaltarine G, Perrouin-Verbe B, et al. Chronic neuropathic pain management in spinal cord injury patients. What is the efficacy of pharmacological treatments with a general mode of administration? (oral, transdermal, intravenous). *Ann Phys Med Rehab.* 2009;52(2): 124–41. doi:10.1016/ j.rehab.2008.12.011. Available at: https://www.hal.inserm.fr/inserm-00435410/ document

Mehta S, McIntyre A, Dijkers M, et al. Gabapentinoids are effective in decreasing neuropathic pain and other secondary outcomes after spinal cord injury: a meta-analysis. *Arch Phys Med Rehab.* 2014;95(11)2180–2186. doi: 10.1016/j.apmr.2014.06.010

Vranken JH, Hollmann MW, van der Vegt MH, et al. Duloxetine in patients with central neuropathic pain caused by spinal cord injury or stroke: a randomized, double-blind, placebo-controlled trial. *Pain.* 2011;152(2) 267–73. doi: 10.1016/j.pain.2010.09.005

11. **What medications are used in patients with ventilation weakness, the risk for mucus plugging, and oxygen desaturation?**
Weakness in inspiratory and expiratory muscles impairs ventilation and cough after SCI. Increased parasympathetic activity, not balanced by sympathetic activity, promotes bronchospasm and increases secretion production. Patients with tetraplegia frequently show airway hyperresponsiveness to methacholine during pulmonary function testing, even without a history of reactive airway disease. *Inhaled beta agonists* such as *albuterol* prevent such bronchospasms. *Theophylline* can also reduce bronchospasm and prevent symptomatic bradycardia after acute SCI. Adverse effects of increased secretions are exacerbated if secretions are made more tenacious by anticholinergic agents. Mucolytic agents such as *guaifenesin* and *acetylcysteine* facilitate secretion clearance when combined with adequate hydration and appropriate assisted cough techniques (mechanical insufflator/exsufflator, mechanical vests, cough assist/quad cough). Albuterol is given before acetylcysteine to reduce the risk of bronchospasm during administration by inhalation with a nebulizer. Purulent secretions may respond to inhaled *recombinant human DNase*, which breaks down DNA released by lysed leukocytes.

Britton D, Karam C, Schindler JS. Swallowing and secretion management in neuromuscular disease. *Clin Chest Med.* 2018;39(2):449–457. doi: 10.1016/j.ccm.2018.01.007

12. **What agents are given to attenuate diarrhea from *Clostridium difficile* colitis?**
Colestipol and *cholestyramine* are nonabsorbable, anion-exchange resins that bind *C. difficile* toxin. They may reduce symptoms but do not eliminate an infection. They can be safely prescribed while awaiting the results of a stool toxin test and culture or antibiotic therapy. However, they bind to medications in addition to the *C. difficile* toxin. Therefore, other medications should be dosed 1 hour before or 4 hours after colestipol or cholestyramine.

Probiotics are micro-organisms with beneficial properties to the host. *Lactobacillus* is found in cultured milk products (some yogurts) and creates an environment unfavorable to some bacteria through their production of lactic acid and help reestablish normal bowel flora. *Saccharomyces boulardii* is a nonpathogenic yeast used to prevent antibiotic-associated diarrhea by reconstituting normal colonic flora, but it is not regulated by the Food and Drug Administration (FDA).

The risk for *C. difficile* colitis can be reduced by using H_2 blockers and proton pump inhibitors (PPIs) sparingly and using targeted antibiotic therapy in the least potent dose and minimum duration needed to treat infections.

Czepiel J, Dróżdż M, Pituch H, et al. Clostridium difficile infection: review. *Eur J Clin Microbiol Infect Dis.* 2019; 38:1211–1221. doi:10.1007/s10096-019-03539-6. Available at: https://www.ncbi.nlm.nih.gov/ pmc/articles/PMC6570665

13. **What are the guidelines for prophylaxis against urinary tract infections (UTIs)?**
Residual urine in a neurogenic bladder is a culture medium for bacteria. Those who have neurogenic bladders either perform intermittent catheterization (IC) or have an indwelling catheter. The neurogenic bladder can be colonized with bacteria but does not necessarily indicate a urinary tract infection (UTI). Chronic, low-dose antibiotic chemoprophylaxis is not recommended due to the risk of antibiotic-resistant bacteria.
Methods of prophylaxis:
- Keep well hydrated to avoid concentrated urine
- Avoid allowing the bladder to fill beyond a volume of 400 mL. This should be accomplished by fluid management including timed voiding, intermittent catheterization, and indwelling catheter.
- Daily irrigation of the bladder with normal saline or *renacidin*.
- *Organic proanthocyanidins* (OPCs) in cranberries and blueberries reduce the adhesion of bacteria to the bladder epithelium. However, evidence from clinical trials suggests that cranberry, in juice or supplement form, does not appear to be independently effective in preventing or treating urinary tract infections in the SCI

population, but demonstrates success in healthy, nonpregnant adult women, but not in elderly, female nursing home residents.

Fu Z, Liska D, Talan D, et al. Cranberry reduces the risk of urinary tract infection recurrence in otherwise healthy women: a systematic review and meta-analysis. *J Nutr.* 2017; 147(12):2282–2288. doi:10.3945/jn.117.254961. Available at: https://academic.oup.com/jn/article/147/12/ 2282/4727969

Juthani-Mehta M, Van Ness PH, Bianco L, et al. Effect of cranberry capsules on bacteriuria plus pyuria among older women in nursing homes: a randomized clinical trial. *JAMA.* 2016;316(18):1879–1887. doi:10.1001/jama.2016.16141. Available at: https://www.ncbi.nlm.nih.gov /pmc/articles/PMC5300771/

Krantz J, Schmidt S, Schneidewind L. Current evidence on nonantibiotic prevention of recurrent UTI. *Eur Urol Focus.* 2019;5(1):17–19. doi: 10.1016/j.euf.2018.09.006.

Opperman EA, Cranberry is not effective for the prevention of treatment of urinary tract infections in individuals with spinal cord injury. *Spinal Cord.* 2010;48(6):451–456. doi: 10.1038/sc.2009.159. Available at: https://www.nature.com/articles/sc2009159

14. Why do individuals with SCI or TBI seem to produce more urine at night compared to during the day?
    Although the precise mechanism is unknown, there can often be a loss of the nocturnal component of the diurnal surge of *antidiuretic hormone* (ADH) after neurotrauma. Additionally, after a person has been upright during the day, there is remobilization of fluid in the evening, leading to the production of greater volumes of urine at night. With the use of *desmopressin* as a nasal spray before bedtime, more than 90% of individuals with loss of nocturnal ADH surge are successfully treated. Within only several days, the treatment can cause greater production of urine during the day instead of at night. This is especially beneficial to those performing IC for neurogenic bladder management.

15. How do celecoxib and nonselective NSAIDs used for musculoskeletal pain and fever work, and what are the precautions?
    Nonselective NSAIDs (nsNSAIDs) inhibit prostaglandin synthesis by inhibiting cyclo-oxygenase 1 and 2 (COX-1 and COX-2) isoenzymes and therefore decrease pain, inflammation, and fever. Gastrointestinal effects such as dyspepsia, peptic ulcers, and bleeding are due to the inhibition of gastroprotective prostaglandins. Short-term and chronic use of NSAIDs have been associated with increased risk of cardiovascular events, including myocardial infarction, stroke, and exacerbation of heart failure. Patients who have cardiovascular disease (e.g., a prior cardiovascular event or obstructive coronary artery disease on angiography) should not receive an NSAID, selective or nonselective. Renal effects include acute renal failure, especially in preexisting renal dysfunction due to vasoconstriction.
    Celecoxib is the only selective NSAID currently available as a COX-2 inhibitor in the U.S. However, diclofenac, etodolac, meloxicam, and sulindac all have more COX-2 than COX-1 selectivity. COX-2 is an inducible isoform of the enzyme present at inflammatory sites. Selective inhibition of inflammatory prostaglandins provides anti-inflammatory effects with less interference to the prostaglandins that protect the stomach, resulting in less stomach ulceration than nonselective agents. Analgesic and anti-inflammatory effects are similar between selective and nonselective agents.

Solomon SD, Wittes J, Finn PV, et al. Cardiovascular risk of celecoxib in 6 randomized placebo-controlled trials: the cross trial safety analysis. *Circulation.* 2008;117(16):2104–2113. doi: 10.1161/CIRCULATIONAHA.108.764530. Available at: https://www.ahajournals.org/doi/ epub/10.1161/CIRCULATIONAHA.108.764530

Walker C, Biasucci LM. Cardiovascular safety of non-steroidal anti-inflammatory drugs revisited. *Postgrad Med.* 2018;130(1):55–71. doi: 10.1080/00325481.2018.1412799

16. What are some important metabolic considerations in patients prone to wasting syndrome, or recurrent/poorly healing pressure ulcers?
    - *Nutrition*. Adequate protein intake is imperative for high-density collagen matrix protein synthesis required for wound healing and to fight infection. As the presence of an open wound causes a catabolic state, most sources recommend 1.5 to 2 mg/kg/day of protein.
    - *Appetite megestrol acetate* is FDA approved for appetite stimulation. It is a progesterone and glucocorticoid analog and can therefore cause lean tissue catabolism, hyperglycemia, and adipose weight gain. It can also deplete testosterone levels, thus resulting in decreased endogenous anabolic stimulus for protein synthesis, poor skin turgor, and further risk of skin breakdown, osteoporosis, muscle wasting, and depression.
    - *Anabolism*. *Anabolic hormone analog* agent *oxandrolone* is FDA approved as an adjunct medication to reverse weight loss from a variety of etiologies and has increased lean body mass from enhanced protein synthesis. It also stimulates fibroblasts to produce the collagen that heals wounds. Low albumin is a marker for

malnutrition, and low levels correlate with the presence, severity, and lack of substrate for the healing of pressure ulcers. Oxandrolone is a testosterone analog with anabolic but few androgenic properties. Oxandrolone's anabolic-to-androgenic ratio is 16:1. It should not be given to those with an elevated prostate-specific antigen (PSA). It also will potentiate warfarin.

- **Testosterone.** Low levels can result from a multitude of etiologies such as SCI, advanced age, malnutrition, opioid use, or catabolic stress from pressure ulcers or trauma. PSA must be checked before prescribing testosterone.

Sadeghi M, Keshavarz-Fathi M, Baracos V, et al. Cancer cachexia: diagnosis, assessment, and treatment. *Crit Rev Oncol Hematol.* 2018;127:91–104. doi: 10.1016/j.critrevonc.2018.05.006.

von Haehling, S, Anker SD, Treatment of cachexia: an overview of recent developments. *J Am Med Dir Assoc.* 2014;15(12):866–872. doi: 10.1016/j.jamda.2014.09.007. Available at: https://www.jamda.com/article/S1525-8610(14)00588-X/fulltext

17. What commonly used medications have anticholinergic effects?

- **Oxybutynin** and **tolterodine** are agents used to prevent bladder spasms and decrease urge incontinence. **Tolterodine** is more selective for receptors in the bladder and may cause less dry mouth, constipation, and orthostatic hypotension.
- **Benztropine** is used for extrapyramidal side effects associated with neuroleptic agents such as **quetiapine**, **risperidone**, and **olanzapine**.
- Tricyclic antidepressants such as **amitriptyline**, **imipramine**, **nortriptyline**, and **desipramine** are sometimes used for sleep, migraine headaches, and neuropathic pain. Amitriptyline and imipramine have significant anticholinergic side effects: dry mouth, blurred vision, constipation, urinary retention, as well as orthostatic hypotension. Nortriptyline and desipramine have moderate anticholinergic side effects.
- **Diphenhydramine** and **chlorpheniramine** are used for allergy symptoms and are associated with significant anticholinergic side effects. **Hydroxyzine** and **cyclobenzaprine** are given for anxiety and muscle spasms, respectively, and have moderate anticholinergic side effects.

18. Describe the differences between spasms and spasticity. What medications are available for symptoms?

A **spasm** is a sudden, involuntary contraction of one or more muscle groups, includes cramps, and contributes to contracture. Medications such as **cyclobenzaprine**, **carisoprodol**, and **methocarbamol** are spasmolytic agents intended for short-term use for muscle relaxation. These agents are not effective for spasticity.

Spasticity is increased muscle tone and exaggeration of muscle stretch reflexes. On examination, it is associated with velocity-dependent resistance to initial stretch and sudden relaxation (**"clasp knife" phenomenon**). Medications used for spasticity include the following:

- **Baclofen** is a short-acting $GABA_B$ site analog that is given up to four times a day and is usually the first choice for both spinal and brain-mediated spasticity. The recommended maximum dosing is 80 mg/day in divided doses. Doses above this may exacerbate sleep apnea and respiratory depression. Side effects include fatigue and clouded mental status, although these usually resolve with habituation. To avoid the risk of seizures, do not discontinue abruptly.
- **Diazepam** is a benzodiazepine effective for attenuating spasticity at the $GABA_A$ site.
- **Tizanidine** is an α2-agonist like **clonidine**. Side effects include hypotension, xerostomia, and sedation.
- **Gabapentin**, a GABA analog, is FDA approved as an adjunct for partial seizures but is also used for neuropathic pain and spasticity. Efficacy above 600 mg four times daily has not been shown for neuropathic pain. It has a saturable absorption process per dose and is excreted by the kidneys. Therefore, the dose needs to be adjusted for renal dysfunction.
- **Lamotrigine** is an antiepileptic that can be effective as an adjuvant for spasticity, but a rash is a major side effect that can lead to Stevens-Johnson syndrome. This is minimized by slowly titrating up the dose. If a dose is interrupted for 5 days, it must be retitrated from the beginning to avoid Stevens-Johnson syndrome.
- **Dantrolene** acts intramuscularly and works by decreasing the amount of calcium released from the sarcoplasmic reticulum. Common side effects are flushing and somnolence. Serious side effects include hyperthermia and hepatotoxicity. Baseline liver function needs to be monitored regularly.
- **Botulinum toxin A/B** irreversibly blocks neuromuscular junction transmission by inhibiting presynaptic acetylcholine release. Each injection is effective for approximately 3 to 6 months.
- **Alcohol/phenol nerve blocks** permanently denature protein in nerve fibers, thereby decreasing muscle contraction, although recovery can occur via terminal motor nerve branching.
- An **intrathecal baclofen pump** can be considered when a sustained comprehensive effort to control spasticity with stretching, ranging, bracing, positioning, and maximal oral doses of medications is unsuccessful.

Lanig IS. Optimizing the management of spasticity in people with spinal cord damage: a clinical care pathway for assessment and treatment decision making from the ability network, an international initiative. *Arch Phys Med Rehab.* 2018;99(8):1681–1687. doi: 10.1016/ j.apmr.2018.01.017

19. Describe some specific considerations required to determine whether a patient is a candidate for an intrathecal baclofen pump.

An intrathecal baclofen pump can be considered when a patient is at the maximum dosing of oral baclofen, requires multiple antispasticity medications, has significant systemic side effects from the antispasticity medications, and the intensity of symptoms is very life limiting. The patient must weigh more than 30 lb. Because of the stability of baclofen, it is suggested that the pump be refilled at least every 6 months (and more often if the patient requires higher doses). Patients should be reminded of the symptoms of overdose and withdrawal should the pump malfunction or fail. In case of pump failure, patients should carry a supply of oral baclofen to prevent acute withdrawal and seizures (a life-threatening event).

Available at: https://www.medtronic.com/us-en/healthcare-professionals/products/neurological/intrathecal-baclofen-therapy-systems/synchromed-ii.html

20. How are the pharmacokinetics of renally cleared medications affected in SCI patients?

Due to immobility and disuse atrophy, muscle mass in long-term spinal cord injury patients is reduced compared to age and weight of matched controls. As a result, the serum creatinine level is lower than controls, which may lead to overestimation of renal function. Be cautious when dosing medications based on serum creatinine levels rather than actual creatinine clearance.

Lee JP, Wang Y-J, Testing the predictive ability of the "spinal cord injury equation" in estimating vancomycin clearance. *Am J Health Sys Pharm.* 2013;70(8):669–674. doi: 10.2146/ajhp120329

21. Which commonly used dietary supplements interact with drugs?

Herbal supplements, vitamins, and minerals are used by patients and need to be included in medication reconciliation. Examples include:

- **St. John's Wort** is used for mild to moderate depression and interacts with SSRIs causing elevated serotonin and increasing the risk for serotonin syndrome and decreases **warfarin** its effects as an anticoagulant in INR measurement.
- **Ginkgo biloba** is used to improve blood flow and is an antioxidant. It should be avoided when taking any anticoagulant or platelet inhibitor such as **aspirin**, **warfarin**, and **clopidogrel**.
- **Garlic**, **ginger**, **ginkgo**, and **green tea** can potentiate the effect of warfarin and increase the INR.
- **Ginseng** decreases INR.

Ferguson LR. Nutrigenomic approaches to functional foods. *J Amer Dietetic Assn.* 2009;452–455. doi: 10.1016/j.jada.2008.11.024

Macan, H, Uykimpang R, Alconcel M, et al. Aged garlic extract may be safe for patient on warfarin therapy. *J Nutr.* 2006;136(3):793S–795S. doi: 10.1093/jn/136.3.793S

U.S. Food & Drug Administration. *Dietary Supplements.* 2019 (August). Available at: https://www.fda.gov/ food/dietary-supplements

22. Which topical agents are effective analgesics?

Several agents have evidence to support their effectiveness in reducing pain by at least 50%. These include **nonsteroidal anti-inflammatories** (NSAIDs), which inhibit cyclooxygenase, COX-2 isoform, reducing inflammation, and producing analgesia. **Rubefacients**, including **salicylates**, cause reddening of skin by dilating superficial blood vessels and create a sensation of warmth that may offset pain by the gate control theory. Topical **capsaicin** binds a nociceptor nerve fiber receptor leading to repeated depolarization and reversible degeneration of nerve terminals ("defunctionalization"). **Lidocaine** stabilizes neuronal membranes, decreasing transmission along nociceptive pathways. The formulation is important for efficacy. Acute strains and sprains can be effectively treated with **diclofenac** formulated as plaster or **emulgel**, **ketoprofen** gel, and **piroxicam** gel. For chronic pain, including knee and hand osteoarthritis and lateral epicondylitis, ketoprofen gel and diclofenac in various formulations are effective.

Moore RA, Derry S, McQuay HJ. Topical analgesics for acute and chronic pain in adults. *Cochrane Database Syst Rev.* 2010;(7):CD008609. doi: 10.1002/14651858.CD008609

23. What are suggested anticoagulants for venous thromboembolism (VTE) prophylaxis?

Many guidelines do not define best practices but seek to provide recommendations from which the clinician can choose what is most appropriate for individual patients. Aspirin therapy alone is getting increasing attention as primary prevention in select orthopedic cases.

Venous Thromboembolism (VTE) Treatment

Diagnosis	Duration
DVT, Provoked	3 months
DVT. Recurrent	Indefinite
DVT, Unprovoked	3 months (consider indefinite)
Pulmonary Embolism	6 months

Selected Medications and Their Uses

Drug	Indication	Dosing
Dalteparin		5000 units SC QD (Check anti Xa level if Clcr <30 mL/h)
Direct oral anticoagulants (DOACS): apixaban, rivaroxaban, and edoxaban		dose adjusted for renal dysfunction and contraindicated in Cr Cl <30 mL/min
Enoxaparin	Acute SCI (complete)	40mg SC QD × 12 weeks
	Acute SCI (incomplete)	40mg SC QD × 8 weeks
	Chronic SCI with (LE fracture, febrile illness	40mg SC QD × 12 weeks bedrest >2 weeks, other DVT risk)
	Renal dosing (ClCr <30 mL/min)	30 mg SC QD
	Trauma	30 mg q12h
	Orthopedic Surgery	40 mg QD or 30 mg q12h (knee) ×7–14 days, then **aspirin** 162 mg BID × 5 weeks
Fondaparinux		2.5 mg SC QD if Clcr >30 mL/min for patient with heparin-induced thrombocytopenia
Warfarin		INR goal 2–3

Kahn SR, Lim W, Dunn AS, et al. Prevention of VTE in nonsurgical patients: antithrombotic therapy and prevention of thrombosis, 9th ed: American College of Chest Physicians evidence-based clinical practice guidelines. *Chest.* 2012;141(2 Suppl): e195S–e266s. doi: 10.1378/chest.11-2296. Available at: https://www.ncbi.nlm.nih.gov/pmc/articles/PMC3278052/

Kearon C, Akl EA, Ornelas J, et al. Antithrombotic therapy for VTE disease: CHEST guideline and expert panel report. *Chest.* 2016;149(2):315–352. doi:10.1016/j.chest.2015.11.026. Available at: https://journal.chestnet.org/article/S0012-3692(15)00335-9/fulltext

Ortel, TL, Neumann I, Ageno W, et al. American Society of Hematology 2020 guidelines for management of venous thromboembolism: treatment of deep vein thrombosis and pulmonary embolism. *Blood Adv.* 2020;4(19):4693–4738. doi:10.1182/bloodadvances.2020001830. Available at: https://ashpublications.org/bloodadvances/article/4/19/4693/463998/American-Society-of-Hematology-2020-guidelines-for

Renner E, Barnes GD. Antithrombotic management of venous thromboembolism. *J Am Coll Cardiol.* 2020;76(18):2142–2154. Available at: https://www.jacc.org/doi/pdf/10.1016/j.jacc.2020.07.070

Thrombosis Canada. *Thromboprophylaxis.* 2018. Available at: https://thrombosiscanada.ca/

24. Medications for mental health

Medications for Mental Health Conditions

Drug Class	Examples	Mental Health Indications[a]	Adverse Effects
Antipsychotics (first-generation; "typical")	Chlorpromazine, fluphenazine, haloperidol, perphenazine,	Schizophrenia	Anticholinergic, akathisia, dystonia, Parkinson's, tardive dyskinesia,
Antipsychotics (second-generation; "atypical")	Aripiprazole, clozapine, lurasidone, olanzapine, paliperidone, quetiapine, risperidone, ziprasidone	Schizophrenia, bipolar disorders, depression, borderline personality disorder (quetiapine)	Constipation, weight gain, hyperlipidemia, glucose intolerance[b] sedation
Benzodiazepines	Alprazolam, clonazepam, diazepam, lorazepam,	Anxiety disorders	Beers Criteria (not recommended >65 years of age),
Mood stabilizers	Lithium and some anticonvulsants such as carbamazepine, lamotrigine, valproic acid (divalproex sodium)	Bipolar disorders	Lithium - weight gain, thirst, tremor lamotrigine - rash (Stevens-Johnson syndrome)[c] valproic acid—nausea, vomiting, dizziness, asthenia
Selective serotonin reuptake inhibitor (SSRI) antidepressants	Citalopram, escitalopram, fluoxetine, paroxetine, sertraline	Anxiety disorders, borderline personality disorder (fluoxetine), depression, OCD, PTSD	Sexual dysfunction, insomnia, GI toxicity
Selective serotonin-norepinephrine inhibitor (SNRI) antidepressants	Desvenlafaxine, duloxetine, venlafaxine	Anxiety disorders, depression, OCD (venlafaxine)	Increase BP (venlafaxine), sexual dysfunction, GI toxicity, insomnia
Tricyclic antidepressants	Amitriptyline, desipramine, doxepin, imipramine, nortriptyline	Depression, panic disorder	Anticholinergic, orthostatic hypotension, QTc prolonged, sedation, weight gain
Other antidepressants	Bupropion, mirtazapine, trazodone, vilazodone, vortioxetine	Depression	Bupropion—Insomnia, agitation, mirtazapine—drowsiness, increase appetite and weight gain, vilazodone, and vortioxetine—GI toxicity
Other anxiolytics (anti-anxiety meds)	Buspirone, hydroxyzine	Anxiety disorders	Sedation, dry mouth, dizziness, nausea

[a]This is not an all-inclusive list. Not all drugs in the class are used or preferred for the listed indications, and may or may not be FDA-approved.
[b]Less with aripiprazole.
[c]Lamotrigine, increase dose slowly.

RECOMMENDED READINGS

Baldwin DS, Chrones L, Florea I, et al. The safety and tolerability of vortioxetine: analysis of data from randomized placebo-controlled trials and open-label extension studies. *J Psychopharmacol.* 2016;30(3):242–252. doi:10.1177/0269881116628440

Brunton L, Knollmann BC. *Goodman and Gilman's Pharmacological Basis of Therapeutics.* 13th ed. New York: McGraw-Hill Medical; 2018.

Ciccone C. *Pharmacology in Rehabilitation.* 5th ed. Philadelphia: F. A. Davis; 2016.

Marra MV, Bailey RL. Position of the Academy of Nutrition and Dietetics: micronutrient supplementation. *J Acad Nutr Diet.* 2018;118(11): 2162–2173. doi: 10.1016/j.jand.2018.07.022. Available at: https://jandonline.org/article/S2212-2672(18)31546-6/fulltext

Reichenpfader U, Gartlehner G, Morgan LC, et al. Sexual dysfunction associated with second-generation antidepressants in patients with major depressive disorder: results from a systematic review with network meta-analysis. *Drug Saf.* 2014;37:19–31. doi: 10.1007/s40264-013-0129-4

Schatzberg AF, Nemeroff CB (Eds.). *Textbook of Psychopharmacology.* 5th ed. Arlington: American Psychiatric Association Publishing; 2017.

CHAPTER 24

COMPLEMENTARY, ALTERNATIVE, AND INTEGRATIVE MEDICINE: INCORPORATING DIVERSE APPROACHES TO MAXIMIZE PHYSICAL MEDICINE AND REHABILITATION OUTCOMES

Steven A. Stiens, MD, MS, Jason Allen, ND, MPH, and Bryan J. O'Young, MD, CAc, FAAPMR

KEY POINTS

1. Complementary and alternative medicine (CAM) is the popular phrase used for medical products and practices that have not been a part of standard medical care.
2. Integrative medicine is an active practice of personalized patient care that uses the most effective evidence-based medical treatments and CAM in a dynamic partnership with the patient to address pathophysiology and symptoms with sensitivity to patient culture and preference.
3. Contemporary clinicians actively seek constant development of the practice by updating the most effective evidence-based treatment by exploring conventional medical literature and emerging evidence for methods yet to be fully recognized.
4. Spirituality is an essential aspect of every person and requires medical understanding and a spiritual assessment. Addressing patients' beliefs throughout health care achieves better outcomes.

COLLABORATIVE MEDICINE

> *Collaborative medicine means we take the time to get to know each other so we can work together toward the best health you can achieve. We may decide to use conventional, alternative or integrative approaches, but the decisions are made in a collaborative way.*
>
> Martin Rossman, MD (1945–present) Interview with Martin Rossman, MD by Andrew Weil, MD

1. **What is complementary and alternative medicine (CAM)? How does it differ from integrative medicine (IM)?**

   CAM is the popular phrase used for medical products and practices that have not been a part of standard medical care. The National Center for Complementary and Integrative Health describes complementary medicine as non-mainstream medicine **used together** with conventional medicine, and **alternative medicine** is nonmainstream medicine used **in place of** conventional medicine.

   Integrative medicine (IM) is described as more than just the sum of conventional medicine plus CAM. It is defined as "healing-oriented wholistic medicine that reemphasizes the relationship between patient and physician and integrates the best of CAM with the best of conventional medicine." IM focuses on the preventive maintenance of health by paying attention to all relative components of lifestyle, including diet, exercise, stress management, and emotional well-being. Other terms for IM include holistic, functional, and blended.

Maizes V, Schneider C, Bell I, Weil A. Integrative medical education: Development and implementation of a comprehensive curriculum at the University of Arizona. *Acad Med.* 2002;77(9):851–860.

Snyderman R, Weil AT. Integrative medicine: Bringing medicine back to its roots. *Arch Intern Med.* 2002;162(4):395–397. https://pubmed.ncbi.nlm.nih.gov/12228072/

2. Are there differences within the IM approach?

In general, IM methodologies include preventing illness by optimizing overall health, early detection, using alternative diagnostics, optional therapies, active via varied mechanisms, and long-term therapeutic relationships with patients for participation, practice, prevention, and optimization.

In some cases, an IM approach could be a unique *diagnostic* method, such as muscle testing (applied kinesiology) or an unconventional lab test, such as secretory immunoglobulin A (sIgA) for allergies. In other cases, IM *therapeutics* include specific procedures, such as inserting needles into energy meridians (acupuncture) or adjusting subluxed vertebrae (chiropractic). In other cases, an IM approach could be a paradigmatic whole systems design, such as in functional medicine or naturopathic medicine, which are *systems* of medicine versus procedures.

Institute of Medicine (US) Committee on the Use of Complementary and Alternative Medicine by the American Public. *Complementary and Alternative Medicine in the United States.* Washington (DC): National Academies Press (US); 2005. Available at https://www.ncbi.nlm.nih.gov/books/NBK83799/

National Center for Complementary and Integrative Health. *Complementary, Alternative, or Integrative Health: What's In a Name?* Available at https://www.nccih.nih.gov/health/complementary-alternative-or-integrative-health-whats-in-a-name

Mayo Clinic. *Integrative Medicine.* Available at https://www.mayoclinic.org/tests-procedures/complementary-alternative-medicine/about/pac-20393581

IM. *Forsch Komplementmed.* 2012;19 Suppl 1:7–14. Available at www.karger.com/Article/Abstract/335181

3. What does the clinician discover by exploring alternative therapies and systems of care?

Analyzing standard definitions, patient choice rationale, potential risks, and benefits of IM is essential in contemporary practice. However, the exponential increase in the use of CAM has resulted in risks and consequences. Therefore it is imperative to understand these various approaches and utilize reliable resources in individualizing your care designs to improve patient outcomes. The revelations in patient assessment, pathophysiologic processes, and multiple therapeutic mechanisms can be translated to achieve more potent intervention capability, prevent complications, improve compliance, and reduce costs.

Adams J, Hollenberg D, Lui CW, Broom A. Contextualizing integration: A critical social science approach to integrative health care. *J Manipulative Physiol Ther.* 2009;32:792–798. Available at www.jmptonline.org/article/S0161-4754(09)00270-X/fulltext

4. How is IM different from conventional medicine?

The focus of IM is to assess, maintain, and, where indicated, improve the patient's overall health and well-being. Patient conditions are addressed using a **therapeutic order** starting with the least invasive and most "natural" (e.g., herbs before pharmaceuticals) interventions as possible. Conventional medicine, by contrast, *typically* intervenes once signs and symptoms are overt: *primarily* with pharmaceuticals and surgery. IM can be used to help prevent and manage specific medical conditions and, in many cases, complements conventional medicine, possibly addressing separate, pertinent mechanisms, unresolved symptoms, and unnoticed findings.

Ali A, Katz DL. Disease prevention and health promotion: how integrative medicine fits. *Am J Prev Med.* Nov 2015;49(5 Suppl 3): S230–S240. Available at www.sciencedirect.com/science/article/pii/S0749379715004080

5. How can CAM be classified despite varied philosophies, theories, mechanisms, and methods?

According to the National Institutes of Health (NIH), CAM can be separated into five categories. Some of these individual categories can have many subdivisions.

- *Alternative Medicine Systems* (e.g., naturopathic medicine, homeopathic medicine, Ayurveda, traditional Chinese medicine [TCM], functional medicine)
- *Mind-Body Interventions* (e.g., meditation, yoga, biofeedback)
- *Biologically Based Treatments* (e.g., botanicals, nutrients, supplements, IV's)
- *Manipulative and Body-Based Therapies* (e.g., chiropractic, massage, Rolfing, craniosacral)
- *Energy Therapies* (e.g., reiki, chi gong, tai chi, magnetic therapy)

Eisenberg DM. The Institute of Medicine report on complementary and alternative medicine in the United States—personal reflections on its content and implications. *Altern Ther Health Med.* 2005 May–Jun;11(3):10–15. Available at https://pubmed.ncbi.nlm.nih.gov/15943128/

6. Why is the taxonomy of CAM such a conundrum?

Common examples of IM that you have probably heard of and that your patients are likely aware of or already using include acupuncture and TCM, aromatherapy, Ayurveda, chiropractic therapy, naturopathic medicine, osteopathic medicine, use of dietary supplements, electromagnetic therapies, massage, homeopathy, cryotherapy, chi gong, reiki, craniosacral therapy, and a whole host of other therapies. The taxonomy of IM can be confusing. As the spectrum of modalities is wide, the certification and licensure (if any) are variable from state-to-state and the vast array of practitioners and evidence-based rationale can be confusing. **Operational definitions** by well-trusted sources have helped alleviate this taxonomic conundrum by categorizing IM into several relatively discrete categories.

Cochrane Complementary Medicine: Operational definition of complementary medicine. Available at https://IM.cochrane.org/operational-definition-complementary-medicine

7. Why do patients choose to use CAM?

Evidence suggests that patients may seek CAM because of dissatisfaction with conventional medicine. This dissatisfaction may stem from the frustration with medication's side effects, lack of collaboration and communication of the conventional providers, or lack of provider open-mindedness to alternative approaches. In addition, patients may find complementary therapies as more acceptable and consistent with their lifestyles and attitudes toward health and life and place more emphasis on respecting the body's natural abilities to heal. Furthermore, the internet has provided numerous cases of successful personal anecdotes using CAM. CAM is often outside the training, scope, and priorities of conventionally trained providers and would require seeking experience, accepting responsibility, and self-education to guide patients. The clinician must integrate the magnitude of health risks, the potency of therapies, and the patients' chosen activities to sustain compliance and achieve outcomes.

Ventola CL. Current issues regarding complementary and alternative medicine (CAM) in the United States. Part 1: The widespread use of CAM and the need for better-informed health care professionals to provide patient counseling. *P T*. 2010 Aug;35(8):461–468. Available at https://www.ncbi.nlm.nih.gov/pmc/articles/PMC2935644/

8. What is the prevalence of patient use of alternative medicine and CAM?

A comprehensive study in *JAMA* suggested a 47.3% overall increase in total visits to complementary medicine practitioners between 1990 and 1997. The number of visits to complementary medicine practitioners in 1990 was greater than to all primary care doctors. A total of 89% of the visits were not prescribed by a physician, and 72% of patients did not discuss CAM visits with their physician. A large recent survey of CAM use by the US Centers for Disease Control and Prevention/National Center for Health Statistics revealed that more than two-thirds of Americans regularly use complementary medicine.

Trends in Alternative Medicine Use in the United States, 1990–1997. Available at https://jamanetwork.com/journals/jama/fullarticle/188148

Trends in the use of complementary and alternative medicine in the United States: 2002–2007. Available at https://pubmed.ncbi.nlm.nih.gov/21317523/

9. What questions should your patients ask CAM and IM providers?

Many patients have questions about if/how IM approaches could augment existing care plans, and they may seek your guidance in evaluating incorporating IM into their treatment. Many patients may already be seeing IM providers. These are some essential questions that they should be considering:
- Is there evidence of efficacy and safety of the treatment?
- What is the provider's experience with the treatment?
- How many treatments will be needed? Treatment frequency and dosing?
- What is a reasonable time frame for a "fair" trial of the treatment?
- What are the costs, and are they reimbursed by insurance?
- What are the toxicity, safety risks, and adverse effects of the treatment?
- Will the CAM provider communicate with the patient's conventional physician?
- Are there any potential adverse interactions between CAM and conventional provider interventions?

Nightingale G, Hajjar E, Guo K, et al. A pharmacist-led medication assessment used to determine a more precise estimation of the prevalence of complementary and alternative medication (CAM) use among ambulatory senior adults with cancer. *J Geriatric Oncol*. Sep 2015;6(5):411–417. Available at https://pubmed.ncbi.nlm.nih.gov/26277113/

10. **What pertinent questions should the health care provider ask about CAM?**
    As a provider, of course, you have questions about CAM as well! Some questions may be similar to those of your patients, and some may be provider specialty specific. General questions should include the following (and resources to answer in sections following):
    - How is an IM diagnosis made and pathology defined?
    - How can the proposed mechanisms be scientifically explained?
    - Is the specific CAM treatment safe?
    - Does the CAM therapy prevent the patient from receiving needed medical management?
    - Can CAM therapy be continued in conjunction with conventional treatment?
    - Is conventional medicine falling short in some way that CAM might address?
    - Has the method been considered in clinical guidelines for care?
    - Is the CAM therapy evidence based?

CLINICAL RESEARCH EVIDENCE HIERARCHY

- Systematic reviews and meta-analyses of randomized clinical trial
- Randomized control trials
- Cohort studies
- Case-control studies
- Cross-sectional surveys
- Case reports
- Clinical experience (yours or others')

Stie M, Jensen LH, Delmar C, Nørgaard B. Open dialogue about complementary and alternative medicine (CAM) integrated in conventional oncology care, characteristics and impact. A systematic review. *Patient Educ Couns*. 2020;103(11):2224–2234. Available at https://pubmed.ncbi.nlm.nih.gov/32563705/

11. **What are the most common conditions treated with IM?**
    IM is used extensively in conjunction with conventional care for cancer patients. Other conditions commonly treated by IM practitioners include pain, fatigue, arthritis, headaches, hypertension, dermatologic conditions, anxiety, insomnia, digestive disorders (gastroesophageal reflux disease [GERD], Crohn disease, small intestinal bacterial overgrowth [SIBO], etc.), endocrine disorders (thyroiditis, diabetes, adrenal fatigue, etc.).

Trkulja V, Barić H. Current research on complementary and alternative medicine (CAM) in the treatment of anxiety disorders: an evidence-based review. *Adv Exp Med Biol*. 2020;1191:415–449. Available at https://pubmed.ncbi.nlm.nih.gov/32002940/

Nightingale G, Hajjar E, Guo K, et al. A pharmacist-led medication assessment used to determine a more precise estimation of the prevalence of complementary and alternative medication (CAM) use among ambulatory senior adults with cancer. *J Geriatr Oncol*. Sep 2015;6(5):411–47. Available at https://pubmed.ncbi.nlm.nih.gov/26277113/

12. **What considerations should the clinician and patient utilize in decision-making?**
    The rationale for decision-making requires consideration in the following criteria:
    - **Safety** (infrequent complications, treatment interactions).
    - **Efficacy** (clinically, personally significant effects, scientific evidence, mechanism, demonstrated outcomes).
    - **Treatment options** (full spectrum available, therapeutic order).
    - **Patient preferences** (understandable unique advantages, unique patient characteristics).
    - **Practical availability** (cost/accessibility/quality of life).

13. **How can IM expand the effectiveness of physical medicine and rehabilitation (PM&R) practice?**
    IM and PM&R share a variety of compatible and synergistic perspectives. Patients living with chronic diseases and persistent impairments often have a variety of symptoms mediated through various systems that can be responsive to a constellation of interventions operating through varied mechanisms. IM's approach to prevention includes sensitive surveillance and varied new intervention methods. These alternatives are started early or can be deployed with symptom exacerbations. Prolonged patient self-managed therapy courses can meet objectives of minimizing symptoms, sustaining function, and maintaining quality of life.

Bonus questions and answers are available online.

REFERENCES

Books

Becker RO, Selden G. *The Body Electric: Electromagnetism and the Foundation of Life.* 1st ed. New York: Morrow; 1985:364 p.

Pert CB. *Molecules of Emotion: Why You Feel the Way You Feel.* New York: Scribner; 1997:368p.

Pert CB, Marriott N. *Everything You Need to Know to Feel go(o)d.* Carlsbad, California: Hay House; 2006:xi, 287 p.

Rakel D. *Integrative Medicine.* 4th ed. Amsterdam: Elsevier; 2017:1152pgs.

Watkins A. *Mind-Body Medicine: A Clinicians Guide to Psychoneuroimmunology.* London: Churchill Livingston; 1997.

Journals

Journal of Complementary and Alternative Medicine. Available at: https://home.liebertpub.com/publications/journal-of-alternative-and-complementary-medicine-the/26/overview

Journal of Natural Products. Available at: https://pubs.acs.org/journal/jnprdf

Phytomedicine. Available at: https://www.sciencedirect.com/journal/phytomedicine

American Journal of Chinese Medicine. Available at: https://www.worldscientific.com/worldscinet/ajcm

Acupuncture in Medicine. Available at: https://journals.sagepub.com/home/aim

Journal of Traditional and Complementary Medicine. Available at: https://www.journals.elsevier.com/journal-of-traditional-and-complementary-medicine/

BMC Complementary and Alternative Medicine and Therapies. Available at: https://bmccomplementmedtherapies.biomedcentral.com/

Complementary Therapies in Medicine. Available at: https://www.sciencedirect.com/journal/complementary-therapies-in-medicine

WEBSITES

National Institutes of Health, National Center for Complementary and Integrative Health NCCIH. Available at: https://www.nccih.nih.gov/health/herbsataglance

Office of Dietary Supplements, NIH. Available at: http://ods.od.nih.gov/factsheets/dietarysupplements.asp

CHAPTER 25

REGENERATION AND REHABILITATION MEDICINE: INNOVATION THROUGH SYNERGY

Xiaoning (Jenny) Yuan, MD, PhD, Alfred C. Gellhorn, MD, Carmen M. Terzic, MD, PhD, Steven A. Stiens, MD, MS, and Christopher J. Visco, MD

Nature has an incredible capacity for regeneration and growth, but we can't experience it if we stay fearful and focused on lack.

Frances Moore Lappé (1944–)

Death, is not an end, but a transition crisis. All the forms of decay are but masks of regeneration—the secret alembics of vitality.

Edwin Hubbel Chapin (1814–1880)

KEY POINTS

1. "Regenerative rehabilitation" is a patient-centered, precision medicine approach, integrating rehabilitation science with regenerative medicine to achieve renewal of body structures and enhancement of function through synergistic interventions.
2. Prolotherapy consists of injections of irritant solution into multiple sites at ligamentous and tendinous insertions, or peri-articularly, to stimulate a localized inflammatory response and induce the release of growth factors that lead to soft tissue healing.
3. Platelet-rich plasma (PRP) has regenerative, anti-inflammatory, anti-microbial, and analgesic actions on tissues. Clinical data supporting the use of PRP is most robust for the treatment of chronic tendinopathy and osteoarthritis (OA), particularly knee OA.
4. Stem cells are characterized by their ability to produce new stem cells (self-renewal) and their capacity to develop into specialized cell types and generate tissues (differentiation). The promise of stem cell-based therapies is the repair or regeneration of damaged tissues.
5. Future directions in regenerative rehabilitation have enormous potential to improve function and clinical outcomes in patients with disabilities through the synergy of regenerative therapies with rehabilitative interventions.

1. What is regenerative medicine?

Regenerative medicine is the therapeutic process of optimizing biological systems for the growth, development, repair, and replacement of cells, tissues, and organs. The objective is the restoration of function that was lost due to age, disease, injury, or congenital defects. "**Regenerative rehabilitation**" is a patient-centered, precision medicine approach, integrating rehabilitation science with regenerative medicine, bioengineering, cell-based therapies, and nanotechnology to achieve renewal of body structures and enhancement of function through synergistic interventions.

Mason C, Dunnill P. A brief definition of regenerative medicine. *Reg Med.* 2008;3(1):1–5. DOI: 10.2217/17460751.3.1.1

2. What are the mechanisms of inflammation and degeneration after injury?

Tissue injury arises from a myriad of mechanisms, which trigger the healing cascade, beginning with injury arrest and early scaffolding with platelets and fibrin. **Wound healing** occurs in phases of **hemostasis, inflammation, proliferation, and tissue remodeling**. In this microenvironment, the clot serves as a provisional matrix and reservoir of cytokines and growth factors, which are released as platelets and inflammatory cells degranulate and upregulate inflammation. Fibrin guides cell adhesion, endothelial cell migration, angiogenesis, and acts as a temporary extracellular scaffolding during proliferation. Fibroblasts and keratinocytes dissolve the fibrin with plasmin and form scar tissue. Angiogenesis is essential for proliferation by delivering substrate and sustaining cells. During tissue remodeling, wound contraction occurs to minimize requirements for scar tissue bulk.

Nurden AT, Nurden P, Sanchez M, Andia I, Anitua E. Platelets and wound healing. *Front Biosci.* 2008;13:3532–3548. DOI: 10.2741/2947

3. **How can the process of regenerative medicine be utilized to solve the problems of individual patients (personalized medicine)?**

The regenerative medicine process encompasses understanding and utilization of the innate biological mechanisms that drive human development, differentiation, adaptation, deconstruction, reconstruction, and function. In addition, engineering principles, innovative biomaterials, synthetic modules, and amalgams are utilized for problem-focused intervention designs. Biopsychosocial targets span from the genome level to the organelle, cell, tissue, organ, organ system, whole body, and body-environment interaction levels. The overall concept is the structural and functional enablement of each unique patient to live at peak capacity throughout their lifespan.

Rando TA, Ambrosio F. Regenerative rehabilitation: applied biophysics meets stem cell therapeutics. *Cell Stem Cell*. 2018;22(3): 306–309. DOI: 10.1016/j.stem.2018.02.003

4. **What are the current clinical applications of regenerative medicine in PM&R?**

An ever-growing understanding of the tissue injury process, chronic disease pathophysiology, and aging constantly informs rehabilitation teams, with a wide variety of interventions available. Localized procedures to increase or decrease inflammation in the healing process, along with use of varied physical modalities, have enhanced wound, soft tissue, and bone healing. Injection of engineered or enhanced **growth factors**, **scaffolding**, or **autologous patient cells** has produced early, promising results. Many clinical applications of regenerative therapies for musculoskeletal disorders discussed in this chapter are currently considered off-label use, including prolotherapy, platelet-rich plasma, and stem cell-based therapies.

5. **What clinical scenarios suggest a regenerative medicine approach may be necessary and most likely to be effective?**

The primary consideration for a regenerative medicine approach to treatment is the ability to offer non-operative options for patients who have failed conventional therapies, who do not want surgery or who are poor surgical candidates, and for conditions with poor surgical outcomes. Special considerations include the vascularity of the native tissue environment and the severity and fidelity of the remaining tissue. **Tissue environments** that are poorly vascularized, such as tendons in the setting of moderate chronic tendinosis, carry a substantially worse prognosis for spontaneous recovery without intervention. Most regenerative treatments achieve the best clinical outcomes when applied to early- to mid-stage rather than end-stage disease. Moreover, in tissue injuries resulting in total discontinuity between the injured tissue and its original site of attachment, such as a full-thickness rotator cuff tear with retraction, a non-operative regenerative treatment is unlikely to lead to successful reattachment and healing of the injured tissue. Finally, additional considerations include the **chronicity of disease, quantity of volumetric tissue loss,** ability to engage in rehabilitation protocols following treatment, ability to heal and recover from a procedure, and systemic considerations such as systemic illnesses and comorbid conditions.

6. **Can clinicians use regenerative techniques regularly in practice now?**

Regenerative techniques signal and facilitate healing processes that can be selectively activated in tissues and organs. Modalities such as massage, tissue tension, and sustained pressure advance fluid flow at microscopic levels and shift charge distributions on surface structures, creating **piezoelectric effects** that signal cells. Regular skin friction from prescribed exercise at proper doses and frequency builds protective calluses. Wound debridement with **mechanical stimulation** triggers low-level inflammatory processes that activate growth factors to stimulate granulation tissue formation and promote healing. For example, percutaneous needle or **ultrasonic tenotomy** and fasciotomy can be considered regenerative, as they stimulate remodeling of injured tissue.

7. **What is prolotherapy?**

The use of prolotherapy injections, which are thought to enhance the "proliferative" phase of healing, began in the 1930s and was formalized in the 1950s by Dr. George Hackett, a general surgeon. **Irritant solutions (sclerosing agents)** are injected into tissues, where enhancement of inflammation to trigger tissue contraction and scar formation is desired. Prolotherapy is hypothesized to stimulate a localized inflammatory response at sites of injection, inducing the release of growth factors that lead to soft tissue healing and strengthening of the collagen foundation of these structures, thereby decreasing joint laxity and pain.

8. **What are the clinical indications for prolotherapy?**

Prolotherapy was originally described for the treatment of ligamentous and joint laxity resulting from and contributing to recurrent ankle sprains. However, clinical indications have expanded to chronic musculoskeletal conditions such as **tendinopathy, sacroiliac instability, pelvic pain due to ligamentous laxity**, and OA. Case series evidence has supported the use of prolotherapy for joint hypermobility syndrome, including Ehlers-Danlos syndrome.

Hauser RA, Lackner JB, Steilen-Matias D, Harris DK. A systematic review of dextrose prolotherapy for chronic musculoskeletal pain. *Clin Med Insights Arthritis Musculoskelet Disord*. 2016;9:139–159. DOI: 10.4137/CMAMD.S39160

9. What are the components of a prolotherapy injection?

   Prolotherapy typically consists of a series of injections of irritant solution into multiple sites at ligamentous and tendinous insertions, or peri-articularly. **Irritant solutions** include dextrose phenol-glycerin-glucose, and sodium morrhuate. Three to eight treatment sessions separated by 2 to 6 weeks is preferred to optimize collagen synthesis, deposition, and remodeling. The three most common irritant solutions are proposed to act by different mechanisms of action: **dextrose** by causing local osmotic rupture of cells, **phenol-glycerin-glucose** by local irritation of cells, and **sodium morrhuate** by chemoattraction of pro-inflammatory mediators. The most commonly used prolotherapy agent is hypertonic dextrose, ranging from 12.5% to 25% in concentration, which dehydrates localized cells at the injection sites, causing local trauma and stimulating inflammation and wound repair.

Schepker C, Habibi B, Yao KV. Prolotherapy. In *Regenerative Medicine for Spine and Joint Pain*; 2020:87–102. DOI: 10.1007/978-3-030-42771-9_6

10. What are the contraindications to and potential adverse effects of prolotherapy?

    Contraindications to prolotherapy include patients with metastatic cancer, disorders of systemic inflammation, bleeding disorders, hepatic conditions, morbid obesity, inability to perform post-treatment exercises, anatomical defects of the spine, low pain threshold, non-musculoskeletal pain, or whole-body pain.

    Since the mechanism of action of prolotherapy involves initiation of controlled local tissue damage and inflammation, mild pain and post-injection tenderness is expected for 3 to 5 days. Additional potential adverse effects of prolotherapy include stiffness, bruising, lightheadedness, allergic reaction, infection, and nerve damage. Adverse events related to needle injury during prolotherapy treatments for spine disorders have been reported, including spinal headache, pneumothorax, systemic reactions, nerve damage, hemorrhage, non-severe spinal cord insult, and disc injury. The incidence of these adverse events was of the same magnitude as other spinal injection procedures. No serious adverse effects have been reported for peripheral joint indications.

11. What is platelet-rich plasma (PRP)?

    Platelet-rich plasma (PRP) is defined simply as a "volume of autologous plasma that has a platelet concentration above baseline." The composition of PRP contains over 300 growth factors and cytokines. These growth factors include platelet-derived growth factors (**PDGFs**), transforming growth factors (**TGFs**), insulin-like growth factor 1 (**IGF-1**), epidermal growth factor (**EGF**), vascular endothelial growth factor (**VEGF**), and fibroblast growth factor (**FGF**). PRP also contains cytokines with pro- and anti-inflammatory functions.

12. What is the proposed mechanism of action of PRP?

    Clinical interest in PRP lies in its **regenerative** properties, as well as its **anti-inflammatory, anti-microbial, and analgesic actions** on the treated tissue. **Platelets** are anucleate cytoplasmic fragments of megakaryocytes from bone marrow. Platelet activation, adhesion, and aggregation are the initial steps of the inflammatory cascade and wound repair process. After activation, platelets degranulate and release growth factors and cytokines involved in cell proliferation, tissue remodeling, and suppression of inflammation, which play key roles in wound healing and repair.

Andia I, Maffulli N. Platelet-rich plasma for managing pain and inflammation in osteoarthritis. *Nat Rev Rheumatol*. 2013;9(12):721–730. DOI: 10.1038/nrrheum.2013.141

13. What are the clinical indications for PRP?

    Current musculoskeletal applications of PRP include treatment of tendinopathy, osteoarthritis (OA), ligamentous and meniscal injury, muscle injury, and spine disorders. Clinical data supporting the use of PRP is most robust for the treatment of chronic tendinopathy and OA, particularly knee OA. For both indications, PRP injection has been reported to reduce pain and improve function in randomized controlled trials at long-term analysis. Although PRP is considered a regenerative therapy, it is important to note that clinical studies have not yet demonstrated definitive evidence of tissue regeneration in musculoskeletal disorders, and positive clinical results are thought to be due to its anti-inflammatory effects and pain reduction.

Fice MP, Miller JC, Christian R, Hannon CP, Smyth N, Murawski CD, Cole BJ, Kennedy JG. The role of platelet-rich plasma in cartilage pathology: an updated systematic review of the basic science evidence. *Arthroscopy*. 2019;35(3):961–976.e3. DOI: 10.1016/j.arthro.2018.10.125

14. How do I prepare PRP?

    Preparing PRP involves one- or more often **two-step centrifugation protocols.** The first centrifugation separates whole blood into platelet and cell fractions, and the second further refines the platelet fraction. Preparation methods vary by platelet concentration, leukocyte concentration (**leukocyte-rich versus leukocyte-poor**), platelet **activation,** and use of anticoagulant. Platelet concentrations range from a 2.5– to 8–fold increase, as compared to whole blood. Early data supports tailoring PRP preparations to the treatment of specific clinical conditions, such as leukocyte-rich PRP for tendinopathy and leukocyte-poor PRP for OA.

15. **What are the contraindications to and potential adverse effects of PRP?**
    Contraindications to PRP therapy include **cancer** (tumor or metastatic disease), active **infections, thrombocytopenia,** and **pregnancy**.

16. **What are stem cells?**
    All cells and tissues in the body are generated from **stem cells.** The two characteristics of stem cells are **self-renewal,** the ability to produce new stem cells, and **differentiation,** the capacity to develop into specialized cell types and generate tissues. Hematopoietic stem cells from bone marrow, which develop into all blood cell types, were the first to be discovered in the 1960s, leading to the first clinical stem cell therapy: bone marrow transplantation.

NIH Stem Cell Information Home Page. Available at: https://stemcells.nih.gov/

17. **What is a pluripotent versus a multipotent stem cell? What is the difference between embryonic and adult stem cells?**
    Two broad categories of stem cells exist based upon their capacity for differentiation: pluripotent and multipotent stem cells. **Pluripotent stem cells** can differentiate into all tissues of the body, except for the placenta and umbilical cord. **Embryonic stem cells** are present in early development and are pluripotent. They are generated from blastocysts created during *in vitro* fertilization that are not implanted or used. **Multipotent stem cells** can differentiate into some cell lineages, but not all. **Adult stem cells,** or tissue-specific stem cells, are multipotent and capable of differentiation into specific cell types relevant to their native tissue environment or niche.

18. **What are induced pluripotent stem cells? How are they derived and used?**
    In 2006, a team led by Shinya Yamanaka announced the creation of **induced pluripotent stem (iPS) cells,** which are adult cells that are "reprogrammed" to gain pluripotency similar to embryonic stem cells through the introduction of key transcription factors that regulate pluripotency. Since iPS cells are generated from adult cells rather than embryos, the ethical controversy involved in the study and use of embryonic stem cells is therefore bypassed.

    Additional questions available online.

19. **What are "mesenchymal stem cells?" Where do they come from?**
    "**Mesenchymal stem cells**" were originally described in 1991 by Dr. Arnold Caplan, derived from bone marrow and periosteum that were culture-adherent with *in vitro* capacity for expansion and multipotent differentiation into bone, cartilage, fat, and other connective tissue lineages. MSCs are therefore a promising source for tissue regeneration, such as the repair or replacement of damaged cartilage in OA, and for therapeutic immunomodulation in conditions such as autoimmune disorders.

Ha C-W, Park Y-B, Kim SH, Lee H-J. Intra-articular mesenchymal stem cells in osteoarthritis of the knee: a systematic review of clinical outcomes and evidence of cartilage repair. *Arthroscopy.* 2019;35(1):277–288.e2. DOI: 10.1016/j.arthro.2018.07.028

20. **What is the proposed mechanism of action of stem cells in regenerative medicine?**
    The most promising clinical applications are stem cell-based therapies to replace or heal injured tissues by utilizing their ability to differentiate into specific cell types and regenerate tissue. At this time, the majority of stem cell-based therapies utilize adult mesenchymal stem/stromal cells (MSCs).

21. **How do I harvest stem cells for regenerative therapies?**
    Stem cell niches reside throughout the body. Sources of MSCs include the bone marrow, adipose tissue, peripheral blood, cord blood, synovium, meniscus, and ligament. For musculoskeletal applications, the most common sites for MSC harvesting are from the bone marrow and adipose tissue. **Bone marrow aspirates (BMA)** are typically collected from the ilium and centrifuged to generate BMA concentrates (BMAC). **Lipoaspirates** are harvested autologously from the subcutaneous fat.

22. **How many stem cells are in these aspirates?**
    The percentage of MSCs in bone marrow is estimated at only 0.01% to 0.02%, although it has been reported that BMAC enriches bone marrow-derived MSC populations to over 10,000-fold versus control BMA, with over 90% cell viability after processing. The percentage of MSCs in adipose tissue is estimated 0.1% to 0.2% with approximately 95% viability of cells harvested from various sites.

Kern S, Eichler H, Stoeve J, Klüter H, Bieback K. Comparative analysis of mesenchymal stem cells from bone marrow, umbilical cord blood, or adipose tissue. *Stem Cells.* 2006;24(5):1294–1301. DOI: 10.1634/stemcells.2005-0342

23. **What "stem cell therapies" are currently used in clinical practice?**
Stem cell-based therapies have been studied for utility in the treatment of OA, rheumatoid arthritis, SCI, stroke, burns, heart disease, diabetes, and macular degeneration. Currently, bone marrow and lipoaspirates are used in clinical practice, primarily for the treatment of musculoskeletal disorders such as tendinopathy and OA.

24. **What are contraindications to and potential adverse effects of stem cell-based therapies?**
Contraindications to stem cell-based therapies include history of cancer, systemic illness, immunodeficiency, pregnancy, and history of bleeding disorders, as there is no safety data for these populations. Post-procedure pain represents the majority of reported adverse events for patients treated with MSCs for musculoskeletal conditions. Although cancer is a contraindication to stem cell-based therapies, clinical studies have not demonstrated evidence that these therapies increase the risk of neoplasm.

U.S. Food and Drug Administration—Watch Out for Unapproved Stem Cell Therapies!—YouTube. Available at: https://youtu.be/onnl-ZeQlai0

25. **What is the rehabilitation protocol following a regenerative treatment for tendinopathy?**
While details vary for different conditions, post-procedure rehabilitation protocols following a regenerative injection for tendon disease typically follow three phases (Table 25.1). **Phase 1** begins immediately post-procedure with 2 to 7 days of **relative rest,** weight-bearing restriction (depending on the location treated), and activity modification. The goals of this phase are to control post-procedural pain related to increased inflammation. NSAIDs are generally not allowed for 2 to 4 weeks before and to be avoided for 1 month after injection. Instead, pain is controlled with acetaminophen, ice, and other soft tissue modalities. **Phase 2** corresponds with the initiation of a **structured stretching program,** starting most frequently between days 2 and 7 following injection. **Phase 3** transitions to a **progressive strengthening program**, which usually commences at 2 to 3 weeks following injection.

Townsend C, Von Rickenbach KJ, Bailowitz Z, Gellhorn AC. Post-procedure protocols following platelet rich plasma injections for tendinopathy: A systematic review. *PM&R.* 2020;12(9):904–915. DOI: 10.1002/pmrj.12347

26. **How can PM&R contribute to the clinical translation of regenerative medicine protocols that lead to life-changing outcomes for patients?**
PM&R encompasses rehabilitation of neurological, cardiopulmonary, pediatric, burn, post-amputation, and other medically complex disorders, and associated conditions including pressure injuries, speech disorders, and renal dysfunction. Ongoing endeavors show promising results for the recovery of individuals with spinal cord injury (SCI) and neurological disorders, and regeneration of blood vessels, skin, heart, pancreas, vocal cords, muscle, and lungs, in preclinical animal studies and early human trials. Given that rehabilitative interventions such as physical occupational, and speech therapy are commonly prescribed treatments for these conditions, rehabilitation has a significant role in catalyzing regenerative processes and maximizing the success of a multimodal treatment plan. Future advances and interdisciplinary efforts in regenerative rehabilitation have enormous potential to improve function and clinical outcomes in patients with disabilities through the synergy of regenerative therapies with a myriad of rehabilitative interventions, therapeutic exercise and modalities.

27. **Which organ systems and conditions are targets of emerging experimental regenerative medicine protocols?**
Traumatic SCI: Recent approval of the use of MSCs for SCI is encouraging following results from a trial of 13 acute traumatic SCI patients in Japan. Adipose-derived MSCs are currently in early clinical studies for the treatment of traumatic SCI in the United States.

Neurological and neuromuscular disorders: Regenerative medicine therapies, including stem cells, autologous cord blood, and exosomes for the treatment of multiple sclerosis, Parkinson disease, stroke, amyotrophic lateral sclerosis, cerebral palsy and Duchenne muscular dystrophy are the subject of past and ongoing clinical trials but are not yet approved worldwide.

Table 25.1 Rehabilitation Protocols Following Regenerative Medicine Procedures

PHASE	TIMING	ACTIVITY
1	Post-procedure (PP) day 0–7	Relative rest, site-dependent weight-bearing restriction, activity modification
2	PP day 2–7	Initiation of structured stretching program
3	PP week 2–3	Progressive strengthening program

Blood vessels: Engineered human vessels may replace patients' own vessels, with potential for significant impact in patients with disabilities and comorbidities related to vascular and metabolic diseases.

Skin: Human fibroblasts grown on polymer scaffolds act as skin replacement grafts for patients with burn wounds or diabetic skin ulcers.

desJardins-Park HE, Foster DS, Longaker MT. Fibroblasts and wound healing: an update. *Regen Med.* 2018;13(5):491–495. DOI: 10.2217/rme-2018-0073

Heart: Stem cell-derived cardiomyocytes can restore the function of infarcted hearts in preclinical studies.

Charles Murry, MD, PhD—Regrowing heart muscle with stem cells—YouTube. Available at: https://www.youtube.com/watch?v=ZkTH05BOR5M

Pancreas: MSCs have been engineered to secrete insulin for treatment of type 1 diabetes mellitus in early clinical trials.

Vocal cords: Bioengineered vocal cord tissue can potentially be transplanted for voice restoration in patients with voice impairment following promising results in animal models.

Muscle: Volumetric muscle loss (VML) from military blast injuries has responded to the combination of surgically implanted extracellular matrix scaffolds and physical therapy. The structural guidance and stimulated healing provided by the scaffolds, in concert with exercise therapy, increased isometric knee extensor strength in military personnel with chronic quadriceps VML.

Lung transplantation: In proof-of-concept preclinical studies, an engineered cross-circulation system recovered injured human lungs that would otherwise not be suitable for transplantation in efforts to increase donor lung availability.

Columbia University Vagelos College of Physicians and Surgeons—Regeneration of severely damaged lungs. Available at: https://vimeo.com/334694218

Kidney: Three-dimensional bioprinting can engineer functional kidney tissues in the laboratory setting, with future promise of restoring kidney function in patients with end-stage renal disease.

Anthony Atala, MD—Printing a human kidney. YouTube. Available at: https://www.youtube.com/watch?v=bX3C20104MA

28. What is dedifferentiation?

Cell **dedifferentiation** is the process by which cells revert from a more differentiated state to an earlier, less differentiated stage within their lineage. This process has implications for therapeutic application by inducing dedifferentiation to repair damaged tissues. Preclinical studies have demonstrated that cardiomyocyte remodeling is closely related to dedifferentiation, for instance. Dedifferentiation is also implicated in pathological changes in tissues that culminate in disease, such as the similarity between changes that occur during chondrocyte dedifferentiation and the events leading to development of osteoarthritis.

Yao Y, Wang C. Dedifferentiation: inspiration for devising engineering strategies for regenerative medicine. *NPJ Regen Med.* 2020;5(1):14. DOI: 10.1038/s41536-020-00099-8

29. What PM&R concepts and strategies will synergize with and translate regenerative therapies into rehabilitation plans of care in the future?

Modern medicine utilizes multimodal and multidisciplinary treatments for the care of patients limited by chronic disease or disability to minimize complications, increase efficiency, and achieve the best outcomes. Rehabilitation provides and utilizes adaptive equipment, modalities, therapeutic exercise, electrical stimulation, ultrasound, and robotic technologies to direct therapies that support the function and treatment of a patient as a person, not a disease. Examples of synergistic contributions of rehabilitation medicine with traditions of success include the care of orthopedic patients undergoing joint replacements, post-transplant patients in collaboration with surgery, and advances in stroke recovery and adaptation working together with neurology. Future developments to optimize the delivery of regenerative and rehabilitative care include the design of rehabilitation units or clinics with close proximity to scientists, engineers, and laboratories, the training of dedicated interdisciplinary health care professionals for consultation and oversight of appropriate regenerative rehabilitative interventions, and the integration of such interventions into coordinated, practical, and cost-effective clinical pathways for patient care.

Willett NJ, Boninger ML, Miller LJ, Alvarez L, Aoyama T, Bedoni M, … Ambrosio, F. Taking the next steps in regenerative rehabilitation: establishment of a new interdisciplinary field. *Arch Phys Med Rehabil.* 2020;101(5), 917–923. DOI: 10.1016/j.apmr.2020.01.007

30. Are pharmacological agents or physical modalities available that can stimulate stem cell function and tissue regeneration?

Active research is underway to identify pharmacological agents that can enhance stem cell function. Scientists are screening compounds that are already available clinically for their ability to support stem cell renewal and differentiation in preclinical models. **Priming** of mesenchymal stem cells (MSCs) in the laboratory can produce cells with specific phenotypes of interest for treatment of various conditions. **Granulocyte colony stimulating factor** (G-CSF) mobilizes hematopoietic stem cells (HSCs) from bone marrow to peripheral blood and is traditionally used to treat chemotherapy-induced neutropenia or to increase donor HSC numbers prior to stem cell transplantation. G-CSF-mobilized peripheral blood can contain a small percentage of MSCs ($\sim$0.01%), and has been utilized in clinical trials of MSC therapy for osteoarthritis.

Physical modalities such as **electrical stimulation** and **ultrasound** are also under investigation in preclinical studies. **Pulsed electric field stimulation** can stimulate cell and tissue matrix proliferation in animal models of wound and fracture healing, nerve, skeletal muscle, and cardiac tissue regeneration. **Low-intensity pulsed ultrasound** (LIPUS) has been studied for bone fracture healing and nerve regeneration in animal models and has been demonstrated to enhance MSC differentiation *in vitro*. **Extracorporeal shockwave therapy** (ESWT) has enhanced MSC-based therapies in preclinical animal models of spinal cord injury, brain injury, bony defects, and muscle injury. **Photobiomodulation** or laser therapy stimulates cell proliferation, differentiation, and tissue healing in preclinical studies of bone and skin regeneration.

To date, however, no high-level clinical evidence supports the use of specific medications, supplements, or modalities to stimulate stem cell or regenerative activity.

da Silva LP, Kundu SC, Reis RL, Correlo VM. Electric phenomenon: A disregarded tool in tissue engineering and regenerative medicine. *Trends Biotechnol.* 2020;38(1):24–49. DOI: 10.1016/j.tibtech.2019.07.002

Yin JQ, Zhu J, Ankrum JA. Manufacturing of primed mesenchymal stromal cells for therapy. *Nat Biomed Eng.* 2019;3(2):90–104. DOI: 10.1038/s41551-018-0325-8

WEBSITES

Alliance for Regenerative Medicine. Available at: https://alliancerm.org/
Alliance for Regenerative Rehabilitation Research and Training (AR³T). Available at: https://ar3t.pitt.edu/
AR³T Regenerative Rehabilitation YouTube Channel. Available at: https://www.youtube.com/channel/UCfMFL8NilagUaUUZN85fAmQ
Current Physical Medicine and Rehabilitation Reports—Topical Collection on Regenerative Rehabilitation. Available at: https://link.springer.com/search?query=regenerative&search-within=Journal&facet-journal-id=40141
Nature Partner Journals (NPJ)—Regenerative Medicine. Available at: https://www.nature.com/npjregenmed/
NPJ Regenerative Medicine—Regenerative Rehabilitation Collection. Available at: https://www.nature.com/collections/vttmqzzcvs
RegenerativeMedicine.net. Available at: http://www.regenerativemedicine.net/

BIBLIOGRAPHY

1. Atala A, Lanza R, Mikos AG, Nerem RM, eds. *Principles of Regenerative Medicine.* 3rd ed. Cambridge, MA: Academic Press; 2018: 1–1454.
2. Cohen JM, Young M, O'Young B, Stiens SA. *Organ Transplantation and Rehabilitation: Process and Interdisciplinary Interventions.* In Moroz A, Flanagan S, Zaretsky H, eds. *Medical Aspects of Disability for the Rehabilitation Professionals.* 5th ed. New York, NY: Springer Publishing; 2016:412–452.
3. Cooper G, Herrera J, Kirkbride J, Perlman Z, eds. *Regenerative Medicine for Spine and Joint Pain.* 2020:1–268. DOI: 10.1007/978-3-030-42771-9
4. Terzic CM, Preston C, Faustino R, Qu W. *Stem Cell Research and Regenerative Medicine.* In Mitra R, ed. *Principles of Rehabilitation Medicine.* New York, NY: McGraw-Hill Education; 2018:1580–1591.
5. Wyles SP, Hayden RE, Meyer FB, Terzic A. Regenerative medicine curriculum for next-generation physicians. *NPJ Regen Med.* 2019;4(1):3. DOI: 10.1038/s41536-019-0065-8

FUNDAMENTALS OF MEDICAL ACUPUNCTURE: SCIENTIFIC FOUNDATION AND CLINICAL APPLICATIONS

Freda Dreher, MD and Joseph Helms, MD

Maintaining order rather than correcting disorder is the ultimate principle of wisdom. To cure disease after it has appeared is like digging a well when one already feels thirsty, or forging weapons after the war has begun.
~ Nei Jing, 2nd Century BCE

KEY POINTS: MEDICAL ACUPUNCTURE

1. Acupuncture is a practice in which fine needles are inserted through the skin at anatomically identifiable points employing the basic premise that needle stimulation assists the body's mechanisms of physiologic regulation and repair.
2. Current acupuncture research demonstrates a continuum of effectiveness above and beyond placebo with Streitberger (placebo) needling or non-acupuncture point needling, with clearly demonstrated effectiveness in common problems such as low back pain, arthritis, headaches, dental pain, nausea, mood disorders, and insomnia.
3. Acupuncture effects have been shown to work through central nervous system neurotransmitters, using endorphin, enkephalin, dynorphin, GABA, and monoamine dependent mechanisms, and analgesic effects can be reversed with the administration of Naloxone.
4. Current research using fMRI demonstrates a direct correlation of body and microsystem (auricular) acupuncture sites with activity of central nervous system areas, including representative somatosensory cortical areas, limbic structures, and subcortical structures involved with the experience of pain.

When acupuncture is provided by a physician who is thoroughly educated and trained in western medicine as well as medical acupuncture, this treatment modality can contribute to a holistic, comprehensive, and cost-effective way to promote health and well-being.

1. **What is medical acupuncture?**
   Acupuncture is the practice of using fine needles inserted through the skin at specific points on the body to treat pain, injury, and disease, optimize health, and prevent illness. The basic premise is that needle stimulation assists the body's mechanisms of physiologic regulation and repair. Medical acupuncture refers to acupuncture as practiced by a physician and is considered comprehensive as the practitioner has a thorough education and understanding of the practice of medicine. This approach respects the contemporary understanding of anatomy and physiology as well as modern treatment strategies while embracing the classical Chinese medicine concepts of care. Comparatively, a non-physician acupuncturist may have a graduate-level degree and may have studied or practiced medicine in another country. To legally practice acupuncture in the United States, non-physicians must have a license to practice acupuncture (LAc) that is state-specific. LAc training often includes other East Asian practices such as herbalism, acupressure, and energetic exercises such as Tai Chi and Qi Gong.

2. **What is TCM?**
   TCM stands for Traditional Chinese Medicine. The style of acupuncture practice called TCM was developed within the past century in China in an attempt to unify disparate practices throughout the country and to codify terminology. Although any practice of acupuncture may be considered traditional, the term TCM refers to a specific style. There are many styles of acupuncture practice available to physicians, including TCM, Japanese, French Energetics, Five Element, microsystems, modern neuroanatomical, and more.

3. What factors contribute to the therapeutic effect of an acupuncture treatment?

Multiple factors can contribute to acupuncture's therapeutic effects, including needling technique, duration of needle retention, subjective (psychological) factors, and acupuncture point specificity.

Shi G, Yang X, Liu C, et al. Factors contributing to therapeutic effects evaluated in acupuncture clinical trials. *Trials.* 2012;13:42. doi:10.1186/1745-6215-13-42. Available at: https://trialsjournal.biomedcentral.com/articles/10.1186/1745-6215-13-42

4. How many acupuncture points are there, and where are they located?

There are 361 classically described acupuncture points located at specific points on the body, on channels also referred to as meridians. Acupoints generally show a decrease in surface electrical resistance when compared to the surrounding tissue and are sometimes tender to palpation. General anatomic characteristics of acupuncture points include proximity to:
- Neurovascular hilus of the muscle
- Motor or trigger points
- Passage of peripheral nerves through bone foramina
- Penetration of deep fascia by peripheral nerves
- Bifurcation points of peripheral nerves
- Nerve plexuses
- Sagittal plane where superficial nerves from both sides of the body meet

5. What is dry needling?

Dr. Janet Travell used the term "dry needling" when referencing a trigger point treatment using a needle without injecting a substance. In recent years, non-physician practitioners have been employing dry needling as a method of treating myofascial pain. Since there is a significant overlap of points identified as myofascial trigger points and points identified as acupuncture points, dry needling constitutes a local acupuncture treatment. Such treatments should only be done by individuals with thorough training in three-dimensional anatomy as well as how to avoid, identify, and manage complications associated with invasive procedures.

6. How safe is acupuncture, and what are the risks?

When acupuncture is provided by a properly credentialed physician with up-to-date skills and knowledge, the procedure is safe. The acupuncturist must have a keen awareness of three-dimensional anatomy and risks associated with interventional procedures. A 2004 review article on adverse events associated with acupuncture notes that the risk of a serious adverse event is estimated to be 0.05 per 10,000 treatments and 0.55 per 10,000 individual patients. The most common side effects noted were bleeding at the needle site and localized needling pain.

Infection is an uncommon consequence of acupuncture treatment, although bacterial skin infections and ear chondritis can occur. Hepatitis B transmission is extremely rare, and the only reported incidences in the United States literature involve the use of unsterilized needles. There have been no legitimate reports of HIV transmission. The current standard of care dictates the use of sterile, one-use, disposable needles using clean technique. There is no established evidence that a surface swipe of alcohol prior to needle insertion prevents infection.

Pneumothorax is an infrequent complication. Deep needling of the thoracic cage is discouraged, and the small size of an acupuncture needle makes a significant and symptomatic pneumothorax unlikely.

A not uncommon phenomenon to be aware of is "needle shock," a vasovagal response that may occur, usually only after initial treatments. This reaction responds readily to standard maneuvers employed for such events encountered in the use of a hypodermic needle.

White A. A cumulative review of the range and incidence of significant adverse events associated with acupuncture. *Acupunct Med.* 2004;22:122–133. doi.org/10.1136/aim.22.3.122

Xu S, Wang L, Cooper E, et al. Adverse events of acupuncture: a systematic review of case reports. *Evid Based Complement Alternat Med.* 2013;2013:581203. doi: 10.1155/2013/581203

7. What are the contraindications for acupuncture?

Contraindications are similar but less restrictive than those for injection techniques: overlying skin conditions such as cellulitis, severe coagulopathy, and uncontrolled anticoagulation. Therapeutic anticoagulation does not present difficulties, although ecchymoses are more common. Vigorous or deep needling techniques should be avoided in patients with impaired coagulation. Pregnancy is not a contraindication to acupuncture, but certain points are avoided on practical or theoretical grounds, such as points overlying the pregnant uterus and those stimulating the lumbosacral nerve plexuses. It is advised that the pregnant patient seek out an acupuncturist who has had specific training or experience in treating pregnant patients. Contraindications to electrical stimulation of acupuncture needles are the same as for electrical stimulation in general: stimulation of the thorax in patients with pacemakers, pregnancy (safety not established), and carcinoma (unknown effects).

8. Isn't acupuncture just placebo?

Whereas no one can argue that placebo can create a measurable response 30% to 35% of the time, verum (true) acupuncture response rates are much higher. Research confirms that there is a continuum of response beyond that of placebo when sham acupuncture is provided either by using false needles (Streitberger needles) or non-acupuncture point needle locations. Response rates in this group range from 33% to 55%, seemingly confirming the benefits of touch, acupressure, and/or situational interaction above and beyond no treatment or waitlist. Verum acupuncture response rates range from 55% to 85% depending upon the condition of the patient and the practitioner's skill level and area of expertise. Research to prove the validity of acupuncture is limited by the necessary human interaction of a treatment. It is near impossible to completely blind an acupuncturist to the treatment they're performing, and as near impossible to blind a patient to the treatment they're receiving. As many current studies now are focusing on pain reduction as a measure of value, subjective reporting of pain further confounds outcome measurements.

Haake M, Müller MH, Schade-Brittinger C, et al. German Acupuncture Trials (GERAC) for chronic low back pain: randomized, multicenter, blinded, parallel-group trial with 3 groups. *Arch Intern Med.* 2007;167(17):1892–1898.

Streitberger K, Kleinhenz J. Introducing a placebo needle into acupuncture research. *Lancet.*1998 Aug 1;352(9125):364–365. doi: 10.1016/S0140-6736(97)10471-8.

9. What disorders can acupuncture treat?

In 1997, the NIH issued a consensus statement reviewing the rational basis for acupuncture treatment and stating that there is sufficient evidence of acupuncture's value to expand its use into conventional medicine and encourage further studies of its clinical value. Subsequently, the WHO conducted global literature reviews and maintains a list of conditions recommended for treatment by acupuncture. Based on this work, many major US medical centers have incorporated acupuncture into comprehensive care management for specific conditions. Although most acupuncture practiced in the United States focuses on pain management, any primary care indication can be addressed with acupuncture. In 2014, The Department of Veterans Affairs (US), after a systematic review of current acupuncture research publications, published an *Evidence Map of Acupuncture* mapping literature size, confidence, and effectiveness in the realms of pain management, wellness, and mental health. Positive results were noted for chronic pain, headache, insomnia, and mood disorder as well as many other conditions.

Hempel S, Shekelle P, Taylor S, Solloway M, et al. *Evidence Map of Acupuncture: Evidence-Based Synthesis Program.* Washington, DC: Department of Veterans Affairs (US); 2014.

National Institutes of Health. Acupuncture. *NIH Consensus Statement Online.* 1997 Nov 3–5;15(5):1–34. Available at: http://consensus.nih.gov/1997/1997Acupuncture107html.htm

10. What are the most common problems treated by acupuncture for pain management?

The most common problem is chronic pain that has not adequately responded to pharmacologic, surgical, or traditional physical therapies. By location, low back and neck/shoulder pain are the most common, followed by appendicular joint pains and headaches. Although these chronic pain problems are the most commonly treated by medical acupuncturists, they are not necessarily the most effectively treated. Often, the patient seeks out acupuncture as a "last resort." In the challenging chronic pain patient population, if success is not achieved, the patient may conclude that acupuncture doesn't work when, in fact, other treatments have not worked well either. Realistic goal setting by the physician is necessary. In the office of a physiatrist acupuncturist, an array of therapeutic remedies can be offered.

It is well accepted in the medical acupuncture community that acute injuries and straightforward pain complaints can be easily treated with acupuncture, often obviating any need for analgesic prescriptions. The Acus Foundation has established a "Think Acupuncture First" framework while teaching acupuncture to United States Air Force Family Practice Residents. Significant reductions in analgesic and benzodiazepine prescriptions have been noted in the acupuncture patients.

A meta-analysis of randomized controlled trials published in 2018 included 20,827 patients with chronic musculoskeletal pain. Acupuncture was found to be substantially better than standard care and significantly better than sham acupuncture in relieving pain. It has also been noted that treatment effects of acupuncture persist over time and cannot be explained solely in terms of placebo effects.

Crawford P, Penzien D, Coeytaux R. Reduction in pain medication prescriptions and self-reported outcomes associated with acupuncture in a military patient population. *Med Acupunct.* 2017;29(4):229–231. doi: 10.1089/acu.2017.123.

Vickers AJ, Vertosick EA, Lewith G, et al. Acupuncture for chronic pain: Update of an individual patient data meta-analysis. *J Pain.* 2018;19:455–474.

MacPherson H, Vertosick EA, Foster NE, et al. The persistence of the effects of acupuncture after a course of treatment: A meta-analysis of patients with chronic pain. *Pain.* 2017;158:784–793. doi: 10.1097/j.pain.0000000000000747.

11. What are the biological effects of acupuncture?

Acupuncture analgesia is one of the most thoroughly researched areas in medicine. Animal and human experiments that started in China in the 1960s have been subsequently pursued in Europe and the United States. In animal models, acupuncture needle insertion, manipulation, and electrical stimulation have been shown to stimulate endogenous opioid release that can be blocked by Naloxone. Two types of analgesia have been identified:

- Endorphin (and other peptide) dependent analgesia is induced by manipulation of the needle or electrical stimulation at low frequency (2 to 4 Hz). Low frequencies are known to create more lasting effects.
- Monoamine dependent analgesia is induced by electrical stimulation at high frequency (>90 Hz). Its characteristics include rapid onset and local/segmental effects only.

Current research includes work in the following areas:

- In chronic pain, brain imaging has demonstrated increases in opioid receptor binding following verum acupuncture treatment.
- In musculoskeletal pain problems, fMRI has shown diminished somatosensory cortex signaling as a response to acupuncture point stimulation.
- To treat emotional aspects of pain, disease, and trauma, response of limbic areas of the brain has been demonstrated on fMRI.
- Extensive research using imaging and measurements of tensile strength has demonstrated exactly what constitutes an acupuncture point as compared with surrounding tissue and has also identified changes at connective tissues in response to the insertion of a seemingly innocuous acupuncture needle.

There is also convincing evidence to support the use of acupuncture to help with the restoration of healthy sleep patterns, improvements in mood, resolution of post-traumatic stress symptoms, and improvements in motor (not motoric) function. As acupuncture is cost-effective, further research for effectiveness in specific disorders is needed.

Langevin HM, Churchill DL, Wu J, et al. Evidence of connective tissue involvement in acupuncture. *FASEB J.* 2002;6:872–874. doi: 10.1096/fj.01-0925fje.

Witt CM, Jena S, Selim D, et al. Pragmatic randomized trial evaluating the clinical and economic effectiveness of acupuncture for chronic low back pain. *Am J Epidemiol.* 2006;64:487–496. doi: 10.1093/aje/kwj224

12. How is the brain stimulated by acupuncture?

Acupuncture actuates nerve fibers at the local tissues that send impulses to the central nervous system activating three centers (spinal cord, midbrain, and hypothalamus-pituitary) to cause analgesia. Low-frequency stimulation causes release of enkephalins and dynorphins at the spinal level to block incoming messages, and other transmitters are released with high-frequency stimulation. The midbrain uses enkephalin to activate the raphe descending system which inhibits spinal cord pain transmission by a synergistic effect of the monoamines, serotonin, and norepinephrine. The midbrain has a circuit that bypasses the endorphinergic links at high-frequency stimulation. At the level of the hypothalamus and pituitary, beta-endorphins are released into the circulation. The hypothalamus sends long axons to the midbrain and via beta-endorphins to activate the descending analgesia system.

13. Has research shown any other effects?

Needle insertion into tissue causes local changes in collagen and fascia, facilitating physical, chemical, and electrical communication across fascial planes. In muscle, needles trigger a dilation of blood vessels via a reflex action involving sympathetic nerve fibers. Needles inserted into paravertebral muscles result in dilatation of blood vessels in peripheral muscles at the same segmental level through a somatoautonomic reflex whose center is located in the contralateral anterior hypothalamus. Both the local and segmental needling result in muscle relaxation in the symptomatic area. A generalized decrease in peripheral sympathetic tone also has been noted after acupuncture. These findings help explain thermographic studies that show a normalizing increase in the temperature of chronic pain areas from acupuncture treatments given locally or distant to the painful site. Studies on tissue healing have demonstrated a measurable electrical current emanating from acupuncture points after needling. This current has been shown to modulate neurohormonal activity and activate tissue-repair mechanisms.

14. How can a physician become an acupuncturist?

Every state establishes its own requirements for licensure, and those requirements may vary over time. The first comprehensive training available for physicians in the United States, a 300-hour CME program offered by the Helms Medical Institute (HMI), is ongoing. Since HMI began in 1980, other programs throughout North America have been established. The American Academy of Medical Acupuncture (AAMA) was founded in 1987 to represent physician acupuncturists and promotes the integration of concepts from traditional and modern forms of acupuncture with western medical training to synthesize a comprehensive approach to health care. The American Board of Medical Acupuncture (ABMA) reviews acupuncture training programs and provides an opportunity for board certification in medical acupuncture. It has been agreed upon by the World Health Organization that 300 CME training hours is sufficient to assure a safe and capable medical acupuncturist, given their background as a physician.

Shorter courses, such as auricular acupuncture training, are available and often entail a weekend of didactic and hands-on work. Training in such a technique is useful, but the physician completing such a course would not be considered a medical acupuncturist qualified for board certification. Physicians may also attend comprehensive training programs that are designed to train non-physicians.

15. **How can acupuncture be integrated into the practice of a physiatrist?**
    Acupuncture is on a continuum of treatment options available to the physiatrist. The best approach is to gain experience with acupuncture and apply it where it is the most effective while maintaining a standard and responsible physiatric care. Acupuncture is an ideal skill in the hands of a physiatrist who can responsibly treat the patient while assessing the patient from a functional perspective. A physiatrist is well situated to coach the acupuncture patient toward realistic goals and a healthy lifestyle while utilizing active therapies as needed, thus enhancing the overall therapeutic outcome of treatments delivered.

WEBSITES

1. Acutrials
   Available at: www.acutrials.ocom.edu
2. American Academy of Medical Acupuncture (AAMA)
   Available at: www.medicalacupuncture.org
3. ClinicalTrials.gov
   Available at: www.clinicaltrials.gov
4. Helms Medical Institute
   Available at: www.HMIeducation.com
5. The Integrated Structural Acupuncture Course for Physicians
   Available at: www.AcuMed.org
6. National Center for Complementary and Alternative Medicine: Acupuncture
   Available at: www.nccam.nih.gov/health/acupuncture
7. Society for Acupuncture Research
   Available at: www.acupunctureresearch.org

BIBLIOGRAPHY

1. Helms JM. *Acupuncture Energetics: A Clinical Approach for Physicians.* Berkeley, CA: Acupuncture Publishers; 1995.
2. MacPherson H, Hammerschlag R, Coeytaux R, et al. Unanticipated insights into biomedicine from the study of acupuncture. *J Altern Complement Med.* 2016 Feb;22(2):101–107. doi: 10.1089/acm.2015.0184.
3. Stux G, Berman B, Pomeranz B. *Basics of Acupuncture.* 5th ed. New York, NY: Springer-Verlag; 2004.

CHAPTER 27

PERIPHERAL INJECTIONS: MEDICATIONS, JOINTS, BURSAE, TENDON SHEATHS/INSERTIONS, AND APPLICATIONS OF BOTULINUM TOXIN

Gerard P. Varlotta, DO, FACSM and Ib R. Odderson, MD, PhD

Poison and medicine are often the same thing, given in different proportions.
Alice Sebold (1963–present)

INJECTION MEDICATIONS: ANESTHETICS

1. How do local anesthetic medications work in peripheral joint and soft tissue injections?
   Local anesthetics reversibly block nerve transmission by inhibiting ion flux through sodium channels of the axon. As a result, the action potential does not reach the threshold, and nerve transmission ceases, resulting in anesthesia. The speed of onset, depth, and duration of anesthesia is based on characteristics of the nerve, anesthetic dosage, tissue site injected, and structure of the anesthetic module. Once injected, anesthetics are transported within the body by simple mechanical bulk flow, diffusion, and vascular transport. The location of injection, especially in highly vascular areas, affects the drug's absorption, duration of action, and toxicity.

2. How do I choose a local anesthetic?
   The choice of local anesthetic depends on the duration of the desired anesthetic effect. Chloroprocaine has a short duration of action. Lidocaine and mepivacaine have an intermediate duration of action, and bupivacaine, ropivacaine, and etidocaine have the longest duration of action. The duration of action is determined by the amount of drug bound to plasma proteins. Local anesthetics with a high protein-binding capacity have a longer duration of action. Adding vasoconstrictors such as phenylephrine, epinephrine, or norepinephrine also will prolong the effect of local anesthetics by decreasing the local absorption of the drug.

3. Which local anesthetics should be used and in what quantity?
   The anesthetic of choice for most musculoskeletal injections is usually 1% lidocaine without epinephrine. Bupivacaine 0.25% or 0.5% is useful in providing a longer analgesic effect. Longer-acting anesthetic agents should not be used in weight-bearing joints to minimize the potential destruction of an insensate joint. The amount injected depends on the size of the joint. The acromioclavicular, sternoclavicular, and elbow joints can take 1 to 2 mL of 1% lidocaine combined with the corticosteroid. The glenohumeral, knee, and hip joints can take 2 to 4 mL. Bupivacaine is often preferable for non–weight-bearing joints.

4. What are the complications related to local anesthetic use?
   Toxicity from local anesthetics is usually dose-related and is cumulative. It often results from rapid absorption from the injection site or an inadvertent intravascular injection. Peak plasma concentration occurs within 5 to 25 minutes.

5. What are the two organ systems and symptoms affected by local anesthetic toxic effects?
   These two organ systems are the central nervous system (CNS) and cardiovascular system. The CNS effects initially include dizziness, circumoral numbness, tinnitus, and blurred vision. Excitatory symptoms such as agitation, muscular twitching, or tremors precede CNS depression. Ultimately, convulsions, respiratory depression, and cardiac arrest can occur. The cardiovascular system symptoms include peripheral vasodilatation, myocardial depression, angina, bradycardia, arrhythmias, and cardiac arrest.

INJECTION MEDICATIONS: STEROIDS

6. How do glucocorticoids work?
   Glucocorticoids exert their action by blocking prostaglandin and leukotriene synthesis. They bind to specific intracellular receptors upon entering target cells and alter gene expression that regulates many cellular processes. The anti-inflammatory effect of glucocorticoids is due to its immunosuppressive action on leukocyte function and availability. The proposed mechanisms of action of corticosteroids are:

- Decrease synovial fluid complement
- Decrease neutrophil number
- Decrease synovial membrane/vascular permeability
- Decrease synovial fluid acid hydrolases
- Stimulation of synovial lining cell lysosomes
- Decrease number of mast cells in the synovium

7. **What glucocorticoids are available for use in peripheral joints, bursae, and tendon sheaths?**
The most widely used corticosteroids are listed in Table 27.1. These compounds were developed to reduce undesirable hormonal side effects with less rapid dissipation from the joint. None of these corticosteroid derivatives appears to have any superiority over another; however, triamcinolone hexacetonide is the least water-soluble preparation and thus provides the longest duration of effectiveness within the peripheral joint space.

8. **List the absolute and relative contraindications for intra-articular and extra-articular corticosteroid injections.**

Absolute contraindications

Infectious arthritis	Relative contraindications
Bacteremia	Juxta-articular osteopenia
Peri-articular cellulitis	Anticoagulant therapy
Acute injury	Joint instability
Osteochondral fracture	Hemarthrosis
Adjacent osteomyelitis	Joint prosthesis
Uncontrolled bleeding or clotting disorder	Questionable therapeutic benefit from prior injections

9. **What are the potential adverse effects of corticosteroid injection?**
Systemic absorption (more common with repeated injections)
Suppression of the hypothalamic-pituitary-adrenal axis
Iatrogenic Cushing's syndrome
Transient hyperglycemia and glucosuria
Glucocorticoid-induced osteoporosis
Local effects
Iatrogenic joint infection occurs at a rate of 0.0001% in properly prepared joints.
Steroid-induced arthropathy
Destructive arthropathy may occur from post-injection pain relief and overuse of the joint rather than steroid-induced cartilage injury.
Other rare local effects
Iatrogenic joint inflammation may occur if the site is prepared with an alcohol solution and disposable needles are used.
Tendon and ligament rupture can occur with systemic steroid use, frequent injection of weight-bearing joint or periarticular soft tissue, injections directly into tendon or ligament, or injection of a high dose of corticosteroids.
Post-injection flare or true crystal-induced arthropathy can occur in the presence of certain paraben preservatives used in local anesthetic preparations. The acute synovitis is self-limiting and responds well to ice, rest, and nonsteroidal anti-inflammatory drugs (NSAIDs). It can be avoided by using single-dose vials of lidocaine or by using

Table 27.1 Comparison of Commonly Used Glucocorticoid Steroids

AGENT	ANTI-INFLAMMA-TORY POTENCY[a]	PLASMA HALF-LIFE (MINUTES)	DURATION OF ACTION
Hydrocortisone (Cortisol)	1	90	Short
Cortisone	0.8	30	Short
Prednisone	4–5	60	Intermediate
Prednisolone	4–5	200	Intermediate
Methylprednisolone (Depo-Medrol)	5	180	Intermediate
Triamcinolone (Kenalog)	5	300	Intermediate
Betamethasone (Celestone)	25–35	100–300	Long

[a]Relative to hydrocortisone.

longer-acting bupivacaine that does not contain the paraben preservative. It is more common after the use of microcrystalline steroid preparations (triamcinolone hexacetonide).

Skin hypopigmentation and subcutaneous atrophy can occur if the depth of injection is less than 5 mm or the steroid is deposited along the needle tract during withdrawal.

10. **Why is proper implementation of the injections procedure important and can the procedure be done in isolation?**
The proper implementation of procedures results in good patient care, providing safety to the physician, and—most importantly—the patient. The safety of the patient is directly related to the physician's technical skills, knowledge of drug pharmacology, and his or her ability to recognize potential complications. The procedure should not be in isolation but rather integrated into a comprehensive treatment plan, including modalities, activity modification, bracing, oral medications, and physical therapy directed by the physiatrist.

11. **What are the indications for intra-articular steroid injections?**
The most common indications for intra-articular injections of steroids are for articular and periarticular inflammatory conditions and painful arthritic conditions. These include synovitis related to rheumatoid arthritis, osteoarthritis, adhesive capsulitis, meniscal derangement or tears, chondral defects, labral tears, and shearing damage of the articular cartilage as seen in maltracking of a joint.

12. **How much methylprednisolone acetate (depo-medrol) should be injected into a joint and in what frequency?**
Commonly larger joints (hip, knee, and shoulder) require injection of 40 mg, whereas medium-sized joints (wrist, elbow, and ankle) require 20 to 30 mg, and small joints (acromioclavicular, finger, and toe) require 10 to 20 mg. Larger joints can accommodate a volume of 2 to 4 mL, whereas smaller joints accommodate 1 to 2 mL. The most common frequency of injections is every 4 to 6 weeks, with a maximum of three injections. Arthroscopic debridement may be necessary if the patient's pain continues.

13. **Are there harmful effects of intra-articular injections of steroids?**
Since the introduction of hydrocortisone in 1951, there have been anecdotal reports of the deleterious effects of corticosteroid injections, including articular surface damage, osteonecrosis, and periarticular problems. These reports have been disputed, and the reported deleterious effects are transient when the injections are performed under accepted guidelines. Multiple injections beyond the recommended dosage or frequency can interfere with normal cartilage protein synthesis.

14. **Is the risk of infection for total knee arthroplasty increased after corticosteroids or hyaluronic acid injections?**
Perioperative corticosteroid or hyaluronic acid injection prior to 3 months before total knee arthroplasty increased the risk of periprosthetic joint infection by 40%. There is no difference in infection risk between medications or between single or multiple injections.

INJECTION TECHNIQUES

15. **What is the most common technique for intra-articular injections of peripheral joints?**
Most commonly, a 22-gauge 1.5-inch needle is used. The clinician should use slow, directed needle placement, avoiding forceful, sudden thrusts. Aspiration should be performed prior to injection to ensure that there is no blood return that may indicate an intravascular injection. Once the needle is placed in the appropriate location, the injectate should be delivered with a slow and steady force. If there is resistance to the introduction of the solution, the needle should be adjusted prior to continuing the injection. If a larger bore needle is necessary, a lidocaine wheal should be performed prior to the injection. A small amount of lidocaine should be used to flush the corticosteroids prior to its removal to avoid introduction into the subcutaneous skin. Pressure should be applied to the area after injection.

16. **When should vapocoolant spray be used?**
Local application of vapocoolant to the skin may be necessary in apprehensive patients to provide superficial anesthesia. The vapocoolant should be applied prior to the use of a cleansing agent, as the contents are aseptic but not sterile. The delivery is under pressure and should be applied with movement of the stream as to not cause a cryo-burn to the skin.

JOINTS

17. **In which disorders of the shoulder should anterior, superior, lateral, and posterior approaches be used?**
The anterior approach is most commonly used in bicipital tendinitis. The superior approach can be used to enter the acromioclavicular joint and, with further advancement, into the subacromial space. Care should be taken as not to advance the needle into the supraspinatus tendon. If resistance is met with the injection, the needle should

be withdrawn until the resistance is eliminated. The lateral injection can be used when treating supraspinatus tendinitis, especially when there is an enthesopathy or insertional pathology. Once again, care must be taken not to inject into the substance of the tendon. Most commonly, the posterior approach is used to treat supraspinatus tendinitis, subacromial bursitis, labral tears, adhesive capsulitis, and glenohumeral osteoarthritis.

18. **What structures are of concern and should be avoided when injecting the sternoclavicular joint?**
When injecting the sternoclavicular joint, the needle should be placed superficially in the joint to avoid penetration of the brachiocephalic veins.

19. **What is the safest injection technique when performing an intra-articular elbow injection?**
Injection of the elbow is safest when performed from the posterolateral approach. This avoids the major vessels and nerves in the medial and anterior aspect of the elbow.

20. **What specific disorders of the wrist require an intra-articular injection of corticosteroids? How should the injection be performed?**
Rheumatoid arthritis and osteoarthritis are the most common reasons for intra-articular wrist injections. Other wrist pathology includes scapholunate ligament and triangular fibrocartilage complex tears. All injections should be performed from the dorsal aspect of the joint. Because most of the wrist joints have interconnecting synovial spaces, the injection should be placed in the area of maximal tenderness or in the region of the most severe pathology.

21. **When is it necessary to inject the sacroiliac joints? How should the injection be performed?**
Synovitis and dysfunction of the sacroiliac joint may cause pain. The sacroiliac joint is composed of fibrous and synovial portions of the joint. With the patient prone, the fibrous portion can be injected medial to the posterior superior iliac crest. The synovial portion of the joint requires fluoroscopic guidance, with needle placement in the inferior portion of the joint. The results of injections may yield diagnostic information, and the therapeutic benefits are variable.

22. **What are the different approaches when injecting the hip?**
The best approach is the anterior approach performed under radiographic guidance. The anatomic landmarks are 2 cm distal to the anterior superior iliac spine and 3 cm lateral to the femoral artery. The needle is advanced at a 60-degree angle posteromedially until it enters the joint. When performing a hip injection from the lateral approach, a 3 to 4 inch needle needs to be used. Needle placement is just anterior to the greater trochanter.

23. **What are the most common axial joints that can cause a referred pain, mimicking peripheral joint pain?**
The most common axial joints are the facet (zygapophyseal) joints and costovertebral joints. Adjacent pathology should be investigated if the patient's peripheral joint pain is refractory to direct treatment.

24. **When should fluoroscopically guided injections be used when injecting a joint?**
Many small joints require the use of fluoroscopic guidance to ensure accurate placement of the corticosteroids into the joint. The intercarpal joints of the wrist, midfoot (Lisfranc and Chopart) joints, subtalar joints, and interphalangeal joints of the hand and foot may require the use of fluoroscopy. Fluoroscopic guidance of larger and deeper joints such as the hip and glenohumeral joints may be needed to confirm the placement of the medication in the intended location.

BURSAE

25. **Describe the structure and function of bursae.**
Bursae are synovial-lined fluid sacs that are located adjacent to joints. Inflammation within the bursa results from direct trauma or indirectly due to repetitive activities resulting in muscular weakness, musculotendinous contractures, and muscular imbalances altering joint mechanics. Bursae function to reduce friction between muscles, tendon skin, and bone. Most bursae are named by the anatomical structure that they are closest to and protect.

26. **What treatments are required to prevent chronic inflammation of the bursae?**
In addition to injections, other treatments used in bursitis include NSAIDs, therapeutic modalities, stretching, and strengthening exercises. Correction of the improper postural mechanics is essential to avoid chronic bursal inflammation.

27. **What is the most common bursitis in the shoulder? What are the causes?**
Subacromial (subdeltoid) bursitis is the most common bursitis of the shoulder. The bursa is located superior to the supraspinatus tendon, inferior to the acromion, behind the coracoacromial ligament, and beneath the deltoid muscle. Subacromial bursitis is secondary to rotator cuff tendinitis, impingement syndrome, cervical radiculitis/

radiculopathy, suprascapular neuropathy, and repetitive strain disorders of the periscapular muscles that result in scapular rotation with acromial depression.

28. Which approach is most commonly used in injection of subacromial bursitis?
The most common and easiest approach is a posterolateral approach. The needle placement is in the depression below the acromion, with the needle directed in an anterior, medial, and superior direction aiming toward the acromioclavicular joint. The total volume accepted by the bursa is 4 to 6 mL.

29. What is the most common bursitis around the elbow? What are its causes and treatment?
The most common bursitis around the elbow is olecranon bursitis, or Draftsman's elbow. It is usually secondary to direct trauma to the olecranon process of the ulnar bone but can also be seen in rheumatologic disorders such as gout. Aspiration with a larger needle (18 gauge), injection with corticosteroids, and application of a compression dressing are the recommended treatments. The needle insertion point should be proximal to the bursal swelling, as direct injection into the bursa may lead to the development of a chronically draining sinus tract.

30. What are the three most common types of bursitis around the hip?
Greater trochanteric, iliopsoas (iliopectineal), and ischial (Tailor's or Weaver's bottom) bursitis are seen around the hip. In greater trochanteric bursitis, the pain is lateral over the greater trochanteric prominence of the femur bone. The greater trochanteric bursa is located in the lateral, proximal thigh. The iliopsoas bursa is located anterior to the hip joint. The ischial bursa is located over the ischial prominence.

31. What structure can cause medial knee pain that is located inferior to the knee joint line?
The pes anserinus bursa is located on the medial aspect of the knee inferior to the joint line. It is found below the conjoined tendons of the semitendinosus, sartorius, and gracilis muscles. It is found in osteoarthritis, increased femoral anteversion of the hip, excessive pronation, and genu valgum deformities. There is an associated medial hamstring weakness on manual muscle testing of knee flexion seated or prone. An injection of corticosteroids into the bursa combined with heating modalities and a hamstring stretching and strengthening program are most effective in treatment of pes anserinus bursitis.

32. When is Achilles pain not Achilles tendinitis?
The retrocalcaneal (subtendinous) bursa is located between the posterior calcaneus and the Achilles tendon. The subcutaneous (Achilles) bursa is located superficial to the Achilles tendon. Inflammation of the subcutaneous bursa is found from direct pressure from the heel counter, especially with high-heeled shoes that cause plantar flexion of the ankle. The inflammation of the retrocalcaneal bursa occurs with pressure from tight heel counters, Achilles contractures, and in runners overtraining with a sudden increase in mileage. The diagnostic differentiation is made on clinical examination, with no tenderness of the Achilles tendon or the enthesis but tenderness below the Achilles in retrocalcaneal bursitis and superficial to the tendon in subcutaneous bursitis. Treatment consists of avoidance of direct pressure, training modification, anti-inflammatory medications, and physical therapy modalities. For refractory cases, an injection is helpful. Care needs to be taken not to perform the injection into the Achilles tendon, and the angle of the needle should be 15 to 20 degrees anteriorly from a lateral approach.

KEY POINTS: COMMON CAUSES OF BURSITIS AND TENDINITIS

1. Abnormal mechanics of the adjacent joint
2. Muscular weakness
3. Overuse/repetitive strain
4. Poor postural control
5. Proximal problem manifesting its effects distally (i.e., cervical radiculopathy resulting in weakness of the muscle group adjacent to the bursa)

TENDONS/ENTHESOPATHIES

33. What are the function and construct of tendon and tendon sheath? How do they compare to a coaxial cable television cable?
The tendon's function is to transmit the force of muscular contraction to the bone, thereby moving a joint. The organizational unit in a tendon is the collagen fibril, which together forms fascicles and, as a group, composes the tendon itself. Some tendons, especially long ones, are guided and lubricated along their paths by sheaths. The tendon is held close to the bone by a pulley system or fibrous arches. The copper inner core of the cable is the tendon, the white outer covering is the fluid in the sheath, and the tacks that hold the cable to the edge of the baseboard are the pulleys.

34. **What is an enthesopathy?**
The enthesis is the portion of the tendon as it inserts into the bone. Inflammation can occur in this attachment site, resulting in tendinitis pain and weakness of the corresponding muscle.

35. **In which tendon regions should injections be avoided?**
Injections should be avoided into the region of large weight-bearing tendons, including the patellar tendon, quadriceps tendon, and Achilles tendon.

36. **Why are patients prone to tendinitis in the shoulder joint?**
The shoulder is susceptible to the development of tendinitis for three basic reasons. First, the joint is subjected to a wide range of repetitive motions. Second, the space in which the musculotendinous unit functions is restricted by the coracoacromial arch, making impingement a likely possibility with extreme abduction with internal and external rotation. Third, the blood supply to the middle of the tendon is poor, thus making the healing of microtrauma more difficult. The primary cause of shoulder tendinitis is from an impingement of the supraspinatus tendon as it traverses under the acromial arch. With the arm at elevated positions, internal and external rotation causes an abrasion of the supraspinatus tendon. Partial-thickness, full-thickness, and complete tears of the supraspinatus tendon can occur. The cause of bicipital tendinitis is impingement on the biceps tendons at the coracoacromial arch. The onset is usually acute, occurring after overuse or misuse of the shoulder. Impingement can be caused by weakness, laxity, or contracture of the trapezius and periscapular musculature from repetitive use or cervical radiculopathy.

37. **How is bicipital tendinitis diagnosed and where do I inject to relieve the symptoms?**
The pain of bicipital tendinitis is constant, severe, and is localized in the anterior shoulder over the bicipital groove. Diagnosis is made by palpating the proximal and anterior aspect of the shoulder. Tenderness is found when the arm is externally rotated, bringing the bicipital groove under the clinician's finger. When the arm is internally rotated with continued pressure, the pain is absent. A catching moment while ranging the shoulder may accompany the pain and is usually indicative of subluxation of the tendon out of the groove. A positive Yergason's sign can also be found. Speed's test is a more dynamic test to reproduce the patient's symptoms as the tendon glides through the bicipital groove.
The injection of the biceps tendon sheath is performed with the patient seated. The bicipital groove is palpated with internal and external rotation. The needle direction should be at a 45-degree angle. The tendon sheath can accommodate approximately 2 mL of the corticosteroid/lidocaine preparation.

KEY POINTS: MEDICATIONS AND INJECTIONS

1. Avoid injection into Achilles, patellar, and quadriceps tendons.
2. "Say Grace before Tea" is a way to remember the components of the conjoined tendons on the medial aspect of the knee (**S** = **S**artorius, **G** = **G**racilis, **T** = semi**T**endinosis).
3. The *watershed area* is the region of the tendon that is most susceptible to the development of tendinitis due to the poor blood supply.

38. **What is tennis elbow?**
Tennis elbow, or lateral epicondylitis, is an inflammation of the fibrous origin of the extensor digitorum and extensor carpi radialis brevis muscles (the longus portion of the muscle inserts above the elbow). It occurs at the lateral aspect of the elbow usually secondary to excessive or repetitive dorsiflexion forces of the extensor group.
Tenderness over the lateral epicondyle and pain with resisted dorsiflexion are diagnostic of lateral epicondylitis. Cozen's test is done with the elbow in full extension with a passive stretch of the wrist extensors.
Injections of corticosteroids into the lateral epicondylar region are very helpful in pain reduction. Additional treatment, including NSAIDs, relative rest, physical modalities (heat, ultrasound, and electrical stimulation), extensor stretching, and wrist extension strengthening, is necessary to prevent recurrences. The use of a tennis elbow band or strap is helpful in deflecting the wrist extension forces from the insertional site. The location of the brace pressure should be 1 inch below the point of maximum tenderness. In patients playing tennis, reduction in string tension and enlargement of the grip of the racket are helpful in preventing recurrences. Surgery is necessary in cases refractory to the above-mentioned treatment and usually is associated with tears.

39. **What are the treatments for piriformis syndrome?**
The piriformis traverses the posterior pelvis from the sacrum to the posterolateral greater trochanter. Tenderness is found in the muscle belly, with weakness in hip abduction and extension. The most common location of tenderness is 3 cm caudal and lateral to the midpoint of the sacrum's lateral border. It can be associated with sciatica. The muscle functions as an internal rotator of the hip. Treatment includes NSAIDs, relative rest, physical modalities (heat, ultrasound, and electrical stimulation), piriformis stretching, and hip abduction and extension

strengthening. In refractory cases, injection and orthotics may be necessary. Rarely, and in the presence of a taut band, surgery may be necessary.

40. Where do you inject for iliopsoas tendinitis?
The injection is performed in the proximal and medial aspect of the thigh at the insertion of the iliopsoas onto the lesser tuberosity. Fluoroscopy is usually necessary for the accurate localization of the injection.

41. Identify the two locations of ITB tendinitis.
The ITB can become inflamed proximally as it traverses the greater trochanter and distally over the lateral femoral condyle.

42. What test is diagnostic of an iliotibial band contracture? How is it performed?
The Ober test is diagnostic for iliotibial band contracture. It is performed with the patient in the side-lying position with the hip and knee flexed to 90 degrees. The hip is abducted, and then extended with the knee maintained in a flexed position. A leg is then allowed to go toward an adducted position. If the knee remains above horizontal, then there is an ITB contracture.

43. What functional changes are seen in a visual gait analysis of someone with ITB Tendinitis?
Excessive internal rotation of the entire lower extremity is found and results as a tight ITB passes over the greater trochanter and of the distal ITB when there is internal rotation of the tibia on the femur. Pronation, excessive femoral anteversion, torsional abnormalities, and gluteus medius weakness are some of the causes of ITB tendinitis.

KEY POINTS: REHABILITATION

1. Proximal lateral thigh pain that does not resolve with an injection into the greater trochanteric bursa injection usually indicates gluteal tendinitis (in the presence of a positive Trendelenburg sign and hip abduction weakness) or hip arthritis (in the presence of reduced internal rotation of the hip).
2. Heel pain in the absence of tenderness of the Achilles enthesis may represent an injectable pain emanating from the retrocalcaneal bursa.
3. Periscapular pain and weakness are usually a secondary cause of posterior shoulder pain resulting from rotator cuff tendinitis, subacromial bursitis, acromioclavicular arthropathy, subacromial impingement, or cervical radiculopathy but also from a pectoral contracture that needs resolution with a focused physical therapy program.
4. In the diagnosis of anterior knee joint pain, the presence of patellar tendinitis usually represents a rotational malalignment of the lower extremity (femoral anteversion, patellar angle, increased tibial torsion, or excessive pronation), contracture of the thigh musculature (quadriceps and/or hamstring), proximal gluteal weakness, or a combination of the above that needs to be resolved with a combination of treatments (physical therapy, injections, and bracing).

TREATMENT OF MUSCLE OVERACTIVITY WITH BOTULINUM TOXIN

44. What are the applications for botulinum toxin?
Chemodenervation is used successfully for muscle overactivity disorders such as spasticity, dystonia, and dystonic tremor. Other applications include headache, migraine, neuropathic pain (trigeminal neuralgia, phantom pain, and residual limb pain), sialorrhea, and hyperhidrosis. The overall treatment objectives are to address painful conditions, minimize activity limitations by improving active and passive function, and improve quality of life, including reducing disfigurement.

45. What is the mechanism of action of neurotoxins?
The current neurotoxins produce a partial chemical denervation by inhibiting the release of acetylcholine from the neuromuscular and neuroglandular junctions as well as inhibiting other neurotransmitters involved in pain perception. Type A neurotoxins cleave SNAP-25 (synaptosomal-associated protein of 25 kDa, SNAP-25) on the plasma membrane, while neurotoxin B cleaves the VAMP (vesicle associate membrane protein) on the synaptic vesicle.

46. Which product should I use?
There are currently four commercial toxins available in the United States: onabotulinumtoxinA (Botox, onaBoNT/A), abobotulinumtoxinA (Dysport, aboBoNT/A), incobotulinumtoxinA (Xeomin, incoBoNTA/A) and rimabotulinumtoxinB (Myobloc, rimaBoNT/B). They are all effective when injected into the correct muscles or sites with the appropriate amounts. RimaBoNT/B is the only toxin available in a sterile solution with a pH of 5.6. IncoBoNT/A and aboBoNT/A come as a freeze-dried powder, while onaBoNT/A is a spray-dried powder. They all have different potencies, and units of one toxin cannot be compared to or converted to units of another toxin. There are no conversion factors, so if switching from one toxin to another toxin, use the recommended starting dose for the new toxin. However,

there is a body of literature that has reported efficacy and safety at a ratio of 2.5 Dysport units to 1 Botox unit in the treatment of patients who previously received onaBoNT/A therapy.

Full prescribing information for Dysport, Ipsen available at: https://ipsen.within3.com/ipsen-advisor-insight platform/rooms/1426/topics/1555/resources/6107/viewer/8973.pdf. Accessed April 7, 2019.

47. Are there absolute contraindications to Botox injections and should Botox be withheld in an anticoagulated patient with therapeutic INR levels?

Absolute Contraindications

Yes, absolute contraindications are individuals with known hypersensitivity to any ingredient in the formulation, myasthenia gravis, and infection at the injection site.

Use extreme caution when injecting individuals with peripheral motor neuropathic diseases (ALS), conditions interfering with neuromuscular transmission (myasthenia gravis, aminoglycosides), and patients with dysphagia and respiratory compromise.

Adverse reactions are mainly related to the spread of the toxin resulting in dysphagia, aspiration, bronchitis, and pneumonia. This is particularly the case with cervical injections where the toxin may spread to the pharyngeal constrictors but can also result from limb injections. Generalized weakness can be seen with prolonged use.

ANTICOAGULATION

With therapeutic INR levels, the risk is only marginally increased, and chemodenervation should not be withheld regardless of the muscles involved. When injecting into deep-leg compartment, use the smallest gauge needle possible.

Dressler D, Ebke M, Saberi FA, Schrader C. Botulinum toxin therapy in patients with oral anticoagulation: Is it safe? *Toxicon.* 2019;156S1:S26 (54).

48. Is it effective to continue chemodenervation on a long-term basis?

Continued benefits can be expected with chronic therapy. Data from prolonged clinic treatments of muscle overactivity for up to 19 years showed that dosage and duration did not change over time. Other studies have shown an increased dose over time when using data from the first visits and not allowing for a titration period. It is interesting that adverse events tended to decrease over time.

Czyz CN, Burns JA, Petrie TP, Watkins JR, et al. Long-term botulinum toxin treatment of benign essential blepharospasm, hemifacial spasm, and Meige syndrome. *Am J Ophthalmol.* 2013;156:173–177.

Ramirez-Castaneda J, Jankovic J. Long-term efficacy, safety, and side effect profile of botulinum toxin in dystonia: A 20-year follow-up. *Toxicon.* 2014;90:344e348.

KEY POINTS: CHEMODENERVATION WITH BOTULINUM TOXINS

1. All available toxins are effective when injected into the correct muscles or sites with the appropriate amounts.
2. Anticoagulation: With therapeutic INR levels, the risk is only marginally increased, and chemodenervation should not be withheld regardless of the muscles involved.
3. A clinical test for non-responders: Inject the EDB (extensor digitorum brevis) and compare atrophy and function to the non-injected side. A more dramatic response can be seen when injecting the frontalis or brow muscle.

Bonus questions and answers available online.

JOINT

49. What are the different visco-supplementation that can be used in osteoarthritis of the knee and their intended benefits?

Numerous visco-supplementation products are available: Hyaline G-F 20 (Synvisc & Synvisc- One), and sodium hyaluronate (Hyalgan, Supartz, Euflexxa, Gelsyn-3, Durolane) and Hyaluronan (Orthovisc, Monovisc, Hymovis). Hyaluronate is a component of synovial fluid, which is responsible for its viscoelasticity. The source of hyaluronate is rooster combs. Clinical studies demonstrate that injections of visco-supplementation substances into the joints of osteoarthritic knees result in a reduction of pain and improvement of function in the majority of patients. Prospective clinical data in knee osteoarthritis patients have shown benefit of treatment up to 52 weeks following a single course of injections. Additional injection may be needed every 6 to 12 months depending on the duration of benefit. A comparison of the products is found in Table 27.2.

Table 27.2 Visco-supplementation Products

TRADE NAME	ACTIVE INGREDIENT	# OF INJECTIONS/SERIES	MG/SERIES
Supartz	Sodium hyaluronate (25 mg)	3 or 5 weekly	75 or 125
Synvisc	Hylan g-f 20 (16 mg)	3 weekly	48
Synvisc-One	Hylan g-f 20 (48 mg)	Once	48
Hyalgan	Sodium hyaluronate (20 mg)	3 or 5 weekly	60 or 100
Orthovisc	Sodium hyaluronate (30 mg)	3 weekly	90
Euflexxa	Sodium hyaluronate (20 mg)	3 weekly	60
Monovisc	Hyaluronan (88 mg)	Once	88
Gel-One	Sodium Hyaluronate (30 mg)	Once	30
Gelsyn-3	Sodium Hyaluronate (8.4 mg)	3 weekly	50.4
Durolane	Sodium Hyaluronate (20 mg)	Once	60
Hymovis	Hyaluronan (24 mg)	2 weekly	48

BURSA

50. What is most commonly associated with greater trochanteric bursitis?

The most common etiology of greater trochanteric bursitis is gluteus medius weakness. Pain is localized lateral but also proximal to the greater trochanter. Weakness is found in hip abduction on manual muscle testing in a side-lying position and on single leg standing (Trendelenburg sign). Visual gait analysis reveals a truncal tilt to the affected side (compensated) or tilt to the contralateral side (uncompensated), Trendelenburg gait pattern. Additionally, internal rotation of the hip seated and supine should be tested to determine if limitations are present, indicating hip osteoarthritis. Observation of leg length discrepancies and scoliosis should be noted and treated. Testing for iliotibial band (ITB) contracture with the performance of an Ober maneuver should be done. Injections in isolation without resolution of the gluteus medius tendinitis, ITB contracture, leg length discrepancy, and pronation may lead to a return in pain.

51. How soon after an intraarticular hip injection can a patient have a total hip joint replacement (THR) and similarly, how soon after an intraarticular knee injection can a patient have a total knee replacement (TKR)?

HIP

The postoperative infection rate is increased by 40% if there is an injection into the hip joint within 3 months of the surgery. The infection rate after 1 year was 2.06% in patients who did not receive an injection, but that rate increased to 2.81% in patients who had an injection within 3 months prior to when an injection was administered within 12 weeks before THR. Injections appeared safe (0.87% rate of infection) if performed more than 3 months pre-operatively.

KNEE

The rates of surgical site infection were significantly higher in patients with an injection prior to TKR than those without (4.4% vs. 3.6%), as were the rates of infection requiring a return to the operating room (1.5% vs. 1%). The rate of infection requiring a return to the operating room remained significantly higher for patients receiving injections in the months prior to surgery, with an odds ratio (OR) of 1.8 for an injection within 1 month of surgery, and an OR of 1.4 for an injection 7 months prior to TKR.

Richardson SS, Schairer WW, Sculco TP, Sculco PK. Comparison of infection risk with corticosteroid or hyaluronic acid injection prior to total knee arthroplasty. *J Bone Joint Surg Am.* 2019 Jan 16;101(2):112–118.

Schairer, WW, Nwachukwu, BU, Mayman, DJ, Lyman, S and Jerabek, SA. Preoperative hip injections increase the rate of periprosthetic infection after total hip arthroplasty. *J Arthroplasty.* 2016;31(9 Suppl):166–169

52. Identify a common bursitis associated with the knee and also for the heel and outline the treatment for each.

KNEE

Prepatellar bursitis (housemaid's knee) is found in patients who perform kneeling activities, usually associated with employment (e.g., carpenters). Treatment can include NSAIDs, therapy modalities, and quadriceps stretching.

The injection is performed from the superior and medial approaches. Avoidance of kneeling and the use of knee pads are effective in preventing the return of pain.

HEEL

Calcaneal bursitis is a common cause of heel pain that mimics plantar fasciitis. It occurs after prolonged walking or running, especially in footwear, with poor shock absorption. It is diagnosed by tenderness over the calcaneus without pain on toe-walking or plantar fascial stretch. Shock-absorbing heel cups, Achilles stretching, modalities, and injections are helpful in resolving the pain. Injection into the bursa located more superficially than the plantar fascia is recommended for patients who are refractory to other treatments.

TENDON

53. What is the difference between little leaguer's elbow and golfer's elbow?

The difference is the age of the participants. Little leaguer's elbow/golfer's elbow, also known as medial epicondylitis, is an inflammation of the origin of the flexor carpi radialis and flexor digitorum group. It occurs on the medial aspect of the elbow and is usually secondary to excessive or repetitive volar flexion forces of the wrist. Tenderness over the medial epicondyle and pain with resisted wrist flexion is diagnostic of medial epicondylitis. Injections of corticosteroids into the medial epicondylar region are very helpful in pain reduction. Additional treatment, including NSAIDs, relative rest, physical modalities (heat, ultrasound, and electrical stimulation), flexor stretching, and wrist flexion strengthening, is necessary to prevent recurrences. The use of a tennis elbow band or strap is helpful in deflecting the wrist flexor forces from the insertional site. In children involved in throwing sports, modification of pitching/throwing technique, a reduction of the amount of pitching, and strengthening of the rotator cuff and lower extremities are recommended. In golfers, modification of technique to prevent repetitive wrist motion is recommended. Surgery is necessary in cases refractory to the previously mentioned treatment, and it is usually associated with tears.

54. Describe de Quervain's tenosynovitis, name the diagnostic test and outline a treatment plan.

ANATOMY AND PATHOPHYSIOLOGY

De Quervain's stenosing tenosynovitis is caused by an inflammation and swelling of the tendons of the abductor pollicis longus and extensor pollicis brevis at the level of the radial styloid process. This inflammation and swelling are usually the result of trauma to the tendon from the wrist's repetitive twisting motions. It is commonly seen in pregnant women due to weight gain and swelling within the first dorsal wrist compartment.

DIAGNOSTIC TEST

The diagnostic test for this syndrome is Finkelstein's maneuver. The thumb is placed inside the closed hand, and the wrist is passively ulnar deviated with a reproduction of pain.

TREATMENT

Treatment should include NSAIDs, relative rest, physical modalities (heat, ultrasound, and electrical stimulation), thumb spica splinting, and exercises in a wrist-neutral position. Injections of corticosteroids can be performed into the first dorsal wrist compartment at the level of the radial styloid. Surgery is recommended for cases refractory to conservative care.

55. Identify three common types of tendinitis in the lower extremities, explain how they are acquired, describe the clinical exam, and outline a treatment plan.

HAMSTRING TENDINITIS

Etiology

The knee is subjected to significant repetitive motion under weight-bearing conditions. The relatively poor blood supply of the musculotendinous insertions makes it susceptible to the development of hamstring tendinitis. Inciting factors may include long-distance running, dancing injuries, or vigorous use of lower extremity strengthening exercise equipment. A contracture and weakness of the hamstring are usually found on the ipsilateral side of the tendinitis.

Clinical Exam

Evaluation of patients with constant and severe pain reveals a lurch-type antalgic gait. There is severe pain to palpation over the tendinous insertion onto the tibia, with the medial portion of the tendon more commonly affected than the lateral portion. Crepitus and pain usually are elicited when palpating the tendon while the patient flexes the affected knee. There is usually an associated contracture and weakness of the affected hamstring.

Treatment

Treatment should include NSAIDs, relative rest, physical modalities (heat, ultrasound, and electrical stimulation), hamstring stretching, and open and closed chain hamstring strengthening. Plyometrics and sport-specific exercises should be included prior to return to full activities. Occasionally, foot orthotics with medial posting can be used to reduce stress on the medial hamstring. Rarely, injection of the region around the hamstring tendon is necessary to reduce inflammation.

POSTERIOR TIBIAL TENDINITIS

Etiology

Posterior tibial tendinitis is seen most commonly in athletes and elderly women. Excessive pronation is the usual cause of an excessive stretch to the tendon. Running on soft or uneven surfaces and improper shoe wear has been implicated in the development of chronic stretching of the posterior tibial tendon.

Clinical Exam

The clinical examination of posterior tibial tendonitis includes tenderness posterior to the medial malleolus and pain with resisted inversion of the foot when maximally plantarflexed. There is usually a contracture of the Achilles tendon when the ankle is placed in subtalar neutral position. Subtalar laxity is also found that contributes to the excessive linear stretch of the posterior tibial tendon and the asymmetrical stretch on the medial border of the planter fascia. In viewing the patient from the back while standing, there is an increased calcaneal valgus and a drop of the navicular bone inferiorly. There are other rotational asymmetries that can contribute to posterior tibial tendonitis, including femoral anteversion, genu varum, and tibial torsion.

Treatment

Treatment should include NSAIDs, relative rest, physical modalities (heat, ultrasound, and electrical stimulation), Achilles stretching in subtalar neutral, and inversion strengthening. Foot orthoses are necessary in chronic cases or in patients exerting excessive pronation forces. Rupture is rare, but when it occurs, the only treatment is shoe wear accommodation or subtalar fusion.

PLANTAR FASCIITIS

Etiology

Plantar fasciitis is an inflammation of the tight fibrous band on the plantar aspect of the foot, usually at the insertion onto the calcaneus. It can be found in patients with excessive pronation and Achilles contractures.

Clinical Exam

The clinical examination of plantar fasciitis reveals tenderness on the plantar aspect of the foot at the distal portion of the calcaneus and pain on forced dorsiflexion of the ankle. There is usually a contracture of the Achilles tendon when the ankle is placed in subtalar neutral position. Subtalar laxity is also found and contributes to the excessive asymmetrical stretch on the medial border of the plantar fascia. In viewing the patient from the back while standing, there is an increased calcaneal valgus and a drop of the navicular bone inferiorly. There are other rotational asymmetries that can contribute to plantar fasciitis, including femoral anteversion, genu varum, and tibial torsion.

Treatment

Treatment should include NSAIDs, relative rest, physical modalities (heat, ultrasound, and electrical stimulation), Achilles stretching, and gastrocnemius strengthening. The use of foot orthotics and a night dorsiflexion splint may be helpful in pain reduction. The use of padded or gel heel pads is usually not effective. Injections of corticosteroids into the site of the insertion of the plantar fascia are helpful in refractory cases. Correction of other intrinsic or extrinsic biomechanical factors is helpful in pain reduction.

Botox

56. What are the risks for developing neutralizing antibodies to Botox and what are the clinical tests for non-responders?

Risks

All protein-based products are potentially immunogenic. Generally, the larger the protein load over time (total amount injected and the frequency of injections), the greater the risk. Antigenic protein load is highest for rimaBoNT/B (10.7 ng/vial); significantly lower for onaBoNT/A (0.8 ng/vial), and incoBoNT/A (0.6 ng/vial) and unknown for aboBoNT/A)A. IncoBoNT/A is a purified neurotoxin without complexing proteins (including hamagglutinating and non-hamagglutinating proteins). The lack of complexing proteins seems to reduce the antigenicity of incoBoNT/A. So far, there have only been two patients worldwide who developed neutralizing antibodies to incoBoNT/A. If patients develop suboptimal therapeutic benefit, they can be switched to a lesser immunogenic toxin. In general, avoid booster injections, and inject the lowest dose needed.

With long-term use of neurotoxins for about 15 years, the risk of neutralizing antibodies was up to 30% to 40%. Interestingly, all patients in the study had at least a partial response to therapy.

Clinical Tests for Non-Responders

The Frontalis Antibody Test, FTAT, or the Unilateral Brow Injection, UBI, where botulinum toxin is injected unilaterally into the frontalis or corrugator muscles. If the patient is resistant to the toxin, there will be no unilateral paralysis, and the patient remains able to raise both eyebrows. For a less demonstrative muscle, use the EDB (extensor digitorum brevis) and compare atrophy and function to the non-injected side.

Jankovic J. Botulinum toxin: State of the art. *Mov Disord.* 2017;32:1131–1138.

Kamm C, Schümann F, Mix E, Benecke R. Secondary antibody-induced treatment failure under therapy with incobotulinumtoxinA (Xeomin®) in a patient with segmental dystonia pretreated with abobotulinumtoxinA (Dysport®). *J Neurol Sci.* 2015;350:110–111.

Albrecht P, Jansen A, Lee J-I, Moll M, Ringelstein M, et al.: High prevalence of neutralizing antibodies after long-term botulinum neurotoxin therapy. *Neurology.* 2019;92:e48–e54.

57. What are the best injection techniques to use: EMG, ultrasound, or E-Stim?

The three most important points for chemodenervation are location, location, location. Ultrasound, electromyography, and electrostimulation are superior to manual needle placement, and end-plate injections improve outcomes compared to multisite quadrant injections.

EMG guidance is recommended for all muscle injections except for facial muscles, where only surface anatomy is used. In addition to locating the muscle, the intensity of the auditory EMG signal is an excellent guide to estimate the amount of neurotoxin needed for the individual muscle and to locate the best site within the muscle.

Ultrasound guidance with EMG provides a tremendous advantage for deeper muscles as well as for smaller muscles. Without EMG guidance, the intensity of muscle contraction is lost, which makes dosing challenging to assess.

Audio-only EMG. This may cause the less-experienced injector to mistake the sound of muscle denervation potentials for motor units.

E-stim is particularly useful if the muscle spasms are dynamic and only present when reflexes are elicited, such as during gait with an upgoing toe or other activities, as well as for specific muscles in focal dystonia (writer's cramp) where contractions only occur with activity. E-stim may be the only way to locate the appropriate muscle and avoid the weakening of nearby muscles.

Location. Target the mid-belly of the muscle where the majority of motor endplates are found. For larger muscles, more injection sites such as 2 to 4 sites provide a better distribution of the toxin. Motor endplates are generally spread throughout the muscle with a few exceptions where they are located linearly across the muscle near the middle (biceps, brachialis, flexor carpi ulnaris, and pronator teres).

58. Do neurotoxin volume and dilution matter?

High-volume injections distant from the endplate are more efficacious than low volumes closer to the endplate. However, smaller muscles such as cervical muscle are limited in terms of total volume that can be injected, and a higher concentration may be needed. Higher volumes injected in the center of a smaller muscle may spread beyond the muscle boundaries. This author, therefore, recommends a 1:1 or 1:2 dilutions (100 u or 50 u per 1 cc saline) for cervical muscles (onaBoNT/A, incoBoNT/A), and higher volumes (1:4, 25 u per cc saline) for larger muscles in the limbs and trunk.

Chan AK , Finlayson H, Mills PB. Does the method of botulinum neurotoxin injection for limb spasticity affect outcomes? A systematic review. *Clin Rehabil* 2017;31:713–721.

Ramirez-Castaneda J, Jankovic J, Comella C, Dashtipour K, et al. Diffusion, spread, and migration of botulinum toxin. *Mov Disord* 2013;28:1775–1783.

BIBLIOGRAPHY

Balch HW, Gibson JMC, el Ghobarey AF, et al. Repeated corticosteroid injections into knee joints. *Rheumatol Rehabil.* 1997;16:137–140

Bedard, NA, Pugely, AJ, Elkins, JM, et al. Do intraarticular injections increase the risk of infection after TKA? *Clin Orthop Relat Res.* 2017;475:45–52.

Czyz CN, Burns JA, Petrie TP, Watkins JR, et al. Long-term botulinum toxin treatment of benign essential blepharospasm, hemifacial spasm, and meige syndrome. *Am J Ophthalmol.* 2013;156:173–177.

Dreyfuss P, Cole AJ, Pauza K. Sacroiliac joint Injection techniques. *Phys Med Rehabil Clin North Am.* 1995;6:785–813.

Finkelstein D, Smith MK, Faden R. Informed consent and medical ethics. *Arch Ophthalmol.* 1993;111:324–326.

Full Prescribing Information for Dysport, Ipsen. Available at: https://ipsen.within3.com/ipsen-advisor-insight-platform/rooms/1426/topics/1555/resources/6107/viewer/8973.pdf. Accessed April 7, 2019.

Geiringer SR, Bowyer BL, Press JM. Sports medicine. The physiatric approach. *Arch Phys Med Rehabil.* 1993;74:S428–S432.

Gray RG, Gottlieb NL. Intra-articular corticosteroids. An updated assessment. *Clin Orthop.* 1983;177:235–263.

Gray RG, Gottlieb NL. Intra-articular corticosteroids, basic science, and pathology. *Clin Orthop Rel Res.* 1983;177:235–263.

Lennard TA, ed. *Pain Procedures in Clinical Practice.* 2nd ed. Philadelphia: Hanley & Belfus; 2000.

Marks MR, Gunther SF. Efficacy of cortisone injection in treatment of trigger fingers and thumbs. *J Hand Surg*. 1989;14A:722–727.

Mazanec DJ: Pharmacology of corticosteroids in synovial joints. *Phys Med Rehabil Clin North Am*. 1995;6:815–821.

Micheo WF, Rodriques RA, Amy E. Joint and soft-tissue injections of the upper extremity. *Phys Med Rehabil Clin North Am*. 1995;6: 823–840.

Millard RS, Dillingham MF. Peripheral joint injections: Lower extremity. *Phys Med Rehabil Clin North Am*. 1995;6:841–849.

Nirschl RP. Elbow tendinosis/tennis elbow. *Clin Sports Med*. 1992;11:851–870.

Pfenninger JL. Injections of joints and soft tissues: Part II. Guidelines for specific joints. *Am Fam Physician*. 1991;44:1690–1701.

Price R, Sinclair H, Heinrich I, et al. Local injection treatment of tennis elbow—hydrocortisone, triamcinolone, and lidocaine compared. *Br J Rheumatol*. 1991;30:39–44.

Ramirez-Castaneda J, Jankovic J. Long-term efficacy, safety, and side effect profile of botulinum toxin in dystonia: A 20-year follow-up. *Toxicon*. 2014;90:344e348.

Stefanich RJ. Intra-articular corticosteroids in treatment of osteoarthritis. *Orthop Rev*. 1986;15:65–71.

Strichartz, GR. *Neural Physiology and Local Anesthetic Action*. In MJ Cousins, PO Bridenbaugh (Eds.). *Neural Blockade in Clinical Anesthesia and Management of Pain*. 2nd ed. Philadelphia, JB: Lippincott; 1988:25–45.

Young ER, MacKenzie TA. The pharmacology of local anesthetics—A review of the literature. *J Can Dent Assoc*. 1992;58:34–42.

CHAPTER 28

PHYSIATRIC IMAGE-GUIDED SPINE INTERVENTIONS: AGGRESSIVELY TREATING THOSE PATIENTS WE CAN IMPROVE

Michael B. Furman, MD, MS, FAAPMR, Shannon L. Schultz, MD, MPH, FAAPMR, Caitlin Cicone, DO, Ninad Durganand Sthalekar, MD, and Frank J.E. Falco, MD, FAAPMR

Grant me the courage and skill to aggressively treat those patients that I can improve, ...the strength and serenity to be conservative with those I cannot, ...and the wisdom to know the difference.
Adapted by Michael Furman from Reinhold Niebuhr's Serenity Prayer

KEY POINTS

1. In an extraforaminal (far lateral) lumbar disc herniation, the superior spinal nerve will be affected (e.g., extraforaminal herniation of L4–5 disc will affect the L4 spinal nerve). In a central lumbar disc herniation, the inferior spinal nerve root will be affected (e.g., central herniation of L4–5 disc will affect the L5 spinal nerve). In the cervical spine, because eight cervical spinal nerves exit more horizontally, the C7 nerve transits and exits between the C6–C7 intervertebral foramen. The C8 nerve transits and exits between the C7 and T1 intervertebral foramen, etc.
2. Preservative-free, non-particulate steroid preparations are recommended as the sole injectate for cervical and thoracic transforaminal epidural steroid injections and first-line treatment for lumbar transforaminal epidural steroid injections.
3. The major risk associated with cervical transforaminal epidural steroid injections is an inadvertent steroid injection of the vertebral artery.
4. When patients are taking anticoagulants, lower-risk procedures, including medial branch blocks, disc stimulation and radiofrequency ablation have decreased potential for bleeding complications.
5. All Z-joints are innervated by two nerve branches: one from the posterior ramus above and one at the same segmental level. For "n" consecutive, ipsilateral Z-joints, $n + 1$ nerves should be blocked.

1. What is interventional physiatry?
   Interventional physiatry integrates a thorough clinical evaluation with diagnostic and therapeutic spinal and musculoskeletal procedures and appropriate rehabilitation for comprehensive care. The focus is to reduce pain and increase function; exercise is medicine. The diagnostic and therapeutic interventions include epidural injections, sacroiliac joint injections, diagnostic nerve blocks, intra-articular injections, nerve ablations, sympathetic blocks, intradiscal procedures, vertebral augmentation, spinal cord, and dorsal root ganglion (DRG) stimulation and much more. This exciting field is ever-expanding and continually focused on optimal non-operative care.

2. How does one differentiate among disc bulge, herniation, protrusion, extrusion, and sequestration on lumbar MRI? In the axial plane, what zones/anatomical landmarks are used to describe the location of disc herniations?
   Disc bulge, herniation, protrusion, extrusion, and sequestration are pathoanatomic classifications of disc displacements, used to describe imaging findings (Table 28.1 and Fig. 28.1a–c). Bulges and herniations are differentiated based on the percentage of disc involvement (Table 28.2 and Fig. 28.2). Herniations are further classified: Protrusions and extrusions are differentiated based on the shape of the disc material. Sequestration describes an extruded disc fragment that has lost all continuity from the disc (i.e., a "free fragment"). Migration identifies the direction an extruded segment has traveled in relation to the parent disc.
   The direction of disc herniations in the axial plane can be more precisely identified by their occurrence in different zones. These zones can be defined as central, right or left central (most common area of herniation as the posterior longitudinal ligament is weakest here), subarticular, foraminal, and extraforaminal [2] (Fig. 28-3). Older terminology texts may describe these areas as posterior-lateral, paracentral, or far-lateral.

Table 28.1 Types of Disc Displacements

TYPE OF DISC DISPLACEMENT	DESCRIPTION
Bulge	Nuclear material extending beyond the vertebral margin but with no annulus defect (*not* considered a type of herniation); can be symmetric or asymmetric
Herniation	Localized or focal displacement of disc material beyond the limits of the intervertebral disc space into or through an annulus defect; further classified as protrusions or herniations
Protrusion	When the distance between the edges of the disc material beyond the disc space is **less** than the distance between the edges at its base
Extrusion	When the distance between the edge of the disc material beyond the disc space is **greater** than the distance between the edges at its base; this can be described as a **"pinch."**
Sequestration	A type of extrusion when no disc tissue bridges the displaced portion and the tissues of the disc of origin; this can be described as a **"free fragment."**
Migration	Describes the direction the disc material from an extruded disc travels away from the parent disc (it may or may not still have continuity)

Adopted from Fardon DF, Williams AL, Dohring EJ, et al. Lumbar disc nomenclature version 2.0: recommendations of the Combined Task Forces of the North American Spine Society, American Society of Spine Radiology, and American Society of Neuroradiology. *Spine J.* 2014;14(11):2525–2545.

The herniations often contact adjacent nerves. At each disc level, a nerve either exits slightly superior to the disc level or traverses centrally and exits inferior to the disc level.

3. In a right foraminal or extraforaminal herniation of the L3–L4 disc, which spinal nerve is involved and should be treated with a more specific selective injection?
   A foraminal or **extraforaminal herniation** contacts the **exiting** spinal nerve superior to that disc level after it exits (laterally) and descends past the disc. Because the L3 spinal nerve exits slightly superior to the L3–L4 disc, a foraminal or extraforaminal herniation would affect the spinal nerve superior to that level. Therefore, a right L3–L4 extraforaminal disc herniation will affect the exiting right L3 spinal nerve.
   Incidentally, **central herniations** affect the **traversing** nerve roots before they exit inferior to that disc level. Therefore, a central L3–L4 disc herniation would affect the traversing L4 nerve prior to its exit through the L4 neural foramen inferior to the disc (Fig. 28.4) [3].

4. In a left C6–7 disc extraforaminal herniation, what spinal nerve is involved and should be treated with a more selective injection?
   Unlike in the lumbar and thoracic spine, an exiting cervical spinal nerve travels superior to the vertebral body for which it is named. Furthermore, in the cervical spine, the nerve exits more horizontally than in the thoracic or lumbar spine. Because of this horizontal trajectory, the exiting nerve does not "transit" down to an inferior level as it does in the lumbar spine.
   Due to these anatomical differences, both a central herniation and extraforaminal cervical disc herniation will affect the exiting spinal nerve. For example, a left C6–7 central and extraforaminal herniation will both contact the left C7 spinal nerve (Fig. 28.5) [3].

5. Which nerves innervate the zygapophyseal (Z)-joints (aka facet joints) in the cervical spine? Lumbar spine?
   All Z-joints, except two (C2–3 and L5–S1 Z joints), are innervated by two medial branches of the dorsal rami. In the cervical spine, C3–4 to C7–T1 receive innervation by medial branches from the dorsal rami above and below the segmental level. For example, the C4–5 joint receives innervation from the C4 and C5 medial branches of the dorsal rami. The C2–3 joint is an exception in the cervical spine as it is innervated solely by the third occipital nerve.
   In the lumbar spine, the Z-joints receive innervation from the dorsal ramus above and the dorsal ramus at the segmental level. The medial branches in the lumbar spine originate from their respective dorsal rami and then course inferiorly (i.e., the medial branch of L4 lies at the junction of the L5 transverse process and superior articular process) as noted in Fig. 28.6a. The numbering nomenclature in the lumbar spine is less intuitive than in the cervical spine, for example, the L4–L5 Z-joint receives innervation from the L3 and L4 medial branches of the dorsal rami nerves. Although the numbering nomenclature at L5-S1 is similar to the other lumbar levels, please note that the L5 nerve is the dorsal ramus as this level does not split into medial and lateral branches. Specifically, the L5–S1 Z-joint receives innervation from the L4 medial branch and the L5 *dorsal ramus.* To reiterate, the innervation to these Z-joints comes

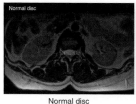
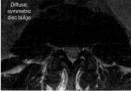
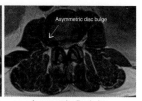

Normal disc

Symmetric disc bulge:
Disc tissue going beyond the edges
of the ring apophyses, throughout
the circumference of the disc

Asymmetric disc bulge:
Asymmetric bulging of a disc < 25%
of the disc circumference

A

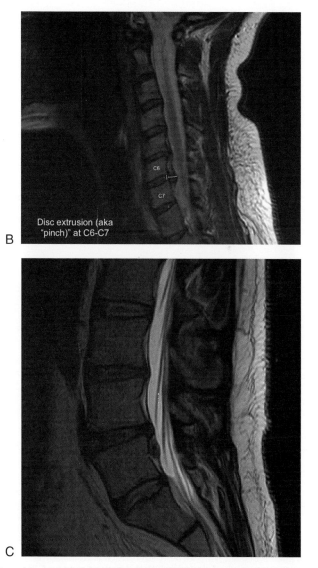

B

C

Fig. 28.1 (A) Normal disc and disc bulge. Disc bulge: Nuclear material extending beyond the vertebral margin, but with no annulus defect; NOT a disc herniation. Classified as symmetric or asymmetric. (Original photos.) (B) Disc herniation. Localized or focal displacement of disc material beyond the limits of the intervertebral disc space into or through an annulus defect; classified as *extrusions (aka "pinch")* or *protrusions.* (Original photo.) (C) Disc sequestration. Sequestration describes an extruded disc fragment that has lost all continuity from the disc (i.e., a "free fragment"). (Original photo.)

Table 28.2 Classification of Disc Bulges and Herniations

DESCRIPTION	DEGREE OF DISPLACEMENT (% DISC CIRCUMFERENCE)
Localized/focal	<25% or <90 degrees
Broad-based	25%–50%
Generalized	>50%

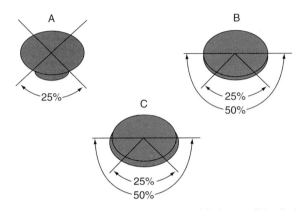

Fig. 28.2 Bulges and herniations can be further described based on the degree of displacement: (A) Localized protrusion; (B) Broad-based protrusion; (C) Generalized protrusion. (Adopted from Fardon DF, Milette PC. Nomenclature and classification of lumbar disc pathology: recommendations of the combined task forces of the North American Spine Society, American Society of Spine Radiology, and American Society of Neuroradiology. *Spine*. 2001;26[5]:E93–E113.)

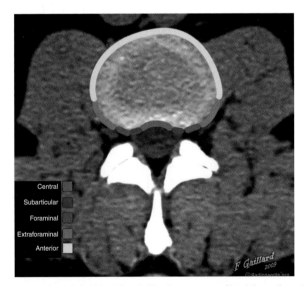

Fig. 28.3 Disc herniation zones can be central, right or left central (most common area of herniation as the posterior longitudinal ligament is weakest here), subarticular, foraminal, and extraforaminal. (Modified from: Case courtesy of A. Prof Frank Gaillard. Available at: Radiopaedia.org, rID: 36344 https://radiopaedia.org/articles/intervertebral-disc-disease-nomenclature?lang=us.)

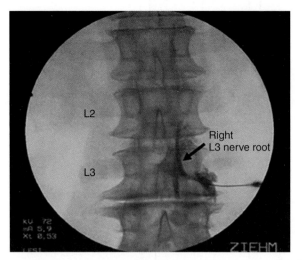

Fig. 28.4 The right L3 nerve can be involved as it traverses centrally past the L2–L3 disc or laterally as it exits the right L3–4 (L3) foramen. (Photo courtesy of: Furman MB, Mehta AR, Kim RE, et al. Injectate volumes needed to reach specific landmarks in lumbar transforaminal epidural injections. *PM&R Journal.* 2010;2[7]:625–635.)

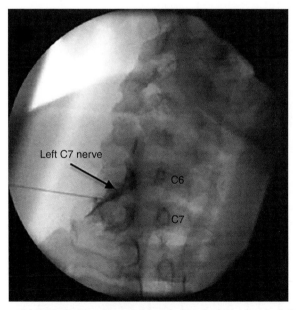

Fig. 28.5 The left C7 nerve can be involved as it traverses centrally past the C6–7 disc or laterally as it exits the left C6–7 (C7) foramen. (Original photo.)

from the medial branch above and at the segmental level (or the L5 dorsal ramus). In addition, the medial branch nerves are named for their originating somatic nerves and are **not** named for the transverse process they cross.

Due to the dual innervation, when performing a single Z-joint (n) block at any level at or inferior to C3–4, two nerves need to be anesthetized ($n + 1$). If two consecutive Z-joints are treated ipsilaterally, then three nerves need to be anesthetized. If one were to treat the L4–L5 and L5–S1 Z-joints, then the nerves to be anesthetized would be the L3 and L4 medial branches and the L5 dorsal ramus. See Fig. 28.6a–b for cervical and lumbar Z-joint innervation [3, 4].

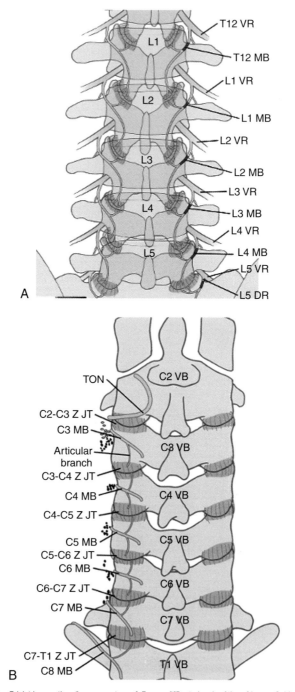

Fig. 28.6 (A) Lumbar spine Z-joint innervation. (Image courtesy of: Furman MB, et al., eds. *Atlas of Image-Guided Spinal Procedures.* 2nd ed. Philadelphia, PA: Elsevier; 2018.) (B) Cervical spine Z-joint innervation. (Image Courtesy of: Furman MB, et al., eds. *Atlas of Image-Guided Spinal Procedures.* 2nd ed. Philadelphia, PA: Elsevier; 2018.)

6. **What should be considered prior to performing a radiofrequency denervation procedure of a lumbar zygapophyseal (Z)-joint?**

Patients should have a confirmed diagnosis of Z-joint pain. This cannot be validly diagnosed by clinical impression, physical exam, or radiographic imaging alone. The recommended method of making this diagnosis and minimizing the large percentage of placebo responders (approximately 30% false-positive rate) is to use a double-block paradigm: A comparative blockade of the medial branch nerves on two different visits using two different anesthetic agents significantly reduces the false-positive response. The patient should have at least 50% to 80% relief following both sets of medial branch blocks to be considered a positive response [4].

7. **What is discitis?**

Discitis is the most concerning complication of an intradiscal procedure or an intervention that enters the disc inadvertently (e.g., infraneural transforaminal epidural steroid injection), with a reported incidence of 0.05% to 1.3% for each disc level. The most common pathogen is *Staphylococcus epidermidis*. Individuals who develop discitis typically present with severe back pain and spasms 2 to 4 weeks after the procedure. Back pain is increased by any activity and relieved by rest. Patients may report fevers and chills and/or have an elevated temperature. The C-reactive protein (CRP) and erythrocyte sedimentation rate (ESR) are usually increased at an average of 20 days, followed by a positive bone scan at an average of 33 days. Although ESR and CRP are highly sensitive, MRI with gadolinium is considered the best means for definitive diagnosis (higher specificity). It may show retrodiscal infection and spondylodiscitis, in which conservative treatment with IV antibiotics is sufficient. In cases of retrodiscal abscess, operative intervention should be considered [5, 6].

8. **What findings on physical exam provide conclusive evidence of sacroiliac joint pathology?**

None. There are several physical exam maneuvers that can help to lead to a suggestive diagnosis of sacroiliac joint pathology. These include the Gillet test, the Gaenslen test, the Patrick or flexion abduction, and external rotation (FABER) test, the posterior shear (POSH), or thigh thrust test, the resisted abduction (REAB) test, and the Yeoman test. Patients may also point to within 2 inches of the posterior superior iliac spine (PSIS) to indicate the site of maximal pain.

Despite providing a high predictive value, it is widely accepted that the physical examination gives valuable but not conclusive information concerning the presence of sacroiliac joint syndrome (SIJS) and that confirmation of SIJS requires a positive sacroiliac joint block [7].

9. **In a lumbar transforaminal epidural steroid injection, what is the "safe triangle"? What structures delineate its borders?**

In a two-dimensional anteroposterior (AP) view, the superior border of the safe triangle is the pedicle, the medial border is the nerve root/dural sleeve, and the lateral border is the vertical portion of the vertebral body (Fig. 28.7).

When performing lumbar transforaminal epidural steroid injections, it is best to avoid directly contacting the dura or spinal nerve. By targeting the safe triangle, the area where the needle tip should be introduced, direct

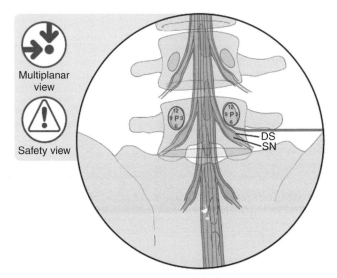

Fig. 28.7 Needle placement for a lumbar transforaminal epidural steroid injection typically targets the "safe triangle." Placing the needle tip in the supraneural "safe triangle" (pedicle superiorly and spinal nerve inferomedially) helps avoid piercing the spinal nerve, but vascular structures may still be encountered in this location. (Image courtesy of: Furman MB, et al., eds. *Atlas of Image-Guided Spinal Procedures*. 2nd ed. Philadelphia, PA: Elsevier; 2018.)

contact with these structures is rare. The safe triangle typically contains only the sinuvertebral nerve and its accompanying vessels. At times, the anterior medullary artery may lie within the "safe triangle," which may increase the risk of embolic phenomena. Hence, this "safe" triangle terminology is a misnomer. It is, therefore, prudent to use live contrast injection and multi-planar imaging to recognize and correct intravascular flow patterns prior to steroid administration [3, 5, 6].

10. When performing a cervical transforaminal epidural steroid, what structures should be avoided? What are the potential complications associated with these structures?
    Neurovascular injury is a primary concern when performing cervical transforaminal epidural steroid injections. The incidence of fluoroscopically confirmed intravascular uptake of contrast has been shown to be as high as 19.4% in cervical transforaminal injections [8]. When intravascular injection of a particulate steroid occurs, it can result in embolism formation and subsequent infarction. There are two major vascular structures to be avoided when performing the procedure:
    The **anterior spinal artery,** which receives supply from the cervical radicular arteries. When injecting a steroid solution such as depot preparations, the particulate material can act as an embolus and theoretically lead to spinal cord infarction or cerebral infarction.
    The **vertebral artery,** which lies adjacent and ventral to the spinal nerve. Local anesthetic injected into the vertebral artery can lead to seizure. Injection of particulate matter could lead to vertebrobasilar thrombosis and brain stem infarction.

11. What is the most common potential complication associated with an interlaminar epidural steroid injection?
    The most common complication is thecal sac puncture, occurring in 2% to 5% of lumbar epidurals. The most notable effect is a spinal headache. Infection, direct trauma to the spinal cord, nerve trauma, intravascular injections, and epidural hematomas (extremely rare) may occur. Severe cases of epidural hematomas present with profound weakness and usually occur in the immediate postprocedural period. These complications may result in devastating sequelae in the cervical or thoracic spine. Most complications can be avoided by using sterile technique, accurate needle placement with multi-planar imaging, and having a thorough understanding of anatomy and flow patterns [5, 6].

12. After a lumbar epidural steroid injection, a patient reports a headache that does not change with position. Would you consider doing a blood patch?
    This scenario is not consistent with a spinal headache. Spinal headaches are exacerbated in the upright position and improve upon lying supine. These headaches occur secondary to an inadvertent puncture of the dura during a spinal procedure. They may begin within an hour to several days after the procedure based on the triggering mechanism. The mechanism of cerebrospinal fluid (CSF) leakage led to the rationale for the several therapeutic methods currently used in the conservative management of spinal headaches. Hydration is instituted with the intent of increasing the production of CSF such that it exceeds its loss through the puncture site, thus restoring the CSF pressure to normal. Caffeine is an optional supplement that seems to be effective because of its vasoconstrictor effect.
    If a spinal headache persists after 24 hours of conservative treatment consisting of rest, IV fluids, and analgesic therapy, an epidural blood patch can be performed. This is done by placing a needle in the epidural space in the vicinity of the dural puncture and aseptically injecting autologous blood. The blood clots and seals the punctured region of the dura [6].

13. What are the indications for implantation of a spinal cord stimulator (SCS)?
    Spinal cord stimulators are used for the treatment of neuropathic pain conditions and involve the placement of stimulator leads with electrodes into the dorsal epidural space. Indications for SCS placement are complex regional pain syndrome, failed back surgery syndrome, peripheral neuropathy, and phantom limb pain. In Europe, it has also been used to treat angina and symptoms of vascular claudication. Outcomes are often better when patients have a more substantial component of appendicular pain, as opposed to axial back pain. Confirmation that there are no treatable causes of the patient's pain as described in imaging or electrodiagnostic studies is recommended. Absolute contraindications for SCS placement are infection, anticoagulation that cannot be stopped, drug abuse, and severe psychiatric illness. Prior to implantation of an SCS, a psychological evaluation is typically required.
    DRG stimulation has more recently been introduced into the field as an alternative neuromodulation technique to the traditional SCS. This type of stimulator acts on the DRG itself, which has been identified as an appropriate target for therapeutic interventions as it houses the primary sensory neurons. DRG stimulation may be more effective in treating localized, discrete areas of chronic neuropathic pain, without involving unaffected dermatomes. [9]

14. Describe the new advances in the field of interventional spine procedures.
    • **Interspinous Process Decompression (IPD):** IPD offers a minimally invasive percutaneous approach to the management of spinal stenosis with neurogenic claudication. This serves as an alternative to surgical decompression in a subset of patients with spinal stenosis (primarily moderate). IPD involves the placement of a stand-alone inter-spinous process spacer device that acts as an extension blocker to decrease the amount

of compression on neural components. This procedure is performed percutaneously and does not require the surgical removal of tissue resulting in less disruption to the normal anatomy when compared with surgical decompression [10].

- **Regenerative Medicine (PRP, mesenchymal stem cell, etc.):** The possibility of applying regenerative medicine to the management of spine pathology continues to expand. Regenerative medicine aims to improve or restore normal function by enhancing cellular migration, replication, and modeling. There continues to be a need for well-designed studies supporting the use of biologics as there are studies out there that both confirm and reject their application. In patients who have failed traditional treatment options, the use of biologics may serve as a reasonable alternative however, additional studies are needed.

- **Basivertebral Nerve Ablation (i.e., Intracept):** Within the vertebral body is a network of nerves referred to as the basivertebral nerve (BVN), which supplies the innervation to the vertebral endplates. The BVN is responsible for the transmission of pain signals, and in degenerated/damaged vertebral endplates, there is an increase in nerve density. Evidence is now suggesting that degenerated endplates can be the source of chronic low back pain, with the BVN being the source of pain transmission [11]. Procedures such as Intracept are minimally invasive procedures that target the BVN and aim to eliminate pain via ablation of this neural network.

15. **What types of steroids are used in epidural steroid injections, and what are the potential side effects?**

Steroids used for interventional spine procedures can be divided into the categories of particulate and non-particulate. Particulate steroids include those such as methylprednisolone, betamethasone, and triamcinolone, whereas dexamethasone is considered to be a much smaller or non-particulate steroid. Particulate steroids have a longer duration of action; however, they have been associated with neurovascular injury due to the formation of aggregates that may result in occlusion of an artery or embolization.

Non-particulate steroids have a small particulate size and do not aggregate, making them a safer steroid by minimizing the risk of neurovascular complications (i.e., spinal cord injury and stroke). While non-particulate steroids may have a shorter duration of action, they have not been shown to be inferior or less effective than particulate steroids.

Another distinction can be made regarding preservative-containing versus preservative-free steroid preparations. While the injection of preservative-containing steroids into the epidural space has not resulted in adverse events, when it has been injected intrathecally, neurological injuries have been reported. For this reason, preservative-free, non-particulate steroid preparations are recommended as the sole injectate for cervical and thoracic transforaminal epidural steroid injections, and first-line treatment for lumbar transforaminal epidural steroid injections. [3]

16. **What are Modic changes, how are they classified, and are they clinically relevant?**

Modic changes are abnormal bone marrow lesions of the vertebral bodies that occur adjacent to a diseased disc. They are placed into one of three categories, as described below, based on characteristic appearance on MRI (Table 28-3 and Fig. 28.8). Type I and type II changes are thought to be associated with pain. These changes may help identify patients with chronic low back pain that have failed conservative management who will respond to newer therapeutic advances in the field, such as basivertebral ablation (as described in question 14) [11].

17. **What factors should be considered regarding ceasing or continuing anticoagulants/antiplatelet (AC/AP) agents when performing interventional procedures?**

The decision to cease or continue AC/AP should be determined on a case-by-case basis to best balance the risk of thrombotic events with that of an epidural (or other) hematoma. Spine Intervention Society (SIS) and American Society of Regional Anesthesia and Pain Medicine (ASRA) have specific guidelines regarding this subject, but even these remain controversial. The following must be understood for each case.

- Why is the patient receiving the AC/AP agent, and what is the risk of stopping it?

Table 28.3 Modic Changes		
TYPE	**MRI APPEARANCE**	**WHAT IS IT ASSOCIATED WITH?**
Modic Type I	Bright on T2; Dark on T1 (Type I = one bright image)	• Inflammatory edema • Associated with disruption/fissuring of the endplate
Modic Type II	Bright on T2; Bright on T1 (Type II = two bright images)	• Fatty infiltration • Result of marrow ischemia
Modic Type III	Dark on T2; Dark on T1	• Sclerosis of vertebral body • Not associated with pain

Adopted from Lotz JC, Fields AJ, Liebenberg EC. The role of the vertebral endplate in low back pain. *Global Spine* J. 2013;3(3):153–164. Doi:10.1055/s-0033-1347298

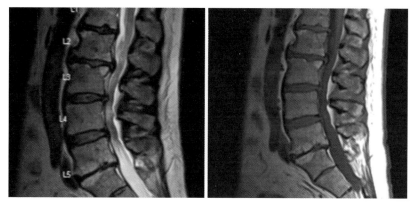

Fig. 28.8 Example of type II Modic changes. (Original photos.)

The reason for and duration of AC/AP should be determined prior to further decision-making. The risk associated with stopping the AC/AP agent is that of a thrombotic event that the medication was intended to prevent. If an interventionist wants to consider discontinuing the AC/AP agent, this should be done in conjunction with the physician prescribing/recommending the AC/AP agent.
- Is the intervention truly warranted, or can it be changed to a less risky procedure?

Lower bleeding risk procedures, including medial branch blocks, disc stimulation, and radiofrequency ablation, have decreased potential for bleeding complications. SIS, ASRA, and others have created risk stratification tables. For example, medial branch blocks have less potential bleeding risks than interlaminar epidural steroid injections.
- What is the risk of performing the chosen intervention without holding the medication?

The main concern would be that of an epidural (or other) hematoma [12, 13].

REFERENCES

1. Elkersh MA, Simopoulos TT, Bajwa ZH. Fundamentals of interventional pain medicine. *Neurologist.* 2005;11(5):285–293.
2. Fardon DF, Williams AL, Dohring EJ, et al. Lumbar disc nomenclature: version 2.0: recommendations of the combined task forces of the North American Spine Society, American Society of Spine Radiology, and American Society of Neuroradiology. *Spine J.* 2014;14(11):2525-2545.
3. Furman MB, Berkwits L, Cohen I, et al., eds. *Atlas of Image-Guided Spinal Procedures.* 2nd ed. Philadelphia, PA: Elsevier; 2018.
4. Manchikanti L, Hirsch JA, Falco FJ, Boswell MV. Management of lumbar zygapophysial (facet) joint pain. *World J Orthop.* 2016;7(5):315–337.
5. Benoist M, Boulu P, Hayem G. Epidural steroid injections in the management of low-back pain with radiculopathy: an update of their efficacy and safety. *Eur Spine J.* 2011;21(2):204–213.
6. Depalma MJ, ed. *iSpine: Evidence-Based Interventional Spine Care.* New York, NY: Demos Medical Publishing; 2011.
7. Zelle BA, Gruen GS, Brown S, et al. Sacroiliac joint dysfunction: evaluation and management. *Clin J Pain.* 2005;21(5):446–455.
8. Furman MB, Giovanniello MT, O'Brien EM. Incidence of intravascular penetration in transforaminal cervical epidural steroid injections. *Spine.* 2003;28(1):21–25.
9. Kumar K, Toth C, Nath RK, Laing P. Epidural spinal cord stimulation for treatment of chronic pain—some predictors of success. A 15-year experience. *Surg Neurol.* 1998;50(2):110–120; discussion 120–121.
10. Nunley PD, Patel VV, Orndorff DG, Lavelle WF, Block JE, Geisler FH. Five-year durability of stand-alone interspinous process decompression for lumbar spinal stenosis. *Clin Interv Aging.* 2017;12:1409–1417.
11. Lotz JC, Fields AJ, Liebenberg EC. The role of the vertebral endplate in low back pain. *Global Spine J.* 2013;3(3):153–164. doi:10.1055/s-0033-1347298
12. Furman MB, Bernstein J, McCormick ZL, Schneider BJ. Concerns regarding "Interventional spine and pain procedures in patients on antiplatelet and anticoagulant medications (second edition)." *Reg Anesth Pain Med.* 2019 Jan 11;44(3):416-417.
13. Furman MB, Plastaras CT, Popescu A, Tekmyster G, Davidoff S, Kennedy DJ. Should antiplatelet medications be held before cervical epidural injections? *PMR.* 2014 May;6(5):442–450.

WEBSITES

1. Spine Intervention Society Available at: https://www.spineintervention.org/
2. American Society of Interventional Pain Physicians Available at: http://www.asipp.org/
3. American Society of Regional Anesthesia and Pain Medicine Available at: http://www.asra.com/

Bonus questions and answers are available online.

REHABILITATION OF PATIENTS WITH SEVERE VISUAL OR HEARING IMPAIRMENTS: INNOVATIONS FOR PERSON-CENTERED FUNCTION

CHAPTER 29

John-Ross Rizzo, MD, Mahya Beheshti, MD, and Stanley F. Wainapel, MD, MPH

Seeing, hearing, feeling, are miracles, and each part and tag of me is a miracle...
From *Leaves of Grass*, Walt Whitman (1819–1892)

KEY POINTS: SEVERE VISUAL IMPAIRMENT

1. About 65% of patients with low vision or blindness are over age 65.
2. Stroke and traumatic brain injury produce frequent and sometimes subtle visual impairments, which will adversely affect outcome if unrecognized and untreated.

1. **What is the prevalence of vision and visual impairment?**
   Worldwide, 1.3 billion people have distance or near vision impairments (VI):188,500,000 have mild impairment; 217 million are moderately to severely impaired; 36,000,000 are blind; and 826,000,000 have near VI.[1]

2. **What are the most common causes of VI?**
   - Older adults: cataract, glaucoma, age-related macular degeneration, diabetic retinopathy.
   - Young and middle-aged adults: diabetic retinopathy, retinitis pigmentosa.
   - Children: congenital (cataract, albinism), neurological (retinopathy of prematurity, anoxic or post-infectious cortical vision loss).
   - In developing countries, infectious causes are major factors in VI across all ages (trachoma, onchocerciasis, mycoses).[2]

3. **How are VI classified nationally and internationally?**
   In the United States, legal blindness is defined as:
   - Corrected visual acuity 20/200 or less in the better eye, or
   - Visual field of 20 degrees or less in the better eye
   - Low vision includes corrected visual acuity between 20/70 and 20/200 or visual fields exceeding 20 degrees from the point of fixation in better eye.[3]
     The World Health Organization (WHO) defines low vision as a person with low vision as one who has impairment of visual functioning even after treatment and/or refractive correction, and has a visual acuity of less than 20/60 (6/18) to light perception, or a visual field of less than 10° from the point of fixation, but who uses, or is potentially able to use, vision for the planning and/or execution of a task. The *International Classification of Diseases 11* classifies VI into distance and near VI.
   Distance VI
   - Mild—visual acuity worse than 20/40 to 20/60
   - Moderate—visual acuity worse than 20/60 to 20/200
   - Severe—visual acuity worse than 20/200 to 20/400 or central visual field 20° or less but more than 10°
   - Blindness—visual acuity worse than 20/400 or central visual field 10° or less
   Near VI
   - Near visual acuity worse than 6/12 or 6/19 with existing correction.[4]

4. **How does VI affect physical function?**
   VI produces deficits in basic and instrumental activities of daily living (ADL) and can be associated with increased risk of falls and resulting hip fractures.[5–8]

5. How can patients access vision rehabilitation services?

An ophthalmologic evaluation documenting the degree of vision loss is sent to a state agency for the blind/visually impaired, which authorizes low vision, vision rehabilitation, and vocational rehabilitation services.

6. What are the fundamental strategies for vision rehabilitation?
   a. Vision Enhancement: devices or techniques that maximize utility of residual visual function
   b. Vision Substitution: technology or techniques not requiring vision, using intact senses such as hearing or touch.[9–11]

7. Name some vision enhancement techniques.

These can be remembered with the mnemonic "IMAGE":

Illumination
Magnification
Altered contrast
Glare reduction
Expanders of visual field

8. Describe common vision substitution techniques.
   - Mobility: Cane, guide dog, sonic devices
   - Tactile: Braille books/devices, raised markings
   - Recorded: Talking books, radio reading services
   - Synthetic speech: Computers with verbal output, talking watches/calculators, Newsline for the Blind (newspapers via telephone)
   - Computer-generated vision systems: computer vision; deep learning and machine learning techniques leveraging robust computational resources from computers or similar technologies
   - Special ADL techniques: Cooking, money identification
   - Vision restoration: gene therapy, genetic editing (CRISPR), retinal prostheses, photoreceptor transplantation.[12–14]

9. Can computers help visually impaired people?

Computers with synthetic speech output, screen reading software, optical character recognition software/scanner/desktop and mobiles, Braille output, or voice-activated operation enhance informational and professional opportunities for those unable to read ordinary-sized print.

10. What are the functional outcomes in patients with visual and neuromusculoskeletal disabilities?

It depends on the disability. A study suggested that 75% of blind amputees became functional prosthetic users, and blind stroke patients have had similar results.[15] However, disparate studies suggest that patients with multisensory impairment in addition to traumatic brain injury have lower functional independence measure, cognitive and motor scores compared to those with little or no sensory impairment.[16,17] Oculomotor dysfunction has been reported in 68% to 90% of patients with stroke and has been negatively associated with quality of life.[18–20]

11. Who provides funding for vision rehabilitation services?

Usually, funding is provided by a state Commission for the Blind rather than standard third-party payers (Medicare/Medicaid). Some occupational and/or physical therapists provide vision rehabilitation, and these may be reimbursed.

12. How many people have hearing impairments?

Approximately 466,000,000 people (over 5% of the world's population) have disabling hearing loss (34,000,000 children and 432,000,000 adults). In the US, 48,000,000 people have significant hearing loss, including 3,000,000 children. Approximately 37,500,000 adults (15%) aged 18 and over report some trouble hearing.[21] As of 2005, about 1 out of 20 Americans were deaf or hard-of-hearing. Nearly 1,000,000 were functionally deaf.[22]

13. When is hearing loss a rehabilitation problem?

Difficulty hearing affects communication, education, exchange of ideas, carrying out orders, and the pure pleasure of listening and responding. Socially incapacitating hearing loss occurs when a pure tone average loss reaches 40 dbHL or greater in the better ear for frequencies of 300 Hz to 3000 Hz (speech frequencies), and in children with hearing loss greater than 30 dB in the better ear.[21] Severe hearing loss is present with 61 dB to 80 dB loss. Hearing loss of more than 81 dB is defined as deafness or profound loss of hearing.[23]

14. Is there a bottom line for hearing aids?

A licensed practitioner should provide hearing aids. Aids ordered via mail, phone, or over the internet may be cheaper but are not likely to be fitted or prescribed for the individual patient's needs, resulting in poor function and compliance. Proper hearing tests include an audiogram performed by a certified audiologist, which identifies hearing loss and its severity, determines whether the loss is conductive or sensorineural, and provides information about inner ear function and the patient's reliability reporting hearing quality.[24]

Bonus questions and answers are available online.

REFERENCES

1. Bourne RRA, Flaxman SR, Braithwaite T, et al. Magnitude, temporal trends, and projections of the global prevalence of blindness and distance and near vision impairment: a systematic review and meta-analysis. *Lancet Glob Health.* 2017;5(9):e888.
2. Bansal S, Grover G, Grover M, et al. Isolated sphenoid mucormycosis presenting as visual impairment: changing trends? *Am J Otolaryngol.* 2010;31(1):64.
3. Varma R, Vajaranant TS, Burkemper B, et al. Visual impairment and blindness in adults in the United States: demographic and geographic variations from 2015 to 2050. *JAMA Ophthalmol.* 2016;134(7):802.
4. World Health Organization. Trachoma; 2018. Available at: https://www.who.int/news-room/fact-sheets/detail/trachoma.
5. Manduchi R, Kurniawan S. Mobility-related accidents experienced by people with visual impairment. *AER J.* 2011;4(2):44.
6. Felson DT, Anderson JJ, Hannan MT, et al. Impaired vision and hip fracture. *J Am Geriatr Soc.* 1989;37(6):495.
7. Klein BEK, Klein R, Lee KE, et al. Performance-based and self-assessed measures of visual function as related to history of falls, hip fractures, and measured gait time: The Beaver Dam Eye Study. *Ophthalmology.* 1998;105(1):160.
8. van Landingham SW, Willis JR, Vitale S, et al. Visual field loss and accelerometer-measured physical activity in the United States. *Ophthalmology.* 2012;119(12):2486.
9. Maidenbaum S, Abboud S, Amedi A. Sensory substitution: closing the gap between basic research and widespread practical visual rehabilitation. *Neurosci Biobehav Rev.* 2014;41:3.
10. Zöllner M, Huber S, Jetter H-C, et al. *NAVI—A Proof-of-Concept of a Mobile Navigational Aid for Visually Impaired Based on the Microsoft Kinect.* In Campos P, Graham N, Jorge J, eds. *INTERACT 2011, Part IV: Human-Computer Interaction.* Berlin: Springer; 2011:584–587.
11. Niu L, Qian C, Rizzo J-R, et al. A wearable assistive technology for the visually impaired with door knob detection and real-time feedback for hand-to-handle manipulation. In *Proceedings of the 2017 IEEE International Conference on Computer Vision Workshops (ICCVW).* New York: IEEE; 2018:1500–1508.
12. Margalit E, Maia M, Weiland JD, et al. Retinal prosthesis for the blind. *Surv Ophthalmol.* 2002;47(4):335.
13. Burnight ER, Gupta M, Wiley LA, et al. Using CRISPR-Cas9 to generate gene-corrected autologous iPSCs for the treatment of inherited retinal degeneration. *Mol Ther.* 2017;25(9):1999.
14. Markowitz SN. State-of-the-art: low vision rehabilitation. *Can J Ophthalmol.* 2016;51(2):59.
15. Wainapel SF, Kwon YS, Fazzari PJ. Severe visual impairment on a rehabilitation unit: incidence and implications. *Arch Phys Med Rehabil.* 1989;70(6):439.
16. Devine N, Olen C. Inpatient physical therapy rehabilitation provided for a patient with complete vision loss following a traumatic brain injury. *Brain Injury.* 2015;29(7–8):993.
17. Jack CIA, McGalliard JN. Rehabilitation in elderly people with visual impairment. *Rev Clin Gerontol.* 1999;9(1):770.
18. McKean-Cowdin R, Varma R, Wu J et al. Severity of visual field loss and health-related quality of life. *Am J Ophthalmol.* 2007;143(6):1013.
19. Varma R, Wu J, Chong K, et al. Impact of severity and bilaterality of visual impairment on health-related quality of life. *Ophthalmology.* 2006;113(10):1846.
20. Vu HT, Keeffe JE, McCarty CA. Impact of unilateral and bilateral vision loss on quality of life. *Br J Ophthalmol.* 2005;89(3):360.
21. World Health Organization. Deafness and hearing loss; 2018. Available at: https://www.who.int/news-room/fact-sheets/detail/deafness-and-hearing-loss
22. Mitchell R. How many deaf people are there in the United States? Estimates from the survey of income and program participation. *J Deaf Stud Deaf Educ.* 2006;11(1):112.
23. Institute for Quality and Efficiency in Health Care (IQWiG). Hearing loss and deafness: normal hearing and impaired hearing; 2017. Available at https://www.ncbi.nlm.nih.gov/books/NBK390300/.
24. National Institute on Deafness and other Communication Disorders (NIDCD). Hearing aids; 2017. Available at: https://www.nidcd.nih.gov/health/hearing-aids#hearingaid_09.

CHAPTER 30

ASSESSING AND TREATING SPEECH AND LANGUAGE IMPAIRMENTS: JOINING THE CONVERSATION

Donna C. Tippett, MA, MPH, CCC-SLP

Communication is the essence of human life...
Light J. "Communication is the essence of human life": reflections on communicative competence.
Augment Altern Commun. 1997;13(2):61–70. DOI: 10.1080/07434619712331277848

KEY POINTS

1. "Speech" (motor production of sounds) and "language" (organization of words to convey meaning) are distinct entities.
2. Disorders of speech, language, and cognition can occur in isolation or in combination across the lifespan.
3. Recognizing and diagnosing comprehension impairments can result in immediate problem-specific communication and functional improvements.
4. Contemporary understandings of the neural basis of language reflect brain interconnectivity and reveal new therapeutic mechanisms.
5. Recognition of specific deficits in interfaces between language and cognition guides immediate patient-centered adaptations and targets contemporary therapies.

1. Define and relate speech, language, and cognition.
    Speech is a motor act involving ventilation, phonation (voice), resonance, articulation, and fluency (rhythm of speech) to produce speech sounds. The functional components of speech are the ventilatory mechanism, laryngeal mechanism, velum (soft palate), pharynx (throat), tongue, lips, face, teeth, and jaw. Language is the organization of speech sounds (or letters) into words and sentences to convey meaning (spoken and written expressive language) and the comprehension of words and sentences by listening or reading (receptive language). Contemporary definitions of language include prosody (i.e., pitch, loudness, stress on syllables and words, rate of speech) which conveys emotion, hence the expression, "it's not just what you say, but how you say it." Higher pitch, louder voice, and faster rate convey positive emotions, such as happiness, whereas lower pitch, soft voice, and slow rate convey negative emotions, such as sadness. Cognition includes attention, perception, memory, organization, problem solving/reasoning, and executive functions.

    Disorders of speech, language, and cognition can occur in isolation or in combination in both children and adults. Speech disorders include **stuttering, dysarthria,** and **apraxia of speech.** Language disorders include impairments in **auditory comprehension, reading comprehension, verbal expression, and written expression,** as in **aphasia.** Cognitive communication disorders can affect attention, memory, organizing, problem solving, reasoning, planning, and insight.

Boroditsky L. *How Language Shapes the Way We Think;* 2018 April 11. Available at https://www.ted.com/talks/lera_boroditsky_how_language_shapes_the_way_we_think?language=en

American Speech-Language-Hearing Association. *What is Speech? What is Language?;* n.d. Available at: https://www.asha.org/public/speech/development/speech-and-language/.

Enderby P. Disorders of communication: dysarthria. *Handb Clin Neurol.* 2013;110:273–881. Available at: https://doi.org/10.1016/B978-0-444-52901-5.00022-8.

National Institute on Deafness and Other Communication Disorders. National Institutes of Health. *Apraxia of Speech.* 2017 Oct 31; https://www.nidcd.nih.gov/health/apraxia-speech.

O'Sullivan M, Brownsett S, Copland D. Language and language disorders: neuroscience to clinical practice. *Pract Neurol.* 2019 Oct;19(5):380–388. Available at: https://doi.org/10.1136/practneurol-2018-001961.

Tippett DC, Ross E. *Prosody and the Aprosodias.* In AE Hillis, ed. *The Handbook of Adult Language Disorders.* 2nd ed. New York: Psychology Press, 2015:518–529

2. Referrals for a speech-language pathology evaluation: who and why?

Anyone with a suspected communication or swallowing impairment should be referred for a speech-language pathology evaluation. The effects of communication and swallowing problems can be minimized, and sometimes eliminated, with proper evaluation and treatment. If there is a question regarding the appropriateness of a referral, speech-language pathologists can perform a screening before giving a lengthy assessment. It is appropriate to obtain a speech-language pathology consultation within 24 to 48 hours after an individual is admitted to the hospital for an acute event, especially if dysphagia is suspected. Indications of dysphagia include drooling, "squirreling" of food in the mouth, gurgly voice after swallowing, and coughing after swallowing. Orders for speech-language pathology consultations are increasingly part of the admitting orders and are **in clinical pathways that address many acute central nervous system insults.**

American Speech-Language-Hearing Association. *Speech-Language Pathology Medical Review Guidelines.* 2015; Available at: https://www.asha.org/uploadedFiles/SLP-Medical-Review-Guidelines.pdf

Capone Singleton N. Late talkers: why the wait-and-see approach is outdated. *Pediatr Clin North Am.* 2018 Feb;65(1):3–29. Available at: https://doi.org/10.1016/j.pcl.2017.08.018.

3. How can clinicians plan to optimize speech and language intervention in the design of patient rehabilitation plans as recovery progresses?

It is difficult to make a definitive statement regarding candidacy for speech-language treatment given the diversity of patient populations and disorders seen by speech-language pathologists. However, it is usually true that treatment should be deferred for patients who are obtunded, sedated, or very ill (Table 30.1). Recovery from aphasia due to stroke is variable and can be prolonged, especially after large left hemisphere strokes. Stroke recovery is influenced by medical interventions to facilitate changes in blood flow in the acute stage; other prognostic variables include lesion site, baseline severity of speech and language impairment, and education level. The role of educational level in recovery is complex. Education may be a marker for "cognitive reserve," healthier lifestyle, or another factor that might positively influence recovery. An important research finding is that stroke survivors and their caregivers are primarily concerned with recovery of higher-level cognitive functions, such as the ability to use written language and to empathize with others, than motor recovery and ability to perform activities of daily living.

Brady MC, Kelly H, Godwin J, Enderby O. Speech and language therapy for aphasia following stroke. *Cochrane Database Syst Rev,* 2012 May 16;(5):CD000425. Available at: https://doi.org/10.1002/14651858.CD000425.pub3

Hillis AE, Beh YY, Sebastian R, Breining B, Tippett DC, Wright A, Saxena S, Rorden C, Bonilha L, Basilakos A, Yourganov G, Fridriksson, J. Predicting recovery in acute poststroke aphasia. *Ann Neurol.* 2018;83(3):612–622. Available at: https://doi.org/10.1002/ana.25184

Hillis AE, Tippett DC. Stroke recovery: surprising influences and residual consequences. *Adv Med.* 2014; Article ID 378263, Available at: http://dx.doi.org/10.1155/2014/378263.

4. Do impairments in language performance suggest specific brain structure malfunction? What is aphasia?

Aphasia is an **acquired language disorder** characterized by impairments in **auditory comprehension, verbal expression, reading comprehension, and/or written expression;** intelligence is not compromised. Aphasia typically results unnecessary from damage to the left hemisphere of the brain, such as stroke, brain tumor, or brain

Table 30.1 Factors Associated With Aphasia Recovery	
FACTOR	**IMPLICATION**
Age	The older the patient, the poorer the prognosis
General health	The healthier the patient, the better the prognosis
Motivation, cooperation	High degrees of motivation and cooperation are favorable prognostic signs
Social support	Family support can facilitate carryover of treatment strategies
Stimulability to cues	Responsiveness to diagnostic therapy is a favorable outcome variable

infection. A stroke affecting the left middle cerebral artery is the most common cause of cortical stroke. Historically, **Broca's area** and **Wernicke's area** were widely considered the primary language centers of the brain. Advances in neuroimaging have shown that, although the left hemisphere shows more activation in the majority of neurotypical adults, both cerebral hemispheres are activated during language tasks as well as distant areas of the cortex, such as inferior and anterior temporal cortex, basal ganglia, and thalamus. This new understanding of the neural organization of language has implications for predictions regarding post-stroke recovery of language.

Stroke Association. *Aphasia and Its Effects;* n.d. Available at: https://www.stroke.org.uk/what-is-aphasia/aphasia-and-its-effects

Crinion JT, Lambon-Ralph MA, Warburton EA, Howard D, Wise RJ. Temporal lobe regions engaged during normal speech comprehension. *Brain.* 2003 May;126(Pt 5):1193–1201. Available at: https://doi.org/10.1093/brain/awg104

Fridriksson J, Morrow L. Cortical activation and language task difficulty in aphasia. *Aphasiology.* 2005;19(3–5):239–250. Available at: https://doi.org/10.1080/02687030444000714

Tippett DC, Niparko JK, Hillis AE. Aphasia: current concepts in theory and practice. *J Neurol Transl Neurosci.* 2014;2(1), 1042.

Wise RJS. Language systems in normal and aphasic human subjects: functional imaging studies and inferences from animal studies. *Br Med Bull.* 2003;65(1):95–119. Available at: https://doi.org/10.1093/bmb/65.1.95

5. Can clinical assessment suggest anatomic location attributed to aphasias and guide treatment?

The "classic aphasia syndromes," associated with the Boston school of aphasia, are Broca aphasia, Wernicke aphasia, conduction aphasia, anomic aphasia, transcortical motor, transcortical sensory, transcortical mixed, and global aphasia. The aphasia syndromes are diagnosed based on impairments in fluency, auditory comprehension, repetition, and naming (Fig. 30.1). Although the usefulness of this classification paradigm has been questioned by some, it remains the standard for planning speech-language therapy and for grouping individuals in aphasia research. In addition to the classic aphasia syndromes, "subcortical aphasias" are proposed: striatocapsular aphasia, thalamic aphasia, and aphasia associated with white matter paraventricular lesions. The specific roles of subcortical structures in language remain controversial. Current theories of aphasia include disruption of cognitive/language operations. The dual stream model is an innovative conceptualization of the complexity of language that includes a ventral stream for mapping sound onto meaning and a dorsal stream for mapping sound onto motoric productions and articulation. This model, unlike classic localization models of language, incorporates the role of interconnections between cortical regions by these two streams. The dorsal stream is left lateralized, projecting from the posterior superior temporal to the inferior frontal cortices. The ventral stream is bilateral and projects from the posterior middle and inferior temporal gyrus to the anterior middle temporal gyrus.

Hickok G. *The Dual Stream Model: Clarifications and Recent Progress;* 2017 January 23. Available at: https://www.youtube.com/watch?v=uLUOzUYC3u4

Hickok G, Poeppel D. Dorsal and ventral streams: a framework for understanding aspects of the functional anatomy of language. *Cognition.* 2004;92:67–99. Available at: https://doi.org/10.1016/j.cognition.2003.10.011

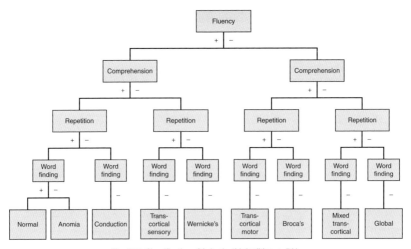

Fig. 30.1 Classification of Aphasia, third edition, p. 541.

Hillis AE. Aphasia: progress in the last quarter of a century. *Neurology.* 2007 Jul 10;69(2):200–213. Available at: https://doi.org/10.1212/01.wnl.0000265600.69385.6f

Kuljic-Obradovic DC. Subcortical aphasia: three different language disorder syndromes? *Eur J Neurol.* 2003;10(4):445–448. Available at: https://doi.org/10.1046/j.1468-1331.2003.00604.x

Tippett DC, Hillis AE. Where are aphasia theory and management "headed"? *F1000Research.* 2017;6(F1000 Faculty Review):1038. Available at: https://doi.org/10.12688/f1000research.11122.1

6. How can a clinician distinguish fluent versus nonfluent aphasia?

The **fluent-nonfluent dichotomy** is central to the widely used Boston school of aphasia classification but can be an elusive concept. **Fluency** refers to the ease of speech production. **Fluent aphasia** is associated with easy articulation, facility with the patterns of sentence structure, and preserved prosody, but with difficulty in word finding, with or without errors of word and sound substitution. These individuals seem to be speaking normally, but upon closer listening, it becomes clear that their speech is lacking in meaning or content. Many words are produced, but little information is conveyed. Fluent aphasias localize to the temporal area of the brain and may not be associated with a hemiparesis. **Wernicke aphasia** is an example of a **fluent** aphasia. Output in nonfluent aphasia, on the other hand, is laborious and contains only few words per breath. **Nonfluent aphasias** are linked to more anterior lesions, near the motor strip, and are usually associated with right hemiparesis. **Broca aphasia** is an example of a **nonfluent** aphasia. Few words are produced, but these words tend to be content words that convey meaning. Determination of fluency is challenging in clinical practice because it is subjective and based on several parameters, including speech rate, signs of struggle, and use of filler words.

National Aphasia Association. *Types of aphasia*; n.d. Available at: https://www.aphasia.org/stories/different-types-aphasia

Goodglass H, Barresi B, Weintraub S. *BDAE-3: Boston Diagnostic Aphasia Examination.* Philadelphia, PA: Lippincott Williams & Wilkins; 2001.

7. What are some of the patterns and names for aphasic utterances? (Table 30.2).

8. Describe the typical communication deficits seen in patients with right cerebral hemisphere damage.

These patients demonstrate relatively **intact language** but **impaired communication abilities.** Key features are **insensitivity to context** (i.e., missing nuances and subtleties), **difficulty organizing information** in a meaningful way (e.g., answering questions with tangential, unnecessary information), **difficulty "reading" facial expressions and gestures**, inability to understand figurative language, **lack of affect,** caustic sense of humor, **impulsivity,** left neglect, denial of deficits, better performance on structured than open-ended tasks, and writing errors (e.g., omission of strokes, letters, or words; perseveration of strokes, letters, and words; failure to dot i's and cross t's; extra capitalization). The right hemisphere plays a vital role in mediating the prosodic and paralinguistic aspects of communication to convey attitudinal and emotional information.

Table 30.2 Selected Aphasia Terminology

TERM	DEFINITION
Neologisms	Substitutions of entirely invented words for correct ones
Semantic paraphasias	Word substitutions belonging to the same semantic class (e.g., chair for table)
Phonemic paraphasias	Substitutions of one sound for another (e.g., fable for table)
Jargon	Fluent but incomprehensible speech due to severity of paraphasias
Telegraphic speech	Speech output which includes substantive words (e.g., nouns, verbs) but omits grammatical modifiers (e.g., articles, conjunctions, pronouns; "girl eat cake")
Agrammatism	Sparse, hesitant, groping speech limited to the most essential content words
Logorrhea	"Pressure of speech;" fluent speech with unnecessary words and neologisms; speech is more abundant than normal speech
Echolalia	Meaningless repetition of other's utterances
Palilalia	Pathologic repetition of syllables or sounds; associated with degenerative brain diseases

Ross ED. Cerebral localization of functions and the neurology of language: fact versus fiction or is it something else? *Neuroscientist.* 2010 Jun;16(3):222–243. Available at: https://doi.org/10.1177/1073858409349899

Tompkins CA. Making it right? Some thoughts about the future of treatment for right hemisphere cognitive-communication disorders. *Semin Speech Lang.* 2016 Aug;37(3):153–157. Available at: https://doi:10.1055/s-0036-1583548.

9. What is primary progressive aphasia?

Primary progressive aphasia (PPA) is a neurodegenerative language condition characterized by predominant impairment in language abilities, particularly word finding. There are **three main variants,** each with specific clinical features, patterns of brain atrophy, and underlying neuropathology: logopenic variant PPA, nonfluent agrammatic PPA, and semantic variant PPA. **Logopenic variant PPA** is characterized by impaired single-word retrieval in spontaneous speech and naming, impaired repetition of phrases and sentences, and left temporo-parietal atrophy. This variant is associated with Alzheimer pathology. **Nonfluent agrammatic PPA** is characterized by nonfluent, effortful speech, and agrammatism, and atrophy in the left posterior frontotemporal area. **Semantic variant PPA** is characterized by impaired object knowledge, anomia, single word comprehension deficits, and atrophy in the anterior parts of the temporal lobe. The variants svPPA and nfaPPA are associated with pathologies in the spectrum of frontotemporal lobar degeneration (FTLD).

Gorno-Tempini ML, Hillis AE, Weintraub S, Kertesz A, Mendez M, Cappa SF, Ogar JM, Rohrer JD, Black S, Boeve BF, Manes F, Dronkers NF, Vandenberghe R, Rascovsky K, Patterson K, Miller BL, Knopman DS, Hodges JR, Mesulam MM, Grossman M. Classification of primary progressive aphasia and its variants. *Neurology.* 2011;76(11):1006–1014. Available at: https://doi.org/10.1212/WNL.0b013e31821103e6

Montembeault M, Brambati SM, Gorno-Tempini ML, Migliaccio R. Clinical, anatomical, and pathological features in the three variants of primary progressive aphasia: a review. *Front Neurol.* 2018;9:692. Available at: https://doi.org/10.3389/fneur.2018.00692

Tippett DC. Classification of primary progressive aphasia: challenges and complexities. *F1000Research.* 2020;9:F1000 Faculty Rev-64. Available at: https://doi.org/10.12688/f1000research.21184.1

Tippett DC, Hillis AE, Tsapkini K. Treatment of primary progressive aphasia. *Curr Treat Options Neurol.* 2015;17(8):362. Available at: https://doi.org/10.1007/s11940-015-0362-5

10. What is speech? How do you recognize apraxia of speech?

Speech is a motor act that relies on intact range, strength, speed, coordination, and accuracy of movement of oral motor structures (see questions 1 and 13). **Apraxia of speech** is a disorder of the execution of learned movement (impaired motor planning and programming) that cannot be explained by weakness, slowness, incoordination, sensory loss, altered muscle tone, or inability to follow directions (as in aphasia). It is associated with left cortical damage and a variety of progressive neurodegenerative disorders. **Developmental apraxia of speech** occurs in children and is present from birth. The etiology of childhood apraxia of speech is not clear, although a genetic component has been reported. Apraxia of speech is characterized by highly variable and unpredictable articulatory breakdown, hesitations, repetitions, and slow, labored output due to **impaired ability to program the positioning of speech muscles and sequence muscle movements.** Apraxia can be distinguished from dysarthria by recognizing irregular articulatory breakdown in the setting of intact muscle function, whereas predictable speech sound errors due to weakness, slowness, incoordination, and alteration in sensation and/or muscle tone are characteristic of dysarthria.

Strand E. *Examples of Different Levels of Severity in Childhood Apraxia of Speech*; 2015 October 20. Available at: https://www.youtube.com/watch?v=cEOy3APLA-g

Basilakos A. Contemporary approaches to the management of post-stroke apraxia of speech. *Semin Speech Lang.* 2018;39(1):25–36. Available at: https://doi.org/10.1055/s-0037-1608853

Hillis AE, Work M, Barker PB, Jacobs MA, Breese EL, Maurer K. Re-examining the brain regions crucial for orchestrating speech articulation. *Brain.* 2004;127(7):1479–1487. Available at: https://doi.org/10.1093/brain/awh172

Josephs KA, Duffy JR, Strand EA, Machulda MM, Senjem ML, Master AV, Lowe VJ, Jack CR, Whitwell JL. Characterizing a neurodegenerative syndrome: primary progressive apraxia of speech. *Brain.* 2012;135(Pt 5):1522–1536. Available at: https://doi.org/10.1093/brain/aws032

Shriberg LD, Lohmeier HL, Strand EA, Jakielski KJ. Encoding, memory, and transcoding deficits in childhood apraxia of speech. *Clin Linguist Phon.* 2012;26(5):445–482. Available at: https://doi.org/10.3109/02699206.2012.655841

11. What is agnosia? How does perception relate to recognition?

Agnosia is a **disorder of recognition** that may occur in any of the major sense modalities despite adequate perception in these modalities (e.g., audition, vision, tactile sensation). An **auditory agnosia** is an inability to match an environmental noise with its sound source. For example, a patient may not be able to recognize a watch from its ticking but can identify a watch placed in his hand. A **visual agnosia** is an inability to identify an object on visual confrontation. For example, a patient may not be able to identify his wife when shown a picture but can describe her appearance (e.g., blonde hair, blue eyes).

Kastner S. *Object Representations in Visual Agnosia*; 2011 June 28. Available at: https://www.youtube.com/watch?v=AAZ7kEuNOAI

Milner AD, Cavina-Pratesi C. Perceptual deficits of object identification: apperceptive agnosia. *Handb Clin Neurol.* 2018;151:269–286. Available at: https://doi:10.1016/B978-0-444-63622-5.00013-9.

Slevc LR, Shell AR. Auditory agnosia. *Handb Clin Neurol.* 2015;129:573–587. Available at: https://doi.org/10.1016/B978-0-444-62630-1.00032-9

12. **What is dysarthria? Can perceivable characteristics point to cause?**
    Dysarthria is a **speech impairment,** not a language impairment like aphasia. Individuals with dysarthria are often difficult to understand and may have "slurred speech." They do not have problems with listening, reading, writing, or spoken language (e.g., vocabulary, grammar). Dysarthria is caused by damage to the central or peripheral nervous system. Dysarthria can be classified by etiology and anticipated course (e.g., developmental, recovering, stable, degenerative); age at onset (e.g., congenital or acquired); or by the speech process and/or functional component which is impaired. The **perceptual classification system** developed at the Mayo Clinic is used extensively in clinical practice by speech-language pathologists. Perceptual deviations can suggest etiology; for example, lower motor neuron dysarthria can be characterized by breathy voice, hypernasality, and imprecise articulation whereas upper motor neuron dysarthria can be characterized by slow rate and strained, harsh phonation. Six types of dysarthrias are described based on perceptual features:
    Flaccid (in bulbar palsy)
    Spastic (in pseudobulbar palsy)
    Ataxic (in cerebellar disorders)
    Hypokinetic (in parkinsonism)
    Hyperkinetic (in dystonia and chorea)
    Mixed (in disorders of multiple motor systems, such as multiple sclerosis)

Strand E. *Differences between CAS and other disorders: examples of phonologic impairment and dysarthria*; 2019 May 9. Available at: https://www.mayoclinic.org/diseases-conditions/childhood-apraxia-of-speech/multimedia/childhood-apraxia-of-speech-and-other-disorders-phonologic-impairment-dysarthria/vid-20169128

Duffy JR. *Motor Speech Disorders: Substrates, Differential Diagnosis, and Management.* St. Louis, MO: Elsevier; 2013.

Spencer KA, Brown KA. Dysarthria following stroke. *Semin Speech Lang.* 2018 Feb;39(1):15–24. Available at: https://doi: 10.1055/s-0037-1608852

13. **How is speech production assessed?**
    Speech-language pathologists perform speech/oral motor examinations to assess the ventilatory mechanism, laryngeal mechanism, velum/pharynx, tongue, lips/face/teeth and jaw in a systematic fashion (Table 30.3). **Speech production** can also be assessed by using commercially available tests. **Speech intelligibility** is rated at single word and connected speech levels. Objective **acoustic measurements** may be obtained using specialized computer software.

14. **How are language and cognition assessed?**
    Comprehensive language batteries, such as the **Western Aphasia Battery** and the **Boston Diagnostic Aphasia Examination**, are administered to survey expressive and receptive language modalities (i.e., listening, reading, speaking, writing). Supplementary tests are administered to probe specific areas, such as naming using the

Table 30.3 Nonspeech and Speech Tests of Oral-Motor Function

COMPONENTS	EXAMPLES OF NONSPEECH TASKS	EXAMPLES OF SPEECH TASKS
Ventilatory mechanism	Breathing at rest	Maximum phonation time
Laryngeal mechanism	Elevation with swallow	Ability to change loudness
Velum/pharynx	Velar position at rest	Maintenance of oral/nasal contrasts
Tongue	Lingual range of movement	Lingual articulation
Lips/face	Facial symmetry	Labial articulation
Jaw	Mandibular strength against resistance	Mandibular assist for articulation

Revised Boston Naming Test or reading using the **Reading Comprehension Battery for Aphasia.** The **Montreal Cognitive Assessment**, a brief screening assessment and Ross Information Processing Assessment, a more extensive battery, are given to examine orientation, attention, short-term memory, and reasoning.

Goodglass H, Kaplan E, Barresi B. *The Assessment of Aphasia and Related Disorders.* 3rd ed. Baltimore, MD: Lippincott Williams & Wilkins; 2001.

Kaplan E, Goodglass H, Weintraub S, Segal O, van Loon-Vervoorn A. *Boston Naming Test (BNT-2).* 2nd ed. Austin, TX: Pro-ed; 2001.

Kertesz A. *Western Aphasia Battery- Revised (WAB-R).* San Antonio, TX: Pearson; 2006.

Lapointe LL, Horner J. *Reading Comprehension Battery for Aphasia (RCBA-2).* 2nd ed. Austin, TX: Pro-Ed; 1998.

Nasreddine ZS, Phillips NA, Bédirian V, Charbonneau S, Whitehead V, Collin I, Cummings JL, Chertkow H. The Montreal Cognitive Assessment, MoCA: a brief screening tool for mild cognitive impairment. *J Am Geriatr Soc.* 2005;53(4):695–699. Available at: https://doi.org/10.1111/j.1532-5415.2005.53221.x

Ross-Swain D. *Ross Information Processing Assessment.* 2nd ed. Austin, TX: Pro-Ed; 1996

15. **How can individuals who have undergone laryngectomy or tracheostomy speak?**
Alaryngeal**,** after laryngectomy, speech can be produced by:
Esophageal speech: Air is trapped in the mouth or pharynx, propelled into the esophagus, and then released. Air flows through the upper esophageal sphincter, resulting in a belch-like sound.
Artificial larynx: There are two types of artificial larynges, an external type that is placed against the neck and an intra-oral type. Both types are battery powered and produce a mechanical sound.
Tracheoesophageal Puncture (TEP): A small puncture is surgically created through the common wall between the trachea and the esophagus. A small, one-way shunt valve is inserted into this puncture. To speak, the individual inhales air through the tracheostoma and into the lungs and then covers the stoma with a finger. Air from the lungs is directed from the trachea, through the shunt valve, and into the esophagus. The esophagus vibrates, creating a sound source for speech.
With all of these methods, sound is shaped into words by the tongue, teeth, lips, and jaw.
Unidirectional speaking valves can restore oral communication for **individuals with tracheostomy.** A unidirectional speaking valve allows inhalation to occur at the level of the tracheostomy and exhalation through the larynx, mouth, and nose. Valve candidates must have generally intact laryngeal structure and function (valves cannot be used with individuals who have had a laryngectomy). The cuff of the tracheostomy tube must be deflated when a valve is used. Some valves are designed to be used in-line with ventilator circuitry. Recent studies have shown that ventilator dependent individuals can achieve excellent oral communication via **leak speech** through partial cuff deflation alone.

Hoit JD, Banzett RB, Lohmeier HL, Hixon TJ, Brown R. Clinical ventilator adjustments that improve speech. *Chest.* 2003;124(4):1512–1521.

O'Connor LR, Morris NR, Paratz J. Physiological and clinical outcomes associated with use of one-way speaking valves on tracheostomised patients: a systematic review. *Heart Lung.* 2019 Jul–Aug;48(4):356–364. Available at: https://doi:10.1016/j.hrtlng.2018.11.006.

Prigent H, Samuel C, Louis B, et al. Comparative effects of two ventilatory modes on speech in tracheostomized patients with neuromuscular disease. *Am J Respir Crit Care Med.* 2003;167(2):114–119. Available at: https://doi.org/10.1164/rccm.200201-0260C

Suiter DM, McCullough GH, Powell PW. Effects of cuff deflation and one-way tracheostomy speaking valve placement on swallow physiology. *Dysphagia.* 2003;18(4):284–92. Available at: https://doi.org/10.1007/s00455-003-0022-x

Tippett DC,ed. *Tracheostomy and Ventilator Dependency: Management of Breathing, Speaking and Swallowing.* New York: Thieme; 2000.

16. **What are some treatment modalities and outcomes?**
Speech-language pathology intervention is evidence-based and patient-centered. The **Life Participation Approach to Aphasia (LPAA)** incorporates personally relevant situations into therapy so that treatment addresses individual concerns and needs**. Melodic Intonation Therapy,** a longstanding therapy technique commonly used to treat Broca aphasia, uses intonation to facilitate speech production. The **Lee Silverman Voice Treatment** is a highly stylized therapy used to treat dysarthria in individuals with Parkinson disease; exercises focus on increasing loudness because low volume voice is often a problem in this population. **Prosthetic stimulation,** such as **transcranial direct cortical stimulation (tDCS),** is an adjunctive approach to behavioral therapy for aphasia due to stroke and neurodegenerative disease. Both anodal and cathodal stimulation have been explored to enhance and inhibit cortical excitability, respectively.

Tspakini K. *tDCS in Primary Progressive Aphasia;* 2017 October 16. Available at: https://www.youtube.com/watch?v=M0CQQ_c-rAc

Duchan R, Linda J, Garcia AK, Lyon JG, Simmons-Mackie N. *Life Participation Approach to Aphasia: A Statement of Values for the Future.* In Chapey R, ed. *Language Intervention Strategies in Aphasia and Related Neurogenic Communication Disorders.* 4th ed. Baltimore, MD: Lippincott Williams & Wilkins; 2001:235–253.

Holland R, Crinion J. Can tDCS enhance treatment of aphasia after stroke? *Aphasiology*. 2012;26(9):1169–1191. Available at: https://doi:10.1080/02687038.2011.616925.

Ramig LO, Sapir S, Fox C, Countryman S. Changes in vocal loudness following intensive voice treatment (LSVT®) in individuals with Parkinson's disease: a comparison with untreated patients and normal age-matched controls. *Mov Disord*. 2001;16(1):79–83.

Sebastian R, Saxena S, Tsapkini K, Faria AV, Long C, Wright A, Davis C, Tippett DC, Mourdoukoutas AP, Bikson M, Celnik P, Hillis AE. Cerebellar tDCS: a novel approach to augment language treatment post-stroke. *Front Hum Neurosci*. 2017;10:695. Available at: https://doi.org/10.3389/fnhum.2016.00695

Sebastian R, Tsapkini K, Tippett DC. Transcranial direct current stimulation in post stroke aphasia and primary progressive aphasia: current knowledge and future clinical applications. *NeuroRehabilitation*. 2016;39(1):141–152. Available at: https://doi.org/10.3233/NRE-161346

Sparks RW, Holland AL. Method: melodic intonation therapy for aphasia. *J Speech Hear Disord*. 1976;41(3):287–297.

BIBLIOGRAPHY

Blake ML. *Right Hemisphere and Disorders of Cognition and Communication (Theory and Clinical Practice)*. 1st ed. San Diego, CA: Plural Publishing; 2017.

Chapey R. *Language Intervention Strategies in Aphasia and Related Neurogenic Communication Disorders*. 5th ed. Philadelphia, PA: LWW; 2008

Haskins EC. *Cognitive Rehabilitation Manual: Translating Evidence-Based Recommendations into Practice*. Vol. 1. Reston, VA: ACRM Publishing; 2012. Available at: https://www.ncbi.nlm.nih.gov/pmc/articles/PMC5367153/

Hickok G. Computational neuroanatomy of speech production. *Nat Rev Neurosci*. 2012;13(2):135–145. doi: 10/1038/nrn3158. Available at: https://www.aphasia.org/aphasia-resources/aphasia-caregiver-guide/

National Aphasia Association, Ford M, Klein R. *The Aphasia Caregiver Guide: Advice for Navigating Aphasia and Your Loved One's Care Without Losing Yourself on the Journey*. Independently published; 2020. Available at: https://pn.bmj.com/content/19/5/380

O'Sullivan M, Brownsett S, Copland, D. Language and language disorders: neuroscience to clinical practice. *Pract Neurol*. 2019;19(5):380–388. doi: 10/1136/practneurol-2018-001961

Swaiman KF, Ashwal S, Ferriero DM, Schor NF, Finkel RS, Gropman AL, Pearl PL, Shevell M. *Swaiman's Pediatric Neurology: Principles and Practice*. 6th ed. St. Louis, MO: Elsevier; 2017.

Webb W. *Neurology for the Speech-Language Pathologist*. 6th ed. St. Louis, MO: Elsevier; 2017.

CHAPTER 31

RECOGNITION, ASSESSMENT, AND TREATMENT OF SWALLOWING IMPAIRMENTS: ENGULFING TRANSDISCIPLINARY SOLUTIONS

Donna C. Tippett, MPH, MA, CCC-SLP, Susan L. Brady, DHEd, CCC-SLP, BCS-S, and Noel Rao, MD

Our professions' futures depend on the effectiveness of our treatments, not on our impressions of their effectiveness.
—Jeri A. Logemann, PhD, CCC-SLP, BCS-S (1942–2014)

KEY POINTS

1. Working knowledge of stages of swallowing and differentiation between laryngeal penetration, aspiration, and silent aspiration is essential in estimation of risk and immediate intervention in patients with swallowing disorders.
2. Bedside swallow, videofluoroscopic swallow study, and fiberoptic endoscopic evaluation each provide specific information used in prevention of aspiration and proactive nutritional planning.
3. Aspiration risks can be reduced through bedside interventions and surgical procedures.
4. Knowledge of the therapeutic indications for compensatory strategies and mechanisms for improving safety of swallowing is essential for staff, patient, and family training.
5. Rehabilitative swallowing strengthening/sensory interventions and novel modalities provide multimodal techniques and when used in therapeutic settings, can further augment safety and nutrition in patients with swallowing problems.

1. Describe the stages of swallowing.
   These traditional arbitrary four stages are often debated.
   - The **oral preparatory stage** is when food is chewed **(masticated)** to break down food particles and start digestion with saliva, which forms a **cohesive bolus**. The bolus is held between the surface of the tongue and the hard palate with the soft palate depressed to prevent premature spillage of the bolus into the airway prior to the swallow.
   - The **oral transport stage** begins after formation of bolus with the anterior to posterior movement of the bolus through the oral cavity into the oropharynx.
   - The **pharyngeal stage** is the most complex and begins with the initiation of the **swallow response.** It lasts approximately 1 second and involves the adduction of the **true vocal folds;** elevation of the pharynx (with simultaneous contraction of the **suprahyoid muscles** elevating the hyoid bone resulting in airway protection by inverting the **epiglottis**); retraction of the **tongue base** to the posterior pharyngeal wall; activation of the **pharyngeal constrictors**; and the opening (relaxation) of the **cricopharyngeal muscle** to open the **upper esophageal sphincter (UES)**.
   - The **esophageal stage** begins as the bolus passes through the UES and ends following the passage of the bolus through the lower esophageal sphincter into the stomach. The expected duration of the esophageal phase is between 8 and 13 seconds.

Martin-Harris B. Anatomy and physiology of swallowing—MBSImP animations. *NorthernSpeech;* June 25, 2019. Available at https://www.youtube.com/watch?v=SBbNxM7g2vg

Shaw ST, Martino R. The normal swallow: muscular and neurophysiological control. In *Dysphagia: Diagnosis and Management* (Editor Kenneth W. Altman). *Otolaryngol Clin N Am.* 2013;46(6):937–956.

2. Describe differences among laryngeal penetration, aspiration, and silent aspiration. Which is most dangerous?
   - **Laryngeal penetration** is when material (i.e., food, liquids, secretions) enters the **laryngeal vestibule (**i.e., laryngeal surface of the epiglottis; the aryepiglottic folds, and the mucosa between the arytenoids to the superior surface of the true vocal folds). Laryngeal penetration is a common clinical observation with individuals with

and without dysphagia. The incidence of laryngeal penetration with healthy individuals has been shown to increase with liquid boluses, bolus size, and age.

- **Aspiration** is when the material enters the airway below the level of the true vocal folds. The presence of aspiration is an abnormal finding on an instrumental swallow exam.
- **Silent aspiration** refers to the absence of any visible distress (i.e., coughing, choking, throat clear) with aspiration. This is the most dangerous situation as clinicians may miss those who aspirate and patients may be placed on an inappropriate regular diet or insufficient supervision, which can lead to pneumonia.

Humbert I. *Penetration-Aspiration Scale Tutorial;* December 22, 2018. Available at https://www.youtube.com/watch?v=hfEYI6ELZos

Allen JE, White CJ, Leonard R, Belafsky PC. Prevalence of penetration and aspiration on videofluoroscopy in normal individuals without dysphagia. *Otolaryngol Head Neck Surg.* 2010;142(2):208–213.

Ramsey D, Smithard D, Kalra L. Silent aspiration: what do we know? *Dysphagia.* 2005;20:218–225.

3. **Does a percutaneous endoscopic gastrotomy (PEG) placement eliminate aspiration and improve outcomes?**
   The PEG is often the long-term preferred route for individuals who are unable to receive adequate oral nutrition. Swallowing difficulties that require placement of a PEG are commonly associated with medical illnesses, including ventilation and liver and renal failure. Neurological diseases such as cerebrovascular accident, acquired brain injury, Parkinson disease, motor neuron disease, and dementia are other indications along with surgical diseases including head/neck and esophageal cancer. Major complications with the PEG may include aspiration pneumonia, peritonitis, massive hemorrhage, and **buried bumper syndrome** (migration of the internal fixation device along gastrostomy tube toward skin surface). Patients with amyotrophic lateral sclerosis (ALS) may experience an overall significant increase in survival duration. There is no evidence to suggest improved long-term survival rates for patients with advanced dementia. The PEG has failed to demonstrate the prevention of aspiration pneumonia in a series of neurologically ill patients.

Bond L, Ganguly P, Khamankar N, Mallet N, Bowen G, Green B, Mitchell CS. A comprehensive examination of percutaneous endoscopic gastrostomy and its association with amyotrophic lateral sclerosis patient outcomes. *Brain Sci.* 2019;9:223. doi:10.3390/brainsci9090223

Park SK, Kim JY, Koh SJ, Lee YJ, Jang HJ, Park SJ. Complications of percutaneous endoscopic and radiologic gastroscope tube insertion: a KASID (Korean Association for the Study of Intestinal Diseases) study. *Surg Endosc.* 2019;33:750–756.

4. **What are the sequences of swallowing assessment, aspiration precautions, and proactive nutritional planning?**
   Patients who demonstrate symptoms such as coughing/choking during meals, **a "wet" vocal quality** when eating or drinking, reduced oral intake/failure to thrive, or unexplained pulmonary infection should be considered for a swallowing assessment. Generally, the first step in the management of patients who may be at risk for aspiration is to complete the **bedside swallow examination** and/or screening. While there is some debate if there is a difference between a bedside swallow examination and a swallow screening, they both involve only the use of clinical skills to determine aspiration risk, the potential for safe oral alimentation, and the need for further evaluation.

   The bedside swallow examination can be completed during a meal where the patient can be given various consistencies to swallow. The **bedside swallow examination/swallow screen** often includes a brief assessment of **cognitive ability** (e.g., alertness level, orientation, ability to follow 1-step commands); **oral mechanism exam** (observe for oral-motor weakness, dentition, oral care conditions); **laryngeal strength** (voice and voluntary cough strength); and patient-reported difficulties with swallowing. The presence or absence of the **gag reflex** is not part of the clinical swallow examination as it is not useful in predicting aspiration. When possible, the patient should be as upright as possible (90 degrees).

   One example of a swallow screen is known as the **3-ounce water challenge** or the **Yale Swallow Protocol**. During this swallow screen, the patient is instructed to drink 3 ounces of water without stopping. The presence of a cough, throat clear, "wet" vocal quality, and/or an inability to consume all 3 ounces at one time suggests aspiration risks.

   While the clinical swallow examination/screening may provide valuable information, it is impossible for the clinician to evaluate pharyngeal or laryngeal anatomy and swallowing physiology (i.e., bolus flow for laryngeal penetration, aspiration, pharyngeal residue). Experienced dysphagia clinicians still miss symptoms of aspiration up to 40% of the time during the clinical examination as compared to an instrumental assessment of the swallow. To definitively diagnose dysphagia and to determine the specific mechanism of the swallowing disorder, the patient needs to undergo an instrumental assessment of the swallow, such as the videofluoroscopic swallow study (VFSS) or the fiberoptic endoscopic exam of the swallow (FEES).

   Swallow assessment results guide appropriate recommendations for optimal route for nutritional support and the need for further evaluation. Oral diets may include thickened liquids or modified solids; compensatory swallow safety strategies; and supervision level. Calorie counts, mini-meals, in-between meal snacks, and strict liquid input/output records may also be recommended to ensure adequate nutrition and hydration. Full or supplemental non-oral alimentation may include intravenous fluids, NG tube feedings (short-term intervention), or PEG tube feedings (long-term intervention).

Leder SB, Suiter DM. *The Yale Swallow Protocol: An Evidence-Based Approach to Decision Making.* Switzerland: Springer International Publishing. 2014:19–28.

Pfeiffer RF. *Neurogenic Dysphagia.* In Daroff R, Jankovic J, Mazziotta J, Pomeroy S, eds. *Bradley's Neurology in Clinical Practice.* 7th ed. Toronto, Canada: Elsevier, Inc.; 2016:148–157.

Shaw ST, Martino R. The normal swallow: muscular and neurophysiological control. In *Dysphagia: Diagnosis and Management* (Editor Kenneth W. Altman). 2013;46(6):937–956.

Speyer R. Oropharyngeal dysphagia: screening and assessment. In *Dysphagia: Diagnosis and Management* (Editor Kenneth W. Altman). *Otolaryngol Clin N Am.* 2013;46(6):989–1008.

5. What is the videofluoroscopic swallow study?

The **videofluoroscopic swallow study (VFSS)**, also known as the **modified barium swallow**, is a dynamic radiographic evaluation of swallow function that allows for the identification of normal and abnormal anatomy and swallow physiology. The VFSS is normally completed by a swallowing clinician (usually a speech language pathologist) and a physician (radiologist or physiatrist). The original VFSS protocol included the presentation of liquids and solid foods impregnated with barium. Today in clinical practice, there are many variations of the original VFSS protocol but most standardized protocols are designed to evaluate the integrity of airway protection; bolus flow; and the effectiveness of bolus modification, postural changes, and swallowing maneuvers to improve swallow safety and efficiency. Impairments of each stage of the swallow should be described during the VFSS and summarized in a written report.

KEY POINTS: INDICATIONS FOR A VIDEOFLUOROSCOPIC SWALLOW STUDY

1. When a swallow impairment is suspected that may involve all four phases of the swallow
2. When the clinical examination is insufficient to answer relevant questions regarding treatment plans (e.g., dietary, compensatory strategies, swallowing rehabilitation interventions)
3. When nutritional and respiratory issues are of concern
4. When medical diagnoses are not established

Fauguier ENT. *Normal Swallow Tutorial with Modified Barium Swallow;* October 22, 2010; Available at https://www.youtube.com/watch?v=xu_YYOAIZEw

Brady S, Donzelli J. The modified barium swallow and the functional endoscopic evaluation of swallowing. In *Dysphagia: Diagnosis and Management* (Editor Kenneth W. Altman). *Otolaryngol Clin N Am.* 2013;46(6):1009–1022. Available at: http://dx.doi.org/10.1016/j.otc.2013.08.001

Martin-Harris B, Jones B. The videofluorographic swallowing study. *Phys Med Rehabil Clin N Am.* 2008;19(4):769–viii. Available at: http://dx.doi.org/10.1016/j.pmr.2008.06.004

Martin-Harris B, Brodsky MB, Michel Y, et al. MBS measurement tool for swallow impairment—MBSImp: establishing a standard. *Dysphagia.* 2008;23(4):392–405. doi:10.1007/s00455-008-9185-9

6. How do we identify and treat esophageal phase swallowing disorders?

When esophageal dysphagia is suspected, a comprehensive patient history is required. Esophageal dysphagia symptoms often present as a fullness or lump in the throat region. Common causes of esophageal dysphagia include stricture, mechanical obstruction/food impaction, eosinophilic esophagitis, achalasia, malignancy, motility disorders (e.g., esophageal spasms), and gastroesophageal reflux disease.

The VFSS protocol may include a brief observation of the esophageal phase of swallowing captured using an anterior–posterior image to assess esophageal clearance in the upright position. This view may provide information regarding incomplete or slowing esophageal clearance and identify the potential risk factors for aspiration of esophageal contents. Common compensatory treatment options for mild slowing of esophageal clearance include reducing eating rate and alternating liquids/solids. While the VFSS is not designed to diagnose esophageal dysphagia, gross abnormalities of the esophagus may be identified that may necessitate a medical referral for further diagnostic evaluation. An upper endoscopy is done to assess for mechanical obstruction or an inflammatory process. High-resolution manometry is used for suspected motility dysfunction. A radiographic esophagram is indicated when the case is unclear.

Martin-Harris B, Jones B. The videofluorographic swallowing study. *Phys Med Rehabil Clin N Am.* 2008;19(4):769–viii. doi:10.1016/j.pmr.2008.06.004

Roden DF, Altman KW. Causes of dysphagia among difference age groups: a systematic review of the literature. In *Dysphagia: Diagnosis and Management* (Editor Kenneth W. Altman). *Otolaryngol Clin N Am.* 2013;46(6):1009–1022. Available at: http://dx.doi.org/10.1016/j.otc.2013.08.008

Triggs J, Pandolfino J. Recent advances in dysphagia management. *F1000Research.* 2019;8:F1000 Faculty Rev-1527. doi:10.12688/f1000research.18900.1

7. **What is the fiberoptic endoscopic evaluation of swallowing?**

The **fiberoptic endoscopic evaluation of swallowing (FEES)** involves the use of a flexible laryngoscope attached to either a halogen or xenon light source. The endoscopist inserts the endoscope transnasally and advances the scope to the hypopharynx that allows for the visualization of the anatomic structures, secretion levels, swallow function, and sensory ability. The direct visualization of the oropharyngeal structures is a distinct advantage of the FEES procedure. For example, during the FEES the examiner can evaluate the effectiveness of a vocal fold medialization procedure for unilateral paralysis on glottal closure to reduce or eliminate aspiration.

During the FEES procedure, there are three segments known as the preswallow, whiteout, and postswallow segment. During the **preswallow segment** the following is evaluated: anatomy and physiology of the laryngeal and pharyngeal structures, premature spillage of the bolus, and laryngeal penetration and aspiration demonstrated before the swallow. During the **whiteout segment,** the examiner is unable to view the hypopharynx because of the light that is emitted from the endoscope during the height of the swallow. Therefore, events that occur during the whiteout segment must be inferred. Finally, during the **postswallow segment** the examiner can evaluate the presence of any airway invasion of the bolus that may have occurred either during or after the swallow as well as the presence of pharyngeal residue. Like the VFSS, during the FEES the examiner can evaluate the effectiveness of various therapeutic interventions (e.g., bolus modification, postural changes, and swallowing maneuvers).

KEY POINTS: INDICATIONS FOR A FIBEROPTIC ENDOSCOPIC EVALUATION OF SWALLOWING

1. When a swallow impairment is suspected that requires an extended assessment for fatigue
2. When the patient presents with both a suspected dysphagia and dysphonia (vocal dysfunction)
3. When difficulty with managing accumulated oropharyngeal secretions is suspected
4. When laryngeal dysfunction (i.e., post-intubation injury, vocal focal paralysis) is suspected along with swallowing dysfunction
5. When exposure to radiation during the VFSS is not recommended (pregnant patient)

Fiberoptic Endoscopy Evaluation of the Swallow—Marianjoy Swallowing & Voice Center; April 19, 2013. Available at https://www.youtube.com/watch?v=M-TbMp_63Yc

Brady S, Leder S. *Chapter 8 Adult Fiberoptic Endoscopic Evaluation of Swallowing*. In Suiter DM, Gosa MM, eds. *Assessing and Treating Dysphagia: A Lifespan Perspective*. New York, NY: Thieme Publishers; 2019:97–110.

Brady S, Donzelli J. The modified barium swallow and the functional endoscopic evaluation of swallowing. In *Dysphagia: Diagnosis and Management* (Editor Kenneth W. Altman). *Otolaryngol Clin N Am*. 2013;46(6):1009–1022. Available at: http://dx.doi.org/10.1016/j.otc.2013.08.001

8. **How much aspiration is too much? Are risks preventable?**

Dysphagia, aspiration, and aspiration pneumonia are distinct but related events modulated by many factors and are dictated by the nature of the patient's illness and accompanying comorbidities. To further complicate the issue, there are various definitions describing the term aspiration pneumonia. Dysphagia and aspiration are necessary, but not always sufficient. Inhaling bacterially contaminated saliva or substance (i.e., food/liquid) is associated with factors including impaired consciousness; older age; functional decline (i.e., dependency for oral feeding/ dependency for oral care); periodontal disease (i.e., number of decayed teeth); tube feeding; multiple medical diagnoses; polypharmacy; smoking; higher levels of accumulated oropharyngeal sections; and refluxed gastric contents causing chemical injury. Many of these risks are preventable. Oral care interventions may significantly reduce the risk for developing pneumonia. Patients who are NPO (nil per os; nothing by mouth) and receiving tube feedings remain at risk for aspiration and should have the head of the bed elevated at minimum 30 degrees.

Langmore SE, Skarupski KA, Park PS, Fries BE. Predictors of aspiration pneumonia in nursing home residents. *Dysphagia*. 2002; 17(4):298–307. Available at: http://dx.doi.org/10.1007/s00455-002-0072-5

Donzelli J., Brady S, Wesling M, Craney M. Predictive value of accumulated oropharyngeal secretions for aspiration during video nasal endoscopic evaluation of the swallow. *Ann Rhino Otolaryngol*. 2003;112:469–475.

Kaneoka A, Pisegna JM, Miloro KV, Lo M, Saito H, Riquelme LF, LaValley MP, Langmore SE. Prevention of healthcare-associated pneumonia with oral care in individuals without mechanical ventilation: a systematic review and meta-analysis of randomized controlled trials. *Infect Control Hosp Epidemiol*. 2015;36(8):899–906. Available at: http://dx.doi.org/1-.01.1017/ice.2015.77

Wirth R, Dziewas R, Beck AM, Clavé P, Hamdy S, Heppner HJ, ... Volkert, D. Oropharyngeal dysphagia in older persons - from pathophysiology to adequate intervention: a review and summary of an international expert meeting. *Clin Interv Aging*. 2016;11:189–208. doi:10.2147/CIA.S97481

9. **What surgical procedures are available to improve glottal closure and reduce aspiration risks?**
Adequate glottal closure is a key component to reducing aspiration risks. Glottal incompetence may be due to **unilateral vocal fold immobility** (VFI) in the lateral or para-medium position, **postintubation insufficiency,** and **bilateral vocal fold atrophy.** Injection laryngoplasty using **vocal fold injectable materials** (e.g., Cymetra, Radiesse voice gel, Gelfoam, Teflon, fat) are used to increase the bulk of the vocal fold to restore glottal competence. Depending upon the material used, the vocal fold injection may last from a few weeks up to 2 years. Another option is **medialization thyroplasty** and is generally reserved for patients with long-standing glottal competency issues (i.e., 9 to 12 months). This procedure involves inserting an implant into the vocal fold and can be completed with or without arytenoid repositioning. Patients with a high-vagal nerve injury may benefit from **pharyngoplasty** that involves reducing the space on the impaired side of the hypopharynx or a **cricopharyngeal myotomy** to increase the opening of the UES.

Giraldez-Rodriguez LA, Johns M. Glottal insufficiency with aspiration risk in Dysphagia. Glottal insufficiency with aspiration risk in dysphagia. In *Dysphagia: Diagnosis and Management* (Editor Kenneth W. Altman). *Otolaryngol Clin N Am.* 2013;46(6):1113–1121. Available at: http://dx.doi.org/10.1016/j.otc.2013.09.004

10. **What modalities are being used by therapists? Are new interventions being evaluated?**
Swallowing treatment modalities can be categorized as **compensatory swallow safety strategies/swallowing maneuvers** (generally used during meals or therapeutic feedings) and **rehabilitative swallowing strengthening/sensory interventions** (generally *not* used during meals). Newer treatment modalities for dysphagia include expiratory muscle strength training, neuromuscular electrical stimulation, laryngeal vibratory stimulation, cryotherapy, and repetitive transcranial magnetic stimulation. Table 31.1 summarizes the various strategies and interventions used in swallowing therapy along with the therapeutic indication.

Table 31.1 Compensatory Swallowing Strategies and Swallowing Maneuvers

STRATEGY	RATIONALE
Chin Tuck	Widens the valleculae and positions the base of the tongue closer to the posterior pharyngeal wall. This posture may be useful to reduce laryngeal penetration and/or aspiration when it occurs before the swallow. This posture may also be useful to assist with pharyngeal clearance.
Chin Up	Upright posture with the patient's head back and neck extended. This may be useful to assist with oral transport of the bolus.
Head Rotation	The unilateral head rotation to the weaker side is used to redirect bolus flow down the stronger side and is used to assist with pharyngeal clearance. The bilateral head rotation is used to assist with increasing the upper esophageal sphincter (UES) opening when residue is present at the level of the UES.
Head Tilt	The head tilt to the stronger side (head to shoulder) is used to redirect the bolus flow to the stronger side via gravity and is used for unilateral pharyngeal residue.
Combination Postural Intervention (e.g., Chin tuck with head rotation)	When a patient demonstrates multiple issues, you can also use a combination of postural interventions such as the chin tuck with the head rotation to address both airway invasion before the swallow and unilateral pharyngeal residue on the weaker side.
Voluntary Throat Clear/Cough	Use of a voluntary throat clear or cough to assist with expelling any airway invasion of the bolus (i.e., laryngeal penetration or aspiration) after each swallow.
Effortful Swallow	Used for pharyngeal residue as it improves base of tongue retraction and pharyngeal constrictor strength contraction.
Supraglottic and Super-supraglottic swallow	Used to improve voluntary airway closure before and during the swallow with use of a breath hold and assist with airway clearance using a voluntary throat clear following the swallow.
Breath Hold	Voluntary breath hold prior to the swallow. This strategy may be used to improve airway protection for an individual who may penetrate or aspirate prior to the swallow.
Liquid Wash/Alternating Liquids and Solids	Used to clear oral, pharyngeal, and esophageal stasis.
Multiple Swallows	Used to assist with oral and pharyngeal clearance.
Oral Hold	Used with liquids to assist with reducing premature spillage of the bolus over the base of the tongue prior to the swallow.

continued

Table 31.1 Compensatory Swallowing Strategies and Swallowing Maneuvers—cont'd

Bolus Modification (e.g. viscosity, volume, sensory enhancement/sour bolus)	Used to improve the safety and efficiency of the swallow. Effectiveness of each type of bolus modification is individualized. The default to use thickened liquids to increase swallow safety is **not** always appropriate. Use of verbal cues to reduce volume/bolus size can be effective.
Adaptive Feeding Equipment	Adaptive feeding equipment (e.g., plate guard, rolling knife, built up utensil grip) to help with feeding independence and bolus size control. Straws may be beneficial with some patients (e.g., spinal cord injury) or may be detrimental (e.g., impulsive patient following a brain injury) and need to be individually evaluated.

Rehabilitation Strengthening/Sensory Treatment Techniques

STRATEGY	RATIONALE
Mendelsohn Maneuver	The Mendelsohn maneuver is a strengthening exercise that can be completed with and without a bolus. It involves the prolonged elevation of the larynx during the swallow as it provides a longer duration of airway closure to reduce the chances of airway invasion. The patient is instructed to keep the larynx elevated in the high position during the swallow for an additional 1–3 s.
Gustatory Stimulation	A sensory stimulation technique to increase swallow frequency in patients who are NPO. A small amount (drop size) of a strong flavored bolus (e.g., sour, sweet, bitter, menthol) to elicit a swallow response.
Ice Chips	A sensory stimulation technique to increase swallow frequency in patients who are NPO. Small ice chips (less than 1 cm) are placed on the tongue of the patient to elicit a swallow response. A FEES should be completed to ensure the patient is able to safely manage small ice chips prior to implementation.
Tongue Hold/Masako Maneuver	Therapeutic exercise to improve base of tongue retraction and is not to be used during consumption of food/liquid. The tip of the tongue is placed between the front teeth and the patient is instructed to swallow.
Shaker Exercise	Head lift exercise that focuses on strengthening the suprahyoid muscles to improve the opening of the UES. The patient lies flat on their back and completes head lifts with the shoulders remaining on the bed. This exercise should not be completed during the consumption of food/liquid.
Thermal Tactical Oral Stimulation	Involves stroking the anterior faucial pillars with a cold probe to heighten oral awareness and improve the timeliness of the pharyngeal swallow response. While this is commonly used, there is limited empiric research to support its use.

Newer Treatment Modalities

STRATEGY	RATIONALE
Expiratory Muscle Strength Training	An indirect swallowing exercise targeting increased anterior suprahyoid activation to improve hyolaryngeal elevation.
Neuromuscular Electrical Stimulation (NMES)	NMES is a therapeutic technique involving the application of electrical stimulation to cause the muscle fibers involved with swallowing to contract. NMES can be applied via a percutaneous (intramuscular) or a transcutaneous (surface/non-invasive) approach. The application of surface NMES to the neck, faucial pillars, palate, and pharynx has been studied. Neck surface NMES has been the most extensively studied with some limited evidence demonstrating a positive treatment; however, further efficacy studies are still required as questions related to dosage, timing, and the use of NMES with different patient populations remain unanswered.
Laryngeal Vibration	A novel non-invasive sensory stimulation technique to increase swallow frequency by providing vibratory stimulation (with no pressure) to the skin over the larynx. This is a promising new therapy approach and further investigation is needed.
Cryotherapy	Involves the use of liquid nitrogen spray for cryoablation under monitored anesthesia for individuals with dysphagia secondary to esophageal cancer. Initial research shows promise as a treatment modality; however, further investigation is warranted to evaluate the synergistic effects of cryotherapy with chemoradiation.
Repetitive transcranial magnetic stimulation (rTMS)	A novel non-invasive treatment approach that delivers cortical stimulation to improve cortical neuroplasticity and swallow function. The evidence regarding rTMS for dysphagia treatment is evolving and no unified treatment approach (i.e., location, frequency, intensity, pulse rate) has been developed. This modality shows promise; however, additional research is needed.

BIBLIOGRAPHY

Brady S, Leder S. *Adult Fiberoptic Endoscopic Evaluation of Swallowing.* In Suiter DM, Gosa MM, eds. *Assessing and Treating Dysphagia: A Lifespan Perspective.* New York, NY: Thieme Publishers; 2019

Brady SL, Wesling MW, Donzelli JJ, Kaszuba S. Swallowing frequency: impact of accumulated oropharyngeal secretion levels and gustatory stimulation. *Ear Nose Throat J.* 2016;95(2):E7–E9. Available at: https://doi.org/10.1177/014556131609500203

Clark H, Lazarus C, Arvedson J, Scholling T, Frymark T. Evidence-based systematic review: effects of neuromuscular electrical stimulation on swallowing and neural activation. *Am J Speech Lang Pathol.* 2009;18(4):361–376. Available at: http://dx.doi.org/10.1044/1058-0360(2009/08-0088).

Hegland KW, Murry T. *Nonsurgical Treatment Swallowing Rehabilitation.* In *Dysphagia: Diagnosis and Management* (Editor Kenneth W. Altman). *Otolaryngol Clin North Am.* 2013;46(6):1073–1085. Available at: http://dx.doi.org/10.1016/j.otc.2013.08.003

Humbert I. *Swallowing Postures and Maneuvers with Videofluoroscopy (Two Healthy Adults).* 2019 April 9; Available at https://www.youtube.com/watch?v=oHoqjTRpBtE

Kamarunas E, Wong SM, Ludlow CL. Laryngeal vibration increases spontaneous swallowing rates in chronic oropharyngeal dysphagia: a proof-of-principle pilot data. *Dysphagia.* 2019;34(5):640–653. Available at: https://doi.org/10.1007/s00455-018-9962-z

Langmore SE, McCulloch TM, Krisciunas GP, Lazarus CL, Van Daele DJ, Pauloski BR, Rybin D, Doros G. Efficacy of electrical stimulation and exercise for dysphagia in patients with head and neck cancer: a randomized clinical trial. *Head Neck.* 2016;38 (Suppl 1): E1221–E1231. doi:10.1002/hed.24197

Papadopoulou SL, Ploumis A, Exarchakos G, Theodorou SJ, Beris A, Fotopoulos AD. Versatility of repetitive transcranial magnetic stimulation in the treatment of poststroke dysphagia. *J Neurosci Rural Pract.* 2018;9(3):391–396. doi:10.4103/jnrp.jnrp_68_18

Raphael LJ, Borden GJ, Harris KJ. *Speech and Science Primer: Physiology, Acoustics, and Perception of Speech.* 6th ed. Baltimore, MD: Lippencott Williams and Wilkins; 2011.

Shah T, Kushnir V, Mutha P, Majhail M, Patel B, Schutzer M, Mogahanaki D, Smallfield G, Patel M, Zfass A. Neoadjuvant cryotherapy improves dysphagia and may impact remission rates in advanced esophageal cancer. *Endosc Int Open.* 2019;7(11):E1522–E1527. doi: 10.1055/a-0957-2798

CHAPTER 32

NEUROGENIC BOWEL DYSFUNCTION: EVALUATION AND ADAPTIVE MANAGEMENT

Steven A. Stiens, MD, MS, Gianna Maria Rodriguez, MD, Lance Goetz, and Jonathan Strayer, MS, MD

This is a fundamental principle of medicine, that whenever the stool is withheld or is extruded with difficulty, grave illnesses result.

—Maimonides (1135–1204)

KEY POINTS

1. Past bowel habits, daily life demands, and successful response to essential components guide *bowel program* design: fluids, diet, medications, exercise, and scheduled bowel care.
2. Neurological demonstration of sensation, pelvic floor strength, reflex responses, and general adaptive mobility and cognition determine the methods for *bowel care*—the individualized procedure for assisted defecation.
3. Clinical attention to patient's frequency of bowel movements, incontinence, symptoms of constipation, medication side effects, and the barriers caused by neurogenic bowel impairments reveals many potentially life-enhancing interventions.
4. Should sustained interdisciplinary interventions prove to be consistently ineffective, surgical interventions such as ostomy should be considered as supported by good documented outcomes.

1. How do the autonomic sympathetic/parasympathetic and somatic systems influence GI function?

The *sympathetic* and *parasympathetic* nervous systems modulate the *enteric nervous system* (ENS). The somatic peripheral nerves innervate the external sphincter permitting voluntary continence. These systems intimately link the brain and GI tract via a complex and organized network of neurons.

The ENS, nicknamed the "brain in the gut," is the evolutionary brain now under autonomic influence. It operates independently as an assembly of highly organized neurons situated in the submucosa (*Meissner's plexus*) and the intramuscular *myenteric* (*Auerbach's plexus*). There are about 500 million neurons in these plexi, plus two to three glial cells per neuron.

Sympathetic nervous system (*T11–L2 Hypogastric nerve*) *stimulation* promotes the storage function by enhancing anal tone and inhibiting colonic contractions, particularly when an individual is physically active, and not prepared to defecate.

The ENS is responsible for local coordination of secretion, peristalsis, and sphincters throughout the GI tract. It maintains repetitive pattern generation and responds through reflex circuits triggered by sensory signals, and synchronizes coordinated motor patterns (migrating motor complex, digestive activity, *giant migratory contractions*).

Kellow JE, Azpiroz F, Delvaux M, Gebhart GF, Mertz HR, Quigley EM, Smout AJ. Applied principles of neurogastroenterology: Physiology/motility sensation. *Gastroenterology*. 2006;130(5):1412–1420. Available at: https://pubmed.ncbi.nlm.nih.gov/16678555/. doi:10.1053/j.gastro.2005. 08. 061

Sharkey KA, Mawe GM. Neurogastroenterology in 2011: emerging concepts in neurogastroenterology and motility. *Nat Rev Gastroenterol Hepatol*. 2011;9(2):74–76. Available at: https://pubmed.ncbi.nlm.nih.gov/22158381/. doi:10.1038/nrgastro.2011.247.

2. What nerves innervate organs pertinent to stool formation, storage, and elimination?

Parasympathetic activity (*Vagus nerve, S2–S4 pelvic nerve*) enhances colonic motility, promotes rectal contraction and relaxation of the internal sphincter, and facilitates defecation. The *vagus* ("vagabond") *nerve* wanders from the brain stem and innervates the gut to the splenic flexure of the colon. The ENS includes unmyelinated fibers from postganglionic parasympathetic ganglia and interneurons that coordinate peristalsis.

Auerbach's (***intramuscular*** or ***myenteric***) ***plexus*** is located between the circular and longitudinal muscle layers, and ***Meissner's*** (***submucosal***) ***plexus*** relays local sensory and motor responses to Auerbach's plexus, pre-vertebral ganglia, and the spinal cord. The ***nervi erigentes*** (***inferior splanchnic nerve***) carries pelvic parasympathetic fibers from the S2–S4 conal levels to the descending colon and rectum. The ***somatic system*** (***S2 to S4 pudendal nerve***) provides voluntary control over the external sphincter, pelvic floor muscles, and defecation (Fig 32.1).

Grundy D, Al-Chaer ED, Aziz Q, Collins SM, Ke M, Taché Y, Wood JD. Fundamentals of neurogastroenterology: basic science. *Gastroenterology.* 2006;*130*(5):1391–411. Available at: https://www.gastrojournal.org/article/S0016-5085(06)00510-5/fulltext. doi: 10.1053/j.gastro.2005.11.060.

3. What is the "law of the intestine"?

    In 1899, two English physiologists, W.M. Bayliss and E.H. Starling, reported that whenever the intestinal wall is stretched or dilated, the nerves in the myenteric plexus cause the muscles above the dilation to constrict and the muscles below the dilation to relax, propelling the contents caudally toward the anus.

Spencer NJ, Hibberd TJ, Travis L, Wiklendt L, Costa M, Hu H, Brookes SJ, Wattchow DA, Dinning PG, Keating DJ, Sorensen J. Identification of a rhythmic firing pattern in the enteric nervous system that generates rhythmic electrical activity in smooth muscle. *J Neurosci.* 2018;38(24):5507–5522. Available at: https://www.jneurosci.org/content/38/24/5507.long. doi: 10.1523/JNEUROSCI.3489-17.2018

4. What is the normal physiologic sequence of steps that lead to defecation?

    Reflex activity:

    a. ***Giant migratory contractions*** start at the cecum and advance stool through the colon to the rectum.

    b. Stool distends the rectum as the internal sphincter relaxes (***rectal inhibitory*** or ***sampling reflex***), which triggers a conscious urge.

    c. Contraction of the internal sphincter retains stool if not ready to have a bowel movement (***holding reflex***).

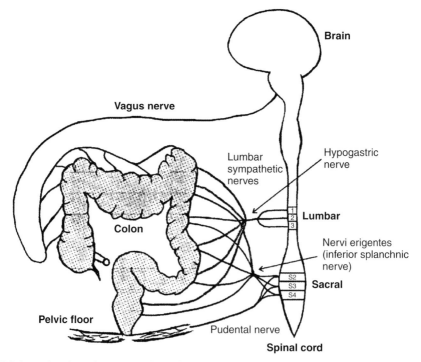

Fig. 32.1 Autonomic and somatic nerve connections to the colon and pelvic floor that mediate stool propulsion, storage, and defecation.

Voluntary activity:

a. Relaxation of the external anal sphincter and puborectalis releases stool.

b. Contraction of the levator ani, external abdominals, and diaphragm, combined with glottic closure, elevates intra-abdominal pressure and propels stool out.

Barleben A, Mills S. Anorectal anatomy and physiology. *Surg Clin North Am.* 2010;90(1):1–15. Available at: https://pubmed.ncbi.nlm.nih.gov/20109629/. doi: 10.1016/j.suc.2009.09.001.

5. What nervous system lesions produce the various patterns of neurogenic bowel dysfunction?

Neurogenic bowel is a term that relates colon dysfunction (constipation), incontinence, and discoordination of defecation due to lack of nerve control.

The **upper motor neuron** (**UMN**) **bowel** results from a spinal cord lesion above the conus medullaris (supraconal) and typically manifests as fecal distention of the colon, overactive and dis-coordinated segmental peristalsis, hypoactive propulsive peristalsis, and a hyperactive holding reflex with spastic external anal sphincter constriction that requires mechanical or chemical stimulus to trigger reflex defecation.

The **lower motor neuron** (**LMN**) **bowel** results from a lesion that affects the parasympathetic and somatic pudendal nerve, cell bodies or axons at the conus, cauda equina, or inferior splanchnic nerve. LMN bowel findings include low descending colonic wall tone and a flaccid pelvic floor and external anal sphincter. No spinal cord-mediated reflex peristalsis occurs. The myenteric plexus alone coordinates slow stool propulsion, and unpredictable incontinence is common when shifting positions. The denervated colon produces a drier, **rounder** (**scybalous**) stool because the prolonged transit time results in increased absorption of moisture.

Stiens SA, Bergman SB, Goetz LL, Neurogenic bowel dysfunction after spinal cord injury: clinical evaluation and rehabilitative management. *Arch Phys Med Rehabil.* 1997;78(3 Suppl):S86–S102. Available at: https://www.archives-pmr.org/article/S0003-9993(97)90416-0/pdf. doi: 10.1016/s0003-9993(97)90416-0.

6. What is the internal anal sphincter? How does it cooperate with the external anal sphincter mechanism and pelvic floor muscles to coordinate continence and defecation?

The **anal sphincter mechanism** includes the internal anal sphincter, external anal sphincter, and the puborectalis muscle that wraps around the distal rectum to kink it forward toward the pubis to maintain continence.

The **internal anal sphincter** is the thick layer of colonic smooth muscle that surrounds the anal canal at the distal rectum. It maintains anal canal closure with a **resting pressure** in response to tonic excitatory sympathetic (T11–L2) discharges. Internal sphincter relaxation is modulated by the parasympathetic system (S2–S4) which facilitates stool evacuation.

Anal dilatation by stool (**rectoanal inhibitory reflex**) or digital stimulation inhibits internal sphincter tone. Highly coordinated synergistic activity between the internal sphincter and external sphincter/pelvic floor muscles (under voluntary control) maintain bowel continence and allow normal defecation. Those experienced in providing bowel care are frequently able to palpate an increase in internal sphincter tone when defecation is complete.

Rao SSC, Bharucha AE, Chiarioni G, Felt-Bersma R, Knowles C, Malcolm A, Wald A. Functional anorectal disorders. *Gastroenterology.* 2016;25:S0016-5085(16)00175-X 10.1053/j.gastro.2016.02.009. Available at: https://www.ncbi.nlm.nih.gov/pmc/articles/PMC5035713/. doi:10.1053/j.gastro.2016.02.009.

7. What must be included in a good history for neurogenic GI dysfunction?

a. Cardinal symptoms

b. Neuromuscular dexterity and mobility

c. GI function

d. Total intake of fluids and type of fluids

e. Diet—include intake of natural fibers, from vegetables and fruits

f. Daily physical activity

g. Comprehensive list of medications

h. Oral and rectal GI medications (current and past)

i. Frequency of BM

j. Stool consistency (use Bristol Stool Scale)

k. Stool amount per BM

l. Times of day of BM; bowel care schedule

m. Specifics of current bowel program including bowel care: technique, initiation method, facilitative techniques, and time requirements

n. Premorbid bowel patterns and presence of disease

o. Presence of abdominal discomfort, bloating, distention
p. Presence of rectal urgency; ability to prevent stool loss
q. Issues with fecal incontinence

Rodriguez G, Stiens SA. *Neurogenic Bowel: Dysfunction and Rehabilitation.* In *Braddom's Physical Medicine and Rehabilitation.* 6th ed. Philadelphia: Elsevier; 2020:407–430.

8. What commonly used medications in rehabilitation can inadvertently contribute to constipation?

Opioid analgesics act at the mu and delta receptors, producing adenylate cyclase, inhibiting calcium channels and blocking neurotransmitter release.

Anticholinergics block acetylcholine signals, reducing peristalsis and secretion.

Antispasmodics, used for control of spasticity (baclofen, diazepam), cause constipation by relaxing muscles through the action of the inhibitory neurotransmitter gamma aminobutyric acid (GABA).

Patel T, Milligan J, Lee J. Medication-related problems in individuals with spinal cord injury in a primary care-based clinic. *J Spinal Cord Med.* 2017;40(1):54–61. doi:10.1179/2045772315Y.0000000055. Available at: https://www.ncbi.nlm.nih.gov/pmc/articles/PMC5376141/

Sharma A, Jamal MM. Opioid induced bowel disease: a twenty-first century physicians' dilemma. Considering pathophysiology and treatment strategies. *Curr Gastroenterol Rep.* 2013;*15*(7):334. Available at: https://pubmed.ncbi.nlm.nih.gov/23836088/. doi:10.1007/s11894-013-0334-4

9. What is the Bristol Stool Scale?

The ***Bristol Stool Scale*** classifies stools into 7 different categories based on form and consistency. It provides information that can indicate stools related to constipation (Types 1 to 2), normal consistency (Types 3 to 4), or diarrhea (Types 5 to 7). When stools remain in the colon too long, they become hard and dry. Normal stools are soft and formed. Diarrhea is characterized by watery, loose stools. These specific descriptions guide management of the neurogenic bowel (Fig. 32.2).

Saad RJ, Rao SSC, Koch KL, Kuo B, Parkman HP, McCallum RW, Sitrin MD, Wilding GE, Semler JR, Chey WD. Do stool form and frequency correlate with whole-gut and colonic transit? Results from a multicenter study in constipated individuals and healthy controls. *Am J Gastroenterol* 2010;105(2):403–411.

10. What must be included in a good physical examination for neurogenic GI dysfunction?

Abdominal evaluation:
a. Observation—signs of malnutrition, dehydration, anemia
b. Inspection—distention, hernias
c. Auscultation—bowel sounds
d. Percussion—listen for tympanitic abdomen
e. Palpation—tenderness, hard stool

Perineal/Anorectal evaluation:
a. Inspection
b. For gaping orifice or puckered anal sphincter
c. Contour of buttocks (hemorrhoids, fissures, bleeding)
d. Visual observation of anal squeeze and perineal relaxation and descent with Valsalva maneuver
e. Evaluate for anocutaneous reflex (anal wink); bulbocavernosus reflex
f. Examination of sensation to light touch and pinprick; sensation to deep anal pressure
g. Digital rectal examination

11. What is the difference between a bowel program and bowel care?

Although the terms are frequently interchanged, the most correct usage is as follows:

The ***Bowel Program*** is the individualized comprehensive management plan for prevention of the problems that come with neurogenic bowel dysfunction. A bowel program has a variety of **components**, which include ***diet, fluid, intake, physical activity, medications,*** and ***consistent***, scheduled bowel care.

Bowel Care is the individualized procedure for initiating and completing a bowel movement. It is the process for assisted defecation. Bowel care may include any or all of the following steps: preparation, positioning, checking for stool, inserting rectal stimulant medications, digital rectal stimulation, manual evacuation, recognizing completion, and clean up.

Stiens SA, Bergman SB, Goetz LL. Neurogenic bowel dysfunction after spinal cord injury: clinical evaluation and rehabilitative management. *Arch Phys Med Rehabil.* 1997 Mar;78(3 Suppl):S86–S102. Available at: https://www.archives-pmr.org/article/S0003-9993(97)90416-0/pdf. doi: 10.1016/s0003-9993(97)90416-0.

Bristol stool chart

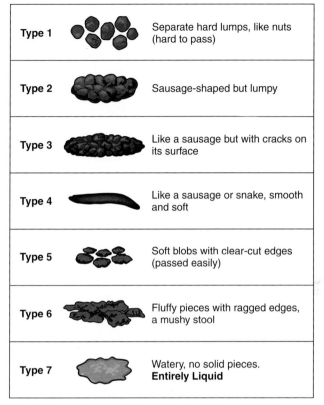

Type 1		Separate hard lumps, like nuts (hard to pass)
Type 2		Sausage-shaped but lumpy
Type 3		Like a sausage but with cracks on its surface
Type 4		Like a sausage or snake, smooth and soft
Type 5		Soft blobs with clear-cut edges (passed easily)
Type 6		Fluffy pieces with ragged edges, a mushy stool
Type 7		Watery, no solid pieces. **Entirely Liquid**

Fig. 32.2 The Bristol Stool Scale is very useful as a standardized visual categorization to guide short-term modulation of the Bowel Program in clinical settings as well as at home.

12. What are the goals of the bowel program?
    1. Regular and adequate passage of stool daily or every other day (at least 3× per week) of moderate to large amounts of stool (approx. 2 to 3 cups)
    2. Bowel evacuation at a consistent time of day (AM or PM)
    3. Complete emptying of the rectal vault with every bowel care session to prevent fecal incontinence
    4. Stools that are soft, formed, and bulky (Bristol Stool Scale 4 to 5)
    5. Completing the bowel care within half an hour (or, at most, within 1 hour)

13. What basic diet modifications can be made to improve bowel movements?
    Drink adequate non-caffeinated fluids and include sufficient fiber in diet. Daily fluid intake of 3 L for males and 2.2 L for females is recommended by the Institute of Medicine.
    A diet that contains at least 38 g of fiber daily for males and 25 g for females is recommended (15 g initially and gradually increase as tolerated). Natural fiber from vegetables, fruits, and grains is preferred, but supplemental fiber can also be useful to improve stool consistency and taken before largest meal to improve weight loss. All fiber sequesters fluid in the gastrointestinal tract and therefore requires free water intake. Caffeine, alcohol, and energy drinks promote diuresis and risk of constipation.

Dahl WJ, Stewart ML. Position of the Academy of Nutrition and Dietetics: health implications of dietary fiber. *J Acad Nutr Diet.* 2015;115(11):1861–1870. Available at: https://jandonline.org/article/S2212-2672(15)01386-6/fulltext. doi: 10.1016/j. jand.2015.09.003.

Popkin BM, D'Anci KE, Rosenberg IH. Water, hydration, and health. *Nutr Rev.* 2010; 68(8):439–458. Available at: https://www.ncbi. nlm.nih.gov/pmc/articles/PMC2908954/. doi: 10.1111/j.1753-4887.2010.00304.x

14. **What is the role of probiotics in neurogenic bowel?**

    The efficacy of probiotic products is both strain-specific and disease-specific. It is vital that the appropriate probiotic is utilized and chosen by matching the strain(s) with the targeted disease or condition, type of formulation, dose used, and the source (manufacturing quality control and shelf-life).

McFarland LV, Evans CT, Goldstein EJC. Strain-specificity and disease-specificity of probiotic efficacy: a systematic review and meta-analysis. *Front Med.* Published online, May 7, 2018. Available at: https://www.ncbi.nlm.nih.gov/pmc/articles/PMC5949321/. doi:10.3389/fmed.2018.00124.

15. **Describe the bowel care used to facilitate reflex defecation for a person with upper motor neuron (UMN) bowel.**

    Persons with spinal cord injury need a scheduled trigger of defecation every 1 to 3 days because they are typically unable to feel the stool in the rectum or to voluntarily initiate defecation. A person with UMN must regularly trigger bowel movements in order to predictably eliminate stool and avoid colonic overdistention. The ***defecation reflex*** is stimulated digitally with a finger (or assistive device) inserted in the rectum (digital stimulation) and/or with appropriate stimulant medication.

    The initializing stimulant medication trigger is typically a suppository, enema, or mini-enema, which is placed against the upper rectal wall and produces a mucosal contact stimulus that initiates conus-mediated reflex peristalsis. After the active ingredients dissolve and disperse, ***first gas*** is expelled and ***stool flow*** begins, augmented as necessary with interval ***digital stimulations***. These stimulations are repeated at least every 5 to 10 minutes to maintain motility. ***End of bowel care*** is signaled by cessation of gas and stool flow, palpable internal sphincter closure, or the absence of stool from the last two digital stimulations. Patients frequently sense the end of defecation. The sensation signaling the end of bowel care is possibly mediated by visceral afferents or partial sacral sparing of anal afferents.

16. **How is digital rectal stimulation performed?**

    Digital rectal stimulation is a technique for inducing reflex peristaltic waves along the colon to evacuate stool. The procedure is performed by getting patient permission and gently introducing the entire gloved and lubricated finger through the anal canal pointing toward the umbilicus. Movement in a circumferential, cone-shaped pattern opens the external anal sphincter by providing a gentle stretch stimulus that reduces spastic tone and outflow resistance. Rotation of the gloved finger in a firm circular manner produces sustained stimulation by maintaining contact with the rectal mucosa and dilating the proximal rectum. It is important to continually maintain mucosal contact and continued rotation until the bowel wall relaxes, flatus passes, and stool comes down.

    This maneuver activates peristalsis locally (coordinated by the myenteric plexus) and stimulates conal-mediated reflex peristalsis. Ideally, digital stimulation can generate peristalsis and stool flow in a minute or less, but the procedure can be continued longer, or repeated every few minutes as needed to initiate and maintain stool evacuation.

17. **What events and intervals mark the progress of bowel care?**
    (Fig. 32.3)

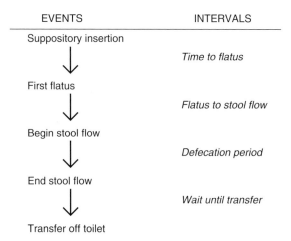

EVENTS	INTERVALS
Suppository insertion	
↓	Time to flatus
First flatus	
↓	Flatus to stool flow
Begin stool flow	
↓	Defecation period
End stool flow	
↓	Wait until transfer
Transfer off toilet	

Fig. 32.3 Events and intervals of bowel care progression. Clinical recognition of the processes that are active during assisted defecation and the signs of initiation and completion guides the frequency of digital stimulations and provides data to use in modulation of the Bowel Program.

18. **What is the gastrocolic response?**
Feeding induces increased propulsive colonic motility mediated by cholinergic motor neurons. Some have referred to this increase in gut motility as the gastrocolic reflex, but the mechanism may not be exclusively neural and has yet to be conclusively defined. Proposals include central vagal mediation, intrinsic colon pathways, and humoral mediation via cholecystokinin or gastrin. This increase in peristalsis is facilitated by a fatty or proteinaceous meal and blunted by atropine. Some investigators have reported that the gastrocolic response is less robust yet still present after SCI.

Callaghan B, Furness JB, Pustovit RV. Neural pathways for colorectal control, relevance to spinal cord injury and treatment: a narrative review. *Spinal Cord.* 2018;56(3):199–205. Available at: https://www.nature.com/articles/s41393-017-0026-2. doi: 10.1038/s41393-017-0026-2.

19. **Describe techniques to produce defecation and maintain continence in those with lower motor neuron (LMN) bowel dysfunction.**
Persons with LMN injuries often retrieve less stool volume with bowel care because low anal sphincter tone prevents accumulation and the absence of spinal reflex peristalsis limits propulsion down the sigmoid colon. Therefore, the rectum must be cleared of stool frequently, usually twice or more per day, to prevent inadvertently passing stool that cannot be retained by the weak internal and patulous external sphincters. Some patients wear tight underwear or bicycle pants to support the pelvic floor and help retain stool. Rectal stimulant medications generally are not used for patients with LMN bowel because the absence of a spinal cord–mediated reflex peristalsis limits their effectiveness to local rectal wall nerve circuits.

The ***LMN bowel care procedure*** usually consists of passive evacuation by removing stool with the finger (***manual evacuation***) and/or flushing the rectum with an enema. Continence is improved by modulation of stool consistency with a high-fiber diet to increase stool bulk and provide stool with formed but pliable texture. Plant fibers such as psyllium hydromucilloid "regularize" stool by absorbing and retaining excess water in order to prevent dry, hard and liquid, loose stool. Adequate and consistent fluid intake is imperative when taking high fiber, or excessive caliber and firmness can cause constipation

20. **What medications are used to augment peristalsis and facilitate overall effectiveness of the bowel program?**
Oral Medications:
- Traditional ***osmotic agents***, such as polyethylene glycol (PEG), docusate sodium, magnesium derivates (milk of magnesia, magnesium citrate, etc.), and mineral oil promote softer stools and movement of stool through the colon. ***Newer osmotic agents*** (e.g., lubiprostone and linaclotide) also increase stool water content by activating chloride channels that facilitate movement of stool through the colon.
- Daily ***fiber supplements*** that contain cellulose, polysaccharide, or psyllium can improve stool consistency by increasing stool bulk formation and plasticity, if adequate fluid intake is maintained.
- ***Oral stimulant laxatives*** that are anthraquinone derivatives, such as senna, aloe, and cascara preparations, stimulate the myenteric plexus and facilitate advancement of stool through the colon.
- ***Mu receptor antagonists*** like naloxegol and methylnaltrexone have been used to reduce constipation without reversing analgesia and or prompting opioid withdrawal (Table 32.1).

Rectal Medications that Trigger Defecation:
- ***Glycerine suppository***—Mild stimulus, lubricating
- ***Bisacodyl*** (phenolphthalein derivative) suppository—A polyphenolic molecule that stimulates colonic mass action on contact and provides a stronger chemical stimulus. May be compounded with a vegetable oil or a potentially faster-acting polyethylene base
- ***Docusate enemas*** are rapid acting. They contain docusate sodium, PEG, and glycerin (with or without benzocaine), which can reduce the incidence of autonomic dysreflexia by locally anesthetizing the rectal wall.
- ***Large-volume enemas*** (300 mL) with glycerin, mineral oil, soapsuds, or milk of molasses vary in how they are used and are poorly studied. Should be reserved for patients who are refractory to other medications.

House JG, Stiens SA: Pharmacologically initiated defecation for persons with spinal cord injury: Effectiveness of three agents. *Arch Phys Med Rehabil.* 1997;78(10):1062–1065. doi: 10.1016/s0003-9993(97)90128-3. Available at: https://www.archives-pmr.org/article/S0003-9993(97)90128-3/pdf

21. **How can diarrhea in patients with neurogenic bowel be evaluated and managed?**
Diarrhea in people with neurogenic bowel is commonly associated with a change in diet, antibiotic use, and external viruses. Diarrhea alternating with constipation may be due to partial bowel obstruction with flow of liquid stool around an impaction. A rectal examination is essential in evaluating these patients and may relieve the obstruction. Right colonic impactions are more common in UMN SCI and can be revealed by stool-filled loops of bowel on plain radiographs and require an osmotic liquid ingestion, usually with magnesium citrate or PEG, to facilitate complete evacuation of the colon.

Table 32.1 Luminally Acting Agents for Constipation

AGENT CATEGORY	MECHANISM OF ACTION	CLINICAL CONSIDERATIONS
Currently Available Agents		
Bulk laxatives e.g., soluble fiber (psyllium, methylcellulose, calcium polycarbophil, partially hydrolyzed guar gum, wheat dextrin) and insoluble fiber (bran, flaxseed, rye)	Increases stool water content to soften stool; increased stool mass might stimulate peristalsis	Use in mild constipation; soluble fiber is more effective than insoluble fiber; psyllium and ispaghula husk most studied; avoid when dyssynergia present
Surfactant laxatives, e.g., docusate sodium, docusate calcium	Anionic detergents lower the surface tension of stool; allows water to penetrate stool	Use in mild constipation; psyllium is more effective than docusate
Osmotic laxatives e.g., PEG, lactulose, sorbitol, magnesium salts	Generation of an osmotic gradient in gut lumen; promotes movement of water into lumen; luminal water softens stool and stimulates secondary peristalsis	PEG and lactulose effective for intermittent and chronic constipation; PEG is more effective than lactulose; might not benefit pain in IBS-C; avoid use of magnesium in patients with renal dysfunction
Stimulant laxatives, e.g., diphenylmethanes (bisacodyl, sodium picosulfate), anthraquinones (senna, cascara), misoprostol, castor oil	Direct colonic wall irritant; stimulation of sensory nerves on colonic mucosa; possible inhibition of water absorption; prostaglandin-induced effects on motility and secretion with misoprostol	Efficacy for intermittent constipation; Diphenylmethanes effective for chronic constipation; long-term safety not established
Chloride channel activation e.g., lubiprostone	Secretion of chloride ions into intestinal lumen through direct activation of C1–C2 chloride channels on enterocytes; results in passive movement of sodium and water into intestine	Short- and long-term efficacy and safety data in chronic constipation and women with IBS-C; main adverse event is dose-dependent nausea
Probiotics e.g., *Bifidobacterium lactis, Lactobacillus paracasei*	Hypothesized effects on gut transit and secretion through alteration of gut microbiota	Possible role in chronic constipation and IBS-C; no long-term efficacy or safety data; quality control issues (regulated as food additives not drugs)
Emerging agents		
Chloride-channel activation e.g., linaclotide, plecanatide	Activation of guanylate cyclase c receptor generating cGMP; secretion of chloride ions into intestinal lumen through cGMP mediated activation of CFTR; results in passive movement of sodium and water into intestine; inhibition of visceral pain fiber firing by cGMP in animals	Effective in chronic constipation and IBS-C in phase II (linaclotide and plecanatide) and phase III clinical trials (linaclotide); main adverse event is diarrhea
Bile-acid analogues e.g., chenodeoxycholic acid	Increases colonic motility; increases luminal secretory activity	Effective in IBS-C as shown in phase 2 trial; risk of abdominal pain and/or cramps
Inhibitors of bile-acid resorption e.g., elobixibat	Partial inhibition of ileal bile acid transporter; increases colonic bile acid concentrations promoting colonic motility and secretion	Effective for chronic constipation shown in phase II trial; dose dependent abdominal pain reported

CFTR, cystic fibrosis transmembrane conductance regulator: *cGMP*, cyclic GMP; *IBS-c*, constipation-predominant IBS; *PEG*, polyethylene glycol.

From Yang H, Tonghui, M. Luminally acting agents for constipation treatment: a review based on literatures and patents. *Front Pharmacol.* 2017;8:418. doi:10.3389/fphar.2017.00418

Laboratory evaluation is used when indicated for infectious causes (including *Clostridium difficile*). Discontinue offending agents.

22. **Which diagnostic tools can be useful in assessment of neurogenic GI dysfunction?**
    - Basic laboratory tests complement the history and physical examination.
    - **Abdominal x-ray**—Can evaluate for degree of fecal loading, assess for impaction, obstruction, megacolon, or ileus.
    - **Abdominal CT**—Can be used to evaluate for detailed structural issues and to identify small or large intestinal lesions and obstructions.
    - **Colonic transit test**—Measures colonic transit time by swallowed radio-opaque markers monitored with abdominal x-rays on subsequent days and are counted as these pass through the right transverse and rectosigmoid segments of the colon.
    - **Wireless Motility Capsule**—Measures segmental gastric, small intestinal and colonic transit times, and whole gut transit time with one procedure, as opposed to standard testing done on separate and multiple days.
    - **Anal Rectal Manometry**—evaluates the pattern of abnormal defecation and pelvic floor dysfunction in neurogenic bowel. It measures rectal and sphincter pressures; coordination of pelvic floor and sphincter muscles and presence of dyssynergia; and anal and rectal sensation.

Bharucha AE, Pemberton JH, Locke GR III. American Gastroenterological Association technical review on constipation. *Gastroenterology*. 2013;144(1):218–38. Available at: https://www.gastrojournal.org /article/S0016-5085(12)01544-2/fulltext. doi: 10.1053/j.gastro.2012.10.028

Rao SS, Rattanakovit K, Patcharatrakul T. Diagnosis and management of chronic constipation in adults. *Nat Rev Gastroenterol Hepatol*. 2016;13(5):295–305. Available at: https://pubmed.ncbi.nlm.nih.gov/27033126/. doi:10.1038/nrgastro.2016.53.

Wald A, Bharucha AE, Cosman BC, Whitehead WE. ACG clinical guideline: management of benign anorectal disorders. *Am J Gastroenterol*. 2014;109(8):1141–1157, 1058(Quiz). Available at: https://acgcdn.gi.org/wp-content/uploads/2018/04/ACG-Anorectal-Disorders-Guideline-Summary.pdf. doi:10.1038/ajg.2014.190

23. **How can complications from neurogenic bowel be prevented?**
    Complications include **hemorrhoids,** fecal overloading (**impaction**), **megacolon,** colonic **diverticuli, rectal prolapse,** and **perirectal abscess**. Consistent adherence to the bowel program system with scheduled effective bowel care, prescribed oral and rectal medications, sufficient fluids, and fiber from the onset is protective. The regular schedule and frequency of bowel care sessions is particularly important, even if stool elimination does not occur each time. Missed bowel care sessions can contribute to excessive stool accumulation, making the stool drier and causing **difficulty with evacuation.** Retained stool can overstretch the colon wall, reducing peristalsis effectiveness and resulting in longer bowel care intervals with poor results. Hemorrhoids can be prevented by minimizing the time necessary for bowel care and by avoiding rectal over-distention. Each patient's unique interdisciplinary bowel program design requires comprehensive revision at least annually to surmount obstacles, innovate for improvements, and adapt to lifestyle.

Adriaansen JJ, van Asbeck FW, van Kuppevelt D, Snoek GJ, Marcel W Post. Outcomes of neurogenic bowel management in individuals living with a spinal cord injury for at least 10 years. *Arch Phys Med Rehabil*. 2015;96(5):905–912. Available at: https://pubmed.ncbi.nlm.nih.gov/25620716/. doi: 10.1016/j.apmr.2015.01.011

Hwang M, Zebracki K, Vogel LC. Long-term outcomes and longitudinal changes of neurogenic bowel management in adults with pediatric-onset spinal cord injury. *Arch Phys Med Rehabil* 2017;98(2):241–248. Available at: https://pubmed.ncbi.nlm.nih.gov/27473299/. doi:10.1016 /j.apmr.2016.07.004

Nielsen SD, Faaborg PM, Finnerup NB, Christensen P, Krogh K. Ageing with neurogenic bowel dysfunction. *Spinal Cord*. 2017;55(8):769–773. Available at: https://pubmed.ncbi.nlm.nih.gov/28290468/. doi: 10.1038/sc.2017.22

24. **What is transanal irrigation?**
    Transanal irrigation (**TAI**) is performed with a retention enema device which includes a rectal catheter and an inflatable rectal retention balloon that creates a sealed system allowing pressure irrigation of the rectum and sigmoid with 500 to 1000 mL of water. This system can facilitate bowel emptying, improve constipation, reduce fecal incontinence, and decrease bowel care time, thereby improving GI symptoms and quality of life.

Christensen P, Krogh K. Transanal irrigation for disordered defecation: a systematic review. *Scand J Gastroenterol*. 2010;45(5):517–527. Available at: https://pubmed.ncbi.nlm.nih.gov/20199336/. doi: 10.3109/00365520903583855

Krassioukov A, Eng JJ, Claxton G, Sakakibara BM, Shum S. Neurogenic bowel management after spinal cord injury: a systematic review of the evidence. *Spinal Cord*. 2010;48(10):718–733. Available at: https://www.ncbi.nlm.nih.gov/pmc/articles/PMC3118252/. doi: 10.1038/sc.2010.14

25. What is a pulsed irrigation enema?

   Pulse irrigation enema (**PIE**) uses a device to provide pulsed, intermittent pressurized water irrigation into the rectum and sigmoid colon, promoting colonic motility and complete colonic emptying. This equipment should be used only by trained and experienced providers in a hospital, clinic, or medically supervised home setting.

Puet TA, Jackson H, Amy S. Use of pulsed irrigation evacuation in the management of the neuropathic bowel. *Spinal Cord.* 1997;35(10):694–699. Available at: https://pubmed.ncbi.nlm.nih.gov /9347600/. doi: 10.1038/sj.sc.3100491

26. What is a continent appendicocecostomy stoma? How does it help bowel care?

   The *Malone*, or *antegrade continence enema* (**ACE**), procedure surgically produces an abdominal catheterizable stoma that enters the cecum for self-administration of antegrade enemas to initiate bowel care. Through an 8 cm incision in the right lower quadrant, the appendix is localized and brought to the surface of the abdomen to form a stoma by amputating the tip to expose the lumen. The appendix is sewn into place and the stoma can be covered with a bandage. Bowel care is performed by catheterizing the cecum through the appendix, then infusing 100 to 400 mL of saline to trigger defecation. Bowel care is completed in the classic manner of repeated digital rectal stimulation in order to promote peristalsis and liberate all the stool and enema liquid. The Malone procedure also has been successful in many patients with spina bifida and a few with SCI.

Yang CC, Stiens SA. Antegrade continence enema for the treatment of neurogenic constipation and fecal incontinence after spinal cord injury. *Arch Phys Med Rehabil.* 2000;81(5);683–685. Available at: https://www.archives-pmr.org/article/S0003-9993(00)90054-6/fulltext. doi: 10.1016/s0003-9993(00)90054-6.

27. What if the bowel care routine becomes less effective, inefficient, newly dependent, or complicated by autonomic dysreflexia or intractable bleeding hemorrhoids?

   Some persons with long histories of SCI may lose the ability to independently perform or manage their own bowel care, develop difficulty in maintaining continence, or evolve excessively time-consuming bowel care routines with insufficient results. A **colostomy** offers many patients independent bowel management, less incontinence, and reduced bowel care time, with an improvement in quality of life. A colostomy is generally an elective procedure and is usually reversible, although people with SCI who elect colostomy seldom have it reversed. Colostomies are also considered if stage 3 to 4 chronic pressure ulcers are present.

Boucher M, Dukes D, Bryan S, Branagan G. Early colostomy formation can improve independence following spinal cord injury and increase acceptability of bowel management. *Top Spinal Cord Inj Rehabil.* 2019; *25*(1):23–30. Available at: https://www.ncbi.nlm.nih.gov/pmc/articles/PMC6368110/. doi: 10.1310/sci18-00026

BIBLIOGRAPHY

Consortium for Spinal Cord Medicine. *Neurogenic Bowel: What You Should Know. A Guide for People With Spinal Cord Injury;* 1999. Available at: https://www.bronx.va.gov/docs/BWLC.pdf

Consortium for Spinal Cord Medicine. *Clinical Practice Guidelines: Spinal Cord Medicine: Injury, Management of Neurogenic Bowel Dysfunction After Spinal Cord Injury;* 2020. Available at: https://pvacf.org/wp-content/uploads/2020/10/CPG_Neurogenic-Bowel-Recommendations.single-6.pdf

Multidisciplinary Association of Spinal Cord Injured Professionals. *Guidelines for Management of Neurogenic Bowel Dysfunction in Individuals With Central Neurological Conditions;* 2012. Available at: https://www.mascip.co.uk/wp-content/uploads/2015/02/cv653n-neurogenic-guidelines-sept-2012.pdf

CHAPTER 33

NEUROGENIC BLADDER

Inder Perkash, MD, MS, FACS, FRCS

The length of a film should be directly related to the endurance of the human bladder.
—Alfred Hitchcock

KEY POINTS

1. The term *neurogenic bladder* refers to organ level dysfunction (impairment) that results from central or peripheral nervous system damage.
2. The pelvic parasympathetic nerve (S2–S4) innervates the detrusor muscle (bladder wall) with motor and sensory fibers. S3 is usually the major nerve.
3. The somatic mixed pudendal nerve (S2–S4) includes motor and sensory fibers and innervates the pelvic floor, which includes the external anal sphincter. S2 is the key nerve.
4. Detrusor–sphincter dyssynergia is the simultaneous contraction of the detrusor (bladder wall) and external urethral sphincter (pelvic floor), which generates excessive bladder pressures (>50 cm H_2O).
5. Detrusor–sphincter dyssynergia occurs with lesions of the spinal cord above the conus. Persistent high-pressure voiding (with pressures beyond 50 cm H_2O) is associated with hydronephrosis and deterioration of renal function over the years.
6. Supraconal bladder dysfunction is associated with bilateral paralysis of toe movement, hyperreflexic phasic stretch reflexes of the gastrocsoleus muscles (SI), and positive bulbocavernosus and anocutaneous reflexes.

1. **How is neurogenic bladder defined?**
   A bladder is considered neurogenic if there are functional impairments that result from abnormalities in the peripheral or central nervous system (CNS). Voluntary control problems include sensory problems, inability to perceive bladder fullness, inability to voluntarily initiate micturition, and incontinence. The result is urinary retention and/or incontinence. Neurologic disorders can affect the brain, brain stem, spinal cord, or peripheral nerves to cause these problems.[1]

2. **What are the neural pathways linking the bladder to the CNS?**
   The organizational center for micturition in the brain is localized in the pontine-mesencephalic reticular formation. Lesions above this level (suprapontine) are usually associated with detrusor hyperreflexia, whereas infrapontine supraconal lesions are always associated with detrusor–sphincter dyssynergia. The micturition center in the spinal cord is localized primarily in the intermediolateral region of spinal cord segments S2–S4, with S3 being the most important nerve root for bladder innervation.
   The bladder is supplied by both the parasympathetic (motor and sensory) and the sympathetic nervous systems. The pelvic parasympathetic nerves (S2–S4) innervate the detrusor muscle and carry both motor and sensory fibers. Preganglionic parasympathetic fibers extend from the spinal cord to the synapse with postganglionic fibers in the bladder wall. The periurethral and external urethral sphincters are innervated by the pudendal nerves (S1–S4). The innervation of most of the striated muscles of the pelvic floor, including those of the periurethral and anal sphincter, is through the pudendal nerve arising from S1 to S4, and provides volitional control.

3. **Describe the physiology of micturition.**
   The first sensation of filling occurs at approximately 100 mL and a feeling of fullness is perceived at 300 mL. This feeling of fullness is registered at the frontal parietal cortex. The filling bladder can be ignored, and micturition is inhibited, or it can be resolved with a voluntary void. The bladder is very compliant and may accommodate high urine volumes of more than 500 mL due to the passive viscoelastic properties and stimulation of beta-adrenergic sympathetic. Therefore, both inhibition and initiation are under voluntary control of the cerebral cortex, and continence is achieved. However, during sudden vigorous activities such as jumping, coughing, or dancing, continence is maintained reflexively via the conus with the local holding reflex.[2]

4. **How does a spinal cord injury (SCI) tip the balance?**
   The pelvic floor becomes spastic, making the holding reflex hyperactive. Complete spinal cord injury above the conus prevents sensory input and voluntary bladder control. As the bladder fills and intravesical pressures rise, sudden reflex detrusor contractions attempt to force urine out. Reflex contractions of the pelvic floor (external urethral sphincter dyssynergia) prevent the voiding, resulting in urine retention or intermittent leakage when the external urethral sphincter intermittently relaxes.

5. **What is the role of sympathetic innervation of the bladder and bladder neck?**

Motor and sensory sympathetic nerves originate in the intermediolateral cell columns of spinal cord segments T11–L2 and promote urine storage and continence. These nerves traverse the paravertebral ganglia through the hypogastric plexus to the bladder wall, bladder neck, and posterior urethra.

The bladder wall (fundus or body) primarily exhibits beta-adrenergic receptors and responds to norepinephrine by relaxing. There is also an abundance of beta-adrenergic receptors at the bladder base, which includes the upper trigone and vesicoureteral junction. This helps bladder storage by relaxing the detrusor muscle.

The bladder neck (vesicoureteral junction) is predominantly supplied with alpha-adrenergic fibers. There is a high density of alpha-adrenergic receptors along the bladder neck, particularly in males. This helps to prevent retrograde ejaculation and helps close the bladder neck during bladder filling. Because alpha-adrenergic activity leads to closure of the bladder neck, alpha-adrenergic blockers (alpha-adrenergic antagonists) usually are used to improve voiding by relaxing the bladder neck.

6. **What basic bedside neurourologic assessments provide initial clinical data for urologic management?**

The patient's history should be elicited for specific impairments in bladder sensation, storage, and voiding. The general neurologic examination should localize the primary neural lesion. Rectal examination is used to evaluate sphincter tone and voluntary strength, bulbocavernosus reflex, and the prostate gland for benign or malignant enlargement. In women, vaginal examination may reveal cystocele, rectocele, uterine support, and the condition of the urethra. Toe plantar flexors (S2) and hip external rotator (S1) strengths provide information about the integrity of sacral spinal cord segments that also supply the external urethral sphincter (S2).

An abdominal examination is important to feel for a distended bladder, before and after attempted voiding. In patients with SCI, attempted voiding can be promoted by suprapubic tapping over the bladder, Valsalva maneuver, and Crede (suprapubic pressure).

Postvoid residual (PVR) measurements are made by allowing the patient's bladder to fill naturally to capacity and then having the patient attempt to void voluntarily in a natural position (standing or sitting). A PVR greater than 100 mL or more than about 20% of the total voided urine is considered abnormal.

7. **How is a routine urodynamic evaluation done?**

The term video urodynamics refers to the simultaneous pressure flow studies with fluoroscopic visualization of the lower urinary tract. Similar studies can also be done using transrectal ultrasonography to simultaneously visualize the lower urinary tract.

Cystometry (CMG) is the recording of intravesical pressures during bladder filling. It requires introduction of a catheter through the urethra and slow filling of 20 to 50 mL/min of water at body temperature. During bladder filling, intravesical pressure usually does not rise above 20 cm H_2O before bladder contraction. Compliance decreases, and pressure increases at smaller volumes in patients with an overactive bladder. Detrusor–sphincter dyssynergia and repeated urinary tract infections (UTIs) can lead to bladder wall stiffness caused by detrusor hypertrophy or fibrosis, which reduces compliance and may contribute to reduced bladder capacity. PVR increases because of outflow obstruction.

8. **What is detrusor compliance?**

Compliance is defined as the increase in bladder pressure per unit of volume introduced and is calculated by the change in volume divided by the change in pressure ($\Delta V/\Delta P$). The detrusor wall is composed of roughly equal amounts of muscle and collagen. When the collagen is more abundant, the elasticity decreases, the detrusor becomes stiffer, and the pressure rises faster during filling. Hypertrophic, spastic (neurogenic) detrusor muscle can lead to reduced compliance as well.[3]

9. **What is detrusor–sphincter dyssynergia and autonomic dysreflexia?**

The normal process of voiding includes a balanced synergy of simultaneous bladder wall contraction and sphincter relaxation. Detrusor–sphincter dyssynergia is a pathologic hyperactive holding reflex characterized by the presence of involuntary pelvic floor urinary sphincter contraction and increased electromyographic (EMG) activity during detrusor (bladder wall) contraction. This is observed in patients with spinal cord lesions below the pons and is absent in those with intracranial lesions. A careful evaluation is required to diagnose detrusor–sphincter dyssynergia in a patient with an incomplete neurologic lesion due to difficulty in differentiating involuntary sphincteric activity such as dyssynergia from voluntary contractions to inhibit micturition.

Autonomic dysreflexia (AD) is a potentially life-threatening medical emergency that affects people with spinal cord injuries at the T6 level or higher. There is a sudden rise in blood pressure and is usually associated with slowing of the heart rate. Most of the spinal injured patients with detrusor–sphincter dyssynergia are prone to AD. It can be triggered with a blocked catheter, UTI, and even loaded rectum. Proper treatment of AD involves administration of anti-hypertensives along with immediate determination and removal of the triggering stimuli.

10. **How are the bulbocavernosus reflex and sacral evoked potential tested?**

The bulbocavernosus reflex is a polysynaptic (S2–S4), crossed sacral withdrawal reflex and a nociceptive reflex of very constant latency. Clinically, it can be tested by squeezing the glans or clitoris and feeling the contraction of the anal sphincter muscle. This reflex is present in all normal persons and in SCI patients with lesions above the conus. The bulbocavernosus reflex can also be recorded objectively by stimulating the dorsal nerve of the penis and picking up the EMG response (50–200 uv) in the anal sphincter muscle or from the perineal striated muscle.

The sacral-evoked response can be obtained either by stimulating the dorsal nerve of the penis with a ring electrode or by placing a stimulating needle on the left or right side of the bulbocavernosus muscle in the perineum to define a unilateral lesion. The first latency (about 12 m/s) can be recorded over T4–L1 on the back, which represents the sensory peripheral conduction time. The central conduction time can be recorded at the scalp, which is usually 50 msec. Patients with previously diagnosed neurologic disease and those with subtle abnormalities on neurologic screening are candidates for this type of evaluation. Sacral-evoked potential testing and somatosensory-evoked potential testing should not be used as screening tests but rather as objective measurements of the location, presence, and nature of afferent penile sensory dysfunction. The findings of such testing can aid in anatomic localization of the lesion as peripheral, sacral, or suprasacral.

11. **Which type of neurourologic dysfunction is typically found in patients with upper motor neuron lesions?**
The pattern of vesicourethral dysfunction depends on the site of the spinal lesion and any preexisting or associated disease, such as diabetes mellitus, radiculopathy, and ethanol abuse, which can reduce detrusor contraction and lead to overdistension of the bladder. Prostatic enlargement and urethral stricture can cause obstruction. After an acute spinal injury, initially there is a widespread autonomic paralysis (spinal shock phase), which often recovers by 3 to 6 weeks but can take longer. The reappearance of reflexes below the level of injury heralds the end of the spinal shock. However, the bladder can easily get overdistended during the acute phase due to areflexia of the detrusor muscles. Later, with the appearance of detrusor–sphincter dyssynergia with intermittent contraction of external urethral sphincter, there is incomplete emptying and retention of urine. Bladder emptying can be accomplished with limiting fluid and intermittent catheterization every 4 to 6 hours. Baseline urodynamic testing is usually performed 6 to 8 weeks after acute injury, when the changes in function associated with possible recovery and return of reflex activity have been stabilized below the level of injury.

Intermittent catheterization can be started as early as 7 to 15 days after injury. Fluid intake may need to be restricted to less than 1500 mL/day. The bladder is emptied with a straight catheter every 4 hours with a target bladder volume of no more than 500 mL. After the establishment of reflex activity, the patient is evaluated objectively with urodynamic monitoring of intravesical voiding pressures (leak pressure). Anticholinergic medications may be required during this phase to achieve continence and help reduce voiding pressures. A cystometrogram (CMG) may need to be repeated to evaluate the effect of anticholinergics on voiding pressures. Persistently high voiding pressures (>40 to 50 cm H_2O) with sustained rise during CMG may necessitate a further increase in the dosage of anticholinergics to prevent both leakage of urine and vesicoureteral reflux. To start, patients are given oxybutynin (Ditropan) 2.5 to 5 mg two or three times per day, to lower intravesical pressure to less than 40 to 50 cm H_2O. Patients who do not tolerate regular oxybutynin, particularly because of dryness of the mouth, can be given either longer-acting oxybutynin or tolterodine. There is some evidence that tolterodine may have less effect on muscarinic receptors in the salivary glands. This helps to achieve continence between catheterizations; therefore, patients do not have to wear external drainage and leg bags.

Patients with multiple sclerosis and incomplete spinal cord injury patients suffering from neurogenic detrusor overactivity and detrusor-sphincter dyssynergia can also benefit with injections of botulinum-A toxin into the detrusor muscles to control detrusor hyperreflexia or injections in the external urethral sphincter to control detrusor sphincter dyssynergia. Thus, bladder drainage can be customized to achieve continence and reduce voiding pressures.[3,4]

12. **What is the best way to provide bladder drainage in patients with acute spinal cord injury?**
During the first 7 to 14 days, an indwelling catheter should be left in the bladder for drainage to prevent inadvertent overdistention. A small catheter (F14 or F16) is recommended, which prevents urethral irritation and allows periurethral secretions to drain easily around it.[5,6]

13. **Which method provides optimal long-term drainage of the neurogenic bladder?**
Patients who have a reflex bladder, particularly tetraplegics, cannot catheterize themselves but can wear an external drainage condom. They need assistance for catheterization. Otherwise, they end up having a suprapubic cystostomy or an indwelling Foley for bladder drainage. Indwelling catheter needs to be taped with a slack to prevent bladder neck stimulation which evokes bladder contractions and AD. These patients could also be considered for surgical reduction of outflow obstruction. Transurethral sphincterotomy (TURS), or stenting of the urethral sphincter, reduces outflow resistance to enable voiding at low pressure. This also helps to reduce the AD triggered by detrusor-sphincter dyssynergia.

A patient with a small retractile penis with reflex bladder may be considered for a penile implant to allow a better water seal of the condom catheter. Other patients who cannot self-catheterize and have a small retractile penis may need an indwelling catheter or suprapubic cystostomy.

In female patients who cannot self-catheterize and are incontinent, vesical or supravesical diversion, such as a suprapubic cystostomy or bowel pouch, may be considered. Continent reservoirs that can be catheterized through sites on the abdomen are also available. Currently, such patients are also considered for dorsal root (rhizotomy) and sacral motor root electrical stimulation to permit functional electric stimulation for voiding.[7,8]

14. Describe the usual protocol for urologic follow-up of patients with spinal cord injury.
Patients with SCI are monitored with annual ultrasounds of the kidneys, ureters, and bladder to detect renal parenchymal loss, hydronephrosis, and stones. The annual risk for bladder stones is 4% with indwelling catheters. Blood urea nitrogen (BUN) and serum creatinine (Cr) levels are compared with previous years. Levels of serum creatinine, which is a muscle metabolite, may be normally as low as 0.5 mg/dL in some tetraplegics who lack muscle mass. Radionuclide renal perfusion imaging is used to evaluate glomerular filtration and renal plasma flow. This is done if needed to further quantify renal function. Glomerular filtration rate (GFR) could be useful to tell how well the kidneys are filtering.

If hydronephrosis of the kidneys or ureters is noted or deterioration of the renal function is found, a full workup, including CT scanning with dye or intravenous urogram and voiding cystourethrogram may be needed. Cystoscopic examination is required to evaluate outflow obstruction and/or to rule out other bladder problems such as tumors. A cystoscopic examination with visualization and biopsy to detect bladder cancer is recommended for patients who have been heavy smokers or who had used chronic indwelling catheters for years.[9,10]

15. What bladder problems are seen in patients with brain injury?
Following head injury or other intracranial lesions, the bladder is hyperreflexic, but there is no dyssynergia. Initially, there may be retention of urine, and patients can be managed with an indwelling catheter followed by intermittent catheterization every 4 to 6 hours. Some patients may be controlled with a small dosage of oxybutynin or tolterodine. In patients with intracranial lesions such as parkinsonism, the bladder also is hyperreflexic. The use of drugs (anticholinergics) to manage tremors may lead to retention of urine. In all such patients with detrusor hyperreflexia, a transurethral resection of the prostate can sometimes result in permanent incontinence. There is also some evidence that oxybutynin is more lipid-soluble and thus may have higher concentration in the brain. This might influence reversible short-term memory problems.[7,11,12]

16. What are the common urinary tract complications of neurogenic bladder? How can they be prevented?
- The earliest changes in the bladder are noticed on voiding cryptographic studies as trabeculations and small diverticulum inside thickened bladder wall.
- Vesicoureteral reflux has been recorded in 10% to 30% of poorly managed patients. The presence of reflux is a serious complication because it leads to pyelonephritis and renal stone disease.
- Severe bladder outflow obstruction can result in bilateral hydronephrosis and hydroureters and an overdistended areflexic bladder.
- Repeated bladder infections can lead to bladder wall changes and marked reduction in the compliance of the bladder.

The bladder wall changes can be prevented to some extent by adequately draining the bladder at a pressure below 40 cm H_2O, either by intermittent catheterization along with the use of anticholinergic drugs or by timely surgical relief of the outflow obstruction.

17. How common are UTIs in patients with SCI?
UTIs and their sequelae are the most frequent medical complications experienced by patients with spinal cord injury. In persons who have long-term indwelling catheters or suprapubic catheters, the presence of bacteriuria is almost universal. The incidence of bacteriuria is reduced significantly in patients who can perform intermittent self-catheterization. Repeated UTIs have been associated with bladder biolayer (like biofilm on ureteral catheters) on the bladder wall.[13–15]

18. What constitutes a significant UTI in a patient with SCI?
A significant UTI is one accompanied by a 1.5°F rise in body temperature with positive urine microbial culture and large number of pus cells. Ordinary spun urine showing greater than 5 to 10 pus cells/high-power microscopic field is considered to be infection. If this is observed in patients on intermittent catheterization, it may require treatment. In the absence of fever, an asymptomatic infection may not be treated in patients with indwelling or suprapubic catheters. The urine culture can be obtained by introducing a new clean catheter to avoid cultures from the old biofilm.[16]

19. What preventive measures can be taken to reduce the risk of UTIs?
Patients wearing external condom drainage with voiding pressures less than 50 cm H_2O, particularly following TURS, are relatively safe from UTIs, but they need to clean the external drainage bag and tubing with 6% bleach. A daily thorough washing will clean the appliances. Personal hygiene with showering and adequate cleaning of the perineum and a daily cleaning of the cushion cover may reduce pelvic floor colonization and subsequent anterior urethral heavy colonization and contamination.

20. List the drugs used in the management of bladder problems and their desired effects.
Options for pharmacologic manipulation of bladder function are outlined in Table 33.1. Tolterodine and oxybutynin as anticholinergics are available to manage detrusor hyperreflexia. Most of the autonomic drugs that change

Table 33.1 Pharmacologic Manipulation of Bladder Function

DESIRED FUNCTIONAL CHANGE	DRUG	MODE OF ACTION
Improve bladder emptying	Bethanechol (clinically used)	Limited indications
Facilitate bladder contraction (muscarinic action)		It should not be used with outlet obstruction or in suspected coronary disease.
		It can be used in selected patients along with alpha-sympathetic blockers and in patients with atonic or hypotonic bladder.
Decrease outlet resistance	Prazosin, terazosin, doxazosin, clinically used	Selective a-1 adrenergic receptor blockers to improve voiding by opening bladder neck.
Reduce bladder contraction	Atropine, propantheline, oxybutynin, tolterodine, Trospium, chloride, darifenacin, Solifenacin, phenylephrine, ephedrine	Anticholinergic action (antimuscarinic action)
Increase outlet resistance		Sympathetic agonist response, alpha-adrenergic receptors
Improve bladder storage and increase outlet resistance	Tricyclic antidepressants	Central and peripheral anticholinergic effects and enhancement of alpha-adrenergic effect on bladder base and proximal urethra

arteriolar tone also seem to have effect on the bladder neck (e.g., alpha agonists constrict the bladder neck, and alpha blockers relax the bladder neck). In selective patients with detrusor hyperreflexia and detrusor sphincter dyssynergia, Onabotulinum toxin (Botox) injection in the bladder wall through cystoscope and directly in the external urinary sphincter has been found to be useful in managing these problems.

In the human bladder (detrusor muscle), there are muscarinic receptors (M2 and M3). M3 receptors, compared with M2, are less in number, but are mainly responsible for bladder contraction. Antimuscarinic drugs (oxybutynin, tolterodine, darifenacin, Solifenacin, and Trospium chloride) are the five major drugs currently available to manage detrusor hyperreflexia and to help reduce bladder voiding pressures. Comparative clinical studies have shown that Oxybutynin and Solifenacin may be marginally more effective than Tolterodine, although the latter seems to be better tolerated. Dry mouth and constipation are still major problems for patient compliance with all of them because of widespread existence of M3 receptors, particularly in the salivary glands.[17]

REFERENCES

1. Przydacz M, Denys P, Corcos J. What do we know about neurogenic bladder prevalence and management in developing countries and emerging regions of the world? *Ann Phys Rehabi Med.* 2017;60:341–346.
2. Altaweel W, Seyam R. Neurogenic bladder in spinal cord injury patients. *Res Rep Urol.* 2015;7:85–99.
3. Wyndaele JJ, Madersbacher H, Kovincha A. Conservative treatment of the neuropathic bladder in spinal cord injured patients. *Spinal Cord.* 2001;39:294–300.
4. Leippold T, Reitz A, Schurch B. Botulinum toxin as a new therapy option for voiding disorders: Current state of the art. *Eur Urol.* 2003 Aug;44(2):165–174.
5. Silver JR, Doggart JR, Burr RG. The *reduced* urinary output after spinal cord injury: a review. *Paraplegia.* 1995;33:721–725.
6. Van Kerrebroeck PE, Amarenco G, Thuroff JW, et al. Dose-ranging study of tolterodine in patients with detrusor hyperreflexia. *Neurourol Urodyn.* 1998;17(5):499–512.
7. Perkash I. Long-term urologic management of the patient with spinal cord injury. *Urol Clin North Am* 20:423–434, 1993.
8. Perkash I. Contact laser sphincterotomy: further experience and longer follow-up. *Spinal Cord.* 1996;34:227–233.
9. Ord J, Lunn D, Reynard J. Bladder management and risk of bladder stone formation in spinal cord injured patients. *J Urol.* 2003; 170(5):1734–1737.
10. Yang CC, Clowers DE. Screening cystoscopy in chronically catheterized spinal cord injury patients. *Spinal Cord.* 1999;37(3): 204–207.
11. Perkash I. Intermittent catheterization failure and an approach to bladder rehabilitation in spinal cord injury patients. *Arch Phys Med Rehabil.* 1978;59:9–17.
12. Sugiyama T, Park YC, Jurita T. Oxybutynin disrupts learning and memory in the rat passive avoidance response. *Urol Res.* 1999;27: 393–395.

13. Garcia-Arguello LY, O'Horo JC, Farrell A, Blakney R, Sohail MR, Evans CT, Safdar N. Infections in the spinal cord-injured population: a systematic review. *Spinal Cord* 2016;1–9.

14. Perkash I. Controlling UTIs in patients with spinal cord injuries: maintaining low intravesical voiding pressures is crucial. *J Crit Illness.* 1996;11(Suppl):41–48.

15. Reid G, Kang YS, Lacerte M, et al. Bacterial biofilm formation on the bladder epithelium of spinal cord injured patients. II: Toxic outcome on cell viability. *Paraplegia.* 1993;31:494–499.

16. Cardenas DD, Hooton TM. Urinary tract infection in persons with spinal cord injury. *Arch Phys Med Rehabil.* 1995;76:272–280.

17. Schwantes U, Topfmeier P. Importance of pharmacological and physicochemical properties for tolerance of antimuscarinic drugs in the treatment of detrusor instability and detrusor hyperreflexia—chances for improvement of therapy. *Int J Clin Pharmacol Ther.* 1999;37:209–218.

CHAPTER 34

SEXUALITY DESPITE DISABILITY: INTIMATE AND REPRODUCTIVE SOLUTIONS

Steven A. Stiens, MD, MS, Rafi J. Heruti, MD, FECSM, Ronit Aloni, PhD, Ruth K. Westheimer, EdD, and Mitchell S. Tepper, PhD, MPH

The body is an instrument which only gives off music when it is used as a body. Always an orchestra, and just as music traverses walls, so sensuality traverses the body and reaches up to ecstasy.

—Anais Nin (1903–1977)

KEY POINTS

1. Demonstrate a positive interest and attitude of acceptance to permissively understanding patients' gender identity, social sex roles, sex orientation, desires, and relationships with partners.
2. Maintain a contemporary and diverse awareness of cultural patterns, physiology, sexual activities, medications, and adaptive equipment to be sexually literate as a service to patients and the interdisciplinary team.
3. Develop and utilize your personal style integrating components of successful models (PLISSIT, ENIGMA) to elicit and implement treatment using the Sexual Rehabilitation Framework.
4. Review process and success with patients and partners utilizing a shared understanding of relationships, aspirations, and adaptions addressing the sexual response cycle: excitement, plateau, orgasm, and resolution.

1. What is sexual literacy?

"***Sexual literacy***" is the ability to obtain, communicate, process, and understand basic sexual health information and services to make appropriate health decisions. The "sexually literate" health professional must be comfortable with his or her own sexuality, able to suspend judgment, and express genuine willingness to pursue understanding and solutions with patients and partners. At the end of a consultation with a patient, the sexually literate clinician should be able to formulate a biopsychosocial problem list with goals that address patient and partner impairments, activity limitations, and barriers to full participation in the relationship.

Centers for Disease Control and Prevention. *What is Health Literacy? Health Literacy.* 17 September 2020. https://www.cdc.gov/healthliteracy/learn/.

Engelen M, Knoll J, Rabsztyn P, Schaaijk N, van Gaal B. Sexual health communication between healthcare professionals andadolescents withchronic conditions inwestern ountries: an integrative review. *Sex Disabil.* 2020;38:191–216. https://link.springer.com/article/10.1007/s11195-019-09597-0. doi:10.1007/s11195-019-09597-0.

2. How does clinical knowledge in sexual literacy guide patient sexuality education?

Sexuality education is often suppressed, delivered in subtherapeutic doses, poorly translated, and offered without thoughtful design for target audiences. A clinician's knowledge of physical and social development, recovery patterns, and the relationships between various impairments and activity limitations allows a ***person-centered curriculum design***. By interviewing patients, life circumstances, self-perceptions, and expectations are revealed.

Patients' needs are met through a variety of educational media, impromptu discussions, a core series of lectures, guided self-discovery assignments, specific suggestions to enhance intimate performance, and demonstrations of equipment. During initial rehabilitation, sexuality should be on the problem list, and one team member should have primary responsibility to orchestrate interdisciplinary efforts to elicit patient concerns and customize response.

Consortium for Spinal Cord Medicine. Sexuality and reproductive health in adults with spinal cord injury. *J Spinal Cord Med.* 2010;*33*(3):281–336. https://www.ncbi.nlm.nih.gov/pmc/articles/PMC2941243/. doi:10.1080/10790268.2010.11689709

Spinal cord medicine: sexuality and reproductive health in adults with spinal cord injury: clinical practice guidelinefor health-care providers https://pvasamediaprd.blob.core.windows.net/prod/libraries/media/pva/library /publications/cpg_sexuality-and-reproductive-health.pdf

3. What is sexuality?

Sexuality is a central aspect of being human throughout life and encompasses: phenotypic sex, gender identities and roles, sexual orientation, intimacy, eroticism, pleasure, and reproduction. It develops through physiologic cues between body systems, experiences of self, maturation, socialization, societal reflection of the person, and intimate relationships. Sexuality, therefore, requires an evolving self-understanding, and ongoing opportunity for communication of self-perception and informed, proactive clinician support for the patient's goals. The clinician's positive anticipation of patients' sexuality as a facet of their roles in relationships is one example of the power of ***therapeutic expectation***.

World Health Organization. *Sexual and reproductive health and research including the Special Programme HRP.* https://www.who.int/teams/sexual-and-reproductive-health-and-research/key-areas-of-work/sexual-health/defining-sexual-health

4. What are the subcomponents of personal sexual expression?
    a. ***Biologic sex***. Phenotypic sex with objective expression and function of secondary sexual characteristics, anatomy, and physiology.
    b. ***Gender identity***. The person's subjective sense of self as man or woman.
    c. ***Social sex role***. Behavior to demonstrate as man or woman, masculinity, and femininity.
    d. ***Sexual orientation***. The focus of desire for sexual relationship; sexual orientation is a fluid continuum ranging from exclusively heterosexual (opposite) to primarily homosexual (same) biological sex.
    e. ***Intention***. Specific interest in sexual fantasy and behavior.
    f. ***Sexual desire***. Amount of interest in a variety of activities, frequency.

5. What is the PLISSIT model of sexual counseling?
    - **P** = **P**ermission to be sexual and to talk about sexual issues
    - **LI** = **L**imited **I**nformation
    - **SS** = **S**pecific **S**uggestions
    - **IT** = **I**ntensive **T**herapy
    This model presents a spectrum of interventional areas that can be addressed, in part, by each member of the interdisciplinary team.

Levine SB. The nature of sexual desire: a clinician's perspective. *Arch Sex Behav.* 32:279–285. https://www.ncbi.nlm.nih.gov/pubmed/591712. doi:10.1023/A:1023421819465

Shively MG, De Cecco JP. Components of exual dentity. *J Homosex.* 1977;3(1):41–48. doi:10.1300/J082v03n01_04

6. Explain the components of the PLISSIT approach.
    - **Permission**
        - Who: All individuals working with the people with disabilities; support and clinical staff.
        - Focus: Acknowledge that talk about sexual areas is okay. Communicate acceptance and understanding that changes in a person's sexual life can be an important issue and that concerns are common.
        - Sensitive questions in history-taking regarding sexual function are ***therapeutic affirmations*** of the patient's sexuality and role in the lives of others. Questions such as, "Are you sexually active?" and, "How has this condition affected your sexual function?" open conversations about sex. Teaching patients and partners range of motion, massage, and management techniques for angina, bronchospasm, autonomic dysreflexia, and prevention of incontinence prepares them for their own problem solving in sexual exploration. Physicians' permission to resume intercourse can often be a prescription for success.
    - **Limited Information**
        - Who: Service providers.
        - Focus: Provide general information related to sexual concerns; dispel sexual myths, refer person, when indicated, to someone with more knowledge about the particular area of concern.
        - All rehabilitation programs should include lectures and discussion that educate the patient about the basic physiology, psychology, and pathophysiology of the sexual response cycles and reproduction. A discussion of the unique effects of a patient's disease or injury should complement this review. This primary education should be the designated responsibility of one rehabilitation team member, with appropriate interdisciplinary and peer referrals.
    - **Specific Suggestions**
        - Who: Professionals with specific knowledge/management skills.

- Focus: Using one's professional knowledge and skills to provide suggestions to manage a specific concern. Obtaining a sexual problem history, definition of the problem, course of the problem, treatment of the problem (e.g., pubococcygeal muscle strengthening,) and ideas about the causes of the problem and goals of treatment.
- Ideally, all team members contribute to successful sexual adjustment and function. For example, training the patient by the primary nurse for skin examination of sores can lead to reflections on body image. A suggestion may include an assignment for the patient or couple to experiment with visual body exploration and survey patient sensation. Such a couple can later be assigned *sensate focus exercises* and then advanced to *body mapping* of new erogenous zones. Physical therapy education for a spouse on transfers and mat mobility might easily be adapted by couples for use in transferring into the Jacuzzi and sexual positioning.
- **Intensive Therapy**
  - Who: Specialist
  - Focus: Interventions may include medication, surgery, counseling, sex therapy including a full sexual history, or a variety of specialized procedures or management techniques. One or a subset of the team providing intervention coordinates the care. Recognition of any problem outside the realm of the usual team intervention requires thoughtful collaborative referral to specialists.

Annon J. The PLISSIT model: a proposed conceptual scheme for the behavioral treatment for sexual problems. *J Sex Educ Ther.* 1976;2:2–15. https://doi.org/10.1080/01614576.1976.11074483

7. **Can taking a sexual history and intervention be made easier?**
   The **ENIGMA process** is a series of steps that clarifies the process:
   - **E**—Engage the patient in conversation by *finding common ground* validating his or her personal aspirations.
   - **N**—Normalize the sexual self-expression by *permissively* exploring interests, activities, and barriers to success.
   - **I**—Inform and *educate* the patient and his or her partner.
   - **G**—Guide them by *mirroring their style* of interaction, validating their success, and suggesting alternatives for next steps. Use their lingo!
   - **M**—Maximize *achievement* by prescribing and providing adjuncts such as educational materials, medication, equipment, therapy, erotic dream programming, and experiences.
   - **A**—Assess and *reassess* by checking on the issue as one in the spectrum of problems addressed on regular visits.

Alexander M, Courtois F, Elliott S, Tepper M. Improving sexual satisfaction in persons with spinal cord injuries: collective wisdom. *Top Spinal Cord Inj Rehabil.* 2017;23(1):57–70. https://www.ncbi.nlm.nih.gov/pmc/articles/PMC5340510/. doi:10.1310/sci2301-57

Elliott S, Hocaloski S, Carlson M. A multidisciplinary approach to sexual and fertility rehabilitation: The sexual rehabilitation ramework. *Top Spinal Cord Inj Rehabil.* 2017;23(1):49–56. https://www.ncbi.nlm.nih.gov/pmc/articles/PMC5340509/. doi:10.1310/sci2301-49

8. **How are the results of the consultation used to design a rehabilitation action plan?**
   Patient and partner behaviors, needs, and expectations can be distributed into the *Sexual Rehabilitation Framework* to guide education, counseling, reassurance, and treatment.
   a. Sexual drive or sexual interest
   b. Sexual functioning abilities
   c. Fertility and contraception concerns
   d. Factors associated with the condition
   e. Motor and sensory influences
   f. Bowel and bladder issues
   g. Sexual self-view and self-esteem
   h. Partnership issues.

Bailey KA, Gammage KL, van Ingen C, et al. Managing the stigma: Exploring body image experiences and self-presentation among people with spinal cord injury. *Health Psychol Open.* 2016;3(1):1–10. https://www.ncbi.nlm.nih.gov/pmc/articles/PMC5193263/pdf/10.1177_2055102916650094.pdf. doi:10.1177/2055102916650094

Ekland M, Lawrie B. How a woman's sexual adjustment after sustaining a spinal cord injury impacts sexual health interventions. *SCI Nurs.* 2004;21(1):14–19.

Potki R, Ziaei T, Faramarzi M, et al. Bio-psycho-social factors affecting sexual self-concept: A systematic review. *Electron Physician.* 2017;9(9):5172–5178. https://www.ncbi.nlm.nih.gov/pmc/articles/PMC5633209/. doi:10.19082/5172

9. How does disability affect body image, sexual self-concept, and adjustment?

Body image is the mind's picture of our bodies, the perception we have of ourselves. It is closely associated with the awareness of our body (the afferent sensory barrage and central processing; the experienced). The expression and practice of sexuality are affected by self-esteem, body image, and interpersonal attachment. It is continually re-evaluated by the self. Despite adaptation to self, individuals are often confronted in society with stigma and risk devaluation by others.

Rehabilitation specialists must strive to help patients become fully self-aware and reconstruct a positive body image that they accept, like, and share. Acceptance of self as desirable and as a source of pleasure emerges with sensual experience of self and perceptions of others. Educational resources, same sex support groups, and involved clinicians are particularly helpful.

10. Is it important to have a relationship first?

Personal relationships begin with our relationship with ourselves. This dynamic process requires self-perception, self-acceptance, self-esteem, sexual-esteem, and self-worth as a potential partner for another. The rehabilitation team must successfully reflect patients' unique personal attributes and reinforce the value of their companionship to others. People who project self-respect and satisfaction are most fully capable of attracting partners, graciously accepting another's attention, and sensitively meeting their needs. People who recognize their capabilities are most able to contribute to a mutually complementary relationship. Consequently, rehabilitation must teach patients the value of recognizing their unique assets and capabilities. With this confidence, they can take the necessary social risks to seek out complementary partners and share sexual empowerment.

Westheimer RK. Partner and relationship issues in the treatment of erectile dysfunction. *Am J Manag Care.* 2000;6(12 Suppl): S639–S640.

11. Would treatment be more effective if a patient's sexual partner is involved? What communication must occur with the patient's partner?

For patients who have a sexual partner, intervention is most effective if the partner is included in any communication between the rehabilitation professional and the patient on matters of sexual functioning. The clinician has the opportunity to provide education to the partner, to receive input on the couple's needs, and to develop a plan of treatment that is mutually acceptable.

Sexual issues must be integrated into the entire rehabilitation plan; life partners need full inclusion in the rehabilitation process. If possible, it is desirable to maintain a separation between the roles of caretaker and sexual partner. This can be achieved by proactively planning for attendant care.

Meesters JJL, van de Ven DPHW, Kruijver E, et al. Counselled patients with stroke still experience sexual and relational problems 1-5 years after stroke rehabilitation. *Sex Disabil.* 2020;38:533–545. https://link.springer.com/article/10.1007/s11195-020-09632-5. doi:10/1007/s11195-020-09632-5

12. What is "fragile partner syndrome"?

Partners often do not have a full understanding of the patient's condition. Without direct, detailed, and specific demonstrations of safe and effective physical interactions with patients, partners may overestimate risk of physical and intimate contact. With patients' permission and guidance, partners should be educated in specific methods for transfers and positions for intimate contact and parameters for the intensity of activity.

Lemon MA. Sexual counseling and spinal cord injury. *Sex Disabil.* 1993;11(1):73–79.

13. What female and male physical signs signal the four stages of the human sexual response outlined by Masters and Johnson?

Excitement, Stage I: Muscle tension, sympathetic activity, nipple erection
- Female: Clitoris swelling, vaginal lubrication
- Male: Penile erection, testes rise

Plateau, Stage II: Heightened excitement, pulse 100 to 160 bpm, sex flush
- Female: Clitoris withdrawals, vaginal vasocongestion
- Male: Testes enlarge, Cowper's secretion

Orgasm, Stage III: (seconds to minutes) Rhythmic muscle contractions
- Female: Uterus, vagina, and anus contract
- Male: Ejaculation, bladder neck closes

Resolution, Stage IV: (minutes to hours) Return to baseline, refractory period.

Westheimer RK. *The Art of Arousal.* Abbeville: New York; 1993.

14. **Describe the physiology of the sexual response in women.**
The uterus and ovaries receive sympathetic innervations from the hypogastric nerve (T10–L2). Sensory messages from the vagina and cervix travel via the pelvic, vagus (parasympathetic), hypogastric, and sympathetic nerves. Clitoral swelling is primarily parasympathetically mediated, and vaginal secretion is primarily sympathetic. At orgasm, the pelvic floor (pudendal nerve) contracts rhythmically. Functional brain MRI studies reveal increased metabolism at the nucleus accumbens.

15. **How do acute neurologic injuries affect female sexual function?**
Menstruation may not occur for three or more months after central nervous system (CNS) trauma. After complete spinal cord injury at level T6 and above, psychogenic subjective arousal does not produce vaginal lubrication via sympathetic pathways. As long as the conus and autonomic connections remain intact, manual clitoral stimulation produces reflex lubrication and increased vaginal pulse amplitude.
  Spinal cord injury, neuromuscular disorders, and connective tissue diseases do not generally affect fertility. Urinary tract infection, pressure ulcers, constipation, and mobility limitations may complicate pregnancy. Labor begins and is driven hormonally. The delivery can be vaginal, but should be anticipated and monitored with autonomic dysreflexia prevention using local anesthesia and preparation for using forceps or Cesarean section.

16. **How do erections occur?**
Erections are initiated by arterial vasodilatation and venous outlet constriction, which result in engorgement of the cavernosal sinusoids. ***Psychogenic*** (imaginative) erections start with arousal in the mind and are mediated by the lumbar sympathetics hypogastric nerve (T12–L1). ***Reflexogenic*** (contact) erection is primarily cholinergic (parasympathetic [S2, S3, S4]) via the inferior splanchnic nerve or nervi erigentes and is augmented by mixed somatic innervation via the pudendal nerve, which contracts the pelvic floor and limits penile blood release. The ejaculation and detumescence process is primarily sympathetic, but a complex interplay of autonomic systems and other neurotransmitters continue to play a role in the process.

17. **Describe the physiology of the sexual response in men.**
Psychogenic stimuli activate the cortex, amygdala, and hypothalamus. Erection and emission containing spermatozoa occur with sympathetic facilitation. ***Emission*** starts with sympathetically (T10–L2 emission center)-driven vas deferens transport of sperm to the posterior urethra to combine with seminal vesicle secretions. ***Ejaculation*** is the forceful delivery of the semen out of the urethra by the pudendal-innervated bulbocavernous and ischiocavernosus muscle contractions. Ejaculation is typically ineffective after complete spinal cord injury and may result in retrograde ejaculation (semen into the bladder). Ejaculation can be triggered with a vibrator (Ferticare) stimulus (2.5 mm amplitude, 100 Hz frequency) under the glans at the frenulum, or inhibited by the ***squeeze technique*** (firm grasp of glans). ***Orgasm*** is the cortical experience of extreme pleasure followed by a feeling of well-being and satisfaction. ***Resolution*** is the blissful exhaustion shared by both sexes.

Goetz L, Stiens S. Abdominal electric stimulation facilitates ejaculation evoked by penile vibratory stimulation. *Arch Phys Med Rehab.* 2005;86(9):1879–1883. doi:10.1016/j.apmr.2005.03.023

Sipski M, Alexander CJ, Gomez-Marin O. Effects of level and degree of spinal cord injury on male orgasm. *Spinal Cord.* 2006;44(12):798–804. https://www.nature.com/articles/ 3101954.pdf. doi:10.1038/sj.sc.3101954

18. **How common is sexual dysfunction in the general population?**
Community samples estimate 25% to 63% of women and 10% to 52% of men have sexual dysfunction. Overlooked causes include medication side effects, hormonal imbalances, inept performance, psychological problems, and exaggerated expectations. Sexual dysfunction for males is largely premature ejaculation, which is mostly associated with psychogenic and functional causes. Another common dysfunction is erectile dysfunction, which is associated with risk factors for coronary artery disease, age, medications, and emotional factors such as anger and depression. For women, common complaints include trouble lubricating, postcoital and urinary tract infections, reduced libido, and psychosocial/relationship issues. Except for trouble with lubrication (which increases with age), these problems are consistently prevalent throughout adolescent and adult womens' lives and require clinical attention.
  Treatments are evaluated for ***efficacy*** (physiologic improvement in randomized controlled trials) and ***effectiveness*** (beneficial in clinical practice). For women, flibanserin and bremelanotide are FDA approved to improve hypoactive sexual desire. Women who are hypogonadal with hypoactive sexual desire have demonstrated increased sexual fantasies, masturbation, and intercourse and report greater well-being while on brief oral estrogen and 300-μg testosterone patch.

Clayton AH, Goldstein I, Kim NN, et al. The International Society for the Study of Women's Sexual Health process of care for management of hypoactive sexual desire disorder in women. *Mayo Clin Proc.* 2018;93(4):467–487. https://www.mayoclinicproceedings.org/article/ S0025-6196(17)30799-1/fulltext. doi:10.1016/j.mayocp.2017.11.002

Heidari M, Ghodusi M, Rezaei P, et al. Sexual function and factors affecting menopause: A systematic review. *J Menopausal Med.* 2019;25(1):15–27. https://www.ncbi.nlm.nih.gov/pmc/articles/PMC6487288/pdf/jmm-25-15.pdf. doi:10.6118/jmm.2019.25.1.15

Heiman JR. Sexual dysfunction: Overview of prevalence, etiological factors, and treatments. *J Sex Res.* 2002;39(1):73–78. doi:10.1080/00224490209552124

Lewis RW, Fugl-Meyer KS, Corona G, et al. Definitions/epidemiology/risk factors for sexual dysfunction. *J Sex Med.* 2010; 7(4 Pt.2):1598–1607. doi:10.1111/j.1743-6109.2010. 01778.x

Wassersug R, Wibowo E. Non-pharmacological and non-surgical strategies to promote sexual recovery for men with erectile dysfunction. *Transl Androl Urol.* 2017;6(5):S776–S794. https://tau.amegroups.com/article/view/15068/17712. doi:10.21037/tau.2017.04.09

19. What are the rehabilitation options for producing erections after neurologic injuries?
    - Without erection, satisfying ***intromission*** can be accomplished with the ***stuffing technique*** (pushing the flaccid penis into the vagina and stimulating the woman with friction and sustained pressure at the introitus) or the use of penile splinting.
    - ***Vacuum tumescence and constriction therapy*** works by engorging and expanding the penis for retention. The corpora expand under negative pressure, and a custom circular rubber-tension ring is slipped around the base of the penis.
    - ***Phosphodiesterase-5 (PDE5) inhibitors*** potentiate erections by preventing the degradation of cyclic guanosine monophosphate (GMP), which is a direct vasodilator. The three currently available compounds have the following onset times and durations of activation: vardenafil, 20 minutes to 12 hours; sildenafil, 30 minutes to 4 hours; and tadalafil, 60 minutes to 36 hours. Use of PDE-5 inhibitors is contraindicated with all nitrate-producing medications and strong vasodilators because of the risk for hypotension.
    - Intracorporal injections with ***papaverine*** or ***prostaglandin E1*** (alprostadil) produce erections by smooth muscle relaxation. Manag side effects such as priapism is treated with observation and needle aspiration of the corpora.
    - ***Penile implants*** may be inflatable or noninflatable (rigid or semirigid) and are used less frequently because of the risk for skin breakdown due to a foreign body.

Yafi FA, Jenkins L, Albersen M, et al. Erectile dysfunction. *Nat Rev Dis Primers.* 2017;2:16003. https://www.ncbi.nlm.nih.gov/pmc/articles/PMC5027992/pdf/nihms815695.pdf. doi:10.1038/ nrdp.2016.3

20. Does spinal cord injury affect male fertility?
    Yes. Deficits in spermatogenesis documented by testicular biopsy have revealed tubular atrophy, spermatogenic arrest, and interstitial fibrosis. Seminal parameters show decreased sperm counts and motility, as well as abnormal morphology and white blood cells. Repeated ejaculation reduces stasis and can improve sperm quality. White blood cell counts can be reduced with short courses of antibiotics covering cultured urinary contaminants.

Brackett NL, Ibrahim E, Lynne CM. *Male Fertility Following Spinal Cord Injury: A Guide for Patients.* 2nd ed. Miami: Miami Project to Cure Paralysis; 2011. https://www.themiamiproject.org/wp-content/uploads/2015/07/male-fertility-booklet-2010-lowres.pdf

21. What are fertility options for males with SCI?
    Though the majority of men with spinal cord injuries can achieve erections and have sexual intercourse, male infertility caused by inability to ejaculate is common. The high threshold for ejaculation has prompted a sequential series of interventions, including penile vibratory stimulation (PVS), electroejaculation, and microsurgical aspiration of sperm from the epididymis and testicular biopsy. PVS uses a custom-designed mechanical vibrator that is placed at the base of the glans penis and induces a reflex ejaculation. This technique works in patients with thoracic and cervical SCI with an intact sacral ejaculatory reflex and is the preferred choice in patients with lesions above T10. With electroejaculation, a low-current stimulation of the ejaculatory organs via a rectal probe is done. Percutaneous Epididymal Sperm Aspiration (PESA) is also a procedure that can retrieve sperm for intracytoplasmic sperm injection (icsi). The semen typically exhibits low sperm count, low motility, and white blood cells. Assisted reproductive techniques such as sperm washing, intrauterine insemination, in vitro fertilization (IVF), and intracytoplasmic injection (ICI) of sperm into eggs can be utilized.

Brackett NL, Ibrahim E, Lynne CM. *Male Fertility Following Spinal Cord Injury: A Guide for Patients.* 2nd ed. Miami: Miami Project to Cure Paralysis; 2011. https://www.themiamiproject.org/wp-content/uploads/2015/07/male-fertility-booklet-2010-lowres.pdf

22. Is there sex after a heart attack?
    Yes! Myocardial infarction, or heart disease in general, need not preclude resuming sexual activity. The metabolic cost of sex in middle-aged married men is no more than five metabolic equivalents (METs; 1 MET = calories/minute at complete rest), equivalent to climbing two flights of stairs. Resting before intercourse, postponing it for 3 hours after meals and alcohol, taking nitrates as needed before intercourse to prevent chest pain, and using familiar positions are all beneficial. However, nitrates are contraindicated with PDE-5 inhibitors. Foreplay may be a

metabolically favorable "warm-up" and training activity. Initial explorations can include masturbation to give the patient full control of the process. The couple then uses successive approximation to achieve mutual exhilaration without excessive exertion.

23. What experiences do women with new neurologic impairments report as they adapt sexually?

The process of sexual readjustment after paralysis varies and may include these experiences:

Cognitive genital dissociation: Making a conscious decision not to deal with their sexuality based on the assumption that sexual pleasure was no longer possible for them because of absence of sensation in their genitals.

Sexual disenfranchisement: Feeling deprived or, more graphically, "robbed" of their sexuality; no longer feeling like whole women; no longer feeling sexually desirable; and no longer feeling sexual pleasure.

Sexual reawakening: Often marked by a significant turning point like a milestone birthday, a new partner, an outside threat to an existing partner relationship, learning new information from other women with disabilities.

Redefining orgasm: Often accomplished with the help of a partner, sometimes a partner with a disability, or with the help of other women with disabilities in peer support groups. Creativity, resourcefulness, and communication were seen as central to accommodating the sexual needs of self and other.

Tepper MS, Whipple B, Richards E, et al. Women with complete spinal cord injury: A phenomenological study of sexual experience. *J Sex Marital Ther*. 2001;27(5):615–623. doi:10.1080/713846817

24. Can erogenous zones change after injury to the CNS?

Recent primate and human data demonstrate central sensory reorganization in response to injuries to the spinal cord or peripheral nerve. People with SCI have reported areas in the zone of partial sensory preservation or hypersensitive zone that are sexually exciting with stimulation. These areas can lead to orgasm with associated tachycardia and flushing above the lesion and can be located with **body mapping** and shared using **sensate focus exercises**.

25. Do experiments sometimes lead to satisfying discoveries?

Yes. Overcoming attitudinal and cultural taboos of interaction transcends barriers. Practices that bring together mutually sensate erogenous zones can become particularly satisfying parts of couples' repertoires. Possibilities for **kissing**, **cunnilingus** (oral and lingual vulva stimulation), and **fellatio** (oral and lingual penile stimulation) should be explored. Unfortunately, a major barrier to sexual fulfillment after disability is fear. Fears of poor acceptance by a partner and issues related to involuntary loss of urinary or bowel control are particularly strong. Planning for sexual encounters reduces anxiety and makes them more achievable.

Westheimer RK, Lieberman L. *Dr. Ruth's Guide to Sensuous and Erotic Pleasures*. Shapolsky: New York; 1991.

26. How does traumatic brain injury affect sexual function?

The sequelae of brain injury are diverse and may include many functional deficits: cognitive, movement, communication, behavior, and emotional expression. Full participation in an intimate and sexual relationship requires the integration of all these capabilities. Sexual functioning is a comprehensive activity that involves the motivation to engage in the activity and appropriate planning, including inhibition of inappropriate behavior. Sexual dysfunction may be the consequence of the primary damage as well as other factors surrounding the survivor such as personal relationships, responses of family to the person, and moral attitudes of the society. Therefore, the sexual dysfunction that follows traumatic brain injury (TBI) may result from the neurologic deficits, survivors' reactions to the injury, premorbid personality, or some combination of these factors. Intervention requires generating and sequentially prioritizing sexually specific goals that may relate to other problems on the problem list (e.g., varied problems with mobility, neurogenic bladder, cognition difficulties, depression) within varied disablement domains, up and down the hierarchy of biopsychosocial systems.

Aloni R, Katz S. *Sexuality Difficulties After Traumatic Brain Injury and Ways to Deal With it*. Springfield, IL: Thomas;2003:20–41.

Baguley IJ, Barden HL, Nott MT. Altered sexual function after central neurological system trauma is reflective of region of injury; brain vs spinal cord. *Brain Inj*. 2020;34(13–14):1732–1740. doi:10.1080/02699052.2020.1832258

Kreutzer JS, Zasler ND. Psychosexual consequences of traumatic brain injury: methodology and preliminary findings. *Brain Inj*. 1989;3:177–186. doi:10.3109/02699058909004550

Latella D, Maggio MG, De Luca R, et al. Changes in sexual functioning following traumatic brain injury: An overview on a neglected issue. *J Clin Neurosci*. 2018;58:1–6. doi:10.1016/j.jocn.2018.09.030

Sander AM, Maestas KL, Pappadis MR, et al. Multicenter study of sexual functioning in spouses/partners of persons with traumatic brain injury. *Arch Phys Med Rehab*. 2016;97(5):753–759. doi:10.1016/j.apmr.2016.01.009

Strizzi J, Landa LO, Pappadis M, et al. Sexual functioning, desire, and satisfaction in women with TBI and healthy controls. *Behav Neurol*. 2015;2015:247479. https://pubmed.ncbi.nlm.nih.gov/26556951/. doi:10.1155/2015/247479

27. How does brain damage relate to sexual function?

Although sexual function is not necessarily directly associated with higher cognitive abilities, severe concentration problems may impair the arousal phase of sexual responses in both survivors and their partners. Cognitive dysfunction can adversely affect the intimate relationship and can cause sexual difficulties due to a loss of mutual interest, role changes, and/or a decline in the survivor's self-esteem. Frontal and temporal lobe damage, impaired judgment, and extreme mood swings can result in inappropriate sexual behaviors that are not tolerated by a partner or society.

Loss of memory and difficulties in concentration may require modification of educational methods and documenting the intervention program. Memory loss can cause the survivor to demand sex repeatedly. Integration of events into a memory book can help. Altered verbal and nonverbal patterns of communication can impede the establishment of new relationships for single survivors or disrupt marital relationships, as they may create misunderstandings and cause frustration, anger, withdrawal, and rejection.

Depression and anxiety may act as inhibitors of sexual desire and function. Emotional regression, mood swings, and irritability can alter a couple's intimate relations through role changes or an inability to predict the partner's reaction to the initiation of sexual activity.

Kaplan SP. Five-year tracking of psychological changes in people with severe TBI. *Rehabil Consel Bull.* 1993;36(3):152–159.

Lezak MD. Brain damage is a family affair. *J Clin Exp Neuropsychol.* 1988;1;10:111–123. doi:10.1080/01688638808405098

28. How can a stoma affect sexuality?

Patients with stomas face many physical, psychological, social, and sexual difficulties. More than 40% have problems with their sex lives. Many patients find it difficult to discuss their sexual feelings, especially after a body image change, causing most of them to leave the hospital distressed and unprepared for sexual life. They lack confidence and are not aware of the anticipated problems, including irregular bowel movements and diarrhea, discharge of gas and unpleasant odor, and diminished sexual and social life. Some of the nerves important for genital sensation and sexual function (lubrication in females; erection and ejaculation in males) may be severed during the operation.

Apart from the physical changes that a stoma and surgery might cause, there are psychosocial aspects concerning self-concept with the change of body image in relation to bodily functions. Patients report restrictions in their level of social functioning. A sensitive and informed approach to discuss sexuality can provide effective support. Patients will more readily adapt to their new body image and way of life if they receive professional counseling concerning sexuality from the preoperative stage through rehabilitation and return to the community.

Albaugh JA, Tenfelde S, Hayden DM. Sexual dysfunction and intimacy for ostomates. *Clin Colon Rectal Surg.* 2017;30(3):201–206. https://www.ncbi.nlm.nih.gov/pmc/articles/ PMC5498165/. doi:10.1055/s-0037-1598161

FURTHER READING

Books

Cooper E, Guillebaud J. *Sexuality and Disability: A Guide for Everyday Practice.* Oxford, UK: Radcliffe Medical; 1999.
Ishak WW, ed. *Textbook of Clinical Sexual Medicine.* Cham, Switzerland: Springer International; 2017.
Kaufman M, Silverberg C, Odette F. *Ultimate Guide to Sex and Disability: For All of Us Who Live With Disabilities, Chronic Pain and Illness.* 2nd ed. San Francisco: Cleis; 2007.
Shuttleworth R, Mona LR, eds. *The Routledge Handbook of Disability and Sexuality.* New York, NY: Taylor & Francis; 2020.
Sipski ML, Alexander CJ. *Sexual Function in People With Disability and Chronic Illness: A Health Professional's Guide.* Gaithersburg, MD: Aspen; 1997.
Westheimer RK, Lahu PA. *Sex for Dummies.* 4th ed. Hoboken, NJ: Wiley; 2019.

Articles

Anderson KD, Borisoff JF, Johnson RD, et al. The impact of spinal cord injury on sexual function: concerns of the general population. *Spinal Cord.* 2007;45(5):328–337. Available at: https://www.nature.com/ articles/ 3101977 doi:10/1038/sj.sc.3101977.
Lamont J. Female sexual health consensus clinical guidelines. *J Obstet Gynaecol Can.* 2012;34(8):769–775. doi:10.1016/S1701-2163(16)35341-5.
Shuttleworth RP. The search for sexual intimacy for men with cerebral palsy. *Sexual Disabil.* 2000;18(4):263–282. Available at: https:// www.researchgate.net/publication/ 227110141_ The_Search_for_Sexual_Intimacy_for_Men_with_Cerebral_Palsy. doi:10/1023/A: 1005646327321
Tepper MS. Providing comprehensive sexual health care in spinal cord injury rehabilitation: implementation and evaluation of a new curriculum for health professionals. *Sexual Disabil.* 1997;15:131–165. Available at: https://www.ncbi.nlm.nih.gov/pmc/articles/ PMC2941243/ doi:10/1023/A: 1024780718488

CHAPTER 35

LOWER LIMB ORTHOSIS

Heikki Uustal, MD

When the sun is shining I can do anything; no mountain is too high, no trouble too difficult.
—Wilma Glodean Rudolph (1940-1994)

KEY POINTS

1. Orthoses are named by the joints and segments of the body that are affected by the brace.
2. By limiting motion at the ankle, AFO will control the knee during stance phase.
3. Most carbon fiber AFOs provide little or no medial/lateral stability to the ankle.
4. A KAFO should be prescribed when there is instability at the knee and ankle.

1. **What are the critical features of an extra-depth orthopedic shoe?**
   Most orthopedic shoes are extra deep to allow room for a custom molded foot orthotic or a plastic AFO. The shoe itself has a heel counter to control varus and valgus motion of the calcaneus. The toe box can be wide or high to accommodate for forefoot deformities such as bunion or hammertoes. The closure of the shoe can be lace or Velcro. A Blucher design allows for easier access of the foot into the shoe with an open throat design. A supportive innersole provides a platform for a foot orthotic or for attachment of a stirrup to a metal brace. The outer sole can be leather or rubber. Orthopedic shoes are available in extra wide sizes to accommodate for edema or foot deformity. Custom molded orthopedic shoes accommodate severe foot deformities.

2. **How does a custom molded foot orthotic protect the diabetic foot?**
   A custom molded foot orthotic protects the diabetic foot by providing cushion and total contact to the plantar surface to capture the entire weight bearing surface of the foot rather than focus pressure at the heel and the metatarsal heads. If there are high risk areas for skin breakdown, then redistribution of pressure is possible with a buildup. An accommodative foot orthotic will capture the current shape of the foot and provide support and protection. A corrective foot orthotic will redistribute pressure away from high risk areas with buildup at the arch or metatarsal shafts, in addition to attempting to correct the foot to a subtalar neutral position. The addition of a metatarsal pad will help to offload the metatarsal heads #2, 3, and 4, while a metatarsal bar will offload all the metatarsal heads. Medial or lateral heel wedging in the foot orthotic will help to control calcaneal varus and valgus deformities.

3. **What are the common indications for Ankle Foot Orthosis (AFO)?**
   Orthoses are named by the joints and segments of the body that are affected by the brace. For example, AFO controls the ankle and foot. The most common indication for an AFO is weakness of the dorsiflexors, resulting in foot drop which may occur due to injury to peroneal nerve, L5 nerve root, or Central Nervous System (CNS). AFO can also control medial lateral instability of the ankle when there is weakness of the inverters or evertors, as well as abnormal movements of the foot and ankle related to spasticity or tone. Amount of support provided by a plastic AFO is determined by the selection of material and trimline of the brace. AFO can also have an ankle joint to provide controlled motion such as dorsiflexion (DF) with plantar flexion (PF) stop.

4. **What are the differences between a metal and plastic AFO?**
   Plastic AFOs are commonly fabricated from a mold of the patient's limb which result in a close fit to the patient's calf and foot. The footplate can fit inside many shoes or sneakers which minimize cosmetic concerns or visibility of the brace. Plastic AFOs can provide control for weakness in DF, PF, inversion and eversion. However, close fit of the brace may be compromised if there is skin breakdown, insensate skin, or fluctuating volume of the limb. A metal AFO is fabricated with double uprights to ankle joint and stirrup which attaches directly to the shoe and it only touches the patient at the shoe and at the calf band. The advantages of a metal AFO are increased durability, increased adjustability, and minimized contact of the skin when there are issues with skin tolerance. A third alternative is carbon fiber AFO which controls foot drop, provides minimal contact to the skin, and provides some forward propulsion to substitute for lack of PF.

5. **How does AFO change gait parameters?**
   By limiting motion at the ankle, AFO will control the knee during stance phase. A rigid or metal AFO locked in neutral will control foot drop during swing phase and will promote knee flexion at initial contact and loading response, and promote knee extension during terminal stance and pre-swing. This can become problematic if the quadriceps

muscle strength is less than 4/5 causing buckling of the knee. An AFO which allows PF motion will have less control at the knee because of the PF motion allowed at the ankle joint during loading response.

6. **What are the trimlines of a plastic AFO?**

The trimlines of an AFO are the degree to which plastic wraps around the ankle and determine the stiffness or stability of the brace relative to foot and ankle motion. A posterior trimline is well behind the malleolus and allows some limited DF and PF. A trimline at the malleolus will give moderate stiffness but yet allow some limited motion. A rigid trimline is anterior to the malleolus and will allow no motion of the ankle in all planes. A more flexible design is often chosen for flaccid conditions of the lower limb, and a more rigid design is often chosen when tone and spasticity are present.

7. **What are the common joints used in metal AFOs?**

There are several types of joints for metal AFOs. A free motion ankle joint will allow unrestricted DF and PF, but will control medial lateral instability at the ankle. A posterior or single channel ankle joint can provide DF assist using a spring and PF stop using a pin. A dual channel ankle joint can provide DF assist, PF stop, and DF stop.

8. **How do the anterior and posterior channels of a metal AFO ankle joint work?**

The posterior channel is present in both single channel and dual channel ankle joints. A compressed spring in the posterior channel will provide dorsiflexion assist, while a steel pin in the posterior channel will provide plantarflexion stop. A dual channel ankle joint can perform all of the same functions in the posterior channel, but also has an anterior channel. Providing a pin in the anterior channel limits dorsiflexion during stance phase. This is sometimes difficult to understand, but imagine the forward progression of the tibia through mid-stance and terminal stance as dorsiflexion of the ankle joint. If there is instability of the knee or weakness of the quadriceps muscle, then forward progression of the knee may lead to buckling. Using a pin in the anterior channel will limit the forward progression of the tibia and therefore provide inherent stability to the knee and prevent buckling. A dual channel ankle joint can lock the ankle in any defined position when pins are used in both anterior and posterior channels.

9. **How does a carbon fiber AFO differ from plastic and metal AFOs?**

A carbon fiber AFO is similar to other AFOs by providing dorsiflexion assist for foot clearance during swing phase. It may also provide some propulsion to replace weakness of the calf muscles. However, most carbon fiber AFOs provide little or no medial/lateral stability to the ankle. Most carbon fiber AFOs today are prefabricated and therefore have limited adjustability when there is edema or deformity present.

10. **How can a knee orthosis stabilize an Anterior Cruciate Ligament (ACL) or Posterior Cruciate Ligament (PCL) deficient knee?**

With ACL or PCL deficiency, there is anterior or posterior translation of the femur on the tibial plateau during walking, running, or stair climbing. The ACL and PCL normally act as a check rein to limit this anterior/posterior translation. With disruption of the ligaments, the patient may feel a sense of slipping or buckling of the knee during activities. A properly designed hinged knee orthosis with a rigid frame can control the anterior and posterior translation of the femur on the tibial plateau to minimize further destruction of the cartilage and sense of instability.

11. **What knee joint options are available for Knee Ankle Foot Orthosis (KAFO)?**

There are many choices for knee joints when prescribing a KAFO. The least restrictive knee joint is a free motion joint which allows unrestricted flexion but with extension stop at neutral and provides knee medial lateral stability. A posterior offset knee joint allows unrestricted flexion with extension stop while providing some stability because the axis of the knee joint is located posterior to the center of gravity of the body. This is most effective when the knee joint is in full extension to approximately 20 degrees of flexion. The drop lock knee joint is still the most commonly ordered joint. In the unlocked position, the joint has unrestricted flexion, but in the locked position, it maintains full extension of the knee. The term drop lock is a misnomer since we cannot rely on gravity to simply pull the lock into a closed position. This must be done manually to lock and unlock. There are spring-loaded locking mechanisms such as the trigger lock and bail lock. These 2 joints will lock automatically from the flexed to fully extended position, but still require manual unlocking for sitting.

12. **What are the common indications for a KAFO?**

A KAFO should be prescribed when there is instability at the knee and ankle which may be due to muscle weakness, hyperextension, or ligamentous disruption. KAFOs can also be used to control abnormal motion such as spasticity during standing or walking activities. KAFO with a proximal weight-bearing thigh shell or brim can also be used to partially offload distal segments.

13. **What are the common material and design features available for KAFOs?**

The most common materials used are plastic and metal. The uprights and joints are commonly made of metal but the thigh shell, calf shell and footplate are most commonly fabricated of plastic which is custom molded. Aluminum or carbon fiber thigh bands and calf bands can also be used if total contact with plastic is not desirable due to underlying skin conditions or edema. If foot contact is to be avoided, then metal stirrup from the ankle joint can be attached directly to an orthopedic shoe.

14. **How does a stance control KAFO work to normalize gait and conserve energy?**
   A stance control orthosis is designed with electronic or mechanical locking of the knee during stance phase and unlocking of the knee during swing phase which prevents circumduction, vaulting, or hip hiking that are common gait deviations experienced with a locked knee KAFO .

15. **How does reciprocal gait orthosis (RGO) improve ambulation in patients with paraplegia?**
   RGO is a specialized design of a bilateral Hip Knee Ankle Foot Orthosis (HKAFO) with a linkage or cable from one hip joint to the other. As one hip joint is flexed, using trunk or pelvic motion, then the cable or linkage creates extension at the opposite hip joint, therefore creating a reciprocal gait pattern which conserves energy and improves forward progression. RGO braces are an improvement over traditional bilateral HKAFOs; however, they are still quite cumbersome and difficult to don and doff. The energy cost is still very high and the use of an assistive device, such as crutches or walker, are still required. RGO braces are most commonly used for exercise rather than functional mobility.

16. **How do you assess a lower limb orthosis?**
   Any orthosis prescribed should be followed up with an assessment visit which should include careful inspection of the orthosis to ensure that it complies with prescription and with high quality standards for fabrication and fit. The skin should be inspected for any areas of redness, irritation, or pressure. Make sure the patient can don and doff the orthosis appropriately and independently. Instructions on wearing time and further follow-up should also be provided. Physical therapy training is sometimes required to learn appropriate use of the orthosis.

BIBLIOGRAPHY

Uustal H: Prosthetics and Orthotics. In Cuccurullo S (ed): Physical *Medicine and Rehabilitation Board Review*, Fourth Edition. New York, NY: Demos, 2018.
Uustal H, Hennessey WJ: Lower Limb Orthotic Devices. In Cifu DX (ed): Physical *Medicine and Rehabilitation*, 5th Edition. Philadelphia, PA: Elsevier, 2015.

CHAPTER 36

UPPER LIMB ORTHOSIS

Heikki Uustal, MD and Chun Ho, MD

The hand is the tool of tools

—Aristotle

KEY POINTS

1. An orthosis can be static to limit motion or dynamic to increase motion.
2. Upper limb orthoses can often be fabricated from low-temperature thermoplastic materials or from prefabricated kits that are available from suppliers.
3. If there is increased tone or spasticity of the upper limb, treatment for controlling the spasticity should be considered before an upper limb orthosis is prescribed.
4. If there is no function of the hand, but there is some function of the shoulder and elbow, then a hybrid "prosthesis" can be used.

1. What is an upper limb orthosis and how are orthoses named?
   An upper limb orthosis is a splint or brace that supports a segment or joint of the upper limb. An orthosis can be static to limit motion or dynamic to increase motion. Orthoses are named by the joints or segments that they cross. As an example, WHO is a wrist hand orthosis. Orthoses may cross multiple joints, and it is important to specify whether the orthoses are static or dynamic across each of these joints.

2. What functional goals should be considered when prescribing an upper limb orthosis?
   The primary function of the upper limb is for prehension, grasping, and manipulating an object. The upper limb can also be used for lifting, pushing, pulling, or carrying. The goal of an upper limb orthosis is to restore these functions which may be impaired by disease or injury. Upper limb orthoses are used to correct or prevent deformity, control abnormal movements or augment motion, and restore prehension of the hand. They are also sometimes used following surgery or injury for stabilization and healing.

3. What are the biomechanical considerations when prescribing an upper limb orthosis?
   The biomechanical design of an orthosis must take into account the potential force applied by the device and the tissue tolerance from that force. Every orthosis uses a three-point control system across each joint involved, and the location of the force application should be a pressure tolerant area. There are more pressure intolerant areas on the hand compared to the foot. Therefore, the risk of skin breakdown must be taken into consideration when designing an orthotic device for the upper limb that includes the hand. If there is increased tone or spasticity of the upper limb, treatment for controlling the spasticity should be considered before an upper limb orthosis is prescribed. Fitting an upper limb with significant spasticity may cause increased pressure against the brace and result in pain or skin breakdown.

4. What are the common indications for upper limb orthoses?
   Common indications include trauma such as fracture or strain, weakness or paralysis, spasticity, disease such as rheumatoid arthritis, contracture, surgical procedures, or for protection.

5. How are static and dynamic orthoses different?
   A static orthosis is designed to limit or stop all motion across a joint to allow healing to occur or stabilize a joint following disease or weakness. A dynamic orthosis is designed to increase motion across the joint that is weak or contracted. A hybrid orthosis may cross multiple joints and therefore provides static control at some joints and dynamic motion at other joints.

6. What is the common recommended wearing schedule for an upper limb orthosis?
   Because the hand is more sensitive and there is relatively little soft tissue padding on the fingers, any device on the hand or finger should be worn only 2 hours on and 2 hours off to prevent skin breakdown and pain. An orthosis above the wrist can be worn for longer periods with less risk due to increase in soft tissue and padding. The skin should be inspected for redness or irritation following every use of the orthosis. If redness persists greater than 20 minutes, then modification or adjustment of the device or wearing schedule will be needed. If the device is used for the purposes of stretching a contracture, then a combination of static positioning device may be used for a longer period of time, while a dynamic stretching device should be used for a much shorter period of time.

7. What are the special considerations for wearing an upper limb orthosis compared to lower limb?

The functional purpose of upper limb orthoses is significantly different from lower limb orthoses. For example, a lower limb orthosis provides stability at the foot and ankle to prevent footdrop or mediolateral instability during weightbearing. Lower limb orthoses require a much more rigid or durable material selection to tolerate weight-bearing. Upper limb orthoses can often be fabricated from low-temperature thermoplastic materials or from pre-fabricated kits that are available from suppliers. This is because the weight tolerance of the material is much lower for prehension than it is for weightbearing. In addition, there are multiple joints involved in the fingers and hand, and each joint must be addressed when an orthosis is prescribed that will cross the fingers and hand.

8. How can finger orthoses help control progressive deformities of the fingers in rheumatoid arthritis?

The two most common deformities of the fingers in rheumatoid arthritis are boutonniere's deformity and swan-neck deformity. Swan neck deformity is hyperextension of the PIP and hyperflexion of the DIP, while boutonniere's deformity is the opposite, with hyperflexion of the proximal interphalangeal joint (PIP) and hyperextension of the distal interphalangeal joint (DIP). Both of these deformities can be controlled with a ring finger orthosis, which crosses only one interphalangeal (IP) joint with 3 points of control to prevent the deformity. They must be sized appropriately and are commonly fitted by a hand therapist or orthotist. The ring orthoses are often required long term to control these deformities of the finger and allow appropriate grasping with the hand and fingers. See Fig. 36.1.

9. What is a short opponens orthosis and what is it used for?

A short opponens orthosis is any hand finger orthosis that maintains the thumb opposite the fingers and maintains the webspace. This type of device is commonly used for median nerve injury or for disease at the base of the thumb, such as rheumatoid arthritis or tendonitis. A short opponens orthosis may be fabricated from plastic and maintains a static positioning of the thumb or may be dynamic across the base of the thumb. See Fig. 36.2.

10. What type of upper limb orthosis is used for radial nerve injury?

Radial nerve injury causes weakness of the wrist and finger extensors. The patient essentially has wrist drop and finger drop. The patient is unable to open the hand to grasp an object, and the wrist falls into flexion when the fingers are flexed resulting in poor grip. A wrist hand finger orthosis (WHFO) with static support at the wrist in neutral position and dynamic extension of the fingers and thumb will restore the ability to grasp and hold objects. This is a hybrid design with static stabilization at the wrist and dynamic extension of the digits using outriggers and finger loops.

11. What type of orthosis is used for median nerve injury?

The median nerve injury causes weakness of the thumb. A short opponens orthosis is a hand thumb orthosis that stabilizes the thumb opposite the fingers to restore grasp. Each of the digits should be able to touch the tip of the thumb to restore fine pinch and gross grasp. A short opponens orthosis does not need to cross the wrist but simply stabilize the thumb opposite the fingers.

12. What type of orthosis is used for ulnar nerve injury?

Ulnar nerve injury causes weakness or paralysis of the intrinsic muscles of the hand which results in poor fine motor skills and hyperextension of the MCP joints. With significant hyperextension of the metacarpophalangeal

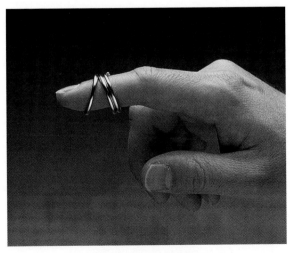

Fig. 36.1 Ring finger orthosis

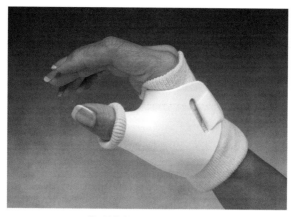

Fig. 36.2 Short opponens orthosis

(MCP) joints, finger flexion fails to occur appropriately which results in loss of pinch and grasp. A dynamic orthosis across the MCPs to improve MCP flexion will help to restore the finger function. This type of orthosis is commonly called a knuckle bender. See Fig. 36.3.

13. What type of orthosis is used for contractures of the hand and fingers?

Contracture of the fingers caused by tight collateral IP ligaments or joint capsule can be treated with a dynamic finger orthosis across the tight IP joint. The three-point control concept is applied using a spring wire dynamic orthosis with small pads at the joint (primary force) and pads proximal and distal to the IP joint (counterforce). This can be adjusted by bending the spring wire to adjust the tension. Finger contracture caused by tight long flexor tendons requires a hybrid wrist hand finger orthosis (WHFO) with static support across the wrist in neutral position and outriggers for dynamic extension or traction to the fingers to stretch the long flexor tendons. In addition, a block at the MCP joints is necessary to prevent hyperextension at the MCP. When multiple joints are crossed, dynamic activity should only occur at the one primary joint and others should be stabilized statically. See Fig. 36.4.

14. How is an orthosis used for finger flexor or extensor tendon repair?

Following flexor tendon repair, the rehabilitation protocol will require a hybrid wrist hand finger orthosis with static stabilization of the wrist in neutral position and progressive motion of the fingers from a fully flexed position to fully extended position over 6 to 12 weeks. Initially, only 30 degrees of motion are allowed across the surgically repaired tendon to prevent adhesions of the tendon within the tendon sheath while minimizing any tension across the repaired segment. The amount of extension allowed is slowly increased as the tendon repair heals.

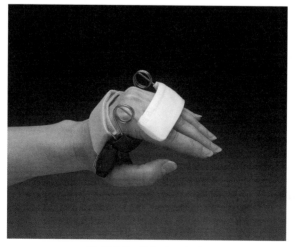

Fig. 36.3 Knuckle bender orthosis

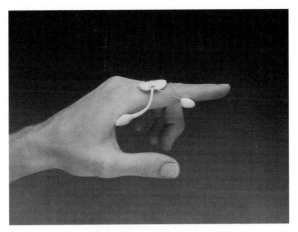

Fig. 36.4 Dynamic finger orthosis

This type of device should be worn 24 hours a day to prevent accidental rapid extension of the digits which may disrupt the surgical repair. See Fig. 36.5.

15. **How should you choose an off-the-shelf or custom-made upper limb orthosis?**
    Unlike lower limb orthoses where custom-made high-temperature thermoplastic designs are most commonly used, there are many more off-the-shelf options for upper limb orthoses. Because of the lower demands of force on the upper limb orthoses, there are kits available with low-temperature thermoplastic material that can be heat molded with a heat gun or heating pan and fitted directly to the patient. There are also premade devices that cross a variety of joints including the wrist hand fingers that can be adjusted with minimal modification using padding or straps to maintain static or dynamic support. If there is significant deformity or significant force that will be applied to the soft tissue, then the recommendation is to consider custom-made upper limb orthoses rather than off-the-shelf.

16. **How would an elbow orthosis help to stabilize an injury or fracture at the elbow but still prevent contracture during the healing period?**
    A: A progressive static or progressive dynamic elbow orthosis will gradually increase the range of motion of the elbow joint while maintaining stability. A progressive static device may initially start in one position and gradually move to another position with modifications to the device, while a progressive dynamic elbow orthosis will slowly increase the range of motion allowed with an adjustable joint while wearing the device. This will prevent adhesions or contractures within the joint or injury area and slowly allow increasing range of motion as the bony injury slowly heals. See Fig. 36.6.

17. **How would you stabilize the shoulder following injury or surgery?**
    The shoulder is a very unstable joint, particularly at the glenohumeral joint. Following surgical stabilization, the surgeon will likely recommend a desired position for healing, and the orthosis should maintain that position. If the

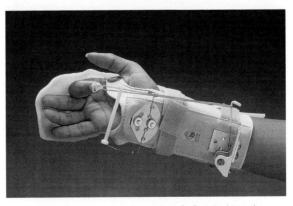

Fig. 36.5 Hybrid wrist hand finger orthosis for flexor tendon repair

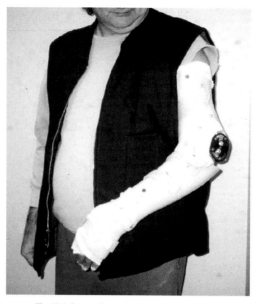

Fig. 36.6 Progressive static elbow wrist hand orthosis

arm is to be abducted 90 degrees, then a static airplane splint is recommended. If the arm is to be held close to the trunk, then a gunslinger orthosis will be used and can be adjusted to a variety of degrees of abduction from 0 to 45 degrees as needed.

18. What type of orthosis will help with prehension or grasping for a patient with C6 level of quadriplegia?

A patient with C6 level of quadriplegia has lost the ability to grasp with either hand and therefore, prehension is lost which results in the patient being dependent in all self-care. However, functioning of C6 muscles such as the wrist extensors, biceps, pectoralis, and proximal muscles of the upper limb will be maintained. The tenodesis effect takes advantage of wrist extension to promote prehension of the fingers against the stationary thumb. This is augmented using a tenodesis orthosis, which relies on 4/5 strength for wrist extension to bring the fingers down against a stationary thumb using a three-part orthotic device. There is a cable or cord that connects the three components of the tenodesis orthosis that slowly pulls the fingers down as the wrist is extended. The opening of the hand or grasping capability can be adjusted by adjusting the length of the cord. See Figs. 36.7 and 36.8.

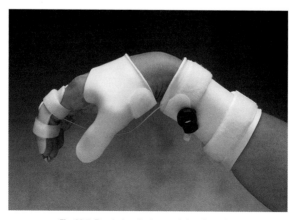

Fig. 36.7 Tenodesis orthosis open (relaxed) position

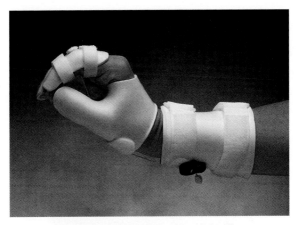

Fig. 36.8 Tenodesis orthosis closed (grasping) position

19. How does a ball-bearing feeder or balanced forearm orthosis help a patient with C5-level quadriplegia?

In a patient with C5-level quadriplegia, the intrinsic muscles of the hand, the flexors of the fingers and wrist, and the extensors of the elbow are plegic while the biceps and the pectoralis are spared. The ball-bearing feeder, also called a balanced forearm orthosis, helps balance the weight of the forearm on a pivot point that allows the use of pectoralis to bring the elbow down while bringing the wrist and hand up. The biceps can be used to bring the hand toward the mouth for feeding or other self-care tasks. Since the patient has no grasp, a universal cuff must be strapped onto the hand with an adapted utensil or device inserted into the universal cuff. A swivel spoon, a fork, or a rocker knife can be used for the patient with C5-level quadriplegia to perform self-feeding activities following setup.

20. How can an electronic upper limb orthosis help with prehension following cerebrovascular accident (CVA) or brain injury?

There are wrist hand finger orthoses that use an electronic signal to create contracture of the fingers against the thumb for prehension. These motions can be triggered with an electronic signal from an existing muscle in the upper limb that is still under voluntary control, or it can be triggered externally by a device or a pushbutton. This type of orthosis will help to restore prehension for an individual that has lost function of the hand but still has some function at the elbow and shoulder to bring the object to the mouth for feeding or self-care.

21. Are there upper limb orthotic options for patients with paralysis of the hand after brachial plexus injury?

If there is no function of the hand, but there is some function of the shoulder and elbow, then a hybrid "prosthesis" can be used. This will use orthotic componentry proximally to help stabilize the shoulder and possibly stabilize the elbow with a lock mechanism. In addition, there will be a forearm shell that will act like the socket of an upper limb prosthesis with a wrist unit for terminal device that is positioned near the palmar surface of the hand. The terminal device, such as a hook or hand, can be activated with a figure-9 harness for the purpose of grasping, holding, and manipulating objects. Prehension is restored with this type of device. See Fig. 36.9.

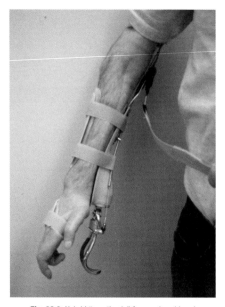

Fig. 36.9 Hybrid "prosthosis" for paralyzed hand

BIBLIOGRAPHY

1. Webster J, Murphy D. *Atlas of Orthoses and Assistive Devices.* 5th ed. Philadelphia, PA: Elsevier; 2019
2. Redford JB. *Orthotics: Clinical Practice and Rehabilitation Technology.* New York, NY: Churchill Livingstone; 1995

CHAPTER 37

SPINAL ORTHOSES: PRINCIPLES, DESIGNS, INDICATIONS, AND LIMITATIONS

Paul S. Jones, DO, Heikki Uustal, MD, and Steven A. Stiens, MD, MS

Never slouch, as doing so compresses the lungs, overcrowds other vital organs, rounds the back, and throws you off balance.
—Joseph H. Pilates (1883–1967)

KEY POINTS

1. Spinal orthoses stabilize and maintain alignment, prevent and correct deformity, relieve pain, and provide kinesthetic feedback.
2. Spinal orthotic prescription requires applied knowledge of regional spine planes of motion, mechanisms of specific pathology, points of support for stabilization, and adaptive patient responses.
3. The Halo Fixator Cervical Thoracic Orthosis is most effective in limiting motion of upper cervical vertebrae but requires regular pin cleaning and maintenance of pin pressure with torque measurements.
4. The "Clam Shell" or plastic Thoracic Lumbar Sacral Orthosis (TLSO) provides flexion, extension, and rotatory control thereby effectively immobilizing stable T10–L2 burst fractures of neurologically intact patients.
5. Spinal orthotics that guide active posture and overcompensate for deformities during development may guide spinal adaptive growth utilizing compressive and distractive forces. The Heuter-Volkmann Law states: "compressive stresses slow growth, whereas tensile stresses hasten growth."

1. What is a spinal orthosis?

The word *orthosis* is derived from the Greek word meaning, "straightening." Spinal orthoses or braces are appliances used in an attempt to correct and support the spine.

Smith GE. The most ancient splints. *Br Med J.* 1908;1(2465):732–736.2. doi:10.1136/bmj.1.2465.732. Available at: https://www.ncbi.nlm.nih.gov/pmc/articles/PMC2436247/pdf/brmedj07954-0008.pdf

2. What is the advantage of interdisciplinary collaboration with an orthotist?

The **orthotist** is an integral contributor due to skills in measurement, customized fabrication, fitting, support of compliance, and repair of orthoses. Synergistic collaboration comes with interactive sharing of patient problems and therapeutic ideas specific to patient needs that translate into individual life contexts. Integration of orthotists into regularly scheduled interdisciplinary patient care clinics with evolving agendas facilitates the best outcomes.

Orthotist & Prosthetist. Available at: https://www.abcop.org/individual-certification/get-certified/orthotist-prosthetist/overview

3. What are the clinical situations that suggest spinal orthotics?

- Stabilization and maintenance of spinal alignment
- Prevention and correction of spinal deformities
- Relief of pain by limiting motion or weight-bearing
- Reduction of axial loading of the spine
- Provision of effects such as heat, massage, and kinesthetic feedback

Cholewicki J. The effects of a 3-week use of lumbosacral orthoses on proprioception in the lumbar spine, *J Orthop Sports Phys Ther.* 2006;36(4), 225–231. Available at: https://www.jospt.org/doi/pdf/10.2519/jospt.2006.36.4.225

4. **What are the spinal anatomical and kinesiological considerations involved in the axial skeleton?**
   There are 33 spinal vertebrae divided into five regions: cervical, thoracic, lumbar, sacral, and coccygeal. The plane of facet joint alignment guides regional motion.

5. **How do spinal orthoses work?**
   Spinal orthoses, when applied to the body, exert forces on the spine. This is accomplished in one or more of the following ways:
   - Three-point pressure system
   Orthotic systems are designed utilizing a minimum of three contact points that distribute aligning forces around a movement axis (Fig. 37.1. Forces Diagram).
   - Circumferential support
   - Irritation that triggers active alignment
   - Skeletal fixation

Lantz SA, Schultz AB. Lumbar spine orthoses wearing: effect on trunk muscle myoelectric activity. *Spine.* 1986;11:838–4234

Pritham, C. Knee orthoses: biomechanics. *Clin Prosthet Orthot.* 1981;5(4):5–7.

6. **What are the potential complications or side effects of spinal orthoses?**
   Patients may become dependent physiologically and psychologically on the use of the orthotic devices. There may be potential weakening of axial muscles, development of soft tissue contractures, and skin ulcerations. The devices could actually limit activities of daily living.

Norbury JW, Mehta SK, Davison A, Felsen GS. *Spinal Orthotoses.* In David C, ed. *Braddom's Physical Medicine and Rehabilitation.* 6th ed. Philadelphia: Elsevier; 2021:248–260

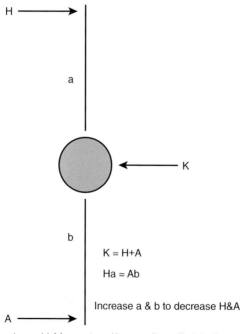

$$K = H + A$$
$$Ha = Ab$$

Increase a & b to decrease H&A

Fig. 37.1 Three-point pressure system model. A force vector and lever arm diagram illustrates the requirement of a minimum of three points of contact for realignment. Recognize the length of the lever arm (a and b) increases leverage and reduces the force requirement (A and H), and that this is a simplification as the spine actually moves at a variety of axes.

7. What are some complications that occur with cervical orthoses?

Cervical orthoses can cause difficulty with swallowing, coughing, breathing, and vomiting. Pressure on the marginal mandibular nerve can result in paralysis of the depressors of the lower lip. It has been reported to increase intracranial pressure.

Camara R, Ajayi OO, Asgarzadie F. Are external cervical orthoses necessary after anterior cervical discectomy and fusion: a review of the literature. *Cureus.* 2016;8(7):e688. doi: 10.7759/cureus.688. Available at: https://www.ncbi.nlm.nih.gov/pmc/articles/PMC4980205/

Herget G. Spinal orthoses: the crucial role of comfort on compliance of wearing-monocentric prospective pilot study of randomized crossover design. *Acta Chir Orthop Traumatol Cech.* 2017;84(2):91–96. Available at: http://www.achot.cz/dwnld/achot_2017_2_091_096.pdf

Woster C. Placement of a cervical collar increases the optic nerve sheath diameter in healthy adults. *Am J Emerg Med.* 2018;36(3):430–434 Available at: https://www.ncbi.nlm.nih.gov/pmc/articles/PMC4790142/

8. What factors are considered when prescribing the most appropriate orthosis for a specific spinal problem?
   a. Baselines: growth rate, spine maturity, deformity, pathophysiology measures.
   b. Pertinent diagnoses, age, bone development, deformity causes, prognosis.
   c. Patient body habitus?
   d. Regions that need to be controlled.
   e. Biomechanical planes of motion that require restriction.
   f. Intended mechanism and results from orthotic.
   g. Projected patient requirements for adherence.
   h. Complications or loss of function that may result.
   i. Orthotist fabrication: availability, ease of use, weight, forces translated, material (strength, flexibility, durability) cosmetic appearance, and cost.

Sypert GW. External spinal orthotics. *Neurosurgery.* 1987;20(4):642–649

Mireille N. Mechanisms of action of lumbar supports: a systemic review: *Spine.* 2000;25(16):2103–2113.

9. How are spinal orthoses classified?

Spinal orthotic devices are named using the convention of the ***body region they cross.*** They also go by other eponyms. Orthotics may be rigid, semi-rigid, or flexible depending on the purpose or amount of control desired from the orthotic device.
   Named by the body region that they cross or by eponyms:
   CO: Cervical Orthosis; HCO: Head cervical orthosis (Soft cervical collar, Rigid cervical collar (Philadelphia, Aspen, Miami J, Newport)
   CTO: Cervicothoracic orthosis (Halo, Sterno-occipital mandibular orthosis, Minerva)
   CTLSO: Cervicothoracolumbosacral orthosis (Milwaukee)
   TLSO: Thoracolumbar orthosis (CASH, Jewett, Custom-molded body jacket. Knight Taylor TLSO)
   LSO: Lumbosacral orthosis (Chairback, Knight, corsets/binders)
   SO: Sacral orthosis (Trochanteric belt, sacral belt, sacral corset)

Harris EE. A new orthotics terminology. *Ortho Prosthet.* 1973;27:6–10. Available at: http://www.oandplibrary.com/op/1973_02_006.asp

Edmonson, AS. Spinal orthotics. *Ortho Prosthet.* 1977;31(4):31–42. Available at: http://www.oandplibrary.org/op/1977_04_031.asp

10. Are there functional limitations with the use of CO/CTO?

CO and CTO limit cervical motion. These may limit the ability to look down to see and perform bowel and bladder care. It may also adversely affect advanced wheelchair skills and transfer activities.

11. What are the relative percentage restriction of motion by the various COs?

Restriction of Motion % by Orthosis

Device	Flexion/Extension	Lateral Bending	Rotation
Halo	96	96	99
Minerva	78	51–90	84–88
Four-Post CTO	79–88	54	73
SOMI	61–72	18–34	29–66
Miami J	60–76	52	65–77
Vista -Aspen	69–90	34–48	74
Philadelphia	59–75	12–34	27–56
Soft Collar	8–26	8	10–17

Harrington A. *Chapter 43: Spinal Orthoses.* In S Kirshblum (Ed.). *Spinal Cord Medicine.* New York: Springer; 2019:744–753.

12. What are some commonly utilized types of COs? What is the limited motion afforded by the device? For what diagnoses are they utilized?

    Soft cervical collar: Provide warmth, psychological reassurance, and a kinesthetic reminder to limit motion. Unfortunately, it may not actually reduce the intensity or duration of pain (Fig. 37.2 Soft Collar).

    Semirigid Collars: Miami J Collar/VISTA Collar/Malibu Collar: May be utilized for fractures, post-operative care, and strains. Various designs restrict particular movements (Fig. 37.3A and B).

13. What is the head to trunk orthotic that is more effective in restricting cervical motion than conventional cervical orthoses?

    The Halo fixator device (Fig. 37.4 Halo Fixator Device).

Evan N. A 3D motion analysis study comparing the effectiveness of cervical spine orthoses at restricting spinal motion through physiological ranges. *Eur Spine J.* 2013;22(Suppl 1):S10–S15. doi:10.1007/s00586-012-2641-0. Available at: https://www.ncbi.nlm.nih.gov/pmc/articles/PMC3578513/

14. What is a halo fixator vest orthosis?

    This CTO consists of two parts: the halo and a vest that encircles the trunk. This device provides the most rigid fixation of the cervical spine and is the orthosis most widely used after upper cervical fractures. It requires pins placed 1 cm above the lateral rim of the orbits (Fig. 37.5 Skull Safe Zone). Complications include pin site infection, scarring nerve injury (supraorbital, supratrochlear, and abducens nerve), dural penetration,

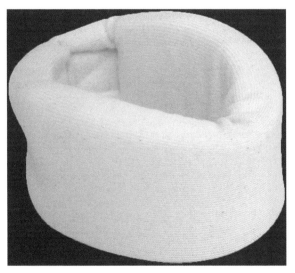

Fig. 37.2 Soft collar: covered compressible foam.

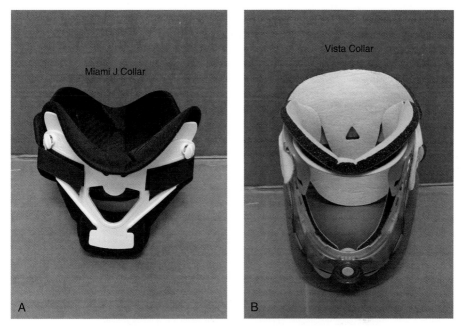

Fig. 37.3 (A) Miami J collar: rigid adjustable plastic. (B) Vista collar: rigid adjustable plastic

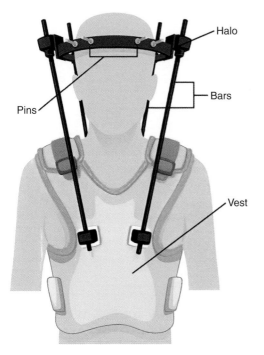

Fig. 37.4 Halo fixator device: cervical thoracic orthosis

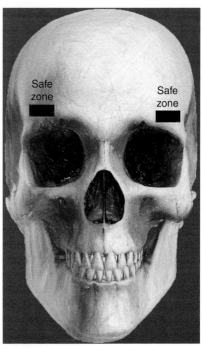

Fig. 37.5 Skull safe zone: anterior pin sites for halo

intracranial abscess, temporal artery dissection, and seizures. The pins need to be **torque adjusted** to prevent puncturing the skull table. They also require **scheduled cleaning techniques**.

Bono C. The halo fixator. *J Am Acad Orthop Surg.* 2007;15(12):728–737. doi: 10.5435/00124635-200712000-00006. Available at: https://journals.lww.com/jaaos/Fulltext/2007/12000/The_Halo_Fixator.6.aspx

Botte MJ, Byrne TP, Abrams RA et al. The halo skeletal fixator: current concepts of application and maintenance. *Orthopedics.* 1995; 18(5):463–471.

Bransford R. Halo vest treatment of cervical spine injuries, a success and survivorship analysis. *Spine.* 2009;34(15):1561–1546. doi:10.1097/BRS.0b013e3181a9702d

Mangum S. A comprehensive guide to the halo brace. Application, care, patient teaching. *AORN J.* 1993;58(3):534–546. doi: 10.1016/s0001-2092(07)68439-7

15. Is there a less invasive alternative to the halo fixator device?
The **Minerva Body Jacket** (Fig. 37.6 Minerva). It is lighter than the Halo, it has no pins and has less risk of infection or slippage. There is less control of Atlanto-occipital motion than the Halo Fixator device. However, intersegmental control may be better overall.

Karimi MT, Kamali M, Fatoye F. Evaluation the efficiency of cervical orthoses on cervical fracture: a review of literature. *J Craniovert Jun Spine.* 2016;7(1):13–19.doi: 10.4103/0974-8237.176611.13-9. Available at: https://www.ncbi.nlm.nih.gov/pmc/articles/PMC4790142/

16. What are the most commonly used TLSOs? How should I approach the type of orthoses based upon biomechanical control desired?
Flexion control (Fig. 37.7 CASH Orthosis, Fig. 37.8)
    Cruciform Anterior Spinal Hyperextension Brace (CASH) (no effect on "reimbursement")
Flexion-extension control
    Taylor Brace: (Fig. 37.9 Taylor TLSO)
Flexion-extension-lateral control

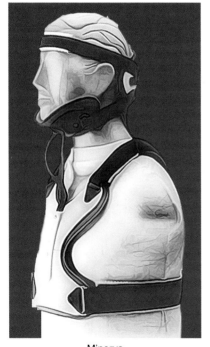

Minerva

Fig. 37.6 Minerva: cervical thoracic orthosis

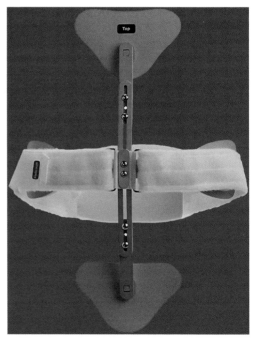

CASH TLSO

Fig. 37.7 Cruciform anterior spinal hyperextension brace (CASH): thoracic lumbar sacral orthosis (TLSO)

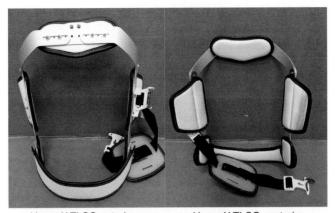

Hyper X TLSO anterior   Hyper X TLSO posterior

Fig. 37.8 The Hyper X TLSO is the Jewett hyperextension brace: three points of support. *TLSO,* Thoracic lumbar sacral orthosis

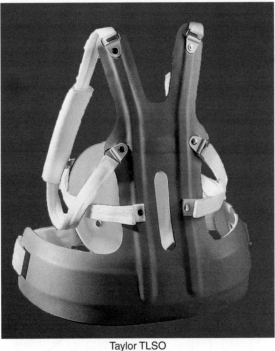

Taylor TLSO

Fig. 37.9 Taylor: thoracic lumbar sacral orthosis (TLSO)

Knight-Taylor TLSO: (Fig. 37.10 Knight Taylor TLSO)
Flexion-extension-lateral-rotary control
   Body Jacket (Fig. 37.11 Clam Shell or Plastic TLSO)

17. What are the types of lumbosacral orthoses (LSO'S)?
   Flexible LSO such as corsets or binders (Fig. 37.12. Soft LSO)
   Chairback TLSO
   Williams flexion LSO
   Knight LSO

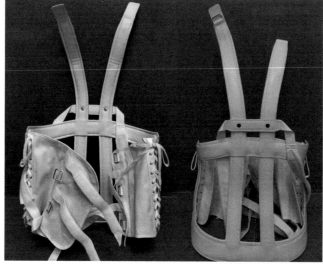

Knight taylor TLSO
anterior

Knight taylor TLSO
posterior

Fig. 37.10 Knight Taylor: thoracic lumbar sacral orthosis (TLSO)

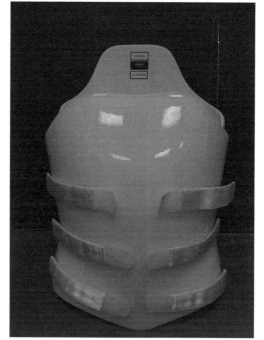

Plastic TLSO

Fig. 37.11 "Clam shell" or plastic TLSO

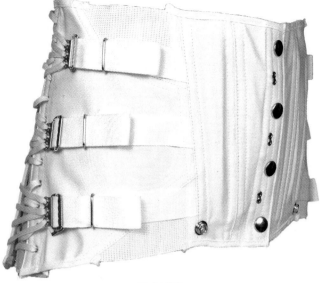

Soft LSO

Fig. 37.12 Soft lumbosacral orthosis (LSO): circumferential support

Custom-molded LSO
Flexion-extension control
   Chairback TLSO
   (Fig. 37.13. Chairback or Knight TLSO)
Extension-lateral control
   Williams Flexion LSO (Fig. 37.14. Williams Brace)

18. **What are the proposed mechanisms for use of LSOs?**
In 1961, Morris hypothesized that elevated intra-abdominal and intrathoracic pressure reduced the net force applied to the spine during the act of lifting a weight from the floor. The spinal column is linked to the rib cage and theoretically can be hydraulically supported by pressure in the abdominal cavity. Active muscle

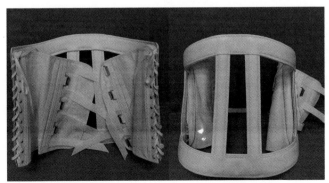

Knight TLSO
(no shoulder straps)
anterior

Knight TLSO
(no shoulder straps)
posterior

Fig. 37.13 Chairback or Knight thoracic lumbar sacral orthosis (TLSO)

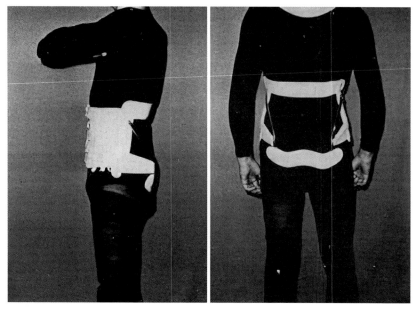

Fig. 37.14 Williams brace: facilitates flexion, limits extension (From: Edmonson AS. Spinal orthotics. *Orthot Prosthet.* 1977;31(4):31–42.)

contraction supports these chambers with rigid walls. This results in decreasing the load on the spine itself. The problem with abdominal corsets is that they may reduce the activity of the abdominal muscles. However, Nachemson and Morris demonstrated in 1964 that a tight inflatable corset reduced disc pressure about 25%. Lantz showed variable effects on myoelectric activity of abdominal muscles and extensor muscles of the spine.

Lantz S. Lumbar spine orthosis wearing II. Effect on trunk muscle myoelectric activity. *Spine.* 1986;11(8):838–842

Morris JM, Lucas DB, Bresler B. Role of the trunk in stability of the spine. *J Bone Joint Surg Am.* 1961;43:327–351.

Nachemson A, Morris JM. In vivo measurements of intradiscal pressure: discometry, a method for the determination of pressure in the lower lumbar discs. *J Bone Joint Surg Am.* 1964; 46:1077–1092.

19. What are the types of "SO"? What does it do?
    Sacro-iliac joint (SIJ) belts or pelvic stabilization orthoses (Fig. 37.15 Sacroiliac Belt) are devices that surround the pelvis allowing forced closure of the sacroiliac joint. It provides support and proprioceptive feedback allowing inflammation to resolve and ligaments to heal.

Don Tigny RL. Function and pathomechanics of the sacroiliac joint. A review. *Phys Ther.* 1985;65(1):35–44.

Forst S. The sacroiliac joint: anatomy, physiology and clinical significance. *Pain Physician.* 2006;9:61–68. Available at: https://www. painphysicianjournal.com/current/pdf?article=NTI5&journal=27

Sichting F. Pelvic belt effects on sacroiliac joint ligaments: A computational approach to understand therapeutic effects of pelvic belts. *Pain Physician* 2014;17:43–51 Available at: https://www.painphysicianjournal.com/current/pdf?article=MjA0Mg%3D%3D &journal=80

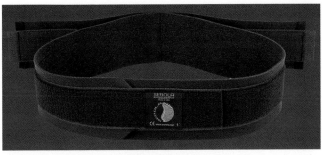

Sacral orthosis

Fig. 37.15 Sacroiliac belt: circumferential pelvis compression

20. How are stable T10–L2 burst fractures treated in the neurologically intact patient?
TLSO treatment as compared to surgical treatment revealed less disability, lower pain scores, higher physical functioning scores, and less complications with lower cost. The functional outcomes at 2 years were similar for surgical and non-surgical treatment.

Li-Yang D. Conservative treatment of thoracolumbar burst fractures: a long-term follow-up results with special reference to the load sharing classification. *Spine*. 2008;33(23):2536–2544. doi: 10.1097/BRS.0b013e3181851bc2.

Shen WJ, Liu TJ, Shen YS. Nonoperative treatment vs. posterior fixation for thoracolumbar junction burst fractures without neurological deficit. *Spine*. 2001;26(9):1038–1045. doi: 10.1097/00007632-200105010-00010.

Wood KB, Buttermann GR, Phukan R, et al. Operative compared with nonoperative treatment of a thoracolumbar burst fracture without neurological deficits: a prospective randomized study with follow-up sixteen to twenty-two years. *J Bone Joint Surg Am*. 2015;97:13–19. doi:10.2106/JBJS.N.00226

21. How are unstable T10-L2 burst fractures treated?
Unstable thoracic-lumbar fractures require acute surgical neuro decompression and fusion. Thereafter, a custom clam-shell TLSO is applied for up to 3 months. The patient is instructed to always wear this, removing it only one half hour at a time for purposes of hygiene and when the spine is supported supine or prone in bed.

Benzel EC, Larson SJ. Postoperative stabilization of the post traumatic thoracic and lumbar spine: a review of concepts and orthotic techniques *J Spinal Disord*. 1989;2(1):47–51

22. WHAT ARE SOME ORTHOTIC DEVICES USEFUL AFTER STABLE VERTEBRAL COMPRESSION FRACTURES AND THEIR TREATMENT MECHANISMS?
Posture-training supports (PTS) (Fig. 37.16. PTS)
Spinomed orthosis (Thoracolumbosacral orthosis) (Fig. 37.17. Spinomed Orthosis)

23. Are there strategies for using spinal orthoses for low back pain in spite of the risk of complications?
There have been controversies about the use of lumbar spinal orthoses for low back pain. The majority of the studies do not support the use of spinal orthotics for acute or chronic low back pain. There may be some limited benefit during the subacute phase of pain within the first 3 weeks of onset. There is no harm or side effects with short-term or intermittent use of LSOs for pain control, spasm reduction, and splinting of painful structures to maintain overall activity. However, long-term full-time use of lumbar orthoses can potentially detract from the treatment plan by reducing flexibility, core muscle strength, and endurance.

Cholewicki J, Alvi K, Silfies SP, et al. Comparison of motion restriction and trunk stiffness provided by three thoracolumbosacral orthoses (TLSOs). *J Spinal Disord Tech*. 2003;16(5):461–468. doi: 10.1097/00024720-200310000-00005.

Qaseem A, Wilt TJ, McLean RM, et al, Noninvasive treatments for acute, subacute, and chronic low back pain: a clinical practice guideline from the American College of Physicians. *Ann Intern Med*. 2017;166(7):514–530. Available at: https://www.acpjournals.org/doi/full/10.7326/M16-2367?rfr_dat=cr_pub+ +0pubmed&url_ver=Z39.88-2003&rfr_id=ori%3Arid%3Acrossref.org

van Duijvenbode ICD, P Jellema, van Poppel MNM, van Tulder MW. Lumbar supports for prevention and treatment of low back pain. *Cochrane Database Syst Rev*. 2008;16(2):CD001823. doi:10.1002/14651858.CD001823.pub3. Available at: https://www.ncbi.nlm.nih.gov/pmc/articles/PMC7046130/

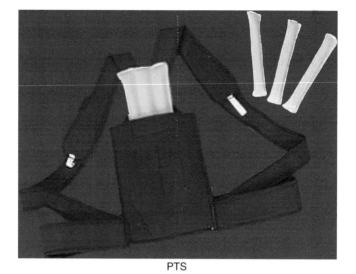

PTS

Fig. 37.16 Posture-training supports (PTS): minimizes overuse, strengthens compensation. Bracing is designed to resist undesired posture and promote extension and strengthening of muscle groups cued with compression. Proprioceptive reinforcement of the desired posture results from corrective muscle contraction and resulting laxity of support with improved posture, reduced pain, and greater endurance for activity.

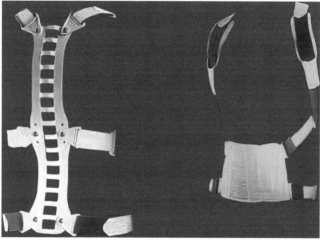

SpinoMed TLSO

Fig. 37.17 Spinomed orthosis: prevents flexion, biofeedback cued extension. The posterior padded metal band is bent to follow the spine and cue extension. The band resists flexion and maintains upright posture. *TLSO,* Thoracic lumbar sacral orthosis

24. **Why would a surgeon use an orthosis after surgical fusion with hardware?**
Surgeons opt to utilize postoperative orthoses for many reasons beyond stability. Orthoses support early mobilization, ADL training, therapy, community participation, and discharge. In the spinal cord patient with loss of sensation, the orthosis can substitute for pain to limit motion. Proprioceptive feedback from an orthosis may remind the patient to be careful with activities and limit range of motion. Spinal orthotics postoperatively provide pain control by dampening movement in the operative field, protecting closed incisions, and reducing muscle spasm. These orthotic devices are often worn for 4 to 12 weeks.

25. **What are my choices of orthotics in scoliosis?**
Determining the span and flexibility of the primary as well as compensatory curves specifies bracing options. High thoracic scoliosis requires cervical control in addition to thoracolumbar.
    The Milwaukee brace fits from neck to pelvis. Curves with apices at T-8 or lower may be treated with orthotics that can be under the arm: the Boston Brace (Fig. 37.18. Boston TLSO) or the Wilmington orthosis (Fig. 37.19. Wilmington Orthosis).

26. **What is the Charleston bending brace? Can curve over-compensation be therapeutic?**
This is a nighttime only TLSO used to treat scoliosis and relies on overcorrecting the patient's curve and unloading the vertebral end plates on the concave side of the curve. Asymmetrical bone growth is thereby decreased. It takes advantage of the ***Heuter-Volkmann Law*** that states, "compressive stresses slow growth, whereas tensile stresses hasten growth." It is worn only at nighttime for 8 to 10 hours per day. If tolerated, combining this treatment with conventional daytime bracing and exercise may improve outcomes (Fig. 37.20).

27. **What is the Milwaukee brace?**
This classic CTLSO consists of a custom plastic girdle supporting two posterior and one midline anterior vertical, body-contoured aluminum bands. A cervical ring is attached to the uprights and has pads that rest 20 to 30 mm inferior to the occiput and mandible. Side support pads rigged from the upright bands are positioned to compress the chest at the apex of the primary and compensatory curves (Fig. 37.21).

Winter R. Orthotics for spinal deformity. *Clin Orthop Relat Res.* 1974;102:72–91

28. **What are the principles of treatment of scoliosis with orthotics?**
    • Large curves are more readily straightened by elongation.
    • Smaller curves are more readily straightened by applying lateral forces.
    • A pad below the apex of the curve directs a lifting and straightening force.

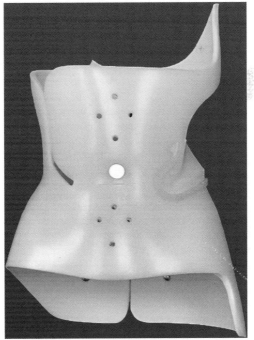

Boston TLSO

Fig. 37.18 Boston brace: bivalve thoracic lumbar sacral orthosis (TLSO) with side extensions

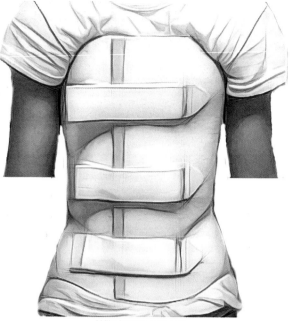

Wilmington orthosis

Fig. 37.19 Wilmington orthosis: thoracic lumbar sacral orthosis

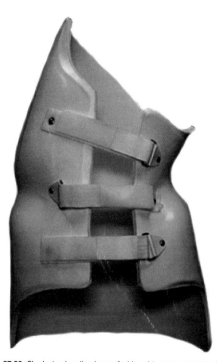

Fig. 37.20 Charleston bending brace: fashioned to over-correct scoliosis

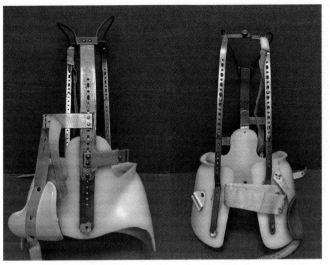

Milwaukee anterior   Milwaukee posterior

Fig. 37.21 Milwaukee thoracic lumbar sacral orthosis

- In the supine position, the TLSO is more effective with the deforming forces of gravity eliminated.
- Elongating the curve and reducing lumbar lordosis results in flattening the thoracic kyphotic curve.

Van Poppel MN, De Loose MP, Koes BW, et al. Mechanisms of action of lumbar supports: a systemic review. *Spine.* 2000;25(16):2103–2113.

29. When do I use an orthotic device for scoliosis?
    - Supple curves (20° to 40°)
        - 20° to 30° use posture, stretching, and exercises initially, if curve progresses by 5°, then add night brace
        - 30° to 40° prompt use of orthosis
        - 40° to 50° requires surgery, but orthoses may retard progression long enough to allow further trunk growth prior to fusion
        - Indicated Risser ≤2

30. How long and how actively do you need to wear the device for scoliosis?
    - 16 to 20 h/day until skeletal maturity
    - Optimum is 23 h/day
    - Correction of the curves includes exercises combining "stretching, strengthening, and breathing in reverse directions of all existing abnormal curvatures, designed to counteract the patient's unique spinal deformation."

31. How does the patient wean from a device for scoliosis?
    - A slow wean with goal to allow only up to 3 degrees of loss.
    - Requires exercises designed to shift an individual's specific spinal curve toward a normal pattern, static posture, and dynamic use.
    - Off 2 hours per day then repeat X-ray in 3 months
    - Off 4 hours per day then repeat X-ray in 3 months
    - Off 8 hours per day then repeat X-ray in 3 months
    - Off 12 hours per day then repeat X-ray at 3 months
    - Use the TLSO at night only for minimum of 1 year

Park J-H. Effects of the Schroth exercise on idiopathic scoliosis: a meta-analysis. *Eur J Phys Rehabil Med.* 2018;54:440–449. doi:10.23736/S1973-9087.17.04461-6

Redford JS, Patel AT. Orthotic devices in the management of spinal disorders. *Phys Med Rehabil State Art Rev.* 1995;9:709–724.

Zarghooni K, Beyer F, Siewe F, et al. The orthotic treatment of acute and chronic disease of the cervical and lumbar spine. *Dtsch Arztebl Int.* 2013;110(44):737–742. doi: 10.3238/arztebl.2013.0737. Available at: https://www.ncbi.nlm.nih.gov/pmc/articles/PMC3831239/

BIBLIOGRAPHY

Chui K. *Orthotics and Prosthetics in Rehabilitation.* 4th ed. St. Louis: Elsevier; 2020.

Lusskin R, Berger N. *Prescription Principles.* In American Academy of Orthopedic Surgeons, ed. *Atlas of Orthotics: Biomechanical Principles and Applications.* St. Louis: Mosby; 1975:105–129.

Webster J. *Atlas of Orthoses and Assistive Devices.* 5th ed. Philadelphia: Elsevier; 2019.

CHAPTER 38

AMPUTATION REHABILITATION: RISK, PHYSIATRIC APPROACH, AND LOWER EXTREMITY PRINCIPLES

Rebecca A. Speckman, MD, PhD, Jeffrey T. Heckman, DO, and Kevin Hakimi, MD

It's an objective fact that I am a double amputee, but it's very subjective opinion as to whether that makes me disabled.
—Aimee Mullins

KEY POINTS

1. There are 1.9 million people (prevalence) living with limb loss in the United States.
2. Over 80% of incidental limb loss in the U.S. is lower limb, while nearly 60% of congenital limb deficiency is upper limb.
3. Ulcers are a risk factor for amputation in persons with diabetic neuropathy.
4. The use of a rigid dressing such as a cast or off-the-shelf rigid removable dressing after transtibial amputation shortens time from amputation to fitting of the prosthesis.
5. Microprocessor knees are associated with greater self-reported well-being and quality of life compared to non-microprocessor knees.

1. **How common is limb loss in the United States?**
   The incidence (new cases annually) of all amputations is estimated to be 185,000 based on hospital discharge statistics. There are 1.9 million people (prevalence) living with limb loss in the United States.

   Sheehan, T. Rehabilitation and prosthethic restoration in upper limb amputation. In: Braddom RL, ed. *Physical Medicine and Rehabilitation*. 4th ed. Philadelphia, PA: Elsevier Saunders; 2011:257.

2. **What are the major reasons for limb loss in the United States? What are the lower limb amputation levels?**
   Over 80% of incidental limb loss in the U.S. is lower limb, while nearly 60% of congenital limb deficiency is upper limb. Dysvascular disease and diabetes combined are the predominant etiology of lower limb amputations, followed by trauma and cancer. Trauma is the predominant etiology of upper limb acquired limb loss. Lower limb amputation levels are described in Table 38.1.

   Dillingham TR, Pezzin LE, Mackenzie EJ. Limb amputation and limb deficiency: epidemiology and recent trends in the United States. *South Med J*. 2003;95:875–879.

3. **What are the risks of re-amputation and mortality after lower limb amputation?**
   In elderly patients, the risk of ipsilateral re-amputation by one year is more than 30% following toe or partial foot amputation, 20% following transtibial amputation, and 10% following transfemoral amputation. The risk of contralateral amputation is about 10% per year. One-year mortality among Medicare beneficiaries is more than 20% following toe or partial foot amputation, 35% following transtibial amputation, and more than 50% following transfemoral or bilateral amputations. Risk factors for re-amputation include sepsis, body mass index over 30, ongoing tobacco use, and end-stage renal disease.

   Dillingham TR, Pezzin LE, Shore AD. Reamputation, mortality, and health care costs among persons with dysvascular lower-limb amputations. *Arch Phys Med Rehabil*. 2005;86(3):480–486.

4. **What contributes to risk of foot ulcer and amputation in persons with diabetes, and what are recommended interventions for prevention?**
   Loss of motor neurons leads to atrophy of foot intrinsic muscles and loss of the normal foot architecture with displacement of protective fat pads and exaggerated or new bony prominences (commonly referred to as claw foot

Table 38.1 Lower Limb Amputation Levels

LEVEL	DESCRIPTION	COMMENTS
Partial toe	Excision or any part of one or more toes	
Toe disarticulation	Disarticulation at the metatarsophalangeal joint	If multiple toes are amputated, consideration should be given to pan-toe disarticulation with goal to prevent further toe ulcerations and amputation by improving shoe and orthosis fit
Partial ray resection	Resection of toe with part of the adjoining metatarsal (can be multiple)	Increases forces on remaining metatarsal heads, predisposing to future amputation
Transmetatarsal	Amputation of the forefoot through all of the metatarsals	Should be fit with custom orthosis with toe filler; consider full-length foot plate or ankle-foot orthosis
Syme's	Ankle disarticulation; preserves the distal end of tibia	Preserves a distal bony weight-bearing surface; socket fit is challenging and there is limited space for prosthetic foot
Transtibial amputation (below knee)	Transects the tibia and fibula	Short is <20% of tibial length, standard is 20%–50% of tibial length
Knee disarticulation	Amputation with disarticulation of knee joint	Results in prosthesis knee being more distal than contralateral knee; subischial socket may work
Transfemoral (above knee)	Transects the femur	Short is <35% of femoral length, standard is 35%–60% of femoral length.
Hip disarticulation	Amputation through hip joint, pelvis intact	Ambulation with prosthesis is very challenging, typically with "bucket"-type socket
Hemipelvectomy	Resection of lower half of pelvis	
Hemicorporectomy	Amputation of both lower limbs and pelvis below L4, L5 level	

deformity). Loss of sensation contributes to repetitive small trauma and may lead to wounds being undetected by the patient. Immune system function and autonomic function is impaired in diabetes. Peripheral arterial disease (PAD), which can occur on its own or in conjunction with diabetes, impairs wound healing and at its most severe can lead to spontaneous, non-healing wounds. Edema or chronic kidney disease predispose to wounds and impair wound healing.

Ulcers are a risk factor for amputation in persons with diabetic neuropathy. Persons with diabetic neuropathy and foot deformities, previous ulcer or amputation, or PAD should be prescribed diabetic footwear and custom foot orthoses, and should avoid walking without footwear. Pre-ulcerative signs (calloused, ingrown or thickened nails, fungal infections) should be managed by a professional. If an ulcer is present, arterial status should be ascertained and the patient referred to vascular surgery if there is PAD. Neuropathic ulcers (over a bony prominence, surrounded by callous) should be managed by offloading (total contact casts, offloading boots), debridement, and local wound care until healed, with consideration of new footwear and orthosis to prevent recurrence. Some patients may require long-term offloading with a Charcot Restraint Orthotic Walker (CROW boot).

Schaper NC, Van Netten JJ, Apelqvist J, et al. Prevention and management of foot problems in diabetes: a summary guidance for daily practice 2015, based on the IWGDF guidance documents. *Diabetes Metab Res Rev.* 2016;32(Suppl 1):7–15.

5. What are the phases of amputation rehabilitation and key goals for each phase?

Pre-operative phase: Consult with patient and surgical team to provide input on expected rehabilitation course including functional expectations, which may differ by the amputation levels being considered.

Immediate post-operative phase (patient on acute care service): Initiate residual limb post-operative management strategy, physical therapy and occupational therapy evaluations, determine setting for rehabilitation.

Pre-prosthetic or non-prosthetic phase: Rehabilitation goals should include modified independence with single-limb mobility and activities of daily living for *every* person with lower limb loss, as even prosthesis users will have times that they are unable to use a prosthesis. Rehabilitation team must consider if home and community environment match the patient's single-limb functional potential. Evidence supports subacute or acute inpatient rehabilitation.

Prosthetic training phase: Rehabilitation goals include gait training, community integration, and vocational and recreational activities.

Follow-up: Patients may require frequent follow-up over the first several years due to limb maturation. Lifelong care with an amputation rehabilitation team is recommended.

VA/DoD Clinical Practice Guideline for Rehabilitation of Individuals with Lower Limb Amputation, September 2017, 2008. Available at: https://www.healthquality.va.gov/guidelines/Rehab/amp/VADoDLLACPG092817.pdf

6. What is best practice for residual limb postoperative management?

The use of a rigid dressing such as a cast or off-the-shelf rigid removable dressing after transtibial amputation shortens time from amputation to fitting of the prosthesis. The goals of rigid dressing are surgical site protection, edema control, and limb shaping.

Churilov I, Churilov L, Murphy D. Do rigid dressings reduce the time from amputation to prosthetic fitting? A systematic review and meta-analysis. *Ann Vasc Surg.* 2014;28(7):1801–1808.

7. What factors predict that a person will be able to use a prosthesis?

Not every person with limb loss will be able to use a prosthesis. Risk factors for not using a prosthesis include transfemoral amputation, residual limb factors (pain, contractures, delayed healing), cognitive or neurological deficits, not ambulating prior to the amputation, and impaired cardiopulmonary status. Transfemoral prosthesis use is particularly challenging due to proximal socket discomfort, difficulty donning and doffing, contralateral limb bearing most of the weight during sit-to-stand transfers, and higher energy cost to ambulation. Many elderly transfemoral amputees use a wheelchair all or part of the time, and a handheld assistive device if they ambulate with a prosthesis.

Fortington LV, Rommers GM, Geertzen JH, et al. Mobility in elderly people with a lower limb amputation: a systematic review. *J Am Med Dir Assoc.* 2012;13(4):319–325.

8. How does standing differ between persons without amputation, persons with transtibial amputation, and persons with transfemoral amputation?

When persons without amputation transfer from sitting to standing, the dominant foot bears slightly more load than the non-dominant foot. In persons with transtibial amputation, the asymmetry is increased. In contrast, in persons with transfemoral amputation, the amputated leg with a prosthesis experiences less than 20% of the loading. Therefore, a transtibial prosthesis may be helpful for the functional goal of sit-to-stand transfers, while a transfemoral prosthesis is unlikely to aid with sit-to-stand transfers.

Burger H, Kuzelicki J, Marincek C. Transition from sitting to standing after trans-femoral amputation. *Prosthet Orthot Int.* 2005;29(2): 139–151.

9. How does energy expenditure differ between dysvascular and traumatic amputees during ambulation?

Comfortable walking speed is slower and the O_2 consumption higher for the dysvascular transtibial amputee than for the traumatic transtibial amputee and for dysvascular transfemoral amputee compared to traumatic transfemoral. Dysvascular transfemoral amputees have a higher metabolic energy expenditure rate than more distal amputees or traumatic amputees. If able to walk, elderly transfemoral amputees have a very slow walking speed and an elevated heart rate if crutch assistance is required.

Czerniecki JM, Morgenroth DC. Metabolic energy expenditure of ambulation in lower extremity amputees: what have we learned and what are the next steps? *Disabil Rehabil.* 2017;39(2):143–151.

10. What are treatments for phantom limb pain (PLP)?

There is evidence to support the use of gabapentin, which has possible side effects of somnolence, dizziness, headache, and nausea. Morphine has been shown to be effective in short-term pain intensity reduction but is avoided due to the risk of side effects such as constipation, sedation, and respiratory problems. Ketamine and dextromethorphan, both in the N-methyl D aspartate (NMDA) receptor antagonist family, have been shown to reduce PLP. The serotonin-norepinephrine reuptake inhibitor duloxetine and tricyclic antidepressants such as nortriptyline are considered second line. Pregabalin has been shown to be effective in reducing post-surgical pain including post-amputation pain. Non-pharmacologic management for PLP can include gentle massage of the residual limb, prosthesis use, gentle pressure on the residual limb using wraps, compressive socks, or prosthetic liners. Mirror therapy, transcutaneous electrical nerve stimulation (TENS), and psychological approaches to chronic pain such as mindfulness meditation or cognitive behavior therapy can be used, if the PLP is neuroma-mediated, interventions such as steroid injection, radiofrequency ablation, or surgical resection can be considered. Lumbosacral radiculopathy, which can mimic PLP, should be considered in the differential diagnosis depending on clinical context.

Alviar MJ, Hale T, Dungca M. Pharmacologic interventions for treating phantom limb pain. *Cochrane Database Syst Rev.* 2016;10(10):CD006380.

van Seventer R, Bach FW, Toth CC, et al. Pregabalin in the treatment of post-traumatic peripheral neuropathic pain: a randomized double-blind trial. *Eur J Neurol.* 2010;17(8):1082-9.

11. What are potential skin and soft tissue problems for amputees?

Table 38.2 Residual Limb Skin and Soft Tissue Problems, Causes, and Treatment

PROBLEM	CAUSE	TREATMENT
Hyperhidrosis (excessive perspiration)	Lack of evaporation	Antiperspirants, wicking "liner liner" socks, botulinum toxin, heat-dissipating liners
Tinea dermatitis	Secondary to increased moisture	Moisture management; antifungal shampoo or topical medication
Nonspecific dermatitis	Moisture, irritation from liner	"Liner liner" socks
Folliculitis, cysts, furuncles	Hair follicle and sweat gland occlusion, with staphylococcal infection	Clean limb and prosthetic liner often; surgical cleanser for refractive cases. Reduce pressure and friction. Recurrent or severe cases may require incision and drainage, systemic antibiotics.
Open ulcer	Pressure, shear	Discontinue prosthesis use Local wound care Barrier cream to reduce shear force Address underlying contributor (socket fit, alignment)
Neuroma-mediated pain	Neuroma (in itself, a naturally-occurring phenomena)	Desensitize by tapping, local injection, surgical excision, targeted muscle reinnervation
Choke syndrome (distal negative pressure changes including edema or verrucous hyperplasia, with cracking and weeping of skin)	Repeated distal negative pressure, as can occur with pistoning or distal limb not being in total contact with socket	Restore total contact with new socket (if socket is too tight) and/or suspension optimization

Skin and soft tissue problems (Table 38.2) can negatively impact a person's ability to use a prosthesis, perform household tasks, engage in social functions, and participate in sports.

Meulenbelt HE, Dijkstra PU, Jonkman MF, et al. Skin problems in lower limb amputees: a systematic review. *Disabil Rehabil.* 2006;28(10):603–608.

12. What are the key components for a prosthesis prescription?

Medicare requires that physicians prescribe prostheses and include information on diagnosis, anticipated functional potential with optimum prosthesis prescription and rehabilitation ("K level," see Table 38.3), comprehensive history and medical examination, and medical justification and plan for prosthetic requirements based on medical assessment.

Socket: The socket fits around the residual limb and helps to transmit forces from the body through the prosthetic limb. Sometimes, the socket can also provide suspension.

Table 38.3 K-Levels and Medicare Coverage of Prosthetic Components

K-LEVEL	FUNCTIONAL ABILITY OR POTENTIAL	FOOT/ANKLE COMPONENTS	KNEE COMPONENTS
K0	Does not have ability or potential to ambulate or transfer	Not eligible for prosthesis	Not eligible for prosthesis
K1	Household ambulatory (level surfaces, fixed cadence)	Solid-ankle cushion heel foot or single-axis foot	Constant friction knee Single or polycentric axis Weight activated stance control Manual lock
K2	Limited community ambulator	Flexible keel foot, multi-axial foot	Same as K1
K3	Community ambulator with ability to traverse most environmental barriers.	Energy storing feet, multi-axial ankle/feet, or dynamic response feet Energy storing foot, dynamic response foot with multi-axial ankle, microprocessor-controlled ankle foot system, shank foot system	Fluid and pneumatic control knees, including microprocessor
K4	Child, active adult, or athlete	Same as K3.	Same as K3. High activity knee control frame.

Suspension: Suspension is the means by which the prosthesis is suspended on the prosthesis user. It is sometimes integrated with the interface.

Interface: An interface is a material between the socket and the skin. There can be multiple interfaces.

Structural style: exoskeleton or *endoskeleton.* An exoskeletal prosthesis has an inner socket and an outer shell, which attaches directly to distal componentry. An exoskeletal prosthesis is sometimes called "double-walled." Exoskeletal prostheses are strong, but difficult to adjust. An endoskeletal prosthesis uses pylons to provide structure between the socket and prosthetic foot or other components.

Knee. A transfemoral or knee disarticulation prosthesis usually has a prosthetic knee.

Foot. A prosthetic foot and ankle mimic to some extent human foot and ankle function.

The brim of a socket is the upper edge of the socket. Sometimes, offset plates are used to offset the position of one component relative to another. A cosmetic cover mimics the shape of the amputated limb (e.g., the calf of the leg), and does not provide structural support.

Medicare. *Medicare Letter to Physicians.* 2013. Available at: https://www.cgsmedicare.com/jb/mr/pdf/dear_physician_artificial_limbs.pdf

13. What are key transtibial socket designs?

The patellar-tendon bearing (PTB) socket is a transtibial socket design in which *pressure tolerant* areas (the patellar tendon, flat surfaces of bones, and muscle compartments) are loaded, and *pressure sensitive* or *pressure intolerant* areas (the hamstring tendons, nerves, and bony prominences) are offloaded. The total surface bearing (TSB) socket is a transtibial socket design that aims to equally load the total surface of the residual limb. In modern practice, many sockets are likely a hybrid of these two designs. Suprapatellar/supracondylar sockets extend higher and around the femoral condyles and the patella, and can be used to help control residual limb motion in the case of knee instability, knee hyperextension, and/or short residual limbs.

Krajbich JI, Pinzur MS, Potter BK, eds. *Atlas of Amputations and Limb Deficiencies.* 4th ed. Rosemont, IL: American Academy of Orthopaedic Surgeons; 2016.

14. What are the differences between an ischial containment transfemoral socket and a quadrilateral socket?

The *quadrilateral* socket ("quad socket"), the predominant post-WWII socket type, was wider in the mediolateral dimension than the anteroposterior dimension, and contained an "ischial seat" on the medial brim. Gait with the quad socket was characterized by a lurch, or a trunk lean over the prosthetic side in stance. The ischial containment socket is intended to improve gait by holding the femur in a normal anatomically adducted position in contrast to the typical abducted position of the femur in the quad socket. The ischial containment socket is narrower in the mediolateral dimension than the quad socket ("narrow ML"), and the brim comes medial to the ischium and lateral to the greater trochanter.

15. **What are different types of prosthetic suspension and interfaces?**

Suction suspension uses natural negative pressure to suspend a prosthesis, and is usually achieved using a one-way air valve and a closed air system. This closed system can be achieved by a sleeve ("suction with sealing sleeve"), gaskets around a gel or silicone liner ("seal-in suction"), or a seal made from having the residual limb skin directly against the socket interior or an inner flexible liner to the socket ("skin-fit suction"). Suction with a sealing sleeve, commonly prescribed for transtibial amputees, allows the use of a prosthetic liner (silicone, gel, or urethane) to be used as a cushion, and for prosthetic socks to be used to adjust for residual limb volume changes.

Elevated vacuum suspension is similar to suction suspension but achieves negative pressure using a manual or electronic pump.

In **pin-lock** and **lanyard suspension,** a locking pin or a lanyard (strap) is attached to a prosthetic liner, which stays on the limb by friction. Both pin-lock and lanyard suspension allow the use of prosthetic socks for volume adjustment.

Anatomic suspension denotes use of the socket shape to suspend the prosthesis. In any joint disarticulation amputation, a socket that "comes in" superior or proximal to the bulbous or protruding bony portion of a limb will hold the socket in place. Fitting the socket over the bony prominence may be achieved with doors, windows, or removable brims or with a closed cell foam socket insert that fits over the bony prominence.

Auxiliary suspension is any suspension method used as a supplement to the primary means of suspension. For example, in transfemoral patients with short residual limbs, a total elastic suspension belt (TES belt) could be used to ensure that the prosthesis does not fall off the patient should the primary suspension fail.

A **thigh corset** attaches to a transtibial socket by metal side joints, which bypasses about 50% of the force that would be transmitted through the knee and socket-limb interface. Clinical indications include severe knee degenerative joint disease, chronic residual limb skin or other complications, and knee instability.

16. **What are the characteristics of prosthetic knees?**

Axis. A **single-axis** knee has a single center of rotation, akin to a door hinge. A **polycentric axis** knee's complex hinge joint creates an instantaneously variable center of rotation, which is high and posterior relative to the knee in 0 to 10 degrees of knee flexion. This creates a relative knee extension moment in early stance, which promotes stance stability. Polycentric knees also shorten in flexion, aiding toe clearance in swing phase and improving cosmesis in sitting.

Swing control. Swing control is a mechanism that controls movement of the pylon and foot during swing phase to aid clearing of the toe and completion of swing phase in sufficient knee extension to safely enter stance phase. In **constant friction** swing control, typically used in single axis knees, a band or clamp around the single axle creates a constant amount of friction that controls the foot and pylon's swing. This does not allow a response to cadence changes. **Pneumatic** swing control uses a closed cylinder filled with air to provide resistance to knee extension in swing phase. **Hydraulic** swing control uses a closed cylinder filled with fluid for knee extension resistance. Pneumatic and hydraulic resistance (together called "fluid controlled") allow variable extension speed within a given swing cycle and in response to changes in cadence.

Stance control. Stance control is any mechanism that prevents the knee from buckling during stance phase and thus provides stability in prosthetic stance phase. Types of stance control mechanism include: (A) a polycentric axis, (B) a manual locking knee, in which a spring mechanism locks the knee into full extension and is unlocked by pulling on a cord, (C) weight-activated stance, in which an axial load while the knee is in extension triggers a friction brake, (D) hydraulic stance control, in which a hydraulic (oil-filled) cylinder creates resistance to knee flexion. A locked knee remains extended during swing phase, which causes gait deviations (circumduction, hiphiking, or vaulting). Polycentric axis, weight-activated stance control, and hydraulic stance control allow for the knee to break into flexion for swing phase. Hydraulic stance control is the only mechanism that allows yielding which is loading of the knee while it is progressively flexing. Most knees with weight-activated stance control are single axis with constant friction swing control. A lock mechanism can be used as the sole stance control mechanism or in conjunction with a more advanced stance control mechanism, which allows for the lock to be used for early gait training, then disengaged as the patient "graduates" to another stance control mechanism. Hydraulic stance control is often paired with hydraulic swing control, and there are single axis and polycentric axis knees with hydraulic stance and swing control.

NOTE: Pneumatic resistance is used for swing control but not stance control, whereas hydraulic can be used for swing and/or stance control.

17. **What are microprocessor knees?**

Microprocessor knees have an on-board computer that collects real-time information from sensors to guess the *environment* of the patient ("is the person in stance phase?"), then instantaneously modifies the characteristics of the knee to match the environment. For example, the knee's sensors and computer might detect a stumble, then quickly increase the knee's resistance to flexion slowing the patient's descent and allowing for increased time to prevent a fall. Most microprocessor knees are hydraulic swing and stance control knees. Microprocessor knees are associated with greater self-reported well-being and quality of life compared to non-microprocessor knees. While the total cost of a given prosthesis with a microprocessor hydraulic knee is greater than the cost of a non-microprocessor knee, the overall total costs of prosthetic rehabilitation are similar. Microprocessor knees have been shown to reduce the incidence of falls in elderly transfemoral amputees and may improve negotiation of environmental obstacles.

Powered knees have motorized knee extension and flexion.

Sawers AB, Hafner BJ. Outcomes associated with the use of microprocessor-controlled prosthetic knees among individuals with unilateral transfemoral limb loss: a systematic review. *J Rehabil Res Dev*. 2013;50(3):273–314.

18. What are the classes of prosthetic feet and ankles?

Solid-Ankle Cushion Heel (SACH) foot: The SACH foot has a cushion heel to slow the progression of the center of pressure from the heel to the midfoot in early stance phase. Indications are: low-level ambulator, or patient who needs a lightweight, durable, and inexpensive foot.

Single-axis foot: A single axis foot has an articulated joint that allows movement in the sagittal plane (i.e., allows dorsiflexion and plantarflexion). The single axis foot has faster foot flat than other types of prosthetic feet, which moves the center of pressure anterior earlier in stance phase and creates a relative knee extension moment in early stance. Indications are a patient prone to instability from the knee buckling in stance phase, for example, a low-mobility transfemoral amputee.

Multi-axis foot: Has an articulated joint that allows movement in multiple directions, such as sagittal, coronal, and transverse plane. This foot type can be used to accommodate uneven terrain, but some patients may prefer a foot with less movement.

Flexible keel: Has a flexible keel (the portion of the foot parallel to the ground), which allows roll-over.

Energy storing/return, also called **dynamic response**: "spring"-like foot that stores energy in early stance and returns energy in late stance to provide some "push-off." Most energy-storing feet are carbon fiber and shaped like the letter "L" or the letter "C." This foot type is appropriate for higher mobility users, especially those who may use the foot for activities including running. Some energy storing feet are designed to be stable for lower mobility users.

Hydraulic ankle. A hydraulic ankle (usually attached to a carbon fiber keel) allows dorsiflexion and plantarflexion with hydraulic resistance for control. A hydraulic ankle can be thought of as a sophisticated version of a single-axis foot by allowing relatively early foot flat with the accompanying early stance stability. Hydraulic ankles allow a heel-toe gait pattern on slopes and can reduce risk of falls by maintaining the ankle dorsiflexion from late stance throughout swing phase.

Microprocessor hydraulic ankles use a microprocessor to modify hydraulic resistance in real time.

Powered ankles provide motorized dorsiflexion or motorized dorsiflexion and plantarflexion. The push-off force generated by a motorized plantarflexion ankle is greater than the push-off achieved by other prosthetic feet and ankles.

CHAPTER 39

WHEELCHAIR PROVISION: A PERSON-CENTERED INTERDISCIPLINARY PROCESS

R. Lee Kirby, MD, Cher Smith, OT, MSc, Rory A. Cooper, PhD, and Michael L. Boninger, MD

As newly abled (people) reconstructing their sense of self… the wheelchair becomes a vehicle of freedom of mobility and independence…

Christina Papadimitriou. Becoming en-wheeled: the situated accomplishment of re-embodiment as a wheelchair user after spinal cord injury. Disability & Society 2008;23(7):691-704.

KEY POINTS

1. The wheelchair is arguably the most important therapeutic tool in rehabilitation with benefits for the user's health, activity, and participation.
2. However, wheelchairs can cause problems due to improper fit, maintenance and repair issues, over-use injuries, and acute injuries.
3. To optimize the benefits of wheelchair use and minimize the problems, the World Health Organization (WHO) has advocated an 8-step service-delivery process for which there is a growing body of supporting research evidence.
4. Obtaining an appropriate wheelchair and learning how to properly use and care for it through the WHO process has the potential to optimize activity and participation, to improve safety, and to prevent overuse injury.

1. What is a wheelchair?

At its simplest, a wheelchair is a chair on wheels. The wheels allow the user to get from one place to another to carry out everyday activities. The "chair" component provides postural support in the sitting position and a platform for other assistive technology (e.g., communication aids).

2. How prevalent is wheelchair use?

The World Health Organization (WHO) has estimated that about 1% of the global population would benefit from the use of appropriate wheelchairs, although many such persons in less-resourced settings do not have access to them.

World Health Organization. *Guidelines on the Provision of Manual Wheelchairs in Less Resourced Settings.* 2008. Available at: http://www.who.int/disabilities/publications/technology/wheelchairguidelines/en/

3. How common are the different types of wheelchairs and how are they propelled?

In more-resourced areas (like most of North America), about 70% of wheelchairs are manual and may be self-propelled or pushed by caregivers. The remainder are about equally divided between battery-powered wheelchairs and scooters. In less-resourced settings, almost all wheelchairs are manual and many of them are arm-crank-propelled tricycles.

4. Discuss the importance of wheelchairs to rehabilitation.

The most substantial functional benefits due to rehabilitation are not due to the reversal of impairments, but to substitution of new ways of meeting functional needs, especially through the provision of assistive technology. Although the types of assistive technology are myriad, for people with serious mobility limitations, the wheelchair provides the most dramatic improvement in function. In terms of the WHO's International Classification of Function (ICF), wheelchairs can have a positive impact on health (e.g., through the prevention of falls while walking), activity (e.g., through improved mobility), and participation (e.g., through return to work).

WHO International Classification of Function. Available at: http://www.who.int/classifications/icf/en/.

5. What problems can users experience due to wheelchair use?
   Wheelchairs can cause problems due to improper fit, maintenance and repair issues, and acute injuries (e.g., due to tipping over). Also, long-term use of wheelchairs can adversely affect the health of users due to chronic or repetitive stresses—for instance, affecting shoulders, peripheral nerves, and skin.

Worobey L, Oyster M, Nemunaitis G, Cooper R, Boninger ML. Increases in wheelchair breakdowns, repairs, and adverse consequences for people with traumatic spinal cord injury. *Am J Phys Med Rehabil.* 2012;91:463–469.

Nelson AL, Groer S, Palacios P, Mitchell D, Sabharwal S, Kirby RL, Gavin-Dreschnack D, Powell-Cope G. Wheelchair-related falls in veterans with spinal cord injury residing in the community: a prospective cohort study. *Arch Phys Med Rehabil.* 2010;91:1166–1173.

Paralyzed Veterans of America Consortium for Spinal Cord Medicine. Preserving upper limb function in spinal cord injury: a clinical practice guideline for health-care professionals. *J Spinal Cord Med.* 2005;28:434–470.

6. What is the process that should be used by rehabilitation practitioners when providing a wheelchair for a person who needs one?
   To optimize the benefits of wheelchair use and minimize the problems, the WHO has advocated an 8-step service-delivery process for which there is a growing body of supporting research evidence. The WHO steps are: (1) **referral and appointment**, (2) **assessment**, (3) **prescription**, (4) **funding and ordering**, (5) **product preparation**, (6) **fitting**, (7) **user training**, and (8) **follow-up, maintenance, and repairs**. This process should be a person-centered one that includes input from members of an interdisciplinary team (including, for instance, a physician, therapist, equipment provider, and social worker) with subspecialty expertise in the provision of wheeled mobility.

World Health Organization. Guidelines on the provision of manual wheelchairs in less resourced settings. 2008. Available at: http://www.who.int/disabilities/publications/technology/wheelchairguidelines/en/

7. What are the advantages of cross-braced versus rigid-frame manual wheelchairs?
   Cross-braced wheelchairs are generally less expensive and more likely to be used by people who use wheelchairs part-time. Such wheelchairs fold side-to-side. The flexibility of the cross-brace leads to a more comfortable ride and makes it more likely that all four wheels will remain in contact with uneven terrain. Such wheelchairs are also more likely to be fitted with footrests that can be moved out of the way for standing up (e.g., to transfer to another surface) or for foot propulsion. Rigid-frame wheelchairs (of which there are various types) are generally lighter and have a customized fit. They can be made smaller by folding the backrest forward onto the seat. They provide a responsive feel to wheelchair propulsion and turning because the applied forces are not dampened by the frame flexing. A rigid frame also allows more precise wheel alignment, which reduces the forces required for mobility.

8. What options are available for the rear wheels of manual wheelchairs?
   Rear wheels come in different diameters, but 60 cm is the most common. Solid tires work well on smooth indoor surfaces and are maintenance-free. Pneumatic tires are lightweight but need to have air added every few weeks. On uneven surfaces they absorb vibrations that make for a comfortable ride and spare axial loading that may harm the spine. Wider tires with treads are useful on soft surfaces. Hand-rims that differ in their shape and friction-enhancing coating can enhance grip. Spokes may be made of metal (that require more maintenance), plastic, or fiber composite and may be radial or overlapping (that provide a softer suspension) in orientation. Quick-release axles allow the rear wheels to be easily removed for transportation.

9. How does rear-axle position affect a manual wheelchair?
   Raising the rear axles lowers the seat height, tilts the wheelchair backwards, lowers rear stability, raises forward stability, and causes a cambered wheel to toe out. Lowering the rear axles has the opposite effects. Moving the axles back lengthens the wheelbase, raises rear stability (limiting the ability to "pop" the casters transiently or into a full wheelie to manage obstacles), interferes with the user's ability to grasp as much of the push-rim, reduces traction, raises rolling resistance, and raises downhill-turning tendency. Moving the rear-axles forward has the opposite effects. Changes in axle position may require compensatory adjustments (e.g., to wheel locks and/or caster-stem angle).

Kirby RL, Smith C, Seaman R, Macleod DA, Parker K. The manual wheelchair wheelie: a review of our current understanding of an important motor skill. *Disabil Rehabil Assist Technol.* 2006;1:119–127.

Cowan RE, Nash MS, Collinger JL, Koontz AM, Boninger ML. Impact of surface type, wheelchair weight, and axle position on wheelchair propulsion by novice older adults. *Arch Phys Med Rehabil.* 2009 Jul;90(7):1076–1083.

10. What is "camber" and how does camber angle affect the wheelchair?
    Camber, usually in the 0 to 3 degrees range except for sport wheelchairs, is present when the distance between the tops of the rear wheels is less than that at the bottoms. Camber provides a natural angle for the

arms to address the wheels during propulsion, protects the user's hands (e.g., from door frames), increases the ease of turning, and increases lateral stability. However, increasing the camber angle widens the wheelchair and induces many mechanical effects (e.g., toe out) for which compensations may need to be made.

Trudel G, Kirby RL, Bell AC. Mechanical effects of rear-wheel camber on wheelchairs. *Assist Technol.* 1995;7.2:79–86.

Trudel G, Kirby RL, Ackroyd-Stolarz SA, Kirkland S. Effects of rear-wheel camber on wheelchair stability. *Arch Phys Med Rehabil.* 1997;78:78–81.

11. What are casters? How do the options available for manual wheelchairs affect performance? About how much weight should be on the casters?

Casters are wheels that are free to swivel about a vertical axis. Solid, smaller diameter, and narrower casters tend to sink into soft surfaces and allow the wheelchair to tip forward more easily. Pneumatic casters provide a more comfortable ride. Larger casters and casters with greater "trail" (the extent of offset of the axle from the vertical swivel axis) may strike the feet as they swivel. Generally, 10% to 30% of the total weight should be on the casters (the lower end of the range for more active users).

Kirby RL, MacLean AD, Eastwood BJ. Influence of caster diameter on the static and dynamic forward stability of occupied wheelchairs. *Arch Phys Med Rehabil.* 1992;73:73–77.

12. Why do many wheelchair users remove the rear anti-tip devices of manual wheelchairs?

Most rear anti-tip devices interfere with maneuverability (e.g., by "grounding out" during incline transitions, or by preventing a wheelchair from being tipped back sufficiently to get the casters up a curb or get into the wheelie position). Caregivers pushing a wheelchair often remove them due to unpleasant contact with feet or shins.

Kirby RL, Thoren F, Ashton B, Ackroyd-Stolarz SA. Effect of the position of rear antitippers on safety and maneuverability. *Arch Phys Med Rehabil.* 1994;75:525–534.

Kirby RL, Corkum CG, Smith C, Rushton P, MacLeod DA, Webber A. Comparing performance of manual wheelchair skills using new and conventional rear anti-tip devices: randomized controlled trial. *Arch Phys Med Rehabil.* 2008;89:480–485.

13. What are the considerations in choosing a wheelchair cushion?

Virtually all personal wheelchairs should be fitted with removable cushions for pressure distribution, shock absorption, and/or positioning. The choice of cushion materials and shape depend on the user's impairments (e.g., of sensation, balance, range of motion, strength), financial resources, and pattern of use.

14. What is the appropriate seat width for a manual wheelchair?

The seat should be wide enough to accommodate the wheelchair user's widest sitting dimension without undue pressure on the lateral tissues or allowing them to rub against the rear wheels (a problem that can be prevented by "clothing guards"). A seat that is too wide can promote truncal instability (by the lack of positioning support), can create problems getting through narrow spaces (due to the increase in the wheelchair's overall width), and makes it more difficult for the wheelchair user to reach the hand-rims for propulsion.

15. What is the appropriate seat depth for a manual wheelchair?

If the user is sitting correctly in the wheelchair (i.e., with the buttocks as far back as possible, the lumbar spine contacting the back support and the feet on the footrests), then the front edge of the seat should be 2 to 3 cm behind the bent knees. This allows the knees to be flexed for transfers or foot propulsion. Other than that, the more of the thigh that is supported the better.

16. What is the appropriate seat-plane angle of a manual wheelchair?

The **seat-plane angle** (the angle of the seat plane relative to the horizontal) is typically 5 to 10 degrees up at the front end of the seat. The advantages of increasing the seat-plane angle are to reduce extensor spasticity, to reduce the tendency for the user to slide forward on the seat, to bring the pelvis firmly against the back support, and to reduce lumbar lordosis. However, an accentuated seat-plane angle can make transfers more difficult and increase the pressure on the ischial tuberosities.

17. What is the appropriate seat height for a wheelchair?

Typical seat height for manual wheelchairs, about 50 cm above the floor at the front edge (excluding the cushion), is a trade-off between the ability to reach a great enough contact angle on the hand-rims for effective propulsion and access to objects high in the environment (e.g., light switches, tables). A lower seat height (often called "hemi-height") is usually needed for foot propulsion. Seats that can be elevated by the user (an option available on some powered and manual wheelchairs) are useful for reaching high objects (e.g., in a store) and for communicating eye-to-eye with standing people. Stand-up options can be used for the same purpose. Seats that can be lowered may be useful for children playing at floor level.

Heinrichs N, Kirby RL, Smith C, Russell K, Theriault C, Doucette S. Effect of seat height on manual wheelchair foot propulsion, a repeated-measures crossover study: Part 1—wheeling forward on a smooth level surface. *Disabil Rehabil Assist Technol.* 2019; 14(4):391-409. Available at: https://doi.org/10.17483107.2018.1456566.

18. What is the appropriate height of the back support for a manual wheelchair?

For users who manually propel their wheelchairs with at least one upper extremity, the upper border of the back support should be at least a few cm lower than the inferior angle of the scapulae to minimize irritation from rubbing. For the user who does not propel his/her wheelchair independently or who uses a tilt-in-space or reclining wheelchair, higher back supports (sometimes with an added headrest) provide more support and more area for pressure distribution. Back supports that do not extend above the lumbar region are commonly used by active users because they permit greater freedom of upper body and trunk movement, but the bottom of the back support should at least make contact with the top third of the pelvis.

19. What is the appropriate back support angle?

The back support is commonly angled back about 8 degrees from vertical (i.e., ~95 degrees from the seat plane). Active users may prefer to increase the seat-plane angle and reduce the back-support-to-seat-plane angle. Such a **"squeezed" position** can assist the user in applying force to the wheels by preventing the trunk from being pushed backward with each arm thrust. For the user with weak trunk muscles, increasing the back-support-to-seat-plane angle ("recline") can decrease the likelihood of falling forward onto the lap, obviating the need for a chest strap in some cases. Recline reduces the pressure on the ischial tuberosities in proportion to the extent of recline. However, because the mechanical axis of a back support with variable recline is usually below and behind the anatomical axis of the user's hip joint, there are shear forces produced due to the relative movement of the chair and user's backs. The back support angle can also be "tilted" backward. Tilt is a change in the seat's orientation in space with no change in the thigh-to-trunk angle. Tilt obviates the shear problem of recliners and is less likely to trigger spasms. Tilt also reduces the pressure on the ischial tuberosities in proportion to the extent of the tilt.

20. What options are available for armrests?

Many active users do not use armrests. Most armrests are padded and can be moved out of the way (by removing them, swinging them to the side, or flipping them up) to access tables or transfer to the side. Longer armrests can assist during a sit-to-stand transfer. Some armrests can be varied in height. Arm position can be maintained with the help of straps and/or shaped troughs or trays.

21. What are the pros and cons of elevating footrests?

Elevating a footrest may be necessary if the wheelchair user is unable to flex a knee (e.g., due to a plaster cast) and can help to prevent pedal edema if combined with other positioning measures (e.g., recline). For users with high tone and or hamstring contractures, elevating footrests may cause the user's buttocks to creep forward and subject the user to the risk of coccygeal or sacral pressure injuries. Elevating the footrests also decreases forward stability of the wheelchair and increases the turning radius. Also, there can be relative movement (and shear) between the elevating footrest and the user if the axes of the footrest and knee joints are not co-linear. Some elevating footrests prevent or compensate for shear by using a gooseneck attachment (to raise the mechanical axis) or a telescoping mechanism that lengthens the footrest as it is elevated. Elevating footrests also add weight, a consideration in manual wheelchairs.

Kirby RL, Atkinson SM, MacKay EA. Static and dynamic forward stability of occupied wheelchairs: Influence of elevating footrests and forward stabilizers. *Arch Phys Med Rehabil.* 1989;70: 681–686.

22. What are the pros and cons of positioning the knees in flexion?

Although the usual "hanger angle" is about 70 degrees (0 degrees being full knee extension) for manual wheelchairs, some wheelchairs position the knees in more flexion (up to 90 degrees or more). This has several benefits: reduced wheelchair length, closer forward access to objects like tables, foot protection, ease of wheelchair transport, inhibition of spasticity, tighter turns, and easier turns. However, such footrests are less effective as forward anti-tip devices. The hyper-flexed position may occlude circulation, pressure injuries may occur under the points where pressure is applied to achieve the hyper-flexed position, and a smaller caster diameter and trail may be needed to avoid having the casters swivel into the footrests or heels when changing direction. A person using **hemiplegic-pattern propulsion** (one arm and one leg) may benefit from a hanger angle of 60 degrees for the non-propelling foot to keep it out of the way during propulsion.

MacPhee A, Kirby RL, Bell AC, MacLeod DA. The effect of knee-flexion angle on wheelchair turning. *Med Eng Phys.* 2001;23: 275–283.

23. What is the most appropriate footrest height for wheelchairs?

The lowest point on the footrests should be at least 5 cm above the floor to avoid being caught on obstacles and incline transitions. Also if the footrests are too low, the front edge of the seat may bear more weight than appropriate, with the potential for pressure injury under the distal thighs. If the footrests are too high, the thighs are lifted from the seat, increasing the pressure on the ischial tuberosities. Also, high footrests are less effective as forward anti-tip devices.

24. What is a "power assist" for manual wheelchairs?

For some users of manual wheelchairs who are experiencing difficulties propelling their wheelchairs for longer distances or when they encounter higher rolling resistance (e.g., on carpets, grass or inclines), an option is to use an add-on device that assists with propulsion. There are three types of devices currently in common use. One solution is to replace the rear wheels with ones that have hub-mounted motors activated by instrumented handrims (push-rim-activated, power-assisted wheelchairs or PAPAWs). The other is a mid-line motorized wheel between and behind the rear wheels that is usually attached to the camber tube of a rigid-frame wheelchair and is controlled by tapping a wrist bracelet that wirelessly sends messages to the motor's controller. The third is a front-end attachment that lifts the casters and is controlled with a set of bicycle-like handlebars. All such devices convert the wheelchair into a hybrid between a manual and powered wheelchair. The main disadvantages of such devices are that they are expensive and heavy, and their batteries need to be recharged.

Best KL, Kirby RL, Smith C, MacLeod DA. Comparison between performance with a push-rim-activated power-assisted wheelchair and a manual wheelchair on the Wheelchair Skills Test. *Disabil Rehabil.* 2006;28:213–220.

25. When should one consider using a powered rather than a manual wheelchair?

If the extent of the user's impairments preclude independent all-day use of a manual wheelchair, then a powered wheelchair should be considered for at least part of the day. In addition to the powered wheelchair's capacity to allow a user to get around in his/her environment, many powered wheelchairs have options for positioning (e.g., tilt, recline, seat elevation, standing, footrest elevation), environmental control, and augmented communication. The main disadvantages of powered wheelchairs are that they are expensive, heavy, difficult to transport, and their batteries need to be recharged.

26. What are the types of powered wheelchair controls?

Analogue devices (e.g., joysticks) allow the user to generate a continuous control command of the wheelchair's speed and direction; the greater the deflection of the joystick, the greater the change. Switched devices (e.g., controlled by sipping or puffing on a straw or a change in head position) provide discrete on-off commands to the wheelchair, typically forward, backward, left, and right.

27. How does the performance of rear-, front-, and mid-wheel-drive powered wheelchairs differ?

Rear-wheel-drive powered wheelchairs (with front casters) provide good directional stability (i.e., less tendency to wander to the left or right), enhanced rider comfort, and control over uneven terrain but are subject to downhill-turning tendency on side slopes. **Front-wheel-drive wheelchairs** (with rear casters) provide better leg clearance for users with hamstring contractures and closer access to objects (e.g., tables) at the expense of directional stability and uphill-turning tendency unless compensating software is used. **Mid-wheel-drive wheelchairs** (with both front and rear casters) minimize the turning radius and ease maneuvering in tight spaces but may have difficulties with directional control. Also, because the drive wheels are positioned right under the seat, such wheelchairs can cause a "bumpier" ride over rough ground. Individualized programming of the controls is key to successful use of all power wheelchairs.

28. How do powered wheelchairs and motorized mobility scooters differ?

Motorized mobility scooters are similar to powered wheelchairs in many ways. However, they are steered differently (using a tiller instead of a joystick), and they do not have as many options for positional control or truncal support. They are typically used by people with good upper-limb function and who are able to stand and walk short distances independently.

29. How important is wheelchair-skills assessment and training?

Wheelchair skills assessment (for instance, using the **Wheelchair Skills Test**) should be used as part of the initial provision process and later during follow-up to confirm the appropriateness of the prescription and to guide training. Wheelchair-skills training is one of the most important steps in the WHO wheelchair-provision process. For instance, manual wheelchair users using two-handed propulsion should be taught proper propulsion technique—wheelchair users should use a long smooth stroke that utilizes as much of the push-rim as possible, letting the hands swing back below the rim during the recovery phase. Manual wheelchair users using hemiplegic-propulsion pattern (one arm and one leg) should proceed in the backward direction whenever high rolling resistance is encountered (e.g., when ascending inclines). Wheelchair users and caregivers should be taught to negotiate curbs (Fig. 39.1), ramps, small obstacles, and maneuvering in compact spaces. Powered wheelchair users need to be

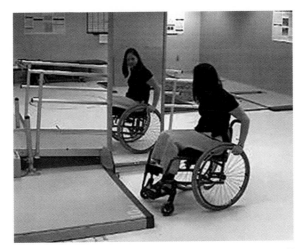

Fig. 39.1. Using a mirror to provide feedback while practicing popping the casters onto a 10 cm curb.

taught how to best use the **user-adjustable controls** to overcome environmental challenges. There is now clear research evidence that a formal approach to such training is more efficacious than an ad-hoc approach.

Keeler L, Kirby RL, Parker K et al. Effectiveness of the Wheelchair Skills Training Program: a systematic review and meta-analysis. *Disabil Rehabil Assist Technol.* 2019;14:391–409.

30. **Is there any relationship between how well a wheelchair user can perform wheelchair skills and broader positive outcomes?**
There is growing evidence of an association between wheelchair skills capacity and participation (as defined in the WHO's ICF) as well as for an association between capacity and such economically important benefits as return to work, maintenance of independent living, and avoidance of institutional care.

31. **Are there readily available and free resources to support health-care personnel interested in the training of wheelchair users, caregivers, and practitioners?**
The **Wheelchair Skills Program** and the **Wheelchair Maintenance Training Program** are sets of free online protocols to assist practitioners in their assessment and training of wheelchair users and caregivers. Specialized training for rehabilitation practitioners can be accessed through the Rehabilitation Engineering and Assistive Technology Society of North America (RESNA) and the International Society for Wheelchair Professionals (ISWP).

BIBLIOGRAPHY

Books
Batavia M. *The Wheelchair Evaluation: A Clinician's Guide.* 2nd ed. Sulbury, MA: Jones and Barlett Publishers; 2010.
Cooper RA. *Wheelchair Selection and Configuration.* New York: Demos Medical Publishing, 1998:410 pgs.
Kirby RL. *Wheelchair Skills Assessment and Training.* Florida: CRC Press, Taylor and Francis, 2016. Hard cover ISBN #9781498738811.

Websites
International Society for Wheelchair Professionals (ISWP). Available at: https://www.wheelchairnet.org/.
Rehabilitation Engineering and Assistive Technology Society of North America (RESNA). Available at: https://www.resna.org/
Waugh K, Crane B, Taylor SJ et al. *A Clinical Application Guide to Standardized Wheelchair Seating Measures of the Body and Seating Support Surfaces.* Revised Edition. Paralyzed Veterans of America and Assistive Technology Partners, University of Colorado, Anschutz Campus, August 2013. Available at: https://www.ncart.us/uploads/userfiles/files/GuidetoSeatingMeasuresRevisedEdition.November2013.pdf/.
Waugh K. Glossary of Wheelchair Terms and Definitions. Version 1.0. Paralyzed Veterans of America and Assistive Technology Partners, University of Colorado, Anschutz Campus, December 2013. Available at: https://www.ncart.us/uploads/userfiles/files/glossary-of-wheelchair-terms.pdf/.
Wheelchair Maintenance Training Program. Available at: http://www.upmc-sci.pitt.edu/node/924/.
Wheelchair Skills Program Manual. Available at: https://wheelchairskillsprogram.ca/en/.

Articles
Akbar M, Balean G, Brunner M, Seyler TM, Bruckner T, Munzinger J, Grieser T, Gerner HJ, Loew M. Prevalence of rotator cuff tear in paraplegic patients compared with controls. *J Bone Joint Surg Am.* 2010;92:23–30.

Auger C, Demers L, Gelinas I, Jutai J, Fuhrer MJ, DeRuyter F. Powered mobility for middle-aged and older adults: systematic review of outcomes and appraisal of published evidence. *Am J Phys Med Rehabil.* 2008;87:666–680.

Charbonneau R, Kirby RL, Thompson K. Manual wheelchair propulsion by people with hemiplegia: within-participant comparisons of forwards vs. backwards techniques. *Arch Phys Med Rehabil.* 2013;94:1707–1713.

Cowan RE, Nash MS, Collinger JL, Koontz AM, Boninger ML. Impact of surface type, wheelchair weight, and axle position on wheelchair propulsion by novice older adults. *Arch Phys Med Rehabil.* 2009 Jul;90(7):1076–1083.

Giesbrecht EM, Mortenson WB, Miller WC. Prevalence and facility level correlates of need for wheelchair seating assessment among long-term care residents. *Gerontology.* 2012;58:378–384.

Kilkens OJE, Post MWM, Dallmeijer AJ, van Asbeck FWA, van der Woude LHV. Relationship between manual wheelchair skill performance and participation of persons with spinal cord injuries 1 year after discharge from inpatient rehabilitation. *J Rehab Res Dev.* 2005;42:65–74.

Kirby RL, Rushton PW, Routhier F, Demers L, Titus L, Miller-Polgar J, Smith C, McAllister M, Theriault C, Matheson K, Parker K, Sawatzky B, Labbé D, Miller WC. The extent to which caregivers enhance the wheelchair skills capacity and confidence of power wheelchair users: a cross-sectional study. *Arch Phys Med Rehabil.* 2018;99:1295–302.

Kirby RL, Smith C, Seaman R, Macleod DA, Parker K. The manual wheelchair wheelie: a review of our current understanding of an important motor skill. *Disabil Rehabilit. Assist Technol. 2006*;1:119–127.

Lin YS, Boninger M, Worobey L, Farrokhi S, Koontz A. Effects of repetitive shoulder activity on the subacromial space in manual wheelchair users. *Biomed Res Int.* 2014;2014:583951.

Nelson AL, Groer S, Palacios P, Mitchell D, Sabharwal S, Kirby RL, Gavin-Dreschnack D, Powell-Cope G. Wheelchair-related falls in veterans with spinal cord injury residing in the community: a prospective cohort study. *Arch Phys Med Rehabil.* 2010;91:1166–1173.

Paralyzed Veterans of America Consortium for Spinal Cord Medicine. Preserving upper limb function in spinal cord injury: a clinical practice guideline for health-care professionals. *J Spinal Cord Med.* 2005;28:434–470.

Worobey L, Oyster M, Nemunaitis G, Cooper R, Boninger ML. Increases in wheelchair breakdowns, repairs, and adverse consequences for people with traumatic spinal cord injury. *Am J Phys Med Rehabil.* 2012;91:463–469.

Xiang H, Chany A-M, Smith GA. Wheelchair related injuries treated in US emergency departments. Injury Prevention 2006;12:8–11.

SOFT TISSUE AND MUSCULOSKELETAL INJURY: DIAGNOSIS AND REHABILITATION

Matthew Mitchkash, MD, Ryan J. Roza, MD, CAQSM, R-MSK, and Joanne Borg-Stein, MD

Injury taught me I need to learn how to face challenges.
—Shawn Johnson, former USA Gymnast (1992-Present)

KEY POINTS

Skin, subcutaneous tissue, fascia, muscle, tendon, myotendinous junctions, entheses, and ligaments are all important structures involved in soft tissue and musculoskeletal injury.

1. The initial evaluation of an injury should identify the nature and location of complaint, mechanism of injury, and associated disability. Life- and limb-threatening conditions should be ruled out first.
2. Most soft tissue injuries can be managed conservatively with supervised progression from initial immobilization and pain control to ultimate return to activity after range of motion (ROM), strength, proprioception, endurance, and overall function are restored.
3. Extra consideration has to be given to the management of adaptive patients for whom "relative rest" becomes more difficult, and surgical management may dramatically compromise function.
4. Targeted injury prevention programs are effective. Injury prevention can be seen as the final phase of recovery from soft tissue or musculoskeletal injury.

1. **What are the soft tissues involved in musculoskeletal injury?**
   Soft tissues to be considered in musculoskeletal injury include skin, subcutaneous tissue, fascia, skeletal muscle, tendons, myotendinous junctions, entheses, and ligaments.

2. **What are the most common causes of musculoskeletal injury?**
   Most musculoskeletal injuries are caused by trauma or overuse. In trauma, the injured structure is acutely overloaded, resulting in failure. Trauma may result in injuries such as fracture, dislocation, and ligamentous or tendon tearing. A previous injury that has incompletely or improperly healed may increase the risk for tissue failure. In contrast, overuse injuries are thought to be the result of cumulative microtrauma and resultant inflammation that can progress to a chronic phase of injury. Examples include tendinitis/tendinopathy and bone stress injury.

3. **What is the difference between a sprain and a strain?**
   A sprain is an injury to a ligament. A strain is an injury to a muscle, myotendinous junction, or tendon. Both types of injuries are often assigned "grades" to indicate the severity of injury (Table 40.1).

4. **How is tendonitis different from tendinopathy?**
   Tendonitis is an acute phase of tendon injury in which there is a pathologic inflammatory response, but the tendon internal structure is unchanged. Tendinopathy is a chronic phase of tendon injury marked by tenocyte and extracellular matrix degeneration and failure of normal tendon remodeling.

5. **What is bursitis?**
   Bursae are fluid-filled sacs with a synovial lining that facilitate gliding of tissue planes during motion. Bursitis is inflammatory pathology involving the bursa. Acute bursitis is typically the result of direct trauma, friction, or prolonged pressure. However, bursitis can be secondary to infection (septic bursitis) or associated with an underlying systemic disorder, such as gout, pseudogout, and rheumatoid arthritis.

6. **What is a muscular contusion?**
   A muscle contusion, or bruise, is characterized by muscle cell disruption, capillary rupture, and hematoma formation that is most often seen after blunt trauma to the extremities. Clinically, contusions present as pain, swelling, decreased ROM of joints spanned by the affected muscle(s), and occasionally as a palpable mass. Recovery is usually complete and takes around 2 to 3 weeks. Treatment is typically conservative and involves early mobilization. One important potential complication is myositis ossificans, which has been shown to be related to the initial grade of injury.

Table 40.1 Classification of Sprains and Strains

GRADE	SPRAIN	STRAIN
I	Partial tear of a few ligament fibers Mild swelling No laxity or joint instability	Partial tear of a few muscle/tendon fibers Mild disability Patient can produce strong muscle contraction
II	Partial tear of a moderate number of ligament fibers Ligament remains functional Moderate swelling Mild ligamentous laxity $+/-$ joint instability	Partial tear of a moderate number of muscle/tendon fibers Muscle-tendon unit remains intact Moderate disability Patient can weakly contract the muscle, limited by pain
III	Complete tear/rupture Severe swelling Definite ligamentous laxity Joint instability	Complete tear/rupture of the muscle-tendon unit Severe disability Extremely limited/absent voluntary contraction of muscle

7. **What are potential injuries and complications associated with abdominal blunt trauma?**
   Blunt abdominal trauma can injure both the abdominal wall and abdominal viscera through a direct blow, displaced rib fractures, or via the abrupt deceleration caused by the blow. Injuries to the abdominal wall include muscular contusions and rectus sheath hematomas. Rectus sheath hematomas are caused by rupture of the epigastric vein/artery and may require surgical ligation or excision. Renal injuries typically present with flank pain with or without hematuria and warrant urgent medical evaluation. Splenic and hepatic injuries may present with left or right upper quadrant (LUQ/RUQ) pain respectively, that can rapidly progress to shock in a higher-grade injury. Splenic and hepatic injuries can be life-threatening and warrant emergent transfer to the nearest hospital.

8. **What is myofascial pain, and what is a "trigger point"?**
   Myofascial pain syndrome (MPS) is a painful condition characterized by the presence of myofascial trigger points (MTrPs) in skeletal muscle. MTrPs are focal, taut bands of skeletal muscle that are hypersensitive to palpation with characteristic pain referral patterns. Pain is typically characterized as dull, deep, aching, and poorly localized. Additionally, MTrPs classically contract sharply in response to palpation or needling, referred to as the "twitch response." MTrPs may occur insidiously or after an injury. They are often associated with postural stress, muscle imbalance, and overuse.

9. **What is the rehabilitation approach to treating MPS and trigger points?**
   Successful treatment of MPS and MTrPs typically requires a multifaceted approach beginning with patient education. Providers should recognize the influence that psychosocial factors can have on pain sensitivity and emphasize the importance of restful sleep, stress reduction, and cardiovascular fitness. Providers should empower patients to self-manage their symptoms with manual techniques. Pharmacologically, there is evidence to support topical non-steroidal anti-inflammatory drugs (NSAIDs), lidocaine patches, and tizanidine. Proper stretching and progression to an exercise program should be incorporated into every treatment plan. Stretching helps lengthen shortened, taut bands of muscle, improves ROM, and decreases pain. Then, strengthening exercises can help establish new movement patterns, correct predisposing muscle imbalances, and improve muscle endurance. Finally, needling therapy can be considered for persistent MTrPs and/or when pain precludes participation in an effective exercise program.
   (MPS is further addressed in Chapter 70.)

10. **What is the process of evaluation after an acute soft tissue and musculoskeletal injury?**
    Evaluation of any injury begins with a thorough history and physical examination. The history should identify the specific nature and location of the complaint, mechanism of injury, severity of pain, and any associated neurological or functional deficits. The physical exam should survey for open injuries, gross deformities, soft tissue swelling, range of motion, and tenderness. Additionally, a thorough neurovascular examination should be performed to rule out emergent and potentially life- or limb-threatening conditions such as spinal cord injury, arterial injury, or compartment syndrome.
    Additionally, imaging is often used to further aid in the diagnosis and management of an injury. The modality used depends on the nature of the injury. Nerve conduction studies (NCS) and electromyography (EMG) can also assist in evaluating nerve injury.

11. **What are the roles of various imaging modalities in the evaluation of soft tissue and musculoskeletal injury?**
    X-ray: Often initially used in the setting of trauma to rule out bony injury. Radiographs can also provide limited soft tissue assessment and can demonstrate joint effusions. They can be performed either non-weight-bearing or stressed/weight-bearing. They can be static or dynamic (fluoroscopy). Fluoroscopy is often used to guide contrast injections for CT or MR arthrography.

CT: Ideally used for detailed evaluation of bony structures and soft-tissue calcification where it provides excellent spatial resolution. 3D rendered formatting can be used for surgical planning and guidance. However, CT has relatively poor differentiation of soft tissue structures compared to ultrasound or MRI.

Ultrasound (US): US offers a fast, dynamic, real-time assessment of muscles, tendons, cartilage, ligaments, nerves, and other structures without the use of radiation. Evaluation of bone is limited. Hardware advances now allow visualization of muscular architecture at a greater resolution than MRI. Power Doppler assessment can also be performed and provide evidence of neovascularization. Furthermore, US can be used immediately after an injury when edema might otherwise obscure important structures on MRI. Modern US machines are often portable and can be accessible on the sidelines. Finally, US is widely used to guide interventional techniques.

MRI: Enables the visualization of soft tissues with excellent contrast, high spatial resolution, and in multiple planes. MRI is considered better suited for the assessment of deeper structures where the resolution of US becomes limited. MRI is also considered superior for the evaluation of cartilage. Detailed evaluation of internal joint structures can be obtained by combining MRI with gadolinium arthrography (MR Arthrography).

12. What variables affect prognosis after soft tissue and musculoskeletal injury?

Prognosis is affected by several biomedical factors, including age, gender, presence of other medical comorbidities, type of tissue injured, severity of the injury, appropriate diagnosis and treatment, and compliance with a complete rehabilitation program.

Additionally, psychosocial factors can influence recovery. These psychosocial factors include depression, fear-avoidance beliefs, and recovery expectations. Patients with depression and psychological distress tend to have worse outcomes after an injury. Fear-avoidance beliefs are the patients' belief that physical or work-related activities will make the injury worse. Patients with fear-avoidance beliefs also have worse outcomes following an injury. Interestingly, the degree of recovery expectations has been shown to be predictive of recovery. Patients who expect to have a good recovery tend to have better outcomes compared to those who have lower expectations of recovery.

13. What is the rehabilitation approach to treatment of general soft tissue and musculoskeletal injuries?

Most soft tissue injuries can be managed conservatively. The typical approach could be thought of as phases rather than concrete timelines. The timeline will vary greatly depending on the structure involved and the severity of the injury (Table 40.2).

14. Are targeted injury prevention programs effective?

Yes! The FIFA 11+ is a 20-minute alternative warm-up program that has been demonstrated to reduce general lower extremity injury in soccer and basketball players. The Nordic hamstring exercise has been demonstrated to reduce hamstring injuries in soccer players. ACL injury prevention programs have been shown to reduce the risk of ACL injury by 52% in female athletes and by 85% in male athletes.

15. Are there general principles in determining readiness to "Return to Play" after injury?

Return to Play/exercise programs are typically the final phase of recovery. These programs are often sport or exercise specific, designed to progressively restore motion, function, and confidence. In general, the criteria include being pain-free and having full functional ROM, adequate static/dynamic stability, and strength greater than 90% compared to the uninjured side.

16. Are there special considerations regarding the management of soft tissue and musculoskeletal injury in the adaptive athlete?

Growing evidence suggests that the rates of injury and anatomic locations of injury may differ in athletes with disability. Let's use wheelchair athletes as an example. Because manual wheelchair athletes use their arms not just for propulsion during sport, but also for general mobility and activities of daily living, they have an increased risk of upper extremity

Table 40.2 Phases of Rehabilitation	
PHASE	**DESCRIPTION**
Passive Rehabilitation	Activity restriction to prevent further injury Control pain and inflammation
Active Rehabilitation	Restore passive and active range of motion Progressive strengthening (isometric to concentric) Proprioceptive training
Functional Rehabilitation	Activity or sport-specific training Improve endurance
Prevention	Injury prevention programs

overuse injuries including rotator cuff injury, subacromial impingement, and focal entrapment neuropathies of the upper extremity, such as carpal tunnel syndrome and cubital tunnel syndrome.

In the adaptive athlete, successful non-operative management is even more critical as surgical intervention may result in a more dramatic impact on everyday function compared to an otherwise non-disabled person. For example, an otherwise independent paraplegic who undergoes rotator cuff arthroscopy and repair may suddenly be dependent on another caregiver for 4 to 6 months.

Successful non-operative intervention is usually multifaceted and begins with the prevention of injury. The wheelchair-athlete interface is often the first target of intervention. Wheelchair weight and rolling resistance should be kept to a minimum. Seating should maximize balance for the user and provide an efficient base for propulsion and control. Wheels should be brought closer to the body to allow the arms to maintain a more neutral position. Anatomically, maintaining muscle balance around the shoulder complex and normal body weight may also reduce the risk of injury.

If an injury does occur, the initial treatment is often conservative, such as with "PRICE" and various analgesics. One must remember that "relative rest" often becomes more difficult. However, it is plausible that the patient may limit non-essential transfers and other repetitive activities while they recover. Underlying biomechanical contributions to the injury should be addressed, and physical therapy is often helpful. If conservative treatments fail, orthobiologic interventions hold promise.

17. What are some of the regenerative therapies available for soft tissue and musculoskeletal injuries?

Prolotherapy is an injection of non-biologic material (usually dextrose) designed to create a local inflammatory response that includes the production of a variety of different growth factors.

Platelet-rich plasma (PRP) uses an autologous plasma derivative in which platelets are concentrated above baseline blood levels and injected into the affected area. There, platelets are thought to release growth factors from alpha granules, which have been theorized to augment the healing process.

Mesenchymal stem cells (MSCs) are derived from perivascular cells called pericytes and can be autologously harvested in abundance from either bone marrow or adipose tissue. Both bone marrow aspirate concentrate (BMAC) and adipose-derived stromal/stem cell (ADSC) are thought to have anti-inflammatory, immunomodulatory, and paracrine effects that promote and support a healing response.

18. Are alternative treatment options available for soft tissue and musculoskeletal injuries?

Percutaneous ultrasonic tenotomy (PUT) utilizes ultrasonic energy to produce low-amplitude, high-frequency longitudinal oscillations of a hollow tip needle to cut through tendon and emulsify tendinopathic tissue with the goal of simultaneously removing tendinopathic tissue while also stimulating a healing response.

Extracorporeal shockwave therapy (ESWT), first introduced into clinical practice in the 1980s for urinary stone lithotripsy, has also been used to treat a variety of musculoskeletal conditions, including fasciopathies, various recalcitrant tendinopathies, medial tibial stress syndrome, and in cases of non-union or delayed union long bone fractures. The exact mechanism of action for ESWT is not fully understood. Still, it is theorized to help stimulate tissue remodeling through the promotion of tenocyte proliferation, stimulation of osteoprogenitor differentiation, promotion of neovascularization at the tendon-bone junction, and stimulation of increased collagen synthesis.

BIBLIOGRAPHY

Adam J, De Luigi AJ. Blunt abdominal trauma in sports. *Curr Sports Med Rep.* 2018;17(10):317–319.

Barnes DE, Beckley JM, Smith J. Percutaneous ultrasonic tenotomy for chronic elbow tendinosis: a prospective study. *J Shoulder Elbow Surg.* 2015;24:67–73.

Beiner JM, Jokl P. Muscle contusion injuries: current treatment options. *J Am Acad Orthop Surg.* 2001;9:227–237.

Booth-Kewley S, Schmied EA, Highfill-McRoy RM, et al. A prospective study of factors affecting recovery from musculoskeletal injuries. *J Occup Rehabil.* 2014;24:287–296.

Borg-Stein J, Iaccarino MA. Myofascial pain syndrome treatments. *Phys Med Rehabil Clin N Am.* 2014;25:357–374.

Borg-Stein J, Osoria HL, Hayano T. Regenerative sports medicine: past, present, and future (adapted from the PASSOR Legacy Award Presentation; AAPMR; October 2016). *PM R: J Injury Func Rehabil.* 2018;10(10):1083–1105.

Cooper RA, De Luigi AJ. Adaptive sports technology and biomechanics: wheelchairs. *PM R: J Injury Func Rehabil.* 2014;6:S31-39.

Finnoff JT. Preventive exercise in sports. *PM R: J Injury Func Rehabil.* 2012;4(11):862–866.

Gerwin RD. Diagnosis of myofascial pain syndrome. *Phys Med Rehabil Clin N Am.* 2014;25:341–355.

Guermazi A, Roemer FW, Robinson P, et al. Imaging of muscle injuries in sports medicine: sports imaging series. Radiology. 2017;282(3):646–663.

Longo UG, Loppini M, Berton A, et al. The FIFA 11+ program is effective in preventing injuries in elite male basketball players: a cluster randomized controlled trial. *Am J Sports Med.* 2012;40(5):996–1005.

Malanga G, Abdelshahed D, Jayaram P. Orthobiologic interventions using ultrasound guidance. *Phys Med Rehabil Clin N Am.* 2016;27:717–731.

McCarty EC, Walsh WM, Hald RD, et al. Musculoskeletal injuries in sports. In: Madden C, Putukian M, McCarty EC, et al. *Netter's Sports Medicine.* 2nd ed. Philadelphia, PA: Elsevier; 2018:42:317-321.e1.

Moen MH, Rayer S, Schipper M, et al. Shockwave treatment for medial tibial stress syndrome in athletes; a prospective controlled study. *Br J Sports Med.* 2012;46:253–257.

Peck E, Jelsing E, Onishi K. Advanced ultrasound-guided interventions for tendinopathy. *Phys Med Rehabil Clin N Am*. 2016;27:733–748.
Peck E, Jelsing E, Onishi K. Advanced ultrasound-guided interventions for tendinopathy. *Phys Med Rehabil Clin N Am*. 2016;27:733–748.
Pope T, Bloem HL, Beltran J, et al. Musculoskeletal Imaging. 2nd ed. Philadelphia, PA: Elsevier Saunders; 2015.
Reilly D, Kamineni S. Olecranon bursitis. *J Shoulder Elbow Surg*. 2016;25:158–167.
Reilly JM, Bluman E, Tenforde AS. Effect of shockwave treatment for management of upper and lower extremity musculoskeletal conditions: a narrative review. *PM R: J Injury Func Rehabil*. 2018;10(12):1385–1403.
Silvers-Granelli H, Mandelbaum B, Adeniji O, et al. Efficacy of the FIFA 11 + injury prevention program in the collegiate male soccer player. *Am J Sports Med*. 2015;43(11):2628–37.
Slocum C, Blauwet CA, Anne Allen JB. Sports medicine considerations for the paralympic athlete. *Curr Phys Med Rehabil Rep*. 2015;3(1): 25–35.
van der Horst N, Smits D-W, Petersen J, et al. The preventive effect of the Nordic hamstring exercise on hamstring injuries in amateur soccer players: a randomized controlled trial. *Am J Sports Med*. 2015;43(6):1316–23.
Wang C-J. Extracorporeal shockwave therapy in musculoskeletal disorders. *J Orthop Surg Res*. 2012;7:11.
Wascher DC, Bulthuis L. Extremity trauma: field management of sports injuries. *Curr Rev Musculoskeletal Med*. 2014;7:387–393.
Wilk KE, Simpson CD, Williams RA. Comprehensive rehabilitation of the athlete. In: Madden C, eds., et al. *Netter's Sports Medicine*. 2nd ed. Philadelphia, PA: Elsevier; 2018:322-329.e1.

WEBSITES

FIFA Medical Network. FIFA 11 +. Available at:
https://www.fifamedicalnetwork.com/lessons/prevention-fifa-11/. Accessed July 8, 2020.
OrthoInfo. Sprains, Strains and Other Soft-Tissue Injuries. Available at:
https://www.orthoinfo.org/en/diseases—conditions/sprains-strains-and-other-soft-tissue-injuries/. Accessed July 8, 2020.

CHAPTER 41

MYOPATHY: DIAGNOSIS AND REHABILITATION

Michelle Stern, MD, Stanley J. Myers, MD, and Fabreena Napier, MD

Symptoms, then, are in reality nothing but a cry from suffering organs.
—Jean-Martin Charcot (1825–1893)

KEY POINTS

1. A myopathy is a disorder of muscle characterized by symmetric, predominantly proximal weakness. Myopathies can be either genetic or acquired.
2. Inflammatory myopathies are acquired disorders of skeletal muscle associated with inflammation on biopsy and may be immune-mediated, associated with collagen vascular disease, paraneoplastic, or associated with infection.
3. Muscular dystrophy is a large group of genetic muscle disorders that are slowly progressive, starting after the age of 2 and associated with abnormal muscle biopsies.
4. The protein defect found in Duchenne muscular dystrophy is absent dystrophin, and in Becker muscular dystrophy is reduced dystrophin.
5. By the age of 12, most Duchenne patients are wheelchair dependent.
6. Rehabilitation interventions play a crucial role in improving the quality of life for patients with myopathies. An exercise program for the myopathic patient should be submaximal in intensity, avoid overfatigue, and be carefully supervised.

1. What is myopathy?

A myopathy is a disorder of striated muscle affecting either the structure, channels, or metabolism of the muscle fiber. It is clinically characterized by symmetric, predominantly proximal weakness. Other symptoms, such as cramps, stiffness, and myalgias, may also be present. Elevated creatinine phosphokinase (CPK) accompanies most myopathic disorders. Myopathies can be acquired or hereditary. Acquired myopathies are acute to subacute in presentation and are generally related to immune-mediated dysfunction, toxins, or infection. Hereditary myopathies are typically chronic and progressive, and their major categories include muscular dystrophies, congenital myopathies, and disorders of metabolism. See Table 41.1 for specific categories of myopathy.

Barohn RJ, Dimachkie MM, Jackson CE. A pattern recognition approach to the patient with a suspected myopathy. *Neurol Clin.* 2014; 32(3):569–611.

Gelfus, C. Chapter 42 myopathy. In: Cifu DX, ed. *Braddom's Physical Medicine and Rehabilitation.* 5th ed. Philadelphia, PA; Elsevier; 2016.

Table 41.1 Major Categories of Myopathies

ACQUIRED	EXAMPLES
Inflammatory myopathies	Polymyositis, dermatomyositis, inclusion body myositis
Toxic myopathies	Statins, steroids
Endocrine myopathies	Hypothyroidism, hyperthyroidism
Infectious myopathies	HIV, trichinosis
Myopathies associated with systemic disease	Critical illness myopathy
HEREDITARY	
Muscular dystrophy	Duchenne, facioscapulohumeral, limb-girdle, myotonic
Congenital myopathies	Nemaline, centronuclear
Channelopathies	Hypokalemic periodic paralysis
Metabolic myopathies	McArdle, phosphofructokinase
Mitochondrial myopathies	Kearns–Sayre syndrome

2. Describe the examination of the myopathic patient.

Inspection of the myopathic patient may reveal atrophic or pseudohypertrophic muscle. Proximal limb weakness, usually sparing extraocular muscles, is the hallmark presentation of myopathy. Neck flexion, bulbar, and respiratory weakness may also be evident the latter two potentially affecting morbidity and mortality. Scoliosis, flaccid abdominal muscles, or exaggerated lumbar lordosis may be present with axial weakness. Camptocormia, a stooped posture while walking, can occur with severe axial muscle weakness. A Trendelenburg or waddling gait is common in severe lower extremity involvement and is a compensation for gluteus medius weakness. Scapular winging or dysmorphic faces may be present in genetic myopathies and can help narrow the differential. Contractures are common and progress more rapidly when a wheelchair is used. Uncovering subtle weakness with functional activities, such as heel and toe walking, hopping, jumping, squatting, and stair climbing may be necessary. The Gower maneuver is another functional test, that when positive, is indicative of severe proximal lower extremity weakness. When asked to arise from the floor, the patient first assumes a prone position, then proceeds to obtain the upright position by climbing up their legs with the use of the hands (see Recommended reading).

Muscular Dystrophy Gowers Maneuver—YouTube. Available at: https://www.youtube.com/watch?v=Ye8jYA08K60

3. What differential diagnoses may be considered in myopathy?

Myopathy is a pure motor syndrome that is symmetric and diffuse. Other neurological conditions affecting the peripheral nervous system, which may mimic myopathy, include disorders affecting the neuromuscular junction (i.e., myasthenia gravis, Lambert–Eaton myasthenic syndrome), disorders of the motor neuron (i.e., spinal muscular atrophy), or motor-predominant demyelinating polyneuropathy (i.e., chronic inflammatory demyelinating polyneuropathy).

4. List helpful ancillary testing in myopathy.

CPK is elevated in muscle disorders associated with necrosis. Aside from identifying a myopathic pattern of weakness, an elevated CK is the first clue that myopathy is present. Needle electromyography (EMG) is also useful in identifying muscle fiber injury in myopathy patients. A myopathic recruitment pattern on EMG comprises short-duration, low-amplitude motor units with an early and full recruitment. A variety of abnormal spontaneous discharges may be seen on needle EMG depending on the underlying cause. If an acquired myopathy is suspected, antibody testing is useful in identifying subtypes of inflammatory myopathy. If a genetic myopathy is suspected, genetic testing is commercially available and can identify many of the genes responsible for genetic muscle diseases. Muscle biopsy may be valuable in the evaluation of myopathy when antibody testing and genetic testing are inconclusive. Neuroimaging with MRI and ultrasound is useful in determining the pattern of muscle involvement, aiding in distinguishing between types of myopathy and in guiding muscle biopsy.

5. What are inflammatory myopathies?

Inflammatory myopathies are acquired disorders of skeletal muscle associated with inflammation on biopsy. Inflammatory myopathies may be immune-mediated, associated with collagen vascular disease, paraneoplastic, or associated with infection. Idiopathic inflammatory myopathies (IIMs) are a subgroup of disorders which are immune-mediated primarily affecting skeletal muscle but may also involve lung, heart, or skin. The four main subtypes of IIMs include dermatomyositis (DM), polymyositis (PM), immune-mediated necrotizing myopathy, and inclusion body myositis.

McGrath ER, Doughty CT, Amato AA. Autoimmune myopathies: updates on evaluation and treatment. *Neurotherapeutics*. 2018;15: 976–994.

6. Describe DM and PM.

DM and PM are associated with subacute progression of proximal muscle weakness with myalgias, elevated CK, and inflammatory infiltrate on muscle biopsy. In DM, a muscle biopsy displaying perifascicular atrophy is pathognomonic. Patients with DM or PM may be idiopathic, paraneoplastic, or as part of an overlap syndrome with a collagen vascular disease. Cardiac dysfunction and interstitial lung disease may be present. DM is commonly associated with skin changes, including heliotrope rash, Gottron's papules, mechanic hands, and shawl rash (see Fig. 41.1). Antibody testing may uncover myositis specific or myositis associated antibodies, which can help confirm a diagnosis with or without a muscle biopsy. Uncovering anti-synthetase antibodies in myositis is associated with a higher incidence of interstitial lung disease. Treatment for DM and PM is with immunosuppression. Rehabilitation goals are determined by the severity of weakness. Patients with severe weakness are relegated to rest and passive range of motion exercises, while those with mild weakness can participate in isometric and isotonic exercise, though cautiously to prevent over fatigue.

7. What are causes of toxic myopathy?

Common toxins to muscle include cholesterol-lowering medications (i.e., statins), corticosteroids, hydroxychloroquine, colchicine, D-penicillamine, anti-retroviral therapy, and illicit drugs (i.e., heroin, cocaine).

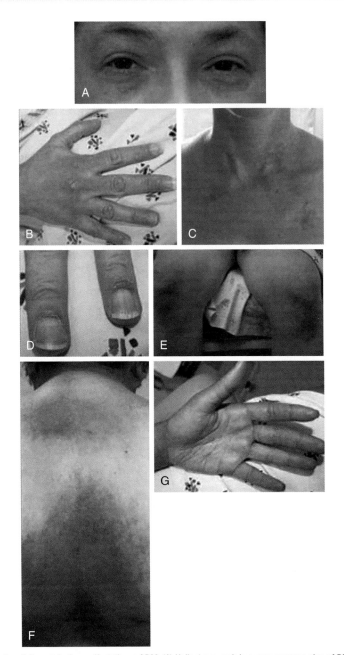

Fig. 41.1 Examples of dermatologic manifestations of DM. (A) Helioptrope rash is a very common sign of DM. It can become more confluent and involve the entire face. (B) Gottron papules, another characteristic manifestation, are symmetric macular violaceous erythema with or without edema overlying the dorsal aspect of the interphalangeal or metacarpophalangeal joints, olecranon process, patella, and medial malleoli. (C) Other characteristic manifestations include the V sign that can occur on the neck and upper chest. (D) Image showing cuticular erythema and hypertrophy. Other characteristic findings include nail fold telangiectasias, cuticular overgrowth, and prominent periungual erythema, which are frequently seen in patients with DM. (E) Gottron sign, also called Gottron papules, is observed in more than 80% of patients with DM. Gottron papules are violaceous flattopped papules and plaques located over the dorsal aspect of the interphalangeal or metacarpophalangeal joints. (F) Shawl sing, another characteristic manifestation, occurs on the nape of the neck, shoulders, and upper back. (G) Raynaud phenomenon occurs in approximately 25% of patients with DM.

8. **What is muscular dystrophy?**

Muscular dystrophy is a term that describes a large heterogeneous group of genetic muscle disorders that are slowly progressive, starting after the age of 2 (though usually in the first to second decades of life) and associated with abnormal muscle biopsies. There are several genetic disorders of specific muscle proteins, which can lead to various muscular dystrophies. Muscular dystrophies are of autosomal hereditary or sporadic. The proteins affected usually involve maintenance of the sarcolemma, function of the nucleus, or structure of the extracellular matrix resulting in diffuse weakness. Rehabilitation in patients with muscular dystrophy is centered around preventing contractures and providing a program that involves submaximal exercise to avoid overuse.

9. **What are some notable forms of muscular dystrophy?**

- Facioscapulohumeral dystrophy (FSHD) is characterized by facial and scapulohumeral patterns of weakness. Scapular winging is asymmetric. Weakness of the biceps, anterior tibial, and pelvic girdle muscles occur with progression. Mutations of chromosome 4q35 as well as epigenetic methylation impairment to this portion of DNA leads to FSHD.
- Limb-girdle muscular dystrophy is a group of genetic disorders of muscle which presents in the second to third decades with proximal weakness involving the shoulder and hip girdle. The progression of weakness is slow over the decades. The vast majority of LGMD are associated with elevated CK, and many are associated with cardiac involvement. Genetic testing is useful for the diagnosis of particular types. LGMD is generally categorized as type 1 and type 2, which are autosomal dominant and autosomal recessive, respectively. These two groups are then further subdivided into specific disease types based on protein abnormalities.
- Emery-Dreifuss Muscular Dystrophy: The clinical triad is gradually progressive proximal weakness, contractures, and cardiomyopathy with conduction defects. Contractures may develop before weakness, especially of the elbows, Achilles tendons, and spine. Pacemaker insertion is often done early to prevent sudden death. Inheritance may be X linked, autosomal dominant, or recessive.
- Dystrophinopathy (see question 10).
- Myotonic Dystrophy (see question 22 in the on-line text section).

10. **What is a dystrophinopathy?**

Dystrophin is a large cytoskeletal protein in the subsarcolemmal lattice that stabilizes the muscle membrane during muscle contractions. Loss of dystrophin leads to an unstable cell membrane and causes muscle fibers to degenerate. Dystrophinopathies are X-linked disorders of dystrophin, leading to progressive proximal muscle weakness associated with markedly elevated CK, cardiac dysfunction, and cognitive impairment. Males are the primary gender affected. However, female carriers may be mildly symptomatic and should be screened for cardiac dysfunction. The two subtypes of dystrophinopathies are Duchenne muscular dystrophy (DMD) and Becker muscular dystrophy (BMD). Dystrophin is absent in DMD and reduced in BMD, and thus DMD and BMD are both dystrophinopathies at different points on the spectrum. Due to the absence of dystrophin in DMD, the natural history of the disease is more severe. BMD has a later onset and a slower rate of progression. Death in both DMD and BMD is usually a result of respiratory and cardiac complications. Rehabilitation goals include nighttime splinting, a submaximal exercise plan, and devices to help the patient adapt in performing activities of daily living.

11. **Identify key features of Duchenne muscular dystrophy**

DMD presents in boys by age 2 to 5 with leg weakness but is progressive and gradually involves nearly all skeletal muscles, sparing extraocular muscles. Other associated features include cognitive impairment, pseudohypertrophy of calf muscles, cardiomyopathy with fibrosis, scoliosis, restrictive pulmonary disease, and orthopedic deformities. Scoliosis occurs between the ages of 13 and 15. Wheelchair ambulation occurs by age 12. Medical therapy with the use of oral corticosteroids by the age of 5 prolongs ambulation and reduces the need for scoliosis surgery. Steroids may also preserve respiratory and cardiac function. Noninvasive respiratory assistive devices are the preferred form of pulmonary support. Life expectancy is generally to the 20s to 30s. To date, there are four FDA approved anti-sense oligonucleotide therapies for DMD, involving exon skipping specifically for eligible Duchenne patients with confirmed mutations at exons 45, 51 and 53. The therapies produce partially functional dystrophin protein, potentially leading to slowed progression of disease.

Current Treatment of Adult Duchenne Muscular Dystrophy. Available at: https://www.sciencedirect.com/science/article/pii/S0925443906001232.

Wagner KR, Lechtzin N, Judge DP. Current treatment of adult Duchenne muscular dystrophy. *Biochim Biophys Acta*. 2007;1772:229–237.

12. **What are congenital myopathies?**

Congenital myopathies are genetic disorders that present before the age of 1. If present at birth, may exhibit the hypotonic (floppy) infant phenotype. The congenital myopathies are relatively nonprogressive muscle conditions diagnosed by genetic testing or muscle biopsy. Examples of congenital myopathies include congenital fiber-type disproportion, central core myopathy, nemaline myopathy, and centronuclear myopathy.

13. What are the benefits of rehabilitation in the myopathic patient?
    - Maximize functional mobility.
    - Maintain or improve strength and endurance.
    - Maximize independence for activities of daily living.
    - Minimize immobility and deconditioning.
    - Prevent and minimize joint contractures.

14. What should a rehabilitation program avoid and include?
    Aerobic exercise, strengthening, and stretching are beneficial in the myopathic patient. Moderate-intensity aerobic exercises may improve cardiovascular performance. However, exercise for strengthening must be submaximal, and overfatigue must be avoided. High-intensity eccentric muscle contracting may cause increased CPK and muscle soreness. Concentric contractions are preferred. Warning signs of overwork weakness include feeling weaker 30 minutes after exercise, excessive muscle soreness 24 to 48 hours after exercise, severe muscle cramping, and prolonged shortness of breath.

Abresch RT, Carter GT, Han JJ, et al. Exercise in neuromuscular diseases. *Phys Med Rehabil Clin N Am.* 2012;23(3):653–673.

15. Identify the benefits of orthoses for patients with muscle disease.
    Lower extremity night splints are often used to provide passive stretch in the lower extremities. In addition, orthoses can prove useful in supporting weak muscles and aiding in ambulation. They can also improve bony alignment and provide joint stability. However, caution must be used in prescribing lower extremity orthoses. Braces which are too heavy to be carried by weak limbs can affect ambulation. In addition, orthotics which change the joint alignment and biomechanics may rob the patient of compensatory gait mechanisms and actually arrest ambulation.

16. What is the role of orthopedic surgery for contractures?
    One must consider benefit versus risk when contemplating elective surgery for contracture release. Surgery may be successful in improving joint alignment and range of motion. However, risks of surgery include anesthesia complications (including ventilator dependence), deconditioning postoperatively, and the potential need to learn new compensations for biomechanical abnormalities. If a lower extremity contracture release procedure is performed in a neuromuscular patient, proper therapy with lower extremity bracing must be initiated quickly to prevent further disuse atrophy and contractures of the already weakened muscle.

17. How do gait aids and standers help the myopathic patient?
    Gait aids reduce lower limb loading and may assist balance but require sufficient upper extremity strength for use. Bilateral canes help stabilize the Trendelenburg gait. As the patient weakens further, advancement to bilateral forearm crutches or a platform walker may be required. Standers (such as parapodiums) allow patients with severe lower extremity weakness to be upright, providing support to bilateral lower extremities and trunk.

18. When are wheelchairs appropriate in the myopathic patient?
    When ambulation becomes unsafe or requires too much energy consumption, a wheelchair or scooter can be liberating. For wheelchairs, it is essential that the height of the seat be adjusted to permit both arm and leg propulsion. The advantages of a manual chair include lower cost, lighter weight, and ease in transport and maintenance. However, if upper extremity strength is not sufficient for propulsion, then a power-assist manual wheelchair, power wheelchair, or scooter may be alternative options, provided that the patient has adequate perceptual safety awareness.

Bakker JPJ, De Groot IJM, Beelen A, et al. Predictive factors of cessation of ambulation in patients with Duchenne muscular dystrophy. *Am J Phys Med Rehabil.* 2002;81:906–912.

Brooke MH. *A Clinician's View of Neuromuscular Diseases.* 2nd ed. Baltimore, MD: Williams & Wilkins; 1986.

WEBSITES

1. Muscular Dystrophy Association. Available at: www.mdausa.org
2. National Organization of Rare Diseases. Available at: www.rarediseases.org
3. Neuromuscular Disease Center. Available at: https://neuromuscular.wustl.edu

RECOMMENDED READINGS

Amato AA, Russell JA. *Neuromuscular Disorders.* New York, NY: McGraw Hill; 2008.
Narayanaswami P, Weiss M, Selcen D, et al. Evidence-based guideline summary: Diagnosis and treatment of limb-girdle muscular dystrophy and distal dystrophy. *Neurology.* 2014;83:1453–1463.
Marascoa E, Cioffi E, Cometi L, et al. One year in review 2018: idiopathic inflammatory myopathies. *Clin Exp Rheumatol.* 2018;36:937-947. Available at: https://www.clinexprheumatol.org/article.asp?a=13127.

Bonus questions and answers are available online.

CHAPTER 42

OSTEOPOROSIS: DIAGNOSIS, MEDICAL MANAGEMENT, AND REHABILITATION

Jad Georges Sfeir, MD, MS, Charles Edward Levy, MD, and Robert J. Pignolo, MD, PhD

The tragedy of osteoporosis is that it's largely avoidable.
 —Robert P. Heaney, MD, in Surgeon General's Report on Bone Health: Prevention is Key, 2004

KEY POINTS

1. Osteoporosis is a treatable, preventable, progressive disease that affects both men and women.
2. Development of a fragility fracture can be the first manifestation of osteoporosis.
3. Dual energy x-ray absorptiometry (DXA) is the single standard by which to assess bone density and fracture risk.
4. Exercise, gait training, home modifications, and fall prevention are essential in reducing the risk of fractures and enhance bone health and quality of life.
5. Secondary prevention programs are essential in preventing subsequent fractures.

1. **What are metabolic bone diseases?**
   Metabolic bone diseases (MBDs) comprise a large number of disorders of bone modeling, remodeling, and mineralization. The most commonly encountered MBD is osteoporosis, which represents the end-result of menopause (in women) and age-related bone loss. Other MBDs include renal osteodystrophy, osteitis fibrosa cystica, osteomalacia, Paget disease of bone, and many others.

2. **What are bone modeling and remodeling?**
   Bone modeling refers to the new deposition of bone upon a bone surface that has not undergone any prior bone resorption. This deposition impacts the shape and size of the skeleton. In contrast, bone remodeling is a very tightly orchestrated process involving multiple cell lines, predominantly osteoclasts that resorb preexisting bone surfaces and osteoblasts that deposit new bone at the same location, without impacting the size or shape of the bone. The concomitant resorption and formation are "coupled" in part due to cross-talk between osteoblasts and osteoclasts.

3. **What is peak bone mass ? When is it achieved?**
   During childhood and adolescence, the skeleton undergoes maximal bone accrual due to growth, modeling, and remodeling. The bone mass then reaches a plateau known as the peak bone mass (PBM) by the end of the second, or early in the third, decade of life.[1] However, the timing and amplitude of PBM vary between sexes and ethnicities: men tend to achieve higher PBM than women; age-adjusted mean PBMs in African-American women are 10% to 20% higher than US Caucasian women.[2] Furthermore, environmental factors such as exercise and mechanical bone loading also impact the amplitude of PBM.

4. **What happens to PBM with age?**
   During young adulthood, there is a balance between the resorptive and formative volumes of bone such that no permanent bone mass is lost. Shortly thereafter, aging results in a number of processes that lead to a decrease in the volume of bone formation during remodeling. This results in an overall 0.3% to 0.5% loss of bone mass per year, starting around the fourth decade of life. In men, this loss continues at the same rate to reach a cumulative loss of approximately 30% of PBM. In women, perimenopausal loss of estrogen causes a significant increase in the rate of bone loss due to osteoclastic resorption, leading to 1% to 2% loss of bone mass per year for approximately 5 to 7 years, before returning to premenopausal rate. The cumulative loss of bone mass in women is up to 50% between the ages of 50 and 80 years.

5. **How is bone mass measured?**
   - Dual energy x-ray absorptiometry (DXA): DXA remains the World Health Organization's (WHO's) gold standard for bone density assessment. A central DXA scan measures BMD at the lumbar spine (L1 to L4) and hips (total hip and femoral neck). BMD measurement is two dimensional and is expressed in g/cm^2 and then compared against a young-adult mean BMD. The risk of fracture doubles for every standard deviation (SD) decreases in BMD.
   - Quantitative ultrasound (QUS): measurement of BMD using ultrasound technology is an alternative to DXA. However, there is significant variability among available systems in terms of transducer size and technique.

The recommended skeletal site of measurement is the calcaneus. WHO criteria to diagnose osteoporosis cannot be applied to QUS measurements.
- Quantitative computed tomography (QCT): Computed tomography (CT) technology provides the advantage of three-dimensional (3D) measurement of BMD as well as the differential measurement of cortical and trabecular bone. It can be used on central (spine and hips) or peripheral (e.g., distal radius and tibia) sites. There is higher radiation exposure than standard DXA and limited availability of software analysis to major tertiary care or research centers.
- Magnetic resonance imaging (MRI): MRI techniques have provided means for noninvasive 3D assessment of trabecular and cortical bone that may provide correlations between microarchitecture and biomechanical properties.

6. What is the utility of bone biopsy?
A bone biopsy is useful to perform a histologic examination of a bone specimen obtained from iliac crest biopsies. It is an invasive technique but also a well-established tool in the evaluation of MBDs. Its clinical use is limited to situations where it can provide diagnostic or therapeutic information such as renal osteodystrophy or mineralization defects (osteomalacia).

7. How is osteoporosis defined?
Using DXA-derived measurements, an individual patient's BMD is compared against young-adult mean BMD and expressed in terms of an SD, known as T-score. Using the lowest T-score, in postmenopausal women and men age 50 years or older, the WHO defines the following:
- Normal: T-score ≥ -1.0
- Osteopenia: T-score between -1.0 and -2.5
- Osteoporosis: T-score ≤ -2.5

However, the occurrence of a fragility fracture (see questions 9 and 10) indicates the presence of osteoporosis, irrespective of BMD T-scores.

8. How is osteoporosis different in men?
The incidence of fracture in men increases dramatically after the age of 70, with vertebral and hip fractures being the most common. This pattern is very similar to that seen in postmenopausal women, although it begins approximately 10 years later in life.[3,4] The lifetime risk of fracture is more than 40% for women older than 50 years but is lower in men, with age-adjusted hip fracture incidence being less than one-third that of women.[5]

However, the burden of fractures tends to be much higher in elderly men, with a higher risk of death and disability following a hip fracture. Men are 2 to 5 times more likely to have a second fracture compared with women, due to a larger number of comorbidities (i.e., secondary causes for bone loss) compared with women at a given age.[6]

9. What is the difference between osteoporosis and osteomalacia?
Osteoporosis refers to the loss of bone mass secondary to age, menopause, or other factors impacting bone remodeling (resorption and formation). The existing bone is normally mineralized. In contrast, osteomalacia refers to decreased mineralization of bone without reference to its volume. A common etiology for osteomalacia is vitamin D deficiency.

10. What is a fragility fracture?
A fragility fracture is defined as any fracture that occurs following a fall from standing height or less. The most common sites of injury are the hips, spine, and distal forearms or wrists. Clinically silent fractures, commonly vertebral fractures, are also considered to be due to underlying fragility of bone. The occurrence of a fragility fracture is indicative of poor bone strength and can be the basis of an osteoporosis diagnosis. The major contributors to bone strength are mineral content and bone microarchitecture.

11. What is the burden of fractures?
In the United States, approximately 17.5% of women and 6% of men will ultimately sustain a hip fracture. In 2005, 2 million osteoporosis-related fractures occurred in the United States, with direct costs totaling $17 billion. These numbers are expected to increase by 50% by 2025.[7] Mortality following a fragility fracture increases twofold in women and up to three-fold in men. Following a hip fracture in adults aged 50 years or older, the 1-year mortality is approximately 17% in women and greater than 30% in men.[8]

12. What are the risk factors for fragility fractures?
There are a number of modifiable and nonmodifiable risk fractures for osteoporosis and fractures. These include age, comorbid conditions, and family history but also medications, nutritional, and lifestyle choices. A comprehensive list is included in Table 42.1.

Risk calculators that take into account the relative risk of individual variables and ethnic differences are available and can provide 5- and 10-year risk estimates for hip and major osteoporotic fractures. The Fracture Risk Assessment Tool (FRAX; available at https://www.sheffield.ac.uk/FRAX/) and the Garvan Institute bone fracture risk calculator (available at https://www.garvan.org.au/promotions/bone-fracture-risk/calculator/index.php) are the most commonly used tools in clinical practice.

Table 42.1 Conditions, Diseases, and Medications that Cause or Contribute to Osteoporosis and Fractures.

Lifestyle factors	Genetic diseases	Miscellaneous conditions and diseases
Alcohol abuse	Cystic fibrosis	AIDS/HIV
Excessive thinness	Ehlers-Danlos	Amyloidosis
Excess vitamin A	Gaucher disease	Chronic metabolic acidosis
Frequent falling	Glycogen storage diseases	Chronic obstructive lung disease
High salt intake	Hemochromatosis	Congestive heart failure
Immobilization	Homocystinuria	Depression
Inadequate physical activity	Hypophosphatasia	End-stage renal disease
Low calcium intake	Marfan syndrome	Hypercalciuria
Smoking (active or passive)	Menkes steely hair syndrome	Idiopathic scoliosis
Vitamin D insufficiency	Osteogenesis imperfecta	Posttransplant bone disease
	Parental history of hip fracture	Sarcoidosis
	Porphyria	Weight loss
	Riley-Day syndrome	
Endocrine disorders	Gastrointestinal disorders	Neurologic and musculoskeletal risk factors
Central obesity	Celiac disease	Epilepsy
Cushing syndrome	Gastric bypass	Multiple sclerosis
Diabetes mellitus (types 1 and 2)	Gastrointestinal surgery	Muscular dystrophy
Hyperparathyroidism	Inflammatory bowel disease	Parkinson disease
Thyrotoxicosis	Malabsorption	Spinal cord injury
	Pancreatic disease	Stroke
	Primary biliary cirrhosis	
Hematologic disorders	Hypogonadal states	Rheumatologic and autoimmune diseases
Hemophilia	Androgen insensitivity	Ankylosing spondylitis
Leukemia and lymphomas	Anorexia nervosa	Other rheumatic and autoimmune diseases
Monoclonal gammopathies	Athletic amenorrhea	Rheumatoid arthritis
Multiple myeloma	Hyperprolactinemia	Systemic lupus
Sickle cell disease	Panhypopituitarism	
Systemic mastocytosis	Premature menopause (<40 years)	
Thalassemia	Turner and Klinefelter syndromes	

Medications
Aluminum (in antacids)
Anticoagulants (heparin)
Anticonvulsants
Aromatase inhibitors
Barbiturates
Cancer chemotherapeutic drugs
Depo-medroxyprogesterone
  (premenopausal contraception)
Glucocorticoids
GnRH (gonadotropin-releasing
  hormone) agonists
Lithium
Cyclosporine A and tacrolimus
Methotrexate
Parental nutrition
Proton pump inhibitors
Selective serotonin reuptake inhibitors
Tamoxifen (premenopausal use)
Thiazolidinediones
Thyroid hormones

AIDS, Acquired immunodeficiency syndrome; *HIV,* human immunodeficiency virus.
Osteoporos Int DOI 10.1007/s00198-014-2794-2

13. How does one diagnose a fracture?

Most fractures present clinically with pain and/or physical impairment and can be diagnosed using plain radiographs or more advanced imaging such as CT scan. However, vertebral fractures can be silent. Loss of height and/or progressive kyphotic posture may indicate underlying vertebral complete or incomplete fractures. Fractures of the spine occur most commonly in the low thoracic (T8 to T12) or upper lumbar (L1 to L2) vertebrae. Each complete compression fracture causes approximately 1 cm loss in height. In severe cases with multiple fractures, height loss maybe 10 to 20 cm.

It is thus recommended that individuals at high risk be screened for fractures using plain films of the entire spine or a vertebral fracture assessment (VFA), which is a specific DXA technique to obtain comprehensive and objective spinal height measurements.

14. Are there clinical pathways for the secondary prevention of fragility fractures, and what are some of the programs reinforcing these clinical pathways?

Yes. Because of the high burden of fragility fractures and the increased risk for subsequent fractures, clinical pathways that ensure optimal care and secondary fracture prevention have been recommended by the American Association of Orthopedic Surgeons and the American Society for Bone and Mineral Research. Fracture liaison services have been established in a number of institutions, some of which achieved 80% to 90% postfracture assessment rates and increased the percentage of patients (up to 50% to 90%) who have been started on treatment.

15. Classify pain mechanisms caused by compression fractures.

Pain mechanisms in osteoporosis can be classified as mechanical or chemical:

Mechanical causes

- Bone or joint distortion because of direct or indirect structural disruption
- Compression of nerves or soft tissue
- Mechanical stress on weak bone

Chemical causes

- Local endogenous algesic mediators such as histamine, serotonin, quinine, and substance P may be released and activated because of vertebral collapse or microfractures.

16. How do patients with osteoporosis present?

Osteoporosis is largely asymptomatic until the occurrence of a fragility fracture. Hip fractures cause significant mobility impairment and pain. Fractures of isolated vertebral bodies at T4 or higher are unusual and may suggest malignancy. Vertebral compression fractures (VCFs) can cause postural deformities and pain. Accumulation of multiple VCFs may lead to:

- Dorsal kyphosis and exaggerated cervical lordosis ("dowager's hump")
- Chronic thoracic or low back pain, nuchal myalgia
- Abdominal protrusion, gastrointestinal discomfort
- Restricted excursion of the thoracic cage, leading to pulmonary insufficiency and increasing the risk of pneumonia

17. Describe the history and physical examination for osteoporosis.

Assess risk factors (see Table 42.1): menopausal status, amenorrhea, nutritional status (ask about calcium intake), endocrine or gastrointestinal disease, lifestyle choices (particularly alcohol consumption and smoking habits), medications, etc. Ask about height change over time and parental history of a hip fracture.

On exam, measure height and calculate body mass index (BMI). Look for anorexia, features of cortisol excess, hypogonadism, and inflammatory disease (particularly rheumatoid arthritis). Examine the spine carefully; look for kyphosis and/or scoliosis, and measure the space between the lower anterior rib cage and the hip.

18. What laboratory tests are warranted?

Up to one-third of patients may have a previously unknown or subclinical MBD.[9] Testing is thus aimed at evaluating bone health but also at identifying secondary causes of bone fragility. The extent of the medical work-up should be dictated by an individual patient's presentation and a provider's clinical suspicion. An initial work-up could include:

- Serum electrolytes (including calcium, magnesium, and phosphorus), as well as liver, kidney, and thyroid function tests, are considered initial screening laboratory studies.
- Complete blood count is obtained to look for hematologic conditions.
- Vitamin D status and parathyroid function are evaluated using 25(OH) vitamin D and parathyroid hormone (PTH) measurements, respectively.
- Calcium homeostasis is evaluated using 24-hour urinary levels of calcium.
- Serum and urine markers of bone resorption (e.g., bone-specific alkaline phosphatase or N-telopeptide) are not routinely recommended.

19. What are the indications for measurements of bone density?

The National Osteoporosis Foundation (NOF) recommends measurement of BMD[10] in:

- Women age 65 and older and men age 70 and older
- Postmenopausal women and men older than age 50 to 69, based on risk factor profile
- Postmenopausal women and men age 50 and older who have had an adult age fracture, to diagnose and determine the degree of osteoporosis

20. **What about falls?**
    - In history, check for:
      - The number, frequency, circumstances, and environment of falls
      - Posture, balance, weakness
      - Sensory deficits
      - Status of sensorium
      - Medications (e.g., sedatives, psychotropic medications); polypharmacy (>3 medications)
      - Urinary incontinence
      - Visual deficits
      - Need for ambulatory assistive device
      - Poor footwear
      - Home safety profile (area rugs, uneven floors, poor lighting, etc....)
      - Depression/agitation
    - In the physical exam, check for:
      - Orthostatic blood pressures
      - Cardiac arrhythmias
      - Weakness
      - Proprioception/position sense
      - Posture (e.g., forward-leaning) contractures
      - Gait and balance impairment
      - Memory and concentration
      - Inflammatory or degenerative disease
    - Additional assessment tools:
      - Timed Up and Go test: The patient is asked to stand up from sitting position and walk for 10 feet (3 m) while being timed.
      - Functional reach test: The patient is asked to stand by a wall with a yardstick placed at shoulder height. The patient is then asked to flex the shoulder at 90 degrees along the yardstick and reach forward without moving their feet. The length of the farthest reach is recorded.
      - Grip strength

21. **What home modifications should be considered?**
    - Elimination of throw rugs
    - Nonskid tape of different colors on the outer edges of steps
    - Improved lighting
    - Stair rails
    - Removal of loose cords and clutter
    - In the bathroom and shower: Nonskid mats, grab bars, transfer tub benches, raised toilet seats, toilet safety frames
    - Ingress, threshold, and egress ramps and rails
    - Anticipating emergencies: Easy access to emergency phone numbers, a fire exit plan, fire and smoke alarms, and alarm bracelets
    - Smart technology for safety and environmental control: Smartphones, and smart speaker-based voice assistants. Other strategies and devices to reduce vertebral compressive forces include:
    - Carrying heavy items at waist height and close to the body (consider backpacks)
    - Repositioning desks, files, and telephones closer to spare trunk flexion
    - Slower pacing of activities
    - Alternating tasks that demand sitting with those that require standing
    - Wheeled carts
    - Rotating platforms (e.g., "lazy Susans")
    - Swiveling, wheeled office chairs with a lumbar support
    - Perching stools
    - Electronic can openers, knives, and mixers
    - Lightweight cups and bowls
    - Levered door closures
    - Long-handled reachers, shoehorns, sock aids, and sponges

22. **How is exercise used as a preventative measure in osteoporosis?**
    Physical activity may: (1) enhance bone strength by attenuating bone loss, (2) increase or preserve muscle mass, and (3) reduce the risk of falling. Frost's mechanostat theory provides a basis for the benefits of exercise, noting the relationship between the intensity of bend or strain on bone and the adaptation of bone to that stimulus. In this model, whenever activity is below a certain threshold, bone resorption exceeds bone formation. In contrast, net gains of bone occur only when the intensity of loading is increased to greater than the physiologic loading zone. This model accounts for the bone loss observed during immobilization and the increased bone mass of elite athletes.[11]

23. **What is the relationship between immobilization and osteoporosis?**

The lack of mechanical loading can significantly impact the skeleton. Following extended immobilization, evidence of decreased bone mass can be noted on imaging as early as 2 months.

24. **Describe exercise considerations for osteoporosis.**

There is limited evidence that exercise can prevent fractures in osteoporosis. However, the impact of exercise and physical activity on BMD, spinal alignment, and falls reduces the risk of fractures. Moderate- or high-intensity multimodal progressive resistance training in older women and men for 12 to 18 months has been shown to be of particular utility. The NOF Scientific Advisory Board's Position Paper on Exercise and Osteoporosis (1991) describes five important principles of therapeutic exercise for osteoporosis:

- Principle of specificity: Activities should stress sites most at risk for fracture, and skeletal protection should be provided for those areas with severe loss of bone mass.
- Principle of progression: A progressive increase in intensity is required for continued improvement.
- Principle of reversibility: The positive effects of an exercise program will be lost if the exercise regimen is abandoned.
- Principal of initial values: Those with an initial low capacity will have the greatest functional improvement.
- Principle of diminishing returns: There is a limit to improvements in function, and as the limit is approached, greater effort is needed for increasingly smaller gains.

Exercise programs in the elderly should improve muscle strength and balance and be safe, frequent, regular, and sustained. A program of walking, sitting, and standing exercises or water aerobics provides a good start. The height of a bicycle seat, saddle style, and handle-bar height and style should be adjusted for an upright spinal alignment. Swimming is unlikely to improve BMD but provides chest expansion, spinal extension, and low-impact cardiopulmonary fitness. A home exercise program should include deep breathing, back-extension exercises, pectoral stretching, and isometric exercises to strengthen the abdomen and avoid kyphosis.[12]

An example of an exercise chart provided to patients at the Mayo Clinic is shown in Table 42.2. Patients are given a visual chart depicting the different positions along with specific instructions on type, intensity, and frequency of the exercises based on the provider's assessment.

25. **What back exercises should be avoided?**

Exercises that place the spine in flexion predispose osteoporotic women to VCFs (as do sudden rotational movements such as an overly vigorous golf swing or tennis serve).

26. **What are the benefits of tai chi?**

It has been suggested that tai chi may impact bone health; however, the quality of the evidence is poor. The most significant benefit from tai chi is improvement in balance, although there may also be a benefit in attenuating bone loss over a 24-week period, particularly in older adults, perimenopausal and postmenopausal women, breast cancer survivors, and women with osteoarthritis.[13]

Table 42.2 Mayo Clinic Osteoporosis Exercise Chart.	

Easier Exercises[a]	1. Walking and standing posture:
	  a. Walking purpose: to strengthen legs and heart and improve balance.
	  b. Standing posture purpose: to learn to stand properly which will improve posture
	2. Wall arch: to stretch shoulders and calves and tone the back and abdomen
	3. Chin tuck: to help straighten head and shoulders
	4. Chest stretch: to stretch chest and improved back posture
	5. Upper back extension: to stretch chest, strengthen upper back muscles and improve back posture
	6. Pelvic tilt: to strengthen lower back and abdominal muscles
	7. Back and shoulder stretch: to stretch upper back and shoulders

Intermediate Exercises[a]	8. Back posture exercise: to flatten upper back, stretch chest and improved posture 9. Sitting stretch: to stretch calf and thigh muscles and improve muscle tone of legs 10. Calf stretch: to stretch back of thighs and calf muscles, improved posture and stretch heel cords 11. Upper back lift: to strengthen back muscles 12. Abdomen strengthening: to strengthen abdomen 13. Shoulders strengthening: to help strengthen shoulder and back muscles 14. Spine and hip exercise: to strength in arms spine and hips and improve muscle tone

[a]Type, intensity, and frequency of the exercises are individualized by the treating physician or physical therapist.

Modified from Mayo Clinic Osteoporosis Exercise Chart, Mehrsheed Sinaki, Stephen Hodgson, patient education booklet MIC200054. Used with permission of Mayo Foundation for Medical Education and Research. All rights reserved.

27. **Are there benefits to yoga?**

The potential benefits of yoga have stimulated recurring enthusiasm for the exercise. The aging population seems to have a particular interest in yoga, with 21% of yoga practitioners in the United States aged greater than 60 years.[14] Indeed, it has been reported that moderate-duration yoga exercises improved balance and were effective in fall prevention in the elderly.[15,16]

However, yoga-related injuries are not uncommon. Indeed, yoga-associated spinal flexion exercises increase torque pressure and compressive mechanical loading applied to the individual vertebral bodies, thus increasing vulnerability to fractures.[17] Importantly, in the elderly population, age-related degenerative changes in the intervertebral discs further amplify this mechanical loading.[18]

28. **Why is bracing used for VCFs? What bracing options are available?**

For acute pain, the reduction of spinal motion allows paraspinal muscles to cease painful guarding and also provides a physical barrier to reinjury, allowing earlier resumption of activity after injury.

For chronic back pain, bracing substitutes for weak muscles reduces ligamentous strain and offers some protection against the occurrence of new fractures. Bracing options, from least to most restrictive, include:

- Elastic binders, which act as a reminder to restrict motion and also increase intra-abdominal pressure
- The heat-moldable plastic thoracolumbar orthosis (TLO), shaped to the patient's contours and then applied in an elastic support, fabricated by a physical therapist; this takes only minutes to fabricate and is generally a less expensive option
- The hyperextension thoracolumbosacral orthosis (TLSO), such as the Jewett and cruciform anterior sternal hyperextension (CASH)
- Custom-molded plastic body jacket

Continued use of spinal orthoses is discouraged because of the increased likelihood of weakening of trunk muscles, decreased spinal mobility, and unloading of the spine. Posture-training supports (small pouches containing weights up to 2 lb suspended by loops from the shoulders), positioned just below the inferior angle of the scapula to counteract the tendency to bend forward, are worn for 1 hour twice a day.

29. **Discuss the options for pain control for VCFs.**

Back pain resulting from a VCF usually resolves in 4 to 6 weeks. Bed rest, although it may be helpful initially, should be limited. Modalities such as moist heat and massage may alleviate symptoms.

Nonsteroidal antiinflammatory drugs (NSAIDs) and cyclooxygenase-2 (COX-2) inhibitors are often helpful but carry risks of peptic ulcers, renal and cardiac complications, as well as the potential for fracture nonhealing. If used, smaller doses are often appropriate for elders. Opioids offer acute pain relief, but slow gastrointestinal motility, cause constipation, can impair cognition (fall risk) and create drug dependence. Topical anesthetics in the form of a patch (e.g., lidocaine) and applied locally can also be helpful.

Nasal calcitonin has been used acutely following fractures to help with pain control. However, the skeletal benefits are limited. If used in this setting, the duration of treatment should be limited because prolonged use has raised concerns of increased cancer rates.

30. **How much calcium and vitamin D should be consumed daily according to age?**

The Institute of Medicine recommends for:

- Adults age 19 to 50 years and men age 50 to 70: Calcium 1000 mg/day and vitamin D 600 IU/day
- Women age 50 to 70 years: Calcium 1200 mg/day and vitamin D 600 IU/day
- Adults 70 years or older: Calcium 1200 mg/day and vitamin D 800 IU/day

These recommendations consider total calcium intake from all sources (i.e., food and supplemental). A total daily calcium intake not exceeding 2000 to 2500 mg is considered safe by the NOF and the American Society for Preventative Cardiology.

31. **What are selective estrogen receptor modulators (SERMs)?**

SERMs are a class of drugs that bind the estrogen receptor with high affinity and have estrogen agonist and antagonist properties that vary depending upon the individual target organ. They can improve BMD and decrease the risk of vertebral fractures.

32. **What are bisphosphonates? How do they work?**

Bisphosphonates are synthetic analogs of inorganic pyrophosphate; they have a high affinity for calcium crystals (hydroxyapatite) and accumulate in the bone where they decrease osteoclast function or survival and thus reduce bone resorption. They have been the mainstay of treatment of osteoporosis and fracture risk reductions for the past two decades. The most common currently used bisphosphonates are alendronate (given orally once a week) and zoledronate (given as an intravenous infusion once a year). Both have shown a significant reduction in rates of vertebral and nonvertebral fractures. In addition, zoledronate may reduce all-cause mortality in patients with hip fractures.

There have been concerns regarding the long-term use of bisphosphonates given the potential for the development of osteonecrosis of the jaw or atypical femoral fractures. Both side effects are extremely rare.

33. **Describe the benefits of denosumab.**

Denosumab is a monoclonal antibody against RANKL, which is an important molecule in the cross-talk between osteoclasts and osteoblasts. It has a significant antiresorptive effect with reduction in vertebral and nonvertebral fractures. Patient compliance with therapy is extremely important while taking denosumab given that there can be a rebound increase in vertebral fracture rate following discontinuation of therapy.

34. **What precautions should be taken before prescribing bisphosphonates or denosumab?**
In addition to appropriate patient selection and education, it is important to ensure calcium and vitamin D sufficiency before initiating either bisphosphonates or denosumab, to avoid the development of hypocalcemia.

35. **What medications can increase bone formation?**
- PTH analogs: Teriparatide (PTH 1-34) and abaloparatide (PTHrP) both act on the PTH receptor to stimulate bone formation with reduction in vertebral and nonvertebral fractures.
- Antisclerostin antibody: Romosozumab is a monoclonal antibody that binds sclerostin, a protein that typically inhibits osteoblast function, promoting an increase in bone formation rate, and significant increases in both spine and hip BMD and reduction in vertebral and nonvertebral fractures.

REFERENCES

1. Baxter-Jones ADG, Faulkner RA, Forwood MR, et al. Bone mineral accrual from 8 to 30 years of age: an estimation of peak bone mass. *J Bone Miner Res.* 2011;26(8):1729–1739.
2. Nam HS, Kweon SS, Choi JS, et al. Racial/ethnic differences in bone mineral density among older women. *J Bone Miner Metab.* 2013;31(2):190–198.
3. Orwoll ES, Adler RA. Osteoporosis in men. In JP Bilezikian (Ed.). *Primer on the Metabolic Bone Diseases and Disorders of Mineral Metabolism.* 9th ed. John Wiley & Sons, Inc., 2019:443–449. doi.org/10.1002/9781119266594.ch56.
4. Orwoll ES, Vanderschueren D, Boonen S. *Chapter 32—Osteoporosis in Men: Epidemiology, Pathophysiology, and Clinical Characterization.* In R Marcus et al. (Ed.). *Osteoporosis.* 4th ed. San Diego: Academic Press. 2013:757–802.
5. Office of the Surgeon General (US). Bone Health and Osteoporosis: A Report of the Surgeon General. Rockville (MD): Office of the Surgeon General (US); 2004.
6. Ismail AA, Pye SR, Cockerill WC, et al. Incidence of limb fracture across Europe: results from the European Prospective Osteoporosis Study (EPOS). *Osteoporos Int.* 2002;13(7): 565–571.
7. Burge R, Dawson-Hughes B, Solomon DH, et al. Incidence and economic burden of osteoporosis-related fractures in the United States, 2005–2025. *J Bone Miner Res.* 2007;22(3):465–475.
8. Orwig DL, Chan J, Magaziner J. Hip fracture and its consequences: differences between men and women. *Orthop Clin North Am.* 2006;37(4): 611–622.
9. Bours SP, et al. Secondary osteoporosis and metabolic bone disease in patients 50 years and older with osteoporosis or with a recent clinical fracture: a clinical perspective. *Curr Opin Rheumatol.* 2014;26(4):430–439.
10. Cosman F, de Beur SJ, LeBoff MS, et al. Clinician's guide to prevention and treatment of osteoporosis. *Osteoporos Int.* 2014;25(10):2359–2381.
11. Frost HM, Bone's mechanostat: a 2003 update. *Anat Rec A Discov Mol Cell Evol Biol.* 2003;275(2):1081–1101.
12. Sherrington C, Whitney JC, Lord SR, et al. Effective exercise for the prevention of falls: a systematic review and meta-analysis. *J Am Geriatr Soc.* 2008;56(12): 2234–2243.
13. Zou L, Wang C, Chen K, et al. The effect of Taichi practice on attenuating bone mineral density loss: a systematic review and meta-analysis of randomized controlled trials. *Int J Environ Res Public Health.* 2017;14(9):1000.
14. 2016 Yoga in America Study. 2016, Ipsos Public Affairs; Yoga Alliance; Yoga Journal: www.yogaalliance.org.
15. Schmid AA, Van Puymbroeck M, Koceja DM. Effect of a 12-week yoga intervention on fear of falling and balance in older adults: a pilot study. *Arch Phys Med Rehabil.* 2010;91(4): 576–583.
16. Youkhana S, Dean CM, Wolff M, et al. Yoga-based exercise improves balance and mobility in people aged 60 and over: a systematic review and meta-analysis. *Age Ageing.* 2016;45(1): 21–29.
17. Sinaki M. Yoga spinal flexion positions and vertebral compression fracture in osteopenia or osteoporosis of spine: case series. *Pain Pract.* 2013;13(1):68–75.
18. Sfeir JG, Drake MT, Sonawane VJ, et al. Vertebral compression fractures associated with yoga: a case series. *Eur J Phys Rehabil Med.* 2018;54(6): 947–951.

CHAPTER 43

FALL, FRACTURE, AND JOINT REPLACEMENT REHABILITATION: SYNCHRONIZING INDEPENDENT PREVENTIVE STRATEGIES TO REEQUILIBRATE PATIENT FUNCTION

Steven A. Stiens, MD, MS, Tarek Shafshak, MD, PhD, and Levi (Levan) Atanelov, MD

We don't stop playing because we grow old. We grow old because we stop playing.
— George Bernard Shaw (1856–1950)

KEY POINTS

1. Falls frequently result in injury but are preventable with treatment of balance, gait, strength, vision defects, and environmental hazards.
2. Vertigo contributes to falls and is treatable with the Dix-Hallpike maneuver adapting the vestibuloocular reflex and habituation to provoking maneuvers.
3. Joint replacement rehabilitation requires prerehabilitation for balance, strength, and endurance.
4. Postoperative care is guided by a clinical pathway preventing pneumonia, decubiti, deep vein thrombosis, delirium, and falls. Early mobilization, quadriceps neuromuscular stimulation, and alternated aerobic and resistance training enhance outcomes.

---

1. **What is the leading cause of fatal and nonfatal injuries of persons older than 65?**
   Falls result in medical treatments or activity restrictions in 38%, result in serious injuries in 25%, and contribute to risk for nursing home placement (where fall risk is 3 times that of community living adults).

   Van Voast Moncada L, Mire LG. Preventing falls in older persons. *Am Fam Physician.* 2017;96(4):240–247. Available at: https://www.aafp.org/afp/2017/0815/p240.html

2. **What are the three most significantly modifiable risk factors for falls?**
   Balance, gait, and strength impairments. Other significant risks are **tripping** or slipping hazards, **lighting** problems, and **vision** deficits. Patients at risk should be screened by asking when they last fell and why and how often it happens. The **Stay Independent Self-Risk Assessment Brochure** available from the Centers for Disease Control and Prevention (CDC) Stopping Elderly Accidents, Deaths & Injuries (STEADI) program targets risks.

   CDC. Available at: http://www.cdc.gov/steadi/patient.html

3. **Are cancer patients at increased risk of falls?**
   Results of a single-site, retrospective cohort study of 304 patients aged 65 or older with hematologic, gastrointestinal, urologic, breast, lung, and gynecologic cancers showed that 35.8% had at least one fall in the preceding 6 months. Early interventions to address metabolic complications is essential.

   Zhang X, Sun M, Liu S, et al. Risk factors for falls in older patients with cancer. *BMJ Support Palliat Care.* 2018;8(1):34–37. doi:10.1136/bmjspcare-2017-001388. Available at: https://www.researchgate.net/profile/Xiaotao_Zhang/publication/319403553_Risk_factors_for_falls_in_older_patients_with_cancer/links/5a709d47aca272e425ed2943/Risk-factors-for-falls-in-older-patients-with-cancer.pdf

4. What are some of the novel approaches to detect older adults at risk of future falls?
A recent study used wearable sensors to analyze gait-related variables in patients with diabetic peripheral neuropathy and showed that **gait initiation variables** (posture, stance, foot swing and strike patterns) and **dynamic balance** may be more sensitive indicators than **gait speed**. Static **posturography** is also a sensitive screen.

Kang GE, Zhou H, Varghese V, Najafi B. Characteristics of the gait initiation phase in older adults with diabetic peripheral neuropathy compared to control older adults. *Clin Biomech (Bristol, Avon)*. 2020;72:155–160. doi:10.1016/j.clinbiomech.2019.12.019

5. Is there a systematic approach to take when evaluating an older adult at risk of falls?
The CDC has developed a practical algorithmic approach for identifying and managing older adults at risk of falls called the **Stopping Elderly Accidents, Deaths & Injuries (STEADI)**. The STEADI fall risk screening and prevention strategies among older adults in the primary care setting reduced fall-related hospitalizations in a large study in upstate New York. The protocol classifies patients with one traumatic fall or two nontraumatic falls a year with gait and balance deficits to be at high risk of falls and recommends screening for **vision deficits, polypharmacy, somatosensory deficits, foot and ankle problems,** and **vitamin D and B12 deficiency**. It also recommends a **physical therapy (PT) evaluation** with focus on balance and initiation of a strengthening protocol, close follow-up within a month and community-based (e.g., at senior centers) **fall prevention programs** as needed.

Johnston YA, Bergen G, Bauer M, et al. Implementation of the stopping elderly accidents, deaths, and injuries initiative in primary care: an outcome evaluation. *Gerontologist*. 2019;59(6):1182–1191. doi:10.1093/geront/gny101

Centers for Disease Control and Prevention. Available at: http://www.cdc.gov/steadi/patient.html

6. What are some foot and ankle–related immediate and intermediate risk factors for falls?
Person-related immediate, intrinsic factors include foot and ankle deformity, pain, range of motion limitation, and weakness; as well as **extrinsic factors,** such as footwear and orthotics use, which are directly linked with fall risk. A current study found plantar skin/soft tissue and sensory deficits connected via **intermediate** (contribute to immediate) **factors** to fall risk.

Neville C, Nguyen H, Ross K, et al. Lower-limb factors associated with balance and falls in older adults: a systematic review and clinical synthesis [published online ahead of print, 2019 Nov 19]. *J Am Podiatr Med Assoc*. 2019. doi: 10.7547/19-143. Available at: https://pubmed.ncbi.nlm.nih.gov/31743051

7. How do clinicians recognize vertigo when patients complain of dizziness and intervene for disequilibrium with a balance prevention program?
Dizziness, a frequent complaint of the elderly, may suggest **vestibular dysfunction** is confirmed by **vertigo** (illusionary sense of motion) and imbalance associated with gaze and postural instability. Screen for treatable causes such as vertebrobasilar insufficiency. **Vestibular therapy** is a program of exercises to adapt the **vestibulo-ocular reflex**, habituate the patient to movement, and teach sensory substitution for balance and postural control. **Habituation** is utilized by practicing a provoking maneuver repetitively to develop tolerance and compensatory responses.

Kundakci, B, Sultana, A, Taylor, A, Alshehri, MA. The effectiveness of exercise-based vestibular rehabilitation in adult patients with chronic dizziness: a systematic review. *F1000Research*. 2018;7:276. doi: 10.12688/f1000research.14089.1. Available at: https://www.ncbi.nlm.nih.gov/pmc/articles/PMC5954334/

8. What are some of the parts of the examination to be included for a patient in multifactorial fall risk assessment?
Vision, cognition, strength foot alignment, and cardiovascular stability should be evaluated in lying and sitting.
    A dynamic evaluation for **vertigo, postural hypotension**, **stability in stance** with **Rhomberg** and for **nystagmus** with the **Dix-Hallpike test**. The patients' eye movements are observed with the patient seated, head bent sideways 45 degrees toward the shoulder. Then the patient is assisted to lie back quickly, ending with the neck extended 30 degrees below the examining surface. The examiner watches for nystagmus. Gait assessment with **Timed Up and Go (TUG) Test** provides an opportunity to assess footwear function, coordination, self-monitoring, and speed of performance.

STEADI Webinar Fall Prevention. Available at: https://www.youtube.com/playlist?list=PLWqeMoseZ2MwwznjB-TFrq4dtHX8hPsSE

Whitman, GT. Examination of the patient with dizziness or imbalance. *Med Clin North Am*. 2019;103:191–201. doi: 10.1016/j/mcna.2018.10.008. Available at: https://www.medical.theclinics.com/article/S0025-7125(18)30130-5/fulltext

9. Are primary clinicians at large fully successful in preventing falls? How can rehabilitation clinicians support care and prevention?

No. Older adults (older than 75 years) died from falls in 2016 almost 3 times more frequently than in 2000. Primary care physicians and nurse practitioners did not review medications 40% of the time, did not recommend exercise 48% of the time, and did not refer patients to a vision specialist 62% of the time when caring for older adults with fall risk. Aging society, clinical systems, and prevention success demand **early intervention** and rehabilitation driven **secondary prevention**.

Hartholt KA, Lee R, Burns ER, van Beeck EF. Mortality from falls among US adults aged 75 years or older, 2000–2016 [published correction appears in JAMA. 2019 Sep 17;322(11):1108]. *JAMA*. 2019;321(21):2131–2133. doi:10.1001/jama.2019.4185. Available at: https://www.ncbi.nlm.nih.gov/pmc/articles/PMC6549288/

Burns ER, Haddad YK, Parker EM. Primary care providers' discussion of fall prevention approaches with their older adult patients-DocStyles, 2014. *Prev Med Rep*. 2018;9:149–152. Published 2018 Jan 31. doi:10.1016/j.pmedr.2018.01.016. Available at: https://www.ncbi.nlm.nih.gov/pmc/articles/PMC5840836/

10. What mistakes should a clinician avoid to prevent falls? How do you choose to provide care wisely?

Do not prescribe bed rest, leaving patients confined to bed, unless absolutely necessary and with provision for positioning and toileting

Do not use physical restraints without trial of alternatives

Do not prescribe without conducting **medication reconciliation**

Do not overprescribe demanding exercise programs that do not match patients' capacity for safety and compliance.

Choosing Wisely Learning Network. Available at: https://www.choosingwisely.org/clinician-lists/#keyword=falls

11. What does level of testosterone have to do with falls?

An international study on osteoporotic fractures in men showed that low total serum and bioavailable levels of testosterone are associated with risk of falls in men older than 65 years of age.

Vandenput L, Mellström D, Laughlin GA, et al. Low testosterone, but not estradiol, is associated with incident falls in older men: The International MrOS Study. *J Bone Miner Res*. 2017;32(6):1174–1181. doi:10.1002/jbmr.3088. Available at: https://asbmr.onlinelibrary.wiley.com/doi/full/10.1002/jbmr.3088

12. What interventions have demonstrated to be effective in preventing repeated falls?

Although single interventions such as **strength training** exercise and **balance training** do help, the multi-factorial nature of fall risk is best prevented with a variety of targeted risk reduction, compensation, assistive measures, and environmental safety interventions. In fact, a patient-specific assessment and plan can reduce falls by 25%.

Agency for Health care Research and Quality (Fall prevention Tool). Available at: http://www.ahrq.gov/sites/default/files/publications/files/fallpxtoolkit_0.pdf

13. What interventions are helpful in preventing falls in subacute facilities?

Surprisingly, systematic review and meta-analysis suggested that nonspecific exercise may not play a significant role in fall prevention. However, a different systematic review showed that not all exercise interventions are created equal: Exercise programs combined with **patient-specific risk targeted fall interventions** and challenge **balance training** to improve balance skills do seem to be effective. **Vitamin D supplementation** was also shown to be effective.

Cao PY, Zhao QH, Xiao MZ, Kong LN, Xiao L. The effectiveness of exercise for fall prevention in nursing home residents: A systematic review meta-analysis. *J Adv Nurs*. 2018;74(11):2511–2522. doi:10.1111/jan.13814

Lee SH, Kim HS. Exercise interventions for preventing falls among older people in care facilities: a meta-analysis. *Worldviews Evid Based Nurs*. 2017;14(1):74–80. doi:10.1111/wvn.12193; Available at: https://www.ncbi.nlm.nih.gov/pmc/articles/PMC6148705/

Cameron ID, Gillespie LD, Robertson MC, et al. Interventions for preventing falls in older people in care facilities and hospitals. *Cochrane Database Syst Rev*. 2012;12:CD005465. Published 2012 Dec 12. doi:10.1002/14651858.CD005465.pub3

14. Can pleasant smells help fight the fall epidemic?

It was shown that **lavender aromatherapy** may reduce falls of elderly nursing home residents. The authors suggested that this was most likely due to lavender **decreasing anxiety.**

Sakamoto Y, Ebihara S, Ebihara T, et al. Fall prevention using olfactory stimulation with lavender odor in elderly nursing home residents: a randomized controlled trial [published correction appears in J Am Geriatr Soc. 2012 Nov;60(11):2193]. *J Am Geriatr Soc.* 2012;60(6):1005–1011. doi:10.1111/j.1532-5415.2012.03977.x

15. How do you reduce fall risk of patients after traumatic brain injury (TBI)?

A recent article reported 22% of patients with TBI suffering at least one fall: 53% in the patient's bedroom, and 57% due to loss of balance. Almost all (93%) of fallers had impaired mobility, and 85% **required assistance for transfers.** The authors conclude that "generic falls prevention measures" are insufficient for preventing falls in the TBI rehabilitation population. Falls prevention initiatives should target times of high patient activity by offering **scheduled assistance** and situations where there is decreased nursing capacity to observe patients by adding other technologic options for monitoring and communication.

McKechnie D, Fisher MJ, Pryor J. The characteristics of falls in an inpatient traumatic brain injury rehabilitation setting. *J Clin Nurs.* 2016;25(1–2):213–222. doi:10.1111/jocn.13087

16. Do chair and bed alarms help reduce falls in subacute facilities?

No. A recent retrospective study of 160 patients compared facilities that use these devices with those that do not and concluded the bed/body alarms did not reduce falls in the elderly population. One hypothesis is that bed alarms "alarm" the patient who is "startled" and falls before help arrives.

White H, Cuavers KY. Do alarm devices reduce falls in the elderly population? *J Natl Black Nurses Assoc.* 2018;29(2):17–22.

17. What three theories suggest mechanisms for the demonstrated success of vestibular rehabilitation?

1. **Vestibuloocular adaptation** is promoted by eye/head coordination exercises in active movements while maintaining fixed gaze on a stationary target and reequilibrates sensory motor nerve circuits. Later, patients are trained to perform **saccadic eye movements**, shifting gaze between targets.
2. **Substitution**—includes visual, tactile, and enhanced **vibrotactile feedback**.
3. **Habituation**—includes movement experiences where the patient is exposed to the provoking stimuli. Contemporary utilization of virtual reality has been effective.

Patients with benign paroxysmal postural vertigo are treated with the **otolith repositioning** maneuver, which is very effective at reducing the frequency of vertigo.

Alghadir AH, Zaheen AI, Whitney SL. An update on vestibular physical therapy. *J Chin Med Assoc.* 2013;76:1–8. Available at: https://journals.lww.com/jcma/fulltext/2013/01000/An_update_on_vestibular_physical_therapy.1.aspx

18. Does whole body vibration (WBV) reduce risk of falls and fractures?

WBW is the oscillation (30 to 40 Hz) of a plate patients bear weight through during exercise for 15 to 60 seconds at a time. Muscle tone is increased by triggering the **tonic vibration reflex (TVR)**. WBV reduces fall risk up to 24% and indirectly reduces fracture risk. A meta-analysis showed no overall but some localized increases in bone mineral density within spine and femoral neck.

Marin-Cascales E, Alcarez PE, Ramos-Camop DJ, Martinez-Rodriguez A, Chung LH, Rubio-Arias JA. Whole-body vibration training and bone health in postmenopausal women: a systematic review and meta-analysis. *Medicine.* 2018 Aug;97(34):e11918. Available at: https://www.ncbi.nlm.nih.gov/pmc/articles/PMC6112924/

Wadsworth, D, Lark, S. Effects of whole-body vibration training on the physical function of the frail elderly: an open, randomized controlled trial. *Arch Phys Med Rehabil.* 2020;101:1111–1119. doi: 10/1016/j.apmr.2020.02.009. Available at: https://www.archives-pmr.org/article/S0003-9993(20)30144-1/fulltext#secsectitle0010

Jepsen DB, Thomsen K, Hansen S, Jørgensen NR, Masud T, Ryg J. Effect of whole-body vibration exercise in preventing falls and fractures: a systematic review and meta-analysis. *BMJ Open.* 2017;7(12):e018342. Published 2017 Dec 29. doi:10.1136/bmjopen-2017-018342. Available at: https://bmjopen.bmj.com/content/7/12/e018342

19. What is the prevalence of senior center–based programs for preventing falls in older adults?

Approximately half of senior centers offer evidence-supported, community-based fall prevention programs (e.g., **Stepping On**), and approximately a third do not offer any programs whatsoever. It was also shown that locales with more senior centers are more likely to offer more evidence-based programs.

Hamel C, Hekmatjah N, Hakakian B, et al. Evidence-based community fall prevention programs at senior centers near 10 US academic centers. *J Am Geriatr Soc.* 2019;67(7):1484–1488. doi:10.1111/jgs.15961.

Kulinski K, DiCocco C, Skowronski S, Sprowls P. Advancing community-based falls prevention programs for older adults—The Work of the Administration for Community Living/Administration on Aging. *Front Public Health.* 2017;5:4. doi: 10.3389/fpubh.2017.00004. Available at: https://www.ncbi.nlm.nih.gov/pmc/articles/PMC5289953/

20. What are the four phases of indirect bone healing? Is a callus required?

Direct bone healing occurs in trabecular bone where inflammation occurs and leads directly to **intramembranous ossification**. More complex indirect bone healing of cortical bone requires a **callus**.

I.	Inflammation	0–7 days	**Platelet degradation**. Hematoma transitions to granulation. **Osteoclasts** remove necrotic bone.
II.	Soft callus	2–3 weeks	Progenitor cells differentiate to fibroblasts. Intramembranous ossification in periosteum.
III.	Hard callus	3–4 months	**Endochondral ossification** of soft callus **bone morphogenic protein (BMP)** released by chondrocytes triggers calcification.
IV.	Remodeling		Surface erosion converts **woven bone** to **laminar bone**.

21. How does biomechanical stability promote bone healing?

Healing rate increases with stability and is further enhanced with stable compression with internal fixation devices. **Perren's strain theory** recognizes the mechanical and piezoelectric (change in charge distribution with collagen strain) properties of bone resulting in force deformation signaling increasing mesenchymal cell differentiation into bone. Internal fixation with compression achieving **absolute stability** can produce more rapid **direct bone healing**.

Foster AL, Moriarty TF, Zalavras C, et al. The influence of biomechanical stability on bone healing and fracture-related infection: *the legacy of Stephan Perren. Int J Care Injured.* 2020;11(38). doi: 10.1016/j.injury.2020.06.044. Available at: https://www.injuryjournal.com/article/S0020-1383(20)30551-9/fulltext

22. What is the diamond concept of fracture healing?

It is a four-pillar conceptual framework: (1) fracture stability, (2) growth factors, (3) scaffolds (**porous biomaterials**—allograft trabecular bone, collagen, hydroxyapatite), and (4) mesenchymal stem cells. Bone vascularity and the metabolic state of host are essential.

23. What therapies can achieve healing in situations of fracture nonunion?

Pulsed ultrasound therapy and **focused extracorporeal shock wave** can be successful in 30% to 80% of subjects 3 to 6 months after fixation. Hypertrophic biologically active nonunions are more responsive than atrophic inactive sites. **Electrical stimulation** or **pulsed electromagnetic waves** is less effective and requires longer administration. Operative methods use **autografts** of bone and cells to enhance **osteogenesis** and trials using various allograft of matrix (supporting **osteoconduction**) and cells from growth lines. Future directions include development of hybrid injectable hydrogel-based, bioceramic-based conglomerates administered with immune suppression. Regenerative medicine cell banks may distribute cell lines for specific indications.

Willems A, van der Jagt, OP, Meuffels, DE. Extracorporeal shock wave treatment for delayed union and nonunion fractures: a systematic review. *J Orthop Trauma.* 2019 Feb;33(2):97–103.

Gomez-Barrena E, Rosset P, Lozano D, et al. Bone fracture healing: cell therapy in delayed unions and nonunions. Bone. 2015; 70:93–101. Available at: https://www.sciencedirect.com/science/article/pii/S8756328214002968?via%3Dihub

24. What can physical medicine and rehabilitation (PM&R) contribute to the continuum of care linking balance and joint replacement rehabilitation?

Comprehensive quality care includes prevention, surveillance, education, early intervention, and treatments supported by evidence and reinforced by outcomes. One example of comprehensive care innovation for patients that may need joint replacement was developed in response to **bundled payments** (single reimbursement per procedure). Such mandates provide incentives for alignment of stakeholders to work across specialties to optimize efficiency and quality. To contribute, PM&R clinical and administrators need to be a part of **task forces** that design systems (electronic care pathways), and **implementation teams** adapting treatment protocols and data collection. Resulting designs include **participant scorecards**, early patient/caregiver engagement through **joint camp classes, prehabilitation programs** building balance, strength, endurance, range, pain reduction, and home safety modifications. Establishing a **postacute care partner network** ensures continued rehabilitation and complication prevention.

Schelp, G. The University of Missouri Health Care approach to Comprehensive Care for Joint Replacement. *Arthroplast Today.* 2019;5:152–153. doi: 10.1016/j.artd.2018.10.006. Available at: https://www.ncbi.nlm.nih.gov/pmc/articles/PMC6588682/

25. Can treatment for osteoarthritis prevent falls?
Osteoarthritis increases the risk for falls in proportion to number of affected weight-bearing joints, with three to four increasing risk by 85%. Pain relief with strengthening, alignment, support, and medications improves tolerance. Joint replacement reduces pain and instability, improving function.

Dore AL, Golightly YM, Mercer VS, et al. Lower limb osteoarthritis and the risk of falls in a community-based longitudinal study of adults with and without osteoarthritis. *Arthritis Care Res* (Hoboken) 2015 May; 67(5):633–639. Available at: https://www.ncbi.nlm.nih.gov/pmc/articles/PMC4404178/

26. What are the rehabilitative goals of total knee replacement?
The goals are safe ambulation in the house using an assistive device, active range of motion of the operated knee, approaching full extension and greater than 90 degrees flexion.

27. How does PM&R accomplish the best outcomes and prognosis after hip fracture?
Hip fracture incidence reaches 1% annually by age 80. Complications include pneumonia, pressure ulcers, deep vein thrombosis, delirium, malnutrition, anemia, and falls. Interventions should be interdisciplinarily designed at each center, with consensus on a working **clinical pathway** (chronologic care event map addressing all disciplines and standard treatments). All reviews of hip fracture rehabilitation outcomes were strongly associated with overall ambulation performance. Function success was enhanced by inpatient care, standing, treadmill training, and quadriceps neuromuscular stimulation, with alternated aerobic and progressive resistance training. Early mobilization, intensive therapy, combined occupational therapy (OT)/PT sessions, and early comprehensive discharge planning achieved the safest most efficient outcomes. **Transitions of care** require a discharge checklist, interfacility transfer form, a discharge summary, and verbal explanations of the risks, complications, monitoring, and treatments in progress. All laboratory tests, medication administration durations, physical restrictions, and future appointments for reevaluation need to be clearly documented. Home care PT for up to 12 weeks was associated with superior community mobility.

Chudyk AM, Jutai JW, Petrella RJ, et al. Systematic review of hip fracture rehabilitation practices in the elderly. *Arch Phys Med Rehabil.* 2009;90:246–262. doi: 10/1016/j.apmr.2008.06.036. Available at: https://www.archives-pmr.org/article/S0003-9993(08)01562-1/fulltext

Eslami, M, Tran, HP. Transitions of care and rehabilitation after fragility fractures. *Clin Geriatr Med.* 2014;30:303–315. doi: 10.1016/j.cger.2014.01.017. Available at: https://www.researchgate.net/profile/Daniel_Mendelson/publication/261602189_Fragility_Fractures_Preface/links/5aaf1be7aca2721710fc4f3f/Fragility-Fractures-Preface.pdf#page=132

Ranhoff AH, Saltvedt I, Frihagen F, et al. Interdisciplinary care of hip fractures. Orthogeriatric models, alternative models, interdisciplinary teamwork. *Best Pract Res Clin Rheumatol.* 2019 Apr;33(2):205–226. doi: 10.1016/j.berh.2019.03.015. Epub 2019 Apr 30.

BIBLIOGRAPHY

American Academy of Orthopedic Surgeons. 2014. Clinical Practice Guidelines for Management of Hip Fractures in the Elderly. Available at: https://www.aaos.org/quality/quality-programs/lower-extremity-programs/hip-fractures-in-the-elderly/

Giangarra, CE, Manske, RC. *Clinical Orthopedic Rehabilitation a Team Approach.* 4th ed. Philadelphia: Elsevier; 2018:605 pgs. Available at: https://aaos.org/globalassets/quality-and-practice-resources/patient-safety/clinician-checklists/aaos-hip-fx-prevention-of-secondary-fractures.pdf

Hoppenfeld, S, Murthy VL. *Treatment and Rehabilitation of Fractures.* Philadelphia: Lippincott William & Wilkins; , 2000:624 pgs. Available at: https://www.nice.org.uk/guidance/cg161

National Institute for Health and Care Excellence (NICE); 2013 Jun. Falls in older people: Accessing risk and prevention Available at: https://pubmed.ncbi.nlm.nih.gov/25506960/

Nordstrom, P, Thorngren, KG, Hommel, A, et al. Effects of geriatric team rehabilitation after hip fracture: meta-analysis of randomized controlled trials. *JAMDA.* 2018;19:840–845. doi:10/1016/j.jamda.2018.05.008

Perracini MR, Kristensen MT, Cunningham C, Sherrington C. Physiotherapy following fragility fractures. *Injury.* 2018;49(8):1413–1417. doi: 10.1016/j.injury.2018.06.026. Available at: https://www.aging.senate.gov/imo/media/doc/SCA_Falls_Report_2019.pdf

United States Senate Special Committee on Aging. *Falls Prevention: National, State, and Local Solutions to Better Support Seniors;* 2019 Available at: https://www.aging.senate.gov/imo/media/doc/SCA_Falls_Report_2019.pdf

THE HIP: ANATOMY, EXAMINATION, DIAGNOSES, IMAGING, TREATMENT, AND REHABILITATION

David J. Kolessar, MD, Justin G. Tunis, MD, RMSK, Alberto G. Corrales, MD, MS, and Areerat Suputtitada, MD

Luck is what happens when preparation meets opportunity.

—Seneca the Younger (4 BC–AD 65)

KEY POINTS

1. An early sign of hip arthritis is loss of internal rotation on physical examination.
2. Plain radiographs are the best initial imaging modality to evaluate arthritis.
3. Hip Labral pathology is best demonstrated and diagnosed with intra-articular contrast-enhanced MRI.
4. Pain is best treated by using a multimodal approach.
5. Ultrasonography can identify small effusions, synovitis and guide needles during interventional procedures.

1. **The hip is what type of joint?**
   The hip is a multiaxial ball and socket joint. The spherical femoral head articulates with a hemispherical acetabulum. Labrum is a fibrocartilaginous rim-gasket seal that maintains synovial fluid within the articulation, aids in distribution of contact forces, adds to socket depth, and enhances joint stability.

2. **What are the capsular ligaments of the hip joint?**
   Iliofemoral ligament ("Y" ligament of Bigelow): Location—anterior, extends from anterior superior iliac spine (ASIS) to the intertrochanteric (ITT) line of femur. Function: prevents hyperextension when standing. Strongest ligament in the body.
   Ischiofemoral ligament (ligament of Bertin): Location—posterior, extends from ischium to ITT line. Function: limits internal hip rotation.
   Pubofemoral ligament (pubocapsular): Location—anteroinferior, extends from superior pubis ramus and obturator crest and blends with the joint capsule and the iliofemoral ligament. Function: prevents hyperabduction.

3. **What are the major muscles around the hip? What are their names, function, and innervation?**
   The muscles around the hip region aid in movement and stability of the joint. The iliopsoas is the strongest hip flexor. The gluteus maximus is the chief extensor of the thigh. There are six small muscles that cross the posterior hip joint which aid dynamic stability and external rotation. The gluteus medius and minimus muscles attach to the greater trochanter and are the primary hip abductors in addition to pelvic stabilizers during single leg activity (Table 44.1).[1–3]

4. **What artery supplies the most vascularity to the femoral head?**
   The medial circumflex artery provides the most vascularity to the femoral head. However, the medial and lateral circumflex arteries, which arise from the deep femoral artery, together contribute the majority blood supply to the hip.[2]

5. **What are some characteristic symptoms of hip joint pathology?**
   Articular hip joint pathology often presents as anterior hip and deep groin pain. However, hip pathology can refer pain to any or all the following locations: groin, lateral hip, buttock, thigh, or knee. Knee pain can originate from the hip! Pain produced by palpation often represents extra-articular hip pathology related to bursae, muscles, tendons, or surrounding soft tissues.

6. **What is the most consistent early sign of hip arthritis on physical exam?**
   Loss of internal rotation. Most easily demonstrated with patient supine; the hip and knee are flexed to 90 degrees followed by gentle thigh internal rotation. Limited internal rotation and pain are elicited. "Start-up" pain, stiffness, and abductor lurch upon initial steps of gait are also common.

7. **What is the FABER test, and what is the significance of a positive finding?**
   FABER (or Patrick) test: patient supine, the thigh is placed in **F**lexion, **Ab**duction, and **E**xternal **R**otation while a posterior directed force is applied to the knee. The ipsilateral heel on the contralateral knee creates the "figure 4"

Table 44.1 Hip: Major Muscles, Functions, and Innervations

MUSCLE	ACTION	INNERVATION	NERVE ROOTS
Gluteus Maximus	Extension, External Rotation	Inferior gluteal n.	L5–S2
Gluteus Medius	Abduction, Medial Thigh Rotation	Superior gluteal n.	L4–S1
Gluteus Minimus	Abduction, Medial Thigh Rotation	Superior gluteal n.	L4–S1
Piriformis	External Rotation	Ventral rami	S1, S2
Superior Gemellus	External Rotation	Sacral plexus br.	L4–S1
Obturator Internus	External Rotation	Sacral plexus br.	L5, S1
Inferior Gemellus	External Rotation	Quadratus femoris n.	L5, S1
Quadratus femoris	External Rotation	Quadratus femoris n.	L5, S1
Iliacus	Flexion	Femoral n.	L2, L3
Psoas	Flexion	Femoral n.	L1–L3
Pectineus	Adduction, Flexion, Internal Rotation	Femoral n.	L2, L3
Rectus femoris	Flexion	Femoral n.	L2–L4

or "frog-leg" position. Pain over the anterior aspect of the hip during this test is consistent with intra-articular hip pathology, iliopsoas stain, or iliopsoas bursitis. Pain over the sacroiliac joint is consistent with sacroiliac joint dysfunction or sacroiliitis.

8. What is the FADIR test, and what is the significance of a positive finding?
   FADIR (or impingement) test: Hip **F**lexion, **AD**duction, **I**nternal **R**otation. Nonspecific test. Pain suggests femoral-acetabular impingement (FAI), labral pathology, hip loose bodies, or hip chondral lesion.[2]

9. What is an antalgic gait?
   Antalgic gait is seen when an individual attempts to minimize pain in the affected lower extremity by shortening the duration of the stance phase relative to swing phase. This translates to the stance phase in the unaffected leg being relatively longer than that of the affected leg.[4]

10. What is a Trendelenburg gait (or gluteus medius lurch)?
    This gait is seen when there is functional weakness of the abductor muscles in the weight-bearing limb causing swaying of the trunk over the side of the affected hip during the opposite limb's swing phase. This can be caused by gluteal nerve injury, gluteus tendon tear, poliomyelitis, or myopathy.[4]

11. What is a Trendelenburg sign?
    This is seen as positive when the pelvis in the non–weight-bearing limb drops while the opposite limb is in stance phase. Indicates weakness in the hip abductor muscles (gluteus medius and minimus: superior gluteal nerve) of the stance limb (Fig. 44.1).

12. What does the Thomas test assess, and how is it performed?
    It checks for hip flexion contracture. Patient lies supine on exam table. To test left hip, instruct patient to passively flex the contralateral hip and knee as far as possible toward chest. A positive test is present if the ipsilateral thigh elevates upward off the table indicating hip flexion contracture. Alternatively, place examiner's hand under patient's lumbar spine. Then push down on patient's thigh. If the lumbar lordosis increases (arches away from examiner's hand), the pelvis is flexing with the downward thigh pressure indicating an ipsilateral hip flexion contracture.

13. What is the Ober test used to evaluate?
    The Ober test is used to evaluate tightness in the tensor fascia lata (TFL) and iliotibial band (ITB). The patient lies on side with ipsilateral hip and knee flexed to flatten the lumbar curve. The examiner stands behind the patient, stabilizes the pelvis with one hand and flexes and abducts, then extends the patient's hip with the knee flexed to 90 degrees with the other hand. The examiner then slowly lowers the leg to the table while preventing hip internal rotation and any further hip flexion. A positive test occurs when the upper leg remains abducted, which indicates the presence of a tight TFL and ITB.[5]

14. How do hip labral tears arise and present?
    Labral tears may arise traumatically from twisting, pivoting movements or extreme hip range of motion (ROM). FAI may lead to labral abnormalities. Most patients with labral tears complain of groin or anterior hip pain. On examination, patients may have pain with the FADIR test.[2]

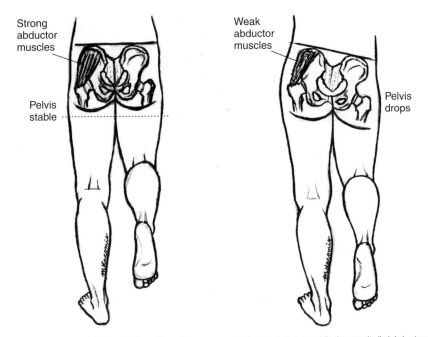

Fig. 44.1 Demonstrates a positive Trendelenburg sign: pelvis on non–weight-bearing limb drops while the opposite limb is in stance phase. Reproduced with permission from Marissa C. Lacomis.

15. **How does traumatic posterior or anterior hip dislocation present?**
    a. *Posterior Dislocation* (most common): hip flexed, thigh adducted and internally rotated. Can be associated with sciatic nerve injury (usually peroneal branch) and knee injuries (Fig. 44.2).
    b. *Anterior Dislocation* (Obturator type): hip flexed, abducted, and externally rotated. Can be associated with femoral nerve injury.
       The vast majority of traumatic hip dislocations due to high-energy etiology are associated with other injuries. Documentation of neurologic examination "pre" and "post" reduction is essential. Osteonecrosis

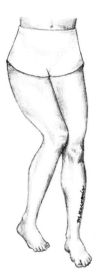

Fig. 44.2 Classic limb posture of posterior hip dislocation: hip and knee flexed, limb adducted and internally rotated. Reproduced with permission from Marissa C. Lacomis.

incidence is related to amount of time femoral head remains dislocated. Treatment goal is emergent closed reduction within 6 hours. Perform postreduction computed tomography (CT) scan in all traumatic native hip dislocations.[6]

16. How are hip fractures classified and treated?

Hip fractures are classified by anatomic location:
- Femoral neck (Garden classification).
- ITT (Kyle classification).
- Subtrochanteric (Seinsheimer classification).

Garden classification of femoral neck fractures:

I. Incomplete or impacted fracture: inferior neck trabeculae still intact.
II. Complete fracture without displacement.
III. Complete fracture with partial displacement.
IV. Complete fracture with full displacement.

Treatment of femoral neck fracture: determined by degree of displacement, bone quality, age, and activity level of patient. Options: multiple screws versus hemiarthroplasty versus total hip arthroplasty (THA).

Femoral neck fracture, Garden type I and II (nondisplaced):
- Internal fixations with multiple screws, especially for patients younger than 65 years.
- Weight-bearing status: usually partial weight bearing ×6 weeks, influenced by degree of fracture stability and bone quality.

Femoral neck fracture, Garden type III and IV (displaced):
- Attempt reduction and internal fixation in patient less than 65 years old.
- Hemiarthroplasty for patients 65 years or older with low functional demands.
- THA for cases with preexisting advanced arthritis or active patients 65 years or older.
- Weight-bearing status: Weight bearing as tolerated (WBAT) for arthroplasty procedures.

Kyle classification of ITT hip fractures:

I. Nondisplaced stable ITT fracture without comminution (two part).
II. Displaced stable ITT fracture with minimal comminution (three part).
III. Displaced unstable ITT fracture with extensive posteromedial comminution (four part).
IV. Displaced unstable ITT fracture with extensive posteromedial comminution and subtrochanteric extension.

Treatment of ITT fracture:

Stable ITT fracture (type I and II):
- Reduction/fixation with dynamic hip screw with side-plate device, or intramedullary (IM) nail.
- Weight-bearing status: WBAT is almost universal.

Unstable ITT fracture (type III and IV):
- Reduction and fixation with IM nail.
- Weight-bearing status: WBAT is almost universal when fixation with IM nails.

17. What is the difference between hemiarthroplasty versus total hip arthroplasty (THA)?

A hemiarthroplasty only replaces femoral head and neck. A THA replaces acetabular surface in addition to femoral head and neck.

18. What is hip osteonecrosis?

Hip osteonecrosis results from ischemia due to obstructed intraosseous femoral head circulation. Femoral head is most common location for osteonecrosis. Steroids and alcohol account for the vast majority of hip osteonecrosis in patients younger than 50 years old. Pain can commence before plain radiographic abnormality is appreciated. A magnetic resonance imaging (MRI) scan is the most valuable imaging study if there is high index of suspicion and plain x-rays are normal. Most patients develop bilateral involvement. Symptomatic subchondral fracture and collapse are debilitating and often lead to THA (Table 44.2).[7]

19. What is Legg-Calvé-Perthes (LCP) disease?

LCP disease is an idiopathic osteonecrosis of the proximal femur which results from disruption of the femoral head blood supply. After vascular insult, growth arrest occurs at the proximal femoral physis. Over time, the femoral head undergoes a period of bone resorption which may result in collapse of the articular surface. Eventually, bone growth resumes. The condition is most common in males 4 to 8 years old. Typical presentation is a painless limp. Treatment is controversial. Protected weight bearing and close observation are critical to ensure the femoral head remains properly seated in the acetabulum during the remodeling phase.[8]

20. What is slipped capital femoral epiphysis (SCFE)?

Typically seen in overweight adolescent males more than females. Hormonal influence on physeal plate development has been suggested as etiologic factor during growth spurt. Common presentation: insidious onset, hip stiffness, limp, pain, and progressive external rotation of lower limb. However, it may at times present with only knee symptoms. Plain x-rays are often diagnostic, revealing a widened physeal growth plate or displacement of epiphysis relative to the femoral neck. This is considered a surgical emergency due to morbidity associated with progression of displacement. Assessment of contralateral hip is necessary.[9]

Table 44.2 Risk Factors for Osteonecrosis

DIRECT RISK FACTORS	INDIRECT RISK FACTORS
Trauma (Fracture or Dislocation)	Corticosteroid Use
Sickle Cell Anemia	Alcohol Abuse
HIV Infection	Systemic Lupus Erythematosus
Radiation	Organ Transplantation
Myeloproliferative Disorders	Renal Failure
Gaucher Disease	Coagulation Abnormalities
	Pregnancy
	Genetic Factors
	Caisson Disease

HIV, Human immunodeficiency virus.

21. **What are the common causes of hip arthritis and risk factors for osteoarthritis (OA)?**
    The common pathology of hip arthritis is articular cartilage damage or loss (Table 44.3).[10]

22. **What can cause a snapping hip syndrome (SHS)?**
    Iliopsoas bursitis, iliopsoas tendonitis (internal SHS), or TFL/ITB (external SHS) can cause SHS.

23. **What is meralgia paresthetica?**
    It is also known as lateral femoral cutaneous neuropathy. Patient may experience pain, hyperesthesia, burning, or numbness over the anterolateral thigh. It is associated with obesity, compression from tight clothing, trauma, repetitive hip flexion (cyclists), mass effect (tumor), or scar tissue from previous surgery.[11]

24. **What radiographs should be ordered to evaluate osteoarthritis (OA)?**
    Plain radiographs are the best initial imaging modality to evaluate arthritis. X-rays: A well centered anteroposterior (AP) pelvis, AP hip, cross-table lateral hip (frog lateral), and false profile view.

25. **What are the radiographic features of OA progression?**
    Sequential progression of osteoarthritic changes on plain radiographic generally include: joint space narrowing, subchondral sclerosis, periarticular osteophytes, subchondral cysts, and structural bone erosion.

26. **What is the role of CT scan in evaluating hip pathology?**
    CT scans are best at evaluating bony structures because they provide more detail than plain radiographs. Subtle fractures, bone tumors, very complex fracture patterns, and FAI are demonstrated well. Three-dimensional reconstructions improve bone pathology visualization.

27. **What is the role of MRI in evaluating hip pathology?**
    MRI is useful for evaluating soft tissue such as cartilage, muscle, tendons, and ligaments. MRI can demonstrate early hip osteonecrosis, stress reactions, or bone contusions by identifying bone edema. MRI arthrogram is excellent for evaluating labrum.

Table 44.3 Risk Factors for Osteoarthritis

RISK FACTORS FOR PRIMARY OA	RISK FACTORS FOR SECONDARY OA
Older age	Trauma
Female gender	Avascular necrosis
Increased BMI	Rheumatoid Arthritis
Higher bone mass	Septic Arthritis
Genetics	Gout
Certain sports (soccer)	Diabetes Mellitus
Occupation requiring heavy lifting	Hypothyroidism
Prolonged standing	Hemochromatosis

BMI, Body mass index; *OA,* osteoarthritis.

28. What is the role of ultrasonography in evaluating hip pathology?

Ultrasonography (US) of hip can detect joint effusion and synovial hypertrophy, changes within the bursa, and abnormalities of muscle and tendons. Additionally, ultrasound can direct needle insertion during aspirations and injections around vital structures.

29. What are the advantages of US?

Advantages: noninvasive, absence of radiation, cost effective, rapid side-to-side comparison, and dynamic real-time evaluation of anatomic structures in multiple planes.[12]

30. What exercises are good for treating hip arthritis?

Nonimpact, gentle, low intensity, and light resistance exercises reduce pain and symptoms associated with arthritis.

31. What are the primary indications for hip arthroscopy? Who are the best candidates? What are the relative contraindications?

Primary indications for hip arthroscopy: loose body removal, labral repair, and treatment of FAI. Best candidates: patients without infection, age younger than 55 years, and 2 mm or greater of joint space remaining.

Relative contraindications:
- age older than 55 years
- significant arthritis with less than 2 mm joint space on radiograph
- hip dysplasia with lateral center edge angle less than 25 to 30 degrees
- Body mass index (BMI) greater than 30 kg/m^2
- concomitant low back injury

32. What are the indications and goals for THA?

Indications for THA: painful advanced hip degenerative joint disease unresponsive to conservative treatments over 3 to 6 months, and concomitant radiographic disease consistent with the patients' symptoms. Principle goals of THA: relieve pain, correct deformity, reestablish proper hip mechanics, and restore ROM and function.

33. What is hip resurfacing?

The femoral head is resurfaced with a metal cap. The acetabular component is metal: thus metal-on-metal articulation. Affords larger head sizes reducing dislocation risk and preserving bone stock. Concerns includes metal ion toxicity and femoral neck fracture. Hip resurfacing has declined to less than 0.5% of THA procedures.[13]

34. What is the most common method of THA implant fixation in bone?

Cementless press-fit textured metal on-growth or porous in-growth surfaces are the dominant methods for acetabular shell and femoral stem component fixation.

35. What are the bearing surface options available for THA?

Ceramic prosthetic head on polyethylene acetabular liner is most common.
Metal head on polyethylene liner—concerns are polyethylene wear and trunnionosis.
Ceramic head on ceramic liner—concerns are squeaking and ceramic fracture.
Metal head on metal liner—concern is metal ion toxicity.

36. What is the best method of pain management for THA patients?

Use multimodal approach to reduce pain while minimizing opioid medications through a combination of preemptive medications, peripheral nerve blocks, intraoperative periarticular capsular injections, and postoperative non-narcotic regimens. In addition, preoperative education, setting expectations, and early mobilization have all proven beneficial.

37. What are the most common nerve injuries during THA surgery?

Depends on surgical approach:
Posterior approach: sciatic nerve (peroneal branch most common).
Anterior approach: lateral femoral cutaneous nerve (pure sensory nerve).[14]

38. What is the time-table for THA rehabilitation?

Immediate WBAT is the norm following uncomplicated primary and revision THA. Currently, accelerated or rapid recovery programs promote immediate mobilization and ambulation on the day of surgery. Rehabilitation programs prior to surgery are encouraged. Therapy is individualized based on patient tolerance. General tenets include:

Postoperative Day (POD) #0: Day of Surgery
- Educate/encourage self-performed exercises.
- Quadriceps and gluteal muscle isometrics.
- Active ankle pumps: dorsiflexion/plantar flexion.
- Sit up on edge of bed, active knee extensions, sit to stand as tolerated with WBAT.
- Walk with WBAT in room and/or hall with crutches or walker, based on patient tolerance.
- If being discharged same day as surgery, add stair climbing exercises.
- Educate patient regarding hip precautions if applicable.

POD 1
- Review all education from previous day.
- Dependent on patient comprehension, include additional sitting/standing exercise to home program (hip flexion marching to 90 degrees, hip abduction, hip extension: all slow, controlled motions).
- Progressive gait training, including stair climbing (goals: ambulate 300 feet and climb 12 steps).
- Give written education on home program, fall prevention/home safety, on-line program.
One Week
- WBAT with walker/crutches.
- Convert to cane when abductors strength adequate, minimal limp, safe and confident.
Recovery time varies by individual. Most patients reach maximum functional level by 3 months post operation. Preoperative condition influences postoperative recovery time and outcome. Peak maximal medical improvement can take up to 12 months in deconditioned individuals.

39. **In what hand should a cane be used for a painful hip during gait?**
The cane is used in the hand opposite the affected hip. This decreases the workload on the ipsilateral abductor muscles and reduces joint forces. The also decreases pelvic drop on the side opposite the affected hip. The cane is advanced with the affected side. This upper extremity movement is consistent with normal gait.[15]

40. **What is proper technique for negotiating stairs with recent hip surgery?**
Just remember "Up with the Good. Down with the Bad."
- Going up steps: the unaffected, "good" leg advances up the stair first.
- Going down steps: the affected "bad" leg advances down the stair first with the crutch or cane.[15]

41. **What lower limb positions are associated with THA dislocations?**
Direction of dislocation correlates with surgical approach.
Risk for posterior dislocation: excessive flexion, adduction, and internal rotation.
Risk for anterior dislocation: hyperextension, adduction, and external rotation.

42. **What is the risk associated with lower lumbar spine stiffness or fusion and THA?**
Increased risk of THA dislocation. Lumbar spine pathology alters the biomechanics of spinopelvic mobility. Lumbosacral spinal fusions prior to THA increase the risk of dislocation within the first 6 months. Fusions involving the sacrum with multiple levels of lumbar involvement substantially increased the risk of THA dislocation.[16]

43. **What are some early postoperative complications after THA?**
Urinary retention, nerve injury, postoperative ileus (paralytic ileus), deep infection, deep vein thrombosis (DVT), pulmonary embolism (PE), or dislocation.

44. **Do all patients need DVT prophylaxis after THA?**
Yes! There are numerous treatment choices. Utilizing risk stratification scales helps choose the most appropriate chemoprophylaxis. Adjuvant mechanical prophylaxis includes pneumatic lower extremity compression devices and compression stockings. THA DVT prophylaxis is typically used for 35 days post operation.

45. **What are the initial laboratory screening tests for suspected infected THA?**
Serum erythrocyte sedimentation rate, C-reactive protein (CRP), and D dimer. If any abnormality, a hip aspiration is recommended to obtain synovial fluid. Analysis of the fluid includes a cell count with differential (absolute white blood cell [WBC] count and percentage neutrophils), α-defensin, CRP, leukocyte esterase, Gram stain, and microbiologic cultures.[17]

46. **When can patients begin to drive after THA?**
Two to 4 weeks. Improved surgical techniques, pain management, and accelerated rehabilitation programs have allowed some patients to safely return to driving as early as 2 weeks following THA. Drivers must be off narcotic medications, otherwise driving is unsafe and illegal. The most critical factor is braking reaction time which has been shown to return in approximately 80% of patients by 2 weeks. After contemporary left-sided THA, 1 week may be adequate for resuming driving.[18]

47. **What is the difference between primary (index, first) and revision (redo) THA?**
Complication risks after revision THA are all greater, including rates of infection, dislocation, fracture, and nerve injury. Functional and weight-bearing status may vary depending on the complexity of revision surgery. Factors include osteotomies performed, bone quality, and fixation methods.

48. **How do femoral osteotomies affect postoperative THA rehabilitation?**
Osteotomies are controlled bone cuts usually involving an extended trochanteric osteotomy. Cerclage wires/cables or plate/screw fixation aid in maintaining the osteotomized bone in its original position while healing. Osteotomies are more common in revision THA surgery. Limitations on postoperative weight bearing depend on the bone and fixation quality and typically last for 6 to 12 weeks or until radiographic evidence of bony union begins.

49. Are there restrictions regarding exercise and sports after THA recovery?

Despite improvements in surgical techniques and enhancements of implant material quality and durability, high-impact activities such as running and jumping are not recommended. Low-impact sports such as walking, hiking, cycling, swimming, golf, bowling, doubles tennis, and light weight exercise machines are considered acceptable.

50. What is FAI?

FAI is pathologic impingement of the femur and acetabulum. Two broad categories: cam type, which is due to lack of concavity of the femoral head-neck junction, and pincer type, which is caused by acetabular over coverage.[19]

51. What is extracorporeal shock wave therapy (ESWT)?

ESWT is a noninvasive therapy, using a high-energy acoustic wave for pain relief and improved blood circulation.

52. What are some established uses for ESWT around the hip?

Greater trochanteric pain syndrome, persisting pain after partial or total joint replacement, primary osteoarthritis, and early-stage osteonecrosis.[20,21]

REFERENCES

1. Birnbaum K, Prescher A, Hessler S, et al. The sensory innervation of the hip joint—an anatomical study. *Surg Radiol Anat.* 1997;19:371–375.
2. Brukner P, Khan K., et al.: *Clinical Sports Medicine.* 4th ed. North Ryde: McGraw-Hill; 2012: 510–575.
3. Sharrard W. The segmental innervation of the lower limb muscles in man. In: *Arris and Gale Lecture* delivered at the Royal College of Surgeons of England; 1964:106–122.
4. O'Dell MW, Lin CD, Panagos A. The physiatric history and physical examination. In: Cifu DX, Kaelin DL, et al., eds. *Braddom's Physical Medicine and Rehabilitation.* 5th ed. Philadelphia, PA: Elsevier; 2016:19.
5. Armstrong AD, Hubbard MC, eds. *Essentials of Musculoskeletal Care.* 5th ed. Rosemont, IL: American Academy of Orthopaedic Surgeons; 2016.
6. DeLee JC. Fractures and dislocations of the hip. In: Rockwood CA, Green DP, Bucholz RW, et al., eds. *Rockwood and Green's Fractures in Adults.* 4th ed. Philadelphia–New York, Lippincott: Raven; 1996:1659-1826.
7. Mont MA, Cherian JJ, Sierra RJ, et al. Nontraumatic osteonecrosis of the femoral head: Where do we stand today? A ten-year update. *J Bone Joint Surg Am.* 2015;97:1604.
8. Karkenny AJ, Tauberg BM, Otsuka NY. Pediatric hip disorders: slipped capital femoral epiphysis and Legg-Calvé-Perthes disease. *Pediatr Rev.* 2018;39(9):454-463.
9. Hansen PA, Willick SE. Musculoskeletal disorders of the lower limb. In: Cifu DX, Kaelin DL, eds. *Braddom's Physical Medicine and Rehabilitation.* 5th ed. Philadelphia, PA: Elsevier; 2016:795.
10. DeWeber P. Hip joint disorders: osteoarthritis and avascular necrosis. In: Miller MD, Hart J, eds. Essential Orthopeadics. W.B. Saunders Philadelphia, Pennsylvania; 2010:559-565.
11. Craig A, Richardson JK. Rehabilitation of patients with neuropathies. In: Cifu DX, Kaelin DL, eds. *Braddom's Physical Medicine and Rehabilitation.* 5th ed. Philadelphia, PA: Elsevier; 2016:936-937.
12. Payne JM. Ultrasound-guided hip procedures. *Phys Med Rehab Clin N Am.* 2016;27:607–29.
13. American Academy of Orthopaedic Surgeons/Fifth AJRR Annual Report (2018) on Hip and Knee Arthroplasty Data. Retrieved from www.aaos.org/ajrr.
14. Woodward JL. Lateral femoral cutaneous neuropathy. In: Frontera S, ed. *Essentials of Physical Medicine and Rehabilitation: Review and Assessment.* Philadelphia, PA: Hanley & Belfus, Inc.; 2003:127-128.
15. Houglum PA. Ambulation and ambulation aids. In: Houglum PA, ed. *Therapeutic Exercise for Musculoskeletal Injuries.* 4th ed. Champaign, IL: Human Kinetics; 2016:341-342.
16. Salib CG, Reina N, Perry KI, et al. Lumbar fusion involving the sacrum increases dislocation risk in primary total hip arthroplasty. *Bone Joint J.* 2019;101-B(2):198–206.
17. Parvizi J, Tan TL, Goswani K, et al. The 2018 definition of periprosthetic hip and knee infection: an evidence-based and validated criteria. *J Arthroplasty.* 2018;33:1309-1314.
18. Hernandez VH, Ong AC, Orozco F, et al. Returning to driving following total hip arthroplasty. *American Academy of Orthopaedic Surgeons 2015 Annual Meeting,* Las Vegas, Nevada, March 24, 2015.
19. Beaule PE, Byrd JW, Wilkins GP, et al. Nonarthroplasty joint-preserving surgery for hip disorders. In: Mont MA, Tanzer M, eds. *Orthopaedic Knowledge Update: Hip and Knee Reconstruction 5.* Rosemont, IL: American Academy of Orthopaedic Surgeons; 2017:327-328.
20. Korakakis V, Whiteley R, Tzavara A, et al. The effectiveness of extracorporeal shockwave therapy in common lower limb conditions: a systematic review including quantification of patient-rated pain reduction. *Br J Sports Med.* 2018;52(6):387-407.
21. Schmitz C, Császár NB, Milz S, et al. Efficacy and safety of extracorporeal shock wave therapy for orthopedic conditions: a systematic review on studies listed in the PEDro database. *Br Med Bull.* 2015;116:115-138.

CHAPTER 45

THE SHOULDER: ANATOMY, PATHOLOGY, AND DIAGNOSIS

Michelle A. Poliak-Tunis, MD, Brandon Bukovitz, MD, Matthew Cowling, DO, Michael J. Young, MD, MPhill, and Mark A. Young, MD, MBA, FACP, FAAPMR, DABPMR

Each generation of scientists stands upon the shoulders of those who have gone before.
—Owen Chamberlain (1920–2006)

ANATOMY AND BIOMECHANICS

1. **What makes up the shoulder girdle complex?**
   Due to the complexity and interrelationship of the shoulder and its surrounding structures, the term *shoulder girdle* is now preferred terminology over *shoulder joint*. It consists of the following six joints that contribute in various ways to its structure and function: glenohumeral (GH) joint, sternoclavicular joint, acromioclavicular (AC) joint, sternocostal joint, scapulocostal joint, and costovertebral joint (Fig. 45.1).

2. **What muscles are involved in the primary movements about the GH joint and scapulothoracic interface?**
   The muscles articulating the GH joint provide a wide range of motion (ROM), the most of any joint in the body. The primary muscles involved in articulation of this joint, and the motions they evoke, are:
   - Pectoralis major: flexion, internal rotation, adduction.
   - Anterior deltoid: flexion.
   - Posterior deltoid: extension, external rotation.
   - Latissimus dorsi: extension, internal rotation, adduction.
   - Teres major: internal rotation and external rotation, adduction.
   - Subscapularis: internal rotation, adduction.
   - Infraspinatus: external rotation.
   - Supraspinatus: abduction.
   - Deltoid: abduction.

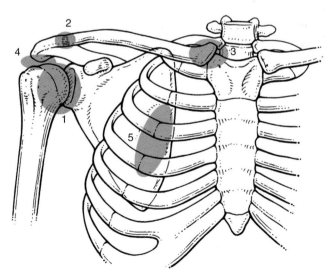

Fig. 45.1 1. Glenohumeral joint. 2. Acromioclavicular joint. 3. Sternoclavicular joint. 4. Subacromial joint. 5. Scapulothoracic joint. (Ombregt L. *A System of Orthopaedic Medicine*. 3rd ed. Edinburgh: Elsevier; 2013.)

The scapulothoracic interface displays much smaller and difficult to measure movements. The primary muscles that play a role in these motions, as well as their respective movements, are:
- Trapezius (whole): retraction, upward rotation.
- Upper trapezius: elevation.
- Lower trapezius: depression.
- Rhomboids: elevation, retraction, downward rotation.
- Pectoralis major: depression, protraction, downward rotation.
- Levator scapulae: elevation, downward rotation.
- Latissimus dorsi: depression.
- Serratus anterior: protraction, upward rotation.

3. What muscles comprise the rotator cuff?

The rotator cuff is composed of the **s**upraspinatus, **i**nfraspinatus, **t**eres minor, and **s**ubscapularis, often remembered through the mnemonic *SITS*. Dynamically, these muscles contract to abduct and forward flex the arm, contracting isometrically in the dependent arm to prevent subluxation. At rest they work to stabilize the GH joint (Fig. 45.2).

4. What muscles are considered the primary scapular stabilizers, and what exercises can be used to strengthen them?
- **Levator scapulae:** Seated press-ups, shoulder shrugs.
- **Rhomboids:** Prone arm lifts, standard rows, low rows.
- **Serratus anterior:** Punches, push-ups with a plus.
- **Teres major:** Pull-downs.
- **Trapezius:** Train/target complete scapular rotation.

5. Describe the importance of the scapula in shoulder function and rehabilitation.

GH articulation and motion use the scapula as a platform. Because of this, it is very common that the prime scapular stabilizers (the serratus anterior and lower trapezius) are reflexively inhibited after an injury to the shoulder. The result is a retracted and downwardly rotated scapula, which can exacerbate the primary shoulder pathology (e.g., rotator cuff disease or impingement). Initial rehabilitation steps usually include neuromuscular reeducation of the serratus anterior and lower trapezius, as well as strengthening.

6. Damage to which nerves and muscles causes scapular winging?

Muscle/Nerve	Resulting Scapula Position
Rhomboids/dorsal scapular	Protracted and upwardly rotated
Serratus anterior/long thoracic	Retracted and downwardly rotated
Trapezius/spinal accessory	Protracted and downwardly rotated

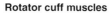

Rotator cuff muscles

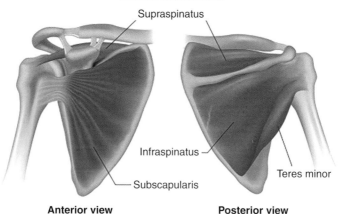

Supraspinatus

Infraspinatus

Subscapularis

Teres minor

Anterior view   **Posterior view**

Fig. 45.2 Rotator cuff musculature. (Source: Micallef J, Pandya J, Low AK. Management of rotator cuff tears in the elderly population. *Maturitas.* 2019;123:9–14.)

7. From which shoulder injuries do peripheral nerve syndromes originate? How do they manifest clinically?
   See Table 45.1.

8. Which anatomic structures of the shoulder are most commonly involved in shoulder impingement syndrome?
   - Biceps tendon
   - Supraspinatus
   - Subacromial bursa

9. What work-related factors affect the development of subacromial shoulder impingement?
   - Amount of weight lifted
   - Frequency of repetitions
   - Position of arm

10. What are the forces resisted by the AC and coracoclavicular (CC) ligaments?
    Normally, the CC ligaments resist axial and superior forces, while the AC ligaments resist anterior and posterior forces. However, excessive forces beyond normal physiologic loads may injure the AC joint and alter these roles; as AC ligaments fail to adequately resist anterior/posterior forces, the CC ligaments bear a greater than normal proportion of anterior/posterior forces, thereby increasing the susceptibility of the CC ligaments to damage as well.

Table 45.1 Shoulder Girdle Complex Peripheral Nerve Syndromes

JOINT	NERVE	MUSCLE(S)	CLINICAL MANIFESTATIONS	COMMON CAUSES
Scapulothoracic	Dorsal scapular n	Rhomboids, Levator scapulae	Protracted and upwardly rotated scapula, weakness of abduction (>90 degrees)	Scalene injury
	Accessory n (CN XI)	Trapezius	Protracted and downwardly rotated scapula, weakness of abduction	Radical neck dissection, direct trauma
	Long thoracic n	Serratus anterior	Retracted and downwardly rotated scapula	Neuralgic amyotrophy, trauma, compression, stretch or traction from repetitive activities
Glenohumeral	Axillary n	Deltoid and Teres Minor	Weakness of shoulder abduction (15–90 degrees) and external rotation; sensory loss over lateral shoulder	Shoulder dislocation, humerus fracture, neuralgic amyotrophy, anesthesia
	Suprascapular n	Supraspinatus and infraspinatus	Weakness initiating shoulder abduction and external rotation; ± shoulder pain	Entrapment at suprascapular notch or spinoglenoid notch, trauma, stretch or traction from repetitive movement, ganglion cyst or tumor
	Musculocutaneous n	Coracobrachialis, biceps brachii	Weakness of elbow flexion, supination, and flexion, adduction and abduction of shoulder	Trauma, shoulder dislocation, strenuous exercise, anesthesia
	Radial n	Triceps brachii (long head)	Sensory loss over posterior arm, forearm and dorsum of hand, wrist drop, weakness of shoulder adduction	"Saturday night palsy," fracture of midhumerus

CLINICAL PRESENTATION

11. What clinical tests suggest the diagnosis of a complete torn rotator cuff tear? How can the diagnosis be confirmed?

While a complete tear cannot be confirmed through any physical examination test, it is indicated clinically by the inability to rotate the arm externally, the inability to abduct the arm from dependency, and a positive **drop arm test**. Confirmation of the tear and evaluation of tendon damage can be aided by magnetic resonance imaging (MRI).

12. Can a complete rotator cuff tear be determined by another test besides faulty shoulder abduction?

Yes. Inability to externally rotate the arm indicates a complete rotator cuff. A complete tear would affect the portion of the rotator cuff represented by the tendinous insertion into the tuberosity from the supraspinatus and infraspinatus muscles, preventing external rotation.

13. How are shoulder impingement and rotator cuff disease indicated on MRI?
- Signal abnormalities of the rotator cuff.
- Subacromial fluid.
- AC arthropathy with downward-projecting osteophytes.
- Anterior acromial enthesophytes (Fig. 45.3).

14. After a traumatic anterior shoulder dislocation, what are common radiographic findings?

Traumatic shoulder dislocations involve a Bankart lesion (detachment of the anterior-inferior glenoid labrum from the glenoid rim) or injury to the anterior–inferior GH joint capsule (middle GH ligament or anterior band of the inferior GH ligament). A **bony** Bankart lesion can occur if there is a fracture of the anterior-inferior glenoid rim, whereas a **Hill-Sachs defect** happens when there is a compression fracture of the posterolateral aspect of the humeral head (Fig. 45.4).

15. What special maneuvers can clinically confirm an AC joint injury? Which other special tests evaluate injury to the shoulder girdle complex?
- **Cross body adduction test**—The patient flexes the arm forward with a fully extended elbow. The clinician then passively adducts the arm across the body's midline (Fig. 45.5).
- **AC shear testing**—The clinician places one hand on the scapula and pushes anteriorly; the other hand is placed on the midclavicle and simultaneously pushes posteriorly (see Fig. 45.6).
- **Active compression test**—There are two parts to the active compression test. The first part is similar to the "empty can" test; the patient's shoulder is flexed to 90 degrees with the elbow fully extended and the arm internally rotated so that the thumb points toward the ground. The patient then resists the clinician pulling the arm downwards (Fig. 45.7). The second part is identical to the first, except the patient supinates the arm so that the palm is facing up (Fig. 45.8).

16. What role does musculoskeletal ultrasound (MSK US) play in shoulder evaluation?

By using high-frequency sound waves (1 to 20 MHz) to produce high-resolution images of soft tissue structures, including ligaments, muscles, bursa, tendons, nerves, and bony surfaces, MSK US is a valuable evaluation technique.

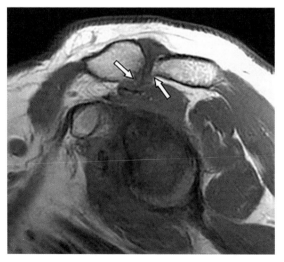

Fig. 45.3 Acromioclavicular joint osteophytes. The white arrows are pointing toward joint osteophytes. (Source: Tuite MJ. Magnetic resonance imaging of rotator cuff disease and external impingement. *Magn Reson Imaging Clin N Am.* 2012;20[2]:187–200.)

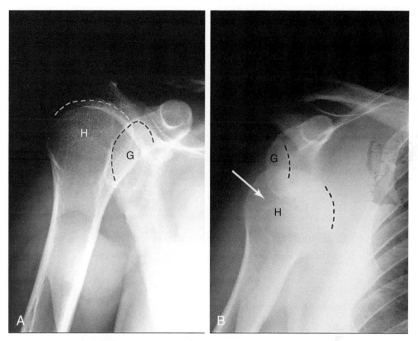

Fig. 45.4 Anterior dislocation of the shoulder. (A) In the normal anteroposterior view of the shoulder, the humeral head (H) is located lateral to the glenoid (G) with a small amount of overlap. (B) With anterior dislocation, the humeral head goes inferiorly and medially with respect to the glenoid (arrow).

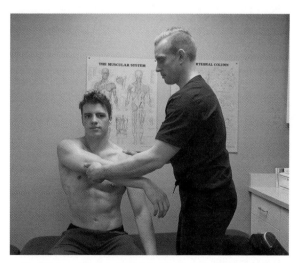

Fig. 45.5 Acromioclavicular joint injury clinical tests. Cross body adduction.

Advantages of MSK US include no ionizing radiation, portability, low-cost, dynamic imaging ability, minimal artifact from metal implant, providing physiologic information, cost, allowing real-time "side-to-side" comparison, and optimized interaction between the examiner and the patient. Potential disadvantages of US include nonpenetrance of bony structures, not being able to identify intramedullary lesions, and inability to penetrate bone and calcific tissue. It is most appropriate to use US when the patient's symptoms are relatively localized. Skill of the examiner determines the quality of the image.

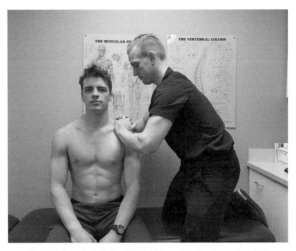

Fig. 45.6 Acromioclavicular (AC) joint injury clinical tests. AC shear test.

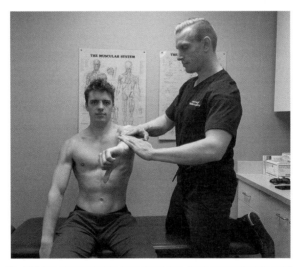

Fig. 45.7 Acromioclavicular joint injury clinical tests. Active compression test, part 1.

DIFFERENTIAL DIAGNOSIS

17. What are the stages of adhesive capsulitis ("frozen shoulder")?
    While adhesive capsulitis traditionally has three stages, these represent a fluid progression of the disease as opposed to distinct phases:

Stages of Adhesive Capsulitis

Stage I: "The painful phase"	Spontaneous shoulder pain with ensuing stiffness; lasts 2.5–9 months
Stage II: "The stiff phase"	Continued shoulder stiffness but improved pain; lasts 4–12 months
Stage III: "The resolution phase"	Gradual functional recovery with a progressive increase in shoulder range of motion; lasts 5–26 months

18. What are the two types of shoulder impingement?
    - **Primary outlet impingement** is more common in patients 40 years of age or older and involves extrinsic compression of the rotator cuff and/or biceps tendon by the acromion or coracoacromial ligament. This can be

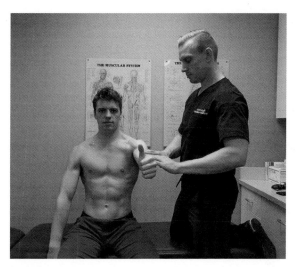

Fig. 45.8 Acromioclavicular joint injury clinical tests. Active compression test, part 2.

exacerbated by an exaggerated thoracic kyphosis, hooked acromion, subacromial osteophyte, and/or protracted and downwardly rotated scapula.
- **Secondary (internal or glenoid) impingement** is more common in young athletes who participate in frequent overhead-throwing motions. It involves irritation of the articular (glenoid) side of the rotator cuff tendons.

19. **What are the types of AC joint separation and how are they treated?**
The Rockwood classification is summarized as follows:

Rockwood Classification of AC Joint Separation

Type	*Treatment*
I. AC ligament sprain	Nonoperative
II: Torn AC and sprained CC ligaments	Nonoperative
III: Torn AC and CC ligaments; CC space is 25%–100% widened	Controversial (tending toward nonoperative)
IV: Type III with clavicle displaced posteriorly	Operative
V: Type III with CC space widened > 100% and deltoid and trapezius are detached from distal clavicle	Operative
VI: Type III with clavicle displaced inferiorly through or behind the biceps tendon	Operative

AC, Acromioclavicular; *CC*, coracoclavicular.

20. **Describe the mechanism, diagnosis, and management of shoulder subluxation.**
Shoulder stability is maintained by the GH capsule and the rotator cuff muscles. Subluxation is partial GH dislocation, resulting from direct trauma or acute stroke, the latter of which invokes frailty in the supraspinatus muscle. It can be managed through mechanical or electrical contraction of the supraspinatus muscle or proper positioning to avoid downward traction.

21. **Besides rotator cuff disease, what other differential diagnoses must be considered when evaluating shoulder pain?**

Differential Diagnosis of Shoulder Pain

Suprascapular nerve entrapment	Bicipital tendinopathy
Shoulder instability	Gallbladder disease
AC degenerative joint disease	Cervical radiculitis
Cardiac ischemia	Cervical facet syndrome (cervical spondylosis)
Diaphragmatic irritation	Upper lobe/pleural irritation
Capsulitis (frozen shoulder)	

AC, Acromioclavicular.

TREATMENT

22. List the six phases of general shoulder rehabilitation.
    1. Pain and inflammation management
    2. Motion restoration
    3. Neuromuscular strengthening and retraining
        a. Scapular stabilizers (generally the first to be rehabilitated)
        b. Rotator cuff muscles
        c. Prime movers
    4. Proprioceptive training
    5. Endurance training
    6. Task-specific or sport-specific activity reinstatement

23. How is rotator cuff tendinitis treated?
    Treatment begins with restriction of painful motion, consistent ice application, 4 to 6 weeks of nonsteroidal anti-inflammatory drugs (NSAIDs), and physical therapy (PT) exercises within a pain-free range. To avoid a loss of motion, the focus should be placed on stretching, followed by activation and strengthening of the scapular stabilizers and rotator cuff (if necessary). Subacromial corticosteroid injection may help with consistent pain.

24. How is a frozen shoulder best treated?

KEY POINTS: TREATMENT OF A STIFF SHOULDER

1. Aggressive passive (then active-assisted) ROM
2. Medications for pain relief (especially before stretching):
    a. NSAIDs and/or nonnarcotic and narcotic analgesics orally
    b. Intra-articular steroids or oral steroids
3. Manipulation under anesthesia
4. Arthroscopic or open surgical evaluation and adhesion release, followed by aggressive PT
5. Hospitalization with an indwelling interscalene catheter and aggressive PT.

25. What is the treatment for severe arthritis of the shoulder?
    Treatment focuses on maintaining ROM through ice and heat application, stretching, and NSAIDs. If nonoperative treatment is unsuccessful, joint replacement of either the humeral head (hemiarthroplasty) or the humeral head and socket/glenoid (total shoulder replacement) is the best surgical option. Reverse prosthesis can be used to treat severe arthritis with rotator cuff tears. A one- or two-night hospital stay is typical, and rehabilitation begins the day after surgery (Table 45.2).

26. What is the treatment for shoulder instability?
    Careful positioning and muscle strengthening may be enough to control shoulder instability in some cases. If necessary, open-incision or arthroscopic surgery can be used to repair the torn labrum to the glenoid rim (Bankart repair) and shorten the ligaments (capsular shift). Following surgery, the arm is put in a sling for 3 weeks to tighten the ligaments. Rehabilitation is similar to the open procedure (Table 45.3). While shifting has been described, is it only currently used in specific cases.

27. List the types of potential therapeutic and/or diagnostic shoulder girdle complex injections and their anatomic sites.

Complex Injections

Injection Location	Anatomic Structure
Anterior	• Acromioclavicular joint
	• Glenohumeral joint
	• Sternoclavicular joint
	• Biceps tendon sheath
Lateral/posterolateral	• Subacromial bursa (Subdeltoid bursa)
Posterior	• Glenohumeral joint

28. How can active-passive shoulder movement be initiated?
    Pendulum (Codman) exercises initiate active-passive motion of the GH joint. These are simple exercises and involve the patient bent forward, with the arm in the dependent (pendular) position and the body "actively" moving to "passively" move the pendular arm.

29. What is the rehabilitation process following shoulder replacement?
    While elevation in front of the body can be instituted soon after surgery, external rotation should be avoided for 6 to 8 weeks. Stiffness is common, and strength-building exercises are important. However, most patients do not entirely regain normal motion. Infection is the most serious complication and is often indicated if there is still

Table 45.2 Rehabilitation After Total Shoulder Replacement.

DURATION	TREATMENT	PRECAUTIONS
Phase 1		
0–3 weeks	• Gentle passive and active ROM to full flexion as tolerated, abduction to 90 degrees, internal rotation and external rotation • Pendulum exercises • Isometric strengthening as tolerated • One-handed ADLs	• No weight bearing • Sling worn at all times, except with exercise • Avoid active abduction, extension >0 degrees, and external rotation
3–6 weeks	• Vigorous isometrics as tolerated • Active-assisted progressing to active ROM • "Wall-walking" with hand used as stabilizer	• Continue sling at night and non–weight bearing • May begin active abduction
Phase 2		
6–12 weeks	• Vigorous isometrics • Progressive isotonics • Active-assisted ROM and active ROM past 90 degrees • Two-handed ADLs encouraged	• May lift up to 2 lb • Discontinue sling • Discontinue ROM precautions in external rotation • Can begin to work on external rotation
Phase 3		
>12 weeks	• Active ROM exercises, progressive resistance, strengthening • Stretching in flexion, abduction, and rotation	Discontinue ROM precautions

ADLs, Activities of daily living; *ROM*, range of motion.

Table 45.3 Rehabilitation After Bankart and Capsular Shift (Open), Bankart and Shift (Arthroscopic), and Thermal Capsulorraphy[a]

DURATION	TREATMENT	PRECAUTIONS
Phase 1		
0–3 weeks	• Passive ROM in abduction in scapular plane • Passive ROM in ER to operative limit • Pendulum exercises • Begin scapular retraction and depression exercises • Active flexion as tolerated • After 1 week, add active-assisted ROM for ER to operative limit • Gradually progress to isometric flexion and ER without weight below shoulder level	• No weight bearing • No active ER Wear immobilizer to sleep and for most of the day for 2 weeks, then just to sleep
Phase 2		
3–6 weeks	• Progressive isotonic exercises (e.g., elastic-tubing exercises) as tolerated • Full ROM forward flexion, abduction • Progressive ER as tolerated after 4–6 weeks	May lift objects up to 2 lb
6–9 weeks	• Progressive isotonic exercises as tolerated • Emphasis on gently regaining ER	• Discontinue night bracing • May lift objects up to 5 lb
Phase 3		
9–12 weeks	• Begin isokinetic IR/ER/FF, abduction • Active ROM exercises, progressive resistance, strengthening • Stretching in flexion, abduction, and rotation	Discontinue all ROM precautions

[a]In thermal shift, motion of the shoulder is not begun for 3 weeks.
ER, External rotation; *FF*, forward flexion; *IR*, internal rotation; *ROM*, range of motion.

drainage from the wound 4 to 5 days post surgery. If the subscapularis tendon repair fails, dislocation of the prosthesis can occur.

30. **What does post–rotator cuff repair rehabilitation entail?**
    See Table 45.4.

31. **How is shoulder arthroscopy indicated?**
    Although shoulder arthroscopy indication is often for diagnostic purposes, the following conditions can be arthroscopically assessed and treated: rotator cuff disease, shoulder instability, biceps tendon and labral pathology, impingement, GH and AC joint arthritis, adhesive capsulitis, and loose bodies.

32. **How are burners (stingers) managed?**
    Initially, strength is improved with eccentric and concentric loading. Chest-out posturing maximally opens the neural foramina, thereby reducing the weight of the head on the nerve roots. As pain-free mobility is restored, sport-specific activities and correction of suboptimal techniques are encouraged. Protective equipment is necessary to reduce the risk of recurrence after recovery.

33. **What is the treatment for shoulder pain following spinal cord injury?**
    First line treatment for shoulder pain in the context of spinal cord injury is generally conservative, consisting of minimizing overuse in tandem with modification and optimization of activities of daily living. Therapeutic exercises yield improved long-term results. This may entail a 12-week course which focuses on incremental isometric exercises which strengthen the rotator cuff muscles. Some patients require corticosteroid injections to tolerate PT/occupational therapy (OT) exercise sessions. Surgical repair may be indicated in limited cases refractory to conservative measures in which spinal cord injury is complicated by tendinous injury.

Finnoff J. *Musculoskeletal Ultrasound of the Shoulder.* Available at: https://www.uptodate.com/ contents/ musculoskeletal-ultrasound-of-the-shoulder. Updated April 2018.

Mettler FA Jr. Skeletal system. In: *Essentials of Radiology.* 4th ed. Philadelphia, PA: Elsevier; 2019.

Youmans J, Winn H. *Neurological Surgery.* 7th ed. Philadelphia, PA: Elsevier; 2017.

Van Straaten MG, Cloud BA, Zhao KD, et al. Maintaining shoulder health after spinal cord injury: a guide to understanding treatments for shoulder pain. *Arch Phys Med Rehab,* 2017;98(5):1061–1063.

Waldman SD, Campbell RSD. *Imaging of Pain.* Philadelphia, PA: Saunders; 2010.

Table 45.4 Rehabilitation After Rotator Cuff Repair.

DURATION	TREATMENT	PRECAUTIONS
Phase 1		
0–3 weeks	• Elbow, wrist, finger ROM • Passive ROM in abduction in scapular plane • Passive ROM in forward flexion • Pendulum exercises • Begin scapular retraction and depression exercises	• No weight bearing • No active ROM above table level • Sling or immobilizer at all times except exercise Avoid arm adduction across body and internal rotation; avoid shoulder extension and external rotation as dictated by surgeon
Phase 2		
4–6 weeks	• Start active-assisted ROM in flexion and abduction • Active ROM of flexion less than 90 degrees	• Start active ROM No lifting of objects causing axial distraction
6–8 weeks	• Continue active-assisted ROM • Isometric strengthening as tolerated by pain in flexion, extension, and internal and external rotation	Patient allowed to use arms in front of body, below shoulder level
8–10 weeks	• Progressively more vigorous isometrics • Progressive isotonic exercises	
Phase 3		
10–12 weeks	• Active ROM exercises, progressive • Discontinue ROM precautions, resistance, strengthening • Stretching in flexion, abduction, and rotation	

ROM, Range of motion.

ACKNOWLEDGEMENT

The authors wish to thank Drs. Harrast, Caillet, McFarland, Chao, and Tasaki for their wonderful work on the previous edition of this chapter.

CHAPTER 46

THE ELBOW: ANATOMY, PATHOLOGY, AND MANAGEMENT

Asad Riaz Siddiqi, DO, Christopher S. Ahmad, MD, and Michael Lee Knudsen, MD

You have to have sharp elbows if you want to change something.

—James Carville

KEY POINTS

1. The humerus forms a hinge joint with the ulna to facilitate flexion/extension and a pivot joint with the radial head to facilitate supination/pronation.
2. The coronoid process of the ulna is an important structure for elbow stability, serving as a bony restraint against posterior translation and varus stress, and an attachment site for the medial ulnar collateral ligament and anterior joint capsule.
3. Overuse injuries of the elbow are initially managed conservatively with rest, activity modification, and therapeutic exercise, while surgery is indicated in cases where elbow stability is grossly compromised.

ELBOW ANATOMY AND BIOMECHANICS

1. Which bones comprise the elbow joint, and how do these articulations facilitate movement?
   The distal humerus articulates with the proximal ulna and radius individually, allowing for flexion/extension of the elbow and supination/pronation of the forearm.

   The ulna articulates with the distal humerus and the trochlear notch, and flexion/extension primarily occurs at this synovial hinge joint (Fig. 46.1).

   The radius articulates with the distal humerus at the capitellum, and supination/pronation occurs through the longitudinal axis of rotation at the radial head at this synovial pivot joint.

   The proximal radius and ulna also articulate via a synovial pivot joint.

Laratta J, Caldwell J-M, Lombardi J, et al. Evaluation of common elbow pathologies: a focus on physical examination. *Phys Sportsmed.* 2017;45(2):184–190.

2. What is the total elbow range of motion (ROM), and what is the functional ROM required for activities of daily living?
   The ranges of motion are found in the following table.

Motion	Total Range	Functional Range
Flexion/Extension	0–140 degrees	30–130 degrees
Pronation	75 degrees	50 degrees
Supination	85 degrees	50 degrees

The muscles facilitating these motions are found as follows.

Movement	Muscle	Nerve Supply
Flexion	Biceps brachii	Musculocutaneous (C5, C6)
	Brachioradialis	Radial (C5, C6)
	Brachialis	Musculocutaneous (C5, C6)
Extension	Triceps brachii	Radial (C6–C8)
	Anconeus	Radial (C7, C8)
Supination	Biceps brachii	Musculocutaneous (C5, C6)
	Supinator	Radial (C5, C6)
Pronation	Pronator quadratus	Median (anterior interosseous) (C8, T1)
	Pronator teres	Median (C6, C7)

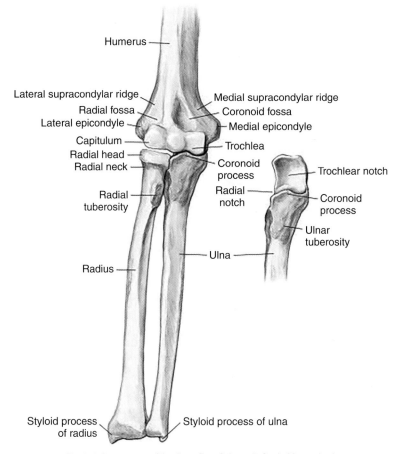

Fig. 46.1 Bony anatomy of the elbow. (From Orthopaedic Surgical Approaches.)

3. What is the normal anatomic elbow angulation?
   The measure of normal anatomic valgus elbow alignment (cubitus valgus) known as the "carrying angle" is the angle between the upper arm and forearm when the elbow is fully extended. This angulation allows the forearm to clear the hip when standing and walking, which is important for carrying objects. The carrying angle measures 5 to 10 degrees in males and 10 to 15 degrees in females. Greater than 20 degrees is considered abnormal.

ANTERIOR ELBOW

4. Describe the role of the coronoid process in maintaining elbow stability.
   The coronoid process acts as a bony restraint against the posterior translation of the ulna and varus elbow stress and serves as the attachment site of the anterior joint capsule, brachialis muscle, and medial ulnar collateral ligament (UCL) (a primary stabilizer against valgus stress).

Source: Hull JR, Owen JR, Fern SE, Wayne JS, Boardman ND. Role of the coronoid process in varus osteoarticular stability of the elbow. *J Shoulder Elbow Surg*. 2005;14(4):441–446.

LATERAL ELBOW

5. **What is lateral epicondylosis (tennis elbow)?**

   Tennis elbow is a common overuse injury in middle-aged individuals who participate in repetitive wrist extension activities, leading to angiofibroblastic hyperplasia at the origin of the extensor carpi radialis brevis (ECRB) on the lateral epicondyle. It is the most common cause of elbow symptoms in patients with elbow pain. Pain worsens with resisted wrist extension or gripping activities and palpation of the ECRB origin (a few millimeters distal to the tip of the lateral epicondyle). Plain radiographs are usually normal, and MRI is not necessary for diagnosis. Treatment involves rest, analgesics, bracing, progressive loading with physical therapy, and ergonomic optimization. Injections and surgery may be indicated in refractory cases. Confounding diagnoses include radioulnar or radiohumeral bursitis, annular or collateral ligament sprains, osteoarthritis of the radioulnar joint, or radial nerve entrapment at the supinator or arcade of Fröhse.

Shiri R, Viikari-Juntura E, Varonen H, Heliövaara M. Prevalence and determinants of lateral and medial epicondylitis: a population study. *Am J Epidemiol.* 2006;164(11):1065–1074.

6. **What is valgus extension overload? What causes it?**

   Valgus extension overload is seen in the dominant arm of throwing athletes, particularly baseball pitchers, due to the generation of excessive shear forces at the medial elbow, compression at the radiocapitellar joint, and tensioning of the medial UCL with the forceful valgus moment created by throwing. This can lead to osteophyte formation at the olecranon tip and posteromedial humerus, cartilage injury, osteochondral lesions of the capitellum, loose body formation, and attenuation of the medial collateral ligament (MCL) with repetitive strain.

Paulino FE, Villacis DC, Ahmad CS. Valgus extension overload in baseball players. *Am J Orthop (Belle Mead NJ).* 2016;45(3):144–151.

7. **What is osteochondritis dissecans of the elbow?**

   This condition is characterized by idiopathic injury to and eventual separation of the articular cartilage and subchondral bone of the capitellum, resulting in elbow pain, loss of elbow extension, and catching/locking symptoms if loose bodies are present (late symptom). It typically affects adolescent gymnasts and throwers and is thought to result from a repetitive compression-type injury to the immature capitellum. Stable lesions are typically managed with activity cessation, and unstable lesions are managed surgically.

Churchill RW, Munoz J, Ahmad CS. Osteochondritis dissecans of the elbow. *Curr Rev Musculoskelet Med.* 2016;9(2):232–239.

MEDIAL ELBOW

8. **What is medial epicondylosis (golfer's elbow)?**

   Medial epicondylosis is an overuse injury affecting the enthesis and tendinous origin of the flexor-pronator mass. Similar to lateral epicondylosis, this condition typically affects middle-aged adults. Pain is present with hand grip and resisted wrist flexion/pronation with the elbow extended. Poor ergonomics in occupational or sports activities involving gripping, pulling, and lifting may contribute to pain and histologic change. Treatment involves rest, analgesics, bracing, progressive loading with physical therapy, and ergonomic optimization. Injections and surgery may be indicated in refractory cases.

Shiri R, Viikari-Juntura E, Varonen H, Heliövaara M. Prevalence and determinants of lateral and medial epicondylitis: a population study. *Am J Epidemiol.* 2006;164(11):1065–1074.

9. **What is little leaguer's elbow?**

   Little leaguer's elbow refers to a spectrum of medial elbow overuse injuries in children and adolescents, where throwing sports result in a repetitive valgus stress to the skeletally immature medial elbow. The spectrum of injuries can include medial epicondyle avulsion fractures, UCL injuries, and flexor-pronator mass strains. Presentation is pain and tenderness over the medial elbow, associated with decreased throwing speed, accuracy, and distance. Radiographs may show physeal widening or avulsion of the medial epicondyle. MRI may show increased edema of the medial epicondyle apophysis (apophysitis). The mainstay of treatment is rest and activity modification; however, surgical intervention is indicated for displaced medial epicondyle avulsion fractures. Enforcement of pitch counts, avoiding year-round participation in throwing activities, and counseling to not throw through arm pain are important preventative strategies.

10. Which forearm flexor is not involved in medial epicondylosis?
    Palmaris longus.

POSTERIOR ELBOW

11. What is olecranon bursitis? How is it treated?
    Olecranon bursitis is inflammation or irritation of the olecranon bursa, which can result in pain and swelling over the olecranon process. In septic olecranon bursitis, the infected bursa may cause the posterior elbow to become red or warm and can result in systemic signs of infection. A septic bursa is ruled out by aspiration, Gram stain, and culture. Radiographs can rule out osteomyelitis and bone spurs. Treatment of septic bursitis includes antibiotics, aspiration, and surgery, while treatment of aseptic olecranon bursitis includes elbow rest, protective padding, nonsteroidal antiinflammatory drugs (NSAIDs), maintenance of functional ROM, aspiration (often unsuccessful), or local cortisone injection. Complication rates for corticosteroid injections in aseptic bursitis are reported as high as 20%, with skin atrophy seen more commonly. Surgical intervention is very rarely required for aseptic bursitis and is associated with a higher rate (16%) of iatrogenic infection.

Sayegh ET, Strauch RJ. Treatment of olecranon bursitis: a systematic review. *Arch Orthop Trauma Surg.* 2014;134:1517–1536.

NERVE PATHOLOGY

12. Describe the major nerve entrapment syndromes about the elbow, including involved nerves, locations of compression, and associated impairments.

PRONATOR SYNDROME (MEDIAN NERVE)

- Location of compression: (1) Ligament of Struthers; (2) Between the heads of pronator teres; (3) Flexor digitorum superficialis; (4) Lacertus fibrosis.
- Sensory impairment: Paresthesias/Numbness in the volar forearm and digits 1 to 3.
- Motor impairment: Weakness of the wrist and finger flexors.

POSTERIOR INTEROSSEOUS NERVE SYNDROME (DEEP BRANCH OF THE RADIAL NERVE)

- Location of Compression: (1) Between brachialis and brachioradialis; (2) Proximal edge of supinator (arcade of Fröhse); (3) Distal edge of supinator; (4) Lateral edge of ECRB; (5) Recurrent radial vessels (leash of Henry).
- Sensory impairment: None.
- Motor impairment: Weakness of the wrist.

CUBITAL TUNNEL SYNDROME (ULNAR NERVE)

- Location of Compression: (1) Between the heads of flexor carpi ulnaris (FCU); (2) Arcade of Struthers; (3) Between Osborne ligament and medial ulnar collateral ligament (MUCL); (4) Anconeus epitrochlearis (anomalous accessory muscle found in 28% of cadavers).
- Sensory Impairment: Paresthesias/Numbness in the ulnar aspect of the forearm and digits 4 to 5.
- Motor Impairment: Weakness of grasp, pinch, and finger abduction/adduction.

Lubahn JD, Cermak MB. Uncommon nerve compression syndromes of the upper extremity. *J Am Acad Orthop Surg.* 1998;6:378–386.

Staples JR, Calfee R. Cubital tunnel syndrome: current concepts. *J Am Acad Orthop Surg.* 2017;25(10):e215-e224.

Nellans K, Galdi B, Kim HM, Levine WN. Ulnar neuropathy as a result of anconeus epitrochlearis. *Orthopedics.* 2014;37(8):e743-745.

13. What is radial tunnel syndrome, and how is it different from posterior interosseous nerve syndrome?
    While both purportedly involve compression of the posterior interosseous nerve, radial tunnel syndrome is characterized only by pain along the dorsoradial aspect of the arm without weakness of the wrist and finger extensors. Compression occurs at the same sites as in posterior interosseous nerve (PIN) syndrome, but electromyography (EMG) findings are typically normal in radial tunnel syndrome.

ELBOW TRAUMA

14. What is a Galeazzi fracture?
    It is a fracture of the distal third radial shaft with an injury (dislocation or subluxation) of the distal radioulnar joint (DRUJ). Radial shaft fractures occurring closer to the wrist (<7.5 cm from the wrist joint) have a greater chance of concomitant DRUJ instability.

15. What is a Monteggia fracture?

It is a fracture of the proximal third of the ulna with concomitant dislocation of the radial head. It is classified based on the direction of dislocation of the radial head, with anterior dislocation being the most common.

Adams JE. Forearm instability: anatomy, biomechanics, and treatment options. *J Hand Surg Am*. 2017;42(1):47–52.

RECOMMENDED READINGS

1. Kuremsky MA, Cain EL, Dugas JR, Andrews JR. Elbow anatomy and biomechanics. In: Miller MD, Thompson SR, eds. *DeLee & Drez's Orthopaedic Sports Medicine*. 4th ed. Philadelphia, PA: W.B. Saunders; 2015: 715–720.
2. Kuremsky MA, Cain EL, Dugas JR, Andrews JR. Elbow tendinopathies and bursitis. In: Miller MD, Thompson SR, eds. *DeLee & Drez's Orthopaedic Sports Medicine*. 4th ed. Philadelphia, PA: W.B. Saunders; 2015:750-760.
3. Chin TY, Chou H, Peh WCG. The acutely injured elbow. *Radiol Clin North Am*. 2019;57(5):911–930.

WEBSITES

1. American Academy of Physical Medicine and Rehabilitation. Available at: https://www.aapmr.org/about-physiatry/conditions-treatments.
2. The American Medical Society for Sports Medicine website created by the computer geek. Available at: https://www.sportsmedtoday.com/elbow-ct-12.htm.
3. OrthoInfo. Available at: https://www.orthoinfo.org/en/search/?q=elbow.

Bonus questions and answers are available online.

CHAPTER 47

THE KNEE: ANATOMY, PATHOLOGY, DIAGNOSIS, AND REHABILITATION

Michael Frederick Saulle, DO, FAAPMR, CAQSM, Bryan J. O'Young, MD, CAc, FAAPMR, and Robert G. Trasolini, DO

Never, never, never give up.

— Winston Churchill (1874–1965)

KEY POINTS

1. Diagnosis is the key to correcting knee pain. A thorough history and physical exam are crucial.
2. Instability of the knee requires a detailed workup and should not be ignored.
3. Always evaluate the joints above and below the knee for dysfunction or pathology
4. The knee is a complex joint that is responsible for the stability of the leg. To best understand and diagnose knee pathology, one must first master knee biomechanics.

1. **How does one view the knee from a musculoskeletal viewpoint?**
   It is helpful to evaluate the knee by categorizing it as anterior, medial, lateral, posterior, and intraarticular anatomical divisions. See Fig. 47.1.

2. **What are the two primary joints of the knee?**
   - Tibiofemoral: Largest joint in the body; provides a great range of motion (ROM) in flexion and extension, limited rotation, and minimal adduction and abduction
   - Patellofemoral: Protects the anterior knee; provides a mechanical advantage for the quadriceps unit

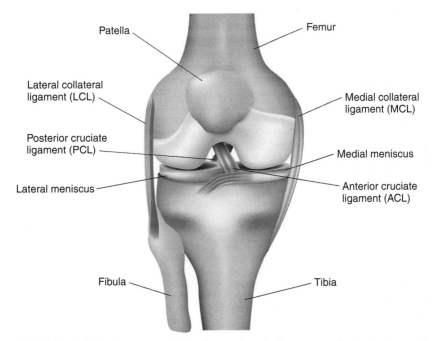

Fig. 47.1 Anterior view of the knee and its structures. (Obtained from https://www.osgpc.com/anatomy-of-the-knee/)

3. What is the normal range of motion of the knee and how is this measured?

ROM should be measured from the lateral side of the patient's leg with a goniometer. Full-extension, an angle between the femur and tibia of 0 degrees, should be recorded as 0 degrees. Full flexion is recorded as a positive number, somewhere between 0 and 135 degrees. If the patient's leg cannot be fully extended, the number of degrees possible short of full extension is recorded as a positive number. For example, the patient who lacks 10 degrees of full extension but can flex to 100 degrees should be recorded as having a ROM +10 to 110 degrees. If the patient's knee comes to hyperextension, the amount past 0 degrees should be recorded as a negative number. For example, if the patient hyperextends approximately 5 degrees and flexes to 100 degrees, the ROM is recorded as −5 to 100 degrees.

4. Describe the basic kinematics of patella.

- The patella facilitates knee extension by acting as a fulcrum to optimize quadriceps function. The efficiency of the extensor muscles is increased by 150% due to the mechanical advantage provided by the patella
- The patella also acts as a centering force for the pull of the four converging quadriceps muscles (rectus femoris vastus lateralis, vastus medialis, and vastus intermedius).

5. What is the "screw home mechanism" of the knee?

- Key element to knee stability
- "Screw" refers to the rotation between the tibia and femur. External rotation occurs during the terminal degrees of knee extension and results in the tightening of both cruciate ligaments, which locks the knee. The tibia is then in the position of maximal stability with respect to the femur.
- It occurs at the end of knee extension, between 20 degrees of knee flexion and full extension (0 degrees).
- The tibia rotates internally during the open-chain movements (swing phase) and externally during closed chain movements (stance phase).

6. Describe how open and closed chain movements affect the knee.

- Open chain:
  - *Extension*: Tibia glides anteriorly on the femur. At 20 degrees of knee flexion through full extension, the tibia rotates externally.
  - *Flexion*: Tibia glides posteriorly on the femur, and from full knee extension to 20 degrees flexion, the tibia rotates internally.
- Closed chain:
  - *Extension*: femur glides posteriorly on the tibia. From 20 degrees knee flexion to full extension, the femur rotates internally on the stable tibia.
  - *Flexion*: femur glides anteriorly on the tibia, and from full knee extension to 20 degrees flexion, the femur rotates externally on the stable tibia.

7. What is extensor lag?

Extensor lag refers to the inability to fully extend the knee actively, although a passively full extension is possible. This results from lengthening of the extensor mechanism or weakening of the quadriceps. Component malposition may also produce this problem.

8. What is the significance of Q angle on the knee joint?

- The **quadriceps angle (Q angle)** or **patellofemoral angle** is the angle formed between a line drawn from the anterior superior iliac spine (ASIS) to the midpoint of the patella and a line drawn from the tibial tubercle to the midpoint of the patella with the hip and foot in a neutral position.
- A normal angle is 13 to 18 degrees (although if the quadriceps is contracted, the normal angle is 8 to 10 degrees).
- The angle in men tends to be smaller than in women. Larger angles may produce added biomechanical stress during vigorous or repetitive activities using the knee.

9. What are rehabilitation strategies to improve excessive Q angle?

The most effective way **to decrease a high Q angle** and lower the biomechanical stresses on the knee joint is to prevent excessive pronation with orthotics. Stretching of tight muscles and strengthening of weak muscles should be included in the therapeutic program. Muscles commonly found to be tight include the quadriceps, hamstrings, iliotibial band, and gastrocnemius muscles. Closed-chain exercises (such as wall squats), performed only to 30 degrees of flexion, are currently recommended.

10. When evaluating knee alignment, what are genu valgum, varum, and recurvatum?

- Genu Valgum: term for knock-kneed appearance. May be seen with larger Q angles. More common in women.
- Genu Varum: term for bow-legged appearance. May have disproportionate stress on the medial compartment of the knee
- Genu Recurvatum: Knee hyperextension or back-kneed.

11. What is the purpose of the knee meniscus?

The meniscus is a half-moon–shaped piece of cartilage that lies between the weight-bearing joint surfaces of the femur and the tibia. It is triangular in cross-section and is attached to the lining of the knee joint along its periphery. There are two menisci in a normal knee; the outer one is called the lateral meniscus and the inner one is the medial meniscus. Their purposes include lubrication, load sharing, proprioception, and reducing contact stresses at the articular surface. Only the peripheral 25% to 30% of menisci are vascular.

12. List the ligaments of the knee and their function.
   - Anterior cruciate ligament (ACL):
     - Primary: Prevents anterior displacement of the tibia on the femur
     - Secondary: Prevents hyperextension. Limits varus/valgus stress and rotation.
   - Posterior cruciate ligament (PCL):
     - Primary: Prevents posterior displacement of the tibia on the femur.
     - Secondary: Assists in the screw home mechanism and limits varus/valgus stress.
   - **Medial collateral ligament (MCL):** Provides ~80% of valgus stability (resists knee valgus). There are superficial and deep layers with the latter sharing fibers with the medial meniscus.
   - **Anterolateral Ligament (ALL):** Importance and function are controversial. Thought to play a role in anterolateral rotational stability of the knee
   - **Lateral collateral ligament (LCL): Also known as** the fibular collateral ligament. It provides ~70% varus stability.

13. What anatomic structures may cause referred pain to the knee?
   Lumbar spine, hip joint, sacroiliac joint, femur, ankle joint, and/or foot.

ANTERIOR KNEE

14. What is the differential diagnosis for anterior knee pain?
   See Table 47.1

15. Identify two key abnormal positions of the patella.
   - Patella alta: Superior position of patella on femur. Decreased patellofemoral contact area leading to chondromalacia. May also be seen in cerebral palsy and spasticity.
   - Patella baja: Inferior location relative to femoral trochlea; often results from soft tissue contracture (scarring) and hypotonia of the quadriceps muscle (abnormally weak function) after surgery or trauma to the knee. Patella baja typically leads to a stiff and less functional knee.

16. Describe the typical signs and symptoms of patellofemoral pain.
   - Anterior knee pain with a gradual onset that worsens with repetitive knee flexion.
   - Pain with prolonged sitting (positive theater sign or "movie-goer's knee").
   - Pain with squatting descending/ascending stairs and sustained running.

17. Why does stairway ascent or descent cause pain in patellofemoral disease?
   There are significant differences in patellar reaction forces with ascending or descending stairs that depend on the location of the center-of-gravity (CG). Predicted force values for ascent range from 1.8 to 2.3 × body weight (BW), compared with 2.9 to 6 × BW for stair descent. The increased values with stair descent are due to the CG being moved further behind the patellofemoral joint, increasing the lever arm to maintain balance.

18. What is the relationship between knee flexion and patellofemoral pressure?
   - The patella is usually out of contact with the trochlea in full extension. The most inferior portion of the patella gains contact with the trochlea of the femur between 10 to 20 degrees of flexion and moves proximally as flexion increases.
   - The patella settles into the deepest portion of the trochlea beyond 30 degrees of flexion.

Table 47.1 Differential Diagnosis for Anterior Knee Pain Other Than Meniscal and Ligament Injury

COMMON	LESS COMMON	SPECIFIC POPULATIONS	NOT TO BE MISSED
• Patellofemoral pain • Patellar tendinopathy • Degenerative Joint Disease)	• Quadriceps tendinopathy • Patellofemoral instability • Synovial Plica • Fat pad impingement • Pre-patellar bursitis • Infrapatellar bursitis	• Osgood-Schlatter • Sinding-Larsen-Johansson Lesion • Stress fracture of the patella • Tenoperiostitis of the upper tibia	• Referred pain from the hip • Osteochondritis dissecans • Slipped capital femoral epiphysis • Perthes disease • Tumor

- Contact area is greatest at 70 to 90 degrees of knee flexion, after which a linear reduction occurs.
- Patellofemoral reaction forces: Walking $= 0.6 \times$ BW, jogging 7.7 $\times$ BW, and jumping is 20 $\times$ BW.

19. What are rehab treatment strategies for patellofemoral pain?
- Physical Therapy to enhance knee mechanics and stability with a focus on strengthening the core, hip abductors, and quadriceps. Initially, full-arc quadriceps exercises (0 to 90 degrees) should be avoided, and isometric closed-chain exercises with short-arc activities (0 to 45 degrees) emphasized.
- Patellofemoral taping can be helpful. Ridged McConnell taping versus flexible Kinesio taping.
- Once quadriceps strength and flexibility are achieved, increased ROM exercise, such as bicycling, can be initiated.
- Kinetic chain evaluation—Assess excessive pronation or supination of the foot and determine if orthotics are necessary.
- In runners, evaluate foot strike preference. Changing from primary heel striker to forefoot striker may reduce pain.
- Surgical indications
  - Recurrent patellar instability
  - Traumatic loose body formation

20. How do you diagnose and treat patellar tendinopathy?
- Non-contrast MRI or musculoskeletal ultrasound. Areas of tendinopathy correspond with areas of increased signal on MRI and hypoechoic regions (dark areas) on ultrasound.
- Nonoperative measures: protection, rest, ice, compression, elevation (PRICE)
- NSAIDs such as aspirin or ibuprofen in the early phases.
- Eccentric strengthening program of the quadriceps and hamstring flexibility (take the pressure off the anterior structures of the knee).
- Given the refractory response to many initial treatments, consider nitric oxide transdermal patches, tenotomy, sclerosing injections, tendon scrapping, platelet-rich plasma therapy, whole blood injections, and extracorporeal shock wave treatment (See chapter 25 on Regeneration and Rehabilitation Medicine: Innovation through Synergy).
- Cortisone injections should be avoided in the treatment of tendinopathy due to their inhibition of collagen synthesis, increased risk for tendon rupture, and poor long-term outcomes.
- Surgery is reserved for patients who experience pain for 6 to 12 months despite close adherence to treatment and for those who have suffered a complete tendon rupture.

21. Differentiate housemaid's knee versus Vicar's knee.
- Both conditions are due to irritated bursae about the knee.
- Housemaid's knee results from prolonged kneeling and involves the prepatellar bursa located between the skin and the patella. It is the most commonly injured bursa.
- Vicars knee involves the superficial infrapatellar bursa located between the skin and the tibial tuberosity. This is associated with kneeling in an upright position.
- Anteriorly, the knee also has the suprapatellar bursa, which typically communicates with the knee joint and is a frequent target for ultrasound-guided knee aspiration/injections.
- The deep infrapatellar bursa located between the patellar tendon and the tibia and may show fluid on imaging.

MEDIAL KNEE

22. What are common conditions that may cause medial knee pain?
See Table 47.2.

23. What is pes anserinus syndrome?
Pes anserinus is a confluence of three muscles, sartorius, gracilis, and semitendinosus (**pneumonic: Say Grac**e before **Te**a) that inserts on the anteromedial tibia to collectively flex the knee and resist valgus strain. These tendons and their associate bursa can become injured with increased valgus stress and repetitive friction, causing

Table 47.2 Differential Diagnosis for Medial Knee Pain

COMMON	LESS COMMON	NOT TO BE MISSED
• Medial Collateral Ligament Sprain • Osteoarthritis • Medial meniscus abnormality • Minor tear • Cyst • Degenerative change • Pes anserine bursitis/tendinopathy	• Insufficiency fracture • Patellofemoral syndrome • Referred pain lumbar spine • Saphenous neuropathy	• Referred pain from the hip or sacroiliac joint • Medial tibial plateau fracture

tendinopathy and or bursitis (pes anserinus syndrome). It is an uncommon cause of knee pain though seen more in cyclists, swimmers (breaststroke), and runners. Symptoms may mimic medial meniscal injury, and diagnosis may be made with MRI or MSK US.

Treatment: PRICE principle and PT focusing on stretching the medial hamstrings and strengthening the core and lateral hip musculature. Ultrasound-guided cortisone injections to the bursa can help with the pain. Intratendinous injections should be avoided. Regenerative options such as PRP may also be considered (see chapter on regenerative medicine).

24. What are the degrees of MCL strains?
    - Grade 1 (first degree): Valgus stress results in medial pain but no increased laxity; laxity = 0 to 5 mm
    - Grade 2 (second degree): Valgus stress demonstrates increased laxity, and an endpoint is appreciated; laxity = 6 to 10 mm
    - Grade 3 (third degree): Valgus stress demonstrates increased laxity with no appreciable endpoint, indicating rupture of the ligament and the surrounding capsular structures; laxity = 11 to 15 mm

25. When can an athlete return to competitive sports after an MCL grade 1 strain?
    When the patient's strength is near normal (90%), and the valgus instability is reduced to the point that a brace is no longer required. The patient should be able to perform one-legged hopping, jumping rope, and climbing stairs before returning to the playing field.

26. Describe the MCL and LCL stress test.
    The patient is supine, and the knee is examined at neutral and at 30 degrees. Valgus and varus stress are applied at both degrees. Valgus stress examines the MCL, and varus stress examines the LCL. The posterior capsule is relaxed at approximately 30 degrees of knee flexion. The maneuver can also be completed by rotating internally and externally the tibia while palpating the joint space.

LATERAL KNEE

27. What are the causes of lateral knee pain?
    See Table 47.3.

28. What is iliotibial band friction syndrome (ITBFS)? Describe the treatment approach.
    Clinical presentation
    - An overuse injury where typically distance runners, military recruits, endurance athletes, and cyclists complain of lateral knee pain worsened with activity in a predictable manner (in cycling ITBFS accounts for 15% to 24% of overuse injuries).
    - Mechanical compressive irritation between the fibrous ITB at the lateral femoral condyle. Biomechanical issues may be ITB tightness, excessive tibial rotation, proximal hip weakness, genu valgus, and poor rearfoot mechanics.
    - Physical exam is notable for tenderness at the lateral femoral epicondyle, approximately 3 cm proximal to the joint line. Soft tissue swelling may be present. Ober's test may reveal ITB tightness. Imaging is not necessary, though both ultrasound and MRI show ITB thickening and fluid collection deep to the ITB at the femoral epicondyle.
    Treatment
    - Initial pain management includes activity modification, protection, relative rest, ice, compression, elevation (PRICE), NSAIDs, cryotherapy, gluteal trigger point injections, and dry needling along the ITB. Ultrasound-guided corticosteroid injection deep into the ITB may also provide pain relief.
    - Rehabilitation must focus on correcting hip and foot biomechanics through physical therapy. Flexibility of the ITB is at times overemphasized, and more significant gains may be seen with stretching of the iliopsoas, gluteus maximus, quadriceps, and gastrocsoleus muscles.
    - Strengthening of hip external rotators and abductors.

Table 47.3 Differential Diagnosis for Lateral Knee Pain

COMMON	LESS COMMON	NOT TO BE MISSED
• Lateral Collateral ligament sprain	• Excessive lateral pressure syndrome	• Insufficiency fracture
• Osteoarthritis	• Biceps femoris tendinopathy	• Fibular fracture
• Iliotibial band friction syndrome (see question 8)	• Superior tibiofibular joint sprain	• Common peroneal nerve injury
• lateral meniscus abnormality	• Synovitis of the knee joint	• Slipped capital epiphysis
• Minor tear	• Referred pain lumbar spine	• Perthes disease
• Cyst		• Osteochondral defect
• Degenerative change		

29. What is biceps femoris tendinopathy?
    - An overuse injury due to frequent acceleration/deceleration activities such as running and cycling.
    - Presenting with posterolateral knee pain that initially improves with exercise. Morning stiffness and pain are common the day following exercise, and as symptoms persist, pain does not abate with exercise and can impair performance.
    - The pain can be produced on the exam with resisted knee flexion and palpation of the biceps femoris tendon as it inserts onto the fibula. Treatment approach is similar to the treatment of tendinopathy, and physical therapy (pt) focuses on eccentric strengthening.

POSTERIOR KNEE

30. What are some common conditions that can cause posterior knee pain?
    See Table 47.4.

31. What causes a Baker's cyst?
    In children, Baker's cyst is usually congenital. In adults, it is usually secondary to underlying articular pathology or trauma. By definition, it is a herniation of synovial tissue through a weakening posterior capsular wall that causes swelling in the popliteal fossa (popliteal cyst). The general population is susceptible. It is a response to events happening in the anterior aspect of the knee.

INTRAARTICULAR

32. Name three types of knee effusions.
    Synovial, hemarthrosis, and purulent

33. What should be done when evaluating an edematous knee?
    If the patient has a history of an acute, hot edematous knee, it is crucial to obtain Gram stain crystals and culture before injecting it with steroids.

MENISCAL TEARS

34. Describe McMurray's test.
    McMurray's test is useful for diagnosing meniscal injury. The test is performed with the patient lying supine with the knee and hip maximally flexed. The examiner stabilizes the thigh and rotates the tibia either medially or laterally. With medial rotation, the presence of a loose fragment in the lateral meniscus can cause a snap or click that is often accompanied by pain. With lateral rotation, the presence of a loose fragment in the medial meniscus can be similarly detected. By repeatedly adjusting the amount of flexion, the examiner can test the entire posterior aspect of the meniscus from the posterior horn to the medial component. The anterior half of the meniscus is not as easily examined because the pressure exerted on the meniscus is not as great.

35. Describe the Apley maneuver.
    The Apley maneuver is another commonly used test for diagnosing meniscal injury. The patient lies prone with the knee flexed 90 degrees. While the examiner stabilizes the thigh, the tibia is rotated medially and laterally with downward pressure. Joint-line tenderness with this movement is considered positive.

36. Can meniscal injuries be treated without surgery?
    Yes. Initially, the **PRICE** regimen is prescribed. One could change the pneumonic to **CRISP** (compression, rest, ice, steroid intra-articular injection, and protection) if conservative care is failing. In fact, most meniscal tears can be treated without the need for surgical intervention.

Table 47.4 Differential Diagnosis for Posterior Knee Pain

COMMON	LESS COMMON	NOT TO BE MISSED
• Baker's cyst	• Adductor tendinopathy	• Popliteal artery aneurysm
• Osteoarthritis	• Referred pain from the lumbar spine	• Deep vein thrombosis
• Posterolateral or posteromedial meniscal tear	• Popliteus Tendinopathy	• Posterolateral corner tear
• Distal hamstring tendinopathy	• Posterior cruciate ligament tear	
	• Proximal gastrocnemius strain or tear	
	• Sciatic neuropathy	

37. What are the surgical indications for meniscus injury?
    - Mechanical related symptoms: locking, effusion, instability, and limitation of motions secondary to biomechanics
    - Pain symptoms: Joint line tenderness, positive provocative physical exam signs including McMurray's or Appley tests and limitation of motion secondary to pain
    - Failure to respond to non-surgical treatment

38. What are the types of meniscus tears?
    - Longitudinal
    - Horizontal
    - Oblique
    - Radial

39. What are the three zones of the meniscus, and what is the blood supply?
    - Medial and lateral geniculate artery
    - Red-Red zone: peripheral 1/3 of the meniscus that receives the most blood supply
    - Red-White zone: middle 1/3 of the meniscus, and is the junction between vascular and avascular portions of the meniscus
    - White-White zone: central 1/3 of the meniscus, avascular portion of the meniscus

40. When is a partial meniscectomy Vs meniscus repair indicated?
    - **Meniscectomy**: tears in the white-white zone; complex tears, degenerative tears, repair failure greater than two attempts, older age, diffuse cartilage damage
    - **Meniscus repair**: red-red zone tears, vertical longitudinal tears, radial tears, horizontal tears, root tears, in conjunction with ACL reconstruction and younger age (<25 ideally)

41. How should one approach the patient with an ACL injury?
    Patients typically develop a rapidly developing effusion (hemarthrosis) and "pop" sign, usually during a pivot motion. The most common tests are the Lachman, anterior drawer sign, and pivot shift test. In an acute injury, depending on the size of effusion, ACL injury may be difficult to assess. The gold standard imaging study is MRI (magnetic resonance imaging) of the knee. To prevent anterior subluxation of the tibia, rehabilitation should focus on the strengthening of the hamstrings and proprioceptive training. To prevent patellofemoral pain, a frequent occurrence after an ACL injury, quadriceps should be strengthened through terminal-range squats. ACL reconstruction is considered depending on the patient's age, level of activity, expectations, degree of instability, and associated injuries.

42. Name and describe three common tests for an ACL injury.
    - Lachman test: Patient lies supine. Knee is flexed approximately 20 degrees, and the proximal tibia is pulled forward to assess excessive translation (more than 5 mm).
    - Anterior drawer test: Patient lies supine. Knee is flexed at 90 degrees, and the hip is flexed at 45 degrees. The proximal tibia is pulled anteriorly to assess excessive translation (more than 5 mm).
    - Pivot shift test: Patient lies supine. Knee is placed in extension. The examiner supports the leg by the upper tibia and flexes the knee while applying a slight valgus stress to the knee (pushing the knee toward the midline) and internal rotation stress about the femur. In a knee with an ACL injury, the femur sags backward on the tibia (or conversely, the tibia moves forward on the femur), creating a subluxation of the lateral tibiofemoral compartment. At approximately 30 degrees of flexion, the subluxated tibia suddenly reduces and externally rotates about the femur. The subluxation and the sudden reduction of the knee joint during flexion are termed the pivot shift.

43. Does a positive Lachman test always mean ACL injury?
    No. Laxity may also be present in the other knee. Knee clinical examination requires comparing both knees. One can also have a false negative Lachman's test in the acute setting when there is significant knee swelling, and the patient is guarding.

44. What are graft options for ACL reconstruction?
    - Bone patellar tendon-bone autograft
    - Hamstring autograft
    - Quadriceps tendon autograft
    - Allograft

45. Identify the cause and acute signs of PCL injury. Discuss a treatment approach.
    The most common mechanism of injury of the PCL is the so-called dashboard injury (while the knee bent, an object forces the tibia backward). Another mechanism of injury is hyperflexion of the knee, with the foot plantarflexed. The acute signs include swelling in the popliteal space with bruising present during the first 36 to 48 hours and no effusion as a result of the extra-articular nature of the PCL. Pain and instability are also common. Rehabilitation should concentrate on regaining ROM and substituting the lost function of the PCL by strengthening the quadriceps. Surgery is reserved for refractory cases or with concomitant ligamentous/meniscal injury.

46. Name and describe common tests for PCL injury.
    - Posterior drawer test: Patient lies supine. Knee is flexed at 90 degrees, and the hip is flexed at 45 degrees. The proximal tibia is pushed posteriorly to assess excessive translation (more than 5 mm).
    - Posterior sag test: Patient lies supine and flexes both hips to 45 degrees and both knees to 90 degrees with examiner supporting both heels. The tibia will drop or sag if there is a PCL tear.
    - Reversed pivot shift test: Patient lies supine. Knee is placed in flexion at 90 degrees. The examiner supports the leg by the upper tibia and extends the knee while applying a slight valgus stress to the knee (pushing the knee toward the midline) and external rotation stress about the femur. In a knee with a PCL injury, the femur moves forward on the tibia (or conversely, the tibia moves backward on the femur). The subluxated tibia will shift into anterior reduction at 20 to 30 degrees.

OSTEOARTHRITIS

47. What are the signs and symptoms of knee osteoarthritis?
    Knee osteoarthritis is characterized by focal or diffuse joint pain, stiffness, tenderness, and decreased ROM. Patients can have swelling, joint effusion, and pain with weight-bearing activity. Physiatric treatment consists of using a cane in the opposite hand, NSAIDs, intra-articular joint injections, a knee brace, and physical therapy.

48. What are the general principles of rehabilitation of arthritis of the knee?
    - Therapy prescriptions may vary based on the location of the greatest arthritis. Strengthening exercises should target the core, lateral hip, and quadriceps.
    - Closed kinetic chain isometric exercises produce the lowest level of shearing stress in the knee and should be an initial approach to strengthening.
    - Hydrotherapy (pool-based) therapy reduces gravitational forces and can improve exercise tolerance.
    - Exercise load should increase each week, and maintenance of cardiovascular conditioning is a must—even before a total joint replacement.
    - Activities of daily living and transfer/ambulatory evaluation are essential and should include evaluation for assistive devices, including raised toilet seats, shower grab bars, reachers, and ambulatory aids to maximize independence and ensure safety in the home environment.

49. What are the types and indications for the use of a knee brace?
    According to the American Academy of Orthopaedic Surgeons, knee braces can be classified as:
    - Prophylactic braces: Intended to prevent or reduce the severity of knee injuries in contact sports; these braces are often not recommended because of excessive preloading of the MCL, limited speed and athleticism, a false sense of security for a previously injured knee, and brace-related contact injuries to other players
    - Functional braces: Designed to provide stability for unstable knees
    - Rehabilitative braces: Designed to allow protected and controlled motion during the rehabilitation of injured knees
    - Patellofemoral braces: Designed to improve patellar tracking and relieve anterior knee pain

50. What are common knee injections in the treatment of knee pain?
    There are three common types of injections with evidence to support their use in the treatment of knee pain due to osteoarthritis:
    - **Viscosupplementation therapy—injectate composed of high molecular weight** hyaluronic acid (HA) that is proposed to improve joint elasticity and viscosity, reduce cartilage friction, and help change the knee joint environment from catabolic to anabolic. Injections are performed in a series of 1, 3, or 5. These injections are more successful in mild to moderate knee osteoarthritis.
    - **Cortisone injections**—can provide meaningful pain relief for inflammatory joint issues such as bursitis, gout, arthritis, and synovitis. Effects may last days to more than 6 months. Cortisone injections can be repeated though recent studies have shown that frequent injections lead to increased loss of intraarticular cartilage when compared to placebo. In general, injections should not be done sooner than 6 weeks apart and no more than three or four times a year.
    - **Platelet plasma injections (PRP)**—Leukocyte poor preparation of PRP. See chapter on regenerative medicine

51. What are x-ray findings of osteoarthritis
    - Joint space narrowing
    - Subchondral sclerosis
    - Subchondral cysts
    - Osteophyte formation

52. What are nonoperative treatments for knee osteoarthritis?
    - Weight loss
    - Anti-inflammatory medications
    - Intraarticular injections

- Lateral wedge insoles
- Unloader braces and assistive devices

53. What are the surgical options for osteoarthritis of the knee?

- Arthroscopic debridement: includes irrigation and removal of loose bodies from the knee (rarely performed).
- Cartilage transplantation: for small isolated areas, portions of autologous articular cartilage can be grafted into the defect.
- Osteotomies of the distal femur or proximal tibia are used for isolated lateral or medial compartment arthritis.
- Unicompartmental knee arthroplasty can be performed for isolated lateral or medial compartment arthritis.
- Patellofemoral replacement replaces just the patellofemoral joint (anterior part of the knee).
- Total knee arthroplasty is used to treat severe tricompartmental arthritis.

54. What are the indications for total knee arthroplasty?

Indications are severe, refractory knee pain, difficulty with activities of daily living, decreased mobility, and failure to respond to conservative measures. The primary goal is to relieve pain caused by arthritis. Secondary goals are to restore functions and correct deformity.

55. Identify one condition in which a patient is at great risk for peroneal nerve palsy after a total knee arthroplasty.

The patient with a valgus knee with a fixed flexion contracture is at high risk of peroneal nerve palsy. The peroneal nerve is at risk when a retractor is placed on the lateral side of the knee during surgery. However, injury from this is not a common occurrence. Neurapraxias more often result from stretching of the nerve with correction of the limb deformity. If a patient presents with a foot drop, then all dressings should be removed, and the knee should be flexed to relieve tension across the peroneal nerve. If there is no resolution of the palsy, surgical exploration and decompression should be considered.

56. What is the weight-bearing status immediately after total knee arthroplasty?

There are different protocols, and it is essential to discuss this with the operating physician. Most commonly, the patient is weight-bearing as tolerated. Patients may be partial weight bearing if complications arise during surgery.

57. Outline a rehabilitation program for the patient with a total knee replacement.

- Day of surgery: deep breathing exercises, active ankle ROM
- Postoperative day 1: lower-limb isometric exercises (quadriceps, hamstrings, and gluteal sets), passive and active ROM exercises
- Postoperative day 2: active-assisted ROM
- Postoperative day 3: progressive isotonic and isometric knee and hip muscle strengthening. (Concentrate on terminal knee extension through active knee extension exercises.)

58. What muscles should be targeted after total knee arthroplasty?

The quadriceps muscles are significantly weaker after total knee arthroplasty. This is, in part, related to the exposure required. Tourniquet and ischemic time also may play a role in muscular weakness. The quadriceps are important for stability during the stance phase of gait. Isometric strengthening and active ROM should begin immediately after surgery and continue for the first 6 weeks. Resisted isokinetic or isotonic strengthening should be added. Other muscles that should be strengthened after total knee arthroplasties include the hamstrings, gastrocsoleus, and ankle dorsiflexors.

59. List the usual sequence of ambulatory aids after a total knee replacement.

- Parallel bars in inpatient physical therapy
- Crutches or a walker, depending on patient stability and comfort
- One crutch or cane
- Most patients do not require assistive devices by 6 to 12 weeks postoperatively

WEBSITES

Available at: www.emedicinehealth.com/articles/9051–1.asp
Knee Pain Info. Available at: www.kneepaininfo.com
Knee Guru. Available at: www.kneeguru.co.uk
Verywell Health. Available at: http://orthopedics.about.com

RECOMMENDED READINGS

Brukner P, Clarsen B, Cook J, et al. *Brukner & Khan's Clinical Sports Medicine*. 5th ed. New South Wales: McGraw-Hill Education Australia; 2016
Cheng OT, Souzdalnitski D, Vrooman B, Cheng J. Evidence-based knee injections for the management of arthritis. *Pain Med (United States)*. 2012;13(6):740–753. doi:10.1111/j.1526-4637.2012.01394.x.

Christian RA, Rossy WH, Sherman OH. Patellar tendinopathy—recent developments toward treatment. *Bull Hosp Jt Dis* (2013). 2014; 72(3):217–224.

DeJong G, Hsieh CH, Gassaway J, et al. Characterizing rehabilitation services for patients with knee and hip replacement in skilled nursing facilities and inpatient rehabilitation facilities. *Arch Phys Med Rehabil.* 2009;90:1269–1283.

de Lange-Brokaar BJ, Ioan-Facsinay A, Yusuf E, et al. Association of pain in knee osteoarthritis with distinct patterns of synovitis. *Arthritis Rheumatol.* 2015;67(3):733–740.

Ellen MI, Young JL, Sarni JL. Musculoskeletal rehabilitation and sports medicine. III. Knee and lower extremity injuries. *Arch Phys Med Rehabil.* 1999;80:S59–S67

Flandry F, Hommel G. Normal anatomy and biomechanics of the knee. *Sports Med Arthrosc Rev.* 2011;19(2):82–92. doi: 10.1097/ JSA.0b013e318210c0aa.

Foley A, Halbert J, Hewitt T, et al. Does hydrotherapy improve strength and physical function in patients with osteoarthritis—a randomized controlled trial comparing a gym based and a hydrotherapy based strengthening program. *Ann Rheum Dis.* 2003;62:1162–1167.

Frey M, O'Young B, Marulanda G, Mont M, Seyler T. The Knee: Anatomy, Pathology, Diagnosis, Treatment, and Rehabilitation. In O'Young B, Young M, Stiens S (eds), *Physical Medicine and Rehabilitation Secrets.* 3rd ed. Philadelphia, PA: Elsevier; 2007:376-391.

Hott A, Brox JI, Pripp AH, et al. Effectiveness of isolated hip exercise, knee exercise, or free physical activity for patellofemoral pain: a randomized controlled trial. *Am J Sports Med.* 2019;47(6):1312–1322.

Jin J, Jones E. Patellofemoral pain. *JAMA.* 2018;319(4):418. doi:10.1001/jama.2017

Laible C, Stein DA, Kiridly DN. Meniscal repair. *J Am Acad Orthop Surg.* 2013 April;21(4):204–213.

Magee DJ. *The Knee.* In: Quillen W, ed. *Orthopedic Physical Assessment.* 6th ed. Philadelphia: W.B. Saunders. 2014:372–447.

Musahl V, Herbst E, Burnham JM, Fu FH. The anterolateral complex and anterolateral ligament of the knee. *J Am Acad Orthop Surg.* 2018;26(8):261–267.

Quinn RH, Murray JN, Pezold R, Sevarino KS. Surgical management of osteoarthritis of the knee. *J Am Acad Orthop Surg.* 2018;26(9):e191–e193.

Sheon RP, Moskowitz RW, Goldberg VM. *Soft Tissue Rheumatic Pain: Recognition, Management, and Prevention.* 3rd ed. Baltimore: Williams & Wilkins; 1996.

Snyder R. *Essentials of Musculoskeletal Care American Academy of Orthopedic Surgeons.* Rosemont, IL: American Academy of Pediatrics; 2016

Bonus questions and answers are available online.

ACKNOWLEDGMENT

The authors would like to acknowledge the contributions of Drs. Michael Frey, Bryan O'Young, German Marulanda, Michael Mont, and Thorsten Seyler, who authored the previous version of this chapter which served as a strong foundation for the updated chapter.

THE FOOT AND ANKLE: CLINICAL PRESENTATION, DIAGNOSIS, AND TREATMENT

Karen P. Barr, MD, Bethany Honce, MD, and Marta Imamura, MD, PhD

The human foot is a masterpiece of engineering and a work of art.

— Leonardo Da Vinci

KEY POINTS: ANKLE AND FOOT DISORDERS

1. Eccentric calf strengthening has been found to be helpful to treat both the pain and the tendon abnormality of Achilles tendinosis.
2. The anterior talofibular ligament is the most commonly injured ligament in an ankle sprain.
3. Foot fractures at high risk for non-union include navicular and metaphyseal-diaphyseal fifth metatarsal fractures.
4. Plantar fasciitis is typically seen in two distinct populations: sedentary patients with high BMI, and runners who have increased their training.
5. Morton's neuroma is a benign enlargement of the fibrotic layer around the digital nerve in the third interspace that is irritated by tight footwear.

1. **For clinical discussions, how are the regions of the foot divided? What structures are in each region?**
   The foot is generally divided into three regions: the hindfoot, which consists of the calcaneus, talus, and related soft tissues; the midfoot, which consists of the cuneiform, navicular, cuboids, and related soft tissues; and the forefoot, which consists of the metatarsals and phalanges. See Fig. 48.1.

2. **What ligaments are injured in a common ankle sprain?**
   Ankle sprains typically occur as a result of an inversion movement of the ankle. The most commonly involved ligament is the anterior talofibular ligament (ATFL), followed by the calcaneofibular ligament (CFL), and lastly the posterior talofibular ligament (PTFL). These ligaments form the lateral ligament complex. See Fig. 48.2.

3. **What are the two tests used to detect injury and instability of the lateral ankle ligament complex?**
   a. The anterior drawer test evaluates the ATFL and is performed with the ankle in slight plantar flexion and applying forward stress at the ankle while stabilizing the tibia.
   b. The talar tilt test evaluates the CFL and is performed with the ankle in neutral and applying inversion stress while stabilizing the tibia. The degree of translation is noted.

4. **What are the Ottawa ankle rules?**
   These are used to determine if an ankle x-ray series is required. They are pain in the malleolar zone, plus:
   i. Tenderness at the posterior edge or tip of the lateral malleolus
   or
   ii. tenderness at the posterior edge or tip of the medial malleolus
   or
   iii. inability to bear weight both immediately and in the emergency department for four steps.

5. **How are ankle sprains most commonly graded?**
   a. Grade I (mild): ligament sprain or strain and no increase in translation on stress testing. Mild tenderness and swelling.
   b. Grace II (moderate): partial ligament tearing and minimal increase in translation on stress testing. Moderate swelling and tenderness.
   c. Grade III (severe): complete tearing of one or both of the lateral ligaments and no endpoint noted on stress testing. Significant tenderness and swelling.

6. **What is the role of exercise in the treatment of ankle sprains?**
   Multiple studies have shown that exercise improves self-reported function after an acute strain and in chronic ankle instability. Exercise can prevent the recurrence of sprains. Supervised rehabilitation has been shown to be

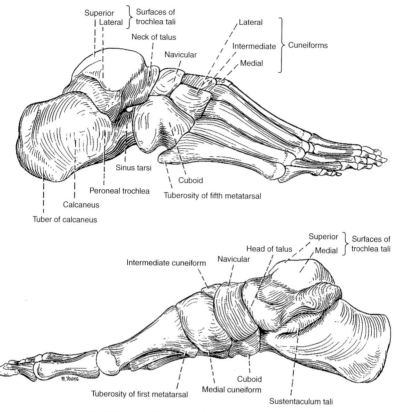

Fig. 48.1 Bones of the foot from the lateral and medial sides.

superior to an unsupervised home exercise program for greater gains in ankle strength and joint position sense and less pain and subjective instability. A typical exercise protocol would include stretching of ankle dorsiflexion, strengthening exercises including resistance of inversion, eversion, dorsiflexion, and plantar flexion, and ankle proprioceptive exercises such as tracing the alphabet with the foot. Once weight-bearing is pain-free, single-leg balance exercises are initiated to focus on balance and restore proprioceptive control of the injured ankle. After achieving pain-free status on weight-bearing, rehabilitation efforts focus on return to sports activities.

Doherty C, Bleakley C, Delahunt E, Holdesn S. Treatment and prevention of acute and recurrent ankle sprain: an overview of systematic reviews and meat-analysis. *Br J sports Med.* 2017 Jan; 51(2):113–125.

Feger MA, Herb CC, Fraser JJ, Glaviano N, Hertel J. Supervised rehabilitation versus home exercise in the treatment of acute ankle sprains: a systematic review. *Clin Sports Med.* 2015 Apr; 34(2):329–346.

7. How many degrees of dorsiflexion at the ankle joint are required for normal gait?
   A minimum of 10 degrees of ankle dorsiflexion is required for normal gait.

8. What diagnosis should be considered in patients with chronic non-healing ankle sprains?
   Osteochondral lesion of the talus is a common condition that is associated with an ankle injury. Symptoms are nonspecific and include pain, swelling, stiffness, and mechanical symptoms of locking and catching. Prolonged weight-bearing or high-impact activities often exacerbate these symptoms. MRI is the imaging method of choice and has 96% sensitivity and 96% specificity for the diagnosis.

Rungprai C, Tennant JN, Gentry RD, Phisitkul P. Management of osteochondral lesions of the talar dome. *Open Orthop J.* 2017 Jul 31; 11:743–761.

Gianakos AL, Yasui Y, Hannon CP, Kennedy JG. Current management of talar osteochondral lesions. *World J Orthop.* 2017 Jan 18;8(1): 12–20.

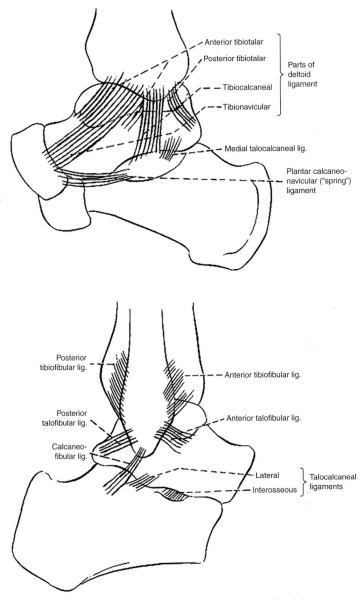

Fig. 48.2 Ligaments of the ankle and subtalar joints in medial and lateral views.

9. What are the treatment methods for osteochondral lesions of the talus?

In patients with nondisplaced lesions of the talus, conservative management includes rest, non-weight-bearing in a short leg cast, and NSAIDs for 3 to 4 months. This is followed by progressive weight-bearing in a CAM boot and PT for 6 to 10 weeks. The purpose of conservative management is to unload the injured cartilage so that bone edema can be resolved and necrosis be prevented. Operative treatment is indicated after failed conservative treatment or for completely avulsed or displaced fragments.

Rungprai C, Tennant JN, Gentry RD, Phisitkul P. Management of osteochondral lesions of the talar dome. *Open Orthop J.* 2017 Jul 31; 11:743–761.

Gianakos AL, Yasui Y, Hannon CP, Kennedy JG. Current management of talar osteochondral lesions. *World J Orthop.* 2017 Jan 18;8(1):12–20.

10. What kind of physical therapy has been found to help treat Achilles tendinosis?

Eccentric calf-strengthening exercises have been found in multiple studies to treat the pain of Achilles tendinosis and to normalize tendon structure on ultrasound. The mechanism is believed to involve strengthening and hypertrophy of the gastrocnemius muscles, lengthening of the muscle-tendon unit, increased tendon tensile strength, and decreased tendon neovascularity. The important component of this exercise program appears to be the intense, eccentric nature of the exercises and that they are done at an intense level, despite producing pain.

Ohberg L, Lorentzon R, Alfredson H. Eccentric training in patients with chronic Achilles tendinosis: normalized tendon structure and decreased thickness at follow up. *Br J Sports Med.* 2004;38(1):8–11.

11. What are the common diagnoses seen by rehabilitation physicians for each region of the foot?

Some common causes of hindfoot pain include plantar fasciitis, fat pad contusions, and S1 radiculopathy. Causes of midfoot pain include tendinopathies (such as posterior tibialis or peroneal tendon) and navicular stress fractures. Forefoot pain may be caused by metatarsal stress fractures, metatarsalgia, interdigital neuromas, extensor and flexor tendonitis, and first metatarsal phalangeal conditions such as hallux valgus and rigidus.

12. What are the innervations of the foot and ankle?

The sural nerve supplies sensation to the lateral ankle and foot. The saphenous nerve innervates part of the ankle joint, then enters the foot at the medial anterior ankle and supplies sensation to the medial dorsum of the foot. The superficial fibular nerve (formerly known as the peroneal nerve) enters the foot at the anterior lateral ankle and supplies cutaneous innervation to the dorsal ankle and foot. The deep fibular nerve passes deep to the extensor retinaculum at the anterior ankle (an area known as the anterior tarsal tunnel) sends branches to the subtalar joint and supplies a motor branch to the deep peroneal muscle, some motor innervation to the first dorsal interosseous, and cutaneous innervation to the first dorsal web space. The tibial nerve enters the foot posterior to the medial malleolus within the tarsal tunnel, and its branches supply the remaining muscles of the foot and sensation to the plantar surface of the foot and medial heel.

13. How is electrodiagnosis helpful in the management of foot pain?

Electrodiagnostic studies can confirm or refute common sources of foot pain such as peripheral polyneuropathy, entrapment neuropathy such as tarsal tunnel syndrome, and L5–S1 radiculopathy.

Del Toro D, Nelson PA. Guiding treatment for foot pain. *Phys Med Rehabil Clin N Am.* 2018;29(4):783–792. doi:10.1016/j.pmr.2018.06.012

14. How is plantar fasciitis diagnosed?

Plantar fasciitis is typically a clinical diagnosis and imaging is unnecessary. It typically occurs in two distinct populations: (1) sedentary people with high BMI, and (2) runners and other athletes, often after an increase in training. These patients often complain of heel pain that is worse first thing in the morning and after prolonged standing and walking. Physical exam reveals pain with palpation over the plantar medial calcaneal tubercle, sometimes pain with palpation of the rest of the fascia and the lateral heel, and no pain with medial-lateral squeezing of the calcaneum (this suggests stress fracture). A thorough neurological and musculoskeletal exam of the foot will exclude competing diagnoses.

15. What are evidence-based treatments for plantar fasciitis?

Stretching of the plantar fascia and Achilles tendon and supportive footwear such as prefabricated or custom-molded orthoses are the first line of treatment. Steroid injections can give some minimal short-term relief. For refractory cases, extracorporeal shock wave therapy and surgery have been shown to be effective. More experimental injections such as prolotherapy and platelet-rich plasma require further study to show their efficacy.

16. Are plantar heel spurs a source of heel pain?

There is no clear relationship between heel spurs and heel pain which is one reason why plain x-rays are not typically indicated in the workup of heel pain if a fracture is not suspected. Evidence that heel spurs are not a cause of heel pain include: between 16% and 30% of asymptomatic heels have bone spurs. When spurs are present, there is no correlation between the size of spurs and the symptoms in patients. In patients with unilateral foot pain and heel spurs, spurs are typically seen bilaterally. There is an increased incidence of heel spurs in patients with increased age, obesity, diabetes, and osteoarthritis. It is likely that the spur itself is not a source of pain, but an indicator of associated conditions that cause foot pain. In the past, it was thought that heel spurs were caused by tight fascia pulling on the bone, but multiple recent studies have found that spurs are typically not in the fascial layer, but superior to the fascia in the intrinsic muscles.

Schneider HP, Baca JM, Carpenter BB, Dayton PD, Fleischer AE, Sachs BD. American college of foot and ankle surgeons clinical consensus statement: diagnosis and treatment of adult acquired infracalcaneal heel pain. *J Foot Ankle Surg.* 2018;57(2):370–381. doi:10.1053/j.jfas.2017.10.018

17. What is a "not to be missed" cause of mid-foot pain in runners?
Navicular stress fractures are common in runners, particularly jumpers, sprinters, and middle-distance runners. They are at high risk for non-union if the patient continues to bear weight, so prompt diagnosis is important. The physical exam is characterized by tenderness over the dorsal aspect of the navicular bone (the "n spot") and pain with push-off. MRI can confirm the diagnosis.

Harrast MA, Colonno D. Stress fractures in runners. *Clin Sports Med.* 2010;29(3):399–416. doi:10.1016/j.csm.2010.03.001

18. What is the "too many toes sign" on a physical exam, and what does it mean?
When viewed from behind, more toes are visible on the pathological foot. This is a sign of forefoot pronation and abduction and increased hindfoot valgus angulation caused by posterior tibialis tendon dysfunction. This is the most common cause of acquired flat foot in adults. Other symptoms and signs of this include the progressive collapse of the medial arch, pain and swelling over the tendon, and weakness of heel raises.

19. How useful are x-rays in diagnosing metatarsal stress fractures?
Imaging devices have varying levels of usefulness. Plain films may remain normal for 3 to 6 weeks after a stress fracture. The first sign usually seen is subperiosteal bone formation. Bone scans will be positive in 20% to 40% of cases in which clinical suspicion is high, but plain films are normal. MRIs are very sensitive in showing stress fractures. Some clinicians consider MRIs to be too sensitive because MRIs sometimes show a bony reaction in asymptomatic athletes. Grading scales have been developed to correlate MRI changes with prognosis.

Arendt E, Agel J, Heikes C, et al. Stress injuries to bone in college athletes: a retrospective review of experience at a single institution. *Am J Sports Med.* 2003;31(6):959–968.

20. What is a Jones fracture? What can cause it? If not significantly displaced, how can it be treated?
A Jones fracture is located at the metaphyseal–diaphyseal junction of the fifth metatarsal (within 1.5 cm distal to the tuberosity of the fifth metatarsal) and often results in delayed healing if untreated. This injury is usually caused by stress placed across the bone when the heel is off the ground and the forefoot is planted. Treatment of an acute Jones fracture that is not significantly displaced consists of a non–weight-bearing cast for 6 to 8 weeks and progressive ambulation after removal of the cast. Fractures about the base of the fifth metatarsal are termed avulsion type fractures and will usually heal with a stiff-soled shoe.

American Academy of Family Physicians: Fractures of the Proximal Fifth Metatarsal. Available at: www.aafp.org/afp/990501ap/2516.html (Accessed February 17, 2020).

21. What are bunion and bunionette deformities?
A bunion, or hallux valgus deformity, develops when the great toe deviates laterally and the first metatarsal head develops a medial prominence. Conversely, a bunionette, or tailor's bunion, arises when a similar process develops laterally or the fifth metatarsal head.

22. What are some of the most common etiologies of bunion deformities?
Congenital bunions often occur in family lines. Certain foot types, such as flatfeet, are prone to pathologic changes by causing an imbalance of the tendons that control the great toe, which results in abnormal motion about the metatarsophalangeal joint (MTPJ). Shoes with a narrow toe box may also create similar tendon imbalances, which may contribute to a bunion deformity over time. Other causes include inflammatory arthritides and trauma.

23. Which joint is the most common location for a gout attack?
The most common location for a gout attack is the first MTPJ. This is called podagral.

24. What is an interdigital neuroma?
Often misunderstood as a tumor, this pathology is actually a benign enlargement of the fibrotic layer surrounding one of the common plantar digital nerves. This enlargement is typically the result of inflammation and irritation caused by shearing forces between the metatarsal heads or entrapment from a tight or enlarged deep transverse intermetatarsal ligament.

25. Where is the most common location for an interdigital neuroma, otherwise known as Morton's neuroma, to occur?
The most common location for Morton's Neuroma is the third interspace.

26. How do plantar calluses and warts differ?
See Table 48.1.

Table 48.1 Calluses Versus Plantar Warts

CHARACTERISTICS	CALLUSES	PLANTAR WARTS
Localization	High shear/friction area	Any location
Skin lines	Cross through the lesion	Pass around the lesion
Satellite lesion	No satellite lesions	Multiple daughter lesions
Local tenderness/pain	Pain on direct compression	Pain on side-to-side squeeze
Punctuate hemorrhages	Central core with punctuate	Hemorrhages around the base
Age	Common in elderly	Rare in elderly

Table 48.2 Biomechanical Effect of Pronation or Supination

BODY PART	PRONATION RESPONSE	SUPINATION RESPONSE
Hindfoot (coronal)	Eversion	Inversion
Forefoot/midfoot (sagittal)	Dorsiflexion	Plantar flexion
Forefoot (transverse)	Abduction	Adduction
Ankle	Dorsiflexion	Plantar flexion
Tibia	Internal rotation	External rotation
Knee	Flexion, valgus	Extension, varus
Femur	Internal rotation	External rotation
Hip	Flexion	Extension
Leg length	Shortened	Lengthened
Effect during gait	Absorbs impact, adapts to uneven terrain	Provides solid leverage for push off

Adapted from Wernick J, Volpe RG. *Lower Extremity Function and Normal Mechanics.* In R Valmassy, ed. *Clinical Biomechanics of the Lower Extremities.* St. Louis: Mosby; 1996:2–57.

27. What is the biomechanical effect of pronation or supination?
    See Table 48.2.

28. How are hallux rigidus (HR) and hallux limitus (HL) treated?
    First, determine if the condition is primary or secondary. Secondary HL is caused by the following:
    • Dorsiflexed first ray in excessive pronation, collapsed medial longitudinal arch from neuroarthropathy, foot orthosis with excessively high medial arch support, or surgery.
    • Tethering the flexor hallucis longus (FHL) after an ankle fracture, deep posterior compartment syndrome of the leg, or diabetes mellitus Charcot joint.
    Treat underlying causes (e.g., lengthening exercise of the gastric soleus muscle, lowering the arch of foot orthosis). Footwear modifications (rocker sole with steel shank, toe-spring, or Springlite carbon plate) are often helpful.

THE HAND AND WRIST: TOP 25 QUESTIONS THAT YOU WERE AFRAID TO ASK

Francis Lopez, MD, Jason L. Zaremski, MD, Ryan Roza, MD

Hands have their own language.

— Simon Van Booy

KEY POINTS FROM CHAPTER

1. Trigger fingers lock. Mallet fingers cannot extend. Jersey fingers cannot flex.
2. Swan-neck deformity: In this deformity, flexion occurs at the MCP joint, hyperextension at the PIP joint, and flexion at the DIP joint.
3. Boutonnière deformity: In this deformity, hyperextension occurs at the MCP joint, flexion at the PIP joint, and extension at the DIP joint.

1. What are the names of the carpal bones?
   One mnemonic is: "So Long To Pinky, Here Comes The Thumb
   S = **S**caphoid (1)   **T** = **T**rapezium (5)
   L = **L**unate (2)   **T** = **T**rapezoid (6)
   T = **T**riquetrum (3)   **C** = **C**apitate (7)
   P = **P**isiform (4)   **H** = **H**amate (8)
      Fig. 49.1.

2. What are the dorsal compartments of the extensor wrist?
   The extensor tendons of the hand are divided into six dorsal compartments. From radial to ulnar, they are as follows:

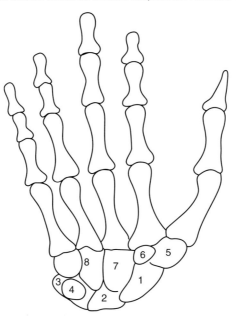

Fig. 49.1 Bones of hand and wrist.

I. Abductor pollicis longus, extensor pollicis brevis
II. Extensor carpi radialis longus, extensor carpi radialis brevis
III. Extensor pollicis longus
IV. Extensor digitorum communis, extensor indicis proprius
V. Extensor digiti minimi
VI. Extensor carpi ulnaris

3. What are the key actions of the interossei muscles?
   - **DAB** = **D**orsal interossei **AB**duct and assist in metacarpophalangeal (MCP) flexion
   - **PAD** = **P**almar interossei **AD**duct and assist in MCP flexion

4. How is lumbrical muscle function related to its anatomy?
   The lumbrical muscles originate from the tendons of the flexor digitorum profundus and insert into the extensor hood tendons. Their main action is flexion of the MCP joints and extension at the interphalangeal (IP) joints.

Conolly B, Prossor R. Functional anatomy and assessment. In: Prossor R, Conolly B, eds. *Rehabilitation of Hand and Upper Limb*. Butterworth-Heinemann. New York, NY, 2003.

5. How do you test the integrity of the flexor digitorum profundus (FDP) and superficialis tendon (FDS)?
   FDS:
   > For this test, the examiner holds the adjacent fingers in full extension while the patient flexes the problematic finger (Fig. 49.2). If there is no injury or tear in the flexor digitorum superficialis tendon, the patient is able to flex the PIP joint, while the distal interphalangeal (DIP) joint remains in extension or neutral.

   FDP:
   > In this test, the MCP and PIP joints are held in extension by the examiner while the patient flexes the DIP joints. If the patient can flex, then the long flexor of the FDP to that finger is intact.

Hoppenfeld S. *Physical Examination of the Wrist and Hand*. In: Hoppenfeld S, ed. *Physical Exam of the Spine and Extremities*. Norwalk, CT: Appleton & Lange; 1999:100–101.

6. How is the Finkelstein test performed?
   The patient flexes the thumb into the palm of the hand and flexes the fingers over the thumb. The examiner then ulnarly deviates the wrist. In de Quervain disease (stenosing tenosynovitis), pain is reproduced over the radial wrist (Fig. 49.3).

Cailliet R. *Common Tendonitis Problems of the Hand and Forearm*. In Cailliet R, ed. *Hand Pain and Impairment*. 4th ed. Philadelphia: F.A Davis; 1994.

7. How is de Quervain tenosynovitis treated?
   Conservative management includes activity modification, therapeutic modalities (Coban wrap for edema, ice massage over the radial styloid, iontophoresis), and gentle passive and active ROM, thumb spica splint, nonsteroidal inflammatory drug (NSAIDs), and corticosteroid injection. If surgical decompression is required, IP joint motion starts immediately after surgery.

8. What is the TFCC and what is the course of treatment?
   The triangular fibrocartilage complex (TFCC) is a confluence of soft tissue structures that provides stability to the distal radiolunar joint during supination and pronation. A type 1 tear is traumatic in nature and type 2 is degenerative.

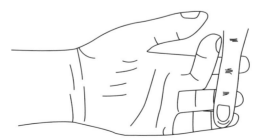

Fig. 49.2 The test for integrity of the flexor digitorum superficialis tendon.

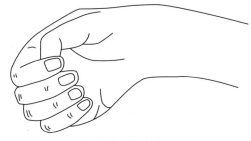

Fig. 49.3 The Finkelstein test.

On physical exam there is tenderness over the ulnar aspect of the wrist. Instability may be reproduced by translational movement of the radius in relationship to the ulna reproducing pain or "clicking." The "TFCC grind" or passive ulnar deviation with the wrist in pronation may reproduce pain. If a patient experiences ulnar-sided wrist pain after pushing up from sit to stand out of a chair ("press test"), then there would be concern for TFCC injury.

The current gold standard TFCC evaluation is arthroscopy. However, x-rays of the wrist are helpful to evaluate for fracture or degenerative changes, or an "ulnar positive variance."

Treatment in a symptomatic patient may initially be conservative including bracing and wrist strengthening. However, instability is best treated with surgical repair. If sporting activity is of importance, a steroid injection may allow for temporary pain relief.

Madden CC, Putukian M, Young CC, eds. *Netter's Sports Medicine.* 2nd ed. Philadelphia, PA: Elsevier; 2017.

Miller M, Thompson S, eds. *DeLee & Drez's Orthopaedic Sports Medicine.* 4th ed. Philadelphia, PA: Elsevier; 2014.

9. **What are the common sites for ulnar neuropathies?**
   The most common site for an ulnar neuropathy is at the elbow followed by the wrist. Peripheral ulnar neuropathies have multiple causes including compressive cubital tunnel syndrome, fractures to the hook of the hamate, repetitive trauma injuries (e.g., propulsion of manual wheelchairs), ganglia, and direct pressure to the ulnar nerve in Guyon's canal seen in cyclists (aka handlebar palsy).

Murata K, Shih T, Tsai M. Causes of ulnar tunnel syndrome: a retrospective study of 31 subjects. *J Hand Surg Am.* 2003;28:647.

Burnham R, Steadward R. Upper extremity peripheral nerve entrapments among wheelchair athletes: prevalence, location, and risk factors. *Arch Phys Med Rehabil.* 1994;75:519.

10. **What is the Froment sign?**
    In an ulnar neuropathy, the ulnar-innervated adductor pollicis is weakened or paralyzed. To compensate for the adductor pollicis, the patient will use the median-innervated flexor pollicis longus (FPL). A positive Froment sign occurs when the patient uses the FPL to flex the thumb at the IP joint. This is often observed when the patient is asked to grasp a piece of paper between the thumb and the index finger causing flexion of the thumb at the IP joint.

Richardson C, Fabre, G. Froment's sign. *J Audiov Media Med.* 2003;26:1.

11. **What muscles are supplied by the anterior interosseous nerve?**
    Flexor pollicis longus (FPL)
    Flexor digitorum profundus (FDP)
    Pronator quadratus (PQ)
    There are no superficial sensation fibers.

12. **What does the inability to make the "OK" sign mean?**
    The absence of the "OK" sign suggest an anterior interosseous nerve (AIN) palsy. Weakness in the FPL and the FDP leads to the inability to flex the IP joint of the thumb and the DIP joint of the index finger.

Santiago S, Vallarino R. *Median Neuropathy.* In: Frontera WR, Silver JK, eds. *Essentials of Physical Medicine and Rehabilitation.* Philadelphia, PA: Hanley & Belfus; 2002:119–125.

13. What is a trigger finger?

Trigger finger is a painful locking, snapping or triggering of the finger when it is flexed and extended. This is due to the nodular swelling or inflammation of the tendon sheath which makes it difficult for the tendon to glide under the annular ligament (A1 pulley) causing a triggering sensation. Patients who have diabetes and rheumatoid arthritis are at greater risk of developing trigger fingers. Treatment includes trigger splints placed at the MCP joint, local steroid injections, and surgery.

Silver J, Cheng J. *Trigger Finger.* In Frontera WR, Silver JK, eds. *Essentials of Physical Medicine and Rehabilitation.* Philadelphia, PA: Hanley & Belfus; 2002:191–194.

14. What are the two common deformities associated with rheumatoid arthritis in the hands? What is the mechanism of the deformities?

Swan-neck deformity: In this deformity, flexion occurs at the MCP joint, hyperextension at the PIP joint, and flexion at the DIP joint (Fig. 49.4A). Contractures and spasms of the intrinsic muscles cause dorsal subluxation of the tendons that results in hyperextension of the PIP joint. Synovitis further aggravates hyperextension by causing laxity of that joint. Flexion and tension on the long flexor cause flexion of the DIP joint.

Boutonnière deformity: In this deformity, hyperextension occurs at the MCP joint, flexion at the PIP joint, and extension at the DIP joint (see Fig. 49.4B). In patients with rheumatoid arthritis, there is weakness and tearing of the terminal portion of the extensor's hood, which tends to hold the lateral band in place. In this deformity, the lateral bands tend to slip down, flex the PIP joint, and exert tension to hyperextend the DIP joint.

Conolly B, Prossor R. *Rheumatoid Arthritis.* In: Prossor R, Conolly B, eds. *Rehabilitation of Hand and Upper Limb.* New York, NY: Butterworth-Heinemann; 2003.

15. What is the mechanism of ulnar deviation of the fingers in rheumatoid arthritis?

The deformities are secondary to chronic synovitis of the MCP joints, which causes a progressive weakening of the radial collateral ligaments and the fibers of the extensor tendon apparatus. The extensor tendons then displace ulnarly.

Smith R, Kaplan E. Rheumatoid deformities at the metacarpophalangeal joints of the fingers. *J Bone Joint Surg.* 1967;49:31.

Stirrat C. Metacarpophalangeal joints in rheumatoid arthritis of the hand. *Hand Clin.* 1996;12:515.

16. Where are Heberden's and Bouchard's nodes usually found?

Heberdens's nodes are found on the dorsal and lateral surfaces of the DIP joint. Bouchard's nodes are found at the PIP joint.

Hoppenfeld S. *Physical Examination of the Wrist and Hand.* In: Hoppenfeld S, ed. *Physical Exam of the Spine and Extremities.* Norwalk, CT: Appleton & Lange; 1999.

17. What is the pathology in Dupuytren's contracture and indications for surgery?

Dupuytren's disease is a form of proliferative fibroplasias of the palmar fascial bands which displaces the neurovascular bundles. This displacement results in soft tissue and joint contractures in genetically susceptible individuals. Surgical indications are mainly to restore hand function and/or to reduce disability.

Conolly B, Prossor R. *Dupuytren's Contracture.* In Prossor R, Conolly B, eds. *Rehabilitation of the Hand and Upper Limb.* New York, NY: Butterworth-Heinemann; 2003.

18. What is the pathology and treatment of scaphoid fractures?

A scaphoid fracture typically is a result of a hyperextension and radially deviated force on the wrist and hand. Radial-sided snuffbox pain is common. Initial imaging should include a radiographic scaphoid view and a lateral

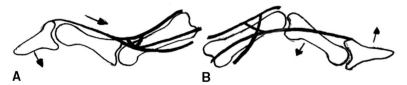

A   **B**

Fig. 49.4 Swan-neck (A) and Boutonnière (B) deformities.

and posterior-anterior (PA) view. Treatment is dependent upon the location of the fracture and whether it is displaced. The scaphoid receives retrograde blood supply; thus a distal pole fracture may be treated nonoperatively. Non-operative management includes a short thumb spica cast for complete immobilization. Proximal pole injuries however, are prone to avascular necrosis and surgical consultation is indicated.

Avery DM, Rodner CM, Edgar CM. Sports-related wrist and hand injuries: a review. *J Orthop Surg Res.* 2016;11:99.

19. What is the Terry Thomas sign?
A PA clenched fist view of the wrist showing a widening of more than 3 mm is known as the Terry Thomas sign. This indicates a potential Scapho-Lunate ligament injury and surgical referral is recommended.

20. What are Boxer's fractures?
Boxer's fractures are associated with a forceful impact with a clenched fist which results in a fracture of the fifth metacarpal (MC) neck. These fractures are most common in young men. Swelling, bruising, and deformity may be present upon presentation. Radiographic imaging is recommended. Non-operative management is indicated if there is up to approximately 30 to 50 degrees of dorsal angulation and no rotational deformity.

Henry MH. Fractures of the proximal phalanx and metacarpals in the hand: preferred methods of stabilization. *J Am Acad Orthop Surg.* 2008;16:10.

21. What is a Bennett's fracture?
Bennett Fractures occur at the base of the first MC and extend into the carpometacarpal (CMC) joint, potentially causing a serious intra-articular fracture or dislocation. They result after a longitudinal axial load is applied to the first MC in the flexed position. This type of a fracture requires surgical intervention.

Huang JI, Fernandez DL. Fractures of the base of the thumb metacarpal. *Instr Course Lect.* 2010;59:343–356.

22. What is Kienböck disease?
Kienböck disease is the osteochondrosis or avascular necrosis of the lunate. The disease occurs frequently in young adults and often affects manual laborers. Contributing factors include vascular, trauma, and/or repetitive loading. If there is clinical suspicion, radiographs are indicated. If the radiographs are negative, MRI and/or bone scintigraphy will be required. If caught early, non-operative management is an appropriate approach. However, if sclerosis, a compression fracture, or collapse of the lunate appear on plain radiographs, surgical referral is indicated.

Allan CH, Joshi A, Lichtman DM. Kienbock's disease: diagnosis and treatment. *J Am Acad Orthop Surg.* 2001;9:2.

23. What are the treatments for first carpometacarpal (CMC) arthritis?
Treatment includes hand therapy, splinting, and a cortisone injection. A short thumb spica splint can restrict the motion of the CMC joint, relieve pain, and avoid an adduction contracture. Hand therapy goals include improving first webbed space range of motion to prevent contracture deformity and strengthening the musculature to improve medial joint stability. In cases of severe arthritis, loss of hand function, and/or failure of non-operative management, surgical referral is recommended.

Van Heest AE, Kallemeier P. Thumb carpal metacarpal arthritis. *J Am Acad Orthop Surg.* 2008;16:3.

24. What is a gamekeeper thumb injury?
A gamekeeper's thumb, also known as a skier's thumb or an MC ulnar collateral ligament (UCL) injury, is caused by forcible abduction with a radial force on an extended thumb. Initially, there is pain with pinch, decreased range of motion, and a reduction in strength. Clinical examination should include valgus stress at 0 and 30 degrees of MCP flexion to assess for laxity. The contralateral thumb should be evaluated for comparison. Radiographs are indicated to assess for avulsion fractures. A stress radiograph may reveal rupture of the UCL. One should be aware of a potential Stener lesion, which is a retraction of the injured UCL that is now proximal and superficial to the adductor aponeurosis. If a Stener lesion is present, this requires surgical referral. Treatment options are dependent upon severity of injury. Grade 1 and 2 injuries may be treated nonoperatively with a thumb spica cast or splint immobilization. Grade 3 injuries require surgical referral.

Goldfarb CA, Puri SK, Carlson MG. Diagnosis, treatment, and return to play for four common sports injuries of the hand and wrist. *J Am Acad Orthop Surg.* 2016;24:12.

25. **What is the difference between mallet finger and jersey finger?**

    A mallet finger is a rupture of the insertion of the extensor tendon at the base of the distal phalanx. The patient is unable to extend the DIP joint, which sits in a flexed position. Treatment for mallet finger is 6 weeks in a volar static splint with the DIP joint in 10 degrees of hyperextension. Afterward, the patient starts on active and passive range of motion at the DIP joint. The patient continues to wear the volar static splint at night for 2 more weeks.

    A jersey finger, also known as an FDP avulsion injury, occurs when the DIP joint is either forced into extension or resisted flexion. Clinically, patient is unable to flex the DIP joint. Physical examination may reveal tenderness or a lump along the FDP tendon. Radiographs can assess for a bony avulsion of the distal phalanx. This injury requires surgical referral.

Bendre A, Harrigan B, Kalainov D. Mallet finger. *J Am Acad Orthop Surg.* 2005;13:5.

Goldfarb CA, Puri SK, Carlson MG. Diagnosis, treatment, and return to play for four common sports injuries of the hand and wrist. *J Am Acad Orthop Surg.* 2016;24:12.

CHAPTER 50

LOW BACK PAIN: CLINICAL, DIAGNOSTIC, AND MANAGEMENT PEARLS

Bosco Francisco Soares, MD, Maury Ruben Ellenberg, MD, Bryan J. O'Young, MD, CAc, FAAPMR and James W. Leonard, DO, PT

When all you have is a hammer, everything you see looks like a nail.
— Abraham Maslow (1908–1970)

KEY POINTS

1. Acute low back pain (LBP) is a symptom or constellation of symptoms and not a disease. Chronic and recurrent disabling pain may be considered a disease in its own right.
2. The natural history of acute LBP is to improve with or without treatment, although certain treatments can hasten the process of recovery and are worthwhile.
3. There is strong evidence that routine imaging for acute/subacute LBP using radiography or advanced imaging is not associated with a clinically meaningful effect on patient outcomes.
4. MRI and CT frequently identify many non-specific abnormalities that may confound diagnosis and treatment.
5. Degenerative changes involving the discs, facet joints, and vertebral bodies are anticipated consequences of aging and often influenced by genetic factors. Degenerative changes from repetitive/non-violent trauma are identical to the changes that occur in the context of normal aging.
6. Often, there is little or no correlation between non-specific degenerative abnormalities seen on imaging and the patient's clinical symptoms or signs.
7. Clinicians should conduct a focused history and physical examination to determine whether a specific underlying spinal condition potentially exists and measure the presence, severity, and level of neurologic involvement.
8. Disability from chronic LBP is a different disorder than acute LBP, and many factors contribute to it. It should be evaluated and treated differently than acute LBP.
9. Although acute and chronic non-specific LBP is evaluated and treated by a wide variety of healthcare professionals, often offering specific treatments that are unique to each discipline or specialty, patient outcomes remain remarkably similar.
10. Special injection techniques are occasionally indicated for short-term treatment in select patients with LBP.

1. Is low back pain (LBP) common?

LBP is a prevalent global health problem and is a leading cause of activity limitation, loss of productivity, disease burden, reduced vocational potential, and healthcare expenditure. About 80% of the general population will experience back pain at some time during their lifetimes. Approximately 30% of adults report having back pain that impacts everyday activities, including sleep. Worldwide prevalence has been rising. Although the prevalence rate for children and adolescents is lower than in adults, it is increasing.

2. What are the more common causes of LBP?

An effective classification of LBP, which can help guide evaluation and management, was initially proposed by a joint effort of the American College of Physicians and American Pain Society in 2007. A focused history and physical examination should assist clinicians in stratifying patients into one of four broad categories:

1. Non-specific (common) LBP (comprises 85% to 90% of adult patients presenting for initial evaluation of LBP, with or without leg pain, in a primary care setting).
2. LBP potentially associated with radiculopathy or spinal stenosis.
3. LBP potentially associated with another specific spinal cause.
4. LBP potentially arising from a non-spinal source.

   Non-specific LBP may be described as LBP, with or without lower extremity pain, that cannot reliably be attributed to a specific, well-understood disease or spinal abnormality. It is the most common cause of LBP across all age groups.

   Specific spinal causes of LBP in adults comprise 10% to 15% of patients presenting to a primary care setting for initial evaluation of LBP and include lumbar radiculopathy (4%), lumbar spinal stenosis (3%), ankylosing spondylitis and other inflammatory spondyloarthropathies (0.3% to 5%), vertebral compression fracture (4%), vertebral infection (0.01%), cauda equina syndrome (0.04%), and malignancy (0.7%).

Spinal metastases are the most common cause of spinal malignancy (97%). The spinal column is the most common site for bone metastasis. Spinal metastatic disease includes vertebral metastases with or without epidural extension (94%), intradural extramedullary metastases (5%), and intramedullary metastases (1%). Most common tumors that metastasize to the spine include prostate, breast, lung, kidney, thyroid, and gastrointestinal tumors. Primary neoplasms of the spinal canal are rare and encompass a range of benign and malignant neoplasms arising from the spinal cord, thecal sac, and spinal nerve roots. The most common myeloproliferative tumors of the spine include lymphoma and multiple myeloma.

Failed back surgery syndrome, post-laminectomy syndrome, or postsurgical spine syndrome is a recognized medical diagnosis (ICD-10 Code M96.1) that is often used to describe persistence or recurrence of back and/or radicular extremity pain of unknown origin in the same topographical distribution, following one more neuraxial surgical interventions. It is a generalized term embracing a constellation of conditions of uncertain origin and is not a true syndrome. Walker concluded in 1992 that 20% to 40% of the patients undergoing lumbar surgery will not experience benefits from the procedure, and that the condition will worsen in 1% to 10%. Despite advances in surgical technology, the incidence has not declined.

LBP may also be a manifestation of a generalized pain disorder such as fibromyalgia and other myofascial pain syndromes. It can also originate from non-spinal causes, especially from genitourinary, renal, gastrointestinal, vascular, and retroperitoneal pathology.

Specific causes of LBP in children and adolescents include spondylolysis, Scheuermann's kyphosis, idiopathic scoliosis, overuse syndromes, vertebral stress fractures, in addition to symptomatic lumbar disc herniation, trauma, tumor, and infection.

Low back, pelvic girdle, and hip pain or discomfort are common in pregnancy. Many can be ascribed to specific conditions associated with pregnancy, including relaxin-induced musculoskeletal changes, lumbar hyperlordosis, transient osteoporosis of pregnancy, round ligament hematoma, direct fetal pressure on lumbosacral plexus, miscarriage, and ectopic pregnancy.

There is increasing evidence that central pain-modulating mechanisms may play a pivotal role in the development and/or persistence and progression of chronic LBP in many patients, and that underlying psychiatric and psychosocial issues (yellow flag conditions) may contribute as primary or significant secondary factors.

Chou R, Qaseem A, Snow V, et al. Diagnosis and treatment of LBP: a joint clinical practice guideline from the American College of Physicians and the American Pain Society. *Ann Intern Med.* 2007;147:478–491.

Walker BF. Failed back surgery syndrome. *COMSIG Rev.* 1992;1:3–6.

3. Can the etiology of LBP be determined by imaging?

Only a minority of individuals will have an identifiable source of pain on spinal imaging that correlates with the history and clinical findings. However, advanced imaging is invaluable for assessing a subset of specific LBP patients and guiding management decisions in the appropriate clinical setting.

Imaging "abnormalities" are present in a high proportion of asymptomatic adults and are inclusive of degenerative, developmental, or adaptive changes that could, in many contexts, be considered clinically normal. Consequently, imaging findings must be interpreted with caution and in the context of the underlying clinical condition.

Provocative discography continues to be a controversial procedure that lacks specificity and a standard against which to compare and is no longer considered the "gold standard" for diagnosing "discogenic pain." Moreover, the diagnosis of "discogenic pain" also remains controversial since degenerative disc changes are frequent in asymptomatic adults across all ages.

4. What is the natural history of non-specific LBP?

Most individuals experiencing their first episode of back pain will predictably improve over a few days to weeks, regardless of treatment. However, up to one-third of patients continue to report persistent pain of moderate or greater severity one year after an acute episode of LBP. Approximately 20% will continue to experience significant limitations and inactivity. Chronic, non-specific LBP is a condition that is quite different from acute LBP. While it can be managed adequately, a "cure" is more elusive.

5. What are the most important tools to assess patients with LBP?

The history and clinical examination remain the mainstays in evaluating LBP and can guide further investigation and management. Imaging and other diagnostic findings should always be interpreted in the context of the history and clinical examination findings.

6. What historical factors are most important?

1. Pain onset and precipitating event(s)
2. Location and radiation, duration, and timing
3. Exacerbating and mitigating factors

4. Associated symptoms such as weakness, sensory impairment, paresthesias (distribution of paresthesias is more specific than the sensory exam in localizing radicular pain), voiding dysfunction, fever, and unintentional weight loss
5. Presence of "red flags"
6. Presence of "yellow flags"
7. Current function/activity level (home, work, recreational)
8. Past medical history including cancer, current/recent infection, recent surgery, prosthetic implant, IVDU, osteoporosis
9. Medications/Allergies
10. Previous treatments and response

The history should help separate spinal from non-spinal causes, and non-specific from specific spinal causes of LBP, as well as identify potentially serious conditions that may require prompt management (red flag conditions), as well as conditions for which specific treatment may be available (e.g., ankylosing spondylitis, vertebral compression fracture). Red flags, if present, indicate a need for further diagnostic testing (Tables 50.1 and 50.2). Yellow flags may identify patients who are at risk for poor outcomes.

Table 50.1 Specific Low Back Pain: Imaging and Diagnostic Tests for Selected Conditions

KEY CLINICAL FEATURES	INITIAL IMAGING	ADDITIONAL STUDIES
Malignancy		
• Hx of CA with new onset LBP or acute/subacute change in chronic LBP	MRI with without contrast	ESR
• Age ≥50 • Unexplained weight loss • Failure to improve after 1 month	Lumbosacral spine x-rays	ESR
• Multiple risk factors present	MRI or L-S Spine x-rays	ESR
Vertebral Infection		
• Fever • Intravenous drug use • Active/recent infection (Urinary tract infection, Resp. tract; skin, prosthetic implant, recent surgery, indwelling catheter)	MRI with without contrast	• ESR • CRP • CBC with differential
Vertebral Compression Fracture		
• Low velocity trauma in older patient[a] • Osteoporosis • Multiple risk factors for osteoporosis[a] • Chronic corticosteroid Rx[a]	Lumbosacral spine x-ray DEXA	AP pelvis or CT (if sacral fracture suspected)
Inflammatory Spondyloarthropathy		
• Pain duration ≥3 months • Younger age at onset (≤40 years) • Prolonged AM stiffness >1 h • Alternating buttock pain • Pain and stiffness worse with inactivity • Improvement with movement/exercise • History of cutaneous Psoriasis/Psoriatic arthritis • Acute onset with recent (~1–4 weeks) hx of non-gonococcal urethritis or infectious diarrhea, asymmetric peripheral arthritis, enthesitis, dactylitis (Reactive arthritis) • Ant. Uveitis	• AP Pelvis + labs (screen) • MR or CT for early/definitive diagnosis (MRI superior for identifying early inflammatory changes)	• ESR • CRP • HLA B-27
Cauda Equina Syndrome		
• Motor +/− sensory deficits at multiple levels • Usually bilateral • Saddle paresthesias or anesthesia • Urinary retention[b] • Fecal incontinence[b]	MRI	

Continued

Table 50.1 Specific Low Back Pain: Imaging and Diagnostic Tests for Selected Conditions—cont'd

KEY CLINICAL FEATURES	INITIAL IMAGING	ADDITIONAL STUDIES
Lumbar Radiculopathy		
• Back pain +/− leg pain • Paresthesias • Weakness • Typical lumbar nerve root distribution • Usually L4, L5, or S1 (>90%) • Positive nerve root tension signs (Straight leg raise test, Crossed straight leg raise test)	None if no significant or progressive neurologic deficit MRI if: • Symptoms present >1 month • Severe or progressive neurologic involvement • Potential candidate for surgery or epidural steroid injection	None Electromyography/Nerve conduction velocity if neurologic involvement present or suspected
Spinal Stenosis with Neurogenic Claudication		
• Older age >65 • Radiating leg pain +/− paresthesias • Pseudoclaudication • Symptoms precipitated by upright posture/ambulation • Unilateral or bilateral • Shopping cart sign	None MRI if: • Symptoms present >1 month • Neurologic involvement • Potential candidate for surgery	None EMG/NCV if neurologic involvement present or suspected

[a]Osteoporosis work-up or appropriate referral.
[b]Urinary retention and/or fecal incontinence = complete cauda equina syndrome = neurologic emergency.
CBC, Complete blood count; *CRP*, C-reactive protein; *ESR*, erythrocyte sedimentation rate; *LBP*, low back pain; *SLR*, straight leg raise test.

Table 50.2 History of Low Back Pain.

GENERAL CHARACTERISTICS	CHARACTERISTICS (OF PAIN)	CHARACTERISTICS OF ASSOCIATED SYMPTOMS	DIAGNOSTIC STUDIES AND TREATMENT	RED FLAGS
Onset Duration Incitin Relation to work, accident, or injury Pending litigation or disability	Intensity Location and radiation Character (aching, burning, sharp, etc.) Relation to position, time of day, or activity Relieving or exacerbating factors	Extremity pain Paresthesias Sensory impairment Motor weakness Perineal paresthesias or anesthesia Bowel or bladder dysfunction	Imaging studies Electromyography Medications taken and benefit Therapy, type and duration Injection procedures Surgical interventions	Fever Significant trauma Hx of Cancer Unexplained weight loss Failure to improve after 1 month Age > 50 IV drug use Recent infection or surgery Risk factors for osteoporosis

7. What are some common "yellow flags" that identify patients less likely to improve?
   • Untreated/inadequately treated mood disorder
   • Psychosocial stressors
   • Somatization
   • Passive coping strategies and attitudes to rehabilitation
   • Catastrophizing
   • Social withdrawal
   • Fear-avoidance beliefs/behavior
   • Reduced activity levels
   • High intake of alcohol or other substances (possibly as self-medication), with an increase since onset of pain

- Job/life dissatisfaction
- Higher disability levels
- Active/disputed compensation claims

8. **What elements should be included in a focused physical examination of a patient with LBP?**

The physical examination should be conducted methodically and efficiently while simultaneously engaging and reassuring the patient. Assure that patient comfort and modesty are maintained throughout the examination. Maintain constant communication with the patient to reassure and briefly explain each step of the examination, especially if it is likely to provoke pain or discomfort.

Key Components:

Posture: Upright coronal and sagittal posture to assess coronal and sagittal plane deviations; bending (Adam's forward bending test).

Gait and balance: Antalgic or pathologic gait pattern, heel and toe walk, squat and rise, tandem gait, and Romberg test.

Range of Motion (ROM):
- Lumbar spine: Forward flexion, extension, lateral flexion, and axial rotation of the upper torso. Assess asymmetric movement, pain generation, flexion or extension preference, and areas of mechanically limited or guarded motion.
- Proximal lower limb joints.

Palpation and percussion: superficial tenderness, paraspinous muscle spasm, percussion tenderness over bony prominences in the back and pelvis; lumbar paraspinous and gluteal muscles/tendons, sciatic notch, or greater trochanter tenderness.

Provocative Tests:

Nerve root tension tests: Straight leg raise and slump test (L5, S1), crossed straight leg raise, femoral stretch (L2–L4) test.

Iliopsoas (Thomas' test), rectus femoris (Ely's test), hamstring (90/90 test), muscle tightness.

Sacroiliac joint (SIJ) provocative tests (FABERE, thigh thrust, Gaenslen test, SIJ distraction, SIJ compression, sacral thrust).

Hip provocative tests (Stinchfield, Scour, FABERE, FADIR).

Note: Patients with back pain may also have co-morbid hip/groin pain, and imaging abnormalities may coexist in the spine and hip, making the diagnosis challenging *(Hip-Spine Syndrome)*. Be aware of non-concordant pain arising from provocative tests.

Peripheral neurologic examination: Examine motor strength, sensation, and muscle stretch reflexes to assess the presence and severity of neurologic involvement and assist with localization. Common upper motor neuron tests in the lower extremities include the plantar response (Babinski) and ankle clonus in addition to hyperreflexia.

Abdominopelvic exam: Examine the abdomen and pelvis if a non-spinal nociceptive source is suspected. Screen for hernia, abdominal, renal, vascular (abdominal aortic aneurysm), and pelvic causes of the back pain.

Vascular exam: peripheral pulses, capillary refill, dependent rubor, chronic ischemic distal lower extremity changes.

Digital Rectal Exam: when cauda equina, conus medullaris syndrome, or spinal cord injury is suspected.

Remember that few physical exam techniques can reliably identify the specific structure or disorder that is the primary source of back pain, especially in isolation, and that asymmetry or abnormality may be non-specific or unrelated to the cause of pain (e.g., scoliosis, sensory loss over the medial leg following medial knee arthrotomy or saphenous vein harvesting for CABG, allodynia or sensory impairment over the anterolateral thigh from comorbid meralgia paresthetica, distal LE weakness and atrophy due to comorbid peripheral neuropathy or muscle injury).

9. **Describe the straight leg raise test.**

The straight leg raise test (SLR) is a clinical sign indicating impingement or irritation of the lower lumbar nerve roots, primarily L5, S1. It is usually performed with the patient supine, hip in a neutral position, and knee extended. One leg at a time is passively raised, and the angle at which the patient has reproduction or exacerbation of radicular pain and/or paresthesias is noted. True tension on the nerve roots occurs between 30 and 70 degrees of hip flexion with the knee extended. Also, indicate whether the crossed straight leg raise is positive (i.e., straight leg raise provokes radicular pain in the contralateral, symptomatic lower extremity). In a 2010 Cochrane review, the SLR test yielded a high sensitivity (92%) but low specificity (28%) for disc herniation, with the crossed SLR yielding a low sensitivity (28%) but high specificity (90%).

10. **How does one clinically differentiate between neurogenic and vascular claudication?**

See Table 50.3.

Table 50.3 Neuro Genic versus Vascular Claudication.

CHARACTERISTIC	NEUROGENIC CLAUDICATION	VASCULAR CLAUDICATION
Pain increases with:	Upright posture/activity	Effort unrelated to posture
Better tolerance to:	Walking uphill	Walking downhill
Walking distance	Variable	Fixed
Pain decreases with:	Sitting/flexion	Standing or sitting
Relief at activity cessation	Delayed	Immediate
Pain pattern	Dull, aching Proximal to distal	Cramping Distal to proximal
Numbness, Paresthesia	Present	Absent
Bicycle riding	Better tolerated	Painful
Pulse	Normal	Reduced or absent
Skin/trophic changes	Absent	Present
Weakness, atrophy	Occasionally	Rarely
Ankle-brachial index	Normal	Abnormal

11. Are routine laboratory and imaging studies helpful for diagnosing non-specific LBP? Should any tests be performed?
    There is strong evidence that routine imaging and/or lab tests for non-specific LBP are not always associated with a clinically meaningful effect on patient outcomes. Imaging studies in adults frequently identify many non-specific and age-related changes that can arouse fear and anxiety in patients and can lead to poor decision-making by practitioners. (Nonetheless, they are widely utilized for medicolegal reasons.) The history, and clinical examination should guide imaging decision.

12. What radiologic studies should be considered in the lumbar spine for evaluation of specific causes of LBP?
    • When used appropriately, diagnostic imaging studies are an invaluable component of patient care in selected individuals with specific low back complaints.
    • Routine imaging, including x-rays for patients with acute non-specific LBP, can be performed parsimoniously as it has not been shown to improve patient outcomes or change treatment decisions.
    • Imaging should always be preceded by a focused history and clinical examination. Since imaging often reveals non-specific degenerative changes or incidental abnormalities in asymptomatic adults, the significance of abnormal findings should always be considered in the context of the underlying clinical condition.
    • Diagnostic imaging and laboratory testing should be considered in patients who have persistent LBP with severe or progressive neurologic deficits, or when history and examination suggest that a serious underlying condition may be present.
    • Patients with persistent LBP and signs and symptoms of radiculopathy or spinal stenosis should be evaluated with MRI if they are potential candidates for surgery or epidural steroid injection.
    • There is insufficient evidence to guide initial imaging or repeat imaging for patients with chronic LBP if the anticipated findings are unlikely to change the diagnosis or guide further management.
    • **X-rays** may be the initial imaging choice for patients with a suspected vertebral compression fracture, scoliosis, spondylolisthesis, or an initial evaluation of surgical spinal hardware. Lateral flexion/extension views may be useful for assessing segmental instability. Oblique views may demonstrate the presence of pars defects. Refer to Table 50.1 for general guidelines for imaging (and additional tests) in suspected specific spinal conditions.

Chou R, Qaseem A, Owens DK, Shekelle P. Diagnostic imaging for low back pain: advice for high-value health care from the American College of Physicians. *Ann Intern Med.* 2011;154:181–189.

Park J, Lui YW. An imaged-based review of the ACR appropriateness criteria for low back pain. *Appl Radiol.* 2016;45(9):9–15. Available at: https://appliedradiology.com/articles/an-image-based-review-of-the-acr-appropriateness-criteria-for-low-back-pain

13. Should MRI or CT be ordered as a definitive diagnostic test?
    MRI is generally preferred over CT because of its high diagnostic accuracy and inter-observer reliability. MRI does not use ionizing radiation and provides better visualization of even slight differences in soft tissue,

including disc abnormalities, ligamentous injuries, vertebral marrow, and the spinal canal and its contents. MRI is also superior for differentiating between normal and abnormal tissue and visualizing inflammatory tissue edema and abscesses. However, like other imaging, the MRI often cannot tell you what findings are relevant (see Question 12). Disadvantages specific to MRI include longer acquisition time. The patient must lie supine and motionless. Open MRIs possess limited magnet strength and provide inferior image resolution. Image acquisition times are also longer compared to closed systems.

CT advantages include lower cost, superior imaging of bone and other calcified tissue, superior delineation of the morphology of vertebral fractures, identifying transverse fracture planes that may be missed on MRI, and imaging of patients with ferromagnetic and certain other metal implants.

14. What other imaging studies may be helpful? When?

- **Nuclear medicine bone scan (bone scintigraphy)**, in combination with laboratory testing, may be useful in selected cases for screening for spinal inflammation, metastases, occult vertebral compression fractures, acute pars fractures, or assessing the acuity of a vertebral compression fracture. Bone scans are sensitive and demonstrate an osseous lesion's physiologic activity; they are not specific and will not identify the morphology of the lesion.
- **Single-photon emission computed tomography (SPECT)** can increase the sensitivity and specificity of planar bone scintigraphy. Like all bone scans, negative scans are clinically useful in ruling out specific pathology. Other diagnoses that can be made or excluded using a bone scan with or without combined SPECT imaging include:
- Early detection of destructive bony lesions. Osteoblastic lesions are generally more readily detectable by bone scan than PET/CT.
- Spinal fractures, including stress/compression fractures, bridging osteophytes, pars interarticularis fracture (may be false negative in 10% of MRIs).
- Sacral, coccygeal, and pelvic fractures.
- Bone metastasis (early lytic disease and lesions <5 mm are generally problematic for all imaging).
- Post-surgical fusion complications (>12 months post-surgery).
- Fusion failure—cold in early post-surgery (<8 months) period, hot in late post-surgery (>18 months) period.
- Sacroiliitis.
- Osteoid osteoma and other benign tumors.
  For selected cases of specific LBP, combining skeletal imaging techniques can permit the physician to relate the superior anatomical detail and morphology provided by plain films, CT, and MRI to the functional information provided by scintigraphy.
- DEXA scans are useful for the evaluation of patients with suspected osteopenia or osteoporosis.
- Because of its invasive nature, **CT myelography** should be reserved for selected cases and surgical planning when MRI is contraindicated, or the presence of surgical hardware obscures adequate visualization.

15. What are the essential anatomic points to observe in a lumbar spine film?
Systematic evaluation of lumbar spine x-rays utilizing ABCDEF format:
A. **A**lignment (coronal and sagittal, global, and segmental).
B. **B**one structures (vertebral body, endplates, pedicles, superior and inferior articular processes, pars interarticularis, facet joints, transverse processes, laminae, spinous process).
C. Bony spinal **C**anal (mid-sagittal diameter from posterior vertebral body to the spinolaminar line [lateral], and interpedicular distance [frontal]).
D. Intervertebral **D**isc spaces.
E. **E**xtraspinal structures (e.g., soft tissues, aortic calcification, renal calculi).
F. Bony neural **F**oramina (lateral view).

16. What are the guiding principles for ordering laboratory tests for a patient with LBP?
Laboratory testing is guided primarily by the history and clinical examination. Reasons may include:
Malignancy—ESR, CRP, Bone specific alkaline phosphatase (ALP), PSA
Malignant melanoma—ESR, SPEP/UPEP, IFE, FLC
Infection—CBC with differential, ESR, CRP, Blood C/S
Inflammatory spondyloarthropathy—ESR, CRP, HLA B-27
Paget's Disease—Bone-specific alkaline phosphatase (ALP)
Pancreatitis—serum amylase and lipase
  *ESR (erythrocyte sedimentation rate); CRP (C-reactive protein); PSA (prostate specific antigen); SPEP (serum protein electrophoresis); UPEP (urine protein electrophoresis); IFE (serum/urine immunofixation electrophoresis); FLC (serum/urine free light chain assay); CBC (complete blood count); C/S (culture and sensitivity)

---

*Glossary of acronyms

17. How do you treat the patient with acute non-specific LBP?

In the vast majority of patients, acute LBP is self-limiting. Patients at low risk for chronic pain and disability may only require reassurance, advice to stay active, education, and guidance on self-management. Education about proper back care is helpful, as are books and handouts that supplement education and self-care measures and/or provide instructions for specific exercises. Pharmacologic treatment may include limited-duration or prn NSAIDs and/or skeletal muscle relaxants (see Question 18).

18. Is bed rest helpful?

There is no evidence that bed rest beyond a day or two helps to relieve back pain; it may even prolong recovery and return to work. Progressive loss of muscle strength and endurance, reduction in bone mass, and DVT can occur with each prolonged period of complete bed rest. Patients should be encouraged to remain as active as tolerable and only avoid/limit activities that result in significant pain increases.

19. What are the main approaches in treating non-specific LBP?

Acute or subacute LBP:

General:

Patient reassurance: over 90% improve spontaneously with or without treatment

Self-care

Advice to remain active

Books, handouts

Superficial heat

Pharmacologic interventions (literature review reveals only a small effect size in most patients with low to moderate strength of evidence):

Acetaminophen

NSAIDs

Skeletal Muscle Relaxants

Non-surgical, non-pharmacologic interventions (literature review reveals only a small effect size in most patients with low to moderate strength of evidence):

Heat

Massage

Acupuncture

Spinal manipulation

Chronic LBP

General:

Patient Reassurance: 85% to 90% of patient population have non-specific LBP

Self-care

Advice to remain active

Educational books, handouts

Pharmacologic interventions: (literature review reveals small to moderate effect on pain and function. Consider limited-duration use for most medications. Medications should not take precedence over non-pharmacologic therapies).

NSAIDs

Serotonin-norepinephrine reuptake inhibitors (SNRI).

Duloxetine

Tramadol (SNRI + weak mu opioid receptor agonism)

Gabapentinoids—Pregabalin (bind to and inhibit alpha2-delta subunit-containing voltage-gated Ca channels [VGCCs])—central and neuropathic pain.

What about acetaminophen? Multiple randomized trials and systematic reviews have led to the recommendation that acetaminophen should no longer be considered a first-line treatment for back pain. A systemic review in 2015 found that, while there was "high quality" evidence that acetaminophen provides a significant, although not clinically important, effect on pain intensity and disability in the short term for hip or knee osteoarthritis, APAP was determined to be ineffective for reducing pain intensity and disability or improving quality of life in individuals with LBP. Nevertheless, because of its safety profile, acetaminophen has often been prescribed for selected patients with limited alternative therapeutic options.

Non-surgical, non-pharmacologic interventions:

Exercise

Motor control exercise

Acupuncture

Yoga

Tai Chi

Mindfulness-based stress reduction

Progressive relaxation

Low laser light therapy

Electromyography Biofeedback

Operant therapy
Cognitive behavioral therapy
Spinal manipulation
Interdisciplinary pain management and rehabilitation (pain and disability)
Work conditioning/work hardening/job retraining (return to work)

Qaseem A, Wilt TJ, McLean RM, et al. Noninvasive treatments for acute, subacute, and chronic low back pain: a clinical practice guideline from the American College of Physicians. *Ann Intern Med.* 2017;166(7):514–530Cherkin DC, Sherman KJ, Avins AL, et al. A randomized trial comparing acupuncture, simulated acupuncture, and usual care for chronic low back pain. *Arch Intern Med.* 2009;169(9):858–866.

Machado GC, Maher CG, Ferreira PH, et al. Efficacy and safety of paracetamol for spinal pain and osteoarthritis: systematic review and meta-analysis of randomised placebo-controlled trials. *BMJ.* 2015;350:h1225.

Chou R, Deyo R, Friedly J, et al. Nonpharmacologic therapies for low back pain: a systematic review for an American College of Physicians Clinical Practice Guideline. *Ann Intern Med.* 2017;166(7):493–505

Chou R, Deyo R, Friedly J, et al. Systemic pharmacologic therapies for low back pain: a systematic review for an American College of Physicians Clinical Practice Guideline. *Ann Intern Med.* 2017;166(7):480–492.

20. Are recurrences preventable?

Many people who experience activity-limiting LBP go on to have recurrent episodes. Few, if any, measures to prevent recurrence and chronicity have proven to be effective. Risk stratification should be routinely implemented to better identify patients at potential risk for poor outcomes and prolonged disability. These patients may require more frequent physician visits, supervised exercise programs, and psychological evaluation. They may also benefit from early involvement in a multimodal, interdisciplinary treatment approach.

21. What are the keys to successful treatment?

- Employ motivational interviewing techniques to encourage collaborative management and treatment compliance.
- Periodically reassess the diagnosis and plan of care.
- Identify and optimize the management of comorbid medical and psychosocial conditions.
- Identify functional impairments and potential barriers to treatment.
- Provide proper patient education, avoiding complex medical terminology; encourage patient engagement; and solicit patient feedback and shared decision making.
- Collaboratively set attainable goals and measurable outcomes.
- Injuries are followed by inflammation and repair. Pain often occurs in the absence of actual or potential tissue injury or may persist and progress beyond the expected duration of recovery. Determine where the patient is in this process.

22. What are the most important points to express to the patient?

- A specific medical or surgical condition has been addressed or ruled out.
- Pain is a sensory and emotional experience and is ideally managed by employing a biopsychosocial model; unless all underlying contributing and amplifying mechanisms are identified and co-managed, there is a high risk of persistence or recurrence.
- There usually is no "magic bullet" or specific treatment for chronic back pain.
- Surgery for back pain is generally appropriate only for less than 2% of patients with back pain and is more successful when the primary objective is to prevent further neurologic injury rather than to relieve pain.
- While chronic back pain may not be curable, it can be appropriately managed with the patient's active participation and compliance with evidence-based self-care and treatment recommendations.

23. What should be done if LBP persists for several weeks after initial treatment?

If comprehensive re-evaluation does not indicate a potential change in diagnosis and/or further investigation, continue reassurance, re-education, and advice to remain active. Consider additional non-pharmacologic interventions that have been shown to be potentially helpful.

Guidelines for further evaluation with imaging have not been established in patients with ongoing back pain if the clinical assessment does not suggest that imaging may lead to a meaningful change in diagnosis and/or management.

If the pain becomes disabling, a psychological evaluation may help identify underlying psychosocial contributors to pain, suffering, and disability. An interdisciplinary pain management approach that includes cognitive, behavioral, and functional restoration therapies in conjunction with other established pain management strategies should be considered early in those identified as high-risk for chronic pain and disability.

Non-pharmacological measures should be considered the mainstay of treatment for non-specific LBP. Pharmacologic therapies have limited benefit in treating nonspecific LBP and are usually tempered by adverse effects and unfavorable risk-benefit profiles, especially with long-term use. Chronic opioid therapy (COT) has been known to be ineffective for non-cancer pain, with unacceptably high risks of misuse, abuse, dependence, diversion, and mortality.

24. What are the alternative decisions when a patient is not progressing?
Answer available in online edition under online bonus questions and answers section -Question 3.

25. Is disability from LBP common?
LBP is the leading cause of disability globally. Despite advances in knowledge of the spine and back pain and diagnostic and treatment approaches, years lived with disability (YLDs) caused by LBP have increased globally by 54% between 1990 and 2015, attributed mainly to population increase and aging. However, the rising prevalence of comorbidities commonly associated with LBP populations, including mood disorders, obesity, sedentary lifestyles, industrialized societies, and iatrogenesis, are also likely contributing factors.

26. How should the patient who is disabled by pain be treated?
Referral for comprehensive interdisciplinary pain management and functional rehabilitation should be considered early to improve outcomes and minimize long-term disability, especially when:
- A specific nociceptive or neuropathic etiology is not identified.
- The underlying pain condition is not amenable to a specific treatment.
- Pain and disability do not respond to standard therapies.
- Significant yellow flag comorbidities are identified.

27. Is LBP usually remediable without surgery?
Non-specific LBP is never a surgical condition. Only a small minority of patients with LBP require surgery. Despite advances in surgical technology, the rates of failed back surgery syndrome have not declined. According to data published by the state of Maine, the best surgical outcomes occurred where surgery rates were lowest; the worst results occurred in areas where rates were highest.

Keller RB, Atlas SJ, Soule DN, et al. Relationship between rates and outcomes of operative treatment for lumbar disc herniation and spinal stenosis. *J Bone Joint Surg Am.* 1999;81(6):752-762.

28. When is surgical referral indicated for LBP?
Prompt spinal surgery referral or transfer to an emergency department with emergent spinal surgery facilities available should be considered in patients presenting with a potential surgical urgency/emergency (e.g., patients with severe or progressive neurologic deficits, suspected cauda equina syndrome, significant trauma, or vertebral infection), especially if associated with neurologic involvement, epidural abscess or spinal instability.
The most common conditions prompting elective spine surgery referrals are symptomatic lumbar disc herniation, lumbar spinal stenosis with neurogenic claudication, and lumbar spondylolisthesis. Surgical outcomes are less favorable when the primary objective is to relieve pain rather than prevent further neurologic injury. The presence of preoperative yellow flag conditions and poor correlation of imaging findings with the history and clinical examination are reliable predictors of poor outcomes.

29. Who should treat patients with LBP?
Despite the vast number of specialists and treatments utilized for LBP, outcomes remain similar across disciplines.
Physiatrists should be considered the first line of specialty referral for all persons with non-urgent, non-emergent LBP. In most cases, a physiatrist would be the ideal "primary physician" for initial evaluation and management and referral decisions for patients with non-urgent or emergent LBP.

30. What are the typical components of a rehabilitation program?
1. Controlling pain and inflammation, minimizing tissue injury.
2. Restoring normal/symmetric ROM and flexibility.
3. Restoring normal/symmetric strength and endurance.
4. Neuromuscular control (proprioception and coordination) retraining.
5. Functional Rehabilitation: Sport-specific activities for return to sport; work conditioning & work hardening for return to work.

31. How should end of healing and maximal medical improvement issues in workers' compensation injury and personal injury cases be approached?
- Diagnosis
- Restrictions (if any)
- Prognosis
- Anticipated time of maximal medical improvement
- Impairment or disability rating (if applicable)
- Future diagnostic and treatment needs (if applicable)
- Conclusions and recommendations must be consistent with evidence-based, objective clinical findings determined by the history, clinical examination, diagnostic studies, and response to treatment.

Bonus questions and answers are available online.

BIBLIOGRAPHY

Brinjikji W, Luetmer PH, Comstock B, et al. Systematic literature review of imaging features of spinal degeneration in asymptomatic populations. American Journal of Neuroradiology 2015;36(4):811-816.

Carey TS, Evans AT, Hadler NM, et al. Acute severe low back pain. A population-based study of prevalence and care-seeking. *Spine*. 1996;21:339-344.

Carragee EJ, Alamin TF, Carragee JM . Low-Pressure positive discography in subjects asymptomatic of significant low back pain illness. *Spine*. 2006;31(5):505-509.

Carragee EJ, Lincoln T, Parmar VS, et al. A gold standard evaluation of the "discogenic pain" diagnosis as determined by provocative discography. *Spine (Phila Pa 1976)*. 2006;31(18):2115-2123.

Chou R, Deyo R, Friedly J, et al. Systemic pharmacologic therapies for low back pain: a systematic review for an American College of Physicians Clinical Practice Guideline. *Ann Intern Med*. 2017;166(7):480-492.

Chou R, Fu R, Carrino JA, et al. Imaging strategies for low-back pain: systematic review and meta-analysis. *Lancet*. 2009;373(9662):463-472.

Chou R, Loeser JD, Owens DK, et al. Interventional therapies, surgery, and interdisciplinary rehabilitation for low back pain: an evidence-based clinical practice guideline from the American Pain Society. *Spine (Phila Pa 1976)*. 2009;34(10):1066-1077.

Chou R, Qaseem A, Owens DK, et al. Diagnostic imaging for low back pain: advice for high-value health care from the American College of Physicians. *Ann Intern Med*. 2011;154:181-189.

Cohen SP: Sacroiliac joint pain: A comprehensive review of anatomy, diagnosis, and treatment. *Anesth Analg*. 2005;101:1440-1453.

da C Menezes Costa L, Maher CG, Hancock MJ, et al. The prognosis of acute and persistent low-back pain: a meta-analysis. *CMAJ*. 2012;184(11):E613–624.

Delitto A, Piva SR, Moore CG, et al. Surgery versus nonsurgical treatment of lumbar spinal stenosis: a randomized trial. *Ann Intern Med*. 2015;162(7):465-473.

Deyo RA, Mirza SK, Turner JA, et al. Overtreating chronic back pain: time to back off? *Am Board Fam Med*. 2009;22(1):62-68. doi:10.3122/jabfm.2009.01.080102.

Deyo RA, Rainville J, Kent D. What can the history and physical examination tell us about low back pain? *JAMA*. 1992;268:760-765.

Duthey B. Priority Medicines for Europe and the World "A Public Health Approach to Innovation". Update on 2004 Background Paper 6.24 Low back pain. 15 March 2013.

Fardon DF, Williams AL, Dohring EJ, et al. Lumbar disc nomenclature: version 2.0: Recommendations of the combined task forces of the North American Spine Society, the American Society of Spine Radiology and the American Society of Neuroradiology. *Spine J*. 2014; 14(11):2525-2545.

Fishbain DA, Cole B, Cutler RB, et al. A structured evidence-based review on the meaning of nonorganic physical signs: Waddell signs. *Pain Med*. 2003;4(2):141-181.

Friedly J, Standaert C, Chan L. Epidemiology of spine care: the back pain dilemma. *Phys Med Rehabil Clin N Am*. 2010;21(4): 659–677.

Genevay S, Atlas SJ. Lumbar spinal stenosis. *Best Pract Res Clin Rheumatol*. 2010; 24(2): 253–265.

Haldeman S. Diagnostic tests for the evaluation of back and neck pain. *Neurol Clin*. 1996;14(1):103-117.

Hartvigsen J, Hancock MJ, Kongsted A, et al. What low back pain is and why we need to pay attention. *Lancet*. 2018;391(10137): 2356-2367.

Hoy D, Brooks P, Blyth F, et al. The Epidemiology of low back pain. *Best Pract Res Clin Rheumatol*. 2010;24(6):769-781.

Jarvik JG, Deyo RA. Diagnostic evaluation of low back pain with emphasis on imaging. *Ann Intern Med*. 2002;137:586-597.

Jarvik JJ, Hollingworth W, Heagerty P, et al. The Longitudinal Assessment of Imaging and Disability of the Back (LAIDBack) Study: baseline data. *Spine (Phila Pa 1976)*. 2001;26(10):1158-1166.

Jensen MC, Brant-Zawadzki MN, Obuchowski N, et al. Magnetic resonance imaging of the lumbar spine in people without back pain. *N Engl J Med*. 1994; 331(2):69-73.

Konin T, Wiksten D, Isear J, et al. *Special Tests for the Orthopedic Examination*. 2nd ed. Thorofare, NJ: Slack; 2002.

Laslett M, Aprill CN, McDonald B, et al. Diagnosis of sacroiliac joint pain: validity of individual provocation tests and composites of tests. *Man Ther*. 2005;10(3):207-218.

Lin IB, O'Sullivan PB, Coffin JA, et al. Disabling chronic low back pain as an iatrogenic disorder: a qualitative study in Aboriginal Australians. *BMJ Open*. 2013;3:e002654. doi: 10.1136/bmjopen-2013-002654.

Maness DL, Khan M. Disability evaluations: more than completing a form. *Am Fam Physician*. 2015;91(2):102-109.

Martell BA, O'Connor PG, Kerns RD, et al. Systematic review: opioid treatment for chronic back pain: prevalence, efficacy, and association with addiction. *Ann Intern Med*. 2007;146(2):116-127.

Pengel LH, Herbert RD, Maher CG, et al. Acute low back pain: systematic review of its prognosis. *BMJ*. 2003;327:323.

Qaseem A, Wilt TJ, McLean RM, et al. Noninvasive treatments for acute, subacute, and chronic low back pain: a clinical practice guideline from the American College of Physicians. Published at Annals.org on 14 February 2017.

Ramírez C, Sanchez L, Oliveira B. Prevalence of sacroiliac joint dysfunction and sacroiliac pain provocation tests in people with low back pain. *Ann Phys Rehabil Med*. 2018;61:e152.

Rubin DL. Epidemiology and risk factors for spine pain. *Neurol Clin*. 2007;25(2):353-371.

Sabharwal S, Kumar A. Methods for assessing leg length discrepancy. *Clin Orthop Relat Res*. 2008;466(12):2910-2922.

Sabharwal S, Zhao C, McKeon J, et al. Reliability analysis for radiographic measurement of limb length discrepancy: Full-length standing anteroposterior radiograph versus scanogram. *J Pediatr Orthop*. 2007;27:46-50.

Toyone T, Tanaka T, Kato D, et al. Patients' expectations and satisfaction in lumbar spine surgery. *Spine (Phila Pa 1976)*. 2005;30(23):2689-2694.

van der Windt DA, Simons E, Riphagen II, et al. Physical examination for lumbar radiculopathy due to disc herniation in patients with low-back pain. *Cochrane Database Syst Rev*. 2010;(2):CD007431.

Verbiest H. *Lumbar spine stenosis*. In: Youmans JR, ed. *Neurological Surgery: A Comprehensive Reference Guide to the Diagnosis and Management of Neurosurgical Problems*. 3rd ed. Philadelphia, PA: Saunders; 1990:2805-55.

Von Korff M, Saunders K. The course of back pain in primary care. *Spine*. 1996;21:2833-2837.

Vroomen PC, de Krom MC, Knottnerus JA. Predicting the outcome of sciatica at short-term follow-up. *Br J Gen Pract*. 2002;52:119-123.

Waddell G. Non-organic physical signs in low back pain. *Spine*. 1980;5:117-125.

WEBSITES

1. AAPMR Knowledge Now. Available at: https://now.aapmr.org/.
2. ACP Clinical Practice Guidelines. Available at: https://www.acponline.org/clinical-information/guidelines.
3. VA/DoD Clinical Practice Guidelines. Available at: https://www.healthquality.va.gov/guidelines/pain/lbp/.
4. NICE Guidelines (Low back pain and sciatica). Available at: https://www.nice.org.uk/guidance/ng59.
5. O'Connell NE, Cook CE, Wand BM, et al. Clinical guidelines for low back pain: a critical review of consensus and inconsistencies across three major guidelines. *Best Pract Res Clin Rheumatol.* 2016;30(6):968-980. Available at: https://doi.org/10.1016/j.berh. 2017.05.001.
6. Park J, Lui YW. An imaged-based review of the ACR appropriateness criteria for low back pain. *Appl Radiol.* 2016;45(9):9–15. Available at: https://appliedradiology.com/articles/an-image-based-review-of-the-acr-appropriateness-criteria-for-low-back-pain.
7. Fardon DF, Williams AL, Dohring EJ, et al. Lumbar disc nomenclature: version 2.0: Recommendations of the combined task forces of the North American Spine Society, the American Society of Spine Radiology and the American Society of Neuroradiology. *Spine J.* 2014;14(11):2525-2545. Available at: https://www.sciencedirect.com/science/article/pii/S1529943014004094.

PATIENT EDUCATION AND SELF-HELP RESOURCES

1. Hanscom D. *Back in Control: A Surgeon's Roadmap Out of Chronic Pain.* 2nd ed. Quicksilver Dr, Dulles VA: Vertus Press - Chelsea Green Publishing; 2016.
2. Deyo RA. *Watch Your Back!: How the Back Pain Industry Is Costing Us More and Giving Us Less—and What You Can Do to Inform and Empower Yourself in Seeking Treatments.* Ithaca, NY: Cornell University Press; 2014.
3. Sarno JE. *Healing Back Pain: The Mind-Body Connection.* Midtown Manhattan, NY: Hachette Book Group; 2010.

Bonus questions and answers are available online.

CHAPTER 51

NECK PAIN: ANATOMY, PATHOPHYSIOLOGY, AND DIAGNOSIS

Andrew J. Duarte, MD, Shailaja Kalva, MD, and Alex Moroz, MD, MHPE

Well, as giraffes say: you don't get no leaves unless you stick your neck out.
—Sid Waddell (1940–2012)

KEY POINTS

1. The cervical spine permits movement of the head in all planes, and the degree of movement decreases with age.
2. Cervical spondylotic myelopathy is the most common cause of cervical myelopathy.
3. The presence of ossification of the posterior longitudinal ligament (OPLL) and diffuse idiopathic skeletal hyperostosis (DISH) increase the risk for spinal cord injury.

1. **What encompasses the functional anatomy of the cervical spine?**
   The cervical portion of the human spine includes the seven rostral vertebrae designated as C1–C7 with a lordotic curvature. The first two vertebrae, C1 (atlas) and C2 (axis), share a fused vertebral body, with C2 having a special process, the odontoid process. The remainder of the cervical vertebra, C3–C7, enable movement in all planes. A functional unit in the spine refers to two contiguous vertebral bodies, with an intervertebral disc, with their corresponding laminae, pedicles, uncovertebral (also known as the Joints of Luschka), and zygapophyseal (frequently referred to as facet) joints. There are two major ligaments that span the vertebral column: the anterior longitudinal ligament and the posterior longitudinal ligament. There are eight cervical nerve roots that arise from the spinal cord, each with a dorsal and ventral root. Each spinal nerve is named for the vertebrae below, with the C8 spinal nerve between C7–T1.

2. **What is the typical range of motion in the cervical spine and its various joints?**
   Typical cervical flexion ranges from 54 to 69 degrees while extension ranges from 73 to 93 degrees. Lateral rotation is approximately 60 degrees in both directions. Lateral flexion ranges from 37 to 43 degrees. These values all decrease as humans age. The majority of cervical rotation occurs at the levels C1/C2, where the odontoid process acts as a swivel for the head to rotate. The flexion and extension of the vertebral bodies in the cervical spine are in the setting of movement at the zygapophyseal joint, the movement of each facet joint is approximately 10 to 20 degrees with the greatest degree flexion and extension occurring at the C4/C5 and C5/C6 levels. **Thus, the anatomic levels that most frequently exhibit degenerative wear are C4/C5 and C5/C6.**

3. **Identify common pain generators in the cervical spine.**
   Cervical pain (cervicalgia) is the fourth leading cause of disability worldwide. The majority of cervicalgia is myofascial in etiology, but there are multiple pain generators in the cervical spine itself. Cervical spondylosis is a common finding that is asymptomatic in a majority of patients but can cause pain. The uncovertebral joints can hypertrophy and are a common culprit in cervical radiculopathy. Zygapophyseal joints are true synovial joints, and as such, contain mechanoreceptors and nociceptors, and when the joint is inflamed, can result in pain. Additionally, there are nociceptive fibers that innervate the posterior longitudinal ligament, dural sheaths of the nerve roots, and intervertebral discs.

4. **Name the provocative maneuvers that should be performed when evaluating someone with neck pain.**
   Spurling's test is a maneuver that was first described in 1943 and involves tilting the head (extension followed by lateral flexion) toward the side with pain, after which an axial load is applied for at least 20 seconds. The test is positive if radicular symptoms are elicited. Later descriptions of Spurling's test include the additional movement of ipsilateral rotation. The test has a sensitivity ranging from 40% to 77% and a specificity ranging from 92% to 100%. The **neck distraction test** involves the patient lying supine and the examiner cephalad; the examiner stabilizes the head holding the occiput and places traction and the patient reports relief of radicular symptoms. This test is considered to be highly specific.

5. **Identify the red flags when evaluating someone with neck pain.**
   So-called "red flag" components of the history are worrisome signs and warrant that the patient be thoroughly evaluated for concerning etiologies of neck pain. When taken in conjunction with the entire clinical picture, urgent workup, including imaging (often MRI) and possible intervention, may be indicated. Traditional red flag symptoms

include a history of malignancy, unintentional weight loss, nocturnal pain, age over 50, bladder dysfunction, bowel dysfunction, extremity weakness, fevers or chills, history of IV drug use, recent trauma, anterior neck pain, and failure to improve after 6 weeks of conservative management.

6. What are the typical radiology studies used to evaluate atraumatic neck pain?

When indicated, radiologic evaluation of a patient's neck pain should be used in conjunction with a thorough history and physical to confirm a diagnosis and synthesize a treatment plan. The American College of Radiology recommends three views for plain films: AP, lateral, and open-mouth to provide a comprehensive view of the vertebral segments. The lateral view arguably provides the most information: alignment, disc spacing, joint arthropathy, including evidence of end-plate sclerosis and osteophytes, and views of the posterior elements. When wanting to view the soft tissue structures, MRI is the study of choice. Various sequences are chosen when anticipating a diagnosis; for instance, fat-suppression sequences can highlight edema in and around the foramen and spinal canal. Common structures evaluated by MRI include discs, spinal cord, neural foramina, the posterior ligamentous complex (interspinous ligaments, ligamentum flavum, etc.), as well as providing additional information for bony abnormalities such as evaluation of metastatic malignancies.

7. What contributes to spondylosis of the cervical spine?

Spondylosis can be defined as encroachment of the spinal canal or foramen. There is a complex multifaceted cascade that occurs over the course of many years that has not completely elucidated. However, it is generally understood that the process starts in the discs and facet joints, and it is the synergistic degeneration that results in spondylosis. With the facet joints, synovitis results in cartilage dissolution and osteophyte formation. In regard to the discs, tears result in disruption of the nucleus pulposus as well as loss of height contributing to vertebral endplate abnormalities. Cervical spondylotic changes essentially include vertebral body osteophytes, facet joint hypertrophy, uncovertebral joint deformity, and disruption of the ligamentum flavum.

8. What are the classic cervical facet referral patterns?

The facet referral patterns were established by a seminal study published in 1990 in which Dwyer et al. injected contrast media into the capsules of facet joints of five healthy volunteers and mapped their pain, see Fig. 51.1.

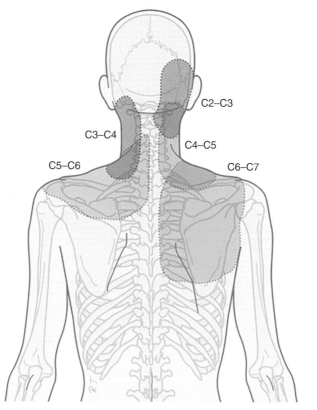

Fig. 51.1 Cervical facet referral patterns. (Illustrated by Rogier Trompert Medical Art. http://www.medical-art.nl.)

Note that the facets are innervated by the medial branches of dorsal rami of that level and the level below. For instance, the facet joint of C4 and C5 is innervated by the medial branches of the C4 and C5 dorsal rami. This is important to distinguish as these dorsal rami are targets for analgesia via medial branch blocks, and if appropriate, radiofrequency (RF) ablations. RF neurotomy often results in sustained analgesia: one study assessed 12 patients with chronic cervicalgia and noted a mean benefit of at least 50% analgesia for 263 days compared to just 8 days in the placebo group.

9. **What is cervical myelopathy and what is in the differential diagnosis?**
Myelopathy is defined as dysfunction of the spinal cord, and its cause can be demarcated into two broad categories: intrinsic and extrinsic etiologies. Intrinsic causes of myelopathy include: infections, syringomyelia, radiation-induced, vitamin deficiencies, and malignancies. Extrinsic etiologies are related to the common mechanism of spinal cord compression: arthritis, malignancy, epidural abscess, ossification of the posterior longitudinal ligament (OPLL) (described later), and cervical spondylosis. Cervical spondylotic myelopathy is the most common cause of extrinsic myelopathy.

10. **What are OPLL and DISH?**
Ossification of the posterior longitudinal ligament, or OPLL, is a multifactorial syndrome that can result in axial pain. The pathophysiology of this disease is not well understood, but it is recognized that there is a defect in the nucleotide pyrophosphatase gene as well as mutations in collagen genes. These aberrations result in ossification of the ligament over time, which can narrow the spinal canal. It is recognized to be on the spectrum of another disease entity known as DISH or diffuse idiopathic skeletal hyperostosis, a condition characterized by a tendency toward ossification of ligament, tendon, and joint capsule (enthesial) insertions. In both disorders, patients may be asymptomatic for some time, but as it progresses, patients can become symptomatic with diminished range of motion and axial pain as the ligaments ossify. If severe enough, it can result in myelopathy. Seventy percent of cases involve C2–C4, and it is much less common in the thoracic and lumbar spine. It is also worth noting that OPLL and DISH increase the risk for SCI as there is less space in the spinal canal for the cord, and it is more likely to be injured.

11. **What is a "stinger?"**
A stinger is a neuropathic pain that results from neuropraxia (transient damage to the myelin along a peripheral nerve resulting in conduction abnormalities) **of nerves in the brachial plexus,** classically the upper trunk. Recall that the brachial plexus stems from the roots of C5–T1. Compression of these nerves by spondylosis in conjunction with certain movements (cervical extension) result in an unpleasant sensation. The clinical presentation is classic among contact sports such as football, rugby, and soccer, but can be the result of any vigorous activity in conjunction. Patients will complain of any or a combination of the following: burning pain, numbness, paresthesias, or weakness. It is important to reassure patients that complain of such symptoms and present with a classic history that their symptoms should spontaneously resolve. If the symptoms don't resolve, the patient should be evaluated for more serious injuries such as nerve root avulsion.

Bonus questions and answers are available online.

BIBLIOGRAPHY

1. Bussières AE, Stewart G, Al-Zoubi F, et al. The treatment of neck pain-associated disorders and whiplash-associated disorders: a clinical practice guideline. *J Manipulative Physiol Ther.* 2016 Oct;39(8):523-564.e27. doi: 10.1016/j.jmpt.2016.08.007.
2. Hoy D, March L, Woolf A, et al. The global burden of neck pain: estimates from the Global Burden of Disease 2010 study. *Ann Rheum Dis.* 2014;73:1309-1315.
3. Kubas C, Chen YW, Echeverri S, et al. Reliability and validity of cervical range of motion and muscle strength testing. *J Strength Cond Res.* 2017 Apr;31(4):1087–1096. doi: 10.1519/JSC.0000000000001578.
4. Manchikanti L, Hirsch JA, Kaye AD, et al. Cervical zygapophysial (facet) joint pain: effectiveness of interventional management strategies. *Postgrad Med.* 2016;128(1):54-68. DOI: 10.1080/00325481.2016.1105092.
5. Lee J, Scott L, Fredericson M. Thoracic outlet syndrome. *PM&R.* 2010;2(1):64-70.
6. Murphy CA, Stockwell E. Cervical Whiplasth. *PM&R Knowledge Now.* May 24, 2021.
7. Lord SM, Barnsley L, Wallis BJ, et al. Percutaneous radiofrequency neurotomy for chronic cervical zygapophyseal-joint pain. *N Engl J Med.* 1996;335:1721.
8. Matsumoto S, Nakamura K, Seichi A, et al. Radiographic predictors for the development of myelopathy in patients with ossification of the posterior longitudinal ligament: a multicenter cohort study. *Spine.* 2008;33:2648-2265.
9. Milne N. The role of zygapophysial joint orientation and uncinate processes in controlling motion in the cervical spine. *J Anat.* 1991;178:189.
10. Theodore N. Degenerative cervical spondylosis. *N Engl J Med.* 2020;383(2):159–168. doi: 10.1056/NEJMra2003558.
11. Voorhies RM. Cervical spondylosis: recognition, differential diagnosis, and management. *Ochsner J.* 2001;3(2):78-84.
12. Yonenobu K, Kozo N, Yoshiaki T. *OPLL.* Springer, 2006. Available at: https://doi.org/10.1007/978-4-431-32563-5.
    Van Zundert J, Vanelderen P, Kessels A, et al. Radiofrequency treatment of facet-related pain: evidence and controversies. *Curr Pain Headache Rep.* 2012;16:19–25 (2012). doi:10.1007/s11916-011-0237-8.

CHAPTER 52

EMERGING MECHANISMS AND METHODS FOR NEUROREHABILITATION: THEORY AND APPLICATION

April D. Pruski, MD, MBA, Albert Recio, MD, PT, and Marlis Gonzalez-Fernandez, MD, PhD

KEY POINTS

1. Constraint-induced movement therapy involves restraining the unaffected opposite extremity in order to promote purposeful use of the involved limb.
2. Locomotor training utilizes a body weight support system over a treadmill with manual assistance for gait movement from trainers.
3. Epidural stimulation involves application of continuous electrical current to the lower part of the spinal cord.
4. Transcutaneous spinal cord stimulation (TSCS) is a non-invasive intervention that stimulates spinal neural circuits using electrodes placed on the skin.
5. Targeted muscle re-innervation (TMR) employs surgical denervation and selective re-innervation of a muscle with a different nerve that can be used for myoelectric control of a prosthesis.

1. What is neurorehabilitation: how can physiatry and neurology help?

Neurorehabilitation is the process of promoting recovery from a nervous system injury and minimizing and/or compensating for any functional alterations by using therapy and a variety of evidence-based and/or emerging interventions. Potentially disabling neurologic conditions (e.g., stroke, spinal cord injury [SCI], and traumatic brain injury [TBI]) can effectively be addressed with neurorehabilitation techniques supervised by physiatrists and neurologists. Functional recovery is dependent on *both* spontaneous neurologic recovery and proactive rehabilitative/physiatric intervention. Physiatrists and neurologists have access to emerging, scientifically supported options to advance neurological recovery, including modalities for neural regeneration, restoration, repair, and dynamic reorganization. Additionally, application of behavioral, neurophysiologic, and learning strategies can amplify favorable outcomes.

2. What is constraint-induced movement therapy (CIMT)?

CIMT, often called "forced use therapy," involves restraining the unaffected opposite extremity in order to promote purposeful use of the involved limb. CIMT is a technique for enhancing hand function in upper extremity hemiparesis. Restraining the able upper extremity is often done by wrapping it in a mitt or sling. Treatment protocols involve repetitive, task-oriented movements (of increasing complexity) performed several hours daily.

3. How is a typical CIMT regimen structured?

- Constraining or using a mitt with non-paretic upper limb to promote use of impaired limb during 90% of waking hours;
- Intensive, task-specific use of affected paretic limb up to 6 h/day over a two-week period;
- Adherence-based behavioral methods designed to translate improvements learned in clinical or lab setting to a patient's habits and routine at home.

Kwakkel G, Veerbeek JM, van Wegen EE, et al. Constraint-induced movement therapy after stroke. *Lancet Neurol.* 2015;14(2):224–234. doi:10.1016/S1474-4422(14)70160-7.

4. Is there evidence of CIMT's efficacy?

CIMT's efficacy was explored in small studies demonstrating benefit for upper extremity (UE) stroke hemiparesis. One landmark randomized control trial (RCT) study focused on a post-3-month stroke (CVA) population. This study suggested that a 2-week program of CIMT for patients more than a year after stroke who maintain some hand and wrist movement can improve upper extremity function that persists for at least one year. Studies have also demonstrated improvements in quality of life and activities of daily living (ADL) proficiency.

Rivas RJ, Doussoulin AP, Saiz JL, et al. Application of constraint induced movement therapy protocol: effectiveness on the quality and quantity of upper extremity movement recovery after stroke. *J Neurol Sci.* 357: e355. doi:10.1016/j.jns.2015.08.1267.

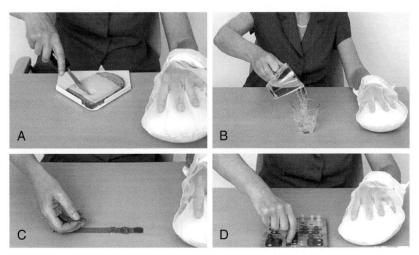

Fig. 52.1 Examples of constraint-induced movement therapy. (A) Patient using affected arm to hold a knife while unaffected arm is re-strained. (B) Patient using affected arm to pour a liquid into another cup while unaffected arm is restrained. (C) Patient using affected arm to pick up coins while unaffected arm is restrained. (D) Patient using affected arm to hold pins while unaffected arm is restrained.

5. **Is neuroplasticity induced by CIMT?**
   Changes in cortical activation patterns (correlating with improved motor abilities in post-CIMT upper-limb CVA paresis) were demonstrated by fMRI and transcortical magnetic stimulation studies.

   Sibin M, Nesin KR, Sabitha AG, et al. Constraint induced movement therapy as a rehabilitative strategy for ischemic stroke—linking neural plasticity with restoration of skilled movements, *J Stroke Cerebrovasc Dis.* 2019;28(6):1640–1653. doi:10.1016/j.jstrokecere-brovasdis.2019.02.028.

6. **How much voluntary motion of the paretic limb is required to begin CIMT?**
   Participants needed a minimum of 10 degrees of thumb abduction/extension or 10 degrees of active wrist exten-sion and at least 10 degrees of extension in two or more other digits.

   Hatem SM, Saussez G, Faille MD, et al. Rehabilitation of motor function after stroke: a multiple systematic review focused on tech-niques to stimulate upper extremity recovery. *Front Hum Neurosci.* 2016;10:442. doi:10.3389/fnhum.2016.00442.

7. **Describe "modified CIMT" (mCIMT).**
   mCIMT is a less intense treatment format that employs the same principles as CIMT but with less intensity (e.g., less time).

8. **When can CIMT therapy be employed after a stroke?**
   Receiving CIMT 3 to 9 months post-stroke results in greater functional gains than delayed training. Although no benefits less than 3 months post-stroke were substantiated, mCIMT has shown larger effects when administered in the acute phase.

9. **What is constraint-induced aphasia therapy (CIAT)?**
   CIAT adapts CIMT for patients with aphasia. Treatment is intensive and involves placing restraints on non-verbal gestures for expressive or receptive aphasia.

   Zhang J, Yu J, Bao Y, et al. Constraint-induced aphasia therapy in post-stroke aphasia rehabilitation: a systematic review and meta-analysis of randomized controlled trials. *PLoS ONE.* 2017;12(8):1–15

10. **Describe locomotor training.**
    Locomotor training, also called body weight-assisted training or body weight-supported treadmill training, in-volves using a body weight support system over a treadmill with manual assistance for gait movement from trainers. It was developed as an experimental intervention to aid in walking recovery following a central nervous system (CNS) injury. A body weight support system consists of a harness supporting the patient's pelvis and trunk, which is attached to an overhead mechanism to precisely maintain the weight support force throughout the gait cycle. Trainers provide tactile postural cues and assist in limb movements.

11. What are the components of locomotor training?

Step training (treadmill), over ground walking/training, and community ambulation training.

What is Locomotor Training? Available at: https://www.christopherreeve.org/research/our-rehabilitation-network/locomotor-training/how-locomotor-training-works.

Joining Forces: Wings for Life and the Christopher & Dana Reeve Foundation – YouTube. Available at: https://www.youtube.com/watch?v=avM54K0AI2s.

12. Describe central pattern generation.

Central pattern generation is the oscillating rhythmical right and left activity of segmental neural circuitry in the spinal cord. They are observed in nearly all vertebrate species and contribute to neural mechanisms responsible for ambulation and swimming. In limb ambulation, the flexors and extensors are activated in an alternating, repetitive pattern independent of supraspinal control. This facilitates alternate swing and stance movement.

Barriere G, Leblond H, Provencher J, et al. Prominent role of the spinal central pattern generator in the recovery of locomotion after partial spinal cord injuries. *J Neurosci.* 2008;28:3976.

Minassian K, Hofstoetter US, Dzeladini F, et al. The human central pattern generator for locomotion: does it exist and contribute to walking? *Neuroscientist.* 2017;23(6):649–663. doi: 10.1177/1073858417699790.

13. What are the differences between locomotor training and current practice for rehabilitation of walking after SCI?

Unlike conventional gait training following SCI, which tends to rely on compensatory strategies (assistive devices such as walkers and braces), locomotor training allows movement of the entire body in (? more natural) gait patterns including arm swing, alternating trunk list, and suspended limb movement.

14. Give examples of robotic treadmill training and its advantages.

Lokomat is a robotic treadmill training system which uses a body weight support system to suspend an individual. The patient's legs are attached to robotic legs that assist with basic walking functions. It allows therapists to focus on the patient and therapy. Conventional BWSTT is very labor intensive. Up to three therapists are often necessary to facilitate upright posture and normal walking patterns. The *Lokomat* is automated so that human assistance to maintain upright posture and provide proper stepping is not needed.

15. What is massed practice as it pertains to SCI?

Massed practice is an intervention that uses repetitive practice as a primary therapeutic intervention. It includes repetitive task-specific and non-task-specific activities, and is repeated multiple times for multiple hours intermittently. Unimanual massed practice (UMP) and bimanual massed practice (BMP) are two such rehabilitation approaches.

Anderson A, Alexanders J, Addington C, et al. The effects of unimanual and bimanual massed practice on upper limb function in adults with cervical spinal cord injury: a systematic review. *Physiotherapy.* 2019;105(2):200–213. doi: 10.1016/j.physio.2018.10.003.

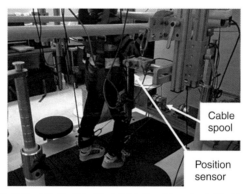

Cable spool

Position sensor

Fig. 52.2 Locomotor training. (Wu M, Kim J, Gaebler-Spira DJ, et al. Robotic resistance treadmill training improves locomotor function in children with cerebral palsy: a randomized controlled pilot study. *Arch Phys Med Rehabil.* 2017;98(11):2126–2133.)

16. **What is task-specific practice as it pertains to SCI?**
   Task-specific practice uses goal-oriented activities repetitively. Task-specific practice should be:
   - Relevant to the patient (tasks in which s/he has a vested interest);
   - Randomly ordered;
   - Repetitive and involve "mass practice";
   - Geared toward reconstructing whole tasks;
   - Provide timely, positive feedback.

17. **What are the benefits of functional electrical stimulation cycling?**
   Increased lower extremity muscle mass and cardiopulmonary function; increased bone mass and reduced risk of osteoporosis and fractures; increased range of motion; reduced risk for skin breakdown, and reduced spasticity.

18. **What is epidural stimulation?**
   Continuous electrical current is applied to the lower part of the spinal cord. The electrical stimulation comes from a microchip implanted over the spinal cord's protective coating (dura).

Rejc E, Angeli CA. Spinal cord epidural stimulation for lower limb motor function recovery in individuals with motor complete spinal cord injury. *Phys Med Rehabil Clin N Am.* 2019;30(2):337–354.

Rejc E, Angeli CA, Bryant N, et al. Effects of stand and step training with epidural stimulation on motor function for standing in chronic complete paraplegics. *J Neurotrauma.* 2017;34(9):1787–1802.

Shah PK, Lavrov I. Spinal epidural stimulation strategies: clinical implications of locomotor studies in spinal rats. *Neuroscientist.* 2017; 23(6):664–680.

19. **What is transcutaneous spinal cord stimulation (TSCS)?**
   Non-invasive intervention that stimulates spinal neural circuits using electrodes placed on the skin.

Gerasimenko Y, Gorodnichev R, Moshonkina T, et al. Transcutaneous electrical spinal-cord stimulation in humans. *Ann Phys Rehabil Med.* 2015;58(4):225–231.

Mayr W, Krenn M, Dimitrijevic MR. Epidural and transcutaneous spinal electrical stimulation for restoration of movement after incomplete and complete spinal cord injury. *Curr Opin Neurol.* 2016;29(6):721–726.

20. **How is the robotic exoskeleton used in locomotion?**
   The exoskeleton is a battery-operated bionic device that enables people with lower extremity weakness and/or paralysis to return to standing and walking.

Louie DR, Eng JJ. Powered robotic exoskeletons in post-stroke rehabilitation of gait: a scoping review. *J Neuroeng Rehabil.* 2016;13(1):53.

Mazzoleni S, Battini E, Rustici A, et al. An integrated gait rehabilitation training based on functional electrical stimulation cycling and overground robotic exoskeleton in complete spinal cord injury patients: preliminary results. *Int Conf Rehabil Robot.* 2017:289–293.

Proietti T, Crocher V, Roby-Brami A, et al. Upper-limb robotic exoskeletons for neurorehabilitation: a review on control strategies. *Rev Biomed Eng.* 2016;9:4–14.

21. **What is blood flow restriction (BFR) training?**
   BFR training involves using cuffs or wraps placed around a limb during exercise that maintains arterial inflow to the muscle but restricts venous return. By limiting blood flow out of the restricted limb or region, the muscle is allowed to be stressed at much lower amounts of force. This is important for those who are paralytic or have neurologic impairment preventing them from using muscles under normal activities.

22. **What are three mechanisms for muscle hypertrophy?**
   1. Mechanical Tension: The amount of weight being lifted;
   2. Metabolite Stress: Lactate response from anaerobic training;
   3. Muscle Damage: Exercise-induced muscle damage.

Everton D, Polito MD. Blood pressure response between resistance exercise with and without blood flow restriction: a systematic review and meta-analysis. *Life Sci.* 2018;209:122–131.

Scott BR, Loenneke JP, Slattery KM, et al. Exercise with blood flow restriction: an updated evidence-based approach for enhanced muscular development. *Sports Med.* 2015;45(3):313–25.

Stavres J, Singer TJ, Brochetti A, et al. The feasibility of blood flow restriction exercise in patients with incomplete spinal cord injury. *PM&R.* 2018;10(12):1368–1379.

23. Describe targeted muscle re-innervation (TMR) and how it improves control of a myoelectric prosthesis.

TMR is a process involving surgical denervation and selective re-innervation of a muscle or muscle segment with a different nerve. This produces a proportionately contracting muscle island that can be used for myoelectric control of a prosthesis. TMR is frequently used for improved prosthetic control following a shoulder or transhumeral disarticulation amputation. The individually controlled muscle islands created by TMR can be volitionally contracted to generate EMG signals that are picked up by the prosthesis and translated into movement. TMR is now also being used for lower limb amputees and is being studied for treatment of phantom limb pain and neuroma.

Cheesborough JE, Smith LH, Kuiken TA, et al. Targeted muscle reinnervation and advanced prosthetic arms. *Semin Plast Surg.* 2015; 29(1):62–72.

Kuiken TA, Barlow AK, Hargrove L, et al. Targeted muscle reinnervation for the upper and lower extremity. *Tech Orthop.* 32(2):109.

24. Following a brain lesion, how can neuroplasticity be facilitated by functional electrical stimulation?

Neuromuscular electrical stimulation (NMES) uses electrical current to produce contractions of paralyzed or paretic muscles and is used for upper motor neuron injury, where lower motor neurons are intact to produce muscle contraction. NMES for stroke rehabilitation is usually applied to elbow, wrist, and/or hand extensor muscles. Improved upper limb function after an NMES device is off is called "therapeutic effect."

Through surface electrodes placed on the forearm over motor points of muscles, cyclic NMES uses a one- or two-channel stimulator to activate wrist and/or finger and thumb extensors in a repetitive fashion. Several RCTs have shown reduced upper limb motor impairments in acute and subacute hemiplegic patients.

NMES is being studied in combination with other emerging therapeutic strategies such as: mirror therapy, rTMS, CIMT, robot-assisted movement therapy, motor imagery, bilateral movement training, virtual relative games, transcranial direct current stimulation (tDCS), and body-weight supported treadmill training.

Khaslavskaia S, Sinkjaer T. Motor cortex excitability following repetitive electrical stimulation of the common peroneal nerve depends on the voluntary drive. *Exp Brain Res.* 2005;162:497–502.

Knutson JS, Fu MJ, Sheffler LR, et al. Neuromuscular electrical stimulation for motor restoration in hemiplegia. *Phys Med Rehabil Clin N Am.* 2015;26(4):729–745. doi:10.1016/ j.pmr.2015.06.002.

Rushton DN. Functional electrical stimulation and rehabilitation—a hypothesis. *Med Eng Phys.* 2003;25:75–78.

Smith GV, Alon G, Roys SR, et al. Functional MRI determination of a dose-response relationship to lower extremity neuromuscular electrical stimulation in healthy subjects. Exp Brain Res. 2003;150:33–39.

25. How else can upper limb function be restored in stroke hemiparesis?

Mirror therapy. Mirror therapy involves placing a mirror on the patient's midsagittal plane and reflecting the non-paretic side as if it were the affected one, creating a visual illusion of normal movements of the paretic limb.
Mental practice with motor imagery. Movement is imagined by the individual.
Non-invasive brain stimulation. Transcranial magnetic stimulation (TMS) and tDCS.

TMS is a high-intensity electric current delivered through a coil done through a single pulse, double pulse, paired pulse, or repetitive pulse. Sessions usually are performed on consecutive days (usually 5 to 10). There is moderate-quality evidence that rTMS, in combination with other rehabilitation techniques, potentiates the effect of rehabilitation treatment (occupational therapy, physiotherapy, motor training) when treating UE impairments.

tDCS is a technique which uses a noninvasive application of a weak electrical current to brain tissue. There are several montages: (1) anodal, (2) cathodal, and (3) bihemispheric. There is low- to moderate-quality evidence for the effectiveness of tDCS versus control for improving ADL performance after stroke.

- *Invasive brain stimulation.* There is insufficient evidence for implanting deep brain stimulation as an adjuvant therapy into stroke rehabilitation when treating upper extremity impairment or disability.
- *Robot-assisted therapy.* Its main advantage is to deliver high-dosage and high-intensity training. Most devices are for elbow and shoulder movements, with a lack of robotic training devices for finger and wrist. Moderate-quality evidence shows robot-assisted therapy for paretic UE to be similar or inferior to standard rehabilitation.
- *Virtual reality.* In virtual reality, the operator is meant to experience a computer-generated environment as if it were part of the real world. Evidence suggests that virtual reality with another rehabilitation treatment appears to be valuable and can be integrated as an adjuvant therapy into stroke rehabilitation to improve UE motor impairment and disability.

Hatem SM, Saussez G, Faille MD, et al. Rehabilitation of motor function after stroke: a multiple systematic review focused on techniques to stimulate upper extremity recovery. *Front Hum Neurosci.* 2016;10:442. doi:10.3389/fnhum.2016.00442.

26. Can non-invasive brain stimulation help aphasia?

TMS and tDCS can modify cortical excitability and aid in the functional recovery of language. fMRI demonstrated neural reorganization and increased activity in the affected side of patients with recovery of aphasia post-stroke. Intensive tDCS over 2 weeks resulted in more significantly improved naming ability that was better maintained 6 months later when compared to the sham group.

Hamilton RH, Chrysikou EG, Coslett B. Mechanisms of aphasia recovery after stroke and the role of noninvasive brain stimulation. *Brain Lang.* 2011;118(1-2):40–50.

27. Can regrowth occur in neurons in the mature CNS?

Most CNS axons in adults do not spontaneously regenerate. However, it does occur in at least two regions: neocortical granule cells are generated in the subgranular zone of the dentate gyrus. It has been observed that granule cell damage can lead to greater recruitment proliferation of new granule cells from resident progenitors. Within the olfactory bulb, new neurons are generated in the subventricular zone in the wall of the lateral ventricle. These neurons migrate rostrally to their destinations and assume the role of interneurons.

There is no current evidence to support the impact of these processes in brain injury recovery. Still, their discovery hints at the possibility of latent self-repairing capabilities in the brain. Some evidence suggests the enhancement of neurogenesis by growth factor application or gene therapy.

Abrahams JM, Gokhan S, Flamm ES, et al. De novo neurogenesis and acute stroke. Are exogenous stem cells really necessary? *Neurosurgery.* 2004;54:150–156.

28. Why is regeneration of injured neurons in the CNS so rare?

Although CNS neurons can extend their axons and participate in branching, the myelin prevents axon growth.

29. How can barriers to CNS regeneration be overcome?

Regeneration involves four factors: (a) survival or replacement of injured neurons; (b) extending damaged or replaced axon processes to the original targets; (c) remyelination of damaged axons; and (d) formation of functional synapses.

Damaged CNS can derive cellular replacement from:

Stem cells and *fetal tissue*: These cells have crucial properties of (1) in vitro propagation, (2) multipotency, (3) the ability to be genetically tagged with therapeutic genes or markers, and (4) direct grafting into the mature CNS. The atypical environment of the injured CNS must not pose a hindrance to the development of the new cells, as they must be able to integrate functionally into the remaining CNS circuitry.

Neurotrophic factor delivery: Neurotrophins (i.e., brain-derived neurotrophic factor [BDNF]) contribute to axon growth and cell survival. They are usually combined with growth-promoting cells or matrices to provide the permissive substrate. BDNF-expressing Schwann cells have been able to facilitate the regrowth of supraspinal axons across a transected spinal cord. Reaching the injured CNS has posed a challenge, as axons struggle to leave the permissive substrate and reach their targets. Some evidence indicates that induction of neurotrophins in the injured tissue may help overcome this barrier.

Axon guidance and *removal of growth inhibition*: Axon guidance, the formation and regeneration of synapses, and activity-dependent plasticity are all dependent on growth-promoting molecules. The formation of a *gliotic scar* following a CNS injury can prevent regrowth molecularly and physically. The normal CNS expresses growth inhibitory molecules (proteoglucan NG2, semaphoring III/collapsing I, keratin, chondroitin sulfate, etc.), which may then be re-expressed in the scar.

Bridging: This can occur in response to a loss of a portion of the CNS, extensive scarring, or the development of a cyst. The bridge guides axons across these barriers and reintroduces axons into intact parenchyma. Current research into the development of artificial substrate to scaffold axon growth is underway.

30. List and explain known mechanisms of CNS neuroplasticity that mediate recovery after injury.

Neuronal regeneration occurs more frequently by the following means:

Collateral sprouting: Following injury to an axon, a nearby axon branches and assumes the injured axon's territory. If the contributing neuron is similar to the lost neuron, recovery can be bolstered. Dysfunction arises when the new sprout transmits a signal that significantly varies from the original. Collateral sprouting has been seen within 8 hours of injury and is usually complete within 1 month in animal studies.

Pruning (actually branching): Re-innervation of the abandoned target occurs through new branch generation from an uninjured axon. Animal studies have shown this process can take several months.

Ingrowth: After injury to an axon, a remote contributing neuron innervates a foreign target. This usually has a maladaptive result and takes months to complete.

31. What is "unmasking" as it relates to recovery of function after brain injury?

Unmasking involves using relatively inactive pathways to take over functional representation of undamaged brain tissue and the neuronal group to assume some of the function of the damaged brain tissue. It involves the shifting of cortical pathways from inhibitory to excitatory, followed by neuronal proliferation and synaptogenesis.

Nahmani M, Turrigiano GG. Adult cortical plasticity following injury: recapitulation of critical period mechanisms? *Neurosci.* 2014;283:4–16.

32. Which medications are used to enhance neurorehabilitation?

- *Serotonergic drugs* (fluoxetine FLAME): A study showed significant gains with arm/leg Fugl-Meyer at 90 days compared with placebo when given within 10 days of ischemic stroke onset.
- *Dopaminergic drugs* (Sinemet): A double-blinded RCT showed 100 mg L-Dopa/day within 6 months of stroke combined with PT was significantly better than placebo + PT on motor recovery using the *Rivermead Motor Assessment.*
- *Amphetamine:* A double-blind, RCT showed no difference between physiotherapy + amphetamine or physiotherapy + placebo. There was no difference in the Fugl-Meyer motor score.
- *Methylphenidate:* Evidence shows therapeutic effects on cognition, motivation, mood, and post-stroke depression.
- *Modafinil:* Evidence shows some improvement in alertness and fatigue in TBI and stroke patients.
- *Donepezil:* There is some improvement in post-stroke aphasia, including improvements in auditory comprehension, naming, repetition, and oral expression.

Borghol A, Aucoin M, Onor I, et al. Modafinil for the improvement of patient outcomes following traumatic brain injury. *Innov Clin Neurosci.* 2018;15(3-4):17–23.

Cramer SC. Drugs to enhance motor recovery after stroke. *Stroke;* 2015;46(10):2998–3005. doi:10.1161/STROKEAHA.115.00743.

Ramasubbu R, Goodyear BG. Methylphenidate modulates activity within cognitive neural networks of patients with post-stroke major depression: a placebo-controlled fMRI study. *Neuropsychiatr Dis Treat.* 2008;4(6):1251–1266.

Zhang X, Shu B, Zhang D, et al. The efficacy and safety of pharmacological treatments for post-stroke aphasia. *CNS Neurol Disord Drug Targets.* 2018;17(7):489–501. doi:10.2174/1871527317666180706143051.

33. What are the uses of modafinil in rehabilitation?

Common uses include self-esteem improvement in individuals with spinal cord acid injury, mood elevation and sleepiness alleviation in myotonic dystrophy, and reduction of fatigue in multiple sclerosis.

34. What are the rehabilitative uses of methylphenidate?

Methylphenidate has proven to be safe and effective for post-stroke depression. In patients with acute TBI, visuospatial attention, working memory, and reaction time were improved by one dose of methylphenidate in another double-blind, placebo-controlled trial. In a 6-week, double-blind, placebo-controlled crossover study on TBI, methylphenidate improved the speed of processing and caregiver ratings of attention.

Burke D, Recio A, Al-Adawi S, et al. Post-stroke depression: medication and rehabilitation, Spaulding Rehab Hospital. In: *Third World Congress of the International Society of Physical and Rehabilitation Medicine.* Bologna, Italy; 2005:7–11.

Whyte J, Hart T, Vaccaro M, et al. Effects of methylphenidate on attention deficits in traumatic brain injury: a multidimensional randomized controlled trial. *Am J Phys Med Rehabil.* 2004;83:401–420.

35. What is virtual reality?

Virtual reality and interactive video gaming include computer-based program designed to simulate real-life objects and events. A Cochrane review from 2017 found virtual reality may not be more effective than conventional therapy. It is a safe intervention for improving arm function and ADL after stroke. Currently, heterogeneity exists between studies, leaving unclear the circumstances in which a virtual reality program is superior.

Chi B, Chau B, Yeo E, et al. Virtual reality for spinal cord injury-associated neuropathic pain: systematic review. *Ann Phys Rehabil Med.* 2019;62(1):49–57.

Laver KE, Lange B, George S, et al. Virtual reality for stroke rehabilitation. *Cochrane Database Syst Rev.* 2017;11(11):CD008349. doi:10.1002/ 14651858.CD008349.pub4.

Villiger M, Bohli D, Kiper D, et al. Virtual reality-augmented neurorehabilitation improves motor function and reduces neuropathicpain in patients with incomplete spinal cord injury. *Neurorehabil Neural Repair.* 2013;27(8):675–83. doi:10.1177/ 1545968313490999.

36. How are BDNF, neuroplasticity, and physical activity related?

Frequent physical activity is associated with an upregulation of a number of genes involved in increased plasticity, including neuronal activity-regulated pentraxin, synaptotagmin 5, and BDNF. BDNF specifically is a key mediator in neuronal connectivity, use-dependent plasticity, and synaptic efficacy in animal studies.

BDNF is neuroprotective and neurotropic:

- Intraventricular infusion of BDNF protects the hippocampus and cortex from ischemic damage and the septal cholinergic neurons from axotomy-induced loss.
- Promotes the differentiation, neurite expansion, and survival in hippocampal, cortical, striatal, septal, and cerebellar neurons.
- BDNF increases neuroplasticity:
- Stimulates synaptophysin and synaptobrevin synthesis.
- Enhances synaptic transmission and long-term potentiation.

Cotman CW, Berchtold NC. Exercise: a behavioral intervention to enhance brain health and plasticity. *Trends Neurosci.* 2002;6:295–301.

Edwards T, Motl RW, Sebastião E, et al. Pilot randomized controlled trial of functional electrical stimulation cycling exercise in people with multiple sclerosis with mobility disability. *Mult Scler Relat Disord.* 2018;26:103–111.

Harkema S, Behrman A, Barbeau H. *Locomotor Training: Principles and Practice.* New York, NY: Oxford University Press; 2011.

Szuhany KL, Bugatti M, Otto MW. A meta-analytic review of the effects of exercise on brain-derived neurotrophic factor. *J Psychiatri Res.* 2015;60:56–64. doi:10.1016/j.jpsychires.2014.10.003.

Umphred DA, et al. Umphred's Neurological Rehabilitation. 6th ed. 2013:191–250.

ACKNOWLEDGEMENT

The authors acknowledge the contributions of Drs. Charles E. Levy and Haim Ring, who authored the previous version of this chapter which served as the foundation for this update.

CHAPTER 53

MOTOR NEURON DISEASE: DIAGNOSIS AND PROACTIVE REHABILITATION

Ileana M. Howard, MD, Nanette Cunningham Joyce, DO, MAS, and Jonathan Strayer, MD, MS

Concentrate on the things your disability does not prevent you from doing well,
Don't regret the things it interferes with,
Don't be disabled in spirit as well as physically.

— Stephen Hawking

KEY POINTS

1. Motor neuron diseases refer to disorders affecting the upper motor neurons (UMN) and/or lower motor neurons (LMN) and generally initially present as weakness without sensory impairment.
2. Amyotrophic lateral sclerosis (ALS) is the most common adult motor neuron disease.
3. Rehabilitation interventions can aid to prevent complications, maintain or improve function, and manage symptoms for persons with motor neuron disease.
4. Spinal muscular atrophy is a familial lower motor neuron disease that most commonly affects infants.

1. **What clinical features suggest motor neuron disease in an adult, and what features suggest an alternative diagnosis?**
   Findings suggestive of motor neuron disease include weakness without sensory changes. Other possible etiologies of these symptoms may include motor neuropathy, neuromuscular junction disorder, or myopathy. Further clues to the diagnosis can be gained by the presence or absence of upper motor neuron signs or bulbar involvement.

   Other clinical features at initial presentation—such as sensory changes, bladder and bowel incontinence, cranial nerve abnormalities involving the non-bulbar cranial nerves 1 to 8, or symmetrical symptoms—may suggest an alternative diagnosis.

2. **What diseases are included under the category of adult motor neuron disease?**
   Amyotrophic lateral sclerosis (ALS) is the most common motor neuron disease in adults. **Primary lateral sclerosis (PLS)** and **progressive muscular atrophy (PMA)** are upper and lower motor neuron predominant variations of motor neuron disease (respectively) that may present along a continuum with "classic ALS" (Fig. 53.1). Although it was once thought that these three disease entities were clearly distinct entities, there is increasing recognition of the phenotypic variability in "classic ALS" that may share significant overlap with PLS and PMA.
   - **Monomelic amyotrophy (Hirayama disease)** describes non-progressive, single upper limb weakness.
   - **X-linked spinobulbar muscular atrophy (Kennedy disease)** is a slowly progressive inherited lower motor neuron disorder (discussed below).
   - **Poliomyelitis** presents as acute flaccid paralysis resulting from a systemic enterovirus infection that targets the anterior horn cell.
   - **Acute flaccid myelitis (AFM)** refers to a polio-like clinical presentation. Like polio, rapid onset of flaccid paralysis results from infection with an enterovirus. Affected individuals often have fever or respiratory illness prior to onset of symptoms. West Nile virus and enterovirus D68 are underlying suspected culprits for AFM. This disease first presented in 2012 in California; 85% of reported cases affected children during that year.

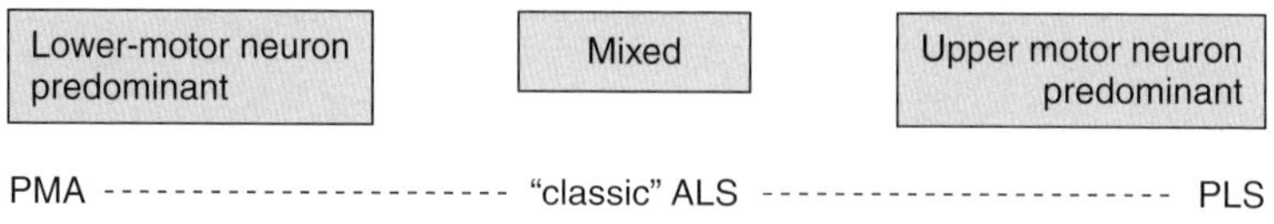

Lower-motor neuron predominant	Mixed	Upper motor neuron predominant

PMA ---------------------- "classic" ALS ---------------------- PLS

Fig. 53.1 Motor neuron diseases along the "ALS spectrum" Lower-motor neuron Mixed Upper motor neuron predominant. *ALS,* Amyotrophic lateral sclerosis; *PLS,* primary lateral sclerosis; *PMA,* progressive muscular atrophy.

- **Spinal muscular atrophy (SMA)** is an inherited lower motor neuron disease. The most severe subtypes (SMA 1, 2, and 3) present in children, however, SMA 4 presents in adulthood. Typical presentation is proximal greater than distal, and lower greater than upper extremity symmetric weakness and hyporeflexia.

Swinnen B, Robberecht W. The phenotypic variability of amyotrophic lateral sclerosis. *Nat Rev Neurol.* 2014;10:661–670.

3. What clinical features are suggestive of Kennedy disease?

A common ALS mimic, Kennedy disease (x-linked spinobulbar muscular atrophy) is an androgen gene receptor abnormality that has a typical clinical presentation of a male older than 30 with slow progression of bulbar and extremity weakness with gynecomastia, tremors, and perioral fasciculations and positive family history suggestive of an X-linked mechanism of inheritance.

Testing a person to confirm a diagnosis of Kennedy disease can provide a reassuring prognosis and valuable genetic information for the individual's family, as individuals with Kennedy disease can expect a normal life expectancy. A genetic test for Kennedy disease is available. This test evaluates CAG triplet repeat expansion on the androgen receptor gene (ARG).

4. What diagnostic tests might be helpful in evaluating an adult patient with suspected motor neuron disease?

There are no set guidelines for laboratory or radiologic testing for a person with suspected motor neuron disease. Instead, diagnostic studies should be selected based upon the patient's presenting symptoms and differential diagnosis.

Common studies used to distinguish competing diagnoses from motor neuron disease based on clinical presentation are reviewed in Table 53.1.

Howard IM, Rad N. Electrodiagnostic testing for the diagnosis and management of amyotrophic lateral sclerosis. *Phys Med Rehabil Clin N Am.* 2018;29(4):669–680.

Table 53.1 Differential Diagnosis and Laboratory Testing for Motor Neuron Disease

Bulbar-onset	Myasthenia Gravis	Acetylcholine receptor and MuSK antibodies
	Brainstem tumor	Brain MRI
Lower Motor Neuron Predominant	Multifocal Motor Neuropathy	GM1 antibodies
	Spinobulbar Muscular Atrophy (Kennedy disease)	Genetic testing
	Spinal Muscular Atrophy	Genetic testing
	Hypothyroidism	Thyroid-stimulating hormone
	Paraproteinemia	Serum protein electrophoresis/immunofixation
	Paraneoplastic	Antibody panel (serum, CSF)
	Inclusion Body Myositis	Muscle Biopsy
	Lyme Disease/West Nile Virus/Polio/Syphilis	Serology
	Tay-Sachs	Hexosaminidase A level
	Heavy Metal Intoxication	24 h Urine Collection for Heavy Metals
Upper Motor Neuron Predominant	Copper Deficiency	Serum Copper and Zinc
	B12 Deficiency	Vitamin B12, methylmalonic acid, homocysteine
	Human Immunodeficiency Virus	HIV
	Tropical Spastic Paraparesis	Human T-cell lymphotropic virus 1 serology
	Adrenomyeloneuropathy	Very long chain fatty acids
	Hereditary Spastic Paraplegia (HSP)	Genetic testing
	Multiple sclerosis	Brain and spine MRI
Mixed	Spine disease	Spine MRI

From: Howard IM, Rad N. Electrodiagnostic testing for the diagnosis and management of amyotrophic lateral sclerosis. *Phys Med Rehabil Clin N Am.* 2018;29(4):669–680.

5. Who should break the news of a diagnosis of ALS to a patient?

Because ALS is primarily a clinical diagnosis, the news of a new diagnosis should be optimally delivered by a clinician who has thoroughly reviewed the patient's clinical presentation and diagnostic studies to exclude alternative diagnoses. A diagnosis of ALS should not be delivered in the EMG lab by a physician unfamiliar with the individual.

In survey-based studies, persons with ALS and their caregivers have reported lack of empathy, insufficient explanation of the diagnosis and prognosis, and lack of resources at the time of receiving their diagnosis. There are several mnemonics available to provide guidance on delivering difficult news to a patient. A commonly used one is "SPIKES," which stands for: Setting, Perception, Invitation, Knowledge, Emotions, Strategy & Summary. Sufficient time should be allotted to provide education, answer questions, and offer resources, such as information in writing, publications from community organizations on the diagnosis, or referral to these community organizations.

McCluskey L, Casarett D, Siderowf A. Breaking the news: a survey of ALS patients and their caregivers. *Amyotroph Lateral Scler Other Motor Neuron Disord.* 2004;5:131–135.

Borasio GD, Sloan R, Pongratz DE. Breaking the news in amyotrophic lateral sclerosis. *J Neurol Sci.* 1998;160(Suppl 1):S127-33.

Baile WF, Buckman R, Lenzi R, et al. SPIKES-a six-step protocol for delivering bad news: application to the patient with cancer. *Oncologist.* 2000;5:302–311.

6. Is exercise safe in motor neuron disease, and what kinds of exercise should be prescribed?

Both animal and human studies have demonstrated no evidence of harm related to low- or moderate-intensity exercise. A recent multi-center randomized controlled trial of low-intensity strengthening, stretching, and endurance exercises for persons with ALS found no evidence of association with increased functional deterioration.

Several small studies have demonstrated benefits such as slowing of functional decline over time (as measured by FIM or ALS-FRS), decreased spasticity, improved quality of life, or preservation of forced vital capacity (FVC) measurements associated with moderate exercise in persons with ALS. This has been observed in moderate home strengthening/endurance exercise protocols, concentric strengthening exercises for muscles with greater than antigravity strength, and home exercise under the direct guidance of a physical therapist. A summary of these findings is presented in Table 53.2.

Table 53.2 Exercise in Motor Neuron Disease: Summary of Evidence

EXERCISE	POPULATION	FINDINGS
Strengthening	ALS	Moderate Endurance/ROM home exercise protocol: Improvements in spasticity (MAS) and function (ALS-FRS) at 3 months over controls[2]
	ALS	Concentric strengthening for muscles with full antigravity ROM: improved function (ALS-FRS, SF-36 physical subscore)[5]
Aerobic exercise		
Mixed exercise	ALS	Mixed stretching, strengthening, and functional home exercise program: preservation of function (ALSFRS), respiratory subscore (ALSFRS-R)[3]
	SMA3	Strengthening and recumbent cycling program x. No change in VO_{2max} or 6 min walk, but improvement in the Hammersmith Functional Motor Scale-Expanded in the intervention group and manual muscle testing

ALS, Amyotrophic lateral sclerosis; *SMA*, spinal muscular atrophy.

However, studies involving animal models of motor neuron disease have demonstrated worse outcomes for high-intensity exercise, therefore it is recommended that persons with motor neuron disease avoid high-intensity aerobic exercises. Practical recommendations for exercise include avoiding exercise to fatigue or exercise that jeopardizes mobility or activities of daily living. Conversely, eccentric strengthening exercises and targeting muscles with less than antigravity strength are avoided due to concern over causing harm

Carreras I, Yuruker S, Aytan N, et al. Moderate exercise delays the motor performance decline in a transgenic model of ALS. *Brain Res.* 2010;1313:192–201.

Clawson LL, Cudkowicz M, Krivickas L, et al. A randomized controlled trial of resistance and endurance exercise in amyotrophic lateral sclerosis. *Amyotroph Lateral Scler Frontotemporal Degener.* 2018;19:250–258.

Dal Bello-Haas V, Florence JM. Therapeutic exercise for people with amyotrophic lateral sclerosis or motor neuron disease. *Cochrane Database Syst Rev.* 2013;2013(5):CD005229.

7. What is the role of rehabilitation for persons with motor neuron disease?

General principles of rehabilitation, including the prevention of secondary complications, remediation of impairments, and provision of compensatory strategies are well-applied to persons with motor neuron disease. A framework applying these principles toward the rehabilitation of persons with degenerative neurological disease has been proposed by Dal Bello-Haas.

Bello-Haas VD, Florence JM, Kloos AD, et al. A randomized controlled trial of resistance exercise in individuals with ALS. *Neurology.* 2007;68:2003–2007.

8. What causes ALS?

Although the specific disease mechanism involved in ALS is still very much an active area of investigation, it is known that the final cause is an activation of genetic programming in scattered motor neuron pools that prematurely (inappropriately) initiates the process of **apoptosis** (genetically programmed cellular death). Broadly ALS can be divided into two groups based on etiology: Familial (FALS)-10%, and Sporadic (90%). Incidence of ALS worldwide runs from 0.3% (China) to 3.6% (Faroe Islands) with a global incidence rate of 2.7/100K; average age of onset: 50 to 65 years; M:F ratio of 1.5:1. Average survival from onset to death is 3 to 4 years, although the range is broad. Factors that raise ALS incidence include: advanced age, genetics, environmental exposures to various toxins, radiation, sports-related head trauma, depression, dementia, Parkinson, epilepsy, and smoking. Specific causative factors include mutations of C9orf72 or superoxide dismutase 1 SOD-1 in FALS. Military service is associated with a nearly two-fold greater incidence of ALS. Favorable signs for increased survival include: predominant UMN signs (PLS, arguably not ALS, though greater than 70% progress to ALS), disease duration greater than 4 years.

Logroscino G, Piccininni M, Marin B, et al. Global, regional, and national burden of motor neuron diseases 1990–2016: a systematic analysis for the Global Burden of Disease Study 2016. *Lancet Neurol.* 2018;17(12):1083–1097.

Mathis S, Goizet C, Soulages A, et al. Genetics of amyotrophic lateral sclerosis: a review. *J Neurol Sci.* 2019;399:217–226.

Committee on the Review of the Scientific Literature on Amyotrophic Lateral Sclerosis in Veterans of the National Academy of Sciences. *Amyotrophic Lateral Sclerosis in Veterans: Review of the Scientific Literature.* Washington, DC: National Academy of Sciences; 2007.

9. What is the initial presentation of ALS, and how does this presentation influence prognosis?

Presentation is generally divided into limb-onset (70%, with combined UMN/LMN signs), bulbar-onset (25%, initial signs dysphagia/dysarthria followed by limb weakness), PLS (pure UMN), and PMA (with purely LMN involvement). Prognosis varies by presentation, with worse prognosis seen in older age of symptom onset, early respiratory muscle dysfunction, and bulbar onset of disease.

Mathis S, Goizet C, Soulages A, et al. Genetics of amyotrophic lateral sclerosis: a review. *J Neurol Sci.* 2019;399:217–226.

10. What are the current diagnostic criteria for ALS?

Typically presenting, or "classic," ALS is primarily a clinical diagnosis, characterized by mixed upper and lower motor neuron signs which extend beyond peripheral nerve or myotomal distribution without sensory loss, sphincter weakness, or eye movement abnormalities (atypical variants have been discussed earlier in this chapter).

The key framework used for establishing a diagnosis of ALS is known as the **El Escorial Criteria,** first designated by the World Federation of Neurology in 1990. The most recent update for these criteria—the Awaji modifications—accept EMG findings as evidence of lower motor neuron involvement (Table 53.3). The Awaji-El Escorial criteria were created to establish a diagnosis of ALS primarily for research recruitment purposes. These criteria should be seen as a guideline but not as exclusionary of the diagnosis, as many persons with ALS will die before ever meeting criteria for "clinically definite ALS."

Table 53.3 World Federation of Neurology–El Escorial Awaji Criteria for Diagnosis of Amyotrophic Lateral Sclerosis

CATEGORY	EXAM AND/OR ELECTRODIAGNOSTIC FINDINGS
Clinically Definite	UMN and LMN findings in ≥3 body regions
Clinically Probable	UMN and LMN findings in ≥2 body regions UMN findings rostral to LMN findings
Clinically Possible	UMN and LMN findings in 1 body region OR UMN findings in ≥2 body regions, OR UMN findings caudal to LMN findings
Clinically Suspected	LMN findings in ≥2 body regions

Body regions: bulbar, cervical, thoracic, lumbar.
Awaji modification: denervation on EMG is equivalent to LMN findings.

11. What are common "ALS mimic diseases" that should be considered when making a diagnosis of ALS?

    In addition to the diseases outlined above in the diagnostic work-up, several "ALS mimic" disorders can possibly be ascertained by abnormal electrodiagnostic findings (Table 53.4). Given the gravity of a diagnosis of ALS, every effort should be made to exclude any other possible diagnosis.

Table 53.4 Electrodiagnostic Findings in Amyotrophic Lateral Sclerosis Mimics

DISORDER	ELECTRODIAGNOSTIC FINDINGS
Multifocal Motor Neuropathy (MMN)	Normal SNAPs Conduction Block Prolonged Latencies Prolonged F-waves Slowed Conduction Velocities +/− Neurogenic MUPs
Myasthenia Gravis	Normal SNAPs and CMAPs Unstable MUPs Decrement with Slow Repetitive Stimulation
Cervical/lumbosacral radiculopathy	Normal SNAPs +/− Decreased CMAPs Neurogenic MUPs in isolated myotome
Inclusion Body Myositis	Normal SNAPs and CMAPs +/− Increased insertional activity Myopathic MUPs
CIDP	Prolonged Latencies Prolonged F-waves +/− Neurogenic MUPs
Hereditary Spastic Paraplegia	Normal SNAPs and CMAPs Normal MUPs
X-linked Spinobulbar Muscular Atrophy (Kennedy's Disease)	Abnormal SNAPs

From: Howard IM, Rad N. Electrodiagnostic testing for the diagnosis and management of amyotrophic lateral sclerosis. *Phys Med Rehabil Clin N Am.* 2018;29(4):669–680.
CMAPs, Compound Motor Action Potentials; *CIDP,* Chronic inflammatory demyelinating polyradiculoneuropathy; *MUPs,* to Motor Unit Action Potentials; *SNAPs,* Sensory Nerve Actional Potentials

12. **What disease-modifying treatments can be offered for patients with ALS?**
Although there are no known cures for ALS, there are two therapeutics approved by the FDA for the treatment of ALS. In clinical trials they were shown to either prolong survival or slow functional decline: **riluzole** (Rilutek) and **edaravone** (Radicava). Approved in 1995, riluzole has been shown to increase survival following disease diagnosis by approximately 60 days. Edaravone, approved in 2017, was shown to slow functional decline when started early in disease; however, its utility is limited by the small portion of the ALS patients ($<$10%) who meet criteria for treatment if based on the inclusion criteria established for the positive clinical trial (FVC $>$80%), disease duration less than 2 years, functionally independent.

Recently, the use of **dextromethorphan/quinidine** (Nuedexta)—an agent typically used to treat pseudobulbar affect in ALS—has shown limited evidence to slow progression of bulbar weakness in persons with ALS, and therefore may also be considered a disease-modifying medication.

There have been several treatment strategies under investigation for drug development, including anti-apoptotic, anti-inflammatory, anti-excitotoxicity, antioxidant, anti-aggression, and neuroprotective treatments.

Dietary supplements have shown limited to no evidence of benefit; among these vitamin E has shown limited evidence in delaying onset and slowing progression of ALS. Vitamin A, creatine, and Pu-erh tea extract have shown variable effects. ALS patients are particularly vulnerable to useless, potentially harmful, and frequently expensive treatments, widely available through the internet. More information on off-label or complementary medicine interventions for ALS is available at www.alsuntangled.org.

Writing Group; Edaravone (MCI-186) ALS 19 Study Group; Abe K, Aoki M, Tsuji S, et al. Safety and efficacy of edaravone in well defined patients with amyotrophic lateral sclerosis: a randomised, double-blind, placebo-controlled trial. *Lancet Neurol.* 2017;16:505–512.

Oskarsson B, Gendron TF, Staff NP. Amyotrophic lateral sclerosis: an update for 2018. *Mayo Clin Proc.* 2018;93(11):1617–1628.

Smith R, Pioro E, Myers K, et al. Enhanced Bulbar function in amyotrophic lateral sclerosis: the nuedexta treatment trial. *Neurotherapeutics.* 2017;14:762–772.

13. **What non-pharmacologic interventions are associated with prolonged survival in ALS?**
Modifiable risk factors associated with acceleration of functional loss include:
- Hypoventilation—exacerbated by smoking, sleep apnea, chronic hypoxia, sialorrhea.
- Poor nutrition—as evidenced by weight loss.
- Dehydration.
- Injuries—specifically falls, fractures.
- Immobility.
Strategies to slow progression of functional loss with ALS.
- Multidisciplinary, problem-focused care is associated with 7 to 11 months greater survival.
- Prevention of weight loss and dehydration through early nutritional support, including placement of feeding tube early in the course of the disease to minimize peri-procedural risk.
- Ventilatory support (either non-invasive ventilatory support [NIVS] or tracheostomy with invasive mechanical ventilation [TIMV]).
- Smoking cessation.
- Secretion management: cough assist, use of bag mask or breath stacking with partner-assisted cough, portable suction, vibration vest.
- Fall prevention with orthotic management, gait aids, assistance, environmental modification, and wheelchair mobility as indicated.
- Functional mobility maximization with prevention of fatigue and adaptive planning for disease progression.
- Environmental designs to maximize active mobility, independent function, socialization, and quality of life.

14. **What formal scales exist for monitoring progression of ALS?**
The **ALS Functional Rating Scale (ALSFRS)**, and the respiratory elaboration, the revised ALSFRS (ALSFRS-R), are used to track the progression and frequently to look at eligibility for research trials and disease-modifying medications. The scale consists of 13 ratings for functional areas including: speech, salivation, swallowing, hand-writing, cutting food, dressing/hygiene, turning in bed, walking, climbing stairs, dyspnea. Orthopnea and respiratory insufficiency are included in the ALSFRS-R. In both scales lower is worse; the ALSFRS ranges from 0 to 40 and the ALSFRS-R from 0 to 48.

The scale is common on the internet; note the version at the University of Massachusetts website will add and produce passable chart copy: www.outcomes-umassmed.org/ALS/alsscale.aspx.

The **ALS-Specific Quality of Life, Short Form (ALSSQOL-SF)** is a brief ($<$5 minutes to complete), validated, and copyright-free outcome measure that provides patient-reported insight into six domains of function, including: physical symptoms, bulbar function, negative emotion, interaction, intimacy, and religiosity. Each domain is measured with a subscore from 1 to 10 (1-lowest, 10-highest) which provides rapid insight into the persons' assessment of their symptom burden and disease impact at a given point in time.

Felgoise SH, Feinberg R, Stephens HE, et al. Amyotrophic lateral sclerosis-specific quality of life-short form (ALSSQOL-SF): a brief, reliable, and valid version of the ALSSQOL-R. *Muscle Nerve*. 2018;58:646–654.

15. **What are common symptoms experienced by persons with ALS that may require medical management?**

Sialorrhea:	**Medications**: atropine drops (sublingual ophthalmic preparation), antihistamines/anticholinergics: glycopyrrolate, amitriptyline, hyoscyamine drops, scopolamine patches. **Injections**: botulinum toxin injections to salivary glands. **Radiation:** to salivary glands.
Spasticity	**Medications:** only baclofen has been studied specifically for ALS; gabapentin, tizanidine, and diazepam may be useful. **Injections:** botulinum toxin.
Fasciculations:	**Modalities** topical heat, massage.
Cramps	**Medications: mexiletine** has been found to be safe and effective for managing cramps in persons with ALS. ECG is recommended prior to treatment initiation. Treatment is contraindicated in the patient with a long QTc interval and should be discontinued if prolongation is observed over time. Annual evaluation of QTc interval is recommended during treatment.
Fatigue	**Non-pharmacologic: Energy conservation** techniques, **Respiratory support** during sleep with non-invasive positive pressure ventilation (NIPPV). **Medications: Neurostimulants**—modafinil has been shown to be effective for fatigue in ALS.
Insomnia	**Medications:** Typical sleep agents: melatonin, trazodone, sedatives used judiciously. **Non-pharmacologic:** non-invasive respiratory support may improve sleep.
Pain	Musculoskeletal pain is common as a result of weakness, and can be managed with modalities, therapies, medications, and injections. Prognosis for functional improvement of pain through strengthening is likely less favorable than persons without neuromuscular disease. A palliative approach to pain management may be employed, with caution in using medications that may decrease respiratory drive.
Bowel	Although not typical neurogenic bowel management, rehabilitation, and nursing management of hydration, constipation, and toileting assistance are frequently needed.
Bladder	When urinary frequency or incontinence is present, obtaining a post-void residual can guide medication management options. However, use of continence aids such as specialized urinals and external and eventually indwelling foley catheters can be useful.
Psychological state	Recognition and participation in life passions and socialization. Review for causes of anxiety and screen for depression.
Pseudobulbar affect	**Medications:** tricyclic antidepressants (TCAs), selective serotonin reuptake inhibitors (SSRIs), dextromethorphan/quinidine (Nuedexta).

Braun AT, Caballero-Eraso C, Lechtzin N. Amyotrophic lateral sclerosis and the respiratory system. *Clin Chest Med*. 2018;39(2): 391–400.

Foster LA, Salajegheh MK. Motor neuron disease: pathophysiology, diagnosis, and management. *Am J Med*. 2019;132(1): 32–37.

Francis K, Bach JR, DeLisa JA. Evaluation and rehabilitation of patients with adult motor neuron disease. *Arch Phys Med Rehabil*. 1999;80(8):951–963.

Weiss MD, Macklin EA, Simmons Z, et al. A randomized trial of mexiletine in ALS: safety and effects on muscle cramps and progression. *Neurology*. 2016;86:1474–1481.

Rabkin JG, Gordon PH, McElhiney M, et al. Modafinil treatment of fatigue in patients with ALS: a placebo-controlled study. *Muscle Nerve*. 2009;39:297–303.

16. **Is cognitive impairment common in ALS?**

Cognitive impairment affects more than half of individuals with ALS although symptoms are generally mild in nature. An expansion in C9orf72 is the most common genetic cause of frontotemporal dementia and familial ALS. Cognitive impairment may impact treatment plans and worsen prognosis. Commonly used cognitive screening tools, such as the MOCA, may not be sensitive to frontotemporal impairments, therefore more specific tools, such as the ALS-Cognitive Behavioral Screen, may be better suited for routine screening purposes.

Depression may contribute to cognitive issues, requiring careful treatment to discriminate between underlying cognitive dysfunction or pseudobulbar affective disorder.

Phukan J, Elamin M, Bede P, et al. The syndrome of cognitive impairment in amyotrophic lateral sclerosis: a population-based study. *J Neurol Neurosurg Psychiatry.* 2012;83:102–108.

Woolley SC, York MK, Moore DH, et al. Detecting frontotemporal dysfunction in ALS: utility of the ALS cognitive behavioral screen (ALS-CBS). *Amyotroph Lateral Scler.* 2010;11:303–311.

17. **What is the most common cause of death in ALS?**

Based upon findings of post-mortem examinations, individuals with ALS most commonly die of aspiration pneumonia. Less common causes of death include respiratory failure, heart failure, and pulmonary embolism.

Burkhardt C, Neuwirth C, Sommacal A, et al. Is survival improved by the use of NIV and PEG in amyotrophic lateral sclerosis (ALS)? A post-mortem study of 80 ALS patients. *PLoS One.* 2017;12:e0177555.

Corcia P, Pradat PF, Salachas F, et al. Causes of death in a post-mortem series of ALS patients. *Amyotroph Lateral Scler.* 2008;9:59–62.

18. **How is ventilatory function quantified in ALS, and what interventions are helpful for maximization?**

The clinical practice guidelines developed by the American Academy of Neurology recommend obtaining FVC, maximal inspiratory pressure (MIP), and maximal expiratory pressure (MEP) at quarterly clinic visits to monitor changes in ventilatory function of persons with ALS. MIP and MEP are earlier indicators of muscle weakness as compared with FVC. Supine, rather than seated, spirometry with FVC measurement may be sensitive earlier to changes in ventilatory function.

Ventilation in persons with ALS is improved by:

- Upright sitting position (rather than laying supine)
- Bronchopulmonary hygiene with a **maximum insufflator/exsufflator** (MIE or cough assist device) can be prescribed when the **peak cough flow** reaches 270 L/min. In the bulbar patient, MIE can cause upper airway collapse and should be used with caution. Other options include assisted cough with **breath stacking** using a bag mask device, or a high-frequency chest percussion device.
- **Non-invasive positive pressure ventilation (NIPPV)** improves quality of life and lengthens survival in ALS. Medicare benchmarks for the initiation of NIPPV are a FVC of 50% predicated, MIP of -60 cm H_2O, sniff nasal pressure of -40 cm H_2O, or evidence of SpO_2 of 88% or below during sleep for a total of at least 5 minutes. Any single abnormality can lead to a covered prescription for ventilatory support. However, earlier initiation has been shown to improve outcomes in patients who successfully transition to use.
- **Tracheostomy with Invasive Mechanical Ventilation (TIMV).** Physicians should discuss the requirements of care and stopping conditions with patients prior to initiation of TIMV. The weakness associated with ALS continues to progress throughout the body, including limb, bulbar, and finally cranial nerve-innervated muscles, and can lead to a locked-in state preventing effective communication in the person with ALS treated with TIMV.

Braun AT, Caballero-Eraso C, Lechtzin N. Amyotrophic lateral sclerosis and the respiratory system. *Clin Chest Med.* 2018;39(2):391–400.

Corcia P, Pradat PF, Salachas F, et al. Causes of death in a post-mortem series of ALS patients. *Amyotroph Lateral Scler.* 2008;9:59–62.

Miller RG, Jackson CE, Kasarskis EJ, et al. Practice parameter update: the care of the patient with amyotrophic lateral sclerosis: drug, nutritional, and respiratory therapies (an evidence-based review): report of the Quality Standards Subcommittee of the American Academy of Neurology. *Neurology.* 2009;73:1218–1226.

19. **What pulmonary interventions might be harmful in ALS?**

Providing supplemental oxygen to a poorly ventilated patient can lead to ventilatory failure. During breathing, fresh air is pulled down through the dead space made up by the pharynx and bronchial tree to the alveoli for gas exchange. As blood traverses the capillaries in the alveolus, the red cell becomes 100% saturated with oxygen one third of the way through due to hemoglobin's active affinity. However, carbon dioxide is passively diffused into the alveolus during the entire length of the capillary at a rate directly related to the difference in partial pressures. Therefore, as less air exchange in the alveolus occurs due to a muscular ventilatory dysfunction, carbon dioxide accumulates first and is buffered by bicarbonate in the serum. Thereafter, blood oxygen saturations fall with further ventilatory deficits. Treating this desaturation due to ventilatory dysfunction with nasal oxygen can decrease ventilatory drive and contribute to worsening hypercarbia and change in mental status. Alternatively, improvement of mechanical ventilation brings free air to the alveolus to resume normalcy for oxygen exchange first and later allows excess carbon dioxide to be "blown off," reducing the requirements for bicarbonate buffering to maintain serum pH.

20. What is the etiology of polio, how is it transmitted, and where does it remain endemic?
Poliomyelitis only affects humans. The polio virus is an enterovirus that is spread via fecal-oral route. The virus divides in the gastrointestinal track, which is where it spreads to the nervous system. 1 in 200 infections lead to paralysis. Five percent to 10% of those with paralytic polio die due to respiratory involvement. Polio remains endemic in Afghanistan, Nigeria, and Pakistan.

Becker BE. Sister Elizabeth Kenny and Polio in America: Doyenne or Demagogue in Her Role in Rehabilitation Medicine? *PM&R*. 2018; 10(2):208–217.

Verville RE, Ditunno JF Jr. Franklin Delano Roosevelt, polio, and the warm springs experiment: its impact on physical medicine and rehabilitation. *PM&R*. 2013;5(1):3–8.

21. What are the most common signs and symptoms of post-polio syndrome (PPS)?
Symptoms required for diagnosis include persistent new onset of progressive muscle weakness, abnormal muscle fatigability, and muscle or joint pain. In addition to having these symptoms, the March of Dimes criteria for the diagnosis of PPS requires a history of paralytic poliomyelitis with evidence of motor neuron loss, partial or complete recovery of neurological function followed by a period of stability (15 years or more), persistent symptoms for at least 1 year, and the exclusion of other causes (medical, orthopedic, or neurologic) that explain the new symptoms. About 78% of those with prior history of paralytic poliomyelitis will eventually develop symptoms of PPS.

The cause of PPS remains incompletely defined; current theories include progressive loss of enlarged motor neurons that had been supporting muscle fibers that lost innervation during the original infection, loss of motor neurons and muscle fibers through the effects of aging, and/or possible inflammatory processes caused by reactivation of the virus or to the virus itself.

Halstead LS. A brief history of postpolio syndrome in the United States. *Arch Phys Med Rehabil*. 2011;92(8):1344–1349.

March of Dimes. *Post-Polio Syndrome: Identifying Best Practices in Diagnosis and Care*. White Plains, NY: March of Dimes; 2001.

22. What are important presenting signs and symptoms that should make a clinician suspicious that a patient has SMA, and how is the diagnosis established?
Hypotonia with a predominance of proximal weakness and the absence of muscle stretch reflexes are common presenting signs in infants with SMA and should trigger the clinician to order genetic testing to confirm the diagnosis. Free genetic testing for spinal muscular atrophy is available through Invitae Corporation. Additional signs commonly observed in early onset SMA include tongue fasciculations, a bell-shaped chest, frog-legged supine posture, and paradoxical rib cage collapse during inspiration.

Children typically appear normal at birth, but weaken and lose motor milestones that they once achieved at disease onset. Earlier symptom onset is associated with a more severe SMA phenotype. Those on the severe end of the spectrum commonly develop failure to thrive, swallowing abnormalities, and breathing difficulties with ventilatory failure related to lower motor neuron weakness. Children and adults with later onset disease often have an initial loss of muscle strength followed by long periods of disease plateau.

Diagnosis is established by confirmation of a disease-related genetic variant. SMA is the leading genetic cause of infant death.

23. What is the most common causative gene abnormality associated with SMA, and what is its inheritance pattern?
While the term SMA is used as a category to describe a set of rare lower motor neuron diseases, the most common cause—for which the moniker is generally considered synonymous—is bi-allelic homozygous mutations of the **survival of motor neuron protein 1 (SMN1)** gene. The SMN1 gene is located at position 13 on the long arm of chromosome 5 (5q13). It is responsible for the primary production of survival of motor neuron protein, which is essential for motor neuron health and survival. The most common SMN1 mutation is a homozygous deletion of exon 7 and/or 8, which results in truncated and dysfunctional protein.

SMA has an autosomal recessive inheritance pattern. The carrier frequency has been reported to be between 1/40 to 1/60 people. The incidence is approximately 1 in 11,000 live births. Sixty percent of those diagnosed with SMA will have an early, severe, infantile onset, categorized as SMA type I.

24. How is SMA classified into sub-types? What are the temporal and motor milestone benchmarks in the traditional SMA classification system?

SMA is a continuous spectrum disorder that, in the traditional classification system, has been divided into four sub-types based on age at onset and motor milestone achievement. The reader should be aware that other classification systems have been proposed to further stratify the disease by severity due to wide variation within each sub-type (Table 53.5).

Table 53.5 Traditional Clinical Classification System for Spinal Muscular Atrophy			
SUB-TYPE	**OTHER NOMENCLATURE**	**AGE AT ONSET**	**MOTOR MILESTONE ACHIEVED**
SMA type I	Infantile; early onset; Werdnig-Hoffman disease	0–6 months	Never attains sitting
SMA type II	Intermediate; later onset	7–18 months	+independent sitting, Never attains independent ambulation
SMA type III	Mild; later onset; Kugelberg–Welander disease	After 18 months	+independent ambulation
SMA type IV	Adult	Second to third decade	+independent ambulation

SMA, Spinal muscular atrophy.

25. How does the SMN2 gene influence disease severity and provide a molecular target for disease-modifying treatments?

On human chromosome 5 position 13 there are two nearly identical genes that participate in the production of survival of motor neuron protein. SMN1 is the telomeric copy that provides nearly all of the necessary protein. The centromeric copy, survival of motor neuron gene 2 (SMN2), provides only a small fraction of full-length protein. The essential difference between the two genes is a single base pair change in exon 7. A thymine in exon 7 of the SMN2 gene, rather than cytosine found in the SMN1 gene, triggers post-transcriptional modification of the SMN2 messenger RNA, deleting exon 7. This results in a shortened, dysfunctional protein. However, about 10% of the time a full-length protein product is transcribed. This discovery has served as the foundation for drug development efforts targeting SMN2 modulation. **Nusinersen (Spinraza)** is the first FDA-approved disease-modifying medication for the treatment of SMA. It is an antisense oligonucleotide that targets the SMN2 mRNA, blocks the excision of exon 7, and results in increased production of full-length survival of motor neuron protein. Treatment is changing the classic phenotypes, as we know them, for many patients receiving therapy. Other SMN2 modulating therapies are in the SMA drug development pipeline.

The SMN2 gene copy number influences the severity of the disease phenotype. Studies have identified anywhere from 0 to 6 copies of the SMN2 gene in SMA patients. In an individual lacking a single competent SMN1 gene, 0 copies of the SMN2 gene is not supportive of life. A recent study by Crawford et al. showed an inverse relationship between genotype and phenotype with increasing SMN2 copy numbers conferring a less severe phenotype. Their data showed mean copy number in subjects with SMA type I of 2.5 (2 to 3 copies), SMA type II of 2.9 (mostly 3 copies), and SMA type III of 3.5 (3 to 4 copies). This relationship was consistent with previously reported studies. Further studies are needed to determine a better understanding of phenotypic influences.

Crawford TO, Paushkin SV, Kobayashi DT, et al. Evaluation of SMN protein, transcript, and copy number in the biomarkers for spinal muscular atrophy (BforSMA) clinical study. *PLoS One.* 2012;7:e33572.

26. What is the role of gene therapy in the management of SMA?

The second drug approved by the FDA (May 2019) for treatment of children with SMA who are younger than 2 years of age is **Onasemnogene abeparvovec-xioi (Zolgensma)**. This drug does not target the SMN2 gene, but rather is an adeno-associated viral vector-based gene therapy, providing a replacement SMN1 gene. Administration is by a single, 60-minute IV infusion, delivered only if laboratory testing is negative for antibodies against the AAV-9 capsid. Pre-dosing with systemic corticosteroids, post-dosing with continuous treatment over 30 days, followed by a 28-day weaning period while monitoring liver function is recommended to prevent acute serious liver injury—a side effect observed during drug development and marked by elevated aminotransferases. Of significance is that outcomes from both FDA-approved disease modifying medications are significantly improved with earlier treatment and are best if treatment is provided prior to the onset of the phenotype. The push toward universal newborn screening in SMA is based on these findings.

A third medication, **risdiplam (Evrysdi)**, is the first oral disease-modifying treatment to be approved by the FDA (August 2020) for all SMA patients 2 months and older. Risdiplam is an SMN2-splicing modifier, designed to increase amounts of full-length SMN protein. It is a liquid solution taken at the same time every day. Weight-based dosing is prescribed until the individual reaches 20 kg and is older than 2 years of age, and then a standard dose of 5 mg is recommended. Fever, diarrhea, rash, upper respiratory tract infection, pneumonia, constipation, and vomiting are the most common adverse reactions

27. In patients with SMA type I, what is the most common cause of death, and what interventions can be offered to prolong life?
The most common cause of mortality in subjects with SMA type I, according to one small observational study, is acute pulmonary infection, followed by airway obstruction and bradycardic arrest. The mean time to death or ventilation has been reported as 8–10 months in patients with SMA type I carrying 2 copies of the SMN2 gene.

Interventions augmenting respiratory function such as NIPPV and tracheostomy with mechanical ventilation improve survival. In addition, gastrostomy placement with enteral nutrition reduces failure to thrive and likely contributes to improved survival in SMA type I and II.

Finkel RS, McDermott MP, Kaufmann P, et al. Observational study of spinal muscular atrophy type I and implications for clinical trials. *Neurology*. 2014;83:810–817.

28. What is the role of clinical video telehealth in providing services to patients with motor neuron disease?
Many patients with motor neuron disease have limited access to specialized interdisciplinary clinics due to distance or disability impacting their ability to travel. A quarter of all persons with ALS in the United States live more than 100 miles from a specialized ALS center. Clinical video telehealth has been studied specifically as a means to provide specialized care to persons with ALS, and has been associated with increased patient satisfaction, decreased hospitalization and ER visits, and similar survival.

Horton DK, Graham S, Punjani R, et al. A spatial analysis of amyotrophic lateral sclerosis (ALS) cases in the United States and their proximity to multidisciplinary ALS clinics, 2013. *Amyotroph Lateral Scler Frontotemporal Degener*. 2018;19(1–2):126–133.

Hobson EV, Baird WO, Cooper CL, et al. Using technology to improve access to specialist care in amyotrophic lateral sclerosis: a systematic review. *Amyotroph Lateral Scler Frontotemporal Degener*. 2016;17:313–324.

29. Why is multidisciplinary care recommended for individuals with motor neuron disease?
Multidisciplinary care describes care provided by multiple specialties in the same clinical area and has been associated with better outcomes, including longer survival, for persons with motor neuron disease. In addition, interprofessional care models are related to decreased burnout for staff.

Howard I, Potts A. Interprofessional care for neuromuscular disease. *Curr Treat Options Neurol*. 2019;21:35.

30. What are the rehabilitation opportunities and responsibilities of patients' public notoriety?
Many people have incurred disabling neuromuscular disease and perhaps all deserve focused attention. Yet, a few have been notable for their prominence, contributions to history, and visibility throughout illness. They can serve as inspiration, evidence for success in adversity, and lessons for the clinician. In contemporary times social media offers other models for **influencers** living with disability as well.

31. Why is ALS called "Lou Gehrig's Disease"?
Lou Gehrig (1903–1941) played 17 seasons as first baseman for the New York Yankees from 1923 to 1940. He was an incredible player by all accounts: All Star (seven times), MVP for the American League (twice), world Series champion (six times) with a career .340 batting average among other accomplishments. Well-loved by many, he was renowned for never missing a game in 14 years, earning him the nickname "The Iron Horse." Emergence of ALS forced him to retire at age 36, with weakness and loss of coordination. His diagnosis was made at the Mayo Clinic, a rarity at a time when most clinicians were unaware of ALS.

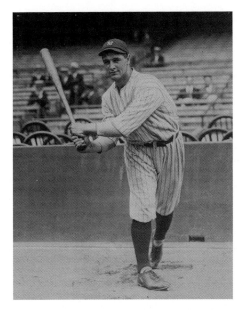

(Wikimedia. Available at https://en.wikipedia.org/wiki/Lou_Gehrig#/media/File:Lou_Gehrig_as_a_new_Yankee_11_Jun_1923.jpg)

32. Should a champion know the truth?

In his farewell speech at Yankee Stadium, Gehrig said, "I consider myself the luckiest man on the face of the Earth… I might have been given a bad break, but I've got an awful lot to live for." As his disease progressed, his family and medical team were very concerned that the unadorned truth could hurt the ballplayer (Brennan, 2012). Gehrig wrote to his medical team requesting the facts, "I feel you can appreciate how I despise the dark, but also despise equally as much false illusions."

Gehrig's ALS progressed to bulbar muscles, and he died in 1941, at age 38, just under 2 years after his diagnosis. Neurological researchers have speculated that perhaps several concussions he suffered in the course of his athletic career contributed to onset of his ALS (McKee, 2010). In one sense the most notable feature of Lou Gehrig's ALS is how his progression resembles that of so many patients nearly 80 years later. In the USA, his fame and popularity have made his name synonymous with ALS, where it is frequently known as "Lou Gehrig disease."

Frank B. The 70th Anniversary of the Death of Lou Gehrig. *Am J Hosp Palliat Care*. 2012;29:512. Originally published online February 23, 2012. DOI: 10.1177/1049909111434635.

McKee AC, Gavett BE, Stern RA, et al. TDP-43 proteinopathy and motor neuron disease in chronic traumatic encephalopathy. *J Neuropathol Exp Neurol*. 2010;69(9):918–929. Available at: https://doi.org/10.1097/NEN.0b013e3181ee7d85.

33. Can the reality of disability be minimized in the persona of a strong leader in war and economic depression and near simultaneously emphasized to support funding for disability charity?

The disability of the 32nd President of the United States, **Franklin Delano Roosevelt (1882–1945)**, was an open secret, known by all, and rarely publicized out of respect. Roosevelt was a rising political figure at the peak of health, when at age 39, on holiday, he became chilled, fatigued, and ill with fever. In the morning he noticed weakness in one leg which progressed to all limbs. Over the next 10 to 14 days he developed an ascending paralysis involving lower limbs greater than upper limbs, facial weakness, and bowel and bladder dysfunction. Expert physicians of the time diagnosed "anterior poliomyelitis," and he received vigorous rehabilitation involving physical therapy, bracing, warm baths, and exercise. Following his political reemergence, he was a strong voice for polio survivors, and promoted the popular fight against polio and toward development of the polio vaccines. FDR became the face of The March of Dimes, sparking millions in donations. Consequently, his image appears on the US 10 cent piece.

34. Did FDR have polio?

In 2003, Goldman et al. applied Bayesian probability theory to the historical features of FDR's illness (Goldman, 2003). They noted that while some aspects were consistent with polio, others were more consistent with Guillain–Barre syndrome (GBS), an inflammatory polyradiculopathy. Factors favoring polio diagnosis included: acute febrile illness followed by flaccid paresis; wide prevalence at the time; permanent paralysis; and lack of objective sensory findings. Factors against polio included: late age of onset (39); relatively symmetrical lower limb involvement; prolonged bladder/bowel involvement; subjective numbness and dysesthesia; and a transient facial weakness. By analyzing these and other factors the authors estimated that the diagnosis had a 31% chance of being polio, versus 51% chance of being GBS.

Subsequent analysis by DiTunno et al. from the point of view of clinicians experienced in polio sequelae concludes that Goldman may have misinterpreted several reports. These included sensory changes, bladder involvement, and other aspects of polio recovery, making poliomyelitis the correct diagnosis. Of course, a complete analysis is impeded by lack of modern testing including CSF analysis and genetic techniques. The truth of the matter is impossible to fully resolve, but does prove an intriguing historical debate, and fodder for academic rumination.

Goldman DA, Schmalstieg FC Jr. What was the cause of Franklin Delano Roosevelt's paralytic illness? *J Med Biogr.* 2003;11(4):232–240. doi: 10.1177/096777200301100412.

Ditunno JF Jr, Becker BE, Herbison GJ. Franklin Delano Roosevelt: the diagnosis of poliomyelitis revisited. *PM R.* 2016 Sep;8(9):883–893. doi: 10.1016/j.pmrj.2016.05.003.

35. Can the progressive restrictions of paralysis contribute to different patterns of thinking and memory that could result in novel scientific discoveries?

English physicist **Stephen Hawking (1942–2018)** demonstrates an exceptional story of overcoming fatal diagnosis and disability and thriving despite (and perhaps because of) his neuromuscular diagnosis. In so doing he beat the survival odds.

Hawking was a 21-year-old undergraduate at University of Cambridge in 1963 when he developed difficulties walking, ultimately leading to a diagnosis of ALS. He was given two years to live and only continued his studies reluctantly. Hawking admits that prior to his diagnosis he was a bright but lackluster undergraduate student. After an initial despondent period, his diagnosis galvanized him to complete his studies and achieve in the lofty world of astrophysics. As he lost physical ability, he developed new ways to think, visualize, develop, and communicate his theories of cosmology.

Professionally, he is credited with developing existing theories of the origin of the universe and the complex mathematics involved. He described the properties of black holes, radiation from which are named after him. He gained notoriety for his work, sharing them in the bestselling "A Brief History of Time." Living with inescapable and unconcealable disabilities, he embraced public life with a keen appetite for fame itself. Despite need for the ventilator, and further physical disability, he maintained residence at home with caregivers, married two times, traveled extensively, and even escaped gravity by flying on NASA's KC-135 "Vomit Comet." He was well known for his engagement with current events and irreverent sense of humor, saying that "Life would be tragic if it weren't funny."

36. How did Dr. Hawking beat the odds?

From a medical perspective, his case is remarkable for several features. First, onset was early at age 21 (rare, but not unique), in a wheelchair in his 30s, losing limb and bulbar function slowly but inexorably. Following a respiratory crisis at age 53, he underwent a tracheotomy to facilitate ventilator breathing, contravening medical advice suggesting hospice. He lost speech in the conventional sense, ultimately operating his communication device using his single remaining voluntary facial muscle. His story illustrates some of the wide spectrum of ALS, slowed progression with early onset, and value in some cases opting for ventilation.

Hawking's survival shows the critical role of family and rehabilitative support and the importance of personal choice. When he died at age 76, 55 years after onset of his first symptoms of ALS, Stephen Hawking had far surpassed possibilities medically, professionally, and personally. As he said, "My expectations were reduced to zero when I was 21. Everything since then has been a bonus."

Hawking S. *My Brief History*. Random House; 2013.

Hawking J. *Travelling to Infinity: My Life with Stephen*. Alma Books; 2014.

BBC Media. *A Brief History of Stephen Hawking, Annotated Article*. Available at https://www.bbc.co.uk/teach/a-brief-history-of-stephen-hawking/z43k382. Accessed May 24, 2021.

37. How can a defensive football player that became a "symbol of recovery" by blocking a punt, later pivot in his life to become a champion for those living with ALS and advocate for care and cure?

Steven Michael Gleason (b. 1977) grew up in Spokane WA and excelled at school in football and baseball, playing for Washington State University, and then a 9-year professional career largely with the New Orleans Saints. As an athlete, Steve was exceptional, performing as a defensive lineman against many larger players.

Perhaps his most remembered athletic feat was the block of a punt early in the Saint's first home game after Hurricane Katrina in 2006, heralding a turnaround and the city's recovery from the storm.

In 2011, he noticed fasciculations and after consultations ranging from naturopaths to neurologists, he announced he had ALS. Steve's affirmation that ALS may "crash my body but not my life" drove him to alternatively explore stem cell therapies and faith healing as well as share adventure travel—"better now than never,"—as he sought to bring "all his relationships in order." His resolution to be public about his life with ALS, to serve his family and those facing ALS, led to formation of Team Gleason ("No White Flags") charity, Gleason House for those with ALS, and opportunities for "pALS" volunteers. The documentary film "Gleason" (2016) shows his life with ALS, family life, rationale for medical decisions, including opting to father children, and later for tracheostomy and ventilation. In 2015 Congress passed "The Steve Gleason Act" to ensure the availability of life-sustaining communication devices. For his advocacy work on behalf of those with ALS, he was awarded the Congressional Gold Medal in 2020.

Gleason Trailer. Available at https://www.youtube.com/watch?v=WgkQU32XSFQ https://teamgleason.org/.

38. What are the clinical lessons to be drawn from shared public experiences of patients?
   1. Despite the grim statistics for those with ALS, each case is individual, and prognosis for any single case is impossible to predict.
   2. Publicity involving celebrities with disabling illness can be important in raising the consciousness of the public to disabling illnesses and disability in general.
   3. Trust with the medical team is vital and valuable; delivering a truthful but bleak message is an important piece of care requiring skill and compassion.
   4. High fitness is not a guarantee of slow progression, though arguably premorbid fitness may slow progression on an individual level.
   5. Youth at onset of ALS can be an advantage to survival, but not a guarantee.
   6. Having and developing an active mental life can literally improve life quality and lifespan.
   7. Although the majority of patients with ALS in the USA choose to avoid tracheostomy, this choice can be viable, given adequate home support, medical care, staffing, equipment, and expectations.
   8. A sense of humor is important to quality of life with a progressive neuromuscular disease and arguably any disability.
   9. Life must be lived despite adversity; choices in response are crucial.

BIBLIOGRAPHY

Becker BE. Sister Elizabeth Kenny and Polio in America: Doyenne or Demagogue in her role in rehabilitation medicine? *PM R.* 2018;10(2): 208–217.

Bello-Haas VD, Florence JM, Kloos AD, et al. A randomized controlled trial of resistance exercise in individuals with ALS. *Neurology.* 2007; 68:2003–2007.

Braun AT, Caballero-Eraso C, Lechtzin N. Amyotrophic lateral sclerosis and the respiratory system. *Clin Chest Med.* 2018 Jun 1;39(2): 391–400.

Burkhardt C, Neuwirth C, Sommacal A, et al. Is survival improved by the use of NIV and PEG in amyotrophic lateral sclerosis (ALS)? A post-mortem study of 80 ALS patients. *PLoS One.* 2017;12:e0177555.

Carreras I, Yuruker S, Aytan N, et al. Moderate exercise delays the motor performance decline in a transgenic model of ALS. *Brain Res.* 2010;1313:192–201.

Clawson LL, Cudkowicz M, Krivickas L, et al. A randomized controlled trial of resistance and endurance exercise in amyotrophic lateral sclerosis. *Amyotroph Lateral Scler Frontotemporal Degener.* 2018;19:250–258.

Committee on the Review of the Scientific Literature on Amyotrophic Lateral Sclerosis in Veterans of the National Academy of Sciences. *Amyotrophic Lateral Sclerosis in Veterans: Review of the Scientific Literature.* Washington, DC: National Academy of Sciences; 2007.

Corcia P, Pradat PF, Salachas F, et al. Causes of death in a post-mortem series of ALS patients. *Amyotroph Lateral Scler.* 2008;9:59–62.

Crawford TO, Paushkin SV, Kobayashi DT, et al. Evaluation of SMN protein, transcript, and copy number in the biomarkers for spinal muscular atrophy (BforSMA) clinical study. *PLoS One.* 2012;7:e33572.

Dal Bello-Haas V, Florence JM. Therapeutic exercise for people with amyotrophic lateral sclerosis or motor neuron disease. *Cochrane Database Syst Rev.* 2013;2013(5):CD005229.

Felgoise SH, Feinberg R, Stephens HE, et al. Amyotrophic lateral sclerosis-specific quality of life-short form (ALSSQOL-SF): a brief, reliable, and valid version of the ALSSQOL-R. *Muscle Nerve.* 2018;58:646–654.

Finkel RS, McDermott MP, Kaufmann P, et al. Observational study of spinal muscular atrophy type I and implications for clinical trials. *Neurology.* 2014;83:810–817.

Foster LA, Salajegheh MK. Motor neuron disease: pathophysiology, diagnosis, and management. *Amer J Med.* 2019;132(1):32–37.

Francis K, Bach JR, DeLisa JA. Evaluation and rehabilitation of patients with adult motor neuron disease. *Arch Phys Med Rehabil.* 1999; 80(8):951–963.

Halstead LS. A brief history of postpolio syndrome in the United States. *Arch Phys Med Rehabil.* 2011;92(8):1344–1349.

Howard I, Potts A. Interprofessional care for neuromuscular disease. *Curr Treat Options Neurol.* 2019;21:35.

Howard IM, Rad N. Electrodiagnostic testing for the diagnosis and management of amyotrophic lateral sclerosis. *Phys Med Rehabil Clin N Am.* 2018;29(4):669–680.

Logroscino G, Piccininni M, Marin B, et al. Global, regional, and national burden of motor neuron diseases 1990–2016: a systematic analysis for the Global Burden of Disease Study 2016. *Lancet Neurol.* 2018;17(12):1083–1397.

March of Dimes. *Post-Polio Syndrome: Identifying Best Practices in Diagnosis and Care.* White Plains, NY: March of Dimes; 2001.

Mathis S, Goizet C, Soulages A, et al. Genetics of amyotrophic lateral sclerosis: a review. *J Neurol Sci.* 2019;399:217–226.

Miller RG, Jackson CE, Kasarskis EJ, et al. Practice parameter update: the care of the patient with amyotrophic lateral sclerosis: drug, nutritional, and respiratory therapies (an evidence-based review): report of the Quality Standards Subcommittee of the American Academy of Neurology. *Neurology.* 2009;73:1218–1226.

Oskarsson B, Gendron TF, Staff NP. Amyotrophic lateral sclerosis: an update for 2018. *Mayo Clin Proc.* 2018;93(11):1617–1628.

Phukan J, Elamin M, Bede P, et al. The syndrome of cognitive impairment in amyotrophic lateral sclerosis: a population-based study. *J Neurol Neurosurg Psychiatry.* 2012;83:102–108.

Rabkin JG, Gordon PH, McElhiney M, et al. Modafinil treatment of fatigue in patients with ALS: a placebo-controlled study. *Muscle Nerve.* 2009;39:297–303.

Smith R, Pioro E, Myers K, et al. Enhanced bulbar function in amyotrophic lateral sclerosis: the nuedexta treatment trial. *Neurotherapeutics.* 2017;14:762–772.

Swinnen B, Robberecht W. The phenotypic variability of amyotrophic lateral sclerosis. *Nat Rev Neurol.* 2014;10:661–670.

Verville RE, Ditunno JF Jr. Franklin Delano Roosevelt, polio, and the Warm Springs experiment: its impact on physical medicine and rehabilitation. *PM R.* 2013;5(1):3–8.

Weiss MD, Macklin EA, Simmons Z, et al. A randomized trial of mexiletine in ALS: safety and effects on muscle cramps and progression. *Neurology.* 2016;86:1474–1481.

Woolley SC, York MK, Moore DH, et al. Detecting frontotemporal dysfunction in ALS: utility of the ALS cognitive behavioral screen (ALS-CBS). *Amyotroph Lateral Scler.* 2010;11:303–311.

Writing Group; Edaravone (MCI-186) ALS 19 Study Group; Abe K, Aoki M, Tsuji S, et al. Safety and efficacy of edaravone in well defined patients with amyotrophic lateral sclerosis: a randomised, double-blind, placebo-controlled trial. *Lancet Neurol.* 2017;16:505–512.

SPINAL CORD INJURY MEDICINE: TRANSLATING SYSTEMS ADAPTATIONS INTO PERSONAL VISIONS

Steven A. Stiens, MD, MS, Henry S. York, MD, Kate E. Delaney, MD, and Lance L. Goetz, MD

Create a compelling vision, one that takes people to a new place, and then translate that vision into a reality.
—Warren Bennis (1925–2014)

KEY POINTS: SPINAL CORD INJURY MEDICINE

1. The spinal cord communicates with all body systems. Disruption results in deficits in perception, voluntary motion, neurogenic organ impairments, and segmental dysfunction.
2. Sacral sparing occurs with central lesions of the spinal cord (contusion, ischemia, tumor). Sensory symptoms tend to descend as the lesion expands, sparing lower segments supplied by tracts closer to the surface of the spinal cord.
3. Brown-Séquard syndrome presents with unilateral paresis and light touch sensation impairment on the side of the spinal cord lesion and contralateral pain and temperature sensation deficit. A classic example is a knife stab causing spinal cord hemisection that interrupts descending motor tracts and ascending spinothalamic tracts that have crossed the spinal cord.
4. The most common primary tumors of the spinal cord are astrocytomas, ependymomas, and oligodendrogliomas.
5. The most common tumors that metastasize to the spine are breast, lung, gastrointestinal, lymphoma/myeloma, and prostate. They all cause extramedullary compression and can be managed with steroids, radiation therapy, and surgical decompression.

National Spinal Cord Injury Statistical Center, Facts and Figures at a Glance. Birmingham, AL: University of Alabama at Birmingham; 2020. Available at https://www.nscisc.uab.edu/Public/Facts%20and%20Figures%202020.pdf

1. **What are the most important long tracts in the spinal cord?**
   See Table 54.1 and Fig. 54.1.

2. **Where in the spinal cord is each of the major long tracts located?**
   Fig. 54.2 shows the somatotopic organization of the major long tracts of the spinal cord. The dorsal columns have lower-extremity fibers (sacral and lumbar) lying medially, whereas the pyramidal and spinothalamic tracts have lower-extremity fibers lying laterally.

3. **What are the differences between *quadri-* and *tetra-*?**
   It is a matter of medical etymology. Both prefixes mean "four" and refer to the loss of function in four limbs from cervical SCI. However, "*tetra*" is derived from Greek, and *quadra* is a Latin root. The Classicists within the SCI community frown on mixing Greek and Latin roots, particularly when compounded with the Greek-derived

Table 54.1 Long Tracts in the Spinal Cord

TRACT	LOCATION	FUNCTION
Gracile	Medial dorsal column	Proprioception from the leg
Cuneate	Lateral dorsal column	Proprioception from the arm
Spinocerebellar	Superficial lateral column	Muscular position and tone
Pyramidal	Deep lateral column	Upper motor neuron
Lateral spinothalamic	Ventrolateral column	Pain and thermal sensation

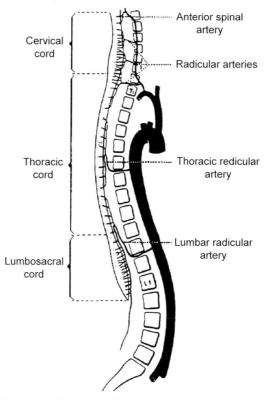

Fig. 54.1 Blood supply of the spinal cord. (From Joynt R. *Clinical Neurology*. Philadelphia: J.B. Lippincott; 1992, with permission.)

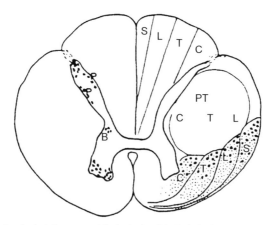

Fig. 54.2 Location of major long tracts. Letters represent the lamination of the Funiculus Cuneatus, Funiculus Gracilis, and corticospinal tracts. *C*, Cervical; *L*, lumbar; *PT*, pyramidal tract; *S*, sacrum; *T*, thoracic. (From Joynt R. *Clinical Neurology*. Philadelphia: J.B. Lippincott; 1992, with permission.)

suffixes -*plegia* (from *plege,* meaning stroke or paralysis) or -*paresis* (letting go), *tetraplegia* is preferred over *quadriplegia*. So be a smart geek, speak Greek!

4. What are the differences between *para-, di-,* and *hemiplegia?*
Paraplegia (*para-* from Greek means "beside," or "adjacent") refers to weakness of the legs (the two limbs next to each other) as the result of damage in the thoracic, lumbar, or sacral (injuries below the cervical spinal cord.) The trunk, legs, and pelvic organs may be involved but not the arms. *Di-* is Greek for "two." Historically, it referred to paralysis affecting symmetrical body parts of the body. It has come to mean the same as paraplegia but is used predominantly in pediatric rehabilitation to classify cerebral palsy. This can all be compared to hemiplegia, which is weakness restricted to one side of the body.

5. What is the International ISNCSCI classification? How are patients' examinations documented?
The International Spinal Cord Society (ISCoS) and American Spinal Cord Injury Association (ASIA) have developed standards for neurologic classification (revised in 2019 for the 8th edition) that quantify impairment through objective recording of sensory and motor findings: the **International Standards for Neurological Classification of Spinal Cord Injury (ISNCSCI) examination**.
    The ISNCSCI examination is used to systematically classify the effects and impairments caused by a spinal cord injury. Providers complete a physical examination, described below, to categorize patients' SCI, which can help explain and predict patients' functional status. The examination is documented on the ISNCSCI Worksheet, which can be found on the American Spinal Injury Association (ASIA) website.
    There is now an expedited version of the ISNCSCI (E-ISNCSCI). This is not intended to replace the full ISNCSCI examination but rather to be available for screening purposes, quick evaluation prior to full ISNCSCI, or monitoring chronic SCI without suspected neurological changes.

ISNCSCI Worksheet: Available at: https://asia-spinalinjury.org/wp-content/uploads/2019/10/ASIA-ISCOS-Worksheet_10.2019_PRINT-Page-1-2.pdf.

ASIA website E-ISNCSCI. Available at: https://asia-spinalinjury.org/expedited-isncsci-exam/

Kirshblum S, Waring W. Updates for the international standards for neurological classification of spinal cord injury. *Phys Med Rehabil Clin North Am.* 2014;25(3):505–517, vii. Available at: www.asia-spinalinjury.org

6. How are sensory levels recognized, defined, and documented with bedside examination of persons with SCI?
To accurately map body sensation with the ISNSCI (ASIA Examination), the examiner starts by testing facial sensation, to which all subsequent sensation testing will be compared. The examiner then proceeds from the C2 **key sensory point** and works down each side, testing **light touch** using a fluffed cotton-tipped applicator. It is essential to avoid inadvertent pressure stimulus. Results are recorded as 0 = absent, 1 = present but abnormal (e.g., feels touch but intensity or character (tingling) of sensation is abnormal), or 2 = normal perception of sensation (as compared with areas above the lesion, such as the face). The majority of paraplegic injuries display normal sensation, then transitional levels (often representing the zone of partial preservation) where sensation is present but abnormal, followed by dermatomes where light touch is completely absent. In people with very incomplete (e.g., AIS D, see below) injuries, the sensation can be patchy, and the testing can become a tedious.
    Next, **pinprick stimulus** (with a clean, unused safety pin) is presented lightly to the skin in the same fashion, and dermatomes are tested sequentially and compared to facial sensation. Results are recorded as 0 = absent, 1 = ability to discriminate sharp/dull sensation is present but abnormal compared with the face, or 2 = normal perception of sensation (compared with the face). If unsure, test 10 times, and if correct 8/10 for pinprick versus dull sensation, it is a 2.
    The **sensory level** for each side is the lowest level at which both light touch and pinprick are intact (2) with normal sensation cephalad. The sensory levels are used in combination with the motor levels to determine the single **neurologic level**, which is the lowest level where all elements, motor and sensory, are normal **bilaterally.**

Kaplan—ASIA assessment—YouTube. Available at: https://www.youtube.com/watch?v=IP_wunjn9lo

7. What are the NLI and the single NLI?
The **Neurologic Level of Injury (NLI)** can be thought of as the summation of the sensory level and motor levels. It is the most caudal spinal cord segment where motor function and sensation to light touch and pinprick are intact. When there is a difference between sides of the body, the NLI can be derived from the four different segments identified in determining the neurological level, i.e., R(ight)-sensory, L(eft)-sensory, R-motor, L-motor. These four segments can be reduced to the **Single NLI**, which is the most rostral of these levels and is used in calculating the ASIA Impairment Scale (AIS).

At spinal cord segments where there is no key muscle with a sensory dermatome intact (high cervical, thoracic, and lower sacral levels), the sensory level determines the motor and neurologic levels.

The 2019 revision of the International Standards for Neurological Classification of Spinal Cord Injury (ISNCSCI)—What's new?. Available at: https://www.nature.com/articles/s41393-019-0350-9

Betz R, Biering-Sorensen F, Burns SP, et al. The 2019 revision of the International Standards for Neurological Classification of Spinal Cord Injury (ISNCSCI)—What's new? *Spinal Cord*. 2019;57:815–817. Available at: https://doi.org/10.1038/s41393-019-0350-9

Kirshblum S, Snider B, Rupp R, Read MS. International Standards Committee of ASIA and ISCoS. Updates of the international standards for neurologic classification of spinal cord injury: 2015 and 2019. *Phys Med Rehabil Clin N Am.* 2020;31(3);319–330. doi: 10.1016/jpmr.2020.03.005

Ho CH, Wuermser LA, Priebe MM, et al.: Spinal cord injury medicine. 1. Epidemiology and classification. *Arch Phys Med Rehab.* 2007; 88(3 Suppl 1): S49–S54. Available at: https://www.archives-pmr.org/article/S0003-9993%2806%2901557-7/fulltext

8. What are the key muscles examined to define the SCI motor level clinically?
   Ten key muscles are examined, representing the C5-T1 spinal cord segments supplying the upper extremities and L2-S1 in the lower extremities. The **motor level** is the most caudal key muscle group graded 3/5 or greater, with the cephalad segment graded normal (5/5) strength. If there is no muscle to test at a particular level (such as C4 or L1), motor information is inferred from the sensory examination; i.e., if the sensation is intact, the motor function is interpreted to be 5, normal.

9. Which examination findings successfully predict and confirm sensory and motor incomplete SCI?
   A patient is classified as **sensory incomplete** if there is sensory function below the NLI that includes S4-5 *or* deep anal pressure sensation and does not meet the criteria for motor incomplete.
      A patient is classified as **motor incomplete** if there is voluntary anal sphincter contraction *or* if there is sensory sacral sparing with sparing of motor function more than three levels below the motor level on one side. The key muscles that define each motor level are listed in Box 54.1. Non-key muscles can also be used for this distinction between sensory incomplete and motor incomplete.

10. Why is the sensation most likely to be spared in the perianal area?
    Sacral sparing is due to **spinal cord somatotopic organization**. Sensory and motor fibers are laminated within the spinal cord tracts, so fibers that serve caudal regions are located laterally and closer to the surface. Contusions and spinal cord ischemia produce relatively more damage to centrally located spinal neurons and axons than those peripherally situated near the surface collateral blood supply.
       In the ISNCSCI examination, the sensation at S4–5, deep anal pressure sensation and voluntary anal contraction are used to determine whether patients have a complete or an incomplete injury. There is a high level of correlation among sensation at S3, deep anal pressure, voluntary hip adduction, toe flexion, and anal contraction. Thus, if an anorectal examination is not feasible, these other examination techniques can be used to predict whether somebody would likely be classified with an incomplete spinal cord injury.
       Motor ZPPs are now defined and should be documented in all cases, including patients with incomplete injuries with absent VAC. The sensory ZPP on a given side is defined in the absence of sensory function in S4-5 (LT, PP) on this side as long as DAP is not present.

Marino RJ, Schmidt-Read M, Chen A, et al. Reliability of S3 pressure sensation and voluntary hip adduction/toe flexion and agreement with deep anal pressure and voluntary anal contraction in classifying persons with traumatic spinal cord injury. *J Spinal Cord Med.* 2019; DOI: 10.1080/10790268.2019.1628496. Available at: https://asia-spinalinjury.org/isncsci-2019-revision-released/

11. What is the ASIA Impairment Scale (AIS)? How are the categories defined?
    The **Frankel classification** was the initial template that pioneered the A through E classification dividing SCI patients based on impairment (A and B) and functional status or disability (C, D, and E). Earlier incarnations of

---

Box 54.1 Index Muscles That Define Each Motor Level

C4—diaphragm	L2—iliopsoas
C5—biceps, brachialis	L3—quadriceps
C6—extensor carpi radialis (longus and brevis)	L4—tibialis anterior
C7—triceps brachii	L5—extensor hallucis longus
C8—flexor digitorum profundus to middle finger	S1—gastrocnemius, soleus
T1—abductor digiti minimi	S2—anal sphincter

the **ASIA Impairment Scale (AIS)** relied on functional descriptors (e.g., AIS D used to be assigned for the ability to ambulate 150 feet), but over time this has been revised using the more objective measurement of muscle strength. It defines distinctions between categories by specifying sensory dermatomes and muscle grades as follows:

- **AIS A:** Complete (no motor or sensory S4–S5 function)
- **AIS B:** Incomplete sensory but no motor function preserved through S4–S5
- **AIS C:** Motor and sensory function incomplete, with the strength of more than half of the key muscles below the neurologic level having a muscle grade less than 3
- **AIS D:** Motor and sensory function incomplete (motor functional), with at least half of key muscles below the neurologic level having a muscle grade of 3
- **AIS E:** Normal motor and sensory function in a patient with known SCI.

12. What is the best way to learn the current ISNCSCI classification?

The two main changes in the 2019 version (8th revision) of the ISNCSCI standards include:

1. Documentation of "non-SCI" related impairments with "*" can affect the scoring, such as pre-existing neurologic injury, pain, or advanced age. These explanations can be entered in the comment box alongside the exam table.
2. The zone of partial preservation (ZPP) should now be defined for incomplete injuries:

   If complete motor (absent voluntary anal contraction, or VAC), you can designate motor ZPP in the presence of sensory incomplete injury.

   If complete sensory (absent sensation at the S4–5 dermatomes), you can designate sensory ZPP in the presence of an incomplete motor injury

   To rapidly locate the sensory ZPP, ask the patient where they are the most numb and work up the body until they recognize a touch or cold stimulus.

ISNSCI standards Revised 2019 Available at: https://asia-spinalinjury.org/international-standards-neurological-classification-sci-isncsci-worksheet/

Available at: https://archive.scijournal.com/doi/abs/10.1310/sci2002-81

American Spinal Injury Association's (ASIA) International Standards Training E Program InSTeP Available at: https://asia-spinalinjury.org/shop/

Betz R, Biering-Sørensen F, Burns SP et al. The 2019 revision of the International Standards for Neurological Classification of Spinal Cord Injury (ISNCSCI)—What's new? *Spinal Cord* 2019;57:815–817. Available at: https://doi.org/10.1038/s41393-019-0350-9; https://www.nature.com/articles/s41393-019-0350-9

13. What is the artery of Adamkiewicz?

The **artery of Adamkiewicz**, also known as the **great anterior radicular artery,** is the major radicular branch that arises from the aorta and enters the cord between **T10 and L3**. It is more accurately known as the great anterior radiculomedullary artery (arteria radicularis magna). Although radicular arteries supply each spinal root, this one large artery typically supplies the low thoracic and lumbar spinal cord via collateral connections with the **anterior spinal artery** from T8 to the conus medullaris. The anterior spinal artery supplies the anterior two-thirds of the spinal cord along the length of the spinal cord. The artery of Adamkiewicz anastomoses with the anterior spinal artery in the lower thoracic region, which is the watershed area of the cord. The most common cause of injury to this artery is iatrogenic. Fig. 54.2 shows the blood supply of the spinal cord.

Taterra D, Skinningsrud B, Pekala PA, et al. Artery of Adamkiewicz: a meta-analysis of anatomical characteristics. *Neuroradiology.* 2019;61(8):869–880. Springer Nature. Available at: https://springer.com/article/10.1007/s00234-019-02207-y

14. What are some of the causes of SCI that occur without trauma?

Nontraumatic SCI (NTSCI) accounts for approximately 30% to 40% of SCI and about 40% to 60% of inpatient rehabilitation admissions for SCI in the US. Common causes of NTSCI include stenosis, ischemia, tumor, infection, and inflammation. Of note, infection comprises approximately 5% of NTSCI in the US but up to 50% of NTSCI internationally. Other causes can include syringomyelia, vitamin B12 deficiency, and radiation myelopathy. Compared to the traumatic SCI population, NTSCI tends to have an older median age, affects men and women at equal rates, and is more likely to be motor incomplete. Patients with traumatic and NTSCI tend to have similar inpatient rehabilitation admission function, Functional Independence Measure (FIM) efficiency, and home discharge rates.

McKinley WO, Seel RT, Hardman JT. Nontraumatic spinal cord injury: incidence, epidemiology, and functional outcome. *Arch Phys Med Rehabil.* 1999 Jun;80(6):619–623.

15. The six SCI syndromes are a fathomable conundrum! What are their lesions, clinical findings, and common causes?

Contemplating these from anatomy to symptom can lead to a diagnosis, even with the most subtle hint!

- **Anterior cord syndrome:** This clinical syndrome includes hyporeflexia, atrophy, and variable motor loss, preserving position sensation but not pinprick (hypalgesia) and temperature sensations. Common causes for these findings are thoracolumbar burst fracture, abdominal aortic aneurysm, and aortic clamping for surgery, which compromises segmental spinal cord circulation.
- **Central cord syndrome:** The clinical constellation includes weakness greater in the arms than legs, lower-extremity hyperreflexia, upper-extremity mixed upper motor neuron and lower motor neuron weakness, and preserved sacral sensation with the potential for preservation of bowel and bladder control. Common causes are extension injury with underlying spinal stenosis, hematoma, expanding intramedullary mass, or syrinx.
- **Brown-Séquard syndrome:** This syndrome presents with hemi- or monoplegia or paresis with contralateral pain and temperature sensation deficit. Although spasticity may compromise total function, there is a good prognosis for motor recovery progressing from the proximal extensors to distal flexors. Causes include knife wounds to the back and asymmetrically oriented spinal tumors.
- **Conus Medullaris Syndrome:** This syndrome presents with bladder and bowel involvement, (e.g., weakness and sensory impairment). Weakness and sensory impairment. The key is that there is a mix of upper and lower motor neuron findings due to injury to the conus of the spinal cord and the nerve roots.
- **Cauda Equina Syndrome:** Injury affects the proximal peripheral nerve roots as they exit the spinal cord in the cauda equina. Thus, this is not the spinal cord and is diagnosed by looking for lower motor neuron injury, i.e., absence of reflexes (note reflexes are not part of the ISNSCI exam).
- **Posterior cord syndrome:** This uncommon presentation manifests with bilateral deficits in proprioception. The potential causes are vitamin B_{12} deficiency (subacute combined degeneration) and syphilis (tabes dorsalis). B_{12} deficiency can be the cause of late deterioration in gait after SCI. This is typically no longer officially recognized by ASIA as a spinal cord syndrome because it is so rare.

Petchkrua W, Burns S, Stiens S, et al. Prevalence of vitamin B_{12} deficiency in patients with spinal cord injury or disease. *Arch Phys Med Rehabil.* 2003;84:1675–1679. Available at: https://www.archives-pmr.org/article/S0003-9993(03)00318-6/fulltext

McKinley W, Santos K, Meade M, Brooke K. Incidence and outcomes of spinal cord injury clinical syndromes. *J Spinal Cord Med.* 2007;30:215–224. Available at: https://www.ncbi.nlm.nih.gov/pmc/articles/PMC2031952/

16. What are some of the important treatments to provide after acute traumatic spinal cord injury (SCI)?

- **Control neurogenic shock** with high-flow isotonic IV fluids, with the goal of maintaining mean arterial pressure (MAP) of 85 to 90 mm Hg with a heart rate of 60 to 100 bpm. This may require the use of vasopressors acutely.
- Place an **indwelling urinary catheter** and maintain a urine output of 30 mL/h or more.
- **Stabilize the spine** in a neutral position and obtain computed tomography imaging of the entire spine to evaluate fractures and ligamentous injuries. Consider MRI imaging if feasible prior to decompression but definitely within the acute period for prognostication.
- Consider performing early surgical decompression (within 24 hours of injury) to avoid secondary injury and improve neurologic recovery. This should be done more urgently in patients with neurologic deterioration.
- Consider urgent distraction and reduction of tetraplegic patients with bilateral locked facets.
- Avoid administering IV methylprednisolone sodium succinate given the lack of evidence supporting clinical benefit and potential for harmful side effects.
- Apply lower limb mechanical compression devices/sequential pneumatic compression early and administer low-molecular-weight heparin once primary hemostasis is established to prevent deep vein thrombosis.
- Evaluate ventilatory function with vital capacity and transcutaneous O_2 saturation, and be aware of the risk of delayed respiratory failure after extubation.
- Early transition to SCI specialty rehabilitation.

Fehlings MG, Tetreault LA, Wilson, JR, et al. A clinical practice guideline for the management of acute spinal injury: introduction, rationale, and scope. *Global Spine J.* 2017;7(2 Suppl):84S–94S. doi: 10.1177/2192568217703387. Available at: https://www.ncbi.nlm.nih.gov/pmc/articles/PMC5684846/

Kirshblum SC, Groah SL, McKinley WO, et al. Spinal cord injury medicine 1. Etiology, classification, and acute medical management. *Arch Phys Med Rehab.* 2002;83:S50–S57. Available at: https://www.archives-pmr.org/article/S0003-9993(02)80014-4/pdf

Consortium for Spinal Cord Medicine. Early acute management in adults with spinal cord injury: a clinical practice guideline for health-care professionals. *J Spinal Cord Med.* 2008;31(4):403–479, Available at: https://doi.org/10.1043/1079-0268-31.4.408. Available at: https://www.ncbi.nlm.nih.gov/pmc/articles/PMC2582434/

17. How should the advancement of gait be prioritized within rehabilitation programs for people with SCI?

Initial rehabilitation following any SCI prioritizes complication prevention and adaptation to injury while maximizing safety and function. Most SCI patients begin learning how to use a wheelchair to achieve mobility and ensure safety even if they are projected to have adequate lower limb strength to ambulate eventually. Selecting appropriate patients for gait training is important because it benefits those who may become ambulators. However, it is essential to balance rehabilitation for ambulation with mastery of high-level wheelchair skills.

Techniques for retraining gait include pre-gait activities such as standing frames, parallel bars, and aquatic therapy. Body weight-supported treadmill training that once relied on a team of therapists to physically mobilize patient's legs has been more recently accomplished using robotic assistance (Lokomat). Underwater treadmill systems, suspended track gait safety systems (Zero-G & Vector), and robotic exoskeletal gait systems (ReWalk, Ekso) offer contemporary options. While all of these devices have been shown to improve function during their use and some exercise benefit, widespread adoption of these devices has been limited by their cost and impracticality. Specialized outpatient centers with this equipment and training experience are increasingly available to meet these needs.

18. What are the principles of bladder management after SCI?

Acute paralysis of toe movement bilaterally suggests neurogenic bladder dysfunction and risk for overdistention and infection. **Indwelling catheter drainage** with a daily urine output of greater than 2 L prevents complications. As spinal shock clears, somatic reflexes return before autonomic in a proximal to distal progression. Reflex bladder tone returns with the return of phasic stretch reflexes at the knees and ankles. **Scheduled intermittent catheter** drainage is initiated if the patient has motor and cognitive capabilities, allowing the bladder to be emptied without a persistent foreign body. Management of expected bacteriuria is accomplished by maintaining an undisturbed mucus lining barrier, preventing vesicoureteral reflux and regular bladder emptying.

Increases in expected pyuria suggest an increased risk for systemic infection and should be addressed with increases in urinary output and catheter irrigation to prevent occlusion. Urinalysis and culture before antibiotic administration can provide sensitivities to guide primary pathogen eradication.

19. What are the mechanisms of motor recovery after SCI?

Motor recovery after SCI occurs rapidly during the first and second week, then recovery continues at a slower pace for the first 4 to 6 months and slows further thereafter. Root impingement may resolve with decompression, spinal alignment, and fixation as needed (Fig. 54.3). Initially, recovery could be mediated by central mechanisms (cortical reorganization), such as the recruitment of latent pathways (unused until injury). Edema and hematomyelia may resolve at the injury site, reducing secondary injury, neurapraxic block, and demyelination. Within the anterior horn, central synaptogenesis may occur in response to denervation hypersensitivity of the anterior horn

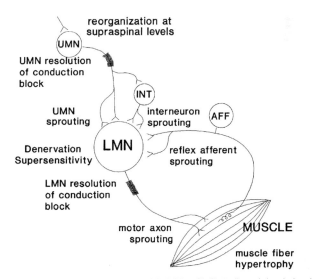

Fig. 54.3 Mechanisms of recovery after spinal cord injury. (From Little J, Stiens SA. Electrodiagnosis in spinal cord injury. *Phys Med Rehabil Clin North Am.* 1995;6:263–296.)

cell. At the muscle level, acetylcholine receptors upregulate in response to denervation and attract sprouting from neighboring alpha motor neurons, producing larger motor units.

Raineteau O, Schwab M. Plasticity of motor systems after incomplete spinal cord injury. *Nature Rev.* 2001;2:263–273.

Donovan J, Kirshblum S. Clinical trials in traumatic spinal cord injury. *Neurotherapeutics.* 2018;15:654–668. Available at: https://. springer.com/article/10.1007%2Fs13311-018-0632-5

20. How do you explain the expected prognosis of SCI with rehabilitation to your patients with new and expected permanent paralysis?

    Spinal cord injury is a prototype for rehabilitation education, reflecting discontinuation of the typical connections between the head and the body. Yet, the nature of humankind is to appreciate, adapt, and control the environment to meet individual life goals. SCI results in impairments in segmental increments, inspiring rehabilitation solutions for self-monitoring and environmental control. Historically, utilizing person-centered spinal cord rehabilitation has successfully prolonged life and reengineered purposeful activity for patients.

    New paralysis may lead to expected and situationally appropriate dysphoria, which can lead to a period of depression, but all is not lost! Patients need to be informed of the nature of their injury and expected prognosis and their ability to regain fulfilling participation in life and work via a shared vision between the patient and the rehabilitation team. Currently, those with SCI can experience prolongation of life to near-normal expected lifespan, full participation in many satisfying life roles, and an expected quality of life that is not proportional to the amount of paralysis. Paradoxically, many patients who have responded to their SCI with resilience say it was one of the most positive turning points in their lives.

Kirshblum S, Fichtenbaum J. Breaking the news in spinal cord injury. *J Spinal Cord Med.* 2008;31(1):7–12. Available at: https://www. ncbi.nlm.nih.gov/pmc/articles/PMC2435037/

21. What is the highest complete SCI level that is consistent with independent living without the aid of an attendant?

    C6 complete tetraplegia: An exceptionally motivated individual with C6 tetraplegia may be capable of living independently in an accessible environment without an attendant's aid. A review of outcomes from a subset of people with motor- and sensory-complete C6 SCI revealed that the following percentages of patients were independent for key self-care tasks: feeding 16%, upper body dressing 13%, lower body dressing 3%, grooming 19%, bathing 9%, bowel care 3%, transfers 6%, and wheelchair propulsion 88%. Feeding is accomplished with a universal cuff for utensils. Transfers require stabilization of elbow extension with forces transmitted from shoulder musculature through the limb as a closed kinetic chain. Bowel care can be performed with a suppository insertion wand and using equipment (e.g., "dil stick") for adaptive digital stimulation.

Gittler MS, McKinley WO, Stiens SA, et al. Spinal cord injury medicine 3. Rehabilitation outcomes. *Arch Phys Med Rehab.* 2002;83:S65–S71. Available at: https://www.archives-pmr.org/article/S0003-9993(02)80016-8/pdf

Consortium for Spinal Cord Medicine. *Outcomes Following Traumatic Spinal Cord Injury: Clinical Practice Guidelines for Health-Care Professionals.* 1999; Available at: https://pva.org/wp-content/uploads/2021/09/cpg_outcomes-following-traumatic-sci.pdf

Bonus questions and answers available online.

WEBSITES

1. www.nim.nih.gov/medlineplus/spinalcordinjuries.html
2. www.ninds.nih.gov/disorders/sci/sci.htm
3. www.spinal-cord.org
4. www.spinalinjury.net

BIBLIOGRAPHY

Bayley JC, Cochran TP, Sledge CB. The weight-bearing shoulder: the impingement syndrome in paraplegics. *J Bone Joint Surg.* 1987; 69A:676–678.

Blackwell T, Krause J, Winkler T, et al. *A Desk Reference for Life Care Planning for Persons with Spinal Cord Injury.* New York: Demos; 2001:1068 pgs.

Eldahan KC, Rabchevsky AG. Autonomic dysreflexia after spinal cord injury: Systemic pathophysiology and methods of management. *Autonomic Neuroscience: Basic and Clinical* 2018;209:59–70.

Garcia-Arguello LY, O'Horo JC, Farrell A et al. Infections in the spinal cord-injured population: a systematic review. *Spinal Cord,* 2016;55: 526–534.

Kirshblum SC, Groah SL, McKinley WO, et al. Spinal cord injury medicine 1: Etiology, classification, and acute medical management. *Arch Phys Med Rehabil.* 2002;83:S50–S57.

Kirshblum SC, Lin V. *Spinal Cord Injury.* 3rd ed. New York: Springer Publishing, Demos; 2019:1006 pgs

McCool FD, Benditt JO. Respiratory manifestations of neuromuscular and chest wall disorders. *Clin Chest* Med. 2018;39(2):i.

McKinley WO, Gittler MS, Kirshblum SC, et al. Spinal cord injury medicine 2. Medical complications after spinal cord injury: identification and management. *Arch Phys Med Rehabil.* 2002;83:S58–S64.

Priebe MM, Chiodo AE, Scelza WM, et al. Spinal cord injury medicine. 6. Economic and societal issues in spinal cord injury. *Arch Phys Med Rehabil.* 2007;83(3 Suppl 1):S84–S88.

Sabharwal S. *Essentials of Spinal Cord Medicine.* New York, NY: Demos Medical Publishing; 2014:453pgs.

Scelza WM, Kirshblum SC, Wuermser LA, et al. Spinal cord injury medicine. 4. Community reintegration after spinal cord injury. *Arch Phys Med Rehabil.* 2007;88(3 Suppl 1):S71–S75.

Stiens SA, Farber H, Yuhas S. The person with spinal cord injury: an evolving prototype for life care planning. In PMR Clinics Lacerte M ed. *Phys Med Rehab Clin N Am.* 2013 Aug;24(3):419-44. Epub May 25, 2013.

Vazquez RG, Ferreiro Velasco ME, Mourelo Farina M, et al. Update on traumatic acute spinal cord injury. Parts 1 & 2 *Med Intensiva.* 2016;41(4):237–247.

CHAPTER 55

MULTIPLE SCLEROSIS: CLINICAL PATTERNS, SYMPTOM MANAGEMENT, AND REHABILITATION

Rosa Rodriguez, MD and Seema Khurana, DO

Our greatest weakness lies in giving up. The most certain way to succeed is always to try just one more time.
— Thomas Edison

KEY POINTS

1. Multiple sclerosis (MS) affects females more than males.
2. A remitting-relapsing course is seen in about 75% of patients.
3. Decreased survival is seen in males, progressive MS, older age at onset, and cerebellar features.
4. MS is characterized by plaques of central nervous system (CNS) white matter demyelination.
5. Spasticity is seen in over 80% of patients with MS.
6. Lower urinary tract symptoms are reported in over 80% of MS patients.

1. **Why is multiple sclerosis (MS) important to physiatrists?**
   MS is an important disease process to recognize and treat not only medically, but with rehabilitation. Rehabilitation can include therapies such as physical therapy, occupational therapy, speech language pathology, neuropsychology, and vocational rehabilitation.

2. **What is the epidemiology and prognosis of MS?**
   MS affects females more than males. A remitting-relapsing course is seen in about 75% of patients. Age of onset is usually between 20 and 50 years. Median survival is greater than 30 years. However, decreased survival is seen in males, progressive MS, older age at onset, and cerebellar features.

Perkin GD, Miller DC, Lane RJM, Patel MC, Hochberg FH. Multiple sclerosis and other demyelinating diseases. In Perkin GD (ed): *Atlas of Clinical Neurology*, Philadelphia, PA: Saunders, 2011:343–359.

3. **What are the demographics of MS?**
   There are approximately 2.3 million people affected by MS according to the Atlas of MS. The distribution of MS favors higher latitudes and decreases progressively towards the equator. Migration from lower to higher latitude increases risk of developing MS. Environmental factors such as vitamin D, sunlight exposure, geographic latitude, and place of birth seem to play a major role. The female-to-male ratio is estimated to be 2.3. In the US, the prevalence of MS was approximately 400,000 individuals. In siblings and dizygotic twins, the risk of developing MS is 3% to 5%, but in monozygotic twins it is 20% to 39%.

MSIF. *Atlas of MS 2013: Mapping Multiple Sclerosis Around the World*, 2013.

Ascherio A, Munger KL. Environmental risk factors for multiple sclerosis. Part I: the role of infection. *Ann Neurol.* 2007; 61(4):288–299.

Wallin MT, Culpepper WJ, Coffman P, et al. The Gulf War era multiple sclerosis cohort: Age and incidence rates by race, sex and service. *Brain.* 2012;135(Pt 6):1778–1785.

Alonso A, Hernán MA. Temporal trends in the incidence of multiple sclerosis: a systematic review. *Neurology.* 2008;71(2):129–135.

Dilokthornsakul P, Valuck RJ, Nair KV, et al. Multiple sclerosis prevalence in the United States commercially insured population. *Neurology.* 2016;86(11):1014–1021.

Sadovnick AD, Armstrong H, Rice GP, et al. A population-based study of multiple sclerosis in twins: update. *Ann Neurol.* 1993;33(3):281–285.

4. **What is the pathophysiology of MS?**
   MS is characterized by plaques of central nervous system (CNS) white matter demyelination, which is most frequently seen in the periventricular white matter, brain stem, and spinal cord, along with lymphocytes and

macrophages. Most evidence suggests it is an inflammatory demyelinating disease caused by environmental and genetic factors. Many environmental and genetic factors have been implicated in the cause of the disease, including autoimmunity, infections, vitamin D deficiency, smoking, and obesity. Loss of tolerance may be the cause of an autoimmune attack to myelin proteins, including molecular mimicry of viral and bacterial peptides. Some of the pathogens considered as potential MS triggers are human herpes virus 6, Epstein-Barr virus, and *Chlamydia pneumonia*. Although not proven to be causative, low vitamin D levels are associated with MS activity and progression. Smoking is associated with MS susceptibility.

Kellerman R, Rakel D. *Conn's Current Therapy*. Philadelphia: Elsevier; 2019.

Daroff R, Mazziotta JC, Jankovic J, Pomeroy SL. *Bradley's Neurology in Clinical Practice*. Lonon, UK: Elsevier, 2016.

Ascherio A, Munger KL, White R, et al. Vitamin D as an early predictor of multiple sclerosis activity and progression. *JAMA Neurol.* 2014;71(3):306–314.

Handel AE, Williamson AJ, Disanto G, et al. Smoking and multiple sclerosis: an updated meta-analysis. *PLoS ONE.* 2011;6(1): e16149

5. **What patterns of disease are seen in MS?**
New consensus has been made since *the 2013 Revisions*, including the addition of Clinically Isolated Syndrome (CIS) and elimination of progressive-relapsing MS. Relapsing-remitting and progressive disease have been retained. Further, all forms are characterized as active or non-active.
Active MS: clinical relapses and/or new lesions over a specified time frame, usually one year.
MS Phenotypes:
- Clinically Isolated Syndrome: term for first clinical event. It is considered to be part of the MS spectrum and course should be followed. If there are magnetic resonance imaging (MRI) findings of MS to suggest a previous episode seen on MRI (demonstrating dissemination in space), then the diagnosis of MS can be made. According to the National MS Society, the risk of developing MS is 60% to 80% in patients with MRI findings of lesions similar to those seen in MS but about 20% in patients without those MRI findings.
- Relapsing-remitting: those with a CIS who have a second relapse or MRI evidence of dissemination.
- Progressive disease: includes primary-progressive and secondary-progressive, which are progressive disability from onset of disease and progressive disability after a relapse, respectively. There are four subtypes:
  - Active and with progression
  - Active but without progression
  - Not active but with progression
  - Not active and without progression

Lublin FD. New multiple sclerosis phenotypic classification. *Eur Neurol.* 2014;72(Suppl. 1):1–5.

Lublin FD, Reingold SC, Cohen JA, et al. Defining the clinical course of multiple sclerosis: the 2013 revisions. *Neurology.* 2014;83(3): 278–286.

Thompson AJ, Banwell BL, Barkhof F, et al. Diagnosis of multiple sclerosis: 2017 revisions of the McDonald criteria. *Lancet Neurol.* 2018;17(2):162–173.

Polman CH, Reingold SC, Banwell B, et al. Diagnostic criteria for multiple sclerosis: 2010 Revisions to the McDonald criteria. *Ann Neurol.* 2011;69(2):292–302.

6. **What diagnostic tools are used to diagnose MS?**
- Brain MRI shows multifocal T2-hyperintense white matter lesions in periventricular, juxtacortical and infratentorial, as well as hypointense lesions on T1.
- Brain and spinal cord lesions may show enhancement with gadolinium contrast.
- Cerebrospinal fluid may provide supportive evidence for MS. Findings would include normal or mildly elevated white cell count and protein, elevated IgG index, and IgG oligoclonal bands not present in serum. Isoelectric focusing and immunofixation is the best method to detect oligoclonal bands, which is found in 90% of patients with MS. However, they can be present in other neuroinflammatory disorders.
- Neuropsychological testing of evoked potentials (EP) can identify clinically silent lesions in visual, sensory, or auditory pathways, indicating dissemination in space and suggesting demyelination.

Brownlee WJ, Hardy TA, Fazekas F, et al. Diagnosis of multiple sclerosis: progress and challenges. *The Lancet*, 2017;389(10076): 1336-1346.

7. Does psychological stress play a role in relapses?

In a prospective study examining relapses in women with MS, it was found that the duration of a stressful event increased the risk of relapse, but type and severity of stress did not (Mitsonis et al. 2008). Another prospective study found that high levels of anxiety were strongly associated with severity and number of stressful life events that increased the likelihood of exacerbations.

Potagas C, Mitsonis C, Watier L, et al. Influence of anxiety and reported stressful life events on relapses in multiple sclerosis: a prospective study. *Mult Scler*, 2008;14(9):1262–1268.

8. What is Lhermitte's sign?

It is an electric shock-like sensation that occurs with flexion of the neck, radiating down the spine and may radiate into the legs, arms, and trunk. It was first described by Marie and Chatelin in 1917 but named after Jean Lhermitte. The sensation is due to the stretching of the hyperexcitable demyelinated dorsal column. It is commonly seen in MS patients.

Khare S, Seth D. Lhermitte's sign: the current status. *Ann Indian Acad Neurol.* 2015;18(2):154.

9. What are important prognostic signs in MS?

MS affects females more than males, a remitting-relapsing course is seen in about 75% of patients, age of onset is usually between 20 and 50 years, and median survival is greater than 30 years. Decreased survival is seen in males, progressive MS, older age at onset, and cerebellar features.

Perkin GD. Multiple sclerosis and other demyelinating diseases: introduction. In *Atlas of Clinical Neurology*, 2011:343–359.

10. What MRI and evoked potential findings are seen in MS?

In nearly all patients with established MS and in over 80% of patients with CIS, there is evidence of MS on brain MRI. MRI typically shows multifocal T2-hyperintense white matter lesions. The typical locations include periventricular, juxtacortical, and infratentorial. T1-weighted MRI shows hypointense lesions. In 80% to 90% of patients with established MS and half of patients with CIS, spinal cord lesions are seen typically in the cervical cord.

With gadolinium lesions, brain and spinal cord lesions typically show enhancement.

EP are able to quantify signal transduction involving sensor and motor pathways. It can provide evidence of multiple sclerosis but is not specific. A well-preserved waveform with a prolonged latency is suggestive of demyelination. EP may be obtained if diagnosis is uncertain.

Brownlee WJ, Hardy TA, Fazekas F, et al. Diagnosis of multiple sclerosis: progress and challenges. *The Lancet.* 2017;389(10076): 1336–1346.

11. What outcome measures are used in MS?

The most widely used MS outcome measures have been the Expanded Disability Status Scale (EDSS) and Functional Systems Scores (FSS). The FSS gathers information from various functional systems and the neurologic examination, which together with some additional information about ambulation, is then used to rate the EDSS. The EDSS was developed in 1983 and has been relatively unchanged, allowing the same scale to be used to compare disease status over many years.

There is also the Multiple Sclerosis Quality of Life-54 (MSQOL-54), which combines general and MS-specific items developed in 1995. MSQOL-54 consists of a physical health composite score, a mental health composite score, and two single-items (satisfaction with sexual function and change in health). This scale is protected by copyright and requires the author's permission to use each time.

Kurtzke JF. On the origin of EDSS. *Mult Scler Relat Disord.* 2015;4(2):95–103.

Vickrey BG, Hays RD, Harooni R, et al. A health-related quality of life measure for multiple sclerosis. *Qual Life Res.* 1995;4(3): 187–206.

12. How do you design a rehabilitation program to maximize beneficial MS outcome with inpatient or outpatient rehabilitation?

Outpatient rehabilitation: A six-week comprehensive multidisciplinary outpatient rehabilitation is effective for improving disability and function as measured by FIM. However, inadequate data exists for self-efficacy, fatigue, depression, or quality of life.

- Inpatient rehabilitation: Although there are limited inpatient rehabilitation studies, there are multiple studies that suggest an inpatient rehabilitation program is beneficial for patients with MS. In a randomized controlled trial in Denmark, patients who had a course of inpatient rehabilitation continued to have reduced decline in health-related quality of life at the six months' mark.

Patti F, Ciancio MR, Cacopardo M, et al. Effects of a short outpatient rehabilitation treatment on disability of multiple sclerosis patients—a randomised controlled trial. *J Neurol.* 2003;250(7):861–866.

Kos D, Duportail M, D'hooghe MB, et al. Multidisciplinary fatigue management programme in multiple sclerosis: a randomized clinical trial. *Mult Scler.* 2007;13(8):996–1003.

Boesen F, Nørgaard M, Trénel P, et al. Longer term effectiveness of inpatient multidisciplinary rehabilitation on health-related quality of life in MS patients: a pragmatic randomized controlled trial—The Danish MS Hospitals Rehabilitation Study. *Mult Scler J.* 2018; 24(3):340–349.

13. Can patients with MS benefit from exercise?

Exercise was previously discouraged in MS patients to avoid exacerbation of MS-related symptoms, including increases in core temperature and fatigue. Programs now are encouraging appropriate levels of exercise to reduce MS-related symptoms and promote general wellness.

A systematic review of physical activity guidelines for multiple sclerosis noted various studies that illustrated the benefits of exercise for MS, including improvement or maintenance of the following: walking ability, aerobic fitness and strength, balance, fatigue, health-related quality of life, depression, chronic disease risk profiles. A meta-analysis from 2013 concluded that moderate-intensity exercise twice per week is effective for increasing aerobic and muscular fitness in patients with mild to moderate disability from MS. Unfortunately, there is limited evidence in patients with severe disability; most studies include patients with mild-to-moderate disability. However, despite there being clear benefits for exercise, most patients with MS are physically inactive.

Sandoval AE. Exercise in multiple sclerosis. *Phys Med Rehabil Clin N Am.* 2013 Nov;24(4):605–618.

Geidl W, Gobster C, Streber R, et al. A systematic critical review of physical activity aspects in clinical guidelines for multiple sclerosis. *Mult Scler Relat Disord.* 2018; 25,200–207.

Latimer-Cheung AE, Pilutti LA, et al. Effects of exercise training on fitness, mobility, fatigue, and health-related quality of life among adults with multiple sclerosis: a systematic review to inform guideline development. *Arch Phys Med Rehabil.* 2013;94(9): 1800–1828.

Edwards T, Pilutti LA. The effect of exercise training in adults with multiple sclerosis with severe mobility disability: a systematic review and future research directions. *Mult Scler Relat Disord.* 2017;16:31–39.

Casey B, Coote S, Donnelly A. Objective physical activity measurement in people with multiple sclerosis: a review of the literature. *Disabil Rehabil Assist Technol.* 2018;13(2):124–131.

14. How can fatigue be assessed and treated in MS?

Multiple sclerosis-related fatigue (MSRF) is reported in 70% to 80% of MS patients. MSRF includes increased weakness after exercise or over the course of the day or lassitude, which is an abnormal feeling of constant tiredness that may be aggravated by heat and humidity. The most widely used assessment tool for assessing fatigue in MS is the Modified Fatigue Impact Scale (MFIS). MFIS is a shortened version of the Fatigue Impact Scale described by Fisk, et al., in 1994. Overall, there is mixed evidence of non-pharmacological interventions in improving MSRF and lack of strong evidence for pharmacological interventions in improving MSRF.

Amantadine, which improves cholinergic and dopaminergic transmission, is the only drug supported by the National Institutes for Health and Care Excellence guidelines for management of MSRF. Limited evidence exists for Prokarin, a proprietary blend of histamine and caffeine. A double-blinded pilot study comparing Prokarin with placebo found significant results in MFIS pre- vs. post-treatment. There is conflicting evidence of modafinil in MSRF. However, a systematic meta-analysis of five randomized control trials from 2000 to 2017 did note that modafinil significantly improved fatigue using MFIS. For non-pharmacological interventions, energy conservation management (ECM) and yoga have the strongest evidence. A systematic review and meta-analysis of ECM found short-term benefits for ECM. However, further research is needed to identify if long-term benefits exist. Most studies regarding Yoga reported statistically significant improvement on fatigue.

Iriarte J, Subirá ML, De Castro P. Modalities of fatigue in multiple sclerosis: correlation with clinical and biological factors. *Mult Scler.* 2000;6(2):124–130.

Miller P, Soundy A. The pharmacological and non-pharmacological interventions for the management of fatigue-related multiple sclerosis. *J Neurol Sci.* 2017;381:41–54.

Fisk JD, Ritvo PG, Ross L, et al. Measuring the functional impact of fatigue: initial validation of the fatigue impact scale. *Clin Infect Dis.* 1994;18(Supplement_1):S79–S83.

Gillson G, Richards TL, Smith RB, et al. A double-blind pilot study of the effect of Prokarin™ on fatigue in multiple sclerosis. *Mult Scler.* 2002;8(1):30–35.

Shangyan H, Kuiqing L, Yumin X, et al. Meta-analysis of the efficacy of modafinil versus placebo in the treatment of multiple sclerosis fatigue. *Mult Scler Relat Disord.* 2018;19:85–89.

Blikman LJ, Huisstede BM, Kooijmans H, et al. Effectiveness of energy conservation treatment in reducing fatigue in multiple sclerosis: a systematic review and meta-analysis. *Arch Phys Med Rehabil.* 2013;94(7):1360–1376.

15. What is Uhthoff's phenomenon?

Uhthoff's phenomenon was first reported in the late 1800s by Wilhelm Uhthoff in patients with optic neuritis who manifested reversible, short, recurrent, and stereotypical visual symptoms. It is seen in MS and other demyelinating diseases and usually triggered by exposure to high temperatures, infection, exercise, menstruation, and psychological stress. All these triggers are related to increased core body temperature. In demyelinated axons, increased temperature results in altered ion-channels that affect action potentials.

Frohman TC, Davis SL, Beh S, et al. Uhthoff's phenomena in MS—clinical features and pathophysiology. *Nat Rev Neurol.* 2013;9(9):535–540.

16. How is spasticity managed in MS?

Spasticity is seen in over 80% of patients with MS, and it can lead to decreased function, pain, contractures, dermal breakdown, and increased burden of care. In MS, there is increased central input to alpha motor neurons that disinhibit reflexes. Additionally, as myelin is damaged, action potentials are not contained in their axons and spread ephatically. Treatment should be multimodal and individualized, and infections should be ruled out, as they are a common precipitator of spasticity.

First-line oral pharmacological treatment is baclofen, a GABA receptor analogue. Dosing is usually started at 5 mg three times per day and titrated up to 80 mg daily as tolerated. Fatigue and sedation are limiting side effects of baclofen. Tizanidine, an alpha-2 central agonist affecting the brain stem and spinal cord, is thought to reduce spasticity by presynaptic inhibition. Dosing is typically started at 2 mg once daily and can be titrated to 12 mg per dose or 36 mg daily. Hypotension and sedation are limiting side effects of tizanidine. Dry mouth is also seen with Tizanidine. Dantrolene, which inhibits calcium release from the sarcoplasmic reticulum, and therefore acts peripherally, may also be used. Dosing is typically started at 25 mg daily and titrated up to 400 mg daily. Hepatotoxicity and weakness may be limiting side effects. Diazepam, a GABA$_A$ agonist, causes presynaptic inhibition. Dosing is typically started at 4 mg daily and may be titrated up to 40 mg daily. Sedation, cognitive impairment, and dependence are some adverse effects. If a single agent is not effective, multiple agents may be used in combination.

Non-oral pharmacologic treatments include chemodenervation, with botulinum toxin or phenol, and intrathecal baclofen. There are a variety of subtypes of botulinum toxin, but only types A (Onabotulinum, Abobotulinum, Incobotulinum) and B (Rimabotulinum) are approved in the United States. Nerve blocks with phenol are typically reserved for less active, more disabled patients that have not responded to other treatments. Phenol may cause loss of sensation. In severely spastic patients, intrathecal baclofen is used for direct infusion into the cerebrospinal fluid (CSF). An intrathecal baclofen trial is performed prior to a permanent pump placement. Initial infusion is with a bolus of 50 to 100 mcg, which is a much lower dosage than oral baclofen treatment.

Cannabinoids may also be used in moderate to severe MS spasticity in patients not responding to the above treatments. Delta-9-tetrahydrocannabinol (THC)/cannabidiol (CBD) are available in oral-mucosal spray. This treatment may be considered in areas where it is legal.

Non-pharmacological modalities include physical therapy, skin cooling, transcutaneous electrical nerve stimulation and massage. These are modalities that should be used prior to or combined with pharmacologic treatment.

Maitin IB, Cruz E. Special Considerations and Assessment in Patients with Multiple Sclerosis. *Phys Med Rehabil Clin N Am.* 2018 Aug;29(3):473–481.

17. When should you suspect bladder dysfunction? What are the patterns of dysfunction and their treatment?

Lower urinary tract symptoms are reported in over 80% of MS patients. Prevalence increases with disease duration and physical disability. One should also suspect bladder dysfunction if patient reports bowel dysfunction or spasticity of the lower limbs. Patients may report symptoms of storage, voiding, or of both phases. However, the patterns of lower urinary tract dysfunction are determined by lesion location. Detrusor overactivity is typically seen in suprapontine lesions and sometimes in suprasacral spinal lesions. Detrusor-sphincter dyssynergia is typically seen in suprasacral spinal lesions. Hypocontractile detrusor is typically seen in infrasacral lesions. Detrusor overactivity is the most frequent bladder symptom in MS. Evaluation should include urinalysis/culture, bladder diary, post-void residual measurements, ultrasonography, renal function assessment, and occasionally a urodynamic study and cystoscopy. Symptoms of detrusor overactivity can be improved with pelvic floor rehabilitation, which may also be combined with neuromuscular electrical stimulation. Commonly used in MS are anti-muscarinics and/or intermittent self-catheterization. However, there is limited data, and its use in MS is interpolated from other neurological disorders. Furthermore, anticholinergics should be avoided in those with cognitive impairment, which is frequently reported in MS as the disease progresses. Oxybutynin, tolterodine, solifenacin, and trospium chloride are anticholinergics. Trospium is the least likely of these medications to cross the blood-brain barrier. Desmopressin, a synthetic antidiuretic hormone, reduces nighttime urinary frequency in patients with MS. In a large, controlled trial with 647 patients with MS, cannabis extract, but not delta-9-tetrahydrocannabinol versus placebo significantly reduced frequency of urge incontinence episodes. In a smaller study, both cannabis extract and delta9-tetrahydrocannabinol reduced urinary frequency and nocturia significantly. In patients with treatment-refractory neurogenic bladder, onabotulinum toxin A or abobotulinum toxin A can be used as intravesicular treatments. Neuromodulation is also used in detrusor overactivity by stimulation of the tibial nerve (percutaneous or transcutaneous stimulation) or S3 sacral nerve root. In certain situations, surgical treatments may be an option. These include augmentation cystoplasty, cutaneous continent diversion, and ileal conduit surgery.

Phé V, Chartier-Kastler E, Panicker JN. Management of neurogenic bladder in patients with multiple sclerosis. *Nat Rev Urol.* 2016; 13(5):275–288.

Mahajan ST, Patel PB, Marrie RA. Under treatment of overactive bladder symptoms in patients with multiple sclerosis: an ancillary analysis of the NARCOMS patient *registry. J Urol.* 2010;183(4):1432–1437.

Panicker JN, Fowler CJ, Kessler TM. Lower urinary tract dysfunction in the neurological patient: clinical assessment and management. *Lancet Neurol.* 2015;14(7):720–732.

De Ridder D, Vermeulen C, Ketelaer P, et al. Pelvic floor rehabilitation in multiple sclerosis. *Acta Neurol Belg.* 1999;99(1):61–64.

McClurg D, Ashe RG, Lowe-Strong AS. Neuromuscular electrical stimulation and the treatment of lower urinary tract dysfunction in multiple sclerosis—a double blind, placebo controlled, randomised clinical trial. *Neurourol Urodyn.* 2008;27(3):231–237.

Madhuvrata P, Singh M, Hasafa Z, et al. Anticholinergic drugs for adult neurogenic detrusor overactivity: a systematic review and meta-analysis. *Eur Urol.* 2012;62(5):816–830.

Zahariou A, Karamouti M, Karagiannis G, et al. Maximal bladder capacity is a positive predictor of response to desmopressin treatment in patients with MS and nocturia. *Int Urol Nephrol.* 2008;40(1):65–69.

Freeman RM, Adekanmi O, Waterfield MR, et al. The effect of cannabis on urge incontinence in patients with multiple sclerosis: a multicentre, randomised placebo-controlled trial (CAMS-LUTS). *Int Urogynecol J.* 2006;17(6):636–641.

Brady CM, DasGupta R, Dalton C, et al. An open-label pilot study of cannabis-based extracts for bladder dysfunction in advanced multiple sclerosis. *Mult Scler.* 2004;10(4):425–433.

18. How does MS affect pregnancy and vice versa?

Overall, MS patients benefit from pregnancy, with immunomodulation being the protective effect, although the mechanism is not fully understood. MS relapse rates increase temporarily in the postpartum period but eventually return to baseline rates.

Voskuhl R, Momtazee C. Pregnancy: effect on multiple sclerosis, treatment considerations, and breastfeeding. *Neurotherapeutics.* 2017;14(4):974–984.

Confavreux C, Hutchinson M, Hours MM, et al. Rate of pregnancy-related relapse in multiple sclerosis. Pregnancy in Multiple Sclerosis Group. *N Engl J Med.* 1998;339(5):285–291.

WEBSITES

1. MS Association of America
   Available at www.msaa.com
2. MS Consortium
   Available at mscare.org
3. The MS Foundation
   Available at www.msfocus.org
4. National MS Society
   Available at www.nationalmssociety.org

CHAPTER 56

MOVEMENT DISORDERS: FUNDAMENTALS OF CLASSIFICATION AND TREATMENT

Philippines G. Cabahug, MD and Kenneth H. Silver, MD

Everything is in motion. Everything flows. Everything is vibrating.

— Wayne Dyer (1940–2015)

KEY POINTS

1. Major motor features of Parkinson disease (PD) include resting tremor, rigidity, akinesia (or bradykinesia) and stooped posture (TRAP).
2. Disabling motor symptoms of advanced PD include impaired walking (slow, shuffling gait, retropulsion-propulsion), increased rigidity as the disease progresses, development of permanent kyphosis, and loss of postural stability, dyskinesias, impaired manual dexterity, speech impairments, and dysphagia.
3. A Rest tremor is a tremor in a body part that is not voluntarily activated and is completely supported against gravity. Action tremors occur while voluntarily maintaining position against gravity (e.g., postural tremor, isometric tremor) or doing voluntary movement (kinetic tremor).
4. Primary symptoms of Tourette syndrome (TS) are motor and vocal tics. Painful motor tics seen in TS may benefit from botulinum toxin injections.
5. Pharmacologic therapies, botulinum toxin injections, and surgical therapies are the main treatment methods for dystonia.

1. ## What are the main clinical features of Parkinson disease (PD)?

   Clinical presentation involves four major domains: motor symptoms, cognitive alterations, behavioral changes, and autonomic nervous system dysfunction. Patients commonly show a **resting tremor, bradykinesia** (slowness of movement), and a form of increased muscular tone called **rigidity.** Other common features include a reduction in facial movements, resulting in **masked facies, stooped posture,** and reduction of the amplitude of movements **(hypometria).** Also seen are changes in speech to a soft monotone **(hypophonia)** and small, less legible handwriting **(micrographia).** Walking becomes slower, stride length is reduced, and pivoting is replaced with a series of small steps (**"turning en bloc"**). See Box 56.1.

2. ## Who gets PD?

   Although PD is a disease primarily found in older people, it is reported that up to 4% of those with PD are diagnosed before age 40. Approximately 2% to 3% of those over age 65 have PD, with an incidence of 20 in 100,000 in the general population. It has a prevalence of almost one million cases in the United States and 10 million globally. The cause of PD is unknown, but likely results from a complex interaction of environmental and genetic factors. People with a history of exposure to pesticides and herbicides (such as farm workers) appear to be at increased risk, and about 15% of individuals with PD have a positive family history. Five identified genes at this time are: pink-1, lrrk-2, park-7, prkn, and snca).[1–3]

3. ## What is the brain pathology of PD?

   PD is a progressive, neurodegenerative disorder characterized by neuronal loss within the substantia nigra pars compacta, causing depletion of striatal dopamine and subsequent increased inhibitory basal ganglia (BG) output

---

Box 56.1 A Mnemonic for Parkinson Disease

Mnemonic: "TRAP"
(Major Motor Features of Parkinson Disease)
1. **T**remor (resting)
2. **R**igidity (possibly with cogwheeling/jerking)
3. **A**kinesia (or bradykinesia)
4. **P**osture (stooped with postural instability)

from the internal globus pallidus and the substantia nigra pars reticulata. Also, there is accumulation in dopaminergic cells of Lewy inclusion bodies composed of α-synuclein. By the time PD symptoms appear, approximately 60% to 70% of neurons in the substantia nigra regions are lost. Non-motor systems are also impaired (e.g., non-BG regions that subserve cognition, mood, impulse control, and autonomic function). Though there is no specific test to diagnose PD, a variety of imaging tests such as MRI, CT, and PET scans help eliminate other disorders. SPECT imaging utilizing a dopamine transporter (DAT) is available, but not widely used.

4. How does PD initially present?

The most common initial symptom, **resting tremor,** usually subsides when the limb is in motion. The tremor often begins in the hands, less often initially in the legs and is usually asymmetrical. Head and voice tremors are rare. Activities that involve other limbs, such as walking, usually increase the tremor. Patients may feel clumsy or weak as well as slow and stiff. They will have noticed that certain normal activities such as dressing (particularly buttoning), shaving, cutting food, and writing are more difficult. Family members may misinterpret the patient's appearance and believe they are depressed. (However, there is increased incidence of depression among PD patients.)[4-6]

5. What is a tremor? How is it classified?

A tremor is defined as an involuntary, rhythmic oscillatory movement of a body part. It is classified along two main axes: clinical features (Axis 1) and etiology (Axis 2). Axis 1 pertains to medical history (age of onset, temporal evolution, family history, and drug or toxin exposure), tremor characteristics (body distribution, activation condition, frequency), and associated signs. Lab tests (e.g., electrophysiological tests, imaging, and biomarkers) may additionally characterize the tremor. Axis 2 refers to whether the tremor is acquired, genetic, or idiopathic.

Body distribution of tremors can be focal, segmental, hemi-tremor (one side of the body), or generalized. Tremor frequencies are categorized as follows: less than 4 Hz (palatal tremor), 4 to 8 Hz (most pathological tremors), 8 to 12 Hz (physiologic tremor), and greater than 12 Hz (orthostatic tremors, for example are 13 to 18 Hz). Myoclonus is typically greater than 8 Hz.[7]

6. What is the difference between a resting tremor and an action tremor?

In Axis 1, activation conditions of tremor are grouped into rest tremor and action tremor. Rest tremor is a tremor in a body part that is not voluntarily activated and is completely supported against gravity. Action tremor (Table 56.1) occurs while voluntarily maintaining position against gravity (e.g., postural tremor, isometric tremor) or doing voluntary movement (kinetic tremor).[7,8]

7. How do physiologic tremors and essential tremors (ET) differ?

A physiologic tremor is a normal finding in the general population. It is a mild, bilateral postural or kinetic action tremor particularly of the hands and fingers. It is exacerbated by stress, anxiety, strenuous activity, exercise, caffeine, or other stimulants. Treatment involves reassurance and avoidance of triggering factors. If severe, β-blockers such as propranolol or primidone may be used.

ET are often misdiagnosed as Parkinson disease and are the most common action tremors in adults. They are also the most common tremors in pediatric patients. The most commonly used medications for ET are propranolol and primidone, which are associated with a 50% reduction in tremor severity in 70% of patients. Second tier medications include benzodiazepines, topiramate, and gabapentin. Botulinum toxin (BoNT) injections have modest benefit. Thalatomy or deep brain stimulation has been used in adults with severe ET, with a 50% to 90% improvement in tremors.[8]

8. What are some disabling symptoms of advanced PD?

Walking becomes impaired as the disease progresses. Postural alterations include increased neck, trunk, and hip flexion which, when coupled with a decrease in righting oneself and equilibrium reactions, lead to balance deficits and an increased risk of falling. Slow gait is typically seen, with difficulty turning and a tendency toward short, shuffling steps. Tripping may occur on irregular surfaces. The patient tends to stagger backward **(retropulsion)** when pushed from the front and forward **(propulsion)** when pushed from behind. Attempts to increase speed result in more rapid stepping but not in increased stride length. Worsening proximal muscle rigidity significantly reduces trunk rotation and arm swing. Postural changes such as stooping with the development of permanent kyphosis can occur after years of Parkinson disease. Loss of postural stability is common in advanced PD, even in the L-DOPA "on" state.

Table 56.1 Types of Tremors		
ACTION	**TREMOR TYPE**	**RELATIONSHIP TO ACTION/MUSCLE STATE**
Kinetic	Simple	Tremor is the same throughout a movement.
	Intention	Increase in tremor as body part approaches a visual target.
	Task-specific	Occurs during a specific task (e.g., writing).
Postural		Seen when maintaining a specific position or posture.
Isometric		Muscle contraction against a rigid or stationary object (e.g., making a fist, squeezing fingers).

More advanced patients may also have loss of action of L-DOPA at times, not just related to end-of-dose **(on-off syndrome)**, which presents as abrupt (freezing). Attempts to improve symptoms by increasing medications seem to overshoot, resulting in involuntary jerking and twisting movements **(dyskinesias)**. Advanced patients move frequently from periods of relative immobility ("off" or akinesia) to normal mobility ("on") to abnormal movements that interfere with voluntary movements ("on" with dyskinesias).

Manual dexterity is invariably impaired as Parkinson worsens, affecting many activities of daily living (ADLs) such as dressing, cutting food, writing, and handling small objects (e.g., coins). This leads to declining efficiency at work and, in many cases, abandoning leisure activities. Social isolation, often caused by changes in physical appearance and impaired function, is common in Parkinson patients. Dementia and depression are common with advanced disease.

Speech impairment in Parkinson patients results in soft, monotonic, virtually mumbled speech. Advanced patients will have **dysphagia** as well and are at risk of silent aspiration. **Drooling** results from a decreased frequency of spontaneous swallowing rather than increased saliva production.

9. How do non-motor symptoms (NMS) impact care for PD patients?
Common side effects of L-DOPA and other PD medications include gastrointestinal upset and dizziness. Virtually all anti-Parkinson drugs can cause confusion, hallucinations, and even psychosis. Cognitively impaired patients and those with psychiatric illness are most at risk. Postural hypotension, in addition to the motor complications, becomes more common with higher doses of levadopa.

NMS includes autonomic dysfunction (bladder incontinence and constipation), pain syndromes, sleep impairment, fatigue, and importantly neuropsychiatric issues including regulation of impulse control, depression, psychosis, and progressive dementia. Also, with increasing age and gait dysfunction, the impact of other comorbidities such as diabetes, cardiac disease, musculoskeletal disorders, and falls/fractures present major challenges for the medical and family care of the PD patient.

10. Which drugs are used to treat PD?
Anti-Parkinson medications work either by replacing dopamine (levodopa), acting as a postsynaptic (dopamine) agonist, or reestablishing the dopamine/acetylcholine balance in the striatum (anticholinergics) (Box 56.2). A guiding principle is to start L-DOPA treatment (still the gold standard after 50+ years) in patients with symptoms that interfere with the performance of ADLs. A resting tremor alone does not usually impede function. L-DOPA emulsion can now be delivered as a more constant supply via pump into the jejunal cavity. In some cases, several of the medications listed in Box 56.2 may be used instead of, or in combination with, levodopa to delay or treat levadopa-related motor fluctuations/dyskinesias.

11. Are there surgical options for treating or controlling PD?
Deep brain stimulation (DBS) is adjunctive therapy to reduce motor fluctuation in advanced PD. DBS improves levodopa-responsive symptoms (tremor, bradykinesia, rigidity) and on–off fluctuations and dyskinesias. Impairments in gait, balance and speech are less likely to improve. DBS targets include the subtahalamic nucleus (STN) or the globus pallidus interna (GPI). Patients with STN stimulation required lower doses of dopaminergic medications. Depression worsened after STN stimulation and improved after GPI. DBS mat have sustained benefit for at

Box 56.2 Drugs Used to Treat Parkinson Disease	
CATEGORY	**EXAMPLES**
Dopaminergic agents	Levodopa/Carbidopa: Extended-release preparations Enteral suspension
Dopamine agonists	Apomorphine/subcutaneous Bromocriptine Pramipexole Ropinirole Rotigotine patch
Catechol-O-methyl transferase (COMT) inhibitors	Entacapone Tolcapone (monitor liver function)
Monamine oxidase B (MAO-B) inhibitors	Rasagiline Selegiline Safinamide
Anticholinergics	Trihexyphenidyl Benztropine
N-methyl-D-aspartate (NMDA) receptor antagonist	Amantadine to reduce dyskinesias

least 10 years. DBS is considered if adequate trials of multiple medications for PD have been unsuccessful. Adverse events include infection (may require device removal and antibiotics) and intracranial hemorrhage (can lead to permanent deficit or death).

Experimental techniques include gene therapy and cell (fetal, stem cell) transplantation.

12. **Which therapeutic exercises are useful for PD patients?**

Maintaining activity is paramount, as physical exertion becomes more difficult with disease progression and the risk of deconditioning increases. Exercises focus on proper body alignment (upright posture) and postural reflexes (response to dynamic balance challenges). Although symptoms caused by the disease itself (rigidity, bradykinesia, and tremor) do not generally respond to specific physiotherapies, secondary manifestations of loss of extremity and axial range of motion (ROM) and deconditioning, which contribute to deficits in gait, balance, and transfers, often improve with physical therapy.

PT and home exercises focus on maintaining hip and upper trunk extension, including pelvic tilt and pectoralis muscle stretching to offset the tendency toward forward trunk flexion and improve postural alignment. A variety of passive and active-assisted stretching exercises for the arm, leg, and trunk, performed either by the therapist or at home, can reduce the loss of joint ROM from rigidity and bradykinesia. Shoulder-girdle exercises with a broomstick handle or a pulley are used to stretch the arms and trunk. Back flexion and extension exercises can be useful in improving balance and posture in sitting and standing. Quadriceps and hip extensor strengthening assist the patient in being able to climb stairs or rise from sitting.

13. **Which exercise strategies can help with gait?**

Frenkel's exercises for coordination of foot placement are helpful to maintain accurate lower-extremity positioning during the gait cycle. Wobble board or balance-feedback trainers can be used to improve body alignment and postural reflexes. The tendency to topple backward can be addressed with heel lifts as well as by assistive mobility devices.

Stationary bicycles, arm ergometers, and treadmills can help restore diminished reciprocal limb motions and increase step length. Proper heel strike should be emphasized as should adequate arm swing and trunk rotation during ambulation. The tendency to freeze in narrow and complicated spaces can be reduced with visual targets, such as the tip of a walking stick or markers on the floor. Some patients prevent freezing by counting rhythmically as they walk or by humming marching music among other visual, auditory, or somatosensory cueing strategies. When frozen, relaxing back on the heels and lifting the toes, as well as raising the arms from the sides with sudden movements, can help restore locomotion. Difficulty in rising from sitting surfaces can be addressed with elevated sitting surfaces (e.g., a chair or toilet) and strategically placed grab rails/bars near a bed and the bathtub. Small mats and rugs that could trip a patient who shuffles should be removed.

The Lee Silverman Voice Training BIG and LOUD programs for PD patients (see also Question 11) is a popular treatment strategy that also addresses motor/gait retraining using increased amplitude limb and body movement with intensive effort. Patients mimic the therapist during intensive, complex, and repetitive core movements that are used in daily living. Alternative exercise programs geared to the PD patient include Tai Chi, dancing, and boxing.

14. **How can the speech therapist assist in PD?**

The hypokinetic dysarthria seen in patients can be addressed with **diaphragmatic breathing exercises** and improved posture and flexibility, which increase vital capacity. Low volume speech may respond to multi-week intensive training with LSVT BIG/LOUD techniques that can improve vocal loudness, intonation, and voice quality. Such strategies also help manage disordered articulation, diminished facial expression and impaired swallowing.

The prevalence and type of swallowing disorder of Parkinson patients varies. They often have trouble with oral bolus formation as well as loss of coordination between oral and pharyngeal stages of swallowing. Tongue and mandibular movement and range are commonly limited. After proper **swallowing assessment,** strategies can include using smaller portions taken more frequently, altering food textures and consistencies to maximize safe oropharyngeal function, optimizing head and neck position during swallow, facilitating oral and pharyngeal movement and reflexes, and performing exercises to increase facial and lingual strength and ROM.

15. **Discuss the use of wheelchairs and walkers for patients with PD.**

The patient may eventually need a wheelchair. An effort should be made to keep the person with PD ambulatory as long as feasible to minimize the development of contracture, stiffness, and deconditioning that follows immobilization. Although wheeled walkers are useful in assisting ambulation—particularly by preventing backward instability—patients with significant postural deficits may prefer more stable devices (such as a shopping cart or walking behind a wheelchair). Some wheeled walkers have been designed specifically for Parkinson patients. They have added weight to lower their center of gravity. Handbrakes are essential in such devices to ensure control, and patients must have the arm-hand dexterity and cognitive ability to use them.

16. **Which occupational therapy (OT) strategies can help those with PD?**

OT can provide vital input for maintaining the home, vocational, leisure, and transportation capabilities of the patient. **Adaptive equipment** is provided when deficits in upper-extremity control limit efficient and safe function. For instance, plate guards or specialized dishes prevent food from sliding off. Plates can be weighted or made more adherent. Cups and utensils can have large handles and may be weighted to dampen excessive motions caused by tremor. Swivel forks and spoons can help compensate for loss of ROM. Smart feeding utensils utilizing position sensors with computerized leveling technology can dampen tremor and compensate for limited extremity ROM. Buttons on clothing can be replaced with Velcro or zipper closures. Stabilizers for handwriting are helpful.

Other **environmental aids** can help keep the person with PD productive at work. Workplace adaptations to accommodate for Parkinson-related impairments and disabilities may include equipment to support writing (built-up pens and forearm supports), typing skills (electronic keyboards and computerized scanning and pointing devices) as well as power mobility devices (scooters or wheelchairs). Many patients can retain driving ability, although slower motor responses as the disease progresses may place these patients at risk when driving. Occupational therapists (or other qualified therapists) can play a critical role in **assessing and retraining of driving skills,** particularly extremity reaction timing and visual field scanning. Families should be counseled to have the patient undergo driver's testing and training earlier, when mobility and ADL performance first begin to decline, rather than later—when accidents are more likely occur.

17. What is the physiology of tics?
Tics are sudden, rapid, recurrent, non-rhythmic motor movement or vocalizations, with a waxing and waning course. They are exacerbated by stress, anxiety, and fatigue and can present with a preceding premonitory sensation (sensory tic: itch, tension in the affected body part) or urge. Tics are classified as clonic (brief), dystonic (sustained), or phonic (vocal); simple (isolated actions such as winking) or complex (speech or coordinated actions). "Blocking tics" manifest as interruptions or slowing of an ongoing motion. Alterations of neurotransmitter systems in the cortical-basal ganglia-thalamo-cortical circuits (CBGTC) are thought to contribute to the expression of tics.[9,10]

18. Can tics be suppressed?
Tics can cause psychosocial difficulties, physical discomfort, and have social consequences. Conscious suppression typically leads to rebound of tics with increased frequency and severity. Behavioral therapy may be effective; however, most require pharmacologic treatment.

Standard and emerging therapies focus on the neurotransmitters in the CBGTC circuits. First-line medications include alpha-adrenergic agonists (clonidine, guanfacine) and anticonvulsants (topiramate). Second-tier medications include atypical antipsychotics (aripiprazole, risperidone, ziprasidone, quetiapine) and typical ones from this group as well (pimozide, fluphenazine, haloperidol). Tetrabenazine is another second-tier medication that is a vesicular monoamine transporter 2 (VMAT2) inhibitor.[11]

19. What is the most socially disabling aspect of Tourette syndrome (TS)?
The primary symptoms of TS are motor and vocal tics. The DSM-V defines TS as a neuropsychiatric disorder with at least one vocal and multiple motor tics, present for over a year with onset beginning before age 18, and not due to another medical condition or substance.

TS is associated with co-morbidities such as attention deficit hyperactivity disorder (ADHD), obsessive-compulsive disorder, anxiety disorder, and depression. ADHD is the most common co-morbidity associated with TS. Coprolalia (involuntary verbal obscenity) and copropaxia (obscene gestures) are the most socially disabling signs. The etiology of TS is unknown; however, those with TS have positive family histories.

20. Are there new treatment options for TS?
Cognitive behavioral interventions for tics can be effective in reducing tic severity by substituting competing behaviors when individuals feel premonitory urges. Education about tics and relaxation techniques are utilized with the hope that the tics, although still present, are reduced to a less socially disabling severity.

Haloperidol, pimozide, and aripiprazole are currently the only FDA approved drugs for TS. However, they have potentially significant side effects such as weight gain, sedation, and muscle stiffness. Other adverse effects of haloperidol and pimozide (both typical antipsychotics) include dystonia, tremor, and cardiac conduction problems.

Despite off-label use, many physicians first use the better tolerated alpha-adrenergic agents such as clonidine and guanfacine. Second line agents include topiramate. Among atypical antipsychotics, aripiprazole, and risperidone have lower risks of extrapyramidal side effects than haloperidol.

Box 56.3 Additional Signs of Dystonia

ADDITIONAL SIGNS OF DYSTONIA	DESCRIPTION
Gestes antagonists (sensory tricks)	Voluntary movements done by the patient to reduce or abolish the dystonic posture or movement (e.g., touching affected body part).
Mirror dystonia	Performing repetitive task at low speed on the contralateral limb (e.g., finger sequence, normal writing) elicits same or similar movement in the more affected limb.
Overflow dystonia	Dystonic movement is accompanied by unintentional contraction in an anatomically distinct neighboring body region.

Painful motor tics in TS can benefit from BoNT injections. There is insufficient evidence for use of cannabinoid-based therapy in TS. Neuromodulation via repetitive transcranial magnetic stimulation and transcranial direct current stimulation are options for TS refractory to standard therapies. Deep brain stimulation is reserved for severe situations that are life-threatening (e.g., whiplash tics causing vertebral artery dissection or myelopathy).[12]

21. **What are the signs of dystonia?**
Dystonia is characterized by sustained or intermittent muscle contractions causing abnormal, often repetitive, movements, postures, or both. Dystonic movements are patterned, twisting, and may be tremulous. Overflow muscle activation is associated with dystonia. Voluntary movement often will initiate or worsen dystonia. Sleep and relaxation lessen or abolish dystonia.
With dystonic posture, continuous muscle contractions force limbs and trunk into sustained postures. The body part is flexed or twisted along its longitudinal axis. Dystonic movements are repetitive, patterned or twisting. These lessen gradually in a preferred posture (often opposite the direction of the dystonic movement). Box 56.3 describes additional physical signs of dystonia.

22. **What are other ways dystonia is classified?**
Dystonia may be classified according to the body region(s) involved, such as focal dystonia (such as neck (torticollis) or arm/hand (writer's cramp) or larger body regions (hemidystonia), or generalized (Box 56.4).[13]

23. **How is dystonia treated?**
Pharmacologic therapies, BoNT injections, and surgical therapies are the main treatment methods for dystonia. Before beginning medical treatment for dystonia, identifiable and treatable causes for dystonia, such as neurometabolic disorders (e.g., dopa-responsive dystonia), heavy metal disorders (e.g., Wilson disease) or acquired disorders (e.g., drug induced—such as neuroleptics; toxins; infections), pseudodystonia (e.g., congenital torticollis) and psychogenic dystonia must be ruled out.
Trihexyphenidyl, an anticholinergic, is a first-line agent. Central side effects (sedation, cognitive slowing, confusion, memory impairment, psychosis, chorea) and autonomic side effects (blurred vision due to mydriasis, dry mouth, urinary retention, constipation) of anticholinergics can limit treatment. Other agents include baclofen, carbamazepine, and benzodiazepines (clonazepam). A mnemonic for the main medications used is "ABCD": **A**nticholinergics, **B**aclofen, **C**lonazepam, and **D**opamine-related medications.
The general treatment strategy is to start at a low dose and titrate up slowly to the lowest effective dose for symptom control without side effects. In children, the rate of upward titration is every 3 to 4 days, while for adults it is every week. If medication is discontinued, a gradual tapering off is recommended to avoid withdrawal symptoms.
BoNT injection is first line treatment in patients with blepharospasm and cervical dystonia. It is also used in focal dystonia such as upper limb dystonia and adductor laryngeal dysphonia. DBS of the internal globus pallidus is the surgical treatment of choice for disabling idiopathic isolated dystonia and inherited generalized dystonia.[13,14]

24. **Can orthotic devices assist in movement disorders?**
Orthotics are traditionally used to improve posture and prevent contractures in dystonia. Orthotics ideally should facilitate functional rehabilitation. Rigid orthoses block or prevent motion of joints involved in residual voluntary or involuntary movements. Soft or semi-rigid braces can aid functional positioning during movement and contain the joint and provide proprioceptive stimulation. Casting or immobilization is thought to deprive dystonic segments of motion and sensation, which could help "reset" the cortical map.[15]

25. **What is proprioceptive rehabilitation?**
Proprioception involves the conscious awareness of body and limbs as well as the unconscious use of proprioceptive signals for postural and tone control. Proprioceptive training is a set of exercises focused on improving these components. Learning based sensorimotor re-education techniques have been used in proprioceptive

Box 56.4 Ways to Classify Dystonias

TYPE	DESCRIPTION
Focal dystonia	Torticollis (neck)
	Blepharospasm (periorbital)
	Oromandibular (mouth or jaw)
	Writer's or occupational cramp (arm or leg)
Segmental dystonia	Cranial
	Brachial
	Crural
Other dystonias	Generalized dystonia (includes dystonia musculorum deformans)
	Multifocal dystonia
	Hemidystonia

rehabilitation in the following situations: electromyography-biofeedback (e.g., in focal dystonia such as writer's cramp), external feedback techniques using visual and auditory cues, muscle vibration (e.g., focal vibration for musician's dystonia, torticollis, and whole-body vibration for PD).

Alternative rehabilitation strategies include Braille reading and discriminative exercises. These are done alone or with selective splinting of dystonic muscles. This has been used in focal hand dystonias; however, the beneficial effect was short lived. Kinesio-taping can reduce pain and modulate sensory function in focal cervical and hand dystonias.

26. **What are other innovations for the proprioceptive rehab of movement disorders?**
Recently developed technologies such as virtual reality systems, gaming consoles, and robotic rehabilitation have been used in stroke rehabilitation and to improve balance, postural control, and arm reach in PD.

Motor imagery (MI) is a complex mental process that generates internal feedback, utilizing mental representation (to feel or see) actions in the absence of overt movement. Action observation therapy (AOT) involves observing different actions combined with repetition of the observed actions. MI and AOT are thought to enhance learning and improve performance of impaired tasks.[16]

27. **Which movement disorder is associated with chronic neuroleptic therapy?**
Tardive dyskinesia (TD) is a condition characterized by involuntary movements of the face, torso, extremities, and at times the respiratory system. TD develops after a minimum of 3 months of neuroleptic treatment in a patient with no other identifiable cause for movement disorders. It may appear as quickly as 1 month in those 60 years or older.

Common movements include tongue protrusion, puckering, chewing, smacking, and grimacing. Choreiform movements of the trunk and extremities can also occur, along with dystonic movements of the neck and trunk. The average prevalence of TD is 20% in patients treated with antipsychotics (dopamine receptor blocking agents [DRBA]). Incidence is higher in first generation (FGA) compared to second generation (SGA) antipsychotics.

TD can be severe and persistent with medical and psychosocial consequences. TD has been associated with poor quality of life and increased mortality. Some risk factors include older age, female sex, pre-existing mood disorder, alcohol/substance abuse, higher doses/longer use of antipsychotic medications, treatment with first generation neuroleptics, use of lithium or antiparkinsonian agents, diabetes, and HIV positivity.

All patients taking antipsychotic medications should be regularly monitored for movement disorders (every 6 months for FGAs and annually for SGAs). Evaluation should include assessment with the *Abnormal Involuntary Movement Scale* (AIMS) tool. Mentoring should continue even after discontinuing neuroleptic medication.[17]

28. **Compare athetosis, chorea, and ballismus (Box 56.5).**

Box 56.5 Comparison

DISEASE	FEATURES
Athetosis	Slow, writhing, repetitious movements. Can lead to bizarre postures. Usually affects face and upper extremities. Often secondary to other neurologic disorders (e.g., stroke, tumor).
Chorea	Nonstereotyped, unpredictable, and jerky movements. Usually involves oral structures, but can occur anywhere. Associated with any central neurologic disease, especially Huntington disease.
Ballismus	Extremely violent flinging of unilateral arm and leg. Usually secondary to bleed or infarct in subthalamic nuclei; less often from abscess or tumor.

REFERENCES

1. Beitz J. Parkinson's disease: a review. *Front Biosci (Schol Ed)*. 2014;6:65–74.
2. Borrione P, Tranchita E, Sansone P, Parisi A. Effects of physical activity in Parkinson's Disease: a new tool for rehabilitation. *World J Methodol*. 2014;4(3):133–143.
3. Oertel W. Recent advances in treating Parkinson's disease. *F1000Res*. 2017;6:260:1–14.
4. Poewe W, Seppi K, Tanner C, et al. Parkinson disease. *Nat Rev Dis Primers*. 2017;23(3):17013.
5. Reich S, Savitt, J. Parkinson's disease: *Med Clin North Am*. 2019;103(2):337–350.
6. Rizek P, Jumar N, Jog M. An update on the diagnosis and treatment of Parkinson disease. *CMAJ*. 2016;188(16):1157–1165.
7. Bhatia KP, Bain P, Bajaj N. Consensus statement on the classification of tremors from the task force on tremor of the International Parkinson and Movement Disorder Society. *Mov Disord*. 2018;33(1):75–87.
8. Miskin C, Carvalho KS. Tremors: essential tremor and beyond. *Semin Pediatr Neurol*. 2018;25:34–41.
9. Augustine F, Singer HS. Merging the pathophysiology and pharmacotherapy of tics. *Tremor Other Hyperkinet Mov*. 2019;8:595.
10. Haq IU, Siddiqui MS, Tate J, Okun MS. *Clinical overview of movement disorders*. In: Winn HR, ed. *Youmans Neurological Surgery*. 7th ed. New York, NY: Elsevier; 2017:573–585.
11. Chadehumbe MA, Brown LW. Advances in the treatment of Tourette's disorder. *Curr Pyschiatry Rep*. 2019;21(5):31.
12. Albanese A, Di Giovanni M, Lalli S. Dystonia: diagnosis and management. *Eur J Neurol*. 2019;26:5–17.
13. Termsarasab P, Thammongkolchai T, Frucht SJ. Medical treatment of dystonia. *J Clin Mov Disord*. 2016;3:19.
14. Garavaglia L, Pagliano E, Baranello G, et al. Why orthotic devices could be of help in the management of movement disorders in the young. *J Neuroeng Rehabil*. 2018;15:118.
15. Abbruzzese G, Trompetto C, Mori L, et al. Proprioceptive rehabilitation of upper limb dysfunction in movement disorders: a clinical perspective. *Front Hum Neurosci*. 2014;8:961.
16. Citrome L. Clinical management of tardive dyskinesia: five steps to success. *J Neurol Sci*. 2017;383:199–204.
17. Correll C, Citrome, L. Epidemiology, prevention and assessment of tardive dyskinesia and advances in treatment. *J Clin Psychiatry*. 2017;78(8):1136–1147.

WEBSITES

NIH U.S. National Library of Medicine/Genetics home reference; Parkinson Disease: Available at: ghr.nlm.nih.gov
Parkinson's Foundation: Parkinson.org
International Parkinson and Movement Disorder Society: Available at https://www.movementdisorders.org/MDS

CHAPTER 57

CEREBROVASCULAR DISEASE

Richard L. Harvey, MD, Preeti Raghavan, MD, Joel Stein, MD, and Richard D. Zorowitz, MD

The secret of your success is found in your daily routine.

— John Maxwell

KEY POINTS

1. Clinical examination of the stroke survivor should correlate with the neuroanatomy observed on imaging (especially MRI). If not, consider diagnoses other than stroke as part of the differential diagnosis.
2. Stroke rehabilitation incorporates both strategies for neurorecovery and compensation for residual impairments.
3. Task-specific training focusing on learning or relearning a motor skill is appropriate for stroke patients with mild to moderate impairment and includes repeated practice, maintaining challenge in practice and selection of goal-oriented activities.
4. Novel technologies, such as robotics and functional electrical stimulation, are emerging as new therapies for stroke rehabilitation.
5. Motor deficits associated with dysphagia after stroke include poor oral bolus control, reduced base of tongue retraction, delayed trigger of pharyngeal swallow, reduced laryngeal elevation, delayed or absent cough reflex, and poor opening of upper esophageal sphincter.

1. What is the epidemiology of stroke?

Approximately 795,000 new strokes occur each year in the United States, with 610,000 being a first stroke and 185,000 a recurrent stroke. Approximately 10% of all strokes occur among individuals age 18 to 50. Just over 140,000 die each year within 1 month after stroke onset, making stroke the fifth leading cause of death in the United States [1]. Stroke deaths have declined over the last two decades due to advances in acute stroke care and expansion of comprehensive stroke centers (CMC). The annual cost of stroke in the US is $ 45.5 billion.

Approximately 7 million Americans are alive today who have survived a stroke. Stroke is the second most frequent cause of disability (arthritis being first), the leading cause of serious long-term disability, and the most common diagnosis among patients on most rehabilitation units. Men have a higher incidence of stroke than do women up until age 80, when the incidence reverses. The lifetime risk of stroke is higher in women than in men. The annual incidence of stroke among blacks and Hispanics is higher than among whites. The global annual incidence of stroke is 16.9 million with an overall prevalence of 80.1 million stroke survivors.

The categories of stroke diagnosed each year are given in Fig. 57.1.

2. What are the risk factors for stroke?

Non-modifiable risk factors for stroke include age, gender, race/ethnicity, and hereditary factors. Adults over the age of 65 make up 65% of individuals hospitalized with a stroke. However, there has been a rising incidence of stroke in individuals younger than 55 years. Although men have a greater incidence of stroke than women, women have a greater lifetime risk of stroke because they have a longer life expectancy. African-Americans and Hispanics show 2.4-fold and 2-fold higher rates of first stroke compared to whites. Genetic screening may allow early identification of genetic determinants for stroke (e.g., homocystinuria, coagulation disorders, sickle cell disease), which could be modified through lifestyle interventions, but this is not yet part of routine clinical practice.

Modifiable risk factors include hypertension, cardiac diseases, diabetes, dyslipidemia, cigarette use, alcohol abuse, physical inactivity, diet, sleep disorders, asymptomatic carotid stenosis, and previous transient ischemic attacks (TIAs). Modifiable risk factors for cardiac disease and stroke and their management recommendations are summarized in Table 57.1.

3. Why is rapid identification and treatment of stroke vital?

The FDA approved an intravenous recombinant tissue plasminogen activator (TPA) in 1996 for treating acute ischemic stroke. Randomized clinical trials of TPA have shown that the effectiveness of TPA declines over time, and the risk of hemorrhage outweighs the benefits just 4.5 hours after onset of initial symptoms. Thus, early administration of TPA within the 4.5-hour window gives better outcomes at 3 months post-stroke (Fig. 57.2) [8].

In 2015, five clinical trials were completed that supported the efficacy of endovascular therapy using stent retrieval devices for patients with acute stroke from large vessel occlusion. Standard of care for acute stroke therefore includes using both TPA and endovascular stent retrieval for patients who meet clinical criteria for these therapies. Notably, patients with anterior circulation large vessel occlusion may be eligible for endovascular therapy beyond 6 hours, and up to 24 hours, with an associated mismatch between the core infarct and

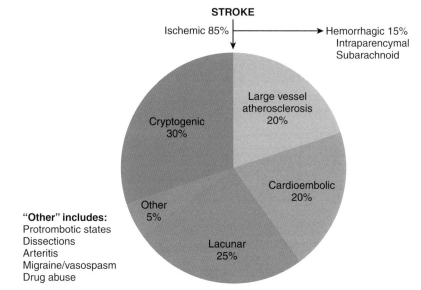

STROKE

Ischemic 85% ──────► Hemorrhagic 15%
Intraparencymal
Subarachnoid

Large vessel
atherosclerosis
20%

Cryptogenic
30%

Cardioembolic
20%

Other
5%

Lacunar
25%

"Other" includes:
Protrombotic states
Dissections
Arteritis
Migraine/vasospasm
Drug abuse

Fig. 57.1 Prevalence of ischemic and hemorrhagic strokes, and their etiologies. (Adapted from Albers G, Amarenco P, Easton JD, et al. Antithrombotic and thrombolytic therapy for ischemic stroke: The Seventh ACCP Conference on Antithrombotic and Thrombolytic Therapy. Chest. 2004;126[3 suppl]:438S-512S.)

Table 57.1 Modifiable Risk Factors for Stroke

RISK FACTOR	ESTIMATED PREVALENCE (%)	ESTIMATED RELATIVE RISK	MANAGEMENT RECOMMENDATIONS
Hypertension	29	2.0–5.0	Regular BP screening, weight control, limit salt intake, antihypertensive drug treatment, BP self-monitoring
Diabetes	9.4	1.5–3.2	Tight glucose control through diet, oral hypoglycemics, and insulin. Strict regulation of BP if hypertensive. Statin treatment, especially in those with additional risk factors
Dyslipidemia Elevated LDL (≥130 mg/dL)	30.3	1.2–1.4	Lifestyle modification, treatment with statins in patients estimated to have a high 10-year risk for cardiovascular events
Low HDL (<40 mg/dL)	18.7	1.0–2.2	
Smoking	15.8	1.5–2.5	Smoking cessation
Physical	21.6	2.0–3.5	Moderate- to vigorous-intensity aerobic physical activity at least 40 min/day, 3–4 days/week
Excess Alcohol (binge drinking in past 30 days)	16.9	1.0–2.2	Up to two drinks per day for men and one drink per day for nonpregnant women
Obesity	39.6	1.3–2.0	Control of weight through diet and exercise
Sleep Disorders (Obstructive Sleep Apnea)	4	1.5–3.2	Screening for sleep apnea and possible treatment using continuous positive airway pressure (CPAP)

BP, Blood pressure; *CHD*, coronary heart disease; *HDL*, High-density lipoprotein; *LDL*; low-density lipoprotein

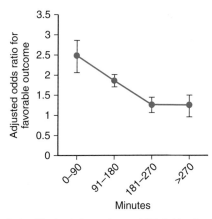

Fig. 57.2 Odds of favorable outcome by time following stroke symptom onset. (Adapted from Lees KR, Bluhmki E, von Kummer, et al. Time to treatment with intravenous alteplase and outcome in stroke: an updated pooled analysis of ECASS, ATLANTIS, NINDS, and EPI- THET trials. *Lancet.* 2010;375:1695–1703.)

cerebral perfusion deficit determined by cranial imaging (CT perfusion and MR diffusion imaging) assuming other criteria for the procedure are met. Endovascular therapy, like TPA, is time dependent. Better outcomes are associated with earlier treatment [13]. (see Fig. 57.3).

The growing complexity of stroke care over the last three decades necessitates the availability of community-based acute stroke systems of care. Acute care hospitals that are prepared to care for stroke are designated primary stroke centers (PMC) or CMC. PMCs can rapidly diagnose stroke and administer TPA. CMCs can administer TPA but also have neurosurgical services, angiography, and interventional care available 24 hours/day. Stroke systems of care now include spokes (PMC) and hubs (CMC) which, ideally, work in tandem with each other often by using telemedicine technology. Some communities have added mobile stroke units containing CT imaging, which can further improve rapid diagnosis. Regardless of the resources available, each community should have an acceptable system of care to optimize the timely management of patients with acute stroke [12].

4. What are common impairments following stroke?
   These are listed in Table 57.2.

5. What are common cognitive and communicative problems after a stroke?
   Stroke can affect any aspect of cognition, and therefore it is impossible to provide a complete list of cognitive functions that may be affected by stroke. A list of some of the main common cognitive consequences of stroke follows, with brief descriptions. Some of these conditions may overlap or have more than one anatomic substrate that can result in similar phenotypes.
   Right hemisphere syndromes
   - *Hemispatial neglect*—Reduced awareness of objects, people, and actions in the neglected left side of the patient's space;
   - *Aprosody*—Loss of normal rhythm of speech;

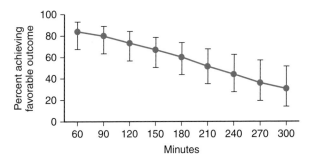

Fig. 57.3 Rate of favorable outcome by time of arrival in ED to cerebral reperfusion with endovascular therapy. (Adapted from Saver JL, Goyal M, van der Lugt A, et al. Time to treatment with endovascular thrombectomy and outcomes from ischemic stroke: a meta-analysis. *JAMA.* 2019;316:1279–1288.)

Table 57.2 Common Neurologic Impairments Following Stroke and Their Frequencies

IMPAIRMENT	ACUTE (%)	CHRONIC (%)
Motor Weakness	90	50
Right Hemiplegia	45	20
Left Hemiplegia	35	25
Bilateral Hemiplegia	10	5
Ataxia	20	10
Hemianopsia	25	10
Visual Perceptual Deficits	30	30
Aphasia	35	20
Dysarthria	50	20
Sensory Deficits	50	25
Cognitive Deficits	35	30
Depression	30	30
Bladder Incontinence	30	10
Dysphagia	30	10

- *Flattened affect*—Loss of normal range of emotional expression;
- *Anosognosias*—Lack of awareness of impairments. May also include loss of recognition of the patient's own body parts on the affected side;
- *Delusions*—Fixed beliefs that are not consistent with reality and not shared by a group.

Left hemisphere syndromes
- *Aphasia*—Loss of the ability to understand or generate language;
- *Apraxia*—Difficulty performing skilled motor activities, such as using a tool;
- *Hemispatial neglect* (less common and more transient than with right hemisphere damage).

Executive Functions
- *Attention deficits*—Difficulty in selecting and maintaining attention;
- *Apathy*—Loss of interest in usual activities and interactions;
- *Abulia*—Severe loss of initiative. In most severe state, can result in akinetic mutism;
- *Disinhibition*—Loss of normal internal checks on appropriateness of behavior.
- *Impulsivity*—Loss of delay in considering actions or acting without considering the consequences.

Visual Functions
- *Prosopagnosia*—Inability to recognize faces;
- *Cortical blindness*—Blindness, often without awareness of inability to see (Anton's syndrome);
- *Visual hallucinations* (rare and usually noted in a fixed location in peripheral vision).

Delirium—A fluctuating global disturbance of cognition affecting multiple domains. Most common early post-stroke.
Memory loss (most typically of short-term memory and new memories).
Behavioral disturbances (e.g., anxiety, depression).

6. What is the typical pattern of motor recovery with stroke-related hemiplegia?
Patients with severe post-stroke hemiplegia initially present with limb flaccidity, defined as less than normal muscle tone. Later, hyperreflexia appears first in the upper limb, then in the lower limb, in a distal-to-proximal direction. Subsequently, hypertonia (or *spasticity*) develops first in muscles crossing the wrist, fingers, and ankle, and later develops in muscles crossing the shoulder, elbow, and hip.

Patients who have voluntary movement of the limbs appearing early post-stroke are less likely to have severe and disabling spasticity. Voluntary movements usually appear first in muscles crossing the hip and shoulder, and later in muscles crossing the hand and foot. As voluntary movements gain strength, *synergy* patterns of movement may develop, which are voluntary mass contractions of a group of muscles producing a stereotypical pattern of limb movement (i.e., joint torques are coupled).

The flexor synergy pattern typically develops first in the upper extremities, and the extensor synergy pattern develops first in the lower extremities (Table 57.3). As recovery continues, movements outside of these synergy patterns, then isolated joint movements are possible. However, motor recovery may stop at any point during this process, and there is considerable variation among stroke survivors.

Table 57.3 Limb Synergy Patterns (dominant patterns in bold)

LIMB	JOINT	FLEXOR SYNERGY	EXTENSOR SYNERGY
UPPER	Shoulder	**Retraction** **Elevation** **Abduction** **External Rotation**	Protraction Adduction Internal Rotation
	Elbow	Flexion	Extension
	Forearm	Supination	Pronation
	Wrist	Flexion	Extension
	Fingers	Flexion	Extension/Flexion
Lower	Hip	Flexion Abduction	Extension Adduction
	Knee	Flexion	Extension
	Ankle	Dorsiflexion	Plantar Flexion Inversion

7. How does neuroplasticity contribute to recovery?

Recovery after stroke reflects the extent to which the body's structures and functions, as well as its activities, have returned to their pre-stroke state. The term "recovery" can be represented in two ways: (1) the change (mostly improvement) of a given outcome that is achieved by an individual between two (or more) time points, or (2) the mechanism underlying this improvement in terms of behavioral restoration or compensation strategies.

Neuroplasticity is the ability of the brain to form and reorganize synaptic connections, especially in response to learning or experience or following injury, all of which have a causal role in recovery of function after stroke. The biological processes underlying neuroplasticity include axonal sprouting, neurogenesis, gliogenesis, and changes in neuronal excitability in peri-infarct tissue [3]. Clinicians alter behavioral activity after stroke by neurorehabilitation, which in turn alters biological processes in specific brain regions. Neurological recovery occurs as an emergent property of the changes in biological processes underlying neuroplasticity and neural repair. The relationships between elemental biological principles and recovery are shown in Fig. 57.4 [7].

8. What is the role of repetitive task practice in motor recovery of the upper limbs following stroke?

Repetitive task practice or task-specific training is focused on learning or relearning a motor skill to improve performance of that action. The key elements of task-specific training are a repeated, challenging practice of functional, goal-oriented activities. Task-specific practice is an aspect of many upper extremity interventions, including constraint-induced movement therapy (CIMT) and neuromuscular electrical stimulation (NMES). Physical rehabilitation interventions have been shown to have a beneficial effect on functional recovery, motor function, balance, and gait velocity after stroke when compared with no treatment or usual care, and their effects persist beyond the intervention period. However, no single physical rehabilitation approach has been found to be more (or less) effective than another [15].

A recent meta-analysis of studies on upper limb function conducted in the first four weeks following stroke concluded that evidence supports using modified CIMT and task-specific training, as well as supplemental use of electromyography (EMG)-assisted biofeedback and electrical simulation during the acute phase post-stroke, but not therapy based on the Bobath approach. Upper limb function can be improved by high-dose and task-specific repetitive use of the arm in individuals with mild-to-moderate weakness. However, this is difficult to achieve in individuals with severe weakness, and new methods of training for this population are needed.

A Cochrane review found that people who practiced functional tasks exhibited small improvements in arm and hand function, walking distance and measures of walking ability that were maintained up to six months, compared with usual care (standard physiotherapy) or placebo groups. However, the quality of the evidence was low for arm function, hand function, and lower limb functional measures, and moderate for walking distance and functional ambulation. The quality of the evidence for each outcome was limited due to poor reporting of study details, inconsistent results across studies, and small numbers of study participants in some comparisons. Therefore, these are areas for further research [7].

9. How does stroke affect gait?

Distance and temporal factors

Hemiplegic stroke survivors require 50% to 67% more metabolic energy expenditure than do healthy people at the same walking velocity. To lower energy expenditure, people with hemiplegia typically ambulate with reduced velocity. In addition to reduced walking speed, hemiplegic gait is characterized by reduced stride and step length, increased step length on the affected lower limb, a moderately wider base of support, and a slightly greater toe-out angle relative to normal gait.

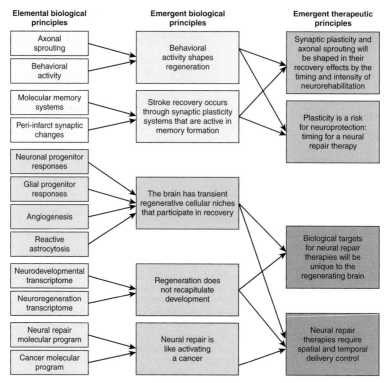

Fig. 57.4 The relationship between elemental biological principles and neurological recovery. (Zorowitz RD, Adamovich BB. Assessment of communication. In: Grabois M, Garrison SJ, Hart KA, Lehmkuhl LD, eds. *Physical Medicine and Rehabilitation: The Complete Approach.* Malden, MA: Blackwell Science, Inc.; 2000:270.)

Temporal aspects of hemiplegic gait are also characterized by increased stride times and reduced cadence. When compared to normal, stance phase times are increased on both lower limbs due to lower walking velocity. The affected lower limb spends less time in stance phase and more time in swing phase, while the unaffected lower limb spends more time in stance phase and reduced time in swing phase. Increased double support time has been observed. The time of single limb support of the affected limb may be less than or equal to the time of that in normal gait, but the time of single limb support of the unaffected limb may be greater than or equal to that of those without stroke.

Joint kinematics

The joint kinematics of the affected limb in the stance and swing phases of gait are different than those of the unaffected limb, but also exhibit significant variability among individuals. During stance phase, hip flexion may be more or less than normal at initial contact. Hip extension at late stance and push-off may be less than normal, and hip flexion may be increased at toe-off. Three types of knee patterns during stance may be present during stance phase:

• Increased knee flexion, particularly at initial contact;
• Reduced flexion during early stance, hyperextension in late stance, and decreased knee flexion at toe-off;
• Increased hyperextension throughout most of stance.

Ankle movements also may vary during stance. At initial contact, the foot may be flat, the ankle may be plantar-flexed, causing initial toe contact, or toe elevation may be moderately decreased. After initial contact, the ankle may move into dorsiflexion, reduced dorsiflexion in mid-stance and push-off, and/or increased plantar flexion during stance. At toe-off, ankle plantar flexion may be reduced.

Swing phase of the affected limb usually is characterized by limited or reduced hip flexion and an upward tilt of the affected hip, lack of or reduced knee flexion, and reduced dorsiflexion or continuous ankle plantar flexion. Increased relative leg length produced by limited hip and knee flexion and reduced ankle dorsiflexion results in reduced floor clearance by the foot during swing, which produces dragging of the toes or vaulting of the unaffected limb. Less commonly, circumduction of the affected limb may be seen.

Other parts of the body are also affected by hemiplegia. Movement of the affected arm may be decreased, with the shoulder relatively fixed in extension and the elbow flexed. Forward flexion of the trunk during stance, which moves the center of gravity anteriorly, can accommodate for hyperextension of the knee. The trunk may shift

weight laterally over the unaffected limb during swing of the affected leg. Three different patterns of truncal and pelvic coordination may occur depending on the velocity of gait:
- Excessive pelvic rotation;
- A lack of normal timing in trunk rotation;
- Difficulty with relative pelvic and truncal rotation.

Muscle activity

The magnitudes and phasic patterns of muscles in affected and unaffected limbs of stroke survivors differ significantly from those without stroke but may still vary considerably among individuals [5]. It has been suggested that the muscles of the lower limbs tend to align into flexor (iliacus, sartorius, tibialis anterior, tensor fascia latae, rectus femoris, and extensor digitorum longus) and extensor (gluteus medius, gluteus maximus, vastus lateralis, tibialis posterior, long head of the biceps, vastus intermedius, medial hamstrings, and soleus) locomotor patterns. One study classified EMG patterns into six categories based on flexor and extensor muscle activity:

1. No activity in the tibialis anterior during stance or swing; continuous activity in the triceps surae;
2. Activity in the tibialis anterior during swing; low activity in the triceps surae during stance and early swing; both muscle groups active during stance and mid-swing;
3. Activity in both the triceps surae and tibialis anterior during stance and the middle of swing, although the magnitude of the triceps surae was less during swing than in stance;
4. Tibialis anterior activity during swing and the first and third parts of stance; activity of the triceps surae during stance phase and terminal swing;
5. Activity in both the triceps surae and tibialis anterior during stance with some reciprocal activity; tibialis anterior active during initial swing;
6. Relatively normal pattern of triceps surae activity in mid-stance; relatively normal pattern of tibialis anterior activity at initial and terminal swing.

10. What therapies can improve walking?

Therapies to improve walking are divided into two major categories: recovery and compensatory approaches. Compensatory approaches seek to improve function without directly improving the underlying motor abilities of the patient; recovery approaches seek to reduce the neurological impairments that underlie the stroke survivor's ability to walk.

Compensatory strategies include long-established walking aids, such as canes, and orthotics. Stroke survivors with sufficiently severe hemiparesis commonly use a straight cane or a four-pronged cane. Occasionally, a hemi-walker may be needed, especially early post-stroke. For stroke survivors with adequate motor strength but impaired balance, walkers or rollators are often useful. Ankle dorsiflexion weakness, which causes foot drop or tonic plantarflexion during stepping, can be managed with an ankle foot orthosis (AFO). The use of functional electrical stimulation (FES) devices is a suitable alternative to AFOs for some patients. Limitations of FES systems include expense, managing batteries, discomfort or skin irritation at the site of electrical stimulation, and unsuitability for patients with substantial spasticity or medial-lateral instability. Research has not demonstrated any benefit of these systems in facilitating recovery of dorsiflexion strength.

Proposed therapies to improve gait include partial body weight-supported treadmill training (BWSTT, also known as locomotor training). Despite encouraging preliminary studies, a large randomized controlled trial failed to demonstrate any benefit of this therapy over more conventional gait and balance training [6]. Robot-assisted gait training has been examined in small studies, without convincing evidence of superiority over traditional approaches. Split-belt treadmill training shows promise in normalizing some parameters of hemiparetic gait, but is not widely available, and definitive clinical trials are lacking. Lastly, very early mobilization after stroke was not found to improve gait outcomes. In fact, one study appears to show that this intervention negatively impacted overall outcomes [2].

11. What is the role of NMES in stroke rehabilitation (i.e., motor training and orthotics)?

NMES involves applying an electrical current via skin surface electrodes to muscles or to nerves supplying the muscle at levels that cause muscle contraction. NMES may be used as an orthotic to compensate for or replace voluntary motion (FES), and/or therapeutically for muscle strengthening and recovery from paralysis as part of stroke rehabilitation (therapeutic electric stimulation, TES) [10].

The WalkAide system (Innovative Neurotronics, Austin, TX) and NESS L300 (Bioness, Valencia, CA) are examples of commercial FES devices for foot drop after stroke. In these devices, surface electrodes for stimulation attach to the leg below the knee by a cuff. Electrical stimulation is given during the swing phase of gait to produce ankle dorsiflexion for foot clearance. Heel contact is detected by a tilt sensor placed with the knee cuff (WalkAide) or by a pressure sensor placed under the insole of a shoe to determine stimulation periods (WalkAide and NESS L300). Reciprocal NMES, which stimulates dorsiflexors and plantarflexors according to the timing of gait, can improve walking ability of patients with stroke. The NESS H200 from Bioness is a widely used commercially available FES device for the upper limb and hand. It has five electrodes to stimulate muscles of the forearm and hand (the extensor digitorum, extensor pollicis brevis, flexor digitorum superficialis, flexor pollicis longus, and thenar muscles) to implement key grip and palmar grasp.

Subthreshold or weak current NMES, which is below the sensory or motor threshold, has been proposed as a supplemental therapy to facilitate sensory and motor function in patients with stroke. This is based on reports that somatosensory input enhances corticomotor excitability to the stimulated body parts. In this approach, NMES is applied in combination with rehabilitation training with the advantages of safety, minimal pain, and usability in various settings. However, it is more common to use NMES to encourage muscle contraction for an intended motion (e.g., to the wrist and finger extensors to enhance voluntary hand opening. EMG-triggered NMES uses intention from the EMG signal to activate electrical stimulation to complete the movement. EMG-triggered NMES alone or in combination with robot-aided rehabilitation has demonstrated improved motor function in patients with stroke. EMG-modulated NMES devices have also been developed to control not only the timing, but intensity of electrical stimulation in direct proportion to the amount of voluntary EMG activity. Contralaterally-controlled FES is being developed to sense the EMD activity from the uninvolved hand to stimulate the muscles of the involved hand for hand opening. Brain computer interface (BCI) systems are also being developed to trigger NMES (EEG-triggered NMES) for upper and lower limb training.

12. **How does stroke affect communication?**

Communication impairments after stroke are generally classified into four types:

- *Aphasia*: Loss of the ability to use language, disproportionate to the impairment of other intellectual functions, manifested by reduced available vocabulary, auditory comprehension, and reading and writing abilities.
- *Apraxia*: An articulatory disorder resulting from impairment due to brain damage of the capacity to program the positioning of speech muscles and the sequencing of muscle movements for volitional production of phonemes.
- *Dysarthria*: A speech disorder resulting from disturbances in muscular control (e.g., weakness, slowness, or incoordination) of the speech mechanism due to damage to the central or peripheral nervous system. The term encompasses coexisting neurogenic disorders of several or all basic processes of speech: respiration, phonation, resonance, articulation, and prosody.
- *Cognitive-Communication Impairment*: A deficit of language, pragmatic, and behavioral function secondary to damage of underlying cognitive processes.

Evaluation of communication begins by conversing with the patient and may be classified as impaired content *(language disorder)* or impaired acoustic features *(motor speech disorder)* (see Fig. 57.4). A patient may exhibit one or a combination of these impairments.

Aphasia results in a multimodal loss that involves all aspects of fluency, comprehension, and repetition, each to a varying degree (Fig. 57.5). Aphasias are classified by the rate of speech: "fluent" normal to rapid *(fluent aphasia)*, or "absent or slow" with labored production *(non-fluent aphasia)*. Evaluation of aphasia should include verbal and written skills as each may be involved differently. Apraxias of speech may involve nonverbal oral postures *(oral apraxia)* such as sticking out the tongue or protruding or puckering the lips, or production of speech *(verbal apraxia)* that is characterized by effortful trial and error, groping articulatory movements, and self-correction. Apraxias not related to speech include an inability to make a proper movement in response to a verbal command *(ideomotor apraxia)*, an inability to coordinate activities with multiple, sequential movements, such as dressing, eating, and bathing *(ideational apraxia)*, and difficulty moving the eyes on command *(oculomotor apraxia)*. An inability to copy, draw, or construct simple figures *(constructional apraxia)* may occur with right brain damage, and likely reflects a visual-spatial deficit rather than a true apraxia.

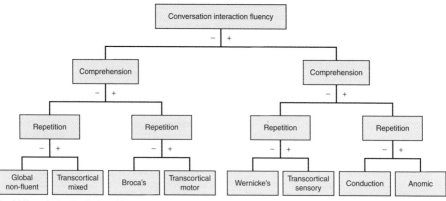

Key: (+) Normal or less involved modality
(–) More involved modality

Fig. 57.5 Bedside Determination of Communication Impairment. (Adapted from Morganstein S. Bedside Examination of Communication Impairment, a Decision Tree; 1990 [unpublished].)

Dysarthrias are classified by pitch characteristics, loudness, vocal quality, respiration, prosody, and articulation. The most common types are lower motor neuron with marked hypernansality *(flaccid),* upper motor neuron with a strained/strangled quality *(spastic),* and cerebellar with excess and equal stress *(cerebellar).*

Cognitive-communication impairment typically occurs with right hemispheric dysfunction (Table 57.4). In addition to the typical problems with memory and attention, stroke survivors may not recognize affective cues, thus appearing rude or indifferent; have difficulties with topic maintenance or taking turns in conversation; or have problems with interpreting humor or abstract concepts, thus appearing apathetic or depressed.

13. Describe right hemisphere dysfunction after stroke.

The right hemisphere is specialized for spatial cognition, self-awareness, and emotional cognitive processing. Right hemisphere dysfunction after stroke leads to spatial neglect of the left hemispace, anosognosia (unawareness of hemiparesis), and emotional processing disorders. It is also associated with longer length of stay in rehabilitation and worse functional outcomes.

Neglect of the left hemispace includes all sensory modalities, including vision, hearing, and tactile sensation as well as motor orientation to the left side. Spatial neglect includes unawareness of left-sided stimuli and extinction to double simultaneous stimulation. Three approaches for treatment that show strong evidence and feasibility are prism adaptation, limb activation, and visual scanning training.

Anosognosia is defined as an unawareness of, denial, or failure to acknowledge motor deficits. The unawareness is not psychological and does not protect the individual from the emotional impact of having had a stroke. In fact, it may increase disability by impairing one's ability to manage the physical limitations. Protocols to treat anosognosia include self-awareness training and spatial neglect intervention, such as vestibular stimulation and self-observation via video feedback.

Table 57.4 Characteristics of Cognitive-Communication Impairment

TYPE	SYMPTOMS OF IMPAIRMENT
Linguistic-Pragmatic	Impaired initiation of conversation Impaired narrative coherence Increased embellishments, irrelevancies Impaired topic maintenance Impaired turn-taking Impaired processing Impaired language organization Impaired expression or comprehension of abstract concepts Impaired prosody Impaired recall, comprehension, or repetition of prosodic or affective material Impaired appreciation of humor
Nonverbal	Altered affect Emotional lability Impaired eye contact Impaired gestures Indifference Denial Motor impersistence
Visual-Perceptual	Hemi-inattention or neglect Impaired perception of objects, faces Altered spatial relationships
Cognitive	Impaired orientation Impaired problem-solving Impaired visual-verbal memory Impaired verbal integration Impaired mathematical computation Impaired attention, concentration Impaired reasoning and judgment Impaired insight

Adapted from Morganstein S, Smith MC. Aphasia and right-hemisphere disorders. In: Gordon WA, ed. *Advances in Stroke Rehabilitation.* Boston, MA: Andover Medical;1993.

Behavioral studies have demonstrated right brain dominance for emotional facial recognition, recall of emotional faces, recognition of emotional prosody in voices, and production of emotional facial expressions. Individuals with right-brain damage have difficulty using stored emotional representations across perceptual domains. Education and explanation of the changes in behavior of an individual is the current standard of care for emotional processing deficits. Facial Affect Recognition (FARS) training, which focuses attention on facial feature configurations, has been shown to improve emotional perception of facial expressions.

14. What are some emerging therapies for stroke recovery?

Recovery from stroke is typically incomplete and often unsatisfactory to stroke survivors despite the best efforts of rehabilitation clinicians. Accordingly, researchers continue to search for new techniques to enhance the ability of the human brain to recover from stroke. Exercise and task-practice remain the mainstays of rehabilitation and perhaps new treatments can be found to enhance the benefits of these approaches.

Non-invasive brain stimulation by transcranial direct current stimulation or transcranial magnetic stimulation (TMS) remains an active area of research. The initial results of a recent clinical trial of repetitive TMS for stroke recovery failed to demonstrate benefit over sham treatment, but other stimulation parameters and strategies have shown preliminary evidence of benefit, and more clinical trials are underway [9]. At present, these are not yet accepted clinical therapies for stroke recovery.

Medications to enhance recovery have been an ongoing area of study, with repeated failures in larger clinical trials of putative therapies. Preliminary studies of dextroamphetamine as a stroke recovery medication were not replicated in larger studies, and this is not a recommended treatment. Similarly, smaller studies of fluoxetine have recently been followed by larger randomized controlled trials of this and other SSRIs, without evidence of benefit [4, 11]. Some evidence of accelerated recovery in patients with brain injury treated with amantadine has been found. However, its use as a therapy in stroke survivors has not been adequately studied at this point.

Stem cell therapies hold the promise of replacing lost cells in the brain, but this remains a distant goal for many reasons, not the least of which are the complexity of brain structure and the absence of any techniques to guide replacement cells to form the proper connections. Phase I and IIa trials of mesenchymal stem cells programmed to deliver neurotrophic growth factors to enhance endogenous recovery have been undertaken, but larger studies remain to be completed to determine if they will prove useful. Stroke survivors would be well advised to avoid offshore clinics providing untested "stem cell" therapies in a poorly regulated environment; more rigorous research needs to be completed using scientific methods.

15. What are common medical complications of stroke?

Stroke is often complicated by a variety of medical complications, some of which result from common comorbid conditions (hypertension), stroke-specific impairments (aspiration pneumonia), immobility (venous thromboembolism), or nosocomial infections (*Clostridium. difficile* colitis). A list of common medical complications is provided below, organized by these categories. Some conditions have multiple contributing causes but are listed only once.

Common comorbid conditions:
- *Recurrent stroke*
- *Atrial fibrillation*
- *Myocardial infarction*
- *Congestive Heart Failure*
- *Uncontrolled hypertension*
- *Uncontrolled diabetes*

Stroke/Stroke impairment-related:
- *Malnutrition*
- *Dehydration*
- *Aspiration pneumonia*
- *Depression*
- *Falls*
- *Fractures*
- *Osteoporosis*
- *Seizures*
- *Hydrocephalus*

Immobility-related:
- *Decubitus ulcers*
- *Deconditioning*
- *Deep venous thrombosis and pulmonary embolism*
- *Urinary retention, incontinence*
- *Constipation*

Nosocomial conditions:
- *C. difficile*
- *Catheter-associated UTIs*
- *IV Phlebitis*
- *Medication side effects and administration errors*

16. **What contributes to dysphagia after stroke?**

Focal injury to either hemisphere or brain stem can lead to disordered swallowing (dysphagia) after stroke. Dysphagia causes aspiration of food and liquid, placing the patient at risk for pneumonia that can delay recovery and lead to unnecessary death. The chief motor deficits within the swallowing mechanism after stroke are:
- Poor oral control of food or liquid bolus resulting in anterior spillage, pocketing, and premature spillage into pharynx.
- Reduced base of tongue retraction.
- Delayed trigger of pharyngeal swallow.
- Reduced laryngeal elevation, anterior hyoid excursion, and incomplete laryngeal vestibule closure, allowing food and liquid to reach larynx with subsequent aspiration.
- Delayed or absent cough reflex following aspiration.
- Poor opening of upper esophageal sphincter leading to pharyngeal residual after swallow.

17. **What conditions cause pain after stroke?**

Approximately 50% to 66% of patients have pain within the first year after stroke. Post-stroke pain leads to worse mood, a reduced quality of life, social life, activities of daily living, and increased disability and dependence. The most common musculoskeletal causes are hemiplegic shoulder pain, joint pain from other arthralgias, spasticity-related pain, and central hypersensitivity.

Causes of hemiplegic shoulder pain can include glenohumeral subluxation, adhesive capsulitis (frozen shoulder), impingement syndromes, rotator cuff tears, brachial plexus traction neuropathies, complex regional pain syndrome, bursitis and tendinitis, and central post-stroke pain. Often, there is either a history of or radiographic evidence for a preexisting or long-standing shoulder problem. It is likely that abnormal mechanical forces from the stroke either exacerbate or make manifest the chronic problem. In some patients, pain and loss of ROM are associated with improper positioning or handling, weakness of the shoulder girdle muscles, or spasticity. Shoulder dysfunction has been found to be significantly more frequent in patients with spastic upper limbs than in those with flaccid upper limbs. Pain and glenohumeral subluxation may occur together or independently, and the extent to which there is a causal relationship between pain and subluxation is unclear.

Central post-stroke pain syndrome occurs in less than 5% of stroke survivors. It causes severe, disabling pain, which usually is described by patients as diffuse, persistent, and refractory to many treatment attempts. The most common descriptions of the pain are "burning and tingling," although many patients experience "sharp, shooting, stabbing, gnawing," and more rarely, "dull and achy." The dysesthesias are often associated with allodynia (pain reaction to mild external cutaneous stimulation) and hyperpathia (exaggerated pain reaction to nociceptive stimulation).

Only about 50% of the patients have thalamic strokes; the remainder have cerebrovascular lesions in a variety of locations. A key characteristic is that all patients have lesions in sensory pathways in the CNS and all have abnormal sensory testing on examination. Clinical management begins with supportive counseling and patient education. Tricyclic antidepressants and anticonvulsant medications (such as gabapentin or lamotrigine) have demonstrated efficacy in central pain management.

18. **What is the frequency of and treatment for post-stroke depression (PSD)?**

The incidence of PSD ranges between 10% and 70%, with the best estimates at around 30%. Major depression occurs in about one-third of those with depression. The pathophysiology of PSD is thought to be related to inflammatory processes, genetic and epigenetic variations, white matter disease, cerebrovascular deregulation, altered neuroplasticity, and changes in glutamate neurotransmission. Participation and functional outcome in rehabilitation may be affected adversely by depression.

Recent meta-analyses of RCTs for treating PSD have demonstrated the efficacy of antidepressants. However, further studies are needed in more representative samples of stroke survivors, and additional study is required to determine the optimal timing and duration of treatment. Early antidepressant treatment of PSD appears to enhance both physical and cognitive recovery from stroke and might increase survival up to 10 years following stroke. Psychosocial therapies may also prevent the development of PSD. However, the studies are not generalizable to all stroke survivors given their narrow inclusion and exclusion criteria. Further research with more rigorous methods is needed to assess the effect of psychotherapy on prevention of PSD [14].

Bonus questions and answers are available online.

REFERENCES

1. Tsao CW, Aday AW, Almarzooq ZI, et al. Heart disease and stroke statistics–2022 update: a report from the American Heart Association. *Circulation*. 2022;145:e153-e639.
2. Bernhardt J, Langhorne P, Lindley RI, et al. Efficacy and safety of very early mobilisation within 24 h of stroke onset (AVERT): a randomised controlled trial. *Lancet*. 2015;386(9988):46.
3. Carmichael ST. The 3 Rs of stroke biology: radial, relayed, and regenerative. *Neurotherapeutics*. 2016;13(2): 348.
4. Dennis M, Mead G, Forbes J, et al. Effects of fluoxetine on functional outcomes after acute stroke (FOCUS): a pragmatic, double-blind, randomised, controlled trial. *Lancet*. 2019;393(10168):265.
5. Dimitrijevic MR, Faganel J, Sherwood AM, et al. Activation of paralysed leg flexors and extensors during gait in patients after stroke. *Scand J Rehabil*. 1981;13:109.

6. Duncan, PW, Sullivan, KJ, Behrman AL, et al. Body-weight–supported treadmill rehabilitation after stroke. *New Engl J Med.* 2011; 364(21):2026.
7. French B, Thomas LH, Coupe J, et al. Repetitive task training for improving functional ability after stroke. *Cochrane Database Syst Rev.* 2016;11:CD006073.
8. Gumbinger C, Reuter B, Stock C, et al. Time to treatment with recombinant tissue plasminogen activator and outcome of stroke in clinical practice: retrospective analysis of hospital quality assurance data with comparison with results from randomized clinical trials. *Br Med J.* 2014;348:g3429.
9. Harvey RL, Edwards D, Dunning K, et al. Randomized sham-controlled trial of navigated repetitive transcranial magnetic stimulation for motor recovery in stroke: the NICHE trial. *Stroke.* 2018;49(9):2138.
10. Knutson JS, Fu MJ, Sheffler LR, et al. Neuromuscular electrical stimulation for motor restoration in hemiplegia. *Phys Med Rehabil Clin N Am.* 2015;26(4):729.
11. Kraglund KL, Mortensen JK, Grove EL, et al. TALOS: a multicenter, randomized, double-blind, placebo-controlled trial to test the effects of citalopram in patients with acute stroke. *Int J Stroke.* 2015;10(6):985.
12. Mokin M, Snyder KV, Siddiqui AH, et al. Recent endovascular stroke trials and their impact on stroke systems of care. *JAMA.* 2016;67:2645.
13. Saver JL, Goyal M, van der Lugt A, et al. Time to treatment with endovascular thrombectomy and outcomes from ischemic stroke: a meta-analysis. *JAMA.* 2016;316:1279.
14. Towfighi A, Ovbiagele B, El Husseini N, et al. Poststroke depression: a scientific statement for healthcare professionals from the American Heart Association/American Stroke Association. *Stroke.* 2017;48(2): e30.
15. Winstein CJ, Stein J, Arena R, et al. Guidelines for adult stroke rehabilitation and recovery: a guideline for healthcare professionals from the American Heart Association/American Stroke Association. *Stroke.* 2016;47(6):e98.

CHAPTER 58

TRAUMATIC BRAIN INJURY: ETIOLOGY, PATHOPHYSIOLOGY, AND COMPLICATIONS

Emma Nally, MD, Emily Ryan-Michailidis, DO, Shailaja Kalva, MD, and Steven Flanagan, MD

If you are always trying to be normal, you will never know how amazing you can be.
— Maya Angelou (1928–2014)

KEY POINTS

1. Falls are the most common cause of traumatic brain injury (TBI) in the United States.
2. The reported incidence of TBI is increasing, likely the result of the aging population and increased awareness of concussion.
3. Men are at higher risk for TBI compared to women.
4. The elderly, very young, adolescents, and young adults are at highest risk for TBI.
5. Primary injury occurs at the time of impact.
6. Cerebral contusions most commonly occur in the inferior frontal and anterior temporal lobes.
7. Diffuse axonal injury is a main pathological feature of TBI, accounting for immediate loss of consciousness, emotional dysregulation, and cognitive impairments.
8. Secondary injury occurs after the initial impact.
9. Increased intracranial pressure (ICP) is the main cause of secondary injury that causes cerebral ischemia.
10. A main goal of acute management of severe TBI is to maintain cerebral perfusion pressure between 60 and 70 mm Hg (CPP = MAP − ICP).

1. **What are the most common causes of traumatic brain injury (TBI)?**

The annual incidence of TBI in the United States is 2.8 million. This underestimates the true incidence as it does not account for those injured who either seek care in non-hospital settings or no care at all. The most common cause of TBI is falls, followed by being struck by or against an object, and then motor vehicle accidents (MVA) (13.7%). MVAs are the leading cause of TBI-related deaths.

The overall incidence represents an increase from reports earlier this century, likely due to a combination of the high rate of falls in older adults, the growth of the aging population, and increased awareness of concussion and sports-related injuries prompting more hospital visits.

Taylor CA, Bell JM, Breiding MJ, et al. Traumatic brain injury-related emergency department visits, hospitalizations, and deaths—United States, 2007 and 2013. *MMWR Surveill Summ.* 2017;66:1–16.

2. **Who is most at risk for TBI?**

Men are two to three times more likely than women to sustain a TBI, although the risk decreases slightly with advancing age. Three age groups share the highest rate of injury, with those aged above 75 having the highest risk, followed by 0 to 4 years, and then 15 to 24 years old. The elderly have the highest rate of TBI-related hospitalization and death. This is in contrast to previously reported data from 2002 to 2006 that found the highest rates of TBI in those aged 15 to 19, which is theorized to be due to a decrease in MVA-related TBI.

3. **What is meant by primary TBI damage?**

Primary injury occurs at the time of trauma and includes diffuse axonal injury (DAI), cerebral contusions, and intracranial hemorrhages. DAI results from acceleration–deceleration and rotational forces applied to the brain and is one of the most important and common pathologic features of TBI. DAI is not readily imaged on standard CT and MRI scans, although its presence can be deduced by petechial hemorrhages. Advanced MR technologies, such as gradient echo (GRE) and susceptibility-weighted imaging (SWI), are sensitive to microhemorrhages associated with DAI. Diffusion tensor weighted MRI (DTI), used experimentally at the present time, assesses the structural integrity of white matter tracts and thus is felt to be a sensitive means to detect DAI.

Contusions occur from impact of cerebral tissue on the rough inner surface of the skull, most commonly affecting the anterior tips of the temporal lobes and inferior frontal lobes. Hemorrhages can occur within the brain parenchyma as well as in the extra-axial spaces. There is also a massive release of excitatory substances within minutes of TBI, predominantly glutamate, that triggers a neuronal influx of sodium, chloride, and intracellular calcium resulting in neuronal and astrocytic cytotoxic (intracellular) edema and death.

4. What is meant by secondary TBI, and how is it treated?

Secondary TBI refers to the damage that occurs after the initial trauma and produces long-lasting effects. It occurs most often from cerebral ischemia resulting from increased cerebral hypertension combined with impaired cerebral vascular autoregulation. As the swelling brain fills the cranial vault, intracranial pressure rises and impedes cerebral circulation. This is exacerbated by impaired cerebral vascular autoregulation resulting in widespread ischemia.

Ventriculostomy with placement of an external ventricular drain permits measurement of ICP. Steps to reduce ICP include CSF drainage, elevating the head of the bed 30 degrees, administration of osmotic diuretics such as mannitol, and treatment of hyperthermia. Inducing a barbiturate coma will lower ICP, but careful monitoring of hemodynamics is critical due to the risk of hypotension, reduced cardiac output, and pulmonary shunting. Short-term hyperventilation can be used as a temporizing measure as sustained hyperventilation adversely impacts cerebral blood flow. Surgical treatment includes evacuation of extra-axial hemorrhages and decompressive craniectomy.

Carney N, Totten AM, O'Reilly C, et al. Guidelines for the management of severe traumatic brain injury, fourth edition. *Neurosurgery.* 2017;80:6–15.

5. How is TBI severity assessed?

The Glasgow Coma Scale (GCS) measures a person's best motor, verbal, and visual response and is widely used to describe injury severity after TBI. Each response is scored, with the combined scores ranging from 3 to 15. GCS classifies TBI into three categories: severe (3 to 8), moderate (9 to 12), and mild (13 to 15). Lower scores are associated with poorer survivals, with the motor subscore the most predictive.

6. What is a concussion?

The vast majority of TBIs are mild and also known as concussions. There are many definitions of concussion with most including components of confusion, disorientation, and/or amnesia surrounding the time of injury. Loss of consciousness is not necessary to diagnose concussion, but if present, it is less than 30 minutes. The length of post-traumatic amnesia (PTA) is no more than 24 hours. GCS is ≥ 13 thirty minutes post-trauma. Symptoms of concussion include headaches, dizziness, mood changes, insomnia, fatigue, vision alterations, and cognitive changes. Most people with a single isolated concussion will make a full recovery. However, a small percentage may develop long-term problems, particularly if there is a history of multiple concussions. Treatments for concussions are geared towards symptomatic relief. A structured sub-symptom threshold aerobic exercise program may facilitate recovery.

Leddy JJ, Haider MN, Ellis MJ, et al. Early subthreshold aerobic exercise for sport-related concussion: a randomized clinical trial. *JAMA Pediatr.* 2019;173(4):319–325.

7. What cognitive changes are commonly seen after TBI, and what pharmacologic interventions can be used to improve function?

Impairments in attention, concentration, processing speed, executive skills, and memory are common after TBI. Catecholaminergic agonists can improve concentration, arousal, and processing speed. Cholinesterase inhibitors may enhance memory. Dopaminergic agonists may improve executive functioning.

8. What behavioral changes are commonly seen after TBI?

People with TBI demonstrate many behaviors, including disinhibition, emotional lability, pseudobulbar affect, psychosis, depression, and aggression. "Post-traumatic agitation" is a subtype of delirium and relates to confusion and PTA. Management is typically multifaceted and tailored to specific individuals, behaviors, and circumstances. These include behavioral modification techniques, environmental modifications, cognitive-behavioral therapy, and judicious use of medications. Medications used to treat these post-traumatic changes are those used for phenotypically similar psychiatric conditions, while others are useful specifically for people with brain injury.

KEY POINTS

1. The GCS is the most commonly used tool to assess acute TBI severity.
2. Most TBIs are considered mild and referred to as concussions.
3. Neurostimulants may be used to improve concentration and arousal. Cholinesterase inhibitors may aid in memory and attention, while dopaminergic agonists may enhance executive skills.
4. There are a variety of post-traumatic behavioral and psychiatric changes after a brain injury.
5. Treatment strategies are often multifaceted, with medication management often derived from similar psychiatric disorders.

9. **What non-pharmacologic strategies can be used for patients with post-traumatic agitation?**
   TBI-related agitation may be an expression of pain, infection, or discomfort in a person who is unable to effectively communicate what they need or are feeling. Therefore, physiological causes of agitation should be sought followed by appropriate treatment. Non-pharmacologic strategies include reducing environmental stimuli by using a private quiet room, removing noxious stimuli, and limiting visitors. Constant observation may be required to protect a person from harming themselves or others. Maintaining a consistent treatment team and schedule, using simple communications, and engaging in appropriately challenging activities that do not overtax abilities will reduce confusion and possibly reduce agitated behavior. Some degree of tolerance towards restlessness can be beneficial, such as permitting someone to ambulate freely rather than insisting they sit still for prolonged periods.

10. **What is the difference between PTA and the post-traumatic confusional state?**
    Behaviors following the period of early recovery following TBI typically include disorientation, sleep–wake disturbances, agitation, cognitive impairments, fluctuating presentations, and psychotic-like symptoms. Traditionally, this period has been referred to as PTA. It is formally measured by the Galveston Orientation and Amnesia Test (GOAT). GOAT scores of ≥75 on 2 subsequent tests separated by at least 24 hours indicate emergence from PTA. The Orientation LOG (OLOG) is another means to measure the length of PTA. Long lengths of PTA correlate to poorer functional outcomes. The post-confusional state (PCS) is a term that some feel more accurately describes the early period of recovery. It is quantified using the Confusion Assessment Protocol (CAP) that assesses seven key behavioral characteristics typically encountered during the early period of recovery. The duration of PCS correlates with functional recovery, injury severity, and with poor cooperation during rehabilitation.

Silva MA, Nakase-Richardson R, Sherer M, et al. Posttraumatic confusion predicts patient cooperation during traumatic brain injury rehabilitation. *Am J Phys Med Rehabil.* 2012;91:890–893.

11. **What does the Rancho Los Amigos (RLA) Levels of Cognitive Function describe?**
    The RLA is a tool that describes common cognitive and behavioral stages of recovery following severe TBI as well as the need people have for assistance to function, ranging from unresponsiveness to being able to live independently in the community. It does not describe motor function. Originally describing eight stages of recovery, the revised RLA has ten stages that incorporates more detailed descriptions at the highest level of functioning. There is no scoring or formal assessment protocol associated with the RLA. Instead, each stage is named for predominate behaviors a person exhibits, with a description of typical behaviors observed for a particular RLA level. Some people may simultaneously exhibit behaviors observed in more than one RLA level, making the tool somewhat imprecise at times. However, it does describe the cognitive and behavioral status of people recovering from TBI that can assist with setting treatment goals and assessing their effectiveness. See Table 58.1 for a description of the RLA levels.

12. **Are people with TBI at increased risk for developing neurodegenerative diseases?**
    Research has revealed relationships between sustaining TBI and an increased risk of developing several neurodegenerative conditions, but a definitive association relationship remains elusive. The relationship between sustaining a TBI and developing dementia remains uncertain, although there is compelling evidence supporting the association. Reports suggest that repetitive concussions may lead to chronic traumatic encephalopathy (CTE), a condition manifested by behavioral, cognitive, and physical problems. Although the clinical presentation and histopathological profiles of CTE reported thus far are similar to other dementias, they are different enough from them to suggest dementia occurring from trauma is a distinct condition from known degenerative conditions.

Dams-O'Connor K, Spielman L, Hammond FM, et al. An exploration of clinical dementia phenotypes among individuals with and without traumatic brain injury. *NeuroRehabilitation.* 2013;32:199–209.

Table 58.1 Ranchos Los Amigos Level of Cognitive Function

I: No response
No response to external stimuli.

II: Generalized Response
Inconsistent non-purposeful response to external stimulation.

III: Localized Response
Responses are directly related to the stimulus with enhanced responses to familiar people.

IV: Confused and Agitated
Hyperactive state with agitated behavior. Impaired cognition.

V: Confused and Inappropriate
Confused with impaired cognition. Behaviors and verbalizations are often inappropriate, but agitation is not a predominant feature.

VI: Confused and Appropriate
Able to follow simple commands consistently with increasing awareness of self and surroundings. Cognitive skills remain impaired.

VII: Automatic and Appropriate
Oriented in familiar environments and able to perform routine daily activities. Often lacks insight, although acknowledges diagnosis. Requires supervision for safety.

VIII: Purposeful and Appropriate, Standby Assistance
Oriented to person, place, and time and able to independently perform familiar tasks in a non-distracting environment. Requires standby assistance in order to compensate for ongoing impairments.

KEY POINTS

1. First-line treatment of agitation is to rule out possible physiologic causes such as pain or infection and to modify environmental stimuli.
2. Medications are a potentially effective treatment for agitation, but side effects must be considered prior to starting treatment.
3. PTA is the period of time post-TBI a person does not have memory of ongoing events.
4. PCS describes the period of recovery from severe TBI manifested by disorientation, fluctuating presentations, agitation, sleep disturbance, daytime arousal impairments, and psychotic symptoms.
5. Longer as opposed to shorter periods of PTA and PCS are associated with poorer recoveries.
6. RLA is a tool that describes ten stages of cognitive and behavioral recovery after TBI.
7. Although there is compelling evidence that TBI is associated with some neurodegenerative conditions, studies are mixed, and a definitive relationship remains elusive.
8. Alzheimer's dementia and cases of suspected TBI-related dementia share similar clinical and histopathological findings but are distinct enough to suggest they are distinct conditions.

13. How are seizures temporally classified after TBI?
Seizures occurring within 24 hours of injury are classified as immediate while those occurring after that time, but within 1 week, post-trauma traumatic seizures are defined as early. These seizures are an acute complication from the injury and are considered provoked, rather than a seizure disorder or epilepsy. Seizures occurring more than 1 week after head injury are known as late post-traumatic seizures. Some clinicians consider immediate seizures limited to the first few minutes after injury with all others occurring within the first week as early seizures.

14. Is seizure prophylaxis effective after TBI?
Anticonvulsant medications are effective in preventing early seizures and are recommended during this period. Routine prophylaxis for late post-traumatic seizures is not recommended due to demonstrated lack of efficacy and the potentially deleterious side effects of many anticonvulsants. The effectiveness of newer antiepileptic drugs has not been evaluated specifically for preventing PTS, but they are frequently used.

15. What is paroxysmal sympathetic hyperactivity (PSH)?
Paroxysmal sympathetic hyperactivity is a condition following severe brain injury manifested by episodic signs of excessive sympathetic discharge. It presents with increased heart rate, hypertension, motor posturing, tachypnea, sweating, and hyperthermia in response to various stimuli. It is a diagnosis of exclusion given the need to rule out etiologies such as infection, pulmonary embolism, and seizures.

Management strategies vary widely, although common components include maintaining adequate hydration, providing appropriate analgesics, and avoiding identified triggers. Other modalities are used inconsistently, and their influence on the outcome is unknown.

Meyfroidt G, Baguley IJ, Menon, DK. Paroxysmal sympathetic hyperactivity: the storm after acute brain injury. *Lancet Neurol.* 2017;16:721–729.

16. What are the recovery mechanisms after TBI?

Recovery of function after brain injury may be explained by several mechanisms. Plasticity occurs via neuronal regeneration/collateral sprouting and cortical re-organization. Reversal of diaschisis (i.e., injury in one area of the brain produces altered function in other areas of the brain) parallels recovery. Functional substitution describes compensatory strategies to substitute for lost function. Redundancy is activation of latent areas that would normally function similarly to the injured areas of the brain. Vicariation involves the ability of uninjured cerebral tissue taking over the function of injured parts of the brain.

Hylin MJ, Kerr AL, Holden R. Understanding the mechanisms of recovery and/or compensation following Injury. *Neural Plast.* 2017; 2017:7125057.

17. How does hydrocephalus manifest clinically after TBI? How is it diagnosed and treated?

Post-traumatic hydrocephalus may present with signs of classic normal pressure hydrocephalus, including dementia, ataxia, and incontinence. More often it presents with nausea, vomiting, headache, papilledema, altered mental status, and arrest or worsening of functional abilities. Atypical features like seizures, emotional problems, and increased spasticity may also be present. Diagnosis is based on neuroimaging findings of enlarged ventricles out of proportion to the sulci with transependymal edema. If the diagnosis is not certain, a high-volume lumbar puncture followed by an assessment of functional abilities may help to confirm or refute the diagnosis. Radioisotope cisternography is rarely needed. Treatment consists of placing a ventricular shunt that drains CSF to other body cavities such as the peritoneal space or atria.

Mazzini L, Campini R, Angelino E, et al. Posttraumatic hydrocephalus: a clinical, neuroradiologic, and neuropsychologic assessment of long-term outcome. *Arch Phys Med Rehabil.* 2003;84:1637–1641.

18. What is the differential diagnosis of hyponatremia in TBI?

Hyponatremia following TBI has several etiologies, including but not limited to the syndrome of inappropriate antidiuretic hormone secretion (SIADH) and cerebral salt wasting syndrome (CSWS). Other causes include the effects of certain medications and other metabolic conditions. Distinguishing SIADH from CSWS is important as fluid status is very different between them, which requires different treatments. It is hypothesized that in CSWS the injured brain releases natriuretic protein, increasing sympathetic activity, and causing changes in the renin-angiotensin-aldosterone system and adrenomedullin. This results in natriuresis, hyponatremia, and hypovolemia, requiring intravascular volume repletion and salt supplementation. In SIADH, hyponatremia results from excessive water resorption from the kidneys as a direct response of antidiuretic hormone and is corrected by fluid restriction.

Leonard J, Garrett RE, Salottolo K, et al. Cerebral salt wasting after traumatic brain injury: a review of the literature. *Scand J Trauma Resusc Emerg Med.* 2015;23:98.

19. What is heterotopic ossification?

Heterotopic ossification (HO) is the formation of mature lamellar bone in soft tissues around joints and is a frequent complication after TBI.

HO presents with joint pain, decreased range of motion, low-grade fever, periarticular swelling, warmth, and erythema. Risk of developing HO is the greatest in the first 3 to 4 months following injury. In decreasing order of frequency, hips, knees, elbows, and shoulders are affected in TBI. Diagnosis requires ruling out other causes of joint pain and erythema. Early radiographs are often unremarkable; thus, a three-phase technetium-99m bone scan remains the most sensitive diagnostic modality. Medication management includes nonsteroidal anti-inflammatory agents and etidronate sodium, although they have limited benefit once HO has formed. Surgical excision of symptomatic HO can be considered if clear functional gains are an anticipated result. Timing of surgical excision is controversial given the risk of reoccurrence. Post-excision low-dose radiation and etidronate can reduce the risk of recurrence.

KEY POINTS

1. Immediate post-traumatic seizure occurs within 1 day.
2. Early post-traumatic seizures occur within the first week.
3. Late post-traumatic seizures occur after the first week.
4. Routine prophylaxis for late post-traumatic seizures is not recommended.
5. PSH is manifested by increased heart rate, hypertension, motor posturing, tachypnea, sweating, and hyperthermia in response to various stimuli.
6. PSH mimics other conditions and is a diagnosis of exclusion.
7. Common components to managing PSH include maintenance of hydration, providing appropriate analgesics, and avoidance of identified triggers.
8. Post-traumatic hydrocephalus often presents with arrest or worsening of functional abilities, with or without nausea, vomiting, headache, papilledema, and altered mental status.
9. SIADH and CSW cause hyponatremia, but their management is very different.
10. Common sites of HO following TBI include the hips, knees, elbows, shoulders, and hands.
11. Etidronate sodium and nonsteroidal anti-inflammatory medications have limited effect once bone has formed.
12. Surgical excision of HO can be considered if functional improvement is anticipated.

Bonus questions and answers available online.

BIBLIOGRAPHY

3. Cifu DX, ed. *Braddom's Physical Medicine and Rehabilitation.* 4th ed. Philadelphia: Elsevier; 2011:1135–1137, 1139–1140.
4. Carney N, Totten AM, O'Reilly C, et al. Guidelines for the management of severe traumatic brain injury, fourth edition. *Neurosurgery.* 2017;80:6–15.
5. Cifu DX, ed. *Braddom's Physical Medicine and Rehabilitation.* 5th ed. Philadelphia: Elsevier; 2016: 963–968.
7. Dams-O'Connor K, Spielman L, Hammond FM, et al. An exploration of clinical dementia phenotypes among individuals with and without traumatic brain injury. *NeuroRehabilitation.* 2013;32:199–209.
8. Leddy JJ, Haider MN, Ellis MJ, et al. Early subthreshold aerobic exercise for sport-related concussion: a randomized clinical trial. *JAMA Pediatr.* 2019;173(4):319–325.
9. Lew HL, Lin PH, Fuh JL, et al. Characteristics and treatment of headache after traumatic brain injury: a focused review. *Am J Phys Med Rehabil.* 2006;85:619–627.
11. Silva MA, Nakase-Richardson R, Sherer M, et al. Posttraumatic confusion predicts patient cooperation during traumatic brain injury rehabilitation. *Am J Phys Med Rehabil.* 2012;91:890–893.
12. Taylor CA, Bell JM, Breiding MJ, et al. Traumatic brain injury-related emergency department visits, hospitalizations, and deaths—United States, 2007 and 2013. *MMWR Surveill Summ.* 2017;66:1–16.

CARDIAC REHABILITATION: LIFESTYLE, EXERCISE & RISK FACTORS MODIFICATION

CHAPTER 59

Matthew N. Bartels, MD, MPH, Yehoshua J. Lehman, MD, and Ira G. Rashbaum, MD

The heart of a fool is in his mouth, but the mouth of a wise man is in his heart.

— Ben Franklin

Suffering has been stronger than all other teaching and has taught me to understand what your heart used to be. I have been bent and broken; but—I hope—into a better shape.

— Dickens

KEY POINTS: CARDIAC REHABILITATION

1. Maximum heart rate (MHR) is best defined as the HR obtained on an exercise stress test but can be estimated by MHR = 220 − age, or MHR = 208 − 0.7 × (age).
2. Target heart rate (THR) for exercise can be found using the Karvonen formula: THR = Resting HR + Percent target intensity × (Maximum HR-Resting HR).
3. Stroke volume (SV) is the amount of blood ejected with each ventricular contraction, and increases with exercise to a maximum, which is 50% over the basal (resting) HR.
4. Cardiac output (CO) = HR × SV. It relates directly to total body oxygen consumption, VO_2, because all O_2 consumed reaches body tissues via the blood.
5. Maximum aerobic capacity, VO_2 max, is the peak rate of O_2 consumption at which a person is capable of metabolizing. It correlates to maximum work output in watts and expressed as L/min or more often as mL/kg body mass/min.

1. **Which categories of patients benefit from cardiac rehabilitation (CR)?**
   Patients with cardiovascular-related physiological, functional, and psychosocial impairments could benefit including those with:
   - Coronary artery bypass graft (CABG) surgery
   - Ischemic heart disease, recent "heart attack" (MI)
   - Percutaneous transluminal coronary angioplasty (PTCA)
   - Receiving a coronary artery stent
   - Congestive heart failure
   - Cardiac transplant
   - Heart valve replacement
   - Heart valve repair
   - Stable angina

   Insurance generally covers patients after a heart attack, stable angina, a transplant, bypass surgery, angioplasty, cardiac valve surgery, and heart failure.

Bartels M, Prince DZ. Acute medical conditions. In: Cifu DX, ed. *Braddom's Physical Medicine and Rehabilitation*. 5th ed. Philadelphia, PA: Elsevier; 2015:571–595.

Bartels MN, Whiteson JH, Alba AS, et al. Cardiopulmonary rehabilitation and cancer rehabilitation. 1. Cardiac rehabilitation review. *Arch Phys Med Rehabil*. 2006;87(3) (Suppl 1):S46-S56.

2. **What are the objectives of CR?**
   - Increase cardiovascular capacity and fitness
   - Reduce myocardial ischemia and the risk of infarction or sudden death
   - Improve exercise tolerance and the ability to improve the activities of daily living (ADL)
   - Create an appropriate patient-directed aerobic exercise program
   - Give guidelines for safe activities and work

- Control risk factors for coronary artery disease (CAD)
- Assist patients in handling stress in their lives
- Show patients how to conserve energy and simplify work activities
- Improve the patient's quality of life
- Reduce hospitalizations

Wenger NK, Froelicher ES, Smith LK, et al. *Cardiac Rehabilitation. Clinical Practice Guideline No. 17.* Rockville, MD: US Department of Health and Human Services, Public Health Service, Agency for Health Care Policy and Research and the National Heart, Lung, and Blood Institute; 1995.

3. Elaborate on the phases of the CR process?

The CR intervention sequence combines medical and/or surgical care needed for any cardiac illness. This entails secondary prevention, acute care, an increasing regimen of subacute care, and rehabilitation.

The CR patient may have had several diagnoses and/or undergo one or more procedure(s): myocardial infarction, CABG, heart failure, coronary artery stent(s), valve surgery (traditional or minimally invasive), left ventricular assist device, or a heart transplant.

CR has three phases:

Phase I: Inpatient phase. Generally from hospital admission to medical/surgical discharge (also called Phase IA). This is followed by acute or subacute inpatient rehabilitation (also termed Phase IB).

Phase II: Outpatient training. This can consist of aerobic conditioning, secondary prevention (e.g., risk factor management, education, and lifestyle changes).

Phase III: Maintenance phase. Patients seek to sustain aerobic exercise and lifestyle modifications. This is often the most difficult aspect of CR.

Bartels M, Prince DZ. Acute medical conditions. In: Cifu DX, ed. *Braddom's Physical Medicine and Rehabilitation.* 5th ed. Philadelphia, PA: Elsevier; 2015:571–595.

4. What are the objectives of Phase I CR?

- Mobility, ambulation, and ADL training supervised by therapists and nurses with cardiac monitoring. Mobility should also be done in the ICU to prevent frailty and deconditioning even if patient requires a ventilator.
- Reduce anxiety and depression.
- Reassure patient so they regain a sense of control of their life.
- Educate patient and family about the reasons for treatment and exercises.
- Evaluate extent of cardiac injury.
- Learn the patient's previous activities (i.e., work and life roles), as well as current personal goals they want to achieve during CR.
- Establish risk factor reduction strategies.
- Assess cardiovascular function and impairments.
- Determine risk of developing complications and rank risks.
- Create guidelines for activity and work after discharge.
- Post-MI heart rate increase with activity should be kept under 20 beats/min of baseline. Systolic BP should remain less than 20 mm Hg of baseline. A decrease of $\geq$10 mm Hg indicates other medical issues and exercise should be halted.
- Phase IB for those needing acute or subacute rehabilitation before discharge. These patients have significant concurrent conditions and/or other situations that interfere with movement and make ADL more difficult to complete. Recommendations are the same as for Phase I patients but with a longer recovery.
- Target intensity by end of Phase I should be at four metabolic equivalents.

Bartels M, Prince DZ. Acute medical conditions. In: Cifu DX, ed. *Braddom's Physical Medicine and Rehabilitation.* 5th ed. Philadelphia, PA; Elsevier; 2015:571–595.

Corcoran JR, Herbsman JM, et al. Early rehabilitation in the medical and surgical intensive care units for patients with and without mechanical ventilation: an interprofessional performance improvement project. *PM R.* 2017;9(2):113–119.

5. What are the primary goals of Phase II (outpatient) CR?

In addition to continuing the goals of Phase I, the main purposes of Phase II are:

- Achieving cardiovascular conditioning and fitness with an aerobic exercise program
- Controlling risk factors that can be changed using psychosocial and pharmacologic interventions and lifestyle changes
- Returning to work as soon as possible.

Phase II is usually three sessions per week for 8 to 12 weeks after a symptom-limited, full-level stress test. Patients learn to self-monitor for their appropriate level of exercise, work, or activities using HR monitoring and/or perceived exertion. They also receive support to reduce anxiety and depression.

This period should result in improvements in VO_2 max, lower HR for exercise or work, and reduced systolic BP. It should also benefit O_2 extraction/utilization by skeletal muscle as well as reduce anxiety and depression by improving coping skills.

Bartels M, Prince DZ. Acute medical conditions. In: Cifu DX, ed. *Braddom's Physical Medicine and Rehabilitation.* 5th ed. Philadelphia, PA: Elsevier; 2015:571–595.

Lakkat TA, Venäläinen JM, Rauramma R, et al. Relation of leisure-time, physical activity and cardiorespiratory fitness to the risk of acute myocardial infarction. *N Engl J Med.* 1994;330:1549–1554.

6. Elaborate on the main interventions of Phase III CR (maintenance).

The maintenance phase of CR is the most important aspect but often receives the least attention. This period has the same goals as Phase II, except the patient and/or their family do the monitoring. The program continues outside the CR center. Often, the patient may choose a community setting or elsewhere.

CR team members (physician, therapist, nutritionist, psychologist, social worker, etc.) should be available to assist and advise the patient as needed. The patient continues the level of exercise achieved and self-monitors them and other activities to avoid overexertion. Patients should perform moderate exercise for at least 30 minutes three times/week or low-level exercise for five times/week in order to keep the benefits of the CR program. Periodic evaluations need to be done to monitor the patient's progress, tolerance, and maintenance of earlier goals. Before beginning or changing the exercise program, the patient should check with his or her physician.

Bartels M, Prince DZ. Acute medical conditions. In: Cifu DX, ed. *Braddom's Physical Medicine and Rehabilitation.* 5th ed. Philadelphia, PA: Elsevier; 2015:571–595

Ornish D, Brown S, Scherwitz L, et al. Can lifestyle changes reverse coronary artery disease? The Lifestyle Heart Trial. *Lancet.* 1990; 336:129–133.

7. When is starting an inpatient or outpatient exercise program not advised?

Although some conditions may delay participation in the exercise portion of CR ("absolute contraindications"), teaching prevention and lifestyle modifications can be done for all patients. "Relative contraindications" are used to identify patients who need closer monitoring and safety screening before beginning CR programs.

Absolute Contraindications	Relative Contraindications
Within 2 days of Acute MI	Left main coronary stenosis
Unstable angina or not stable on medical therapy	Moderate stenotic valvular disease
Uncontrolled arrhythmia with hemodynamic compromise	Electrolyte abnormalities
Acute pulmonary embolism	Severe arterial hypertension (SBP >200 mm Hg and/or DBP >100 at rest)
Active pulmonary infection	Presence of tachyarrhythmia or bradyarrhythmia
Acute myocarditis	Hypertrophic cardiac myopathy
Acute pericarditis	Mental or physical impairment impeding participating in exercise
Acute aortic dissection	A high atrioventricular (AV) block
	Left ventricular dysfunction (Ejection Fraction <20%)

Other conditions that prevent a patient from beginning CR:
- Unstable angina
- Pulmonary arterial hypertension >60 mm Hg
- Resting systolic BP >200 mm Hg
- Resting diastolic BP >100 mm Hg
- Orthostatic BP drop or drop during exercise of >20 mm Hg
- Moderate to severe aortic stenosis
- A systemic illness or fever
- Uncontrolled atrial or ventricular dysrhythmias
- Uncontrolled sinus tachycardia (120 bpm)
- Uncontrolled congestive heart failure
- Third-degree AV block

- Active pericarditis or myocarditis
- A recent embolism
- Thrombophlebitis
- Resting ST displacement that is >3 mm)
- Uncontrolled diabetes
- Neurologic and/or orthopedic problems that preclude exercise

Bartels M, Prince DZ. Acute medical conditions. In: Cifu DX, ed. *Braddom's Physical Medicine and Rehabilitation*. 5th ed. Philadelphia, PA: Elsevier; 2015:571–595.

8. Enumerate the five main components of a CR exercise program.
   - **Modality**: The American College of Sports Medicine recommends that the exercise modality be any activity that uses large muscle groups, can be done for an extended time, and is rhythmic and aerobic.
   - **Intensity**: Prescribed by target HR, subjective rating of exertion, or metabolic equivalents. It is usually either 60% to 70% of VO_2 for CR patients or 70% to 80% of VO_2 for patients who are healthy at the start of a program.
   - **Duration**: Depends on the mode and intensity of exercise. Often 20 to 45 minutes initially and may increase to 60 minutes over time.
   - **Frequency**: While in the hospital daily and at least three times weekly while in the aerobic training and maintenance phases, usually skipping a day between intensive sessions.
   - **Progress**: Depends on the patient's individual tolerance, progress, endurance, needs, and goals.

US Department of Health and Human Services. *Physical Activity Guidelines for Americans*. 2nd ed. Washington, DC: US Department of Health and Human Services; 2018.

9. Why are warm-up and cool-down periods needed?
   The warm-up period usually lasts 5 to 10 minutes and increases the intensity of exercise gradually from rest to the desired level of intensity. Also, it is designed to stretch the major muscles that will be used. A warm-up decreases the risk of cardiovascular problems (e.g., delays onset of angina) and prevents sprains or strains. Patients with cardiac transplants and heart failure need a longer warm-up time before attempting more intensive aerobic exercises.
   A cool-down time gradually reduces cardiac work and redistribution of blood from muscles and extremities to internal organs. A gradual reduction of exercise intensity with continued body movements maintains venous return; prevents pooling of blood in the lower limbs, post exercise hypotension, and end-organ insufficiencies; and promotes continuous dissipation of heat. Patients with heart failure or transplant may need a longer cool-down time.

American College of Sports Medicine. *Guidelines for Exercise Testing and Prescription*. 6th ed. Indianapolis, IN: ACSM; 2000.

10. Elaborate on the connection between the heart rate, stroke volume, cardiac output, aerobic capacity, and anginal threshold.
    - The **maximum heart rate** (HR) is the maximum HR obtained during a stress test. It decreases with age and can be estimated for most people using the equation MHR = 220 − age or MRH = 208 − 0.7 × age.
    - **Stroke volume** (SV) is the amount of blood ejected with each ventricular contraction and increases with exercise to a maximum of 50% above resting (basal) HR.
    - **Cardiac output** (CO) equals HR × SV and directly related to the total body oxygen consumption (VO_2), as all oxygen consumed is delivered to the body via the blood.
    - **Maximum aerobic capacity** is the greatest rate of O_2 consumption a person is capable of metabolizing. It directly corresponds to maximum work output in watts. One way to understand and calculate it is by the formula SV × HR × (arterial O_2 − venous O_2), which takes into account the delivery and extraction of O_2. An increase in CO (the product of SV × HR) and/or an increase in arteriovenous O_2 difference increases the VO_2. Maximum VO_2 decreases with age, inactivity, and after an MI.
    - **Anginal threshold** is the CO at which myocardial O_2 use exceeds the O_2 delivered. An ischemic myocardium is not able to maintain a steady cardiac workload, which results in a fall in CO, VO_2, and/or BP.

American College of Sports Medicine. *Guidelines for Exercise Testing and Prescription*. 6th ed. Indianapolis, IN: ACSM; 2000.

11. Cite the risk factors for atherosclerotic CAD?
    Risk factors for developing CAD are:
    - Age
    - Being male
    - Elevated total cholesterol

- Elevated low-density lipoprotein (LDL) cholesterol
- A low high-density lipoprotein (HDL) cholesterol
- Elevated systolic or diastolic BP
- Diabetes
- Obesity
- Sedentary lifestyle
- Cigarette smoking
- Stress
- Family history of early CAD
- ECG evidence of left ventricular hypertrophy

The Framingham study (1984) showed that modifiable risk factors were hypertension, cigarette smoking, high cholesterol, inactivity, low HDL cholesterol ($<$35 mg/dL), obesity, high triglycerides, diabetes, and stress.

There is strong evidence that reducing risks reverses atherosclerosis. For example, a prospective study of randomized patients and a control group along with single drug therapy using simvastatin, lovastatin, colestipol, or niacin for cholesterol control showed CAD regression, reduced rates of CABG, and lower rates of mortality. Meta-analysis of randomized control trials of CR programs that focused on exercise and lessening risk factors resulted in a 10% reduction in 3-year mortality rates.

American College of Sports Medicine. *Guidelines for Exercise Testing and Prescription*. 6th ed. Indianapolis, IN: ACSM; 2000.

12. Are lifestyle changes for CAD beneficial?

Aggressive lifestyle changes to control hypertension and smoking, dieting with less than 10% of total calories from fat, combined with 3 hours of aerobic exercise per week as well as stress management have been demonstrated to produce clinically significant reduction in coronary atherosclerosis as documented by coronary arteriography. In the Lifestyle Heart Trial Study, patients on the American Heart Association's recommended diet of less rgan30% fat showed worsening of their CAD upon repeat catheterization. These studies suggest that common recommendations for patients with CAD do not reverse or even slow the disease.

A CR dietary program should provide nutrition needed for exercise, reduce risk factors associated with lipids and body fat content, and acclimate the body to minimize cardiac effort in order to maximize functional independence. To achieve this dietary ideal, the quantity and content of the diet need to be calculated.

Lastly, the incidence of MI in depressed patients is significant, and post-MI depression can lead to increased disease and death. Therefore, medical and psychological therapies are important components of CR. Adequate social support also aids recovery and lowers stress.

US Department of Health and Human Services. Physical Activity Guidelines for Americans, 2nd ed. Washington, DC: US Department of Health and Human Services; 2018.

13. Is CR needed for other rehab patients at risk for CAD and cardiac complications?

Patients with peripheral vascular disease and stroke share many risk factors with coronary disease patients. Of course, these patients should receive CR with appropriate precautions. Other patients at risk include geriatric patients, sedentary individuals, and those with a history of stroke and cardiac abnormalities.

Bartels M, Prince DZ. Acute medical conditions. In: Cifu DX, ed. *Braddom's Physical Medicine and Rehabilitation*. 5th ed. 2015; Philadelphia, PA: Elsevier: 571–595.

Pang MYC, Eng JJ, Dawson AS. Relationship between ambulatory capacity and cardiorespiratory fitness in chronic stroke. Influence of stroke-specific impairments. *Chest*. 2005;127:495–501.

14. Do patients with congestive heart failure benefit from CR?

Yes. Stable patients with congestive heart failure are able to increase their functional capacity up to 20%. Slowly increasing the intensity and duration of each exercise session, continued for at least 3 months, and followed by a maintenance program, has demonstrated a significant improvement in functional capacity for these patients.

Forman DE, Sanderson BK, Josephson RA, et al. American College of Cardiology's Prevention of Cardiovascular Disease Section. Heart failure as a newly approved diagnosis for cardiac rehabilitation: challenges and opportunities. *JACC*. 2015;65:2652–2659.

15. How can CR assist cardiac transplant patients?

Due to the loss of nerve innervation of the heart, HR increases only in response to changes in circulating catecholamines. Intervention in transplant recipients includes a longer warm-up, progressive endurance exercise at 50% to 60% of maximum HR, followed by longer cool-down periods. Cardiac transplant recipients need conditioning and CR programs to improve conditioning, improve quality of life, decrease fatigue, and enhance endurance and strength.

Young MA, Stiens SA, O'Young BJ, et al. Rehabilitation of the patient who has undergone organ transplant. In: Braddom R, ed. *Physical Medicine & Rehabilitation.* 4th ed. Philadelphia, PA: Elsevier; 2011:1439–1456.

16. What is appropriate for stroke survivors?

General recommendations: As the risk factors for CAD are identical to those for stroke, it is logical to apply the same exercise-based behavior modification model to them. BP must be maintained and may require more frequent measurement than in patients without a history of stroke. A suitable blood pressure range should be discussed with a neurologist.

Specific recommendations:
- Aerobics: Large-muscle activities such as walking, treadmill use, stationary cycle, combined arm-leg ergometer, arm ergometer, and seated stepper.
  - *Intensity:* 40% to 70% heart rate reserve; 40% to 80% peak oxygen uptake; 55% to 80% of MHR; 11 to 13 (6 to 20 scale) rating of perceived exertion (RPE)
  - *Duration:* 20 to 60 minutes for each session
  - *Frequency:* 3 to 7 days/week
- Strength: Circuit training, weight machines, free weights, and isometric exercise.
  - *Intensity:* 1 to 3 sets of 10 to 15 repetitions of 8 to 10 exercises involving the major muscle groups
  - *Frequency:* 2 to 3 days/week
- Flexibility: Stretching.
  - *Intensity:* 2 to 3 days/week (before or after aerobic or strength training)
  - *Duration:* Hold each stretch for 10 to 30 seconds
- Neuromuscular: Coordination and balance activities.
  - *Duration:* 2 to 3 days/week (on same day as strength activities)

Bartels M, Prince DZ. Acute medical conditions. In: Cifu DX, ed. *Braddom's Physical Medicine and Rehabilitation.* 5th ed. Philadelphia, PA: Elsevier; 2015:571–595.

Billinger SA, Arena CR, Bernhardt J, et al. Physical activity and exercise recommendations for stroke survivors: a statement for healthcare professionals from the American Heart Association/American Stroke Association. *Stroke.* 2014;45:2532–2553.

Please consider: Macko RF, Ivey FM, Forrester LW, et al. Treadmill exercise rehabilitation improves ambulatory function and cardio-vascular fitness in patients with chronic stroke: a randomized, controlled trial. *Stroke.* 2005;36(10):2206–2211.

17. What is the methodology for assessing cardio-respiratory fitness?

Measuring VO_2 during a maximal exercise test.

American College of Sports Medicine. *Guidelines for Exercise Testing and Prescription.* 6th ed. Indianapolis, IN: ACSM;2000.

Skerker RS. Review and update: the aerobic exercise prescription. *Crit Rev Phys Med Rehabil.* 1991;2:257–271.

18. How is the cardio-respiratory fitness of those with chronic stroke and residual disabilities measured?

- Cycle ergometry provides a better estimate of VO_2 than the 6-minute walk test (MWT) because the 6 MWT is also influenced by the balance, strength, and spasticity of these patients. However, in situations where a full cardiopulmonary exercise test is unavailable, the 6-minute walk or a shuttle walk test can provide an estimate of VO_2 max that has 80% to 90% of the accuracy of a lab result.
- A treadmill with harness support is an alternative.

American College of Sports Medicine. *Guidelines for Exercise Testing and Prescription.* 6th ed. Indianapolis, IN: ACSM; 2000.

Pang MYC, Eng JJ, Dawson AS. Relationship between ambulatory capacity and cardiorespiratory fitness in chronic stroke: influence of stroke-specific impairments. *Chest.* 2005;127:495–501.

19. What causes reduced cardiovascular capacity after spinal cord injury (SCI)?

Reduced exercise capacity in SCI patients has multiple elements. These include:
- Impaired autonomic nervous system control of the cardiovascular system
- Altered hormonal effects on the cardiovascular system
- Loss of the muscle pump, causing decreased venous return

- Muscle weakness and/or atrophy
- Altered respiratory system
- Smaller size of cardiac chambers
- More use of Type II muscle fibers than Type I
- Sedentary lifestyle

20. Which aerobic exercises are suited to SCI patients?
- Wheelchair propulsion
- Arm ergometry
- Wheelchair cycling using an arm crank
- Functional electrical stimulation (FES)
- Hybrid exercise (e.g., arm ergometry combined with lower-extremity FES)

WEBSITES

1. American Heart Association. *Heart Attack and Stroke Symptoms.* Available at: www.americanheart.org/presenter. jhtml?identifier=1200000
2. Available at: https://medlineplus.gov/cardiacrehabilitation.html

CHAPTER 60

PERIPHERAL VASCULAR DISEASE AND LYMPHEDEMA; LOCALIZATION AND INTERVENTION

Robert G. Schwartz, MD, Matthew Terzella, MD, and Steven A. Stiens, MD, MS

Angioplasties are a little like potato chips. You can't have just one.

— William P. Castelli, MD (1931-)

KEY POINTS

1. Early prevention with diet, exercise, smoking cessation, cardiac rehabilitation, anticoagulation, antiplatelet and neostatic treatments preserves limbs and prolongs life.
2. Limb ischemia intervention requires early recognition of the **SIX P's**: paresthesia, poikilothermia (polar), pain, pallor, pulselessness, and paralysis.
3. Aggressive utilization of rehabilitation modalities provides increased active and passive mobility, tissue sequential pneumatic compression, and recognition of indications for angioplasty and bypass improve outcomes.

Acute Arterial Occlusion—StatPearls—NCBI Bookshelf. Available at: www.ncbi.nlm.nih.gov › books › NBK441851

---

1. **What elements of the history and examination may suggest peripheral vascular disease?**
   Vascular ischemia may be the root cause of non-responsive pain even when symptoms are presumed to have neuromuscular etiologies. An index of suspicion for vascular disease should be heightened in the presence of diabetes, inflammatory disorders, coagulopathies, peripheral neuropathy, injury, immobility, and obesity.

   While a classical history includes post-exertional leg pain (claudication) relieved by rest, many patients may only report calf or leg tightness, hot or cold sensations, balance problems, numbness, restless legs, or leg pain aggravated by ambulation.

   A peripheral vascular physical examination only takes a moment. Look for signs of pallor, dependent rubor, varicosities, brawny changes, open wounds, edema, decreased peripheral pulses, loss of hair, trophic skin changes, and trophic or fungal nail changes.

Mangione S, Sullivan P, Wagner MS, *The Extremities and Peripheral Vascular Examination, Physical Diagnosis.* Secrets 3rd Edition Ch. 15, Philadelphia, 2021

Kalish, J, Hamdan, A. Management of diabetic foot problems. *J Vasc Surg.* 2010;51:476–486. Available at: https://www.sciencedirect.com/science/article/pii/S074152140901684X

---

2. **Can vascular disorders coexist with common neuromusculoskeletal (NMSK) conditions and confound patient care?**
   Functional vascular disease is much more common than obstructive vascular disease, so the apparent absence of severe disease should not deter the consideration of a vascular component. Sympathetic modulation of blood flow can exacerbate multifactorial pain syndromes and provide a mechanism for treatment. It stands to reason if circulation is impaired, then its impact is compounded.

   Common NMSK conditions that should be considered include fibromyalgia, chronic widespread pain, nerve root ischemia due to compromised circulation at the level of the **vasa nervorum,** cutaneous vasoconstriction associated with dysautonomia-induced RSD/CRPS, ischemia-induced **small fiber neuropathy,** and comorbid pseudo-claudication in failed back syndrome. If there is anything in the history that might suggest altered blood flow, attempts should be made to improve it in an effort to clear inflammation and enhance healing.

Abramson DI, Miller DS. *Vascular Problems.* In: *Musculoskeletal Disorders of the Limb.* New York: Springer-Verlag; 1981.

Albrecht PJ, Hou Q, Argoff CE, et al. Excessive peptidergic sensory innervation of cutaneous arteriole–venule shunts (AVS) in the palmar glabrous skin of fibromyalgia patients: implications for widespread deep tissue pain and fatigue. *Pain Med.* 2013;14:895–915.

2. What tests are available to measure/monitor vascular compromise?
   1. **Ankle-Brachial Index (ABI)**. This is the ratio of the systolic pressure taken at the ankle (dorsalis pedis artery) and the arm (brachial artery). It should be greater than .90 if normal.
   2. **Vascular Plethysmography**. This provides pulse volume waveform analysis to detect atherosclerosis and segmental obstruction. Changes in waveform morphology can be important even when absolute ABI numbers are normal.

      If the ABI is normal but there is a pulse volume drop in any segment, or if there is a pressure change $\geq$30 mm Hg from segment to segment, then consideration for atherosclerotic obstructive disease should be given. The ABI can be normal even when exercise stress examination shows decreasing pressure with exercise (pressure should increase), signifying functional vascular ischemia.

      Stress vascular studies increase the sensitivity of resting measurements. Think of them as functional examinations. Stress studies provide information about vessel wall pulsatility and elasticity. Stress studies may be abnormal even where ABI and resting plethysmography studies are normal. A post-exercise decline of more than 20% or a post-exercise ankle pressure decrease of more than 30 mm Hg can establish the diagnosis of PAD.
   3. **Arterial Duplex studies**. These studies are typically done after plethysmography evaluations. They provide additional information about lumen narrowing and vessel wall elasticity.
   4. **Venous Duplex studies**. While typically used for the assessment of DVT in the hospital setting, venous duplex studies are quite valuable for the evaluation of reflux and post-thrombotic recanalization.
   5. **Arteriography**. Radiographic imaging is indicated for cases being considered for surgical referral. They are also utilized to assess for vascular anomaly or inflammatory arteritis.

Rooke T. Controversies in vascular screening art versus science. *Vasc Med.* 2007;12:235–242. Available at: https://journals.sagepub.com/doi/pdf/10.1177/1358863X07080836

McDermott MM, Guralnik JM, Ferrucci L, et al. Asymptomatic peripheral arterial disease is associated with more adverse lower extremity characteristics than intermittent claudication. *Circulation-J Am Heart Assoc.* 117:2484–2491, 2008. Available at: https://www.ahajournals.org/doi/full/10.1161/CIRCULATIONAHA.107.736108

Mehta A, Sperling LS, Wells BJ. Postexercise ankle-brachial index testing. *JAMA.* 2020 Aug 25;324:796–797.

Figs. 60.1 and 60.2.

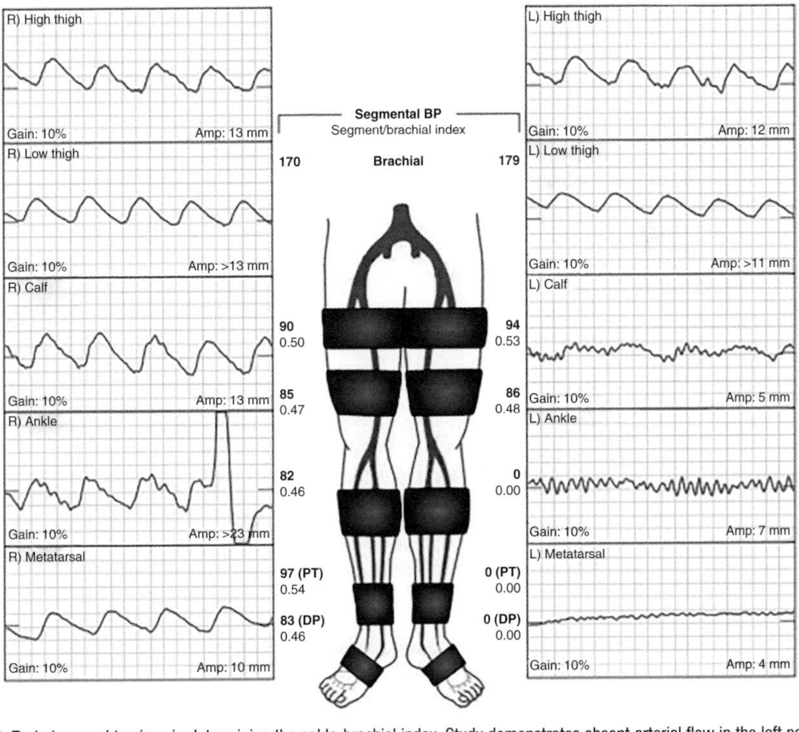

Fig. 60.1 Technique and tracings in determining the ankle-brachial index. Study demonstrates absent arterial flow in the left posterior tibial and dorsalis pedis arteries. *BP,* Blood pressure; *DP,* dorsalis pedis; *PT,* posterior tibial. (Tarek Al-Shafie and Paritosh Suman (2012). Aortoiliac Occlusive Disease, Vascular Surgery, Dr. Dai Yamanouchi (Ed.), ISBN: 978-953-51-0328-8, InTech, Available from: http://www.intechopen.com/books/vascular-surgery/aortoiliac-occlusive-disease.)

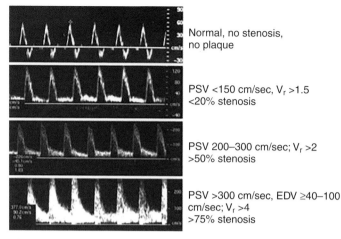

Normal, no stenosis, no plaque

PSV <150 cm/sec, V$_r$ >1.5
<20% stenosis

PSV 200–300 cm/sec; V$_r$ >2
>50% stenosis

PSV >300 cm/sec, EDV ≥40–100 cm/sec; V$_r$ >4
>75% stenosis

Fig. 60.2 Peek systolic velocity definitions for arterial duplex studies. (*Rutherford's Vascular Surgery and Endovascular Therapy.* 9th ed. 2019. Chapter 21, 227–237.e1, Fig. 21.6.)

3. What are the benefits of assessing for vascular disease in NMSK patients?
Reduced blood flow compromises inflammation resolution, exacerbates pain mediators, and impairs regenerative healing. It is an important consideration even in the absence of large vessel disease. Microcirculation is the blood circulation in vessels that are less than 200 microns in diameter. It is the *functional* part of the circulatory system. Like all other systems within the body, the microcirculatory system is self-regulating.
   It is through **sympathetic neural control** (alpha/beta receptors), as well as a complex orchestration of **mechanical sensors (glycocalyx)** and **signaling molecules (nitric oxide)**, that micro-hemodynamics is regulated. Dysfunction within the microcirculation has been recognized as a causal and subclinical manifestation of an increasing number of relevant rheumatic and NMSK diseases.

Gutterman DG. The human microcirculation—regulation of flow and beyond. *Circ Res.* 2016;118:157–172. Available at: https://www.ncbi.nlm.nih.gov/pmc/articles/PMC4742348/

Olutende O, Kweyu IW, Sabiri E. Exercise and chronic diseases. *Int J Sci Res.* 2017;6(10):588–599.

4. What are some easily employed vascular medicine approaches for patient care?
The goals are to increase blood flow, reduce pain, and improve function. Mild (or functional) arterial disease often improves with transitioning to a higher fruit, vegetable, and fish content diet, and supplementing with polyphenols, antioxidants, and omega-3 fatty acids. Medical studies have demonstrated a 47% increase in peripheral blood flow with this change alone. In addition, structured **walking programs** (including treadmill), smoking cessation, antiplatelet and antihypertensive medications, and sympathetic blocks can be helpful, depending upon individual needs. Collaboration and organization of **multidisciplinary vascular teams** integrate care plans efficiently.
   When venous or lymphatic changes are present, consider adding **compression stockings** first. Approaches to reduce venous reflux and prevent thrombosis include anti-fibrinolytic supplements, such as **Bolouke** (an earthworm enzyme extract that breaks down fibrinogen), and anti-inflammatories like **aspirin**. If there are laboratory or imaging signs of fibrin deposition, thrombus, or thrombotic organization, then other anti-coagulants, such as **heparin** or **low molecular weight heparin** compounds, can also be considered.
   Fig. 60.3

Ashor M, Lara J, Siervo M, et al. Exercise modalities and endothelial function: a systematic review and dose–response meta-analysis of randomized controlled trial. *Sports Med.* 2015 Feb;45(2):279–296

Kolte D, Parikh SA, Piazza G, et al. Vascular teams in peripheral vascular disease. *J Am Coll Cardiol.* 2019;73(19):2477–2486. Available at: https://www.sciencedirect.com/science/article/pii/S0735109719345061?via%3Dihub

Nosova EV, Conte MS, Grenon SM. Advancing beyond the "heart-healthy diet" for peripheral arterial disease. *J Vasc Surg.* 2015;61(1):265–274. doi: 10.1016/j.jvs.2014.10.022. Available at: https://www.ncbi.nlm.nih.gov/pmc/articles/PMC4275620/pdf/nihms-636860.pdf

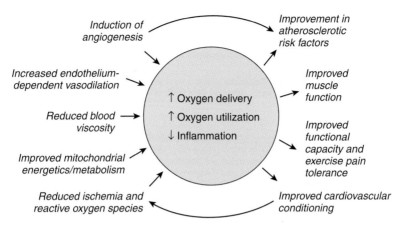

Fig. 60.3 Benefits of exercise in peripheral arterial disease. (From Bonaca MP, Creager MA. Pharmacological treatment and current management of peripheral artery disease. *Circ Res*. 2015;116:1579–1598.)

5. Can vascular disorders present as chronic NMSK pain syndromes?
   1. Yes. **Perino (chilblains)** is a cold-induced vascular disorder associated with red to blue (acute) or brown (chronic) inflammatory skin lesions, burning, and itching.
   2. **Blue Toe Syndrome** presents with blue areas of discolorations, typically in the toes, that are described as petechia. There can be sudomotor changes associated with the disorder—however, it is due to microembolization and is not a manifestation of RSD/CRPS.
   3. **Ischemic foot** is due to arterial occlusion and should not be confused with sympathetic fiber vasoconstriction. Naturally, it can be life-threatening. It is not associated with sudomotor change.
   4. **Thromboangiitis Obliterans (Buerger's Disease)** presents with digital ischemia and is due to vasculitis of small to medium arteries or veins. Smoking increases symptoms, and there are no sudomotor changes.
   5. **Livido Reticularis** is a pattern of red, violet, or blue fishnet-like skin surrounding areas of normal skin. It is aggravated by cold and disappears with warming. It can be due to an atheromatous embolic shower to the dermal vessels.

Seretny M, Colvin LA. Pain management in patients with vascular disease. *Br J Anaesth*. 2016;117(S2):ii95–ii106.

Rooke T. Controversies in vascular screening—art versus science. *Vasc Med*. 2007;12:235–242. Available at: https://journals.sagepub.com/doi/10.1177/1358863X07080836?url_ver=Z39.88-2003&rfr_id=ori:rid:crossref.org&rfr_dat=cr_pub%20%200pubmed

6. Can venous disorders be the source of persistent pain?
   Small venous perforators distally, rubor with dependency, **livedo reticularis,** or simply complaints of calf tightness or limp should raise your index of suspicion that there is a venous component to treat. In addition, when **edema** is present, venous disorders should be considered. This is true with or without brawny changes, rubor, or varicosities.
   Ultrasound Venous Duplex examination can be quite helpful to demonstrate **reflux** and organization of old thrombosis, not just **DVT**.
   Post-phlebitic syndromes that masquerade as NMSK chronic limb pain can be present in the absence of vessel trauma, venous stasis, or coagulopathy (**Virchow's triad**). **May-Thurner syndrome** is due to inferior vena cava obstruction from an over-riding internal iliac artery. Patients present with complaints of groin, thigh, or leg pain that is often positional.

Lamerton AJ, Bannister R, Withrington R, et al. Claudication of the sciatic nerve. *Br Med J*. 1983;286:1785–1786. Available at: https://www.ncbi.nlm.nih.gov/pmc/articles/PMC1548036/pdf/bmjcred00556-0021.pdf

7. What are some common approaches to the treatment of venous disorders?
   1. **Limb elevation,** compression, and **sequential pneumatic compression stockings,** supplements like **Bolouke,** and **low molecular weight medications or heparin** can lead to remarkable results in clearing up trophic changes and reducing pain.

2. Stasis ulcers respond to **local wound care** and cleansers, **hydrotherapy,** hyperbaric oxygen, **una boots,** compression bandages, antibiotics, **cellular therapies, ablation of incompetent superficial vessels,** and surgical debridement.
3. Treatment of May-Thurner can require **anticoagulants, stenting,** or even bypass surgery.

O'Donnel TF, Passman MA, Marston WA, et al. Management of venous leg ulcers: clinical practice guidelines of the Society for Vascular Surgery and the American Venous Forum. *J Vasc Surg.* 2014;60:3S–59S. Available at: https://www.jvascsurg.org/article/S0741-5214(14)00851-9/fulltext

8. Can lymphatic disorders be the source of chronic pain?

Yes. A mild increase in peripheral edema, or simply complaints of limb swelling should be enough to raise your index of suspicion. NMSK conditions like **Thoracic Outlet** and **Shoulder-Hand Syndromes** can cause enough platysma and scalene spasm to impede lymphatic return and contribute to breast, neck, thoracic, and chest wall pain.

Chapman's reflexes are felt to be **neurolymphatic reflex points.** These are tender points located deep in the skin and subcutaneous tissue, frequently in the deep fascia or periosteum of the bone. They are found in specific areas of the body that correspond to visceral dysfunctions (viscerosomatic reflex regions).

Chronic, low-level **compartment syndromes** have been mistaken for MSK pain syndromes as well. While lymphangiomas and angiectasias exist, inflammatory, oncologic therapy, and acquired mechanical etiologies are the most common causes of lymphedema.

Bath M, Nguyen A, Bordoni B. *Physiology, Chapmans's Points.* StatPearls. Available at: https://www.ncbi.nlm.nih.gov/books/NBK558953/

Ward RC. *Foundations for Osteopathic Medicine.* Chap 67: *Chapman's Reflexes.* Baltimore, Williams and Wilkins, 1997:935–940.

9. How is lymphedema diagnosed?

The diagnosis of **lymphedema** is largely a clinical exercise of exclusion. Differential diagnosis includes **lipedema** (due to adipose deposition), **myxedema,** and venous insufficiency. In contrast to edema that occurs secondary to hydrostatic forces (as with congestive heart failure, venous hypertension, and venous insufficiency), **pure lymphatic edema** does not respond to diuretics.

10. Other than physical examination, what tests can help diagnose lymphedema?

Lymphangiography is likely the most common objective assessment. Near-infrared fluorescent lymphography utilizes dermally-injected indocyanine green, which is then monitored with fluorescent spectroscopy. It is most commonly used as an adjunctive tool in lymphatic microsurgeries.

Radionucleotide **lymphoscintigraphy,** which while less sensitive, allows for quantitative analysis. Serial limb volumetric measurement with the use of water displacement or through extrapolation form circumferential dimensions.

Tonometry, the measurement of **tissue dielectric constant,** and **bioimpedance spectroscopy** are newer techniques used to detect subclinical interstitial edema and alterations in tissue water content.

11. What are some common approaches to the treatment of lymphatic disorders?

Hydrostatic regulation with **intermittent pneumatic compression** or **compression stockings** to facilitate lymphatic drainage and the correction of lymphatic filariasis through a host of anti-infective strategies can reduce edema. In more severe cases, the creation of **lymphatic-to-venous anastomosis** and **autotransplantation of vascularized lymph nodes** into the edematous limb to facilitate the restoration of function are surgical techniques that have been tried.

Keep in mind that while rarely life-threatening, lymphedema does escalate the threat of infection, restriction of motion, and loss of function. Treating it can provide significant NMSK relief and restorative benefits to patients. The use of physical and restorative therapies, such as **pulsed electromagnetic frequency currents** and **lymphatic massage,** are popular interventions. Since cell swelling activates NMDA receptors, addressing edema can also decrease neuronal excitability and peripheral, sympathetic, and centralization sensitization.

Fialka-Moser, V, Korpan, M, Varela, E, et al. The role of physical and rehabilitation medicine specialist in lymphoedema. *Ann Phys Rehabil Med.* 2013;56:396–410. Available at: https://www.sciencedirect.com/science/article/pii/S1877065713000456?via%3Dihub

Fig. 60.4

12. Can coagulopathies affect vascular and NMSK disorders? How can they be approached?

Since coagulopathies include abnormalities in the clotting cascade, they can induce vascular ischemia. Examples include von Willebrand disease, factor V deficiency, and protein C and S deficiencies. However, most coagulopathies do not reveal themselves with a severe clinical presentation.

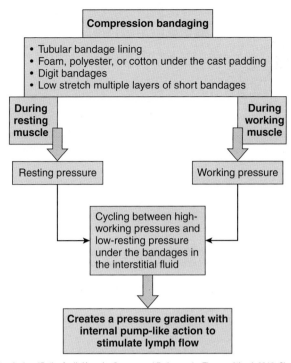

Fig. 60.4 Compression bandaging. (*Rutherford's Vascular Surgery and Endovascular Therapy*. 9th ed. 2019. Chapter 169, 2206–2220.e4, Fig. 169.8.)

Associated ischemia does not have to deprive a large tissue volume to cause chronic pain. Rather, multiple punctate lesions may have a cumulative effect that makes an otherwise easily treatable condition difficult to address. Coagulopathies may result in small punctate lesions. There can be associated vasomotor instability, cold sensitivity, hyperpathia, and dysesthesia—however, sudomotor instability is usually absent.

With coagulopathies, look for objective findings in serum. Treatment options depend upon the underlying reason for the coagulopathy, but addressing hidden infection and other factors that may exacerbate it should be minimized. When coagulopathy is present, efforts to minimize other vascular disorder symptoms should be implemented as well.

BIBLIOGRAPHY

Conte MS, Bradbury AW, Kolh P, et al. Global vascular guidelines on the management of chronic limb-threatening ischemia. *Eur J Vasc Endovasc Surg*. 2019;58:S1eS109. Available at: https://www.jvascsurg.org/article/S0741-5214(19)30321-0/fulltext

Cousin A, Popielarz S, Wieczorek V, et al: Impact of a rehabilitation program on muscular strength and endurance in peripheral arterial occlusive disease patients. *Ann Phys Rehabil Med*. 2011;54:429–444. Available at: https://www.sciencedirect.com/science/article/pii/S1877065711010700?via%3Dihub

Gerhard-Herman, MD, Gornik HL, Barrett C, et al. 2016 AHA/ACC guideline on the management of patients with lower extremity peripheral artery disease. *J Am Acad Cardiol*. 2017;69(11):1465–1508. Available at: https://www.jacc.org/doi/full/10.1016/j.jacc.2016.11.007

Lagattuta F, Langer C, Tipei C, et al. Treatment of small fiber neuropathy with pentoxifylline and alpha lipoic acid. *Int J Endocrinol*. Published online 2012 Jan 26. doi: 10.1155/2012/456279

Tu C, Das S, Baker AB, Zoldan J, Suggs LJ. Nanoscale strategies: treatment for peripheral vascular disease and critical limb ischemia. *ACS Nano*. 2015;9(4):3436–452. doi: 10.1021/nn507269g.

Rathbun S, Heath PJ, Whitsett T, et al. The venoarterial reflex. *Vasc Med*. 2008;13:315–316. Available at: https://hal.archives-ouvertes.fr/hal-00571383/document

Regensteiner JG, Wolfel EE, Brass E, et al. Chronic changes in skeletal muscle histology and function in peripheral arterial disease. *Circulation*. 1993;87:413–421. Available at: https://www.ahajournals.org/doi/pdf/10.1161/01.CIR.87.2.413

Wolberg AS, Aleman MM, Leiderman K, Machlus KR. Procoagulant activity in hemostasis and thrombosis: Virchow's triad revisited. *Anesth Analg*. 2012;114(2):275–285. Available at: https://www.ncbi.nlm.nih.gov/pmc/articles/PMC3264782/pdf/nihms335267.pdf

CHAPTER 61

PULMONARY REHABILITATION: IMPROVING DYSPNEA, ENDURANCE AND WELLBEING

John R. Bach, MD, and Jonathan H. Whiteson, MBBS

The first step to wisdom is to call something by what it really is…for example ventilatory rather than respiratory failure and interface rather than ventilator associated pneumonia
When the breath is unsteady, all is unsteady; when the breath is still; all is still. Control the breath carefully. Inhalation gives strength and a controlled body; retention gives steadiness of mind and longevity; exhalation purifies body and spirit
— Goraksasathakam

KEY POINTS: PULMONARY REHABILITATION FOR OBSTRUCTIVE LUNG DISEASES

1. Chronic bronchitis and emphysema, whilst both classified as chronic obstructive pulmonary diseases (COPD) there are significant pathologic and clinical differences and so must be addressed and managed differently. In many cases of COPD, however, there is significant overlap and a personalized management approach is essential to optimize outcomes.
2. Prognosis in COPD can be directly correlated with Forced Expiratory Volume in 1 second (FEV1) - serial evaluation of FEV1 can help guide appropriate management including care planning and advanced directives.
3. A comprehensive evaluation including clinical exercise stress testing is strongly recommended before starting pulmonary rehabilitation to assist in exercise risk stratification, to individualize the treatment plan and to guide and monitor functional progression.
4. The four essential elements of a pulmonary rehabilitation program include: (1) **exercise**; (2) **nutrition**; (3) **emotional support**; and (4) **education**. The focus of the exercise program includes: (1) **chest therapy** - secretion clearance and breathing re-training; (2) **postural therapy** - to promote optimal chest wall mechanics and balance; (3) **generalized strength training**; and (4) **aerobic conditioning** - to improve endurance focused on functional activities like walking and stair climbing over cycling and rowing.
5. For many patients with obstructive and restrictive lung disorders, access to pulmonary rehabilitation programs and long term adherence to the treatment plan post-program is limited - there is tremendous opportunity for alternative program design and implementation including telehealth monitored home and community based programs.

1. Describe the fundamental categories of respiratory disease.
   Intrinsic versus mechanical, lung tissue versus pump dysfunction and denervation, obstructive versus restrictive.
      Intrinsic, or obstructive disease, results in oxygenation impairment, and patients are normally eucapnic or hypocapnic despite hypoxia until end-state respiratory failure.
      Patients with mechanical dysfunction of respiratory muscles, lungs and chest wall, have ventilatory pump dysfunction (VPD) that initially causes retention of CO_2 and later hypoxia, only secondarily to worsening hypoventilation and ineffective cough flows.

VENTILATORY IMPAIRMENT (CO_2 RETENTION)

2. List the conditions causing primarily ventilatory impairment amenable to physical medicine applications.
   Ventilatory impairment may result from neural, muscular, or skeletal disorders causing a relatively increased work of breathing or increased mechanical work of breathing as with morbid obesity or chest wall disease, without primary oxygenation impairment from lung intrinsic disease (Table 61.1) .

Bach JR, Goncalves MR. Etiologies of ventilatory pump failure. In: Bach JR, Chiou M, eds. *Noninvasive management of ventilatory pump failure: for neuromuscular diseases, spinal cord injury, morbid obesity, and general debility.* Book Vine, 2022:18-31.

Bach JR. Noninvasive respiratory management of patients with neuromuscular disease. *Ann Rehabil Med.* 2017;41(4):1-20. doi: 10.5535/arm.2017.41.4.519.

3. Name two prerequisites to assure benefit from noninvasive respiratory muscle aids for patients with VPD.
   1. The ability to cooperate and learn
   2. A patent upper airway

4. State the seven most common errors in evaluating and managing patients with ventilatory impairment.
   1. Misinterpretation of symptoms which are due to hypercapnia and inspiratory muscle weakness rather than central or obstructive hypopneas.
   2. Failure to do **spirometry** with the patient supine and to monitor **maximum insufflation capacity**.
   3. Use of polysomnography, pulmonary function testing, and arterial blood gas analyses instead of spirometry, cough flow measurements, oximetry, and noninvasive CO_2 monitoring.
   4. Administration of oxygen, continuous positive airway pressure (CPAP), and inadequate spans of bi-level positive airway pressure (BiPAP) when noninvasive respiratory muscle aids are what is needed.
   5. Use of methylxanthines and any other respiratory medications on an ongoing basis without evidence of bronchospasm.
   6. Failure to prevent acute respiratory failure and hospitalization by using oximetry to gauge the effectiveness of noninvasive ventilatory support and mechanical insufflation-exsufflation.
   7. Resort to tracheostomy for any patients with myopathic or lower motor neuron disease.

5. Name the clinical parameters critical for monitoring patients with ventilatory pump failure.
   - Vital capacity (VC) and maximum insufflation capacity (MIC) via spirometry
   - Peak cough flows (PCF), unassisted and assisted
   - Oxyhemoglobin saturation (O_2 sat) via oximetry
   - End tidal Carbon dioxide ($EtCO_2$) via Capnography

Bach JR. Noninvasive respiratory management of patients with neuromuscular disease. *Ann Rehabil Med.* 2017;41(4):1–20. doi: 10.5535/arm.2017.41.4.519.

Bach JR, Gonçalves MR, Hon AJ, et al. Changing trends in the management of end-stage respiratory muscle failure in neuromuscular disease: current recommendations of an international consensus. *Am J Phys Med Rehabil.* 2013;92(3):267–277. doi: 10.1097/PHM.0b013e31826edcf1.

6. What is the MIC?
   The MIC is the maximum volume of air that can be held with a closed glottis. It correlates with bulbar-innervated muscle function and pulmonary compliance. Accumulated with "**air stacking**" (holding in repeated breaths with a closed glottis).

McKim DA, Katz SL, Barrowman N, Ni Andy, LeBlanc C. Lung volume recruitment slows pulmonary function decline in Duchenne muscular dystrophy. *Arch Phys Med Rehabil.* 2012;93:1117-22.

7. What are respiratory muscle aids?
   The devices that act on the body include the **negative-pressure body ventilators** (NPBVs) and the **intermittent abdominal pressure ventilator** which create pressure changes to the thorax and abdomen, **forced exsufflation devices** which apply force directly to the body to mechanically displace respiratory muscles, and devices that apply intermittent pressure changes directly to the airway.

Bach JR. Update and perspectives on noninvasive respiratory muscle aids: Pt 1. The inspiratory muscle aids. *Chest.* 1994;105:1230–1240. DOI: 10.1378/chest.105.4.1230.

Bach JR. Update and perspectives on noninvasive respiratory muscle aids: Pt 2. The expiratory muscle aids. *Chest.* 1994;105:1538–1544. DOI: 10.1378/chest.105.5.1538.

8. What are the ideal methods of noninvasive ventilatory support (NVS) for long term daytime use?
   Mouthpiece intermittent positive pressure ventilatory support (NVS) and the **intermittent abdominal-pressure ventilator (IAPV)** are both very effective. For mouthpiece NVS, a mouthpiece is mounted near the mouth, adjacent to the controls for the motorized wheelchair, where the patient can easily grab it at about 2 to 10 times a minute as needed for up to full ventilatory support (NVS).

   The pneumatic IAPV intermittently inflates an air sac contained in a corset or belt worn beneath the patient's outer clothing. Inflation by a positive-pressure ventilator moves the diaphragm upward, causing a forced exsufflation. During deflation, the abdominal contents and diaphragm fall to the resting position, and inspiration occurs passively.

Bach JR. Noninvasive respiratory management of patients with neuromuscular disease. *Ann Rehabil Med.* 2017;41(4):1–20. doi: 10.5535/arm.2017.41.4.519.

Bach JR, Radbourne M, Chiou M. A mechanical intermittent abdominal pressure ventilator. *Am J Phys Med Rehabil.* (AJPMR-D-18-00526. Submitted and will be in press).

Banfi P, Volpato E, Arcadu A, et al. A new intermittent abdominal pressure ventilator for post-ischemic cervical myelopathy ventilatory failure. *Multidiscip Respir Med.* 2019;14(4). Available at: https://mrmjournal.biomedcentral.com/articles/10.1186/s40248-019-0169-4

9. What are the ideal inspiratory muscle aids for nocturnal use?
   Nasal NVS delivered via nasal interfaces (CPAP masks) is the most popular method of nocturnal NVS. At least three or four different nasal interfaces should be tried by each patient to determine which ones will be most effective and comfortable. Many patients use different styles on alternate nights to vary skin contact pressure. Vented CPAP interfaces must have the holes (portals) sealed to be used with active ventilator circuits for NVS.

   Mouthpiece NVS via lip cover interfaces are more effective but generally less preferred than nasal NVS. **Lip cover NVS** can be delivered during sleep with less insufflation leakage and with little risk of losing the mouthpiece. However, speaking clearly is more difficult.

Bach JR. A comparison of long-term ventilatory support alternatives from the perspective of the patient and care giver. *Chest.* 1993; 104:1702–1706. DOI: 10.1378/chest.104.6.1702

10. How can airway secretions be best minimized and expectorated in this population?
    Over 100 L/m of expiratory flow is necessary to bring airway secretions out of the airways and into the mouth. Therefore, whether using a ventilator or not, patients with ventilatory pump failure are often unable to generate adequate cough peak flows (CPF) without manual or mechanical assistance. With the use of an insufflation to greater than 1.5 L and with a properly timed abdominal thrust, CPF of 180 to over 300 L/m can usually be generated. When scoliosis, abdominal distension, trauma, bulbar muscle dysfunction, or obesity interfere with manually assisted coughing, a **mechanical insufflator-exsufflator** can be used at pressures of 40 to 60 cm H_2O.

Gomez-Merino E, Bach JR. Duchenne muscular dystrophy: prolongation of life by noninvasive respiratory muscle aids. *Am J Phys Med Rehabil.* 2002;81:411–415. Available at: https://www.ncbi.nlm.nih.gov/pubmed/12023596

11. What is a mechanical insufflator–exsufflator?
    The mechanical insufflator-exsufflator provides mechanical insufflation-exsufflation or MIE for full lung inflation and vacuum-assisted exhalation. This clears bronchopulmonary secretions by applying positive pressure to open airways and then rapidly shifts to negative pressure for sudden powerful expiratory flows.

12. Describe the symptoms and signs of hypoventilation (hypercapnia).
    Fatigue, shortness of breath, morning or continuous headaches, sleep awakenings with shortness of breath, poor concentration, frequent nightmares, symptoms and signs of heart failure such as lower limb swelling, irritability, anxiety, decreased libido, frequent arousal from sleep to urinate, impaired intellectual function, depression, excessive weight loss, muscle aches, and memory impairment.

13. Which factors decrease blood oxyhemoglobin saturation (O_2 sat)?
    1. Hypoventilation causing hypercapnia
    2. Fixed or transient airflow obstruction with the latter usually due to mucus
    3. Intrinsic lung disease (such as atelectasis or pneumonia)
       Under normal conditions, hemoglobin in red blood cells rapidly binds oxygen and fully saturates during the first third of the passage through the alveolar capillary system. Impairments that prevent full exposure of the blood to recently inhaled air as it courses through the lungs can prevent normal saturation.
       Oximeters that measure pulse and blood O_2 sat are increasingly inexpensive, and **oximetry should be considered a fourth vital sign**. If airway mucus congestion (especially to the extent that causes oxyhemoglobin desaturation below 95%) is not cleared and O_2 sat not returned to normal (>94%) in a timely manner, pneumonia and/or lung collapse develops.

14. Discuss the use of oximetry in initiating NVS (the oximetry/NVS/MIE protocol).
    Introduction to and use of mouthpiece or nasal NVS can be facilitated by oximetry feedback. An O_2 sat alarm may be set at 94%. CO_2 will normalize and the patient sees that by taking deeper breaths, the O_2 sat will exceed 94%

within seconds. The patient is taught to use oximetry to gauge the depth of breaths needed to maintain normal O_2 sat and thereby, adequate CO_2 levels. If one cannot accomplish this by breathing without assistance, NVS is used until the O_2 sat normalizes. This oximetry feedback protocol facilitates optimal daytime use of NVS which helps to reset central ventilatory drive.

15. What is the difference between noninvasive ventilation (NIV) and NVS?
NIV has come to be synonymous with CPAP and bi-level PAP which are used to treat the central and obstructive apneas and hypopneas that are noted on polysomnograms. However, polysomnography is programmed to interpret all apneas and hypopneas as central and/or obstructive in nature and never due to the respiratory muscle weakness which is the cause for all patients with VPD. NVS utilizes full ventilatory support settings, that is, volume preset at 700 to 1500 mL a rate of 10 to 12 or pressure preset at about 20 cm H_2O to optimally rest and totally support the inspiratory muscles.

16. When do you initiate nocturnal NVS for patients with hypoventilation, e.g., Duchenne muscular dystrophy (DMD)?
You initiate nocturnal NVS for patients with hypoventilation, e.g., Duchenne muscular dystrophy (DMD) when patients have symptoms of ventilatory insufficiency and some combination of the following: hypercapnia ($EtCO_2$ >47 mm Hg) during sleep with diminished VC, a mean SpO_2 greater than 95% for longer than 5 minutes of sleep, multiple episodes of oxyhemoglobin desaturation during sleep, or CO_2 greater than 45 mm Hg when awake. All infants and small children with paradoxical breathing also require sleep NVS to promote lung growth and prevent chest deformity.

Al-Qadi MO. Disorders of the chest wall clinical manifestations. *Clin Chest Med.* 2018;39:361–375. Available at: https://doi.org/10.1016/j.ccm.2018.01.010

Bach JR, Bianchi C. Prevention of pectus excavatum for children with spinal muscular atrophy type 1. *Am J Phys Med Rehabil.* 2003;82(10):815–819. DOI: 10.1097/01.PHM.0000083669.22483.04.

17. What is glossopharyngeal breathing (GPB)? Why is it called "frog breathing"?
The patient is instructed to take a deep breath and then augment it by projecting boluses of air into the lungs with pumping action of the pharynx. The air is pushed by the tongue through the glottis which closes with each "gulp." One breath usually consists of 6 to 8 gulps of 60 to 200 mL each. During training, GPB efficiency is monitored by spirometrically measuring the subsequent exhalation of the air and dividing by the number of gulps to determine the milliliters of air per gulp and breaths per minute. A GPB rate of 12 to 14 breaths/min can provide patients with little or no VC with normal tidal volumes, minute ventilation, and hours of ventilator-free breathing ability. This technique is called **"frog breathing"** because frogs ventilate their lungs in this manner because they do not have diaphragms.

18. When is tracheotomy indicated?
- For chronic ventilatory failure AND when MIE-exsufflation flows are ineffective (generally below 130 L/m) and when O_2 sat is persistently less than 95% in ambient air despite up to continuous NVS (CNVS) and optimal use of MIE (at 40 to 60 cm H_2O pressures). MIE-exsufflation flows are rarely ineffective except for patients with upper motor neuron disease who have inadequate patency of the upper airways.
- For ventilatory support of mentally incompetent or uncooperative patients or who require ongoing heavy sedation or narcotics
- Ventilatory failure due to severe intrinsic lung disease
- Ventilatory failure and substance abuse or uncontrollable seizures
- Ventilatory failure and conditions that interfere with the use of NVS interfaces

Bach JR, Bianchi C, Aufiero E. Oximetry and indications for tracheostomy for amyotrophic lateral sclerosis. *Chest.* 2004;126:1502–1507. https://pubmed.ncbi.nlm.nih.gov/15539719/

19. What are the risks and benefits of oxygen therapy for hypoventilation? What are the alternatives?
Hypercapnia severe enough to result in hypoxia with oxyhemoglobin saturation decreasing below 95% is treated by ventilatory assistance/support, not oxygen. Oxygen exacerbates hypercapnia and hypoventilation. There are no benefits because supplemental O_2 renders NVS ineffective, thereby causing exacerbation of hypercapnia by both the **Haldane effect** and directly by exacerbating hypoventilation. Although oxygen therapy is routinely given to virtually all ventilator users whether or not they are hypoxic, for patients with VPD its use is tantamount to putting a band aid on a cancer. Oxygen therapy depresses ventilatory drive, exacerbates hypercapnia, prevents the use of oximetry feedback to signal hypoventilation, increases hypoventilation symptoms like daytime drowsiness, nightmares, and depression, and can render the nocturnal use of nasal or mouthpiece NVS ineffective. Hypercapnic patients who are treated with oxygen therapy can have their CO_2 levels increase by over 100 mmHg, go into almost immediate respiratory arrest, and require emergency intubation.

O_2 can only be provided safely to hypercapnic patients who are intubated and, thereby, whose alveolar ventilation can be controlled.

The alternative to normalizing O_2 levels for hypercapnic patients is to normalize them by providing up to CNVS and MIE before considering oxygen therapy and intubation.

Chiou M, Bach JR, Saporito LR, et al. Quantitation of Oxygen-induced hypercapnia in respiratory pump failure. *Rev Port Pneumol (Port J Pulmonol)*. 2016;22(5):262–265. doi: 10.1016/j.rppnen.2016.03.005.

20. What is the difference between CPAP and BiPAP?

    Continuous positive airway pressure (CPAP) delivered via a CPAP mask provides a pneumatic splint that maintains airway patency during sleep and allows the patient with obstructive sleep apneas to effectively ventilate using his or her own muscles. **Bi-level positive airway pressure (BiPAP)** permits **independent adjustment of inspiratory (IPAP)** and expiratory positive airway pressures (EPAP): the greater the IPAP/EPAP difference (span), the greater the inspiratory muscle support. Spans of about 20 cm H_2O are required for effective respiratory muscle rest and for ventilatory support (NVS) for patients with normal lung compliance. However, EPAP is always counterproductive for hypoventilation due to neuromuscular weakness so rather than use bi-level PAP of IPAP 24 and EPAP 4 cm H_2O, pressure control of 20 cm H_2O with no EPAP is more comfortable and effective.

21. List five maxims regarding use of intubation and tracheostomy in the rehabilitation of ventilatory failure.

    1. Endotracheal intubation is unnecessary for managing most cases of uncomplicated acute ventilatory failure (acute CNVS and MIE dependence).
    2. Endotracheal suctioning is often less effective than MIE via an invasive airway tube since MIE creates high expiratory flows to clear both lung fields whereas suctioning usually only enters the right mainstem bronchus.
    3. Intubation and tracheostomy are neither needed nor desired by patients with VPD due to myopathic or lower motor neuron disease as opposed to using up to continuous CNVS and MIE to prolong life. For these patients MIE-expiration flows remain effective and CNVS can always be used. Tracheostomies are only needed for ventilatory support when the upper airway is insufficiently patent, and that only occurs for some patients with upper motor neuron disease or disease of the CNS.
    4. Oxygen should never be used as a substitute for NVS and MIE.
    5. Rehabilitation is not complete for any ventilator user who has not been evaluated for tracheostomy tube removal and had the tube removed when MIE-exsufflation flows permit, irrespective of the extent of respiratory muscle failure or ventilator dependence.

    Physical medicine alternatives to the invasive measures of endotracheal intubation, tracheotomy, and airway suctioning are cheaper, safer, more comfortable, and greatly preferred by patients with VPD and deserve wider application.

KEY POINTS: NONINVASIVE PULMONARY REHABILITATION

1. Signs of successful noninvasive pulmonary rehabilitation are decreased respiratory rate and accessory respiratory muscle use, increased chest expansion, normalization of $EtCO_2$ and O_2 sat, relief of dyspnea, and decreased hospitalization rates.
2. Ventilatory impairment and oxygenation impairment need to be evaluated and managed differently.
3. Respiratory muscle aids can substitute for inspiratory and expiratory muscle function but not for the function of bulbar-innervated muscles.
4. Nasal ventilation is introduced to treat symptoms of nocturnal hypoventilation and patients increase its use as needed and can use it continuously for full ventilatory support without ever being hospitalized.
5. Polysomnograms diagnose central and obstructive apneas, not symptoms due to muscle weakness. This is like blaming the brain and throat for what the diaphragm cannot do.

OBSTRUCTIVE DISEASES (OXYGENATION IMPAIRMENT)

22. What causes COPD and how do you diagnose and follow it?

    Obstructive pulmonary diseases are characterized by an obstructive pattern of expiratory airflow limitation on pulmonary function testing. Obstructed expiratory airflow is caused by a narrowing of the respiratory lumen caused by: excess mucus production; bronchial wall inflammation with a resultant thickening, obstructing the lumen; or dynamic expiratory collapse of the wall due to weakness caused by destruction of supporting structures. Expiratory airflow limitation is heard as a **wheeze,** and the airway collapse produces air trapping and **chest hyper-expansion**.

The most common **obstructive pulmonary diseases** are COPD comprising chronic bronchitis and emphysema; asthmatic bronchitis; bronchiectasis; cystic fibrosis.

Causes and "triggers" of COPD exacerbation include:

- Cigarette smoking—#1 cause of COPD in USA
- Air pollutants—smoke
- Genetic—α1-antitripsin deficiency—think "early onset" emphysema or COPD in a non-smoker; multiple genes in cystic fibrosis
- Chronic pulmonary infections—bronchopneumonia; Staph Aureus in children—bronchiectasis
- Other environmental factors—allergens and "cold" in asthma

Smokers are 3.5 to 25 times more likely (depending on the amounts smoked) to die of COPD than non-smokers.

23. What is the difference between emphysema and chronic bronchitis?

Chronic bronchitis is a "clinical" diagnosis based on the volume of daily mucus production over months and years cleared by cough and typified by acute exacerbations, often infective, and relatively quiescent remissions. Excess mucus, resulting from an increased number and size of the mucus-secreting **goblet cells** (**Reid index**—ratio between the thickness of the submucosal mucus-secreting glands and the thickness between the epithelium and the cartilage that covers the bronchi) that are stimulated by elements in tobacco smoke and infection, blocks airways causing obstruction. Mucus plugging leads to ventilation/perfusion mismatching and can progress to significant hypoxemia, marked hypercapnia, pulmonary hypertension and right heart failure—**cor-pulmonale**—the classic "***blue bloater***"—dyspneic, cyanotic and volume overloaded.

Emphysema is a "pathological" diagnosis based on evidence of airway destruction distal to the terminal bronchiole on high resolution lung CT scan or lung biopsy (now rarely done). Elements in tobacco smoke activate proteases that cause destruction of elastins and supportive tissues in the lung interstitium, leaving bronchial walls unsupported and prone to expiratory collapse, causing obstruction. There is no ventilation/perfusion mismatching due to the equal destruction of respiratory epithelium and vasculature, resulting in significant hypoxemia, mild hypercapnia, and air trapping (**pursed lips breathing**) increases internal airway pressure during exhalation to "splint" the airways open to allow exhalation)—the classic "***pink puffer***"—dyspneic, non-cyanotic, barrel chested.

In general practice, patients often display a mixed overlap syndrome of chronic bronchitis and emphysema. Over time, "pure asthma" can progress to develop features of asthmatic bronchitis, which retains some responsiveness to bronchodilators. Bronchiectasis similarly may present with features resembling chronic bronchitis.

24. How can you estimate the prognosis and plan interventions for patients with COPD?

Life expectancy in COPD is strongly correlated with pulmonary function tests (PFTs). The forced expiratory volume in one second (**FEV$_1$**) **is the best predictor:** 30% die within a year with an FEV$_1$ less than 750 cc, and 50% within 3 years.

Survival is also negatively impacted by ongoing **tobacco use, failure to vaccinate** as recommended against flu and pneumonia, **poor nutrition** status and **limited mobility.**

Elevated dyspnea rating, whilst more subjective, has also been shown to correlate with poor survival, as have features of **cor pulmonale** and more extensive disease on chest CT.

Functional prognosis, quality of life and self-rated disability tend to be worse in emphysema than chronic bronchitis.

A negative psychological state and **depression** (common in COPD) also portend poor functional prognosis.

25. Who are candidates for pulmonary rehabilitation (PR)?

Patients with COPD are selected for PR based on symptoms, function and quality of life. For insurance eligibility, a diagnosis of COPD must be confirmed with PFTs indicating the FEV$_1$/forced vital capacity (FVC) $\leq$0.70. Symptoms supportive of the need for PR include dyspnea on exertion, cough, weakness, and limited endurance. Difficulty completing activities of daily living, limited community ambulation, difficulty handling steps, and social isolation strongly support the need for PR. Ideally patients should be "tobacco-free", psychologically oriented, and motivated to comply with the entire program.

Transfer to PR following hospitalization for acute COPD exacerbation is a great opportunity to speed recovery and redesign chronic treatment. PR is very under-utilized with referral rates less than 3% in the 6 months following discharge. Early referral when patients can benefit and change disease and functional course is critical.

Exclusion criteria for outpatient PR include medical instability, physical limitations that preclude participation in the PR program, active smoking with a no-quit plan, and psycho-social barriers, including lack of motivation. Other barriers include failure to refer, availability and accessibility of a PR program, and insurance coverage.

Cornelison SD, Pascual RM. Pulmonary rehabilitation in the management of chronic lung disease. *Med Clin North Am*. 2019 May;103(3):577–584. DOI: 10.1016/j.mcna.2018.12.015

26. Why use clinical exercise testing?

Clinical exercise testing (ET) is ideally done with a treadmill **cardio-pulmonary exercise test (CPET)** and provides PFT, oxygen saturation, EKG/cardiac and metabolic fitness data, including **anaerobic threshold** and

maximal oxygen consumption. Bike and upper body ergometer protocols exist when needed. Standard ET is acceptable if no metabolic cart is available. A **six-minute walk test (6MWT)** is appropriate in patients who cannot tolerate standard ET equipment.

Clinical ET allows for the differentiation of impairment due to pulmonary or cardiac disorders and the degree of physiologic deconditioning present. Safety for exercise can be determined, and the data interpretation enables an initial exercise intensity to be prescribed. Serial ET allows for the documentation of fitness and functional progress and the recalibration of ongoing exercise training intensity.

American Thoracic Society, American College of Chest Physicians. American Thoracic Society (ATS) and the American College of Chest Physicians (ACCP) statement on cardiopulmonary exercise testing. *Am J Respir Crit Care Med.* 2003 Jan 15;167(2):211–217. DOI: 10.1164/rccm.167.2.211

27. What medical strategies are used to manage patients with lung disease and primarily oxygenation impairment?

Adequate oxygenation cannot occur with airway obstruction from mucus plugging or bronchoconstriction. **Secretion clearance** utilizes general oral hydration, humidified air oxygen, mucolytics and expectorants, breathing and coughing techniques, appropriate use of vibratory respiratory devices (chest vest, aerobikA, acapella, and lung flute). Bronchoconstriction is managed with breathing techniques (e.g., pursed lips breathing, bronchodilators), inhaler or nebulizer, anti-inflammatories, and anti-allergic medications. **Oxygen therapy** is indicated if PaO_2 is less than 55 to 60 mm Hg, O_2 sats less than 88% at rest or on exertion. Use caution when ordering oxygen at rest. Hypoxic patients can lose consciousness from CO_2 retention due to reduced hypoxic respiratory drive. Voluntary override and other factors drive respiration during exertion. Therefore, prescribe a flow rate that maintains O_2 sats greater than 88% with rehabilitation training.

28. Outline a sample rehabilitation prescription for a patient with COPD. Name the seven major components.

The rehabilitation prescription for a patient with COPD must start with **patient identification** and medical condition: patient **name, age, sex, diagnoses,** and **comorbidities.**

1. **Goals**—improve strength and endurance, reduce dyspnea at rest and on exertion, enhance secretion clearance, improve tolerance of activities of daily living, increase ambulation distance and promote community integration and resumption of avocational/vocational roles. Psychosocial goals include reduction in anxiety and resumption of interpersonal relationships including intimacy. Long-term compliance with medications/medical regimen, nutrition and exercise plans. Enhanced quality of life and reduced medical burden are also expected.
2. **Precautions**—maintain O_2 sats greater than 88%. Standard indications to terminate exercise therapy include hemodynamic instability, evidence of exercise-induced ischemia, complex arrhythmia, and cardiac failure. Highlight comorbidities that impact safety with exercise—balance, vision, cognition, etc.
3. **Respiratory therapy**—train in the correct use of medication inhalers and nebulizers. Promote secretion clearance through coordination of medication use, coughing and pursed lips, diaphragmatic breathing techniques, and use of secretion-clearing respiratory devices. Integrate breathing techniques during exercise. Titrate ncO2 use to maintain O_2 sats greater than 88%. Educate in "community" use of oxygen—sleeping, at rest, outdoors. Dyspnea management to minimize its psychological impact.
4. **Physical Therapy**—complete an intake evaluation including review of pre-program CPET and gross mobility, including 6MWT, Timed Up and Go Test (TUG) and Berg balance to set initial exercise program and intensity and plan progression. Train in use of Borg Rate of Perceived Exertion Scale (RPE=1 to 20). Reinforce correct use of oxygen and breathing and pacing techniques. Focus on body mechanics, posture and balance training as well as generalized strength training. Progress multi-modality aerobic training with goal of 3x/week, 60 minutes of moderate intensity exercise with RPE goal of 12 to 14.
5. **Occupational Therapy**—educate in energy conservation and pacing techniques. Focus therapy to promote independence in ADLs and IADLs (activities required for independent living). Integrate breathing and relaxation techniques to daily activities and evaluate for cognitive deficits. Promote avocational and vocational activities and psychosocial reintegration and intimacy.
6. **Psychological support**—train in dyspnea and anxiety management. Provide psychosocial support and evaluate for cognitive deficits. Guide peer-group interaction and support. Promote lifelong compliance with healthy lifestyle.
7. **Nutrition therapy**—identify nutritional deficiencies and educate in ideal calorie and dietary composition. Monitor body weight and modify diet throughout the program to promote increased lean strong muscle mass.

29. What methods can be used to assist the patient in airway secretion elimination?

Breathing techniques: coughing; **huff-coughing**—gentle forced expiratory flows through a partially closed glottis; **active cycle of breathing**—a three-phase technique; **autogenic drainage**—"self-drainage" using gravity and air flow to advance mucus.

Chest PT: percussion—tapping, cupping, vibration; postural drainage.

Simple respiratory devices: incentive spirometer to promote deep breathing/chest expansion; oscillating positive expiratory pressure devices—flutter, acapella, aerobikA, lung flute.

Advanced respiratory devices: chest vest—high-frequency chest wall oscillation using an inflatable vest; cough assistance with an insufflator-exsufflator.

Cox NS, Oliveira CC, Lahham A, et al. Pulmonary rehabilitation referral and participation are commonly influenced by environment, knowledge, and beliefs about consequences: a systematic review using the Theoretical Domains Framework. *J Physiother.* 2017 Apr;63(2):84–93. Available at: https://doi.org/10.1016/j.jphys.2017.02.002

30. When should supplemental oxygen therapy be used?

Oxygen therapy reduces mortality when used appropriately in patients with COPD and hypoxemia with PO_2 less than 55 mm Hg or O_2 sat less than 88%.

Long term domiciliary oxygen therapy in chronic hypoxic cor pulmonale complicating chronic bronchitis and emphysema. Report of the Medical Research Council Working Party. *Lancet.* 1981 Mar 28;1(8222):681–686. Available at: https://doi.org/10.1016/S0140-6736(81)91970-X

Increased life expectancy is due to reduction in pulmonary hypertension and right heart failure and is directly correlated with duration of use.

Other benefits include improved strength, reduced fatigue and improved cognitive function.

Nocturnal hypoxemia detected by overnight oximetry should be managed judiciously with supplemental oxygen in patients with documented hypercapnia.

Continuous or nocturnal oxygen therapy in hypoxemic chronic obstructive lung disease: a clinical trial. Nocturnal Oxygen Therapy Trial Group. *Ann Intern Med.* 1980 Sep;93(3):391–398. DOI: 10.7326/0003-4819-93-3-391

31. Should supplemental oxygen be used by COPD patients on commercial airlines?

Commercial airliners are pressurized at 8,000-10,000 feet above sea level and as such, patients with COPD and borderline oxygen saturations at sea level might require supplemental oxygen in-flight. For longer flights, over 5 hours, the more likely the need. If saturations fall less than 92%, oxygen should be started. Typically, in those not using supplemental oxygen at baseline, **1 L is sufficient** to maintain adequate O_2 sats. Otherwise, the rule of thumb is **1 to 2 L over normal flow rates** for patients on chronic oxygen.

Barreiro E, Bustamante V, Cejudo P, et al. Guidelines for the evaluation and treatment of muscle dysfunction in patients with chronic obstructive pulmonary disease. *Arch Bronconeumol.* 2015 Aug;51(8):384–395. DOI: 10.1016/j.arbres.2015.04.011

32. Can ventilatory muscles be trained?

The bellows pump system can be optimized with the fullest range and strength of inspiratory muscles and active expiratory muscle force. Exercise training of weak musculature is most effective in stable well-nourished patients.

Use of **inspiratory resistance loading** in moderate COPD during three, thirty breath sessions per day over a 2-month period increased negative inspiratory force, endurance of aerobic exercise, and tolerance. Supraphysiologic resistance may recruit and strengthen accessory muscles increasing muscle mass for endurance.

Langer D, Ciavaglia C, Faisal A, et al. Inspiratory muscle training reduces diaphragm activation and dyspnea during exercise in COPD. *J Appl Physiol.* Submitted December 8, 2017; accepted in final form March 9, 2018; 125(2):381–392. doi:10.1152/japplphysiol.01078.2017.

33. How should reconditioning exercises be prescribed?

Reconditioning exercises are **"task-specific"** but **cross-training** using different aerobic machines is beneficial for general endurance and all functional tasks. Land-based, anti-gravity exercise produces more significant functional reconditioning than pool-based activities. **Walking and stair climbing** should be the focus of functional reconditioning training in PR for COPD as they translate best into meaningful functional gains. Often basic strength training, using body weight against gravity, resistance bands, free weights, and resistance machines, is required as a prelude to conditioning training. On initiation of PR, brief periods of low intensity exercise interspersed with rest is recommended as endurance is often significantly limited. Duration and intensity are progressed slowly with **a goal of 60 minutes of moderate intensity exercise**—RPE 12 to 14. Adhering to a training heart rate (HR) can sometimes be misleading due to resting sinus tachycardia and the impact of sympathomimetic medications on HR. Frequency of training is two to three times a week on outpatient PR, increasing to four to five times a week after completion. Additionally, patients should be encouraged to continually increase their daily activity through walking and stair climbing.

34. What are the benefits of PR?
    Reduction in dyspnea
    Improved strength and endurance—improved VO$_2$max
    Increased ambulation distance on 6MWT
    Greater independence with ADLs
    Enhanced mood—improved anxiety and depression
    Social re-engagement
    Fewer COPD exacerbations, fewer pulmonary infections
    Reduced health care utilization—office visits, hospitalizations and overall healthcare costs
    Prolonged survival

Pulmonary rehabilitation. Up To Date. Jul 12, 2018. Celli, B. Available at: https://www.uptodate.com/contents/pulmonary-rehabilitation/print

Schroff P, Hitchcock J, Schumann C, et al. Pulmonary rehabilitation improves outcomes in chronic obstructive pulmonary disease independent of disease burden. *Ann Am Thorac Soc.* 2017 Jan;14(1):26–32. DOI: 10.1513/AnnalsATS.201607-5510C

35. What is exercise-induced asthma (EIA)?
    Airflow obstruction can occur during exercise due to **exercise-induced bronchoconstriction (EIB)**, also known as **exercise-induced asthma**. Symptoms include coughing, shortness of breath on exertion, wheezing and chest tightness. Other triggers are pollution, high pollen or allergen counts, irritants, including smoke and fumes, and a recent cold or asthma episode. Close to 90% of people who have asthma will experience EIB. Exercises most likely to trigger EIA include: activities in cold/dry weather (i.e., ice hockey, skiing, ice skating, and snowboarding), sports that need constant activity, long distance running, soccer, etc.

    Symptoms do not occur immediately on initiation of exercise but begin during exercise and may worsen even after stopping exercise, typically **resolving 30 minutes after exercise cessation**. A later phase of less severe symptoms 4 to 12 hours after stopping exercise is observed, **taking up to 24 hours to resolve**.

Kofler T, Daikeler T, Prince SS, et al. "Exercise induced asthma" is not always asthma. *Respir Med Case Rep.* 2018; 24:138–142, Available at: https://doi.org/10.1016/j.rmcr.2018.05.015

Stempel DA. The pharmacologic management of childhood asthma. *Pediatr Clin North Am.* 2003;50:609–629.

36. What is the best available predictor of survival in patients with Cystic Fibrosis?
    The forced expiratory volume in 1 second (FEV$_1$) is the best single predictor of survival. Patients with CF and an FEV$_1$ less than 30% of the predicted value, have a 50% 2-year mortality.

Yankaskas JR, Marshall BC, Sufian B, et al. Cystic fibrosis adult care: consensus conference report. *Chest.* 2004 Jan;125(1 Suppl):1S–39S. DOI: 10.1378/chest.125.1_suppl.1s

    Recently, models for the dynamic prediction for survival of people with CF have been developed using 16 key variables; whilst FEV$_1$ remains the strongest predictor, predictive performance is improved by incorporating additional variables, including body mass index, pancreatic function, and pulmonary infection profile.

Keogh RH, Seaman SR, Barrett JK, et al. Dynamic prediction of survival in cystic fibrosis: a landmarking analysis using UK patient registry data. *Epidemiology.* 2019 Jan;30(1):29–37. DOI: 10.1097/EDE.0000000000000920

BOOKS

Bach JR, ed. *Pulmonary rehabilitation: The obstructive and paralytic conditions.* Hanley & Belfus, 1996.

Casaburi R, Petty TL, eds. *Principles and Practice of Pulmonary Rehabilitation.* Philadelphia: W.B. Saunders; 1993.

Bonus questions and answers available online.

CHAPTER 62

CANCER REHABILITATION: FOCUS ON FUNCTIONAL QUALITY OF LIFE IN THE ONCOLOGIC POPULATION

Franchesca König, MD, Katarzyna Ibanez, MD, and Theresa A. Gillis, MD

You beat cancer by how you live, why you live, and in the manner in which you live.
— Stuart Scott, ESPN Broadcaster (1965–2015)

KEY POINTS

1. Dietz was the first to describe the four models of cancer rehabilitation, including prehabilitation, restorative rehabilitation, supportive rehabilitation, and palliative rehabilitation.
2. Evidence has supported improvement in functional status in patients with brain tumors and those with graft versus host disease undergoing acute inpatient rehabilitation. The most common cause of unplanned transfer has been shown to be infection.
3. Although evidence supports exercise interventions in patients undergoing active treatment in both the inpatient and outpatient settings, immunologic and hematologic effects as well as orthopedic precautions must be considered when prescribing the level of activity.
4. Long term sequelae of cancer treatments are common and can include weight gain, physical inactivity, cardiovascular disease, diabetes, cognitive dysfunction, premature menopause, infertility, osteoporosis, anthracycline-related cardiomyopathy, neuropathy, lymphedema sexual dysfunction, fatigue, second malignant neoplasms, chronic pain, musculoskeletal pain, depression, and anxiety.

1. What is the role of a cancer physiatrist?

A physiatrist specializing in cancer rehabilitation leads a multidisciplinary team including physical, occupational, speech, lymphedema and recreational therapists, nutritionists, social workers, mental health professionals, and nurses, among others, to provide rehabilitative care to patients with cancer throughout the course of their disease. A cancer physiatrist focuses on the assessment and management of musculoskeletal, neuromuscular, and functional complications of cancer and its treatments. Cancer physiatrists additionally work closely with the oncology team to determine achievable functional goals along the continuum of the patient's care.

2. What are the models for rehabilitation at different times during treatment?

Dietz was the first to describe the four models of cancer rehabilitation, including prehabilitation, restorative rehabilitation, supportive rehabilitation, and palliative rehabilitation. Prehabilitation focuses on the optimization of the patient's functional status prior to initiation of treatment, having the potential to decrease treatment-related comorbidities and increase treatment options. Restorative and supportive rehabilitation occurs during the treatment and post-treatment phase to address temporary or permanent functional deficits respectively. Palliative rehabilitation focuses on optimizing comfort and providing caregiver support.

3. What are special considerations for patients on active treatment?

Although evidence supports exercise interventions in patients undergoing active treatment, both immunologic and hematologic effects must be considered regarding the level of activity. For example, a patient with hemoglobin less than 8 g/dL should ideally be participating in short periods of symptom limited interventions with education on energy conservation.[1] Other values to be aware of include vital signs and blood counts (white blood cell count, platelets). There should be a low threshold to obtain ultrasound Doppler studies to rule out deep vein thromboses in patients exhibiting swelling in extremities. This may affect rehabilitation interventions as compression and manual therapies are contraindicated in patients with severe thrombocytopenia and those with thrombotic events that are not on anticoagulation treatment. Both liver and renal function should be considered as this may limit medical treatment with medications such as Acetaminophen and NSAIDs, which can additionally mask fever. In patients undergoing surgical interventions, post-surgical precautions, weight bearing status, and range of motion restrictions must be clarified with the surgeon to establish a rehabilitative plan of care. Furthermore, the use of modalities should be avoided in areas of disease, irradiated tissue, and hardware.

4. **A middle-aged female patient with history of left-sided breast cancer presents for evaluation of a sensation of "pins and needles" in her toes and fingertips after starting Paclitaxel 2 months ago. What is your leading diagnosis and plan for evaluation?**
Chemotherapy-induced peripheral neuropathy (CIPN) is the most common neuromuscular condition associated with cancer. Evaluation includes blood work to evaluate for other reversible causes, including impaired glucose tolerance, hypothyroidism, vitamin and nutritional deficiencies, among others. Additionally, electrodiagnostic studies can be performed, typically revealing a large fiber polyneuropathy. Commonly implicated include vinca alkaloids and taxanes, which disrupt axonal microtubules and result in a length-dependent neuropathy. Platinum-based compounds, such as Cisplatin and Oxaliplatin, exert their toxic effect on the dorsal root ganglia, producing a neuropathy that is not length dependent and predominantly affects large myelinated sensory fibers. Immune checkpoint inhibitors, such as nivolumab and pembrolizumab, have also been associated with generalized acute or subacute neuropathy. Overall, symptoms tend to be dose-dependent and cumulative. Patients typically experience sensory greater than motor symptoms in a symmetric, stocking-and-glove distribution. In many cases, there is gradual improvement over time after chemotherapy has been completed, however, it may continue to progress (described as a "coasting phenomenon" seen with platinum-based agents).

5. **What are neurologic paraneoplastic syndromes?**
A group of non-metastatic syndromes affecting any part of the central and peripheral nervous system that occur in patients with cancer, but not caused by direct invasion. Instead, they are thought to be induced by antigens expressed by tumor cells or as an immune response triggered by the cancer.[2] Clinical presentation often precedes the diagnosis of cancer and treatment of the malignancy may result in improvement of symptoms. Symptoms may include ataxia, pain, paresthesias, numbness, and weakness. Small cell lung carcinoma is one of the most common tumors associated with neurologic paraneoplastic syndromes, associated with Anti-Hu autoantibodies as seen in paraneoplastic encephalopathy and limbic encephalitis. Other examples include Lambert-Eaton syndrome (also associated with small cell lung cancer), myasthenia gravis (associated with thymoma), polymyositis and dermatomyositis (associated with ovarian, breast, and lung cancer) and stiff person syndrome (associated with breast cancer). Of note, patchy neurologic deficits may also manifest with leptomeningeal disease and biologic treatments such as chimeric antigen receptor T-cell therapy and immune checkpoint modulators. Leptomeningeal disease, or leptomeningeal carcinomatosis, refers to metastases to the meninges surrounding the brain and spinal cord.

6. **What are possible neuromuscular impacts of cancer treatment?**

Cancer Treatment	*Neuromuscular Impact*
Chemotherapy (i.e., vinca alkaloids, taxanes, platins)	Neuropathy
	Myopathy (cisplatin, fluorouracil)
Radiation therapy	Myelopathy
	Radiculopathy
	Plexopathy
	Neuropathy
	Myopathy
Oral immunosuppressants (i.e., prednisone)	Myopathy
Immunotherapy	Myasthenia Gravis (exacerbation and de novo)
	AIDP
	CIDP
	Inflammatory myositis
Surgery	Cranial/peripheral nerve and muscle damage (mechanical)

7. **What is radiation therapy? How does it cause radiation fibrosis syndrome (RFS)?**
Radiation therapy focuses on the use of ionizing radiation for the treatment of cancer. The basic unit is the gray (Gy). There are two main forms of radiation therapy (RT) delivery—external beam RT (radiation source distant from tumor, i.e., stereotactic body radiation, intensity modulated radiation therapy) and internal RT (placing radioactive sources inside of tumors, i.e., brachytherapy). Radiation source may be photons (x-rays, gamma rays), electrons, or protons. Radiation can cause direct DNA or indirect tissue damage through the production of reactive oxygen and nitrogen species which, in turn, leads to an inflammatory state within the radiation field, impacting all structures in its path including soft tissue, muscle, nerves, lymphatics, bone, vessels, among others. A well-described presentation of RFS in patients with head and neck cancer is dropped head syndrome (DHS); this is caused by cervical neck extensor weakness, leading to the inability to maintain the head in a normal upright position.[2]

8. You are performing electrodiagnostic studies for a patient with suspected post-radiation brachial plexopathy. What features would help you distinguish this from a plexopathy caused by tumor infiltration?

   Myokymic discharges and fasciculation potentials suggest radiation-induced plexopathy. It has traditionally been described that radiation plexopathies tend to preferentially affect the upper trunk whereas neoplastic plexopathies more commonly involve the lower trunk; however, studies have suggested that plexus involvement may be more diffuse in both etiologies.[2] Clinically, radiation plexopathy is classically delayed in onset with symptoms of weakness and paresthesias usually being progressive. Pain tends to be more common in neoplastic plexopathies. Of note, if recurrence is suspected, imaging, including MRI and/or PET scans, is warranted.

9. You are asked to evaluate a 50-year-old woman with right-sided breast cancer for swelling and heaviness in her right arm. What are common causes and what rehabilitation interventions have been found effective in controlling symptoms?

   Lymphedema is a pathologic condition of the lymphatic system that occurs due to lymphatic blockade secondary to tumor obstruction, surgery, or radiation therapy. It can occur not only in breast cancer, but also in head and neck cancers and gynecological cancers, affecting the face/neck and pelvis/legs, respectively.[2] Prior to starting treatment, other causes of edema should be ruled out, including deep vein thromboses. The standard of care for lymphedema, complete decongestive therapy (CDT), consists of short stretch bandaging with gradual transition to compression garments, and manual lymphatic drainage, a specialized massage technique with the purpose of directing lymph fluid to non-obstructed areas. For patients with significant functional impairment, surgical techniques—including lymphatic revascularization to increase the capacity of the lymphatic system to drain lymph—can be considered.

10. What is post-mastectomy pain syndrome (PMPS)?

    PMPS is described as persistent pain following any breast surgery including mastectomy, lumpectomy, sentinel/axillary lymph node dissection, and breast reconstruction. Diagnosis is one of exclusion in patients experiencing pain for more than 3 months postoperatively. Etiologies of pain include surgical interruption to the intercostobrachial nerve, incisional pain, phantom breast pain, musculoskeletal pain, and neuroma pain. Other differentials to consider include tumor recurrence, infection, rib and sternal fracture, among others.[3] Management of PMPS includes myofascial mobilization, early desensitization techniques, stretching (specifically the pectoralis muscles and latissimus dorsi), range of motion (cervical, shoulder, and scapula), strengthening shoulder girdle muscles, and pharmacologic interventions when indicated. These may include NSAIDs and co-analgesics such as gabapentinoids and anti-depressants. It is important to note, however, the potential drug-drug interaction between Tamoxifen and some anti-depressants, including Duloxetine, which may decrease the effect of Tamoxifen.

11. A patient with breast cancer presents to your clinic for evaluation of diffuse arthralgias. She was recently started on Anastrozole. What is your differential diagnosis?

    Differentials include degenerative arthropathies, inflammatory arthropathies, metastatic disease, fibromyalgia, and aromatase inhibitor (AI) induced arthralgia. AI induced arthralgia is a frequently observed phenomenon in patients taking AIs as part of adjuvant treatment for breast cancer. It can be seen in up to 50% to 82% of patients on treatment.[2] The pathophysiology remains unknown; however, it is thought that the estrogen depletion produced by AI is the most likely underlying mechanism.[2] Patients usually present with diffuse morning stiffness and joint discomfort. Symptom onset is generally observed within the first 2 months of starting treatment and can worsen during the first year of treatment, typically stabilizing thereafter. It is important to rule out other causes, as AI treatment usually lasts from 5 to 10 years. Studies have shown that patients with diffuse symptoms experience relief with physical activity, including yoga and aquatic exercise.

12. What is trismus and how is it treated?

    Trismus, or restricted mouth opening, is often seen in head and neck cancers as a complication of tumor infiltration itself or treatment. This includes surgery and radiation therapy in field including the nasopharynx and oral cavity. Jaw contracture can be severe and lead to difficulty eating, speaking, drinking, and performing oral hygiene. Early recognition is key. Patients benefit from a multidisciplinary approach including physiatry, physical therapy, speech therapy, and dental services. Jaw stretching devices allow for passive prolonged stretch. Dental clearance must be obtained prior to the use of such devices. Botulinum toxin injections have also been found to be of potential benefit.

13. What functional impairments can result after neck dissection?

    There are three main types of neck dissection surgeries. Radical neck dissections clear all ipsilateral lymph nodes as well as the spinal accessory nerve (SAN), internal jugular vein (IJV), and sternocleidomastoid muscle (SCM). Modified radical neck dissections clear all ipsilateral lymph nodes in the neck, but preserve the SAN, IJV, and SCM. Selective neck dissections clear selected lymph node regions, while also preserving the SAN, IJV, and SCM. Functional impairments often include neuropathic and myofascial pain, face and neck lymphedema, decreased cervical range of motion, and trapezius weakness from spinal accessory neuropathy, leading to scapular dyskinesia and rotator cuff impingement.

14. What is graft versus host disease (GvHD)?

GvHD is a T-cell mediated immune response of donor tissue to host occurring in approximately 30% to 70% of patients who receive a hematopoietic stem cell transplantation (HSCT).[3] It can affect multiple organ systems including the skin/fascia, gastrointestinal, pulmonary, hepatic, ocular, and oral mucosal systems. Patients are initially treated with high-dose steroids. Complications of GvHD may include decreased stamina, joint contractures, lymphedema, myositis, myasthenia gravis, among others.

15. You are consulted on a patient admitted to the hospital for GvHD after a bone marrow transplant. The patient is on high-dose glucocorticoid therapy and is experiencing proximal greater than distal weakness in his lower extremities. What is a common complication of high-dose steroid use?

Steroid myopathy is commonly seen in patients on high-dose glucocorticoid immunosuppression. While the pathophysiology is not fully understood, there is a predilection for type 2 skeletal muscle fiber involvement, for which electrodiagnostic studies are typically normal. Risk increases with dose and duration of use. Patients on doses of 40 to 60 mg/day for at least 1 month will experience some degree of muscular weakness.[3] Patients typically experience painless proximal muscle weakness with a tendency to affect the hip girdle muscles followed by the shoulder girdle.

16. What are the most common primary brain tumors? Metastatic tumor?

The most common primary brain tumors in adults are meningiomas and glioblastomas; for children, they are astrocytomas and medulloblastomas. The most common tumors to metastasize to the brain are lung and breast. 80% of brain metastases are supratentorial, while 15% affect the cerebellum and 5% affect the brainstem.

17. What are the most common malignant bone tumors?

Metastatic bone tumors account for more than 40 times more cases than all primary bone tumors combined. Breast cancer accounts for most of these, with an incidence of 50% to 85%. Prostate carcinoma is the most common primary tumor for metastatic lesions in men, with bone metastases occurring in more than 90% of patients with advanced disease. Lung, renal, bladder, thyroid, and gastrointestinal primaries have an incidence of 20% to 40% of bone metastases. Myeloma is the most common primary malignant tumor of bone in adults, arising within the bone marrow from plasma cells. The most predominant primary malignant bone tumors in children include osteosarcoma, Ewing's sarcoma, and primitive neuroectodermal tumors.

18. Discuss the difference between osteoblastic and osteolytic lesions.

Normal bone remodeling involves the synchronous process of osteoclastic bone resorption and osteoblastic bone deposition. Cancerous bone lesions are characterized by the abnormal regulation of this process. Radiographic evidence can help with differentiating the type of lesion.[2]

Osteoblastic Lesions	Osteolytic Lesions	Mixed Lesions
Prostate	Renal cell	Breast
Lung	Melanoma	Gastrointestinal
	Thyroid	

19. When is bone susceptible to pathologic fractures?

Pathologic fractures occur in approximately 9% to 29% of patients with bone metastases, most commonly in patients with multiple myeloma. These types of fractures are more common in osteolytic metastases compared to osteoblastic lesions. Mirels criteria is a weighted scoring system used to quantify the risk of sustaining a fracture.[2] The scoring system is based on 4 parameters—anatomic location of the lesion, severity of pain, size of the lesion relative to diameter of the bone, and nature of the lesion (lytic, blastic, or mixed). Each parameter is assigned a score of 1 to 3 with a maximum total score of 12. Higher scores correlate to greater chance of suffering a fracture. Patients with score greater than or equal to 9 warrant prophylactic surgical fixation.

Mirels Scoring Criteria

Score	1	2	3
Site	Upper Limb	Lower Limb	Peritrochanteric
Pain	Mild	Moderate	Increased with activity
Lesion	Blastic	Mixed	Lytic
Size	<1/3	1/3–2/3	>2/3

20. You are evaluating a patient with multiple thoracolumbar compression fractures related to his primary diagnosis of multiple myeloma. What conservative measures may be helpful for this patient?

If the patient has no neurological deficits or mechanical instability, then initial conservative management is reasonable. Multiple myeloma treatment should help with symptoms as well. Pain medication regimen and overall bone health should be optimized. Bisphosphonates, commonly used in patients with multiple myeloma, reduce the risk of pathological fractures, can assist with pain management, and help control hypercalcemia. Spine bracing helps to achieve postural correction and limit movement. Spine precautions should be reiterated: avoiding spine flexion or extension, twisting, and lifting. Physical therapy for core strengthening and postural training can be helpful.

21. What is the most common initial symptom in patients with spine tumors?
The most common initial symptom is pain, followed by weakness. Localized pain results from tumor causing periosteal stretching and inflammation.[3] It is often worse at night and improves with activity and anti-inflammatory medications, such as corticosteroids. Mechanical pain is exacerbated by movement, changes in position, or axial load on the spine. Mechanical pain is unlikely to respond to steroids or radiation and may require surgical stabilization. Radicular pain indicates nerve root involvement.

22. Discuss the different types of spine tumors.
Spinal tumors are divided into extradural, intradural extramedullary, and intradural intramedullary. Extradural tumors are commonly metastatic in nature. Intradural extramedullary tumors arise outside of the spinal cord itself, but within the dura, such as meningiomas, schwannomas, neurofibromas as well as leptomeningeal disease. Intradural intramedullary tumors are located within the spinal cord parenchyma, most commonly ependymomas and astrocytomas.[3]

23. What workup is required for spine tumors?
History and physical examination should be performed first. MRI with gadolinium contrast is the best imaging modality to diagnose spinal lesions with most of the tumors showing post-contrast enhancement. CT provides detailed bony anatomy. Myelogram may be needed to identify compressed neural structures. Imaging of the chest, abdomen, and pelvis is necessary when metastatic disease is suspected. Labs may include CBC, CMP, PSA, CEA, serum and urine protein electrophoresis. Genetic testing may be needed. Biopsy is needed for diagnosis in patients with or without prior cancer history or unknown primary tumor. Following imaging lumbar puncture may be needed in patients with suspected intradural disease.[3]

24. You are evaluating a 67-year-old male who completed radiation treatment for a thoracic ependymoma 1 month ago. Physical examination is notable for an uncomfortable electrical sensation running down his back with cervical flexion. He is otherwise neurologically intact. What is the most likely diagnosis?
Most likely diagnosis is acute transient radiation myelopathy (ATRM), typically manifesting soon after completion of radiation and resolving over weeks to months.[3] It's presumably caused by dorsal column demyelination. Lhermitte's sign as described in the vignette is typically a sole symptom and indicates dorsal column involvement in cervical and upper thoracic spine. MRI spine should be considered to rule out other causes if clinically indicated.

25. What is "chemobrain" and what can be done about it?
"Chemobrain" or "chemofog" is used by patients to describe cognitive problems potentially persisting long after completion of cancer treatment. Cognitive dysfunction is reported by up to 90% of patients with history of brain tumors, up to 75% of patients treated for breast cancer and up to 30% of patients' post-leukemia therapy. The mechanisms by which chemotherapy affects cognition are still being investigated. Behavioral and pharmacological treatments have shown to result in improved cognition, quality of life, and coping.

26. Describe long-term survivor issues.
Health problems following cancer treatment are common. Long-term side effects vary depending on the type of cancer and treatment modalities used. For example, post-breast cancer treatment long term sequelae include weight gain, physical inactivity, cardiovascular disease, diabetes, cognitive dysfunction, premature menopause, infertility, osteoporosis, anthracycline-related cardiomyopathy, neuropathy, lymphedema sexual dysfunction, fatigue, second malignant neoplasms, chronic pain, musculoskeletal pain, arthralgias related to hormonal therapy, depression, and anxiety. Specific extensive guidelines are available to guide care and surveillance for cancer survivors depending on their cancer type or treatment exposure.

27. A 6-year-old child was referred to you for evaluation of diffuse leg pain and limping ongoing for several weeks without history of trauma. What clinical characteristics would make you worry about malignancy?
While more commonly these symptoms would be due to transient synovitis, reactive arthritis, osteomyelitis, or juvenile idiopathic arthritis, you should include malignancy (most commonly acute leukemia) in your differential diagnosis when evaluating a child with unexplained musculoskeletal complaints. Bone pain is one of the initial symptoms in 25% of children with acute leukemia. Malignancy is more likely when accompanied by nighttime pain, pallor, fatigue, cytopenia (sometimes subtle), recurrent fevers, infections, and organomegaly. Complete history, physical examination, laboratory testing, and imaging help establish the diagnosis. X-rays in a child with acute leukemia may show osteolytic lesions, transverse metaphyseal radiolucent bands, growth arrest lines, or subperiosteal new bone formation.

28. A 7-year-old girl became mute immediately following a gross total resection of medulloblastoma. What is the most likely diagnosis and what other symptoms may also be present?

Posterior fossa syndrome may develop in about 25% of children following surgical resection of infratentorial brain tumors, most commonly medulloblastoma. Symptoms may include mutism or impaired speech (dysarthria, decreased speech production, etc.), ataxia, hypotonia, behavioral changes, and emotional lability. Symptoms improve over weeks to months however, long-standing residual impairments of speech, neurocognitive function, and balance are common.[4] Treatment is supportive, focusing on rehabilitation (physical, occupational, speech and behavioral therapies) and symptomatic management.

29. What are long-term implications of limb salvage versus amputation in survivors of pediatric lower extremity bone tumors?

Limb salvage surgery using endoprosthesis, allografts, or reconstruction is the preferred treatment option when possible. Several studies show that survival, long-term functional outcome, and quality of life are similar between these two groups. Other studies demonstrated that limb-sparing surgery preserved more function than amputation. Small numbers of patients, differences in surgical approaches, and different assessment tools used make direct comparisons difficult.

30. You are evaluating a childhood cancer survivor who wants to start exercising. What are important considerations when recommending an exercise program for this patient?

Childhood cancer survivors are at increased risk for cardiovascular disease, including 15-fold increased risk for congestive heart failure and a 10-fold increased risk of coronary heart disease. Anthracyclines (doxorubicin, daunorubicin) commonly used to treat children with cancer (45%) may result in cardiotoxicity during treatment for many years following treatment. Childhood cancer survivors treated with anthracyclines or with history of radiation in proximity to the myocardium should undergo cardiac function monitoring and avoid intensive isometric exercise and heavy resistance training.[2]

31. Which group of children with cancer is at high risk for developing cognitive dysfunction?

Children with brain tumors, acute lymphoblastic leukemia, and tumors involving head and neck are at high risk for developing cognitive dysfunction. Additional risk factors include young age at diagnosis, cranial irradiation, neurotoxic chemotherapy or HSCT.

Bonus questions and answers available online.

BIBLIOGRAPHY

1. Maltser S, Cristian A, Silver JK, Morris GS, Stout NL. A focused review of safety considerations in cancer rehabilitation. *PMR*. 2017; 9(9S2):S415–S428.
2. Stubblefield M, O'Dell M. *Cancer Rehabilitation Principles and Practice*. New York: Demos Medical Publishing; 2018.
3. Cheville, AL. *Adjunctive Rehabilitation Approaches to Oncology, An Issue of Physical Medicine and Rehabilitation Clinics of North America*. Saint Louis: Elsevier Health Sciences; 2017.
4. Wibroe M, Cappelen J, Castor C, et al. Cerebellar mutism syndrome in children with brain tumours of the posterior fossa. *BMC Cancer*. 2017;17(1):439.
5. Ibanez K, Andrews CC, Daunter A, et al. Pediatric Oncology Rehabilitation. In: Mitra R. eds. *Principles of Rehabilitation Medicine*. McGraw Hill; 2019.
6. Gawade PL, Hudson MM, Kaste SC, et al. A systematic review of selected musculoskeletal late effects in survivors of childhood cancer. *Curr Pediatr Rev*. 2014;10(4):249–262.

CHAPTER 63

RHEUMATIC DISORDERS

Sara Cuccurullo, MD, Sagar Parikh, MD, Laurent Delavaux, MD, MS, and Craig Van Dien, MD

I don't deserve this award, but I have arthritis and I don't deserve that either.
— Jack Benny (1894–1974)

KEY POINTS

1. The use of non-steroidal anti-inflammatory drugs in rheumatologic disease is primarily for anti-inflammatory effect and does not significantly alter disease progression.
2. Distinguishing between non-inflammatory and inflammatory arthritis is an important step that will modify treatment strategies.
3. Pain relief, maintaining joint alignment, and maintaining functional movement are the hallmarks of treatment for most rheumatologic conditions.
4. The natural clinical progression of joint disease in rheumatoid arthritis is stiffness, inflammation, and eventual structural damage.

1. What are the mechanisms of action for non-steroidal anti-inflammatory drugs (NSAIDs) and their common side effects?
   NSAIDs have anti-inflammatory, antipyretic, and analgesic properties. NSAIDs inhibit prostaglandin (PG) production from arachidonic acid through the inhibition of cyclooxygenase (COX) enzyme isoforms. The second isoform (COX-2) is induced in inflammatory states. Specifically, the acetylation of COX-2 produces anti-inflammatory, anti-pyretic, and analgesic effects. The COX-1 isoform is necessary for gastric protection, homeostasis in the lung and kidney, and platelet aggregation. Inhibition of COX-1 may cause adverse effects involving gastric irritation and antiplatelet properties. With the loss of gastric protection, dyspepsia, reflux, and any degree of gastric or intestinal erosions can occur with prolonged exposure to NSAIDs. Although NSAIDs decrease inflammation, they do not significantly alter disease progression in rheumatologic conditions.

2. How are COX-2 selective NSAIDs different from less selective NSAIDs, and how does this dictate their use in treatment?
   NSAIDs are classified by their selectivity to the different isoforms of the COX enzyme. Low-dose aspirin is considered to be a COX-1 selective NSAID (mainly used for its antiplatelet properties). Most NSAIDs used for inflammation (i.e., Naproxen, Ibuprofen, Diclofenac) have varying degrees of selectivity for COX-1 and COX-2 isoforms. Celecoxib is currently the only selective COX-2 inhibitor available in the US.

3. What is the mechanism of action of Aspirin?
   Aspirin is widely used for its antiplatelet effect at low doses but is still used for anti-inflammatory, analgesic, and antipyretic purposes. Aspirin was first created as an acetylated form of salicylic acid. Like other NSAIDs, aspirin irreversibly inhibits the activity of COX, and consequently the formation of PGs and thromboxane-A2—key components in inflammation, swelling, pain, and fever.

4. What is the mechanism of action of corticosteroids and their common side effects?
   Corticosteroids have anti-inflammatory effects. Corticosteroids pass through cell membranes where they bind and form steroid-receptor complexes. These complexes then travel to the cell nucleus where they exact their influence on a genetic level. They have strong immunosuppressive effects and have been known to reduce the production of inflammatory cytokines, suppress the activation of macrophages, and antagonize leukocyte migration (key steps in the inflammatory cascade). Common adverse effects include weight gain, insomnia, elevated blood-sugar levels, emotional variability, and elevated blood pressure. Long-term use of corticosteroids can also cause avascular necrosis of bone, psychosis, and myopathic changes.

5. What are disease-modifying antirheumatic drugs (DMARDs)?
   DMARDs are a group of medications used to prevent or slow joint damage and decrease pain and inflammation. DMARDs take time to exact their effects, typically over a span of weeks to months. DMARDs are not used to treat acute attacks or acute pain. They work to suppress the body's overactive immune and/or inflammatory systems. Two common examples are Methotrexate and sulfasalazine.

6. **What is the mechanism of action of tumor necrosis factor-α (TNF-α) inhibitors and what toxicities are associated with these?**
TNF-α is a cytokine associated with the inflammatory process of rheumatoid arthritis (RA) and other inflammatory arthritides. Inhibitors of TNF-α can help reduce disease progression. Patients on long-term TNF-α agents should be mindful of infections (since TNF-α is important in immune defense) and possible reactivation of dormant tuberculosis. Patients with heart failure should exercise caution due to possible exacerbation. Less common adverse effects include autoimmune antibody creation, pancytopenia, and lupus-like manifestations.

7. **What are the effects of heat and cold on tissue in arthritis?**
Heat and cold modalities are commonly used in physical therapy and by patients. Although these modalities seldom have statistically significant evidence of benefit, there is a high degree of anecdotal evidence to support their efficacy.

Heat therapy is applied either superficially (through moist and electric heating pads) or deep (through paraffin wax, ultrasound, and shortwave diathermy). Heat increases tissue temperature and the elasticity of collagen fibers, thus relieving stiffness and enhancing range of motion during stretching. Heat can also produce analgesia by raising the pain threshold. Cold therapy can also produce analgesia by decreasing tissue temperature and reducing joint swelling. Cold is therefore a preferred modality for an acutely inflamed joint, as heat can increase joint swelling and leukocyte count in joint fluid. Cold can also decrease the overall metabolic demand of a joint structure in the acutely inflamed state. Examples of cold modalities include cold packs, cold air, and cold baths. Cold therapy should be avoided in the setting of Raynaud's disease, as this may exacerbate vascular compromise.

8. **What are the goals around which to design a rehabilitation program for a patient with rheumatic disease?**

9. **What are some techniques for joint protection in rheumatic conditions?**
To maintain joint health in the setting of a rheumatic condition, the patient must adhere to a set of principles and behavioral modifications. The goal is to maintain movement of the joint within reason, strength, and biomechanics to the best of one's ability. A patient should know to stop joint movements when pain is experienced. Using the joints within the available range and maintaining strength will reduce the risk of disuse atrophy. Utilizing the strongest and largest muscle groups and joints for daily tasks and avoiding improper positioning and postures may prevent the progression of any deformity. Patients should know when to rest but should avoid keeping their joints in any one position for prolonged periods of time. They must maintain a balance of movement and rest. Lastly, patients should learn to use tools and modify their behavior to minimize relative force on their most vulnerable joints.

10. **What are the classification criteria for diagnosis of RA and what is the target population?**
Patients should be evaluated by these diagnostic criteria if they have at least one joint with clinical synovitis (swelling), or with synovitis not otherwise explained by another disease. The diagnostic classification represents a score-based algorithm with an additive score $\geq 6/10$ (adding all scores from all categories) needed for a definitive diagnosis of RA. The four categories (and individual points) for RA diagnosis are listed below with corresponding number values given to each answer within each category:
1. Joint Involvement,
   - 1 Large Joint (0 points)
   - 2–10 Large Joints (1 point)
   - 1–3 small joints with or without involvement of large joints (2 points)
   - 4–10 small joints with or without involvement of large joints (3 points)
   - >10 joints (at least 1 small joint) (4 points)
2. Serology (at least one test result is required to be positive in this category),
   - Negative rheumatoid factor (RF) and Negative ACPA (0 points)
   - Low-Positive RF or Low-positive ACPA (2 points)

Table 63.1 Rehabilitation Goals for Rheumatic Diseases

1. Increase or maintain functional performances, including developing skills and knowledge on joint protection and energy conservation.
2. Keep proper joint alignment to prevent joint deformities.
3. Relieve pain and inflammation.
4. Increase or maintain mobility, strength, and endurance.
5. Increase aerobic capacity and bone density.
6. Facilitate successful adaptation to help the patient cope with the natural history of the disease process.
7. Achieve a sense of self-efficacy and well-being.

- High-positive RF or High-positive ACPA (3 points)
  - ACPA = Anti-citrullinated protein antibody
3. Acute-phase reactants (at least one test is required to be positive in this category)
  - Normal C-reactive protein (CRP) and normal erythrocyte sedimentation rate (ESR) (0 points)
  - Abnormal CRP or abnormal ESR (1 point)
4. Duration of symptoms
  - Less than 6 weeks (0 points)
  - Greater than or equal to 6 weeks (1 point)

11. **What are common blood tests to order in the setting of RA?**
    Close to 85% of patients with RA are RF positive, and this is usually associated with increased disease severity. The presence of RF is not specific to RA and can be found in other diseases, including systemic lupus erythematosus, scleroderma, and Sjögren's disease. Patients with RA often also have elevated CRP and ESR. A complete blood count may be useful in identifying an underlying disease and establishing baseline levels prior to treatment with medications that may affect different cell lines. Anti-cyclic citrullinated peptides (anti-CCP) are predictive of erosive arthritis.

12. **What are the three common onset patterns of RA?**
    1. Insidious onset is the most common onset pattern (50% to 70% of cases), with slow onset occurring over weeks to months. Initial systemic signs are diffuse musculoskeletal pain, fatigue, malaise, fever, and chills. Joint involvement is usually symmetrical, but not always. There may be joint swelling, erythema, and morning stiffness lasting more than 1 hour.
    2. Acute onset occurs in 10% to 20% of cases and is marked by rapid onset over several days, severe muscular pain, and involvement of the joints, which is usually less symmetrical.
    3. Intermediate onset occurs in 20% to 30% of cases, usually manifesting over several days to weeks and is marked by more noticeable systemic complaints.

13. **Describe the radiographic findings consistent with RA.**
    Radiographic findings in RA classically involve uniform joint space narrowing in a symmetrical distribution. Smaller joints of the wrist and hand, such as carpal bones, metacarpophalangeal (MCP) and PIP joints, may be involved early and, when progressive, manifest on imaging with radial deviation of the radiocarpal joint and compensatory ulnar deviation of the phalanges. Joints may show marginal bone erosions and juxta-articular osteopenia with evidence of bone washout. A classical x-ray of the wrist may show erosion of the ulnar styloid. The atlantoaxial joint may also be evaluated for possible subluxation; separation greater than 2.5 to 3 mm.

14. **What is the most important element responsible for joint destruction specific to RA?**
    Pannus formation is the primary driving force that leads to joint destruction. Pannus manifests as granulation tissue covering the articular cartilage at joint margins. This tissue is composed of fibroblasts, blood vessels, and various inflammatory cells. Fibroblast-like cells invade and destroy the adjacent cartilage and periarticular bone. This leads to progressive joint destruction and deformity and can eventually result in ankylosis.

15. **What is the natural clinical progression of joint disease in RA?**
    1. Morning stiffness which lasts for more than 1 hour before improving with movement.
    2. Structural inflammation with underlying pannus, manifesting as warmth, swelling, and tenderness of involved distal interphalangeal joint (DIP).
    3. Structural damage as the pannus evolves, and the accompanying inflammatory response leading to cartilage loss and erosion of bone.

16. **What are boutonnière deformity, the mechanism by which it occurs, and treatment options?**
    Boutonnière deformity describes a flexed proximal interphalangeal joint (PIP) and hyperextended DIP; so named because the finger is positioned as if tightly grasping with finger and thumb opposed when fastening a button. This is initially caused by PIP joint synovitis leading to the rupture of the terminal portion of the extensor hood, which holds the two lateral bands in place volar to the joint. When this mechanism fails, the lateral bands of the extensor hood sublux down on each side of the PIP, falling to the palmar side of the joint and becoming flexors of the PIP. The altered pull of these extensor bands on the DIP leads to hyperextension. This deformity can be treated with a Boutonnière ring splint.

17. **What is swan neck deformity and by what mechanism does it occurs?**
    Swan neck deformity, common in RA, is described as MCP flexion contracture, PIP hyperextension, and DIP flexion, resulting in a finger that looks like the profile of a swan's neck. This deformity may be due to synovitis at the MCP, PIP, or, less commonly, the DIP. Resulting flexor tendon tenosynovitis leads to a flexion contracture at the MCP. Accompanying contracture of the lumbrical and interossei muscles pulling on the finger with a fixed MCP contracture leads to the extension of the PIP. Contracture of the deep finger flexors then results in DIP flexion. Treat with swan neck ring splint orthosis.

18. Why should you order preoperative cervical spine flexion-extension x-rays in a patient with RA who is being cleared for surgery, and what finding would you be looking for?
Cervical spine atlantoaxial joint instability/subluxation is common in RA. Tenosynovitis involving the transverse ligament of C1 can lead to weakening or rupture of the ligament and erosion of the odontoid process or the atlas itself. C1 can slide over C2, which might cause pain, myelopathy, or spinal cord compromise. On flexion-extension films, the atlantoaxial (A-A) space should not increase significantly. Any A-A space greater than 2.5 to 3 mm denotes abnormal motion. It is crucial to rule out cervical instability prior to general anesthesia requiring prolonged neck flexion or extension.

19. What positions do the wrist and fingers commonly adopt as a result of RA joint pathology?
Overall, the wrist tends to deviate radially because of the weakening of ECRU, as well as ulnar and radial collateral ligaments. This changes the alignment of the stronger finger flexors, causing them to pull the fingers toward the ulnar side of the wrist and resulting in ulnar deviation of the fingers.

20. What are the extra-articular manifestations of RA?

21. What is Felty's syndrome?
Felty's syndrome describes the evolution of RA with the classic triad of RA, splenomegaly, and leukopenia. This is usually seen in seropositive (RF+) RA, with accompanying cutaneous nodules and/or leg ulcers. Two-thirds of affected patients are women, most often having had RA for more than 10 years, with Felty's syndrome manifesting in the fifth or seventh decade.

22. What is the pathophysiology of osteoarthritis?
Osteoarthritis (OA) involves the degeneration of joints from progressive wear and tear of articular cartilage and bone.
Early Stage: Hypercellularity of chondrocytes and loosening of cartilage collagen framework leads to minimal inflammation.
Later Stage: Progression to cartilage pitting, fissuring, and destruction; in conjunction with chondrocyte hypocellularity, osteophyte formation, subchondral bone sclerosis, cyst formation, inflammation, and synovitis, accompanied by an increase in the water content of joint cartilage.

23. What are the anatomical components of a diarthrodial joint?
Diarthrodial joints, also known as synovial joints, allow a fair degree of movement. They are formed by boney articulations typically surrounded by a joint capsule. The joint capsule is comprised of an outer fibrous layer and an inner layer of synovial membrane. Synovial fluid is found within the joint capsule and between the boney articulating surfaces. The ends of the bones are covered by a thin layer of hyaline cartilage atop a layer of subchondral bone.

Table 63.2 Extra-Articular Manifestations of Rheumatoid Arthritis	
Dermatologic	• Subcutaneous nodules present in 50% of RA patients, usually over tendons, extensor surfaces; may be accelerated by methotrexate. • Vasculitic lesions, palpable purpura
Ocular	• Keratoconjunctivitis • Scleritis: severe inflammation may erode through structures • Episcleritis: self-limiting
Pulmonary	• Interstitial lung disease with rheumatoid nodules or interstitial fibrosis • Pulmonary fibrosis • Pleurisy • Involvement of cricoarytenoid joint leading to dysphagia or dysphonia • Bronchiolitis obliterans
Cardiac	• Pericarditis, manifesting as chest pain, pericardial friction rub, diffuse ST elevations on EKG; can lead to constrictive pericarditis and heart failure • Valvular heart disease
Gastrointestinal	• Xerostomia • Gastritis and peptic ulcer disease secondary to NSAIDs
Renal	• Renal involvement if amyloidosis develops
Neurologic	• Atlantoaxial instability leading to cervical myelopathy • Entrapment neuropathy secondary to synovial inflammation or joint position
Hematologic	• Hypochromic microcytic anemia • Felty's syndrome

NSAIDs, Non-steroidal anti-inflammatory drugs; *RA*, rheumatoid arthritis.

24. **In contrast to RA, what are the radiographic findings typically seen with OA?**
On radiographic evaluation, OA will manifest with asymmetric joint space narrowing. In contrast to findings in RA, erosive or osteopenic changes will not be seen. There will, however, be evidence of subchondral bony sclerosis and new bone formation, especially in the form of osteophytes. There may also be evidence of osseous cysts, microfractures, or loose bodies. The most common joints involved include the first CMC, DIP, and the large joints, such as the knee or hip.

25. **What are the differences between inflammatory and noninflammatory arthritis based on presentation and diagnostic findings?**

26. **What is diffuse idiopathic skeletal hyperostosis?**
DISH is a variant of OA which is characterized by proliferation of spinal osteophytes and ossification in the thoracic or thoracolumbar spine, often leading to progressive ossification of intervertebral discs and associated ligaments, and eventually partial spinal fusion. The hallmark of DISH is ossification of three or more intervertebral discs. Ossification and fusion result in morning and evening stiffness and loss of range of motion. There may be radiographic evidence of ossification of the anterior longitudinal ligament and peripheral involvement and ossification manifesting as calcific enthesopathy. Large cervical osteophyte(s) can lead to dysphagia. DISH is more prevalent in white males after the age of 60, often associated with diabetes mellitus, obesity, hypertension, and coronary artery disease.

27. **What is the overall treatment plan for OA?**
Treatment begins with a conservative patient-driven approach directed at controlling painful symptoms and improving function. Initiate activity modification promoting modest weight loss, moderate exercise, and resistance exercises of the involved joints. This has been shown to reduce pain and improve function, even in severe OA. Acute joint pain can be treated with acetaminophen first line and NSAIDs second line; avoid long-term use of NSAIDs, especially in older patients. Topical treatments with NSAIDs, local anesthetics, or other compounded combinations may be effective as well. Patients who continue to struggle can be offered intra-articular injections with corticosteroids, hyaluronic acid, or other therapeutic agents to control pain; the frequency and total number of injections should be closely monitored. Further symptomatic control may also be obtained through various nerve blocks. For those with severe OA, refractory to conservative, non-surgical options, and total joint arthroplasty can offer relief.

28. **What is gout and what are the pathologic manifestations?**
Gout is a disorder of purine metabolism and monosodium urate-induced arthritis, in which there is a deposition of urate crystals in synovial, bursal, and tendinous tissue. It is characterized by four clinical stages, with the second stage displaying the manifestation of a painful peripheral joint (most commonly the great toe). Patients typically have elevated serum uric acid levels (> 7 mg/dL). Hyperuricemia is intermittent or constant and is often due to underexcretion versus overproduction. In these scenarios, uric acid crystals cluster and form microtophi along the synovial membrane of joints, and once disrupted, can release these crystals into the joint space. Gout attacks are the result of this release of preexisting tissue crystal deposits and not from hyperuricemia alone. Once the crystals are released, an immune-related inflammatory process ensues.

Table 63.3 Presentation and Diagnostic Findings in Inflammatory and Noninflammatory Arthritis

FEATURES	INFLAMMATORY ARTHRITIS	NONINFLAMMATORY ARTHRITIS
Worse pain timing	AM	PM
Erythema	Common	Absent
Swelling	Joint and soft tissue	Bony and or joint
Warmth	Common	Absent
Aggravating factor	Rest aggravates symptoms	Movement aggravates symptoms
Relieving factor	Movement relieves symptoms	Rest relieves symptoms
Morning Stiffness	Longer than 30 min	Less than 30 min
Systemic features	Occasional	absent
Elevated ESR, CRP	Elevated	normal
Synovial fluid WBC	WBC > 2,000	WBC < 2,000
Examples	Septic joint, RA, SLE, gout, psoriasis	OA, trauma, hemarthrosis

CRP, C-reactive protein; ESR, erythrocyte sedimentation rate; OA, osteoarthritis; RA, rheumatoid arthritis; SLE, systemic lupus erythematosus.

The four clinical stages of gout are the asymptomatic period of hyperuricemia, the period of acute gouty arthritis, the intercritical period (after the first gout attack, when the patient appears asymptomatic but is prone to future attacks), and finally, the chronic tophaceous period with the formation of tophi throughout the body. The presentation of gout is typically monoarticular and occurs at night or in the early morning. The joint swelling is quite painful and warm to the touch.

29. **What is the pathogenesis and clinical manifestation of tophaceous gout?**
Tophaceous gout is characterized by the presence of tophi (uric acid crystals encased by inflammatory cells and fibrotic tissue) typically found in peripheral joints, subchondral bone, extensor surfaces of the upper and lower extremity, and the pinna of the external ear. It is considered a later manifestation of gout and caused by constantly-elevated serum uric acid levels. Tophi can be seen on x-ray as erosive, "punched-out" lesions in bone. Physically, these manifestations are yellowish and firm and can break open.

30. **What are some dietary restrictions for an individual diagnosed with Gout?**
Higher levels of meat, seafood, and alcohol consumption are associated with an increased risk of gout, whereas a higher level of consumption of dairy products is associated with a decreased risk. Moderate intake of purine-rich vegetables or protein is not associated with an increased risk of gout.

31. **What are the pharmacologic treatment strategies for patients suffering from gout?**
During acute attacks, NSAID therapy is used for the anti-inflammatory effect. Indomethacin is commonly utilized to alleviate inflammation and pain during acute attacks. Corticosteroid (given as a tapering dose) or oral colchicine (given in doses of 0.6 mg hourly until resolution) are also effective; however, one must be mindful of the side effects of colchicine, including diarrhea and multi-organ injury in inappropriate doses.

32. **What are the differences between the crystal and aspirate found in both gout and pseudogout?**
Monosodium urate crystals are typically found in patients with gout. These crystal deposits are found within the synovial membrane and joint cavity, and joint aspirate will be negatively birefringent on polarized microscopy. Pseudogout is characterized by the presence of calcium pyrophosphate dihydrate (CPPD) crystals which display positive birefringence. The crystals are typically found in hyaline cartilage and fibrocartilage joints.

33. **What is pseudogout and how is it treated?**
Pseudogout is an inflammatory arthritic condition that is a result of the release of CPPD crystals in the articular space. Patients will feel acute onset pain and the swelling of a single, typically large joint. In the event of an acute flare, fluid is aspirated from the affected joint and sent for analysis. Synovial fluid with a high number of polymorphonuclear leukocytes is often seen, and polarized light microscopy reveals the presence of CPPD crystals. Aspirating the affected joint may be all that is needed to relieve pain. NSAIDs, such as indomethacin, or even oral steroids can be used during acute inflammatory attacks. Colchicine has also been shown to have positive effects on both gout and pseudogout.

34. **What are the seronegative spondyloarthropathies?**
Spondyloarthropathies comprise a host of inflammatory disorders/arthritides with similar musculoskeletal (axial spine disease, peripheral arthritis, enthesitis, and dactylitis [acronym SPeED]) and extra-articular/non-musculoskeletal manifestations. Four major relevant arthropathies include psoriatic arthritis, enteropathic arthropathy, ankylosing spondylitis, and reactive arthritis (acronym PEAR). Spondyloarthropathies have a high incidence of human leukocyte antigen-B27 and are RF negative. Current classifications define spondyloarthropathies as axial or peripheral.

35. **What clinical characteristics should raise suspicion for inflammatory back pain?**
There should be increased suspicion for inflammatory back pain if two or more of the following features exist: Back pain of *insidious onset* that persists for *greater than 3 months* in an individual *less than 45 years of age.* Associated characteristics may include *morning stiffness greater than 30 minutes, improvement in pain with exercise but not rest, nocturnal pain,* and *alternating buttock pain.*

36. **What is a pertinent radiographic finding of patients with ankylosing spondylitis?**
Sacroiliitis on plain radiographs is a defining characteristic of ankylosing spondylitis. Magnetic resonance imaging has allowed for the identification of sacroiliitis that may not be evident on plain radiographs.

37. **What is reactive arthritis (formerly known as Reiter's disease), and define the clinical triad typically associated with this disease process.**
Reactive arthritis is an inflammatory arthritis that is preceded by infection, usually enteropathic or uropathic. The classic disease triad is defined by conjunctivitis, arthritis (usually oligoarthritis), and urethritis. Symptoms generally become evident 1-4 weeks after the inciting infectious process.

38. **What is fibromyalgia? How is it different from myofascial pain syndrome?**
Fibromyalgia is a chronic condition characterized by pain in the soft tissue structures without an associated articular disease. Fibromyalgia is non-inflammatory, diffuse in nature, and has an unknown etiology. There are no

associated radiologic or laboratory studies. Patients have characteristic "tender points" and associated findings such as fatigue, sleep disturbances, or mood disorders. The severity of pain may vary daily. Tender points can be found on any soft tissue surface structure but tend to be found on pressure-sensitive areas.

These "tender points" should not be confused with "trigger points" often accompanying myofascial pain syndrome. Myofascial trigger points are typically localized to a specific body region (e.g., the shoulder) and are characterized by a taut band of muscle with a tender palpable nodule. Dry-needling these trigger points will often elicit a "twitch response" of the muscle fibers and is therapeutic. In contrast, dry-needling of a fibromyalgia "tender point" is not indicated and is not an effective treatment strategy.

39. **What are the diagnostic criteria for fibromyalgia?**
    The American College of Rheumatology established diagnostic criteria for fibromyalgia in 2010 with suggested revisions in 2016.
    1. Widespread pain index (WPI) ≥7 and symptom severity scale (SSS) score ≥5 or WPI 4 to 6 and SSS score ≥9.
    2. Generalized pain, defined as pain in various locations throughout the body; in the 2016 revision, this pain is to be located in at least 4 of 5 regions (left upper, right upper, left lower, right lower, axial).
    3. Symptoms have been present at a similar level for at least 3 months.

40. **What are some pharmacological treatment options for fibromyalgia?**
    Though exercise, mood, and lifestyle-based treatment strategies are of the utmost importance in the treatment of fibromyalgia, there are adjunctive pharmacologic options. Gabapentinoid medications, such as pregabalin and gabapentin, have been used with good efficacy and tolerance. In addition, tricyclic antidepressants, serotonin-norepinephrine reuptake inhibitors, and g-hydroxybutyrate have the strongest evidence of efficacy.

Bonus questions and answers available online.

BIBLIOGRAPHY

Aiello PD, Trautmann JC, McPhee TJ, et al. Visual prognosis in giant cell arteritis. *Ophthalmology.* 1993;100(4):550–555.

Aletaha D, Neogi T, Silman AJ, et al. 2010 Rheumatoid arthritis classification criteria: an American College of Rheumatology/European League Against Rheumatism collaborative initiative. *Arthritis Rheum.* 2010;62(9):2569–2581.

Aringer M, Costenbader K, Daikh D, et al. 2019 European League Against Rheumatism/American College of Rheumatology Classification Criteria for Systemic Lupus Erythematosus. *Arthritis Rheumatol.* 2019;71(9):1400–1412.

Benzon HT, Fishman S, Liu S, et al. *Essentials of Pain Medicine.* Philadelphia, PA: Elsevier Inc.; 2011.

Bohan A, Peter JB. Polymyositis and dermatomyositis (first of two parts). *N Engl J Med.* 1975;292(7):344–347.

Bohan A, Peter JB. Polymyositis and dermatomyositis (second of two parts). *N Engl J Med.* 1975;292(8):403–407.

Buttgereit F, Dejaco C, Matteson EL, et al. Polymyalgia rheumatica and giant cell arteritis: a systematic review. *JAMA.* 2016;315(22): 2442–2458.

Choi HK, Atkinson K, Karlson EW, et al. Purine-rich foods, dairy and protein intake, and the risk of gout in men. *N Engl J Med.* 2004;350: 1093–1103.

Choi HK, Atkinson K, Karlson EW, et al. Alcohol intake and risk of incident gout in men: a prospective study. *Lancet.* 2004;363(9417): 1277–1281.

Cifu DX, Braddom RL. *Braddom's Physical Medicine and Rehabilitation.* 5th ed. Philadelphia, PA: Elsevier, Inc.; 2016.

Cuccurullo S. *Physical Medicine and Rehabilitation Board Review.* 3rd ed. New York, NY: Demos Medical; 2015.

Cuccurullo S. *Physical Medicine and Rehabilitation Board Review.* 4th ed. New York, NY: Demos Medical; 2019.

Dasgupta B, Cimmino MA, Maradit-Kremers H, et al. 2012 provisional classification criteria for polymyalgia rheumatica: a European League Against Rheumatism/American College of Rheumatology collaborative initiative. *Ann Rheum Dis.* 2012;71(4):484–492.

Denton CP, Khanna D. Systemic sclerosis. *Lancet.* 2017;390(10103):1685–1699.

Epstein PE, Alguire PC. *MKSAP 14: Medical Knowledge Self-Assessment Program.* Philadelphia, PA: American College of Physicians; 2006.

García-Kutzbach A, Chacón-Súchite J, García-Ferrer H, et al. Reactive arthritis: update 2018. *Clin Rheumatol.* 2018;37(4):869–874.

Hachulla E, Launay D. Diagnosis and classification of systemic sclerosis. *Clin Rev Allergy Immunol.* 2010;40(2):78–83.

Healy PJ, Helliwell PS. Classification of the spondyloarthropathies. *Curr Opin Rheumatol.* 2005;17(4):395–399.

Hunder GG, Bloch DA, Michel BA, et al. The American College of Rheumatology 1990 criteria for the classification of giant cell arteritis. *Arthritis Rheum.* 1990;33(8):1122–1128.

Jennette JC, Falk RJ, Bacon PA, et al. 2012 Revised International Chapel Hill Consensus Conference Nomenclature of Vasculitides. *Arthritis Rheum.* 2013;65(1):1–11.

Lundberg IE, Tjärnlund A, Bottai M, et al. 2017 European League Against Rheumatism/American College of Rheumatology classification criteria for adult and juvenile idiopathic inflammatory myopathies and their major subgroups. *Arthritis Rheumatol.* 2017;69(12): 2271–2282.

Mader R, Verlaan JJ, Buskila D. Diffuse idiopathic skeletal hyperostosis: clinical features and pathogenic mechanisms. *Nat Rev Rheumatol.* 2013;9(12):741–750. doi:10.1038/nrrheum.2013.165. ISSN 1759-4804.

McAllister K, Goodson N, Warburton L, et al. Spondyloarthritis: diagnosis and management: summary of NICE guidance. *BMJ.* 2017;356: j839.

Allen M. *NMS Medicine.* 5th ed. Lippincott Williams & Wilkins; 2005.

Preston DC, Shapiro BE. *Electromyography and Neuromuscular Disorders Clinical-Electrophysiologic Correlations.* 3rd ed. London: Elsevier Saunders; 2013:555.

Salvarani C, Cantini F, Boiardi L, et al. Polymyalgia rheumatica and giant-cell arteritis. *N Engl J Med.* 2002;347(4):261–271.

Steiman AJ, Pope JE, Thiessen-Philbrook H, et al. Non-biologic disease-modifying antirheumatic drugs (DMARDs) improve pain in inflammatory arthritis (IA): a systematic literature review of randomized controlled trials. *Rheumatol Int.* 2013;33:1105.

Strauss KW, Gonzalez-Buritica H, Khamashta MA, et al. Polymyositis-dermatomyositis: a clinical review. *Postgrad Med J.* 1989;65(765): 437–443.

Taurog JD, Chhabra A, Colbert RA. Ankylosing spondylitis and axial spondyloarthritis. *N Engl J Med.* 2016;374(26):2563–2574.

Van den Bosch F, Vander Cruyssen B, Mielants H. Clinical assessment in the spondyloarthropathies, including psoriatic arthritis. *Curr Opin Rheumatol.* 2006;18(4):354–358.

Van den Hoogen F, Khanna D, Fransen J, et al. 2013 Classification Criteria for Systemic Sclerosis: An American College of Rheumatology/ European league against rheumatism collaborative initiative. *Ann Rheum Dis.* 2013;72(11):1747–1755.

Van den Hoogen F, Khanna D, Fransen J, et al. 2013 classification criteria for systemic sclerosis: an American College of Rheumatology/ European League Against Rheumatism collaborative initiative. *Arthritis Rheum.* 2013;65(11):2737–2747.

Vane JR, Botting RM. The mechanism of action of aspirin. *Thromb Res.* 2003;110(5-6):255–258.

Weyand CM, Goronzy JJ. Medium- and large-vessel vasculitis. *N Engl J Med.* 2003;349(2):160–169.

Wigley FM, Flavahan NA. Raynaud's phenomenon. *N Engl J Med.* 2016;375(6):556–565.

Wolfe F, Clauw DJ, Fitzcharles M-A, et al. 2016 Revisions to the 2010/2011 fibromyalgia diagnostic criteria. *Semin Arthritis Rheum.* 2016;46(3):319–329. doi: 10.1016/j.semarthrit.2016.08.012.

Wolfe F, Clauw DJ, Fitzcharles M-A, et al. The American College of Rheumatology preliminary diagnostic criteria for fibromyalgia and measurement of symptom severity. *Arthritis Care Res.* 2010;62(5):600–610. doi:10.1002/acr.20140.

CHAPTER 64

PRESSURE INJURIES (PRESSURE ULCERS): ETIOLOGY, PREVENTION, ASSESSMENT, AND TREATMENT

Michael Priebe, MD, MPH, Constance Strauss, BSN, RN, CWOCN, CFCN, CDE, Mark Finnegan, RN, MSN, and Mayur J. Amin, MD

You don't learn from successes;
you don't learn from awards;
you don't learn from celebrity;
you only learn from wounds and scars
and mistakes and failures.
And that's the truth.

— Jane Fonda (1937–)

KEY POINTS: PRINCIPLES OF PRESSURE INJURY CARE

1. Prevention is paramount and should be addressed continually.
2. Correct the underlying factors that led to the development of the injury.
3. Wounds must be adequately debrided before healing can occur.
4. Maintain a moist wound environment to optimize wound healing.

1. **What is a "pressure injury" and what happened to the term "pressure ulcers?"**
   The National Pressure Ulcer Advisory Panel (NPUAP) redefined Pressure Ulcers as Pressure Injuries in 2016. The term Pressure Injury is inclusive of Pressure Ulcers and Deep Tissue Injuries. Pressure Injury is defined as follows:

   "A pressure injury is localized damage to the skin and underlying soft tissue, usually over a bony prominence or related to a medical or other device."

2. **Why does pressure cause soft tissue injury?**
   When tissues are compressed between a bony prominence and an external surface, capillaries are compressed, and blood flow is obstructed. This leads to soft tissue ischemia, reperfusion injury, infarction, and, ultimately, tissue necrosis.

3. **How much pressure is too much?**
   We don't really know. In general, the more pressure applied, the shorter the duration needed to produce tissue injury. Therefore, rather than relying on absolute pressure measurements, focus on pressure management and perform pressure relief maneuvers frequently.

4. **Which tissues are most sensitive to pressure?**
   Tissues vary in their sensitivity to pressure. Muscle is the most sensitive, whereas skin is most resistant to pressure-induced ischemia. Therefore, pressure-induced injury typically involves the deep tissue first. Superficially, the affected area appears as an area of induration, erythema, and warmth, but with intact skin. This is termed a "Deep Tissue Injury." Within a few days to a week, even with complete pressure relief, the wound may open and reveal a deep crater.

5. **If muscle is so sensitive to pressure, why do surgeons use myocutaneous "flaps" to close large pressure injuries?**
   Myocutaneous "flaps" are used to eliminate dead space. Flaps do not provide a "cushion" but rather provide well-vascularized tissue to fill the dead space left after resection of a pressure injury. Another benefit is that the surgeon may be able to move the suture line away from the site of maximum pressure.

6. **How does shear contribute to pressure injury?**
   Shear is the mechanical force that parallels an area. The presence of significant shear forces lowers by half the threshold pressure needed to disrupt blood flow in the dermis. One theory is that shear forces cause superficial tissue ischemia by kinking dermal capillaries oriented perpendicularly to the surface of the skin. The combination of pressure and shear can result in a superficial pressure injury with significant underlying tissues injury.

7. **What are the major strategies to prevent pressure injuries?**
   Use the acronym: ***PRESS***:
   - (***P***)ressure (***R***)elief: Performing frequent pressure relief maneuvers is the principal prevention strategy.
   - (***E***)ven distribution of pressure: As pressure equals mass/area, pressure can be decreased by increasing the area over which it is distributed. Increase the weight-bearing surface by utilizing body surfaces that can tolerate more pressure for weight distribution (e.g., posterior thigh during sitting).
   - (***S***)upport Surfaces: Use pressure-distributing support surfaces in bed, wheelchair, commode seat, etc. to protect soft tissues.
   - (***S***)hear: Minimize shear through good positioning in a chair or bed (e.g., avoid sitting in semi-inclined or "slouched" positions).

8. **What are the six key elements for assessing and describing a pressure injury?**
   Use the acronym "**ASSETS**":
   (A)natomic location
   (S)tage
   (S)ize (length, width, depth, wound area, undermining, sinus tracts)
   (E)xudate (volume, quality, odor)
   (T)issue type (wound bed quality, slough, necrosis, granulation)
   (S)urrounding tissue (wound margins, induration, erythema, cellulitis)

9. **At what anatomic sites are pressure injuries most likely to develop?**
   Pressure injuries develop most commonly over areas of bony prominence or areas in contact with a medical device (orthosis, cast, chair components, etc.). Tissue caught between a "rock and a hard place" is most vulnerable. The most common sites include the sacrum, coccyx, ischia, trochanter, heel, and malleoli. The locations listed change in frequency depending on the specific patient population (e.g., spinal cord injury [SCI] or geriatric) and the time after injury (e.g., acute SCI or chronic SCI).

10. **What does pressure injury location tell us?**
    The location tells us what caused the pressure injury and allows for focused interventions for treatment and prevention. Location is often predictable and depends on the individual's activity levels. Persons who spend much or all of the day lying in bed most often develop pressure injuries over the sacrum, trochanters, and heels. Persons who are sitting develop pressure injuries over the ischia, coccyx, and trochanters.

11. **How does sitting exert pressure on the trochanters?**
    The trochanters naturally bear weight during sitting. The weight borne is increased when there is pelvic obliquity. These trochanteric injuries tend to develop posterior to the greater trochanter rather than directly lateral to it (which is seen in side-lying injuries). The use of a wheelchair with a sling seat that is overstretched will also contribute to trochanteric pressure injuries.

12. **What is the difference between a sacral pressure injury and a coccygeal pressure injury?**
    Sacral pressure injuries are located over the sacral prominence and are caused by lying supine. Coccygeal pressure injuries are located over the coccyx and are caused by poor posture resulting in increased shear and pressure over the coccyx. These injuries can coalesce into a single pressure injury. Attempts should be made to differentiate them because the etiologies and treatments are different.

13. **How are Pressure Injuries staged?**
    Stage 1 Pressure Injury: Non-blanchable erythema of intact skin, which may appear differently in darkly pigmented skin.
    Stage 2 Pressure Injury: Partial-thickness skin loss with exposed dermis.
    Stage 3 Pressure Injury: Full-thickness skin loss in which adipose is visible in the ulcer and granulation tissue and roll wound edges are often present.
    Stage 4 Pressure Injury: Full-thickness skin and tissue loss with exposed or directly palpable fascia, muscle, tendon, ligament, cartilage, or bone in the ulcer.
    Unstageable Pressure Injury: Persistent non-blanchable deep red, maroon or purple discoloration in area of full-thickness skin and tissue loss where the extent of tissue damage within the ulcer cannot be confirmed due to being obscured by slough or eschar.
    Deep Tissue Injury: Localized area of persistent non-blanchable deep red, maroon, or purple discoloration or dermal separation revealing a dark wound bed or blood-filled blister.

14. **What is the best treatment for a pressure injury?**
    Below are four basic principles in the treatment of pressure injuries. Be mindful to *"Treat the whole patient, not the hole in the patient."*
    - Prevention is paramount.
      Careful attention to risk factors allows early detection pressure injury. Preventive efforts are ongoing and must continue even after a wound is healed.
    - Correct the underlying factors that initially led to the development of the ulcer.

Biologic, psychosocial, and environmental problems must be addressed to maximize healing. A complete evaluation is necessary to determine which of these aspects are most critical to address initially.
- Wounds must be adequately debrided before healing can occur.

It is necessary to remove the dead tissue as the first step in pressure ulcer care to promote healing. Chronic, nonhealing pressure injuries may also benefit from debridement to stimulate the acute wound–healing cascade.
- Maintain a moist wound environment.

Moist environment provides the optimal conditions for cell migration and mitosis. Many products are available to assist in maintaining a moist wound environment.

15. **What is the difference between an eschar and a scab?**
Eschar is the black or brown necrotic devitalized tissue covering a wound. This is necrotic skin and subcutaneous tissue, and not a beneficial natural dressing. An eschar prevents adequate wound staging, harbors bacteria, and prevents the formation of granulation tissue and epithelialization of the wound.

Scab is dried serum that covers a superficial wound. A scab may be the body's way of laying down a natural dressing or a matrix for healing and usually maintains a clean and moist environment for a superficial wound bed. If there is cellulitis, or if it is unclear whether the dry matter is a scab or an eschar, remove it.

16. **What is the fastest way to debride a necrotic pressure ulcer?**
The fastest and often the most effective way is surgical, or "sharp" debridement. Small wounds may be debrided at the bedside, but extensive wounds should be debrided in the operating room, especially if hemostasis will be difficult to maintain, or anesthesia is needed. Debridement is often necessary early in the management of stages III and IV pressure injuries and is mandatory in the face of advancing cellulitis or sepsis.

17. **What is meant by autolytic debridement?**
Autolytic debridement utilizes the body's own enzymes to degrade dead tissue. This is accomplished by placing an occlusive dressing over a superficial, non-infected wound and allowing the wound fluid to collect under the dressing. The wound fluid, which is full of enzymes, helps to soften the eschar and begins the separation of healthy tissue from nonviable tissue, making sharp debridement easier. However, if the wound is infected, an abscess can be created by covering the wound with an occlusive dressing.

18. **When should a "wet-to-dry" dressing be used?**
Unfortunately, the term "wet-to-dry" dressings has been confused with "saline and gauze" dressings. The only indication for "wet-to-dry" dressings is for mechanical debridement. If the wound requires debridement, "wet-to-dry" dressings may be appropriate, but there are drawbacks. The dressing material should be removed dry (not moistened before removal) and any attached matter pulled out of the wound to clean it. These dressings non-selectively debride wounds, meaning that healthy tissue may also be damaged as you remove necrotic tissue. This may also be very painful in the patient with sensation in the wound area. Once the wound is debrided, the focus must change to maintaining a moist wound environment.

19. **How does one select the appropriate type of dressing?**
The choice is usually determined by wound depth and amount of moisture.

20. **What to do if the wound isn't healing after a couple of weeks?**
If a wound shows no signs of healing, it is likely that there are underlying factors that have not been completely addressed. Go back and carefully evaluate each of the factors related to that wound. Usually, the problem is not the use of the wrong dressing, but that there are remaining underlying factors such as malnutrition, wound infection, microvascular disease, or underlying osteomyelitis that have not been adequately managed.

21. **What is the difference between wound infection and colonization?**
Wound infection and bacterial colonization can both interfere with healing. Use the acronym ***NERDS*** to help differentiate.
(***N***)on-healing
(***E***)dema
(***R***)edness
(***D***)rainage
(***S***)mell

Swabbing of wounds will often lead to incorrect identification of organisms. To determine if a wound is infected, a quantitative tissue biopsy is necessary.

Wound infections may need to be treated systemically with antibiotics, whereas wound colonization is always treated locally with debridement, wound cleansing, and frequent dressing changes.

22. **How is osteomyelitis underlying a pressure injury diagnosed?**
The gold standard for diagnosis of osteomyelitis is pathologic findings and culture from bone biopsy which also help guide antibiotic selection. Plain radiographs can be helpful, but changes on x-ray develop late in the course of osteomyelitis. Bone scans are rarely useful because of the high false-positive rate in the presence of

a pressure ulcer. Magnetic resonance imaging has been shown to be highly sensitive for osteomyelitis underlying a pressure ulcer, but specificity varies between studies, thus making the chance of false positives high.

23. Why is serum albumin low even with good nutritional support?
Serum albumin and pre-albumin are acute phase reactants that decrease during times of acute illness and inflammation. Albumin may also be lost through a highly exudative wound. Serum albumin and pre-albumin do not represent nutritional status in persons with pressure injuries. They indicate ongoing inflammation.

24. How much nutrition is needed to heal a pressure injury?
Each patient should have a comprehensive evaluation of nutritional needs and support provided based on that assessment. Recommendations include total energy need, protein needs, hydration, vitamins and minerals. Patients with pressure injuries need 1.5 to 2.0 g of protein/kilogram of ideal body weight per day. Do not simply add but substitute protein calories for carbohydrate and fat calories. Obesity can become a significant problem for patients with decreased activity and increased caloric intake during the prolonged healing time.

BIBLIOGRAPHY

Ayello EA, Cuddigan JE. Debridement: controlling the necrotic/cellular burden. *Adv Skin Wound Care*. 2004;17(2):66–75; quiz, 76–78.

Boyko T, Longaker MT, Yang GP. Review of the current management of pressure ulcers. *Adv Wound Care (New Rochelle)*. 2018;7(2):57–67

Brunel AS, Lamy B, Cyteval C, et al. Diagnosing pelvic osteomyelitis beneath pressure ulcers in spinal cord injured patients: a prospective study. *Clin Microbiol Infect*. 2016;22(3):267.e1–267.e8.

Dinsdale SN. Decubitus ulcers: role of pressure and friction in causation. *Arch Phys Med Rehabil*. 1974;55:147–154.

Fang L, Pandya A, Cichowski A, et al. Deep tissue injury rat model for pressure ulcer research on spinal cord injury. *J Tissue Viability*. 2010;19(2):67–76.

Jones VJ. The use of gauze: will it ever change? *Int Wound J*. 2006;3:79–86.

Kjolseth D, Frank JM, Barker JH, et al. Comparison of the effects of commonly used wound agents on epithelialization and neovascularization. *J Am Coll Surg*. 1994;179:305–312.

Kosiak M. Etiology of decubitus ulcers. *Arch Phys Med Rehabil*. 1961;42:19–29.

Kwon R, Rendon JL, Janis JE. In DH Song, PC Neligan (Eds.). *Pressure sores Plastic Surgery: Volume 4: Lower Extremity, Trunk, and Burns*. 4th ed. London: Elsevier. 2018:350–380.

Litchford MD, Dorner B, Posthauer ME. Malnutrition as a precursor of pressure ulcers. *Adv Wound Care (New Rochelle)* 2014;3(1):54–63.

National Pressure Ulcer Advisory Panel. *NPUAP Pressure Injury Stages*. Available at http://www.npuap.org/resources/educational-and-clinical-resources/npuap-pressure-injury-stages/. (Accessed 2019, March 24).

National Pressure Ulcer Advisory Panel. *NPUAP Pressure Injury Stages*. Available at http://www.npuap.org/resources/educational-and-clinical-resources/npuap-pressure-injury-stages/. (Accessed 2019, March 24).

Posthauer ME, Banks M, Dorner B, Schols J. The role of nutrition for pressure ulcer management: national pressure ulcer advisory panel, European pressure ulcer advisory panel, and pan pacific pressure injury alliance white paper. *Adv Skin Wound Care*. 2015;28(4):175–188.

Priebe MM, Wuermser LA, McCormack. *Medical Management of Pressure Ulcers*. In VW Lin (Ed.). *Spinal Cord Medicine: Principles and Practice*. 2nd ed. New York: Demos; 2010:659–672.

Salcido R, Popescu A, Chulhyun A. Animal models in pressure ulcer research. *J Spinal Cord Med*. 2007;3(2):107–116.

Tedeschi S, Negosanti L, Sgarzani R, et al. Superficial swab versus deep-tissue biopsy for the microbiological diagnosis of local infection in advanced-stage pressure ulcers of spinal-cord-injured patients: a prospective study. *Clin Microbiol Infect*. 2017;23(12):943–947.

Wound, Ostomy and Continence Nurses Society. *Guidelines for Prevention and Management of Pressure Ulcers (Injuries)*. WOCN Clinical Practice Guideline Series 2. Mt. Laurel, New Jersey; 2016:101.

BURN REHABILITATION: GUIDANCE OF HEALING AND OPTIMAL PARTICIPATION

Vincent Gabriel, MD, FRCPC, Jeffrey C. Schneider, MD, and Karen J. Kowalske

Mild physician—putrid wounds (Linur bartskeri gjörir fúin sár)

— Icelandic proverb

KEY POINTS: HYPERTROPHIC SCARRING

1. A hypertrophic scar is red, raised, and fibrotic.
2. Patients with increased skin pigment are at greater risk.
3. Burns that do not heal within 3 weeks are at higher risk.
4. A hypertrophic scar causes joint contractures and impairs function.

1. **What threats do burns pose to the person through damage to the skin?**

   The **integumentary system** makes up the largest organ of the body with its many appendages and intricate tissue interactions. These are derived from **ectoderm** and contain **neural crest** cells, producing sensory receptor organs, enamel, and pigment. Skin maintains homeostasis responding to temperature, light, touch, and injury. It manifests the authentic physical self as it reflects light into the environment and is animated by voluntary and autonomic musculature and circulation.

   Image: Schematic Skin and Appendages in Netter's Essential Histology.

2. **How common are burns?**

   In the United States, more than 1 million burn injuries occur each year. There are approximately 700,000 emergency department visits per year and approximately 45,000 patients admitted to the hospital. Worldwide, 96% of burn related mortality occurs in low to middle income countries, with approximately 265,000 deaths from flame injuries alone.

   Burn Incidence and Treatment in the US. *2016 Fact sheet*. Available at the American Burn Association. www.ameriburn.org/resources_factsheet.php

   World Health Organization. *A WHO Plan for Burn Prevention and Care*. Geneva, Switzerland; 2008.

3. **What are the most common causes of burn injury?**

   Burns are caused by thermal, electrical, chemical, and radiation agents. Scald burns are most common in women, children and the disabled. Flame burns often require treatment at burn centers and occur in house fires, car crashes, and in intoxicated young adults around campfires.

4. **Describe the zones of injury in a full-thickness thermal wound.**

   A burn wound can be divided into three zones:
   - In the **zone of coagulation,** the protein destruction is most severe and cellular necrosis is complete, forming eschar.
   - In the **zone of stasis,** the majority of cells are initially intact, but inflammation can lead to ischemia and necrosis.
   - The most peripheral is the **zone of hyperemia** with increased blood flow and negligible cellular injury.

5. **How are burns classified?**

   Superficial injury only involves the epidermis. Skin is erythematous, painful, but not blistered; heals in 3 to 7 days; and does not scar.

   Partial thickness

   Superficial partial thickness: Includes the epidermis and superficial dermis. Burn may blister, is red and painful, will blanch with pressure, and will heal in 7 to 21 days and may result in pigmentation changes.

   Deep partial thickness: Extends into deeper dermis. Wound is mottled pink to white with poor capillary refill. May heal but will result in significant hypertrophic scarring and is thus usually best addressed with excision and grafting.

Full thickness: Involves entire epidermis and dermis, destroying the regenerative capacity of skin. Eschar is usually present. Central portions of the wound are not painful because of destruction of sensory nerve endings. Depending on the size and anatomic location, the patient will require surgical intervention for best outcomes.

Kowalske, KJ. Burn wound care. *Phys Med Rehabil Clin N Am.* 2011;22(2):213–227.

6. What is the rule of nines?

The rule of nines is a convenient and fairly accurate way of estimating an adult's total body surface area (TBSA) burn percentage (Fig. 65.1). The TBSA is calculated by attributing 9% to the front and back of the head and neck, 9% to the front and back of each arm and hand, 9% to the chest and the stomach, 9% to the upper back, 9% to the lower back, 9% to the front and back of each leg and foot and 1% to the groin area. The rule of nines is not accurate for children who have different proportions, with a proportionally larger head compared to adults (the head represents 19% of the TBSA in an infant).

7. What are the damages caused by electrical injury?

Tissue damage is caused by electrical conduction traversing through the least resistant conduits of the body in blood vessels and nerves. In the distal extremities, current density increases as cross-sectional area decreases, resulting in greater tissue damage. The surface wound may look minor, but the damage to deep structures can be severe, resulting in compartment syndromes and neuropathy. Damage is usually worse on distal extremities due to concentration of current and explosive arch to conductors outside the body. At burn centers, these wounds are labeled as contact points. Currents below 1000 V ventricular fibrillation rarely occur but neurologic complications may still result. Currents driven at greater than 1000 V cause greater nervous and muscular damage. Serum **Creatine Kinase (CK) levels** exceeding 2500 IU, suggest risk for amputation. There is a high prevalence of neuropsychological dysfunction after electrical injury. Cataracts may be a late complication of electrical injury even without contact on the head.

Kelley KM, Tkachenko TA, Pliskin NH, et al. Life after electrical injury. Risk factors for psychiatric sequelae. *Ann NY Acad Sci.* 1999; 888:356–363.

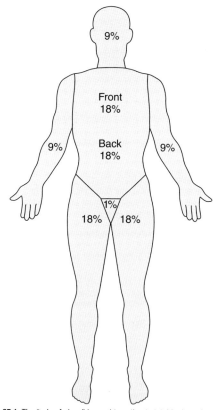

Fig. 65.1 The "rule of nines" is used to estimate total body surface area.

8. What happens to the skeletal muscles in a patient with a large burn?

A lot happens! A large burn results in a **catabolic state** throughout the body, resulting in lean body mass loss. Treatment with anabolic agents, such as oxandrolone, has demonstrated decreased nitrogen loss, increased muscle protein synthesis, increased weight gain, and increased lean body mass. Changes in acetylcholine receptors may impact anesthetic options.

Murphy KD, Thomas S, Mlcak RP, et al. Effects of long-term oxandrolone administration in severely burned children. *Surgery.* 2004; 136:219–224.

9. What factors determine burn injury survival?

Burn depth, percentage of TBSA burned, inhalation injury, patient age, associated trauma, and premorbid health determine survival after a burn injury. Survival in burn centers with adequate infrastructure has increased over time due to improved acute care, as well as early excision, and grafting of severe burns. The **LD_{50} or burn size lethal** to 50% of the population has increased from 65% TBSA in the 1980s to more than 80% TBSA. The **modified Boz score** combines TBSA with age and an additional 15 points for inhalation injury is used to approximate mortality. Patients with a Boz score of over a 100 have a high risk of death, and survival with $>$140 being very unlikely.

Smolle C, Cambiaso-Daniel J, Forbes AA, et al. Recent trends in burn epidemiology worldwide: a systematic review. *Burns.* 2017; 43(2):249–257.

10. How should the rehabilitation clinician think and act when approaching the patient with burns? Can sequenced interventions enhance the system of care throughout the institution and health network?

The conceptual approach begins with the clinical continuum and **prevention** of burns of vulnerable, insensate, immobile, and cognitively compromised patients. At the time of injury, stopping the burn and immediate water flushing reduces tissue. Most burns do not require a surgery, and the burn physiatrist must be prepared to manage acute pain and non-operative wound damage. Inpatient care should bring rehabilitation into the **clinical pathway** at the bedside in the intensive care unit because the injury, healing, scarring, and patient adaptation is a protracted process that requires maintenance of patient mobility and limitation of life limiting scars and contractures. Also, the physiatrist should interview the patient and family to get a good perspective of premorbid function. This evaluation improves the transfer to rehabilitation and long-term survival in the elderly burn survivor. Thereafter, early interdisciplinary team consultation with the patient, family, home health, school, and employer aligns interventions for a predictable discharge as innovations in burn care are continually shortening inpatient remains.

Stoddard FJ, Ryan CM, Schneider JC. Physical and psychiatric recovery from burns. Psychiatric. *Clin N Am.* 2015;38(1):105–120.

Young AW, Dewey WS, King BT. Rehabilitation of burn injuries: an update. *Phys Med Rehabil Clin N Am.* 2019;30(1):111–132.

11. How should the patient be positioned to avoid contracture formation?

- Neck extension
- Shoulder abduction at 80 degrees and flexed at 15 degrees
- Elbows extended and supinated
- Wrists and hands in the intrinsic plus position
- Hips extended, abducted at 10 degrees with no external rotation
- Knees extended
- Ankles in neutral dorsiflexion
    Remember not to leave your patient in this position. Patients need stretching and active exercise!

Dewey WS, Richard RL, Parry IS. Positioning splinting and contracture management. *Phys Med Clin N Am.* 2011;22(2):229–247.

12. How should a burned hand be splinted?

The most common hand deformity is a **claw hand,** with metacarpophalangeal (MCP) extension, proximal interphalangeal (PIP) flexion, and distal interphalangeal (DIP) flexion, and thumb adduction. General splinting guidelines to prevent the claw hand are as follows:

- Wrist in 15 to 30 degrees of extension
- MCP flexion in 60 to 90 degrees
- Proximal and distal IP joints in full extension
- Thumb in radial or palmar abduction

Kowalske KJ. Hand burns. *Phys Med Clin N Am.* 2011;22(2):249–259.

13. How should a hand with exposed tendons be splinted?

Tendons that are exposed should be covered with a moist dressing and maintained in a slack position without tension. Disruption of the extensor tendon at the PIP joint can result in a **boutonnière deformity** (PIP flexion and DIP hyperextension). Damage to the extensor tendon at the DIP joint can result in a **mallet deformity** with DIP flexion. Contractures of the dorsal hand structures can result in a **swan-neck deformity** (PIP hyperextension, DIP flexion).

14. How do partial-thickness burns heal?

Epithelial progenitor cells deep in the dermis (**rete pegs**) will regenerate to epithelialize the wound while local fibroblasts regenerate the collagen strands and extracellular matrix of the dermis.

Franz, Michael G, Steed DL, et al. Optimizing healing of the acute wound by minimizing complications. *Curr Probl Surg.* 2007;44(11):691–763.

15. When are grafts necessary?

Deep partial- and full-thickness burns that are not expected to heal within 21 days are likely to benefit from early excision of nonviable tissue and autologous grafting to reduce pain, length of hospital stay, wound infection, risk of hypertrophic scarring, and medical complications.

Zuo KJ, Medina A, Tredget EE. Important developments in burn care. *Plast Reconstr Surg.* 2017;139(1):120e–138e.

16. What types of grafts are available?

- An **autograft** is taken from a donor site on the patient's body. **Split-thickness skin grafts (STSG)** include the epidermis and superficial dermis. An autograft can be used as a **sheet graft** on functionally important regions or as a **mesh graft** to cover larger areas to promote re-epithelialization. A **full-thickness skin graft (FTSG)** includes the epidermis and entire dermis and is used to graft small areas such as the palm, eyelid, or tip of the nose. An FTSG donor site requires primary closure for healing. An STSG donor site will heal with non-surgical management.
- A **xenograft** is skin from another species and provides a biologic dressing to promote healing and prevent infection.
- An **allograft** is taken from cadavers and also provides a temporary covering that will be rejected by the immune system. If an allograft remains adherent to the prepared wound bed before rejection, an autograft placed on the wound may be expected to survive.
- **Dermal substitutes** are varied and may include bovine collagen in a matrix of shark cartilage covered by silicone. The collagen is vascularized over 2 to 3 weeks. The silicone then is removed, and a thin autograft is placed on the granulated wound bed.
- **Cultured Skin Substitutes:** Autologous cultured epithelium and epithelium in combination with dermal cell cultures are utilized in large burns with inadequate uninjured skin to harvest. This type of tissue is experimental and currently only used in very large burn injuries.

Lucich EA, Rendon JL, Valerio IL. Advances in addressing full-thickness skin defects: a review of dermal and epidermal substitutes. *Regen Med.* 2018;13(4):443–456.

17. Describe the clinical features of hypertrophic scars.

Hypertrophic scars are raised, red, rigid, and itchy, and can result in joint contractures and deformities. The epidermis and dermis are thicker, with fewer epithelial ridges, indistinct collagen fibers, increased water content and mast cells as compared to normal skin.

Kwan P, Tredget E. Biological principles of scar and contracture. *Hand Clin.* 2017;33(2):277–292.

18. How does applying pressure help in treating a hypertrophic scar?

Pressure applied to a burn scar may have a transient effect on limiting burn scar volume. They are expensive and many patients find them uncomfortable. Although still the standard of care at many burn centers, others are using off-the-shelf garments to provide protection and decrease neuropathic pain. Pressure garments may have a benefit in providing an environmental barrier to injury and a socially acceptable covering of the remodeling tissue.

Gabriel V. Hypertrophic scar. *Phys Med Rehabil Clin N Am.* 2011;22(2):301–310.

19. What types of instruments may be used to quantify scar?

Three-dimensional (3D) cameras for area and volume, reflected light devices for pigmentation, high frequency **ultrasound** for thickness and **vacuum devices** applied to the scar for elastic properties.

Lee KC, Dretzke J, Grover L, et al. A systematic review of objective burn scar measurements. *Burns Trauma.* 2016;4:14.

20. What are five common complications of deep facial burns?

Deep facial burns may result in:
- **Hypertrophic scarring** (a dramatic change in appearance, affecting recognition and self-perception)
- **Eyelid ectropion** (when the lower eyelid is everted and pulled downward)
- **Microstomia** with decreased mouth opening (affecting voice, eating, and drinking)
- Nasal deformities with retraction of the alar margin and **nostril stenosis**
- **Alopecia** (remedied with transplant and artfully utilized wigs)

Klein M, Moore M, Costa B, et al. Primer on the management of face burns at the University of Washington. *J Burn Care Rehabil.* 2005;26(1):2–6.

21. What are the risks and treatment for developing heterotopic ossification?

The incidence of heterotopic ossification (HO) after burn injury is reported to be between 1% and 3%. It is difficult to predict, but it is more common in larger burns and in joints with an overlying deep burn. HO after burn injury most commonly develops around the elbows. Treatment requires a combination of ongoing active and passive therapies, nitrogen containing bisphosphonates and selected surgical resection.

Sinha S, Biernaskie JA, Nickerson D, et al. Nitrogen-containing bisphosphonates for burn-related heterotopic ossification. *Burns Open.* 2018;2(3):160–163.

22. Can neuropathies be prevented?

Many neuropathies cannot be prevented and may be caused by heat, scarring or ischemia. The incidence of peripheral neuropathy is estimated at 15% to 30% in burn patients. Neuropathies are more commonly seen in patients with >20% TBSA and electrical burns. Iatrogenic causes include stretch and pressure from improper positioning or tight, bulky dressings.

Schneider JC. Neurologic and musculoskeletal complications of burn injuries. *Phys Med Rehabil Clin N Am.* 2011;22(2):261–275.

23. What is the best approach for the management of pain?

A burn care pain plan is essential. **Background pain** or pain that is present when the patient is at rest is best treated with a continuous infusion of opiates in the intensive care unit or with long-acting opiate medications. **Procedural pain,** such as that experienced during wound care and therapy sessions, can be treated with short-acting opiate pain medications given before and during the treatment. Studies have shown that the use of hypnosis and immersive virtual reality distraction can assist in decreasing procedural pain.

Hoffman HG, Patterson DR, Magula J, et al. Water-friendly virtual reality pain control during wound care. *J Clin Psychol.* 2004;60(2):189–195.

24. What psychological problems are seen in burn patients?

Anxiety, depression, and post-traumatic stress disorder are common in burn patients. Adaptation to body image and community reintegration require interdisciplinary proactive individualized strategies. Meetings with another burn survivor can significantly improve adjustment after injury. Research has demonstrated that the size of the burn does not correlate with psychological outcome.

Wiechman SA. Psychosocial recovery, pain, and itch after burn injuries. *Phys Med Rehabil Clin N Am.* 2011;22(2):327–345.

25. What causes problems with self-image and appearance in burn patients?

Paradoxically, the total body surface area of burn injury does not correlate with the severity of problems with body esteem and self-image. The visibility of the burn scar and variables such as social adjustment, depression, and family support are better predictors of self-acceptance and reintegration.

Lawrence JW, Fauerbach JA, Heinberg L, et al. Visible vs hidden scars and their relation to body esteem. *J Burn Care Rehabil.* 2004; 25(1):25–32.

26. When should children return to school after a burn injury?

After an injury, a child should go back to school as quickly as possible despite splints, scars, and ongoing therapies. Early reintegration promotes a positive body image and prevents disruptive and maladaptive behavior. Many burn centers have school reentry programs involving on-site visits to the school.

27. What barriers and successful interventions need to be part of the formulation of a community-based education and work plan?

Return to school is an urgent rehabilitation goal that needs to be addressed early with a rehabilitation and care with a rehabilitation team liaison with the target educational institution. Person-centered reintroduction with voice contact, followed by custom video and phone telecommunication to adapt coworkers to changes in appearance and adaptive function is recommended. Returning to work involves a complex navigation of barriers with maximization of adaptive personal characteristics, as well as social support with creative rehabilitation interventions. It is important to address psychological issues related to previous employment, self-blame, and discovery of strengths. Success is achieved with early intervention from a vocational counselor, modified duties, adaptations in the work-place, and alternative hours.

Esselman P. Community integration outcome after burn injury. *Phys Med Rehabil Clin N Am.* 2011;22(2):351–356.

28. What three factors increase the likelihood of a burned patient returning to work?
- One study demonstrated that the average time off work after a burn injury is 17 weeks in a population with mean TBSA of 17%, with 66% of individuals with burn injuries having returned to work within 6 months. Predictors preventing returning to work have been investigated in many studies, resulting in varied and inconsistent barriers. However, a desire to go back to work is the best positive predictor, supported by needing an income and enjoying work. Psychologic factors, TBSA and hand burns have small negative predictive values.

Carrougher GJ, Bamer AM, Mandell SP. et al. Factors affecting employment after burn injury in the United States: a burn model system national database investigation. *Arch Phys Med Rehabil.* 2020;101:S71–S85.

The TBSA is calculated by attributing 9% to the front and back of the head and neck, 9% to the front and back of each arm and hand, 9% to the chest and the stomach, 9% to the upper back, 9% to the lower back, 9% to the front and back of each leg and foot and 1% to the genital area.

29. What tools are used to measure burn outcomes?

Global measures of quality of life, such as the **SF-36**, are sometimes used for comparative impact. The **Burn Specific Health Scale** measures patient reported symptoms and concerns such as itching. Other symptom specific scales may also be incorporated.

Meirte J, Van Daele U, Maertens K, et al. Convergent and discriminant validity of quality of life measures used in burn populations. *Burns.* 201;43(1):84–92.

Gerber LH, Bush H, Holavanahalli R, et al. A scoping review of burn rehabilitation publications incorporating functional outcomes. *Burns.* 2019;45(5):1005–1013.

Rapid tissue viability evaluation using methemoglobin as a biomarker in burns.

Leung G, Duta D, Perry J, et al. Rapid tissue viability evaluation using methemoglobin as a biomarker in burns. *Int J Burns Trauma.* 2018;8(5):126–134.Books:

Herndon DN (ed): *Total Burn Care.* 5th ed. Philadelphia: Elsevier; 2018:812.

Burn Evaluation and Management

Schaefer TJ, Szymanski KD. Burn Evaluation And Management. [Updated 2021 Aug 11]. In: StatPearls [Internet]. Treasure Island (FL): StatPearls Publishing; 2022 Jan. Available from: https://www.ncbi.nlm.nih.gov/books/NBK430741/

BIBLIOGRAPHY

Burn and Trauma Branch of Chinese Geriatrics Society,. Ming J, Lei P, et al.Duan JL, Tan JH, Lou HP, Di DY, Wang DY. [National experts consensus on tracheotomy and intubation for burn patients (2018 version)]. *Zhonghua Shao Shang Za Zhi.* 2018;34(11):E006.

Devinck F, Deveaux C, Bennis Y, et al.Deken-Delannoy V, Jeanne M, Martinot-Duquennoy V, Guerreschi P, Pasquesoone L. [Deep alkali burns: Evaluation of a two-step surgical strategy]. *Ann Chir Plast Esthet.* 2018;63(3):191–196.

Eyvaz K, Kement M, Balin S, et al. Acar H, Kündeş F, Karaoz A, Civil O, Eser M, Kaptanoglu L, Vural S, Bildik N. Clinical evaluation of negative-pressure wound therapy in the management of electrical burns. *Ulus Travma Acil Cerrahi Derg.* 2018;24(5):456–461.

Grammatikopoulou MG, Theodoridis X, Gkiouras K, et al. Stamouli EM, Mavrantoni ME, Dardavessis T, Bogdanos DP. AgreeGREEing on guidelines for nutrition management of adult severe burn patients. JPEN *J Parenter Enteral Nutr.* 2019;43(4):490–496.

Johnson SP, Chung KC. Outcomes assessment after hand burns. *Hand Clin.* 2017;33(2):389–397.

Mason SA, Nathens AB, Byrne JP, et al. Ellis J, Fowler RA, Gonzalez A, Karanicolas PJ, Moineddin R, Jeschke MG. Aassociation between burn injury and mental illness among burn survivors: a population-based, self-matched, Longitudinal Cohort Study. *J. Am. Coll. Surg.* 2017;225(4):516–524.

Mehta M, Tudor GJ. *StatPearls* [Internet]. StatPearls Publishing; Treasure Island, (FL): StatPearls Publishing; 2019. Jun 7, 2019. Parkland Formula.

Regan A, Hotwagner DT. *StatPearls* [Internet]. StatPearls Publishing; Treasure Island, (FL): StatPearls Publishing; 2019. Jan 10, 2019. Burn Fluid Management.

Sahin C, Kaplan P, Ozturk S, et al.Alpar S, Karagoz H. Treatment of partial-thickness burns with a tulle-gras dressing and a hydrophilic polyurethane membrane: a comparative study. *J Wound Care.* 2019;28(1):24–28.

Stiles K. Emergency management of burns: part 2. *Emerg Nurse.* 2018;26(2):36–41.

Stiles K. Emergency management of burns: part 2. *Emerg Nurse.* 2018 Jul 03.

Watson C, Troynikov O, Lingard H. Design considerations for low-level risk personal protective clothing: a review. *Ind Health.* 2019 Jun 04;57(3):306–325.

Wu YT, Chen KH, Ban SL, et al.Tung KY, Chen LR. Evaluation of leap motion control for hand rehabilitation in burn patients: An experience in the dust explosion disaster in Formosa Fun Coast. *Burns.* 2019 Feb;45(1):157–164.

CHAPTER 66

ORGAN TRANSPLANTATION: MEDICAL AND REHABILITATION MANAGEMENT

Jeffrey Cohen, MD, Matthew Bartels, MD, MPH, and Samantha Mastanduno, MD

What you leave behind is not what is engraved in stone monuments, but what is woven into the lives of others.
— Pericles (495–425 BC)

KEY POINTS

1. Transplant recipients benefit from pre-transplant rehabilitation focusing on optimizing aerobic capacity, maximizing musculoskeletal strength, and maintaining range of motion to maintain viability for transplantation and to pre-emptively reduce the weakness and limitations they will experience post-operatively.
2. Transplant recipients require immunosuppressant medications for life; typically, a combination of a calcineurin inhibitor (tacrolimus/Prograf or cyclosporine/Neoral), an antimetabolite (mycophenolate mofetil/Cellcept or azathioprine/Imuran), and a steroid (prednisone), all of which limit muscle strength and capacity.
3. Transplant recipients require extremely close monitoring with frequent blood work, including immunosuppressant levels. Laboratory abnormalities may be the first sign of subclinical or acute rejection in a transplant recipient. Calcineurin inhibitors can cause a central demyelination syndrome, which is reversible if medications are changed early, and 5-10% of patients experience tremors and other peripheral nervous symptoms.

INTRODUCTION

1. **How many different transplantable organs are there? What are the most common post-transplant patients seen by physiatrists?**
   Currently, there are 22 organs that can be transplanted. This chapter will focus on the four most common transplantable organs seen in rehabilitation medicine: kidney (most commonly transplanted organ), liver, heart, and lung transplant.
   Hand, face, and penile transplantation have recently been added to the transplantable list. Additionally, tissues such as cornea, skin, heart valves, bone, blood vessels, connective tissues, bone marrow and stem cells, umbilical cord blood, and peripheral blood stem cells can be transplanted. The number of post-transplant patients admitted to acute inpatient rehabilitation is increasing; partly due to the increasing number of transplants being performed each year and long-term survivors experiencing neurological or other events.

2. **Who are the members of the transplant rehabilitation team?**
   The transplant rehabilitation team should ideally consist of a specialty medical team for the organ system transplanted including transplant surgeon, physiatrist, physical therapist, occupational therapist, registered nurse, social worker, case manager, clinical pharmacologist, nutritionist, and psychologist. Transplant surgeon, physiatrist, physical therapist, occupational therapist, registered nurse, social worker, case manager, clinical pharmacologist, nutritionist, and psychologist. The physiatrist's role is to serve as the team leader for functional recovery. He or she will work to coordinate the functional recovery components of patient care in the large interdisciplinary team.

3. **Importance of close communication with the transplant team**
   The physiatrist's continued communication with the transplant team is essential. Transplant recipients require extremely close monitoring with frequent blood work and medication changes. The physiatrist should communicate closely with the transplant surgeon and his or her team to inform them of any clinical changes. It is good practice to notify the transplant team of any medication changes. Becoming a part of the team and attending weekly transplant team selection rounds can facilitate this communication.

GENERAL MEDICAL MANAGEMENT OF ORGAN TRANSPLANT PATIENTS

4. **What are the key medications physiatrists need to be familiar with when managing post organ transplant patients?**
   The key medications physiatrists need to be familiar with in post-transplant patients are immunosuppressant medications and prophylactic antivirals, antifungals, and antibiotics. Immunosuppressant triple therapy is typically a combination of three medications that are taken for life: a calcineurin inhibitor (tacrolimus/Prograf or

cyclosporine/Neoral), an antimetabolite (mycophenolate mofetil/Cellcept or azathioprine/Imuran), and a glucocorticoid steroid. Steroids can often be tapered to a low maintenance level of 5 to 10 mg of prednisone or equivalent per day in 3 to 6 months post-operatively; however, some transplant surgeons may prefer to keep the patient on low-dose steroids indefinitely. It is important to be aware of the multiple drug interactions that can occur with this triple therapy.

IMMUNOSUPPRESSANT MEDICATIONS

Kidney and liver transplant:
These transplants usually require triple immunosuppressant therapy with a calcineurin inhibitor, an antimetabolite, and prednisone. This combination has demonstrated greater than 90% allograft survival at 1 year and acute rejection rates of less than 20%.

Heart and lung transplant:
Similar to liver and kidney transplantation, patients remain on lifelong immunosuppression. The levels of immune suppression are higher in heart patients and highest in lung transplant recipients due to the continued allogeneic characteristic of the lung transplant being in a non-sterile environment causing higher rates of rejection.

MEDICAL MANAGEMENT OF LIVER/KIDNEY TRANSPLANT

LIVER TRANSPLANT

5. What labs need to be followed in post-liver transplant patients, and how frequently?
   - Liver function tests, including aspartate transaminase (AST), alanine transaminase (ALT), gamma-glutamyl transferase (GGT), alkaline phosphatase (ALP), bilirubin, prothrombin time (PT), albumin should be monitored daily.
   - Tacrolimus trough—will need to be checked daily until a steady state is achieved. This level must be drawn before the next dose of tacrolimus. The medications will be adjusted based on the trough.
   - Magnesium levels—tacrolimus use can lead to hypomagnesemia through renal magnesium wasting. Low magnesium levels have been associated with higher mortality and increased cardiovascular events in the general population and in transplant recipients.

6. What are the key signs/symptoms that one needs to be aware of in liver organ rejection and what lab abnormalities may be indicative of organ rejection?
   Acute cell-mediated rejection is not uncommon in the first 3 months following liver transplantation and decreases in frequency with time. Symptoms of mild rejection are nonspecific and may include the following: fatigue, malaise, generalized weakness, and right upper quadrant pain. Clinical signs include low-grade fever, jaundice, right-upper-quadrant tenderness, or generalized abdominal tenderness.
   Diagnosis of acute liver transplant rejection based on clinical symptoms and signs alone is unreliable, and laboratory data is required. The rejection process may be subclinical, with laboratory abnormalities as the only sign of its presence. GGT, ALP, and bilirubin are the most sensitive and convenient tests to check for acute liver transplant rejection. With early detection, most acute rejection episodes can be treated successfully by augmentation of existing immunosuppressive medications or high doses of steroids.

7. What other complications should the physiatrist be aware of in post-liver transplant?
   - Graft ischemia and primary graft nonfunction: signs of graft ischemia are poor bile flow, high transaminase activities, and coagulopathy.
   - Hepatic artery thrombosis-most cases occur within the first 2 weeks. Presentation may be subtle and present as relapsing septicemia following bile duct ischemia. At the other extreme, it may present as a fulminant liver failure with prolonged protime and a massive increase of transaminases.
   - Liver transplant patients are also at increased risk for delayed cognitive recovery and malnutrition.

KIDNEY TRANSPLANT

8. What labs need to be followed in post-kidney transplant patients, and how frequently?
   Basic metabolic panel daily to monitor blood urea nitrogen (BUN) and Cr. Tacrolimus levels should also be monitored daily as mentioned above for hepatic transplants.

9. What medications should be avoided in kidney transplant patients?
   Non-steroidal anti-inflammatory medications should be avoided. In addition, ACE inhibitors and angiotensin receptor blockers should be avoided in the early post-transplant period until renal function stabilizes.

10. What are the key signs/symptoms of kidney transplant organ rejection that one needs to be aware of?
    The incidence of kidney organ transplant rejection has decreased since the advent of calcineurin inhibitors and antiproliferative agents. Acute rejection most often occurs within the first 6 months after transplantation. Most patients with acute rejection are asymptomatic.

Kidney rejection can present as malaise, anorexia, fever, hypertension, increased BUN, kidney enlargement with tenderness at the graft site, decreased urine output, or leukocytosis.

11. **What lab abnormalities may be indicative of kidney transplant organ rejection?**
Subclinical rejection—histologic evidence of rejection but no increase in serum creatinine.
Acute rejection may present with an increase in serum creatinine or proteinuria.

12. **What are specific blood pressure parameters to monitor in kidney transplant patients?**
Post-transplant elevated blood pressure may reflect volume overload, graft dysfunction due to rejection, ischemia, or calcineurin inhibitor toxicity. Treatment of the underlying cause will usually lower the blood pressure.
The blood pressure goal is based on the presence or absence of proteinuria and/or additional co-morbid conditions. In patients without proteinuria, the target blood pressure is <140/90 mmHg. For patients with significant proteinuria, the target blood pressure should be <130/80 mmHg.

13. **What other issues in a post-kidney transplant should the physiatrist be aware of?**
Another consideration to keep in mind when treating a post-kidney transplant patient is the possible need for stress steroid coverage when the patient has an acute illness.

REHABILITATION MANAGEMENT OF LIVER/KIDNEY TRANSPLANTS

PRE-OP

14. **What are the benefits of pre-op rehab in transplant patients?**
The benefit of pre-op rehabilitation in transplant patients is to establish a baseline. It is important to assess a patient's pre-op functional mobility status, use of assistive devices, independence in activities of daily living, cognition, communication, and vocational status. It is also essential to optimize aerobic capacity and maximize musculoskeletal strength and functional endurance prior to organ transplantation.

15. **What specific exercises are recommended pre-op for patients undergoing kidney and liver transplants?**
Patients requiring organ transplantation usually suffer from severe medical problems and are likely less active at baseline. They may experience fatigue, muscle weakness, and decreased endurance due to their co-morbidities. In the pre-op period, progressive range of motion exercises and strengthening exercises are recommended. Exercises to optimize aerobic capacity are initiated. Focusing on balance training and core strengthening will be useful to counteract the weakness and limitations sustained from a post-op incision. It is also important to educate patients on proper form and teach a home exercise program prior to surgery.

16. **What goals are we attempting to accomplish in the pre-op rehab program?**
1. Patient education about postoperative activity expectations-this can help reduce anxiety and increase postoperative compliance.
2. Patient independence with their exercise program.

POST-OP

17. **What specific precautions are needed when prescribing a rehab program for post-op kidney and liver transplant patients?**
In addition to universal precautions, when evaluating a post-transplant patient, one should adhere to immunocompromised precautions.
Immunocompromised precautions—hand hygiene before and after patient contact; avoid contact with animals and cleaning animal stool; fruits and vegetables that will be eaten raw should be washed well with safe water (commercially -bottled water, boiling water, filtered tap water, or distilled water) prior to consumption; peel fruits or vegetables after washing them if they are going to be consumed raw; no unpasteurized milk or dairy products. There are currently no studies to support isolating neutropenic patients in their own rooms to prevent infection.

18. **What are the major components of the rehab program post transplantation?**
The major aim of the post-transplantation rehab program is to provide a progressive increase in function to allow patients to enjoy a more active lifestyle with their new organ.
Another important aim is to provide the patient and caregivers with education and additional resources regarding the transplant process and how it may affect their lives.
In assessing a patient's post-transplant functional status, it is important to note that a patient's posture may be altered due to the incision's location and associated pain. Additionally, a patient's breathing pattern and depth of breath may be decreased to avoid pain. Breathing techniques, energy conservation, cough assist techniques, and endurance training contribute to the recovery.

19. Are there specific goals for the post-op rehab program?

The goals of the postoperative rehabilitation program are to maximize muscle strength, optimize chest wall movement, improve exercise tolerance, and improve functional mobility. This is accomplished through low to moderate level exercises and functional ADL skills training.

Patients are also educated on signs and symptoms of rejection, medication management, and management of co-morbidities such as diabetes.

DISCHARGE PLANNING

20. What are the key factors necessary to prepare the patient for discharge?

Prescription of home therapy or outpatient therapy to continue the rehabilitation program.

Caregiver training.

Psychosocial support/management to address the following: acute stress reaction, adjustment to disability, anxiety leading up to discharge, and support for the family/caregivers.

Coordinating outpatient blood work schedule, as they need close monitoring.

Coordinating medications at home—who will manage this after discharge? It is essential to teach patients the importance of each medication, when to take it, and what to do if they miss a dose.

MEDICAL MANAGEMENT OF HEART AND LUNG TRANSPLANT

HEART TRANSPLANT

21. What labs need to be followed in post-heart transplant patients, and how frequently?

- As in any patient post-transplantation, heart transplant patients need a regular schedule of biopsies and blood measurements of immunosuppressive medication levels. This is particularly important after a first post-operative biopsy 10 to 14 days after transplant and then as dictated by the clinical condition. A noninvasive marker for rejection in these patients is a change in cardiac function seen on echocardiograms, and these will be followed regularly.

22. What special considerations for exercise should be considered in heart transplant patients?

Since the transplanted organ is not innervated by the sympathetic or parasympathetic nervous systems, patients with heart transplantation have an alteration of exercise physiology. Due to loss of direct vagal inhibition, there is an elevated resting heart rate (often around 100 BPM) and a prolonged recovery of resting heart rate after exercise. On the contrary, there is a delayed increase in heart rate and lower peak heart rate due to sympathetic denervation and reliance on circulating catecholamines for heart rate control. This results in a decrease in maximal capacity after transplantation.

23. What lab abnormalities may be indicative of heart transplant organ rejection?

As in all other transplantation patients, kidney dysfunction and liver function should be monitored. Any changes in echocardiogram are also monitored for early signs of rejection.

24. What other complications/issues in a post-heart transplant should the physiatrist be aware of?

Chronic, low-grade humoral rejection in heart transplant patients can lead to accelerated atherosclerosis that is usually seen after about five years post-transplantation. This is a process of the small arteries and arterioles of the grafted heart and is not amenable to either bypass surgery or percutaneous interventions.

LUNG TRANSPLANT

25. What labs need to be followed in post lung transplant patients, and how frequently?

In addition to the close monitoring of immunosuppressive levels, post lung transplant patients benefit from the monitoring of lung function tests. Early signs of rejection are seen with the onset of an obstructive picture on Pulmonary Function Tests. In later rejection, imaging may show more radio-opacity of the lung transplants, and pleural effusions may develop.

26. What precautions are specific to lung transplant patients?

Lung transplant patients need to avoid excessive respiratory exposure. Since the lung transplants are the transplanted organ, it is important to minimize the immunological stimulation in the organ to lower the chance of rejection. Even in the best situations, there is a higher chance of immunogenicity, and these patients run higher immunosuppression than patients with other transplanted organs. Hot tubs and other sources of mold are to be avoided as are working or being in an environment with high levels of aerosols or particulates in the air. If a patient is to be in any of those environments or an area with aerosolized infections, face masks with high efficiency particulate air filtration capacity should be used.

27. What lab abnormalities may be indicative of lung transplant organ rejection?

Pulmonary function testing with the onset of obstructive physiology is seen most commonly. The chronic humoral form of rejection in lung transplant is obstructive bronchiolitis (OB), which is a narrowing of the terminal bronchioles in chronic rejection. There is no treatment for advanced OB besides re-transplantation, and since it is a chronic humoral rejection, once it starts, it may not be able to be slowed in some cases.

28. **What other complications/issues should the physiatrist be aware of in post-lung transplant?**
As in other transplant patients, osteoporosis and side effects of the medications are present but often exaggerated in lung transplant patients. Because of the higher levels of chronic immunosuppression, kidney failure is of particular concern.

Bonus questions and answers are available online.

BIBLIOGRAPHY

1. Azathioprine: Drug Information. UpToDate. Available at: https://www.uptodate.com/contents/azathioprine-drug-information.
2. Braddom RL. Ed. Transplantation of organs: rehabilitation to maximize outcomes. In *Physical Medicine & Rehabilitation*. 4th ed. Philadelphia, PA: Elsevier Saunders; 2011:1439–1456.
3. Brennan DC, Alhamad T, Malone A. *Clinical Features and Diagnosis of Acute Renal Allograft Rejection*. [UpToDate]. Available at: https://www.uptodate.com/contents/clinical-features-and-diagnosis-of-acute-renal-allograft-rejection.
4. Cohen JM, Young MA, Stiens SA, et al. Organ transplantation and rehabilitation. In: Moroz A, Flanagan SR, Zaretsky H, eds. *Medical Aspects of Disability for the Rehabilitation Professional*. 5th ed. Springer Publishing Company; 2017:412–512.
5. Filipovich AH, Weisdorf D, Pavletic S, et al. National Institutes of Health consensus development project on criteria for clinical trials in chronic graft-versus-host disease: I. Diagnosis and staging working group report. *Biol Blood Marrow Transplant*. 2005;11(12):945.
6. Fishman JA, Alexander BD. Prophylaxis of infections in solid organ transplantation. [UpToDate]. Available at: https://www.uptodate.com/contents/prophylaxis-of-infections-in-solid-organ-transplantation.
7. Garnier AS, Duveau A, Planchais M, et al. Serum magnesium after kidney transplantation: a systematic review. *Nutrients*. 2018;10(6):729. Published 2018 Jun 6. doi:10.3390/nu10060729
8. Hickman PE, Potter JM, Pesce AJ. Clinical chemistry and post-liver-transplant monitoring. *Clin Chem*. 1997;43(8):1546–1554. Available at: http://clinchem.aaccjnls.org/content/43/8/1546.
9. Kidney Disease: Improving Global Outcomes (KDIGO) Transplant Work Group. KDIGO clinical practice guideline for the care of kidney transplant recipients. *Am J Transplant*. 2009;9(Suppl 3):S1.
10. Lahart M. Solid organ transplants: inpatient post-operative considerations. *Rehabilitation for Solid Organ Transplant*. 2013. Available at: http://cardiopt.org/csm2013/Rehab-after-solid-organ-transplant.pdf.
11. Leroy C, Rigot JM, Leroy M, et al. *Immunosuppressive drugs and fertility. Orphanet* J Rare Dis. 2015;10:136. Epub 2015 10 21.
12. Mycophenolate mofetil (Cellcept) and mycophenolate sodium (Myfortic): Drug information. UpToDate. Available at: https://www.uptodate.com/contents/mycophenolate-mofetil-cellcept-and-mycophenolate-sodium-myfortic-drug-information.
13. Organ Donation FAQs. *U.S Government Information on Organ Donation and Transplantation*. Available at: https://www.organdonor.gov/about/facts-terms/donation-faqs.html.
14. Prevention & Control—Immunocompromised Persons. Centers for Disease Control and Prevention. Available at: https://www.cdc.gov/parasites/crypto/gen_info/prevent_ic.html.
15. Savitsky EA, Uner AB, Votey SR. Evaluation of orthotopic liver transplant recipients presenting to the emergency department. *Ann Emerg Med*. 1998;31(4):507–517.
16. Soave R. Prophylaxis strategies for solid-organ transplantation. Clin Infect Dis. 2001;33(Suppl 1):S26–S31.

CHRONIC PAIN: ASSESSMENT AND INTERDISCIPLINARY INTERVENTION

Charles Kim, MD, CAc, Bryan J. O'Young, MD, CAc, FAAPMR, Christopher Gharibo, MD, Kiril Kiprovski, MD, John A. Sturgeon, PhD, and Steven A. Stiens, MD, MS

There are two types of pain in this world; pain that hurts you and pain that changes you.

— Anonymous

KEY POINTS

1. Pain is multidimensional and involves an interplay of bio-psycho-social-emotional factors.
2. Chronic pain affects more Americans than diabetes, heart disease, and cancer combined.
3. The main goal of opioid therapy should emphasize maximizing functional goals and minimizing adverse events.
4. Due diligence in prescribing opioids for pain is not an optional responsibility but a duty.
5. Pain treatment should first focus on non-opioid treatments.

1. How is chronic pain defined?

The International Association of the Study of Pain (IASP) has updated its definition of pain as "an unpleasant sensory and emotional experience associated with, or resembling that associated with, actual or potential tissue damage". The components of this definition show the multi-dimensionality of pain, including its bio-psycho-emotional aspects. This definition captures the characteristics of both acute and chronic pain.

Acute pain is (or is expected to be) transient (less than 3 months), typically disappearing with the resolution of the insult, pain generator, or event (e.g., trauma, surgery, acute illnesses). *Chronic pain* is defined as pain persisting for longer than 3 months beyond the healing of an acute injury or insult, frequently recurring over time, or is associated with a lesion or not.

Raja SN, et al. The revised international association for the study of pain definition of pain: concepts, challenges, and compromises. *Pain.* 2020 Sep 1;161(9):1976–1982.

King, W. (2007). Acute Pain, Subacute Pain and Chronic Pain. In: Schmidt, R., Willis, W. (eds) *Encyclopedia of Pain.* Springer, Berlin, Heidelberg, pp 35–36.

2. Is chronic pain a symptom or a disease?

The IASP, in conjunction with the World Health Organization (WHO), classifies chronic pain into two categories:

Chronic secondary pain, in which pain may be at least initially a chronic symptom (e.g., cancer-related, visceral, neuropathic, post-traumatic and post-surgical, secondary headache and orofacial pain, and secondary musculoskeletal pain).

Chronic primary pain syndromes, in which pain can be the sole or leading complaint, and requires special treatment and care (e.g., fibromyalgia or nonspecific low-back pain).

Utilizing this classification system and specific codes in the new edition of the *International Classification of Disease* (ICD-11, 2020) will improve classification and diagnostic coding, thereby advancing the recognition of chronic pain as a health condition in its own right.

ICD-11, 2020. Available at https://icd.who.int/en.

Treede RD, Rief W, Barke A, et al. Chronic pain as a symptom or a disease: the IASP Classification of Chronic Pain for the International Classification of Diseases (ICD-11). *Pain.* 2019;160(1):19–27.

3. How common is chronic pain, and what are its costs in the U.S.?

In 2016, the Centers for Disease Control and Prevention (CDC) analyzed data from the 2016 *National Health Interview Survey* (NIHS) and estimated that 20.4% (50 million) adults had chronic pain, and 8% (19.6 million) of adults had high-impact chronic pain. The total cost of chronic pain in the U.S. In 2010 dollars ranged from $560 to $635 billion. This exceeds that of heart disease ($309 billion), cancer ($243 billion), and diabetes ($188 billion). Pain is a leading cause of disability and a major contributor to health care utilization. Chronic pain affects ***more*** Americans than diabetes, heart disease, and cancer ***combined***.

Gaskin, DJ, Richard P. *Relieving Pain in America: A Blueprint for Transforming Prevention, Care, Education, and Research: Appendix C the Economic Costs of Pain in the United States*. Washington, DC: Institute of Medicine Committee on advancing pain research, care, and education; 2011. Available at https://www.ncbi.nlm.nih.gov/books/NBK92521/.

Interagency Pain Research Coordinating Committee. *National Pain Strategy: A Comprehensive Population Health-Level Strategy for Pain*. Washington, DC: US Department of Health and Human Services, National Institutes of Health; 2016.

Institute of Medicine. *Relieving Pain in America: A Blueprint for Transforming Prevention, Care, Education, and Research*. Washington, DC: National Academies Press; 2011.

National Institutes of Health. *Research Portfolio Online Reporting Tools (RePORT)*. Pain Management. Available at https://report.nih.gov/nihfactsheets/ ViewFactSheet.aspx?csid557.

4. How is chronic pain evaluated?

The interview begins with the chronological details of the pain experience, including associated symptoms, details of previous treatment, and outcomes. Current medications, including over the counter (OTC) meds and other active treatments, are listed. The clinician assesses description of biofeedback, physiotherapy, massage therapy, anesthetic blocks/injections, or surgeries patients may have had, and determines if these treatments are useful, ineffective, or cause intolerable side effects.

Important information can be gained from assessing comorbidities that may influence manifestation of the pain syndrome, and could affect treatment, such as dementia, diabetes, renal failure, cardiovascular disease, sleep disorder, seizure disorder, substance abuse, and psychiatric illness. Other factors (family or cultural issues, personality characteristics, employment history, litigation issues, financial situation, and family and/or community support) are entered in a database.

A comprehensive general physical exam should be done and vital signs should be included with each visit. A directed ***musculoskeletal exam*** and other pertinent systems assessment are performed to address the pain. A ***neurological examination***, including cognitive assessment, cranial nerves, motor, sensory capabilities, reflexes, coordination, and gait, is essential.

5. What characteristics of every pain syndrome must be assessed and documented to describe its presentation and provide a baseline for intervention?

Temporal/ continuous or intermittent: The timing of pain can provide diagnostic clues to pain etiology. Neuropathic pain is often spontaneous and without provocation. Alternately, nociceptive pain, such as osteoarthritis of the hip, is usually not severe unless provoked by use. The typical timing of cluster headaches differentiates it from the "ice pick headache," and the intermittent nature of trigeminal neuralgia distinguishes it from herpes zoster pain of the fifth cranial nerve.

Sensory qualities: Neuropathic pain symptoms include numbness, tingling, pins and needles, electric shocks or shooting pain, and hot or burning pains.

Intensity/ severity: There are several rating scales validated as measures of pain severity and are discussed below.

Location/region/radiation: The different pain sites can be visually represented by having the patient draw their pain on a pain diagram. Neuropathic characteristics can be described simultaneously by using symbols or adding colors to the diagram.

Exacerbating/relieving: Assessing what provokes or relieves the pain provides valuable clues to the diagnosis.

Physical functioning/ recreational functioning: Pain can alter mood and aggravate preexisting mood disorders. Social contacts can be lost, leading to social isolation that worsens pain symptoms, creating a vicious cycle.

Pain rating scales: ***Verbal rating scales*** (VRSs), ***numerical rating scales*** (NRSs), and ***visual analog scales*** (VASs) are often used in pain research and clinical settings. Due to the individuality and subjectiveness of pain; these are usually best used to gauge clinical status and treatment responses.

6. How is chronic pain clinically described and classified?

The description of the pain by the patient and subsequent classification of the type of the pain can help clinicians infer its potential etiology and enhance treatment effectiveness.

Based on the relevant pathophysiology, pain is classified as:

- ***Nociceptive***: Pain initiated or caused by a primary lesion or dysfunction in the ***tissues*** other than the nervous system. The nociceptive pain can be either *somatic* or *visceral*. The patient usually describes this pain as *dull, achy, crampy, or deep*.
- ***Neuropathic***: Pain initiated or caused by a primary lesion or dysfunction in the somatosensory nervous system. Characteristic verbal description of neuropathic pain is *burning, electric shocks, shooting, lancinating, numbness, pins and needles,* and *itching* pain. To identify definite neuropathic pain, it is necessary to demonstrate a lesion or disease involving the nervous system. Some common causes of neuropathic pain are diabetes or other painful polyneuropathies, complex regional pain syndromes (CRPS), postherpetic neuralgia (PHN), radiculopathy, phantom limb pain, and post-surgical scar pain.

- *Mixed*: Pain initiated or caused by a simultaneous lesion or dysfunction in the nervous system and other tissues.
- *Psychogenic*: Pain not initiated or caused by a primary organic lesion.
- *Central pain*: Pain initiated or caused by a primary lesion or dysfunction in the CNS. Examples include post-stroke central pain syndrome due to thalamic syndrome (*Dejerine-Roussy Syndrome)*, multiple sclerosis, trigeminal neuralgia, and central pain syndromes associated with spinal cord injury.

7. What are the clinical presentations of neuropathic pain?
Neuropathic pain can be spontaneous or provoked. Neuropathic pain is recognized by the patient's complaint profile and confirmed with typical findings. They are grouped below:
- *Dysesthesia*: An unpleasant abnormal sensation, whether spontaneous or evoked.
- *Hyperalgesia*: An increased response to a stimulus that is normally painful.
- *Allodynia*: Pain due to a stimulus that does not normally provoke pain. It can be upon contact, temperature, or vibratory stimulus (usually modality-specific).
- *Hyperesthesia*: Increased sensitivity to stimulation, excluding the special senses.
- *Hyperpathia*: Painful syndrome characterized by an abnormally painful reaction to a stimulus, especially a repetitive stimulus, as well as an increased threshold.
- *Neuralgia*: Pain in the distribution of a single nerve or multiple nerves.
- *Autonomic signs*: Local changes in skin color, skin appearance, atrophic skin, subcutaneous edema, skin temperature extremes, excessive sweating, or lack of sweat response.

8. What is the impact of the "opioid crisis" on chronic pain?
Pain as the "5th vital sign" grew out of the *Joint Commission*'s (formerly the Joint Commission on Accreditation of Healthcare Organizations, or JCAHO) call to address pain. Clearly, acute pain associated with trauma, surgery, and inflammation must be proactively managed to match respiration, mobility, and best outcomes. Unfortunately, many chronic pain patients had excessive and escalating doses of opioids that led to unacceptable complications. The number of opioid prescriptions dispensed from U.S. pharmacies increased from about 76 million in 1991 to 219 million in 2011. The timing of pressures from multiple sources, coupled with the growth of synthetic opioids in the U.S., led to unintended consequences. In 2017, there were 70,237 deaths attributable to drug overdoses, with 67.8% of these deaths involving a prescription opioid. Notably, from 2016 to 2017, synthetic opioid-involved overdose death rates increased by 45.2%.

Baker DW. *The Joint Commission's Pain Standards: Origins and Evolution.* Oakbrook Terrace, IL: The Joint Commission; 2017.

Scholl L, Seth P, Kariisa M, et al. Drug and opioid-involved overdose deaths—United States, 2013–2017. *Morb Mortal Wkly Rep.* 2018;67(5152):1419–1427. Available at https://www.ncbi.nlm.nih.gov/pmc/articles/PMC6334822/.

9. What is the primary goal of opioid therapy?
While the main goals of opioid therapy might seem obvious, health care providers and patients often have opposing viewpoints. A 2017 study conducted by Bell et al. showed considerable differences in prioritized outcomes by physician-patient care plans. Of most importance to patients was reducing the intensity of pain, closely followed by diagnosing the cause of the discomfort. Not surprisingly, the most commonly sought-after goal by physicians was functionality, followed by minimizing medication side effects. The physician's emphasis on maximizing functional goals and minimizing adverse events related to opioids is attributable to recommendations made by organizations such as the CDC. Providers and patients often have different levels of understanding concerning pain, which leads to divergent management goals. Although primary goals may differ among providers and patients, no evidence has been found that this difference compromises patient experience.

Henry SG, Bell RA, Fenton JJ, et al. Goals of chronic pain management: do patients and primary care physicians agree, and does it matter? *Clin J Pain.* 2017;33(11):955–961.

10. What options are available to clinicians assessing adherence to long-term opioid therapy?
The perceived limitations for viable substitutes to opioids in managing chronic pain have created unnecessary dependence on this class of medications and essentially created a risk of addiction. Providers have many tools at their disposal to assess dependence on chronic opioid therapy, but none is more important than *prescription drug monitoring programs*. With proper due diligence, a provider can review a patient's controlled substance prescription history and assess signs of opioid misuse or abuse. Evaluating a patient's candidacy for an initial opioid prescription is vital to curbing potential lethal outcomes. Running a thorough check through state monitoring programs opens an avenue for providers to refer individuals to treatment programs if warranted. If no warning signs are uncovered, then *urine drug screening* and *past medical records* should be used to further evaluate candidacy. Once chronic opioid therapy is initiated, patients can be closely monitored through urine and *saliva*

drug testing. Follow-up visits can be utilized to review *medication diaries*, pill counts and reassess provider-patient agreements.

Hudson S, Wimsatt LA. How to monitor opioid use for your patients with chronic pain. *Fam Pract Manag.* 2014;21(6):6–11.

11. What is adjuvant pain medication?

Adjuvant pain medications are drugs with primary indications other than pain, often used *off-label* when treating pain. They are distinguished from opioid and nonopioid analgesics, acetaminophen, and non-steroidal anti-inflammatory drugs (NSAIDs). Adjuvants for chronic pain can include antidepressants, anticonvulsants, central-acting adrenergic agents, and muscle relaxants, among others.

12. What is the role of antidepressants in chronic pain management?

Due to the complexities of chronic pain, antidepressants have a role in treatment. With the psycho-emotional aspects of chronic pain being prominent, research supports their use in managing chronic pain due to their primary analgesic effects.

The best-studied antidepressants for treating chronic pain are *tricyclic antidepressants* (TCAs). The tertiary amine drugs, particularly amitriptyline, are more likely to be effective than secondary amine agents such as nortriptyline. Tertiary TCAs tend to have more side effects (e.g., dry mouth, constipation, orthostatic hypotension, urinary retention, increased heart rate) than the newer secondary TCAs.

Comparing the TCAs to newer selective serotonin reuptake inhibitors (SSRIs) and serotonin norephinephrine reuptake inhibitors (SNRIs), we see a more favorable response in chronic pain conditions with TCAs. In fact, their efficacy for treating chronic pain seems to be better with agents having broader neurochemical effects than more specific ones. In order of efficacy, we tend to see the best response in older TCAs, then SNRIs, with SSRIs being least effective. *Duloxetine* is an SNRI with Food and Drug Administration (FDA) approval for managing diabetic neuropathic pain, fibromyalgia, and chronic musculoskeletal pain.

13. Are anticonvulsant medications also helpful for chronic pain?

Initially developed to treat seizure disorders, these agents have become widely used as a treatment for many pain conditions. *Gabapentin* is the most widely prescribed anticonvulsant for pain. Despite its name, it does not affect Gamma-Aminobutyric acid (GABA) receptors. Its mechanism of action involves *inhibiting the alpha-2-delta subunit of the nerves' voltage-gated calcium channels. Pregabalin*, a newer version of gabapentin with superior bioavailability, has also been more widely utilized. In 2005, the U.S. Drug Enforcement Agency listed pregabalin as a Schedule V drug under the Controlled Substances Act due to 4% of users reporting euphoria after its use in clinical trials. In clinical practice, the gabapentinoids seem to work best for central, neuropathic, and radiculopathic type pains versus other pains (e.g., somatic and visceral).

14. What roles do anti-anxiety and hypnotic medications have in chronic pain treatment?

In many chronic pain patients, we often see comorbid anxiety and sleep disturbances. The use of *benzodiazepines* (BDZs) is quite commonly prescribed for these disturbances, as well as for muscle spasms. In general, none of the BDZs are recommended for pain-related sleep disturbances, and BDZs have poor restoration of sleep architecture (mainly deep stage IV sleep). **Non-BDZ hypnotics (**e.g., zolpidem, eszopiclone) have more *favorable effects on sleep architecture*. Extreme caution should be practiced when a patient is on an opioid or opiate and any of these agents, especially BDZs. In fact, concomitant use of opioids and BDZs have been associated with significantly increased risks of side effects, respiratory depression, and death, even at surprisingly low doses. It is best to *avoid combining these agents with opioids* altogether in the clinical setting. Alternative hypnotics can include TCAs and trazodone (an SSRI).

15. What are nonopioid analgesics?

The main nonopioid analgesics include *acetaminophen* and *NSAIDs*. These agents produce analgesia via both peripheral and central mechanisms. Unlike opioids, the analgesia produced by these agents has a ceiling effect (a dose level above which additional amounts provide no added analgesia). NSAIDs are both anti-inflammatory and analgesic. Aspirin and NSAIDs (e.g., ibuprofen, naproxen) inhibit prostaglandin synthesis. Aspirin is unique in that it irreversibly inactivates cyclooxygenase (COX). Acetaminophen inhibits prostaglandin synthesis in the CNS and is antipyretic but not anti-inflammatory. Concerns related to NSAIDs include gastric issues ranging from abdominal pain and bloating to massive gastrointestinal bleeding. This risk is somewhat lessened with COX-2 specific NSAIDs. All NSAIDs can also impair renal function, including peripheral edema and even acute renal failure. In 2015, the FDA raised its warning about all NSAIDs (prescribed and OTC) concerning an increased risk of causing serious cerebrovascular thrombotic events and possible death, regardless of duration of use. If prescribing any NSAIDs, pretreatment and intratreatment blood pressures are essential monitoring strategies.

16. How about muscle relaxants?

Although BDZs have been used historically as first-line muscle relaxants, their addictive and opioid interaction potentials should be concerning. Alternative muscle relaxants should be utilized as first-line agents. These include *cyclobenzaprine*, *metaxalone*, *methocarbamol*. These agents are centrally acting and do not directly relax skeletal muscle. Tizanidine is an alpha-2-adrenergic agonist and should be used with caution for patients with cardiac issues. **Cyclobenzaprine** is a TCA that should be used cautiously with patients on SSRI and SNRI antidepressants due to the potential for serotonin syndrome, a potentially life-threatening condition. **Baclofen** directly activates GABA-B receptors, although its exact mechanism of action is not fully understood. Care must be taken when stopping baclofen; abrupt cessation can cause seizures. A slow taper schedule is the standard of care. In general, the main side effect of muscle relaxants is sedation and clouded mentation. It is often recommended to take these before bed and start at the lowest dose to achieve acceptable effects.

17. What types of cannabis have medical purposes?

There are two species of the *Cannabis* genus typically used for medical purposes: *Cannabis indica* and *Cannabis sativa*. *Sativa* species tend to produce more psychoactivity, whereas *indica* is more sedating and helpful for pain. The variations in these are based on the ratios of delta 9-tetrahydrocannabinol (THC) and cannabidiol (CBD). THC is more psychoactive, and CBD is more sedating and helpful for pain. Concerning the synthetic variations (dronabinol and nabilone) of THC, the former has an identical structure to THC while the latter is a more potent version of it.

Regarding medicinal uses of cannabis, according to a study in the *British Medical Journal*, found that there was moderate certainty of benefit for chronic pain and multiple sclerosis. They found low certainty of benefit for treatment-resistant epilepsy and for chemotherapy-induced nausea and vomiting. Other often studied medical conditions include glaucoma, HIV/AIDS, and cachexia.

Hillig KW, Mahlberg PG. A chemotaxonomic analysis of cannabinoid variation in Cannabis (Cannabaceae). *Am J Botan.* 2004;91(6): 966–975.

18. Is cannabis safe?

There are short- and long-term adverse effects of cannabis use. Some short-term effects include impaired short-term memory, impaired motor coordination, altered judgment, and, in higher doses, paranoia and psychosis. Long-term use leads to psychological addiction, altered brain development in younger users, cognitive impairments, chronic bronchitis, diminished life satisfaction and achievement, and chronic psychosis.

In general, cannabinoids are well tolerated by most. Several studies have investigated drug interactions with cannabis. Cannabinoids are metabolized via *Cytochrome 450* and *UDP-glucuronosyltransferase*. Theoretically, when combined with other drugs, cannabis use can lead to potentially unwanted effects. Caution should be taken when prescribing any medications when cannabis is also used, especially in the elderly and patients with impaired hepatorenal function. The Mayo Clinic recommends caution when cannabis is used with alcohol, anticoagulants, anti-platelets, CNS depressants, protease inhibitors, and SSRIs.

Volkow ND, Baler RD. Compton WM, et al. Adverse health effects of marijuana use. *NEJM.* 2014;370(23):2219–2227.

19. Is cannabis the solution for the opioid epidemic?

According to most sources, research support for Cannabis's role in Chronic Pain and ameliorating the opioid crisis is insufficient. In February 2016, the *3rd Symposium on Controlled Substances and Their Alternatives for the Treatment of Pain* was held in Boston. Participants and attendees represented the biopsychosocial authorities on chronic pain. The conclusion of this symposium regarding cannabis for chronic pain was that, "we need a better understanding and evidence for its use that is free from cultural bias." They also determined a lack of conclusive clinical utility of cannabis for chronic pain existed, and further research is needed. There is much variability of cannabis preparations (i.e., THC and CBD content) and regulatory/legal issues that impact its further study. We must be certain that we are not jumping from one era of harmful substance use to another.

Freeman TP, Hindocha C, Green SF, et al. Medicinal use of cannabis-based products and cannabinoids. *BMJ.* 2019;365:1141.

Maher DP, Carr DB, Hill K, et al. Cannabis for the treatment of chronic pain in the era of and the opioid epidemic: a symposium-based review of the sociomedical science. *Pain Med.* 2017;pnx143.

Volkow ND, Baler RD, Compton WM, et al. Adverse effects of marijuana use. *NEJM.* 2014:370(23):2219–2227.

20. What is the role of complementary medicine in chronic pain?

In recent years, the epidemic of opioid overuse and abuse has made pain very challenging for clinicians and patients. An increasing number of pain patients are benefitting from complementary medicine as an adjunct to standard medical and surgical and procedural management of pain. For example, there is evidence to support acupuncture's role in promoting endorphin release, thus potentiating the effects of opioids allowing for dose de-escalation. There is a growing need for evidence-based integration of complementary therapies into conventional care. The National Center for Complementary and Integrative Health (NCCIH) at the National Institutes of Health (NIH) was established in 1998 to fund and conduct research into complementary health approaches to assess what works and what does not work. In 2016, the NCCIH published a clinical digest (*Complementary Health Approaches for Chronic Pain*) to summarize evidence-based findings on the efficacy of complementary medicine for fibromyalgia, headache, irritable bowel syndrome, low back pain, neck pain, osteoarthritis, and rheumatoid arthritis.

Mao J, Dusek J. Integrative medicine as standard care for pain management: the need for rigorous research. *Pain Med.* 2016;17(6): 1181–1182. Available at https://www.ncbi.nlm.nih.gov/pmc/articles/PMC4894245/.

NCCIH. *Complementary Health Approaches for Chronic Pain.* NCCIH Clinical Digest; 2016. Available at https://www.nccih.nih.gov/health/providers/digest/complementary-health-approaches-for-chronic-pain.

21. What is the difference between a multidisciplinary approach and an interdisciplinary approach? Why is this relevant?

The **multidisciplinary** approach implies involvement of several health care providers, including physicians, physical therapists, occupational therapists, and psychologists. However, integrating their services, particularly communication, may be limited if they are not in the same facility. Even if they are located together, they may still be considered as providing multidisciplinary care if they pursue treatments with separate goals and do not take into account contributions by other disciplines.

The **interdisciplinary** approach consists of greater coordination of services in a comprehensive program, as well as frequent communication among health care professions providing services with common, shared goals under one roof. Interdisciplinary pain programs have been repeatedly demonstrated to be cost-effective. However, there is reluctance by third-party payers to compensate such care. With the advent of electronic medical records and group video telecommunications, interdisciplinary care has become more feasible with a "cyber-home" location.

Gatchel RJ, Okifuji A. Evidence-based scientific data documenting the treatment and cost-effectiveness of comprehensive pain programs for chronic nonmalignant pain. *J Pain.* 2006;7(11):779–793.

22. How do physical and occupational therapies contribute to the rehabilitation plan for chronic pain?

As members of the physiatry stewarded team, physical therapists and occupational therapists contribute to the collaborative pain team effort through evaluation of the nervous and musculoskeletal systems, education in active physical coping skills, physical rehabilitation processes including exercise (stretching, strengthening, aerobic, balance), manual therapy (aerobic, joint mobilization, mobilization), modalities (electrical stimulation, hot packs, ultrasound, cold), motor re-education, sensory re-education, home exercise program, and assessment of the home and workplace. The goals are to reduce pain and maximize function. This involves a multidisciplinary approach using both active approaches (self-management, education, exercise, sensory and motor re-education) and passive ones (physical modalities and manual therapies). The interdisciplinary team members consistently look to the physiatrist as leaders of the team to render medical and procedural intervention to advance treatment objectives.

Self-management includes instruction on the disease process (chronic pain mechanism and central sensitization), remaining active, and pacing activities. Patients with chronic pain are typically deconditioned. Patients should therefore start their exercise slowly, progress slowly, and stretch before and after exercise. Physical and occupational therapists encourage using exercise in daily life, ergonomics, facilitate exposure to repeated movements as much as possible despite the pain, and reinforce education emphasizing the biopsychosocial model of pain management.

Smith BE, Hendrick P, Smith TO, et al. Should exercises be painful in the management of chronic musculoskeletal pain? A systematic review and meta-analysis. *Br J Sports Med.* 2017;51(23);1679–1687.

Rochman, Deborah Occupational Therapy, and Pain Rehabilitation. Available at https://www.aota.org/ About-OccupationalTherapy/Professionals/HW/Pain%20Rehabilitation.aspx.

23. What role do psychologists play in chronic pain management?

Psychologists play multiple roles in pain management settings, including providing evidence-based psychotherapy and assessing patients' psychological function to determine needs or readiness for specific medical interventions. There are several evidence-based psychological interventions, including cognitive-behavioral therapy; mindfulness-based interventions that help patients learn to manage pain and emotions using meditation; and acceptance and commitment therapy techniques that help patients adjust unhelpful patterns of behavior in the service of attaining meaningful long-term goals.

These interventions show small but reliable reductions in pain and disability, and reduce stress, depression, anxiety, and unhelpful cognitive processes related to pain (e.g., pain-related fear, catastrophic appraisals of pain, and fear of movement) that impair patients' ability to participate and benefit fully from treatment (Kroner-Herwig, 2009; Williams et al., 2020). Psychological screening is a standard of care for patients undergoing interventional device trials, most notably spinal cord stimulators. Identifying patients in need of additional treatment to address high levels of psychological distress (depression, anxiety, and somatization) and poor coping responses to pain can improve the likelihood of optimal response to interventional treatments (Campbell et al., 2013).

Campbell CM, Jamison RN, Edwards RR.. Psychological screening/phenotyping as predictors for spinal cord stimulation. *Curr Pain Headache Rep.* 2013;17(1):307. Available at https://www.ncbi.nlm.nih.gov/pmc/articles/PMC3601592/.

Kröner-Herwig B. Chronic pain syndromes and their treatment by psychological interventions. *Curr Opin Psychiatry.* 2009;22(2): 200–204.

Williams AC, Fisher E, Hearn L, et al. Psychological therapies for the management of chronic pain (excluding headache) in adults. *Cochrane Database Syst Rev.* 2020;8(8):CD007407. Available at https://pubmed.ncbi.nlm.nih.gov/32794606/.

BIBLIOGRAPHY

Ballantyne J, Fishman S, Rathmell J, eds. *Bonica's Management of Pain.* 5th ed. Philadelphia: Wolters Kluwer Health: 2019.
Honorio B, Rathmell J, Wu CL, et al. eds. *Practical Management of Pain.* 5th ed. Philadelphia: Elsevier, 2014.

Bonus questions and answers available online.

CHAPTER 68

CENTRAL PAIN: PATHOPHYSIOLOGY, DIAGNOSIS, AND TREATMENT—A CHALLENGING DIAGNOSIS

Charles Argoff, MD, Ravneet Bhullar, MD, and Evangeline P. Koutalianos, MD

Pain is inevitable. Misery is a choice.

— Christopher Reeve (1952–2004)

KEY POINTS: CENTRAL PAIN

1. The most commonly cited causes of central pain syndromes are spinal cord injury (SCI) pain and central post-stroke pain (CPSP).
2. Most cases of CPSP follow ischemic strokes; thalamic and lateral medullary strokes have the highest incidence of CPSP.
3. Although difficult to treat, several medical and nonmedical treatments are available for patients living with central pain.

1. **What is central pain and what are the most common central pain syndromes?**
   Central pain is pain associated with lesions of the central nervous system (CNS), brain, and/or spinal cord. Central pain syndromes are among the most difficult pain syndromes to evaluate and treat successfully. The International Association for the Study of Pain defines central neuropathic pain as pain "caused by a lesion or disease of the central somatosensory system." The most commonly cited central pain syndromes are central post-stroke pain (CPSP), multiple sclerosis, and spinal cord injury (SCI) pain. Identifying and treating central pain is extremely important, especially in the rehabilitation setting, since ineffective pain management may lead to difficulty with rehabilitation program participation.

Watson JC, Sandroni P. Central neuropathic pain syndromes. *Mayo Clin Proc.* 2016;91(3):372–385. Available at: https://doi.org/10.1016/j.mayocp.2016.01.017.

2. **What causes Central post-stroke pain?**
   CPSP, first described in 1906, occurs in approximately 2% to 8% of stroke patients. CPSP can result from any insult to the CNS, including vascular, demyelinating, infectious, or neoplastic lesions affecting the spinal cord and brain. Of all stroke patients with somatosensory deficits, 18% develop CPSP. This kind of pain is seen in patients with ischemic strokes; thalamic and lateral medullary strokes have the highest incidence. The onset of pain following a stroke can begin as early as 1 to 2 months or as late as 1 to 6 years. Patients often describe their pain in vague terms, sometimes delaying diagnosis.

Oh H, Seo W. A comprehensive review of central post-stroke pain. *Pain Manag Nurs.* 2015;16:804–818. Available at: http://accurate-clinic.com/wp-content/uploads/2016/01/A-Comprehensive-Review-of-Central-Post-Stroke-Pain-2015-no-highlights.pdf.

Meacham K, Shepherd A, Mohapatra DP, et al. Neuropathic pain: central vs. peripheral mechanisms. *Curr Pain Headache Rep.* 2017; 21:28. Available at: https://doi.org/10.1007/s11916-017-0629-5.

3. **Identify the causes of SCI pain.**
   The most common cause of SCI-related pain is trauma (60% to 70% of SCI patients). Other causes of SCI include postsurgical, neoplastic, inflammatory, and vascular conditions, as well as demyelination and congenital abnormalities. The International Spinal Cord Injury Pain group (ISCIP) classifies chronic SCI pain into three tiers based on the origin of pain, subcategories of nociceptive and neuropathic pain, and finally the source of pain.

Hadjipavlou G, Cortese AM, Ramaswamy B. Spinal cord injury and chronic pain. *Br J Anaesth.* 2016;8:264–268. Available at: https://doi.org/10.1093/bjaed/mkv073.

4. Discuss the pathophysiology of central pain syndromes.

There are two main hypotheses explaining the mechanism behind central pain syndromes. The first states there is nociceptive hyperexcitability secondary to a lesion that affects the somatosensory pathways, which leads to increased nociceptive activity. The second states that the pain syndrome results from neuron denervation.

SCI-related pain commonly occurs in patients with lesions of the dorsal or dorsolateral aspects of the spinal cord, resulting in abnormalities of descending pain inhibitory input to the spinal cord. Thalamic areas most commonly involved in CPSP include the ventroposterior inferior and ventromedial nuclei. Cortical processing is also considered to be important in the development of CPSP. Spinal thalamic cortical pathways may be injured following an ischemic or hemorrhagic infarct.

Boivie J, Casey KL. *Central Pain in the Face and Head.* In J Olesen (Eds.). *The Headaches.* Philadelphia: Lippincott Williams and Wilkins, 2006:1063.

Jensen TS, Finnerup NB. Central pain. In: McMahon, SB et al. (eds). *Wall & Melzack's Textbook of Pain.* 6th ed. Philadelphia: Saunders; 2013:990–1002.

5. What are the clinical features of central pain syndromes?

CPSP has a variable presentation, usually involving unilateral facial and or head pain, with impaired sensation in the craniocervical region due to the stroke. Onset of CPSP or SCI-related pain may be delayed months to years after the insult. SCI-related pain may be associated with nerve root lesions, partial or segmental cord damage, more complete cord injury, secondary visceral involvement through connections via the sympathetic nervous system, and injury to the cauda equina. Patients may complain of pain with varying intensity that is persistent or can present with sudden intermittent episodes. Patients with SCI pain may complain of a band-like muscle pain, described as a crushing or aching sensation. Many patients with central pain may complain of abnormal sensations, which are often poorly localized. Living with central pain often leads to development of severe depression. **Allodynia and hyperalgesia** are common in central pain. Patients may also complain of lancinating as well as shooting pain, pins and needles, and sensations of bloating or bladder fullness.

McHenry KW. International association for the study of pain: lessons from my central pain. *Pain.* 2002;10(3):1–6.

6. What are the diagnostic criteria for CPSP syndromes?

According to the International Classification of Headache Disorders, 3rd edition (ICHD-3), the diagnostic criteria for CPSP include the following: facial and or head pain; ischemic or hemorrhagic stroke; pain developed within 6 months after a stroke; brain imaging reveals vascular lesion in appropriate site; and clinical presentation does not fit any other ICHD-3 diagnosis.

The International Classification of Headache Disorders, 3rd edition (beta version). Headache classification committee of the International Headache Society. *Cephalalgia.* 2013;33(9):629–808. Available at: https://www.ncbi.nlm.nih.gov/pubmed/23771276.

7. What are the oral pharmacologic treatment options for central pain?

The following pharmacologic recommendations are made for central neuropathic pain: tricyclic antidepressants (TCAs) are first-line agents; gabapentinoids are second-line agents. However, these agents can be considered as first line in elderly patients or when TCAs are contraindicated. Lamotrigine and opioids are third-line agents secondary to the risk of dependency, addiction, and overdose. When the above medications fail, other medications that treat neuropathic pain syndromes may be attempted. These include phenytoin, carbamazepine, clonazepam, valproate, phenothiazines, SNRIs (i.e., duloxetine), mexiletine, and baclofen.

Multiple randomized clinical trials revealed that amitriptyline (doses titrated to 75 mg daily) and lamotrigine are effective in the treatment of both CPSP as well as SCI-related pain. Of these studies, amitriptyline was considered to be first-line treatment for CPSP. Depending on the location of the pain, certain medications are recommended over others. Carbamazepine, starting at doses of 100 to 200 mg daily (up to 1200 mg), is a good initial therapy for treatment of neuralgic facial pain secondary to stroke.

Kim JS. Pharmacological management of central post-stroke pain: a practical guide. *CNS Drugs.* 2014;9:787–797. Available at: https://link.springer.com/article/10.1007%2Fs40263-014-0194-y.

Oh H, Seo W. A Comprehensive Review of Central Post-Stroke Pain. *Pain Manag Nurs.* 2015 Oct;16(5):804–818. doi: 10.1016/j.pmn.2015.03.002. Available at: https://doi.org/10.1016/j.pmn.2015.03.002.

8. What are some of the options for injected medications?

Anesthetic treatment options such as ketamine, lidocaine, and propofol have been shown to be effective in managing CPSP. There are limited studies on this topic; however, a study in 2001 reported that ketamine, a NMDA antagonist, can decrease allodynia and hyperalgesia in this patient population (Vick & Lamer 2001). Intravenous lidocaine has also been shown to be effective in the management of central pain; however, there are limitations with this treatment option, as it is short-acting and requires repeated doses to maintain its effect. In a randomized controlled study, pain intensity and allodynia was reduced compared to placebo (Attal 2000). Overall, in the same study, 69% of patients receiving intravenous lidocaine, compared with 38% of patients receiving placebo, experienced moderate or complete relief. The use of intrathecal analgesics, including both opioid and nonopioid analgesics, can also be considered in refractory situations.

Attal N, Gaude V, Brasseur L, et al. Intravenous lidocaine in central pain: a double-blind, placebo-controlled, psychophysical study. *Neurology.* 2000;54:564–574. Available at: https://www.ncbi.nlm.nih.gov/pubmed/10680784.

Vick PG, Lamer TJ. Treatment of central poststroke pain with oral ketamine. *Pain.* 2001;92(1–2):311–313. Available at: https://www.ncbi.nlm.nih.gov/pubmed/11323153.

9. What are the nonpharmacologic treatment options for central pain?

Nonpharmacologic treatment options can be considered in cases that are refractory to medication or when medication is not tolerated. Options include spinal neuromodulation, motor cortex stimulation, deep brain stimulation (DBS), cingulotomy, and repetitive transcranial magnetic stimulation (rTMS).

Spinal neuromodulation is effective in treating medically refractory central pain syndromes such as phantom limb pain and CPSP. A study reported that 7 out of 10 patients receiving permanent spinal cord stimulation systems reported significant pain relief on the visual analog scale (VAS) (Aly 2010). Chronic motor cortex stimulation was once considered to provide pain relief; however, the 2016 guidelines from the European Academy of Neurology found poor to moderate-quality evidence that motor cortex stimulation relieves neuropathic pain.

DBS involves the implantation of a medical device into the brain that transmits signals through electrodes targeting specific neural structures. DBS has been shown to be effective in managing chronic pain syndromes. The periventricular matter, ventral posterior lateral region of the thalamus, and the nucleus accumbens are the most effective target structures in patients with CPSP. A meta-analysis showed that of the 45 patients with CPSP, 53% received a permanent DBS implantation and 58% of these patients achieved long-term pain relief (Bittar 2005).

Other surgical techniques such as cingulotomy or direct lesioning of the anterior cingulate cortex have shown to be successful in patients with pain disorders. There are only few cases reported regarding cingulotomy in stroke patients that have shown improvement in their VAS of 51.9% over the first month following the procedure. However, these results are confounded by the fact that these patients also had deep-brain stimulators implanted and these were activated around the same time of the cingulotomy—which makes it difficult to determine whether the benefit is from the DBS or the cingulotomy. Further research is needed in this area to determine whether this is a viable treatment option for CPSP.

rTMS is a treatment in which a coil that transmits a magnetic pulse is placed over the patient's scalp, inducing an electrical current through a particular region of the cerebral cortex. Studies examining rTMS treatment in the CPSP population have shown a significant reduction in VAS with minimal side effects. A recent open-label study from Japan reported that motor cortex stimulation using rTMS over 1 year led to significant reductions in VAS.

Aly M, Saitoh Y, Hosomi K, et al. Spinal cord stimulation for central poststroke pain. *Neurosurgery.* 2010;67(3):206–212. Available at: https://www.ncbi.nlm.nih.gov/pubmed/20679928.

Bittar RG, Kar-Purkayastha I, Owen SL, et al. Deep brain stimulation for pain relief: a meta-analysis. *J Clin Neurosci.* 2005;12(5): 515–519. Available at: https://www.ncbi.nlm.nih.gov/pubmed/15993077.

Brain stimulation therapies for epilepsy. Available at: https://www.ninds.nih.gov/About-NINDS/Impact/NINDS-Contributions-Approved-Therapies/Brain-stimulation-therapies-epilepsy.

Chail A, Saini RK, Bhat PS, et al. Transcranial magnetic stimulation: A review of its evolution and current applications. *Industrial Psychiatry Journal.* 2018 Jul-Dec; 27(2):172–180. Available at: https://www.ncbi.nlm.nih.gov/pmc/articles/PMC6592198/.

Cruccu G, Garcia-Larrea L, Hansson P. EAN guidelines on central neurostimulation therapy in chronic pain conditions. *Eur J Neurol.* 2016; 23(10):1489–1499. Available at: https://onlinelibrary.wiley.com/doi/full/10.1111/ene.13103.

Kim, JP, Chang WS, Park YS, et al. Impact of ventralis caudalis deep brain stimulation combined with stereotactic bilateral cingulotomy for treatment of post-stroke pain. *Stereotact Funct Neurosurg.* 2012;90(1):9–15. Available at: https://www.ncbi.nlm.nih.gov/pubmed/22189908.

Kobayashi M, Fujimaki T, Mihara B, et al. Repetitive transcranial magnetic stimulation once a week induces sustainable long-term relief of central poststroke pain. *Neuromodulation.* 2015;18(4):249–254. Available at https://www.ncbi.nlm.nih.gov/pubmed/25906811/.

Lundstrom BN, Gompel JV, Khadjevand F, et al. Chronic subthreshold cortical stimulation and stimulation-related EEG biomarkers for focal epilepsy. *Brain Commun.* 2019;1(1):fcz010. Available at: https://pubmed.ncbi.nlm.nih.gov/31667473/.

10. What is the role of botulinum toxin and intrathecal baclofen in patients with central pain?

Botulinum toxin injections and intrathecal baclofen are effective treatment options for central pain. A randomized controlled study evaluated 40 patients with SCI-associated neuropathic pain and showed that botulinum toxin A subcutaneous injections provide a significant reduction in pain of 20% or greater.

Intrathecal baclofen—as well as other muscle relaxants (diazepam, dantrolene, tizanidine)— has been reported to reduce severe CPSP. These medications have been shown to effectively treat spasticity-associated pain in CPSP. A recent phase 4, randomized, controlled multicenter study conducted in rehabilitation hospitals evaluated the efficacy of intrathecal baclofen among patients with CPSP and found that there was a significant improvement in both pain and quality of life with this intervention (Creamer 2018).

Creamer M, Cloud G, Kossmehl P, et al. Effect of intrathecal baclofen on pain and quality of life in poststroke spasticity: a randomized trial (SISTERS). *Stroke.* 2018;49:2129–2137. Available at: https://www.ncbi.nlm.nih.gov/pubmed/30354975.

Han ZA, Song DH, Oh HM, et al. Botulinum toxin type A for neuropathic pain in patients with spinal cord injury. *Ann Neurol.* 2016 Apr; 79(4):569–578. Available at: https://www.ncbi.nlm.nih.gov/pubmed/26814620.

BIBLIOGRAPHY

Argoff CE, Dubin A, Pilitsis JG, eds. *Pain Management Secrets.* 4th ed. Philadelphia: Elsevier; 2018.

Ballantyne J, Fishman S, Rathmell J, eds. *Bonica's Management of Pain.* 5th ed. Alphen aan den Rijn: Wolters Kluwer; 2018.

Watson J, Sandroni P. Central neuropathic pain syndromes. *Mayo Clin Proc.* 2016;91(3):372–385.

CHAPTER 69

SPINAL SEGMENTAL SENSITIZATION: DIAGNOSIS AND MANAGEMENT

Bryan J. O'Young, MD, CAc, FAAPMR, Giampaolo de Sena, MD, Marta Imamura, MD, PhD, and Mark A. Young, MD, MBA, FACP, FAAPMR, DABPMR

We need to treat both the disease/injury process in the periphery and the changes it induces or triggers in the CNS. Prevention of central sensitization will substantially eliminate the hyperalgesia and allodynia that patients find so distressing. Spinal neuronal plasticity is shown to be a key contributor to pathologic pain hypersensitivity.

—Clifford J. Woolf, MD

"Clifford Woolf, who can be considered as the "grandfather" of central sensitization (CS), first introduced the concept in 1983 (Woolf, 1983). He suggested that neuroplasticity and abnormal changes in the central nervous could result in an intense enhancement of pain. Since that time, CS mechanisms have been demonstrated in many animal and human studies (Latremoliere & Woolf, 2009; Woolf, 2011). Our evolving understanding of CS has fundamentally changed our view of pain and is now recognized as a major underpinning of many chronic pain disorders (Harte, Harris & Clauw; Woolf, 2011)."

Gatchel R, Neblett R. Central sensitization: a brief overview. *J Appl Biobehav Res.* 2018;23(2) (Special Issue on Central Sensitization):e12138.

KEY POINTS: SEGMENTAL NEUROMYOTHERAPY

1. The system of diagnosis and treatment is based on spinal segmental sensitization (SSS)
2. SSS can be diagnosed only by improved, more sensitive, and precise examination methods.
3. Specific treatments, including special injection techniques, are combined with physical therapy and exercises concentrated on the involved segment.

KEY POINTS: SIGNIFICANCE OF SENSITIZED SPINAL SEGMENT

1. This step indicates that the sensitizing process, which starts at the periphery, has reached the central nervous system
2. Effective management requires treatment of both peripheral and central sensitization.
3. Its presence, along with peripheral tissue sensitization, may escape diagnosis when conventional examination techniques are employed.
4. This condition can be successfully diagnosed by quantitative objective methods with high sensitivity and precision (e.g., algometry, electric skin conductance, tissue compliance measurement).

KEY POINTS: ACCURATE DIAGNOSIS OF PAIN DISTRIBUTION

1. An accurate diagnosis requires the identification of sensitized spinal segment(s).
2. This diagnosis can be achieved only if it is based on the correct dermatomes described by Keegan and Garret (1948).
3. Sensitization of myotomes can be detected only if the correct innervation pattern is kept in mind.
4. Each myotome innervates only part of a muscle, which is covered by the corresponding dermatome.

KEY POINTS: EFFECTIVE TREATMENT OF PAIN

1. Treatment cannot be limited to the alleviation of pain.
2. Identify and remove the causes of pain and address the mechanisms underlying the sensitization.
3. Treatment of spinal segmental sensitization should involve all of its affected components.
4. Treatment consists of desensitization of the involved segment.
5. Long-term results require eradication of irritative foci, which induce sensitization.

1. How has the goal of pain management changed within the past four decades?
   Contemporary pain management has shifted from symptom control to management based on fundamental pathophysiological mechanisms. Among these important mechanisms is the critical concept of **sensitization**. Sensitization is now known to be a key element in the development and perpetuation of pain. To properly treat pain, there must be an understanding that pain develops due to peripheral sensitization leading to central sensitization, necessitating the reduction of both peripheral and central sensitization to allow recovery to occur. This approach has been associated with reduced pain, improved function, and health-related quality of life. One clinical approach based on these principles discussed in this chapter is **segmental neuromyotherapy**.

   Recently, it has been recognized that constant and intense nociceptive sensory information generated by painful, inflamed deep somatic structures produce significant neurochemical and metabolic changes and reorganizations within corresponding spinal cord segments. These changes include increased excitability of dorsal horn neurons producing pain hypersensitivity in a segmental distribution. Together, these neurochemical changes suggest that pain induces—and is partially maintained by—a state of central sensitization in which increased transmission of nociceptive information normally allows non-noxious input to be amplified and perceived as noxious stimuli. Once these complex mechanisms are present, the rationale for treatment approaches should target desensitization mechanisms. It is necessary to note that these spinal cord changes may not be attenuated by blocking the original tissue damage and pain. Diagnosis of central and peripheral sensitization is very important because **spinal cord neurons normally activated by noxious stimuli are now activated by normally non-noxious stimuli (allodynia).**

Woolf CJ, Salter MW. Neuronal plasticity: increasing the gain in pain. *Science*. 2000;288(5472):1765–1769. doi:10.1126/science.288.5472.1765.

2. According to the international association study for the study of pain (IASP) classification, what are the three types of pain mechanisms? Why is nociplastic pain important?
   (a) Nociceptive pain: Pain arising from actual or threatened damage to non-neural tissue and is due to the activation of nociceptors.
   (b) Neuropathic pain: Pain caused by a lesion or disease of the somatosensory nervous system.
   (c) Nociplastic pain: Pain arising from **altered nociception** despite **no clear evidence of actual or threatened tissue damage** causing the activation of peripheral nociceptors **or evidence for disease or lesion of the somatosensory system** causing the pain.
   In 2011, the IASP had two primary mechanistic descriptors for chronic pain states: nociceptive pain and neuropathic pain, as defined above. However, there was no term to describe pain states characterized by clinical and psychophysical findings suggesting altered nociception without clear evidence of actual or threatened tissue damage causing the activation of nociceptors or evidence for disease or lesion the somatosensory system causing the chronic pain. In 2020, the term *nociplastic pain* was introduced in the revised IASP definition of pain and intended primarily for patients suffering from chronic pain conditions unable to be characterized as nociceptive or neuropathic pain. Examples are irritable bowel syndrome, fibromyalgia, visceral pain disorders, complex regional pain syndrome, chronic nonspecific low back pain, and other chronic musculoskeletal pain commonly defined as "functional." The term *nociplastic* was selected to reflect the plasticity of the central nervous system, as evidenced by findings of the cumulative research in the changes of the peripheral and central nervous system in pain pathways.

Raja SN, Carr DB, Cohen M. The revised International Association for the Study of Pain definition of pain: concepts, challenges, and compromises. *Pain*. 2020;161(9):1976–1982. doi:10.1097/j.pain.0000000000001939. Available at: https://journals.lww.com/pain/Abstract/2020/09000/The_revised_International_Association_for_the.6.aspx.

3. What is sensitization?
   Sensitization is a heightened sensitivity to stimuli that may occur in the peripheral or central nervous system. In pain mechanisms, sensitization can be sustained in the nervous system as peripheral and central nervous system function changes in response to nociceptive or neuropathic input. Sensitization may produce pain stimuli in pathological conditions even without clear evidence of actual or threatened tissue damage or identifiable disease or lesion of the somatosensory system causing the pain.

   Sensitization is also a term related to the nervous system's plasticity in which the continuous nociceptive afferent input to the central system "modulates" the central nervous system function, leading to more "sensitivity" to the stimuli. For those mechanisms, this term has been used as a descriptor for two different levels of sensitization: peripheral sensitization, which occurs as hyperalgesia of the peripheral nervous system; and central sensitization, which can be divided between spinal sensitization and supraspinal sensitization. In central sensitization, supraspinal structures in the brain undergo demonstrated changes in specific cerebral structures, connectivity, cerebral activation, and even in certain clinical pain states when adjusted for depression or anxiety.

4. What is peripheral sensitization?

Peripheral sensitization is an "increased responsiveness and reduced threshold of nociceptive neurons in the periphery to the stimulation of their receptive fields," characterized by hyperexcitability (i.e., hyperreactivity) of sensory nerve fibers to stimuli. The clinical manifestations of nerve fiber sensitization include hyperalgesia (increased reaction to painful stimuli, such as scratching or pinprick). The usual mechanism of sensitization consists of local tissue damage producing sensitizing, inflammatory, irritating substances, such as prostaglandins and bradykinin. The sensitized peripheral afferent sensory neuron will then trigger a long-lasting increase in the excitability of spinal cord neurons, profoundly changing the gain of the somatosensory system (i.e., spinal sensitization). A vicious cycle develops between central sensitization and irritative foci, each increasing the sensitization of the corresponding component. Increased sympathetic outflow potentiates the sensitization of peripheral nerves in the acute state. Edema around the tissue damage entraps inflammatory substances along with nerve endings (see Fig. 69.1).

Baron R, Hans G, Dickenson AH. Peripheral input and its importance for central sensitization. *Ann Neurol*. 2013;74(5):630–636. doi:10.1002/ana.24017 Available at: https://pubmed.ncbi.nlm.nih.gov/24018757/.

Mizumura K. Peripheral mechanism of hyperalgesia-sensitization of nociceptors. *Nagoya J Med Sci*. 1997;60:69–87. Available at: https://www.med.nagoyau.ac.jp/medlib/nagoya_j_med_sci/6034/ v60n34p69_87.pdf.

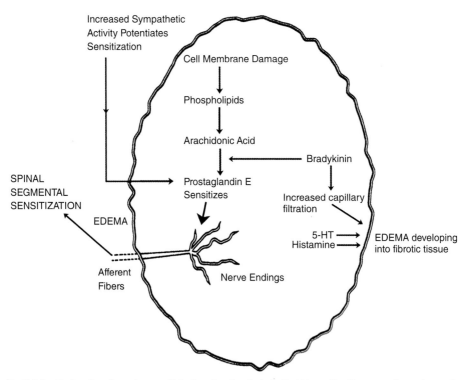

Fig. 69.1 Reaction to cell membrane damage with the formation of prostaglandin E, which sensitizes the nerve endings, subsequently causing spinal segmental and central sensitization. Simultaneously, vasoactive substances cause edema that entraps nerve endings along with the sensitizing substances. In a few weeks, the edema changes into fibrotic tissue forming a chronic irritative focus.

5. Define central sensitization (CS).

Central sensitization is "an enhancement in the function of neurons and circuits in nociceptive pathways caused by increases in membrane excitability and synaptic efficacy as well as reduced inhibition and is a manifestation of the remarkable plasticity of the somatosensory nervous system in response to activity, inflammation, and neural injury". It has long been recognized as a possible consequence of nociceptive or neuropathic pain, leading to increased responsiveness of nociceptive neurons in the central nervous system to their normal or subthreshold afferent input due to hyperactivity in pain pathways from peripheral to central. However, it is increasingly evident that it plays a role in various chronic pain disorders such as fibromyalgia, irritable bowel syndrome, chronic fatigue syndrome, endometriosis, rheumatoid arthritis, chronic low back pain, chronic neck pain, whiplash injuries, chronic tension headaches, migraine headaches, osteoarthritis of the knee, and injuries sustained in motor vehicle accidents or after surgeries—all of which seem to have the common denominator of central sensitization.

Afferent pathways, which carry abnormal information sensation from four different tissues (myofascial, cutaneous and subcutaneous, nervous, and connective tissues), connect with ascending spinothalamic and thalamocortical tracts, relating sensory information to the cortex and the limbic system. Descending tracts, such as cortico-spinal, connect with efferent segmental structures including somatic and visceral motor neurons in the serotoninergic, adrenergic, and internal opioid systems. The hyperexcitability connected with sensitization is increased by sensitized peripheral tissues and descending tract control. In addition to allo-dynia and hyperalgesia, CS is also associated with cognitive deficits, increased levels of emotional distress, particularly anxiety; role behaviors, such as resting and malaise; and pain behavior.

Latremoliere A, Woolf C. Central sensitization: a generator of pain hypersensitivity by central neural plasticity. *J Pain.* 2009;10(9): 895–926. doi:10.1016/j.jpain.2009.06.012.

6. What is segmental spinal sensitization (SSS)?

SSS is a condition characterized by hyperactivity, facilitation, and hyperexcitability of a spinal segment developing in reaction to an irritative focus, constantly bombarding the sensory ganglion with nociceptive stimuli. The irritative focus usually consists of a small area of damaged or dysfunctional tissue where peripheral sensitization or irritation of the nerve fibers generates the continuous nociceptive stimuli, causing sensitization of the CNS.

Sensitization and hyperexcitability spread from sensory to motor components of the segment, inducing hyperto-nicity and tenderness (muscle spasm) and activate TS/TrPs (trigger point) within the myotome. This CS starts with the spinal segment (i.e., SSS is the initial step in CS). This complex clinical picture of associated muscular, cutaneous, and articular innervations has been known for the past 160 years, based on embryological observations of nerve innervation by John Hilton (Hilton's Law embodies the principle that the nerve supplying a joint also supplies both the muscles that move the joint and the skin covering the articular insertion of those muscles).

Fischer AA. *Functional Diagnosis of Musculoskeletal Pain by Quantitative and Objective Methods.* In ES Rachlin, IS Rachlin (Eds.). *Myofascial Pain and Fibromyalgia. Trigger Point Management.* 2nd ed. St. Louis: Mosby; 2002:145–173.

Grzybowski A, Zamachowska M. John Hilton (1805–1878). *J Neurol.* 2021;268(3):1130–1132. doi: 10.1007/s00415-020-09802-7.

7. What is the anatomical and embryological basis of SSS?

During embryonic development, myotome, sclerotome, dermatome develop together in segmental meta-mere, where each spinal segment is a switchboard for several nerve fiber connections. Afferent pathways—which carry information sensation from different tissues—as the first station, reach the wide dynamic range (WDR) neurons in the fifth lamina of the posterior horn of the spinal cord, connecting with ascending spinothalamic and thalamocortical tracts relating sensory information to the cortex. Nobel Prize recipient Eric Kandel demonstrated through his aplysia experiments that WDR 5th lamina sensitization led to sensitization of the anterior horn in the same segment, producing segmental muscle spasm.

Horizontal structures connect the spinal segment with afferent impulses from and efferent signals to different peripheral tissues. Both incoming afferent and outgoing efferent pathways connect the spinal segment with different organs. Descending tracts, such as the cortico-spinal, connect with efferent segmental structures, including somatic and visceral motor neurons. Unlike a telephone switchboard, the spinal segmental connections are dynamic. Their activity and function continuously depend on the balance between excitatory and inhibitory impulses from the periphery and their modulation by higher nerve centers. Sensitized peripheral tissues and descending track control increase hyperexcitability related to sensitization. Steps in peripheral and central sensitization are summarized in Fig. 69.2.

Kandel E, Koester JD, Mack SH, Siegelbaum S, eds. *Principles of Neural Science.* 6th ed. New York: McGraw Hill Education/ Medical; 2021.

Sadler TW. *Langman's Medical Embryology.* 14th ed. Philadelphia: Lippincott Williams & Wilkins; 2018.

Woolf CJ. Dissecting out mechanisms responsible for peripheral neuropathic pain: Implications for diagnosis and therapy. *Life Sci.* 2004;74:2605–2610.

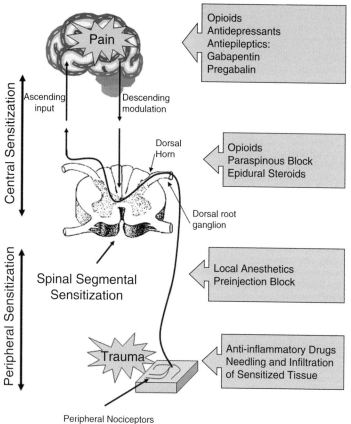

Fig. 69.2 Steps in peripheral and central sensitization and corresponding therapeutic interventions.

8. What are the clinical manifestations of sensitization?
   See Table 69.1.

9. What are the two primary characteristics of central sensitization? and how does the intensity of peripheral sensitization relate to central sensitization?
   - **Temporal Summation:** Consists of increased pain intensity on repeated stimuli such as pinprick or electric stimulation (1/s). This "wind-up" can be explained by the abnormal continuous electrical activity of the sensitized hyperexcitable nerve. Local anesthetic reverses the hyperexcitability and interrupts continuous activity, the basis of sensitization. Once normal sensitivity and reactivity of the nerve have been restored, the condition is maintained until an irritative focus causes its sensitization again.
   - **Spatial Irradiation:** Consists of the hyperexcitability spreading to adjacent areas and tissues and the entire spinal segment. In addition, the spreading of spinal sensitization proceeds vertically to the adjacent cranial and caudal segments.
   - The more intense the peripheral sensitization is in the irritative focus, as manifested by a lower pressure pain threshold, the more intense the local and central sensitization. The signs and symptoms of sensitization (hyperalgesia, allodynia, and augmented electric skin conductance [ESC]) increase exponentially with the progressive sensitization of the irritative focus.

Curatolo M, Arendt-Nielsen L, Petersen S. Evidence, mechanisms, and clinical implications of central hypersensitivity in chronic pain after whiplash injury. *Clin J Pain.* 2004;20(6):469–476. doi: 10.1097/00002508-200411000-00013.

Table 69.1 Diagnosis of Peripheral and Segmental (Central) Sensitization

Findings	Quantification Methods
A. Peripheral Sensitization	
1. *Hyperalgesia of skin:* sharper feeling on scratch and pinch and roll	
2. *Tenderness:* Decreased pressure pain threshold.	Algometer
a. Skin	
b. Subcutaneous	
c. Deep tissues, muscles	
3. *Micro-trophoedema:* Indentation by nail persists	Algometer
4. *Subcutaneous edema:* Thicker skin fold	Caliper, ultrasound
5. *Electric skin conductance:* Increased	Micro-Amp meter
B. Segmental (Central) Sensitization	
1. Dermatomal distribution of peripheral sensitization findings.	See Part A
2. Temporal summation of repetitive stimuli. Use pinprick or electric stimuli repeated 1/s causes gradually increasing pain	Pinprick or electrical stimulation
3. Myotomal distribution of muscle sensitization	
a. Tender spots/trigger points	Algometer
b. Taut bands	Tissue compliance meter
c. Muscle spasm (tender hypertonicity)	Tissue compliance meter
4. Sclerotomal inflammation	
a. Enthesopathy at insertions of taut bands	Algometer
b. Tendinitis, bursitis, epicondylitis	
c. Joint changes, capsulitis	
d. Ligament tenderness	
5. Viscerotome: Segmental organ irritation and dysfunction (see Table 69.2)	Palpation/auscultation of target organs
6. Spatial irradiation: spreading of segmental sensitization proximally and distally	All of the above tools are used to identify spinal segmental sensitization.

From Fischer AA. *Algometry in the Diagnosis of Musculoskeletal Pain and Evaluation of Treatment Outcome: An Update.* In AA Fischer (Ed.). *Muscle Pain Syndromes and Fibromyalgia.* New York: Haworth; 1998:5–32.

10. What are the manifestations of SSS in viscerotomes and other segmental components?
- **Viscerotome:** Pain, local and referred, with symptoms specific to each organ (i.e., gastrointestinal: gastroesophageal reflux disease, nausea, vomiting, irritable bowel syndrome) (see Table 69.2).
- **Myotome:** Tender spots/trigger points, taut bands, spasm. Myotomal deep tissue (muscle) tenderness is assessed by digital pressure and quantified with a pressure algometer. The pressure pain threshold—the minimum pressure that induces pain—is considered abnormal if lower than 2 kg/cm^2 compared to a normosensitive control point.
- **Dermatome:** Skin and subcutaneous tissue tender on pinch and roll and scratch tests, increased electric skin conductance (see Fig. 69.3)
- **Sclerotome:** Tenderness over sclerotome tissues (i.e., ligaments, bursa, entheses, joints) within the involved segment
- **Sympathetic:** Segmental sweating, skin cooling and discoloration, microedema, and increased electric skin conductance over the involved segment (dermatome)

Ballantyne JC, Fishman SM, Rathmell JP. *Bonica's Management of Pain.* 5th ed. Philadelphia: Lippincott Williams & Wilkins; 2018.

Table 69.2 Symptoms and Signs of Spinal Segmental Sensitization Related to Viscerotomes and Other Segmental Structures

VISCERAL ORGAN	INNERVATING SPINAL SEGMENTS	SYMPTOMS	COMPONENTS OF SENSITIZED SPINAL SEGMENT
Lungs	T2–T6	Chest pain	T2–T6 innervated myotomes, including paraspinal and intercostal muscles T2–T6 innervated sclerotomes T2–T6 innervated dermatomes
Heart	T1–T4 C5–C6 C7–C8	Chest pain and tightness Referred pain to upper limb Referred pain to the neck and interscapular regions	T1–T4 and C5–C8 innervated myotomes, including paraspinals, intercostals, pectoralis major/minor, and sternalis T1–T4 and C5–C8 innervated sclerotomes T1–T4 and C5–C8 innervated dermatomes
Upper gastrointestinal (esophagus, stomach, duodenum, small intestine, gallbladder, liver)	T5–T9	Substernal pain, epigastric pain, rib cage pain, mid-thoracic pain, abdominal pain, nausea, emesis, dyspepsia, heartburn	T5–T9, T10–L1 innervated myotomes, including rectus abdominis, abdominal obliques, and iliocostalis T5–T9, T10–L1 innervated sclerotomes, including supra/interspinous ligaments and muscle attachment site on ribs, sternum
Lower gastrointestinal (large intestine, appendix)	T10–L1	Lower abdominal pain, diarrhea, constipation, flatulence (irritable bowel syndrome-like symptoms)	T5–T9, T10–L1 innervated dermatomes
Genitourinary (kidneys, ureters)	T10–L1	Abdominal/pelvic pain, flank pain, groin/scrotal pain	T10–L2 innervated myotomes, including paraspinals, quadratus lumborum, abdominal obliques
Bladder, urethra, prostate, epididymis, testes	T12–L2	Bladder pain, pelvic pain, urinary frequency (e.g., interstitial cystitis)	T10–L2 innervated sclerotomes T10–L2 innervated dermatomes
Pelvic (gynecologic) Ovaries Uterus	T10 T10–L2	Pelvic pain, dysmenorrhea (e.g., chronic inflammatory pelvic disease, chronic endometriosis)	T10–L1 innervated myotomes, including pelvic floor muscles, lower abdominal muscles, and paraspinals T10–L1 innervated sclerotomes T10–L1 innervated dermatomes

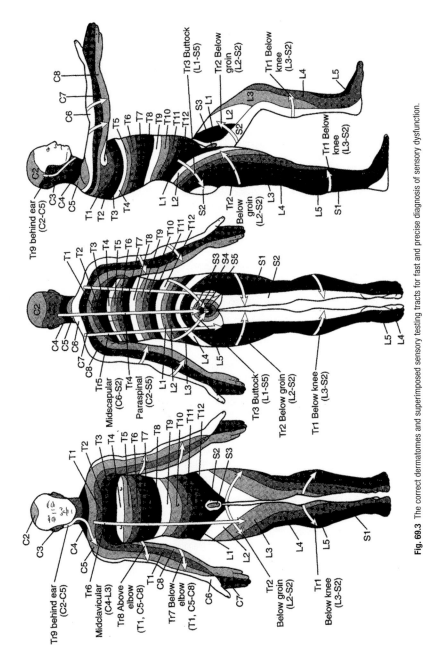

Fig. 69.3 The correct dermatomes and superimposed sensory testing tracts for fast and precise diagnosis of sensory dysfunction.

11. How do you treat peripheral sensitization?

Eliminating irritative foci within the somatic components of the SSS is necessary for effectively treating pain and dysfunction originating in the periphery, *myotome, sclerotome, dermatome*, or the viscerotome. (see Box 69.1). Early effective treatment of peripheral sensitization can prevent the onset of central sensitization and chronicity.

Kraus H. *Clinical Treatment of Back and Neck Pain.* New York: McGraw-Hill; 1970:1–17.

Box 69.1 Management of Peripheral Sensitization and Prevention of Central Sensitization

A. Noninvasive methods
  1. Start treatment as soon as possible.
  2. Do not use RICE (rest, ice, compression, and elevation). Do not rest injured part! Use MECE (move, ethyl chloride spray, compression, and elevation).
     - Use vapocoolant spray to deactivate trigger points, which limit movement. The spray inactivates the trigger points' tender spots and makes relaxation exercises and passive stretching of the involved muscle more effective.
     - No weight-bearing; only use crutches until normal ambulation is possible.
     - Return to activities only when scale test (knee bend, standing on two scales) shows equal weight distribution on both lower extremities.
     - Relaxation and stretching: relax by deep exhalation, eye movement, and activation of antagonist. Stretch passively by gravity.
  3. Medications
     - Take anti-inflammatory drugs, but steroids only as an exception.
     - Use short-acting opiates regularly to desensitize and prevent pain.
     - Do not use medications for early return to activity.
B. Injections: most effective treatment with dramatic, instantaneous pain relief and restoration of function
  1. Pre-injection block preempts the pain and irritation caused by injections of tender areas.
  2. Needling and infiltration breakthrough and eradicates edema, which later becomes fibrotic tissue entrapping nerve endings along with sensitizing substances; eliminate irritative foci.

---

12. What are effective injection techniques for treating irritative foci and damaged tissue to facilitate peripheral sensitization?

- Injection block: Initially, the needle would be inserted and introduce the anesthetic to interrupt sensory impulses from the irritative focus, TS/TrPs, so that needling and infiltration, which follow, can be carried out relatively pain-free. The injection block consists of spreading 1% lidocaine on the side of nerve entry to the treated tissue. Other advantages of injection block include preventing central sensitization caused by needling or injecting a sensitized area. The injection block relieves the neurogenic component of the taut band, shrinking it to about 20% of its original size. A "fibrotic core" located within the taut band is uncovered and is the sole target for N & I.

Needling and infiltration (N & I) of the damaged tissue eradicate the TS/TrPs. These outcomes are confirmed by improved pressure sensitivity quantified by algometry along with pain relief.

Fischer AA. *New Injection Techniques for Treatment of Musculoskeletal Pain.* In ES Rachlin, IS Rachlin (Eds.). *Myofascial Pain and Fibromyalgia: Trigger Point Management*, 2nd ed. St. Louis: Mosby; 2002:403–419.

---

13. What is segmental neuromyotherapy?

Segmental neuromyotherapy is a system of diagnosing and managing pain based on the concept of spinal segmental sensitization. The diagnosis is based on quantified and objective assessment methods distinguished by a higher degree of sensitivity in detecting abnormal neurologic and other tissue dysfunction compared to conventional examination methods. These improved sensory and motor techniques and additional tissue evaluation have led to two clinical pain syndromes described: *SSS and the pentad of vertebrogenic dysfunction* (PVD). The significance of these new pain syndromes is that they are consistently associated with pain of different etiologies. In addition, specific injection techniques promptly relieve pain by rectifying the abnormalities.

The therapeutic approaches employed in SNMT focus on desensitization of the sensitized segment. In the first step, this is achieved by special blocks such as paraspinous (PSB) block and using physical modalities (relaxation, limbering exercises), which decrease sensitization and hyperexcitability of the myotome, dermatome, and other components of the spinal segment.

Fischer AA. *New Injection Techniques for Treatment of Musculoskeletal Pain.* In ES Rachlin, IS Rachlin (Eds.). *Myofascial Pain and Fibromyalgia: Trigger Point Management.* 2nd ed. St. Louis: Mosby; 2002:403–419.

14. What are the components of PVD?
    - Sensitized supraspinous and interspinous ligaments are pressure-sensitive and show micro-edema (impression of fingernail fails to recover for a few minutes). The sensitized ligament acts as an irritative focus causing SSS or contributing to it.
    - Paraspinal spasm, which is part of SSS and its causes.
    - Narrowed neural foramina.
    - Root compression.
    - Narrowed disc space.
    The last two aspects are manifested clinically by narrowed space between the spinous processes. Specific treatment of PVD is N & I of the interspinous/supraspinous ligaments, usually performed in conjunction with paraspinous block using 1% lidocaine at the identical level.

15. What are the basic principles of treatments according to the concept of segmental neuromyotherapy?
    The first principle is to alleviate pain immediately by desensitization of the spinal segment. Segmental desensitization is achieved by four components:
    - Injections: PSB with 1% lidocaine alleviates pain instantaneously by reversing SSS to normal sensitivity; N & I with 1% lidocaine of the supraspinous/interspinous ligament, followed by N & I of muscle TrPs eradicates the irritative foci. This is a prerequisite for long-term relief. Pre-injection blocks preempt the pain and irritation caused by injections of TrPs and tender areas.
    - Specific physical therapy: The healing of the needling is supported by electric stimulation, hot packs, and relaxation exercises. The relaxation exercises should concentrate on all the muscles of the involved myotome. The exercises should be limited to relaxation and limbering, which decrease sensitization and prevent a recurrence. Strengthening exercises in the early stage after an injection has the opposite effect, causing aggravation of the existing sensitization.
    - Removing conditions causing irritative foci (TrPs/TS, inflammation).
    - Medications that induce or support peripheral and central desensitization.

Fischer AA. *New Injection Techniques for Treatment of Musculoskeletal Pain.* In ES Rachlin, IS Rachlin (Eds.). *Myofascial Pain and Fibromyalgia: Trigger Point Management.* 2nd ed. St. Louis: Mosby; 2002:403–419.

Kidd RF. *Neural Therapy: Applied Neurophysiology and Other Topics.* Custom Printers of Renfrew; 2005:24–66.

Maigne R. *Segmental Vertebral Cellulotenoperiosteomyalgic Syndrome.* In WL Nieves (Ed.). *Diagnosis and Treatment of Pain of Vertebral Origin: A Manual Medicine Approach.* 2nd ed. Boca Raton: Taylor & Francis; 2006:103–112.

16. Describe the techniques of PSB and its effect.
    PSB (see Fig. 69.4) is a unique injection technique effectively desensitizing SSS and alleviating pain in the segment. PSB consists of spreading a local anesthetic (1% lidocaine) and the spinous processes and their connection in the supraspinous/interspinous ligaments. PSBs effectively desensitize (reversing to normal sensitivity) the sensitized segment and relieve the segmental pain. This is manifested by normalization of the hyperalgesic dermatome upon scratch, electric skin conductance, and pinch and roll. The TS/TrPs become less tender on motor testing, and spasm within the corresponding myotome is relieved. PSB achieves this effect by blocking the nociceptive impulses from the sprained interspinous ligament(s), which act as an irritative focus, mediating SSS.

Imamura, M., Imamura ST, Targino SA, et al. Paraspinous lidocaine injection for chronic nonspecific low back pain: a randomized controlled clinical trial. *J Pain.* 2016;17(5):569–576. doi:10.1016/ j.jpain.2016.01.469.

17. What are the roles of medications and exercises in the management of SSS?
    - Medications should be used as an adjunct to therapy and consist of anti-inflammatory medications and drugs to reduce central sensitization (antidepressants, anticonvulsants, opiates).
    - Exercises are prescribed to reduce risk factors for recurrence, such as postural correction, restoring cervical and lumbar lordosis, and to relax key postural muscles which lack flexibility. Endurance of the weak key postural muscles should be enhanced but strengthening against high resistance should be employed only in the final rehabilitation stage. Most relaxation exercises are active, slow through a range of motion without resistance, combined with eye movement, deep exhalation, and mild activation of the antagonist muscle(s). This can be followed by passive stretching, preferably by gravity.

Fischer AA. Myofascial pain: update in diagnosis and treatment. *Phys Med Rehabil Clin North Am.* 8(1):53–169. Published in issue: February 1997.

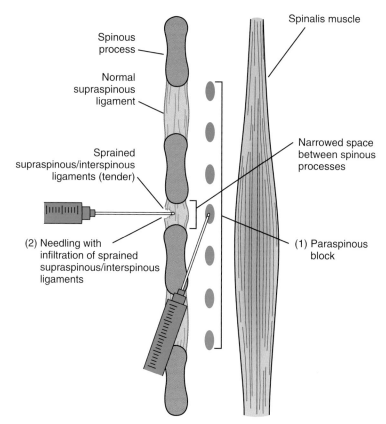

Spinous process

Normal supraspinous ligament

Sprained supraspinous/interspinous ligaments (tender)

(2) Needling with infiltration of sprained supraspinous/interspinous ligaments

Spinalis muscle

Narrowed space between spinous processes

(1) Paraspinous block

Fig. 69.4 Technique of paraspinous block combined with needling and infiltration of sprained supra-spinous/interspinous ligaments.

18. How do you prevent recurrence of SSS?

Remove factors that cause its recurrence such as TrPs, TSs, muscle spasm, and inflammation, all of which cause peripheral sensitization that spreads to the CNS, causing SSS. For this purpose, special injection techniques include N & I of the entire sensitized abnormal tissues to eradicate the underlying pathologic, particularly fibrotic, tissue. Prior to N & I, a pre-injection block is performed, preventing nociceptive and irritative impulses from reaching the CNS and decreasing sensitization at the spinal level.

19. What is the significance of a sensitized spinal segment?

This step indicates that the sensitizing process, which starts at the periphery, has reached the CNS. Effective management requires treatment of both peripheral and central sensitization.

- Its presence, along with peripheral tissue sensitization, may escape diagnosis with conventional examination techniques.
- This condition can be successfully diagnosed by quantitative objective methods with high sensitivity and precision (e.g., algometry, electric skin conductance, tissue compliance measurement).
- SSS is diagnosed by hyperalgesia and pressure pain sensitivity that extends over the sensory, motor, and skeletal areas and viscera supplied by the involved spinal segment (i.e., its dermatome, myotome, sclerotome, and viscerotome).
- Dermatomal hyperalgesia is diagnosed by the following methods:
  - Sensory testing for the diagnosis of SSS: Scratching the skin with the tip of an opened paper clip tests sensitivity to painful stimuli more precisely than a pinprick. The sharp object is slowly dragged across the dermatomal borders. Patients are asked to indicate if the sensation of the paper clip changes and gets sharper or duller. The use of sensory testing tracks allows a more accurate diagnosis and requires only a fraction of the time compared to the conventional pinprick method (see Fig. 69.3).
  - The sensitivity of subcutaneous tissue is tested by the pinch and roll method. This test is performed by picking up the skin between the thumb and forefinger and rolling the tissue beneath. It is the most sensitive test for the diagnosis of sensitization.

- ESC is an objective test of sympathetic dysfunction and can be measured by a microampere meter.

Head H. On disturbances of sensation with especial reference to the pain of visceral disease. *Brain.* 1893;16(1–2):1–133. Available at: https://doi.org/10.1093/brain/16.1-2.1.

Keegan JJ, Garrett FD. The segmental distribution of the cutaneous nerves in the limbs of man. *Anat Rec.* 1948;102(4):409–437. Available at: doi:10.1002/ar.1091020403.

20. Outline an algorithm for diagnosis and management of musculoskeletal pain based on SSS. See Box 69.2.

Kraus H. *Diagnosis and Treatment of Muscle Pain.* Chicago: Quintessence; 1998:9–54.

McKenzie R. *7 Steps to a Pain-Free Life.* 2nd ed. New York: Plume; 2014.

Box 69.2 Algorithm for Diagnosis and Management of Musculoskeletal Pain Based on Sensitized Spinal Segments

Goals

- **Short-term**: to alleviate pain before the patient leaves the office. This is achieved by treating the immediate cause of pain, which most frequently consists of tender spots (TSs), trigger points (TrPs), muscle spasm (MSp), or inflammation.
- **Long-term**: to remove perpetuating and etiologic factors responsible for the immediate cause(s) of pain to prevent the condition's recurrence.

Phase I: Identify the immediate cause of pain: TrPs/TSs, MSp, inflammation

1. Ask the patient to point with one finger to the spot of the most intensive pain.
2. Find the point of maximum tenderness or TrP.
3. Quantify the tenderness (degree of sensitization) with an algometer.
4. Reproduction (recognition) of pain: Press over the maximum tender point and ask, "Is this the pain you are complaining about?"

Phase II: Diagnose the SSS and specify the segment corresponding to the TrP/Ts spot. Diagnoses of SSS:

1. **Sensory**. Diagnose the hyperalgesic dermatomes.
   - Scratching along the sensory diagnostic tracks
   - Electric skin conductance, which objectively documents nerve fiber dysfunction
   - Pinch and roll, which tests sensitization of subcutaneous tissue; can be quantified by a pressure algometer
2. **Motor**. Diagnose the affected myotome.
   - TrP/TSs by palpation and algometry
   - Taut bands (TBs) by palpation and tissue compliance meter
   - Muscle spasm, by palpation and tissue compliance meter
3. **Sclerotome**. Bursitis, tendinitis, epicondylitis, enthesopathy

Phase III: Treatment. Concentrate on the SSS corresponding to the immediate cause of pain (TrPs/TSs, MSp, neurogenic inflammation), the associated supraspinous ligament sprain, and pentad.

1. Injections: for immediate and long-term relief of pain
   - Paraspinous block to desensitize the SSS
   - Injection block to anesthetize the painful, sensitive area to be infiltrated
   - Needling and infiltration of the TB to break up the entire underlying pathology around the TrPs/TSs
2. **Physical therapy**: to promote healing after injections, restore function, and prevent a recurrence
   - Modalities: Heat or cold; electric stimulation (sinusoid surging and tetanizing currents)
   - Exercises: Relaxation exercises and stretching: general and specific for the involved myotome, in which the pain-generating TrPs/TSs, MSp are located. Relaxation by activation of antagonist muscle(s)
   - Postural correction: **Kraus-Weber test** specifically diagnoses dysfunction (weakness or loss of flexibility) in key postural muscles and **Robin McKenzie test**: flexion deficiency of the lumbosacral spine is indicated by knee-chest over 5 cm. Extension deficiency is considered if, on the push-up, pelvic-floor distance is over 2.5 cm. On lateral bending, the shoulder should pass midline. Induce the corresponding correction by specific postural exercises (Robin McKenzie, Hans Kraus).

Phase IV: Diagnosis and removal of perpetuating and etiologic factors

1. Mechanical: overuse, sports injuries, cumulative trauma disorder
2. Postural deficiencies: muscle deficiencies (loss of strength or flexibility)
3. Lab results: endocrine and metabolic tests, electrolytes, vitamins, disorders

REFERENCES

Fischer A, Imamura M, Dubo H, O'Young B, Cassius D. *Spinal Segmental Sensitization: Diagnosis and Treatment*. In B O'Young, M Young, S Stiens (Eds.). *Physical Medicine and Rehabilitation* Secrets. 3rd ed. Philadelphia: Elsevier; 2008:610–625.

Harte S, Harris R, Clauw D. The neurobiology of central sensitization. *J Appl Biobehav Res*. 2018;23(2):e12137.

Latremoliere A, Woolf CJ. Central sensitization: generator of pain hypersensitivity by central neural plasticity. *J Pain*. 2009;10:895–926. Available at: https://doi.org/10.1016/j.jpain.2009.06.012.

Suputtitada A. Myofascial pain syndrome and sensitization. *Phy Med Rehabil Res*. 2016;1(4):71–79.

Woolf CJ. Evidence for a central component of post-injury pain hypersensitivity. *Nature*. 1983;306(5944):686–688. Available at: https://doi.org/10.1038/306686a0.

Woolf CJ. Central sensitization: implications for the diagnosis and treatment of pain. *Pain*. 2011;152:2–15. Available at: https://doi.org/10.1016/j.pain.2010.09.030.

Note on Andrew A. Fischer, MD, Ph.D., credited with several scientific discoveries that have revolutionized the practice of pain management and enhanced functional outcomes of pain sufferers throughout the world. One important basic contribution has been the discovery of the syndrome called *spinal segmental sensitization* (SSS). The significance of SSS is that it is a consistent component of all painful conditions. Furthermore, it can be diagnosed and treated successfully in clinical practice if the particular examination and treatment methods he created are used. This seminal observation led to the segmental neuromyotherapeutic (SNMT) model. SNMT consists of a unique system of objective and quantitative examination methods that detect the basic pathophysiological components of pain. It provides not only a scientifically valid and reproducible diagnosis but also an assessment of the efficacy of various treatment methods. Only the exceptional sensitivity of these methods makes the diagnosis of SSS in clinical practice possible.

Based on the diagnosis of SSS, a more efficacious treatment plan can be formulated. In therapeutic terms, Fischer has pioneered a novel system of safe and efficacious injection techniques, including paraspinous blocks (designed to control pain by reversing the SSS to normal), pre-injection blocks, and needling and infiltration of taut bands, which eradicates the pain generator. His model of diagnosing spinal segmental sensitization and new injection techniques have been successfully employed and gaining acceptance nationally and internationally.

CHAPTER 70

CENTRAL AND PERIPHERAL MANIFESTATIONS OF MYOFASCIAL PAIN SYNDROMES AND FIBROMYALGIA: DIAGNOSIS PATTERNS AND DIVERSE INTERVENTIONS

Steven A. Stiens, MD, MS, David Cassius, MD, Bryan J. O'Young, MD, CAc, FAAPMR, and Jay Shah, MD

Take up one idea. Make that one idea your life—think of it, dream of it, live on that idea. Let the brain, muscles, nerves, every part of your body, be full of that idea, and just leave every other idea alone. This is the way to success.
— Swami Vivekananda (1863–1902)

KEY POINTS: MYOFASCIAL PAIN SYNDROME AND FIBROMYALGIA

1. The precise pattern of pain described by the patient is the most valuable clue to the location of myofascial trigger points (MTrPs) and spinal segmental sensitization (SSS) causing the symptoms.
2. The clinical manifestation of central sensitization is comprised of hyperalgesia of the dermatome, sclerotome, and myotome, along with MTrPs within the myotome of the specific sensitized spinal segment (SSS).
3. The clinical significance of SSS is that it is consistently found when musculoskeletal pain is present, and it is dynamically responsive to treatments that target the "wind-up" of the neural circuit.
4. Treatment that desensitizes the involved spinal segment can often alleviate pain due to MTrPs within the myotome.
5. Fibromyalgia presents a matrix of symptoms requiring treatment via multiple simultaneous mechanisms to restore function, build endurance, rejuvenate with rest, and participate in meeting personal life goals.

MYOFASCIAL PAIN SYNDROME

DIAGNOSIS

1. Define myofascial pain syndrome
   Myofascial pain syndrome (MPS) is a regional muscle pain condition associated with myofascial trigger points (MTrPs) located in muscle fascia or near tendinous insertions. It is characterized by local and referred pain, muscle spasm (Msp), inhibitory weakness, sensory changes, and autonomic symptoms.

Jafri MS. Mechanisms of myofascial pain. *Int Sch Res Notices*. 2014;2014:523924. doi: 10.1155/2014/523924. Available at https://www.ncbi.nlm.nih.gov/pmc/articles/pmc4285362/.

---

2. Describe the differences in palpating TrPs, tender spots (TSs), taut bands (TBs), and Msp
   - **Myofascial trigger points (TrPs)** are tender, hyperirritable areas within palpable TBs of muscle fibers and are painful upon compression, stretch, or muscle contraction. MTrPs have a distinct pain referral pattern called the **referred pain zone (RPZ).**
   - **Tender spots (TSs),** contrary to MTrPs, induce pain locally without referral.
   - **Taut bands (TBs)** consist of a group of tense muscle fibers that are tender and demonstrate hard consistency on palpation. MTrPs and TSs represent the most tender, pressure-sensitive area within the TBs.
   - **Muscle spasm (Msp)** is characterized by tenderness and hard consistency extending over an entire muscle, not limited to selected fibers, such as TBs. Msp is an involuntary, usually painful muscle contraction/shortening. The spasm may be initiated by MTrPs within the same muscle. It may also reflect **spinal segmental**

sensitization (SSS) caused by the nociceptive input of other tissues (muscles, fascia, or joints) within the spinal segment.

3. How do you diagnose TrPs?
   By careful history, assessment, and a skillful, specific physical examination.
   • **Pain diagrams** drawn by the patient assist in identifying the pain distribution and RPZ. The precise patterns and areas of most intense pain described by the patient are the most valuable clues in locating MTrPs. Using pain referral diagrams with MTrP sites (Travell and Simons), and dermatomal charts (Keegan's Dermatomes), help locate and diagnose MTrPs and associated segmental conditions that may have initiated or perpetuated pain cycles.
   • Diagnosing specific areas of SSS by physical exam can quickly guide which muscles within the sensitized myotome(s) need to be examined for MTrPs.
   • Palpate the muscle(s) by flat or pincer palpation to identify TBs. Press over the maximum points or MTrP to produce local pain and a **jump sign,** i.e., a reflexive muscle withdrawal in response to a painful stimulus. Irritate further to elicit the MTrP referred pain. Ask the patient if this reproduces their usual pain complaint(s).
   • Elicit a local twitch response by **"snapping palpation"** across the TB in accessible muscles.
   • Examine for a painful restricted stretch range of motion in the muscles harboring MTrPs.
   • Muscle weakness without atrophy may be present.

4. Name the two most reliable criteria for the diagnosis of MTrPs
   • Point (focal) tenderness
   • Reproduction (recognition) of symptoms (referral pattern) on compression of the point of maximum tenderness

Rivers WE, Garrigues D, Graciosa J, Harden RN. Signs and symptoms of myofascial pain: an international survey of pain management providers and proposed preliminary set of diagnostic criteria. *Pain Med.* 2015;16(9):1794–1805. doi: 10.1111/pme.12780. Available at: https://academic.oup.com/painmedicine/article/16/9/1794/1876647.

Gerwin RD, Shannon S, Hong CZ, et al. Interrater reliability in myofascial trigger point examination. *Pain.* 1997;69:65–73. doi: 10.1016/s034-3959(96)03248-4. Available at: https://citeseerx.ist.psu.edu/viewdoc/download?doi=10.1.1.594.1168&rep=rep1&type=pdf.

5. What are primary and secondary MTrPs?
   • Primary MTrPs are central TrPs caused by direct trauma, acute or chronic overload, or repetitive use of the muscles in which they occur. Subclinical segmental sensitization of the myotome may reduce the threshold for developing an MTrP.
   • Secondary MTrPs develop in a synergist or antagonist of the muscle harboring the primary MTrP. Secondary MTrPs also arise from irritative foci in sclerotomes, ligaments, joints, bursae, tendons, discs, and radicular or visceral tissue. Peripheral nociceptor sensitization with subsequent development of central sensitization and SSS causes secondary MTrPs within the myotome of the involved SSS.

6. What is the difference between an active and a latent MTrP?
   An **active trigger point** causes a clinical pain complaint spontaneously or during movement. A **latent trigger point** is clinically quiescent with no spontaneous pain or pain on movement. Latent TrPs are tender on compression and manifest all findings characteristic of active TrPs, including their location within a TB. Latent TrPs can be activated by compression, overuse of the muscle, or prolonged muscle immobilization in a shortened position. The development of central sensitization can convert latent MTrPs into symptomatic active MTrPs within muscles of the sensitized myotome.

Grieve R, Barnett S, Coghill N, et al. The prevalence of latent myofascial trigger points and diagnostic criteria of the triceps surae and upper trapezius: a cross sectional study. *Physiotherapy.* 2013;99(4):278–284. doi: 10.1016/j.physio.2013.04.002.

7. Are there any tests that can diagnose MPS?
   MPS is a clinical diagnosis. There is no imaging test, laboratory test/blood work, electromyography, or muscle biopsy to diagnose MPS.
   If there are concerns for other comorbidities that may be associated with a patient's MPS, consider screening blood tests for nutritional/mineral deficiencies (including Vitamins B1, B6, B12, and D, as well as iron and magnesium), chronic infections (such as hepatitis C and Lyme disease), and endocrine imbalances (including thyroid, adrenal, estrogen, testosterone, and growth hormones).

Giamberardino MA, Affaitati G, Fabrizio A, et al. Myofascial pain syndrome and their evaluation. *Best Pract Res Clin Rheumatol.* 2011;25:185–198. doi: 10.1016/j.berh.2011.01.002. Available at https://www.sciencedirect.com/science/article/pii/S1521694211000064?via%3Dihub.

8. How do you differentiate central from attachment MTrPs?
   - Central MTrPs are located near the center of the muscle belly and are closely associated with dysfunctional motor endplates.
   - Attachment MTrPs are located at the musculotendinous junction and/or the attachment site of taut muscle bands against bone. They can be associated with **enthesopathies** (inflammation at the insertion sites of ligaments into bone) with tenderness and thickening at the attachment sites. Such changes may be facilitated by the development of a sensitized sclerotome as a component of SSS.

Simons DG. Myofascial trigger points. In: Gebhart GF, Schmidt RF, eds. *Encyclopedia of Pain.* Berlin, Heidelberg: Springer; 2013. Available at https://doi.org/10.1007/978-3-642-28753-4_2567.

9. What are the different therapies to treat MPS?
   Although there are various options to manage MPS, there is no clear established consensus for these interventions. Therapies include:
   - Physical therapy
     - Emphasis on stretching, manual techniques, and physical modalities, including heat, ice, ultrasound, electric stimulation, microcurrent, and laser therapy as the current treatment approach.
   - Dry needling and trigger point injection
     - Minimally invasive and inexpensive
     - Best response is a local twitch response elicited by the needle
   - Medications:
     - Strong evidence for using anxiolytics such as clonazepam, diazepam, and alprazolam combined with ibuprofen, amitriptyline, or tropisetron, but not as monotherapy.
     - Moderate evidence for agents, including methylsalicylate, menthol, and diclofenac patches.
   - In general, avoid opioids in the management of MPS.

Annaswamy TM, De Luigi AJ, O'Neill BJ, et al. Emerging concepts in the treatment of myofascial pain: a review of medications, modalities, and needle-based interventions. *PM&R.* 2011;3(10):940–961. doi: 10/1016/j.pmrj.2011.06.013.

10. What are the perpetuating factors of MPS?
    MTrP therapy will only lead to short-term improvement without the proper identification and rectification of possible perpetuating factors.
    Mechanical stresses include skeletal asymmetry and disproportion (e.g., short leg, hemipelvis), poor posture, and overuse of muscles.
    - Nutritional inadequacies include "low normal" levels of vitamins D3, B_1, B_6, B_{12}, folic acid, and low calcium, magnesium, potassium, iron, and hemoglobin levels.
    - Metabolic and endocrine disorders include hypometabolism due to suboptimal thyroid function, hyperuricemia, and hypoglycemia.
    - Psychological factors include depression, anxiety, and post-traumatic stress disorder.
    - Chronic infection, allergies, and sleep disorders have all been cited as perpetuating factors.
    - Articular, radicular, and visceral disorders and fibromyalgia (FM) may perpetuate MTrPs due to central sensitization and SSS.

Malanga GA, Cruz EJ. Myofascial low back pain: a review. *Phys Med Rehabil Clin N Am.* 2010;21:711–724. Available at https://doi.org/10.1016/j.pmr.2010.07.003.

Gerwin RD. A review of myofascial pain and fibromyalgia—factors that promote their persistence. *Acupunct Med.* 2005;23:121–134. Available at https://doi.org/10.1136/aim.23.3.121.

PERIPHERAL AND CENTRAL SENSITIZATION: PATHOPHYSIOLOGY AND TREATMENT APPROACH TO MPS

11. How can the tenderness of a TS or MTrP be quantified?
    Tenderness is quantified by an algometer. A **pressure algometer** is a pocket-sized force gauge fitted with a disc-shaped plunger with a 1 cm^2 surface. When applied over the maximum TS, a **pain pressure threshold (PPT)** value is established (i.e., the minimum force that induces pain). An abnormal degree of tenderness consists of a

PPT that is 2 kg/cm^2 lower than a normosensitive control point. Algometry procedures have been determined to be valid and reliable.

Fischer AA. Algometry in diagnosis of musculoskeletal pain and evaluation of treatment outcome: an update. *J Musculoskelet Pain.* 1998;6(1):5–32. DOI: 10.1300/J094v06n01_02. Available at: https://www.tandfonline.com/doi/abs/10.1300/J094v06n01_02.

Pelfort X, Torres-Claramunt R, Sanchez-Soler JF, et al. Pressure algometry is a useful tool to quantify pain in the medial part of the knee: an intra- and inter-reliability study in healthy subjects. *Orthop Traumatol Surg Res.* 2015;101:559–563. Available at: https://www.sciencedirect.com/science/article/pii/S1877056815001164?via%3Dihub.

Park G, Kim CW, Park SB, et al. Reliability and usefulness of the pressure pain threshold measurement in patients with myofascial pain. *Ann Rehabil Med.* 2011;35(3):412–417. doi: 10.5535/arm.2011.35.3.412. Available at: https://www.e-arm.org/journal/view.php?doi=10.5535/arm.2011.35.3.412.

12. Describe the pathophysiologic changes leading to the formation of MTrPs and peripheral sensitization

David Simons's integrated hypothesis regarding MTrP formation emphasizes concomitant tissue damage, the release of sensitizing substances, motor endplate dysfunction with excessive release of acetylcholine, and increased electrical endplate noise that cause sustained sarcomere contraction with resultant contraction knots and TBs. An energy crisis develops due to increased metabolic demand and hypoxia/ischemia, causing the enhanced release of activating and sensitizing substances and subsequent peripheral sensitization.

Microanalytical techniques using microdialysis needles to record the biochemical milieu of an active MTrP region in human muscle fibers have shown significantly increased prostaglandins, bradykinin, serotonin, norepinephrine, tumor necrosis factor–α (TNF-α), interleukin 1, calcitonin gene-related peptide (CGRP), substance P, and decreased pH compared to latent TrPs and normal control sites. CGRP is known to increase the release of acetylcholine in the endplate region. Intracellular calcium pumps may become dysfunctional, increasing intracellular calcium in the sarcoplasm, inducing sustained muscle contraction and subsequent development of TBs.

Active MTrPs are dynamic irritative foci of peripheral nociceptor sensitization that can initiate, amplify, and maintain central sensitization.

Gerwin RD, Dommerholt J, Shah JP. An expansion of Simons' integrated hypothesis of trigger point formation. *Curr Pain Headache Rep.* 2004;8(6):468–475. doi: 10/1007/s11916-004-0069-x.

Shah JP, Phillips TM, Danoff JV, et al. An in vivo microanalytical technique for measuring the local biochemical milieu of human skeletal muscle. *J Appl Physiol.* 2005;99(5):1977–1984.

13. What are the hypothesized mechanisms for the pathophysiology of MPS?

Available evidence supports the hypothesis that TrPs are a persistent peripheral source of nociception, contributing to pain propagation and widespread pain. Quintner and Cohen have proposed a plausible alternative. They suggest hyperalgesia secondary to peripheral or central sensitization of nociceptors and the spontaneous firing of nociceptive dorsal horn neurons as the etiology of the pain syndrome. Neurogenic inflammation has been proposed as a possible etiology of this peripheral or central sensitization.

An essential dichotomy in the literature is whether the MTrP is a cause or effect of chronic myofascial pain. The **Integrated Hypothesis** posits that the MTrP is the primary pathologic focus (cause) mediating the clinical manifestations of MPS, and myofascial pain is triggered by an injury of the muscle, either acute or chronic, leading to local contracture as a result of spontaneous release of acetylcholine at a dysfunctional motor endplate.

However, the Integrated Hypothesis does not explain how MPS occurs and persists without muscle tissue damage. Studies have demonstrated that patients suffering from visceral or somatic conditions such as interstitial cystitis/bladder syndrome, chronic pelvic pain, and osteoarthritis also suffer from MPS. In addition, when pressure is applied over an area of tissue damage (e.g., a torn tendon, ligament, or muscle), it causes a withdrawal reflex. This does not typically occur in patients with active MTrPs. Many patients prefer greater pressure (e.g., during manual therapies), a clinical observation incompatible with frank tissue injury.

Emerging research suggests that neurogenic mechanisms may play a foundational role. Apropos, the **Neurogenic Hypothesis** proposes that the dynamic clinical manifestations of chronic MPS are initiated, amplified, and facilitated by central sensitization and neurogenic inflammation in the absence of overload injury to the muscle. Central sensitization is caused by the persistent bombardment of nociceptive impulses from a primary pathologic source, either somatic (e.g., discopathy, degenerative joint, MTrPs, etc.) or visceral (e.g., endometriosis).

An important sequela to central sensitization is neurogenic inflammation, a neuro-inflammatory response caused by the retrograde (antidromic) release of vasoactive and pro-inflammatory neuropeptides, predominantly Substance P, into peripheral tissues (either somatic and/or visceral) via sensory nerves. The Neurogenic Hypothesis suggests that the MTrP is a secondary manifestation (effect) of neurogenic inflammatory mechanisms expressed peripherally within skeletal muscle.

Neuro-segmental links between muscles and joint cartilage have been demonstrated using naturally occurring and experimentally induced spine osteoarthritis models. These findings greatly enhance our understanding of the underlying neuro-inflammatory, neuro-segmental mechanisms in muscle and elucidate the potential physiologic mechanisms contributing to the dynamic clinical manifestations of MPS, central sensitization and spinal segmental sensitization, and the somato-visceral and viscero-somatic disorders commonly observed in clinical practice.

Duarte FCK, Zwambag DP, Brown SHM, et al. Increased substance P immunoreactivity in ipsilateral knee cartilage of rats exposed to lumbar spine injury. *Cartilage.* 2020;11(2):251–261. Available at https://www.ncbi.nlm.nih.gov/pmc/articles/PMC7097978/.

Duarte FCK, Hurtig M, Clark A, et al. Experimentally induced spine osteoarthritis in rats leads to neurogenic inflammation within neurosegmentally linked myotomes. *Exp Gerontol.* 2021;149:111311. Available at https://pubmed.ncbi.nlm.nih.gov/33744392/.

FitzGerald MP, Payne CK, Lukacz ES, et al. Randomized multicenter clinical trial of myofascial physical therapy in women with interstitial cystitis/painful bladder syndrome and pelvic floor tenderness. *J Urol.* 2012;187(6):2113–2118. doi: 10.1016/j.juro.2012.01.123. Available at https://pubmed.ncbi.nlm.nih.gov/22503015/.

Phan VT, Stratton P, Tandon HK, et al. Widespread myofascial dysfunction and sensitization in women with endometriosis-associated chronic pelvic pain: a cross-sectional study. *Eur J Pain.* 2021;25(4):831–840. doi: 10.1002/ejp.1713. Available at https://europepmc.org/article/pmc/pmc4347996#free-full-text.

Quintner JL, Bove GM, Cohen ML. A critical evaluation of the trigger point phenomenon. *Rheumatology (Oxford).* 2015;54(3):392–399. Available at: https://pubmed.ncbi.nlm.nih.gov/25477053/.

Shah JP, Thaker N, Heimur J, et al. Myofascial trigger points then and now: a historical and scientific perspective. *PM R.* 2015;7(7):746–761. doi: 10/1016/j.pmrj.2015.01.024. Available at: https://www.ncbi.nlm.nih.gov/pmc/articles/PMC4508225/.

Srbely JZ. New trends in the treatment and management of myofascial pain syndrome. *Curr Pain Headache Rep.* 14(5):346–352. Available at https://pubmed.ncbi.nlm.nih.gov/20607458/.

Stratton P, Khachikyan I, Sinaii N, et al. Association of chronic pelvic pain and endometriosis with signs of sensitization and myofascial pain. *J Obstet Gynecol.* 2015;125(3):719–728. Available at https://pubmed.ncbi.nlm.nih.gov/25730237/.

14. **What is central sensitization? Explain its role in chronicity.**

Peripheral sensitization causes afferent noxious stimuli from muscle or any other peripheral tissue to bombard the dorsal horn of the spinal cord via C and A-delta afferent nerve fibers. This persistent nociceptive bombardment leads to central nervous system (CNS) sensitization with neuroplastic changes at the spinal cord level. This sensitization state within a spinal segment manifests clinically as hyperalgesia, allodynia, referred pain, motor dysfunction, and autonomic dysfunction. Allodynia develops due to the opening of "silent" nociceptors via A-beta fibers, which emerges because of a phenotype switch from A-beta mechanoreceptors to C fiber-type functional nociceptors. Dorsal horn bombardment via A-beta fibers leads to amplification and maintenance of central sensitization, whereby light touch and low-pressure stimuli become painful. Peripheral sensitization initiates and drives central sensitization and, once established, becomes self-perpetuating because of synaptic and functional changes within the spinal cord.

The transition from acute to chronic pain directly results from persistent peripheral sensitization leading to central sensitization and neuroplastic changes of the CNS, rather than a factor of time alone. Central sensitization may occur within hours after the onset of peripheral sensitization. Still, the development of neuroplastic functional and structural CNS changes requires much longer and, once established, becomes much more challenging to eradicate. Once central sensitization occurs, muscles in the myotome of the involved sensitized segment have a lower threshold to form MTrPs. If active, such MTrPs may be more difficult to deactivate and/or eradicate. A clinical opportunity occurs with the recognition that chronic MPS fails to effectively treat and eliminate MTrPs. Without addressing the central sensitization component. Once sensitization All symptoms should be treated concurrently, achieving improved long-term outcomes.

Ji RR, Nackley A, Huh Y, et al. Neuroinflammation and central sensitization in chronic and widespread pain. *Anesthesiology.* 2018;129:343–366. doi: 10/1097/ALN.0000000000002130. Available at: https://pubs.asahq.org/anesthesiology/article/129/2/343/18003/Neuroinflammation-and-Central-Sensitization-in.

Woolf CJ, Salter MW. Neuronal plasticity: increasing the gain in pain. *Science.* 2000;288(5472):1765–1769. doi: 10.1126/science.288.5472.1765.

15. **Define SSS and its relationship to peripheral and central sensitization**

SSS is a hyperactive facilitated state of the spinal cord that develops due to an irritative focus originating in peripheral sensitized tissues. Hyperexcitability spreads from sensory to motor components in the spinal cord segment, inducing hypertonicity, Msp/shortening, and initiating or activating MTrPs within a myotomal pattern. In the thoracic cord, spread to the intermediolateral column (T1 through L1) leads to sympathetically mediated viscero-somatic and somatic-visceral interrelationships because of the convergence of somatic and visceral afferents at the same spinal segmental level in the dorsal horn (lamina I and V).

The clinical manifestation of central sensitization and SSS involves five functional components of the spinal segment: dermatome, sclerotome, myotome, viscerotome (in the thoracic region), and segmental sympathetic overactivity. A vicious cycle develops between SSS and peripheral irritative foci, each increasing the sensitization of the other. With chronicity, a single SSS may sensitize other adjacent spinal segments, leading to multiple levels of SSS with myotomal spread of MTrPs to distant sites and the development of widespread pain.

16. **What is the relationship between musculoskeletal (MSK) pain and SSS?**
SSS can be diagnosed with objective examination techniques in most patients with MSK pain. Therefore, SSS should be identified or ruled out, regardless of which peripheral tissue pain generator is present. Although TSs/MTrPs are irritative foci sending nociceptive signals to the spinal segment, SSS can antidromically induce sensitization in the periphery (peripheral nervous system and local tissues), creating TSs/MTrPs, Msp, and tenderness within the myotome. SSS may also activate previously latent TrPs or amplify and maintain active MTrPs. This dysfunctional pain processing in the CNS is considered the essential mechanism in chronic MSK pain conditions, including MPS and FM. Failure to recognize, clinically diagnose, and treat SSS early leads to amplified, persistent, and more widespread pain symptoms. Treatment methods that do not dampen or eliminate SSS often fail to eradicate MTrPs by physical therapy and/or MTrP injection procedures targeted at the peripheral MTrPs alone. This may lead to transient benefit with recurrence of MTrP symptoms and dysfunction rather than long-term relief.

The clinical significance of SSS is its consistent association with chronic MSK pain. Desensitization of the involved segment(s) alleviates the symptoms.

Rygh LJ, Svendsen F, Fiska A, et al. Long-term potentiation in spinal nociceptive systems—how acute pain may become chronic. *Psychoneuroendocrinology.* 2005;30(10):959–964. doi: 10/1016/j.psyneuen.2005.04.007.

17. **How is a MTrP deactivated on a peripheral level?**
MOS, due to MTrPs, is often unrecognized, misdiagnosed, and mistreated, causing unnecessary pain, dysfunction, suffering, and disability. As a result, accurate diagnosis is essential. Understanding pain mechanisms and targeting management at the mechanistic levels to inactivate or eradicate MTrPs/TS/TB/sensitized nociceptors is crucial. Table 70.1 summarizes therapeutic techniques focusing on peripheral pain mechanisms.

MTrP release and stretch techniques aim to disrupt the contracture of sarcomeres in the contraction knot of MTrPs. This results in the release of the TBs to relieve pain, regain a full stretch of muscle fibers, and restore function. Needling is an effective treatment regardless of the solution injected, but local anesthetic has the

Table 70.1 Therapeutic Techniques Targeted at Peripheral Pain Mechanisms

MANUAL TRP RELEASE TECHNIQUES	INJECTION/NEEDLING TECHNIQUES OF MTRPS	AUGMENTATION MANEUVERS
Vapocoolant spray and passive stretch or active limbering, relaxation exercises	Injection—deposited in one location as bulk	Directed eye movements
Intermittent ice and stretch	Infiltration—depositing small amount over multiple spots	Coordinated breathing—slow exhalation
TrP pressure release and stretch	Dry needling—repetitive insertion and withdrawal to mechanically break up and disrupt abnormal tissue	PIR
Deep stroking massage of TrP/TB	PIB (Fig. 70.1)	Reciprocal inhibition
Augmentation maneuvers	N&I (Fig. 70.2)	RAA
	Augmentation maneuvers after N&I	One or more maneuvers can be used in combination with manual TrP release or post–TrP injection/needling techniques to enhance relaxation and to achieve more effective muscle stretch.

N&I, Needling and infiltration; *PIB,* preinjection block; *PIR,* postisometric relaxation; *RAA,* relaxation by activation of antagonist; *TB,* taut bands; *TrP,* trigger point.

advantage of decreasing post-injection soreness and allows for more extensive, less painful needling. Botulinum toxin is expensive, unproven to be more effective than local anesthetic or normal saline injection, and is not indicated as a first-line treatment. Steroids provide no added benefit, are myotoxic, and have systemic side effects with multiple injections.

Shah JP, Thaker N, Heimur J, et al. Myofascial trigger points then and now: a historical and scientific perspective. *PM R.* 2015;7(7): 746–761. doi:10.1016/j.pmrj.2015.01.024 Available at: https://www.ncbi.nlm.nih.gov/pmc/articles/PMC4508225/.

18. Name therapeutic techniques that deactivate MTrPs using central pain pathways.
- Acupressure
- Spray and stretch
- Myofascial release
- Manual spinal manipulative/mobilizing techniques (Maigne): Manual spinal techniques are aimed at the pain of spinal origin with segmental effects involving the dermatome, sclerotome, and myotome.
- Intramuscular stimulation (IMS): Dry acupuncture needling provides stimulation of deep paraspinal muscles. This results in the relaxation of shortened muscles and desensitizes hyperalgesic dysfunction of the other components of the spinal segment.
- Preinjection block (PIB): A "coating block" using 1% lidocaine is performed around the TB prior to needling it. This causes the TB to shrink and exposes the remaining "core" tissue where the needling can be focused.
- Paraspinous block (PSB): Blocks afferent nociceptive input to the dorsal horn from the periphery with 1% lidocaine. This immediately desensitizes the hyperalgesic components of the spinal segment (e.g., dermatome, sclerotome, myotome) and reduces the MTrPs of muscles within the myotome.

The beneficial effects of all methods can be observed immediately. Long-term effects require eradicating peripheral irritative foci (i.e., ligamentous and MTrPs), causing or perpetuating the SSS.

Ji RR, Nackley A, Huh Y, et al. Neuroinflammation and central sensitization in chronic and widespread pain. *Anesthesiology.* 2018; 129(2):343–366. doi: 10.1097/ALN.0000000000 002130. Available at: https://www.ncbi.nlm.nih.gov/pmc/articles/PMC6051899/pdf/ nihms935636.pdf.

Sammons TE. *Dry Needling: A Brief History and Demonstration.* Available at: https://youtu.be/wbXNvK7JbP4.

Review of Evidence Base for Trigger Point Treatments. Available at: https://youtu.be/dJnsAl1CpVY.

Woolf CJ. Pain: moving from symptom control toward mechanism-specific pharmacologic management. *Ann Intern Med.* 2004; 140(6):441–451. doi: 10/7326/0003-4819-140-8-200404200-00010.

19. What management techniques can be targeted at both central and peripheral mechanisms?
Segmental neuromyotherapy systematic approach:
Diagnose level of SSS (e.g., C5 or L5).
PSB with 1% lidocaine to desensitize the SSS immediately.
Needling and infiltration (N&I) of supraspinous/interspinous ligament TrP.
Preinjection block to anesthetize the painful, sensitive area for N&I (see Fig. 70.1).
N&I of MTrPs/TS and TBs is necessary for long-term relief (see Fig. 70.2).
Postinjection segmental physical therapy (Box 70.1).
Use modalities to increase blood flow and promote relaxation immediately after treatment.

After dampening or eliminating the SSS and eradicating the peripheral pain generators, begin an exercise program of strengthening and aerobic conditioning. Premature emphasis on strengthening and work hardening leads to acute flare-ups of pain, muscle shortening/spasm, muscle weakness, and in coordination with functional deterioration.

Treatment targeted at pain mechanisms should address central and peripheral sensitization to prevent or reverse long-term pain and dysfunction.

Fischer AA. Treatment of myofascial pain. *J Musculoskelet Pain.* 2010;7:131–142. doi: 10.1300/J094v07n01_13.

20. What is the role of acupuncture in the management of MTrPs?
Acupuncture plays a vital role in the deactivation of TrPs. From a physiologic viewpoint, acupuncture's needling effects on the TrP stimulates the A-delta fibers. At the dorsal horn, the A-delta fibers block the pain-producing activity of the C fibers arising from the peripheral nociceptors. This mechanism also reduces or prevents the sensitization of the spinal cord by suppressing the peripheral nociceptive input.

From a biomechanical viewpoint, acupuncture's solid needle tip minimizes tissue damage compared to the shear effects of the hypodermic needle's sharp, beveled, and cutting tip.

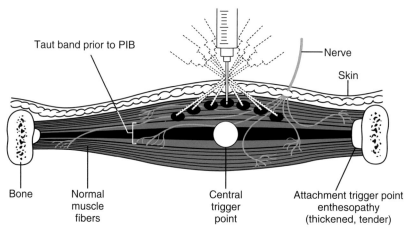

Fig. 70.1 The technique of preinjection block (PIB) is illustrated. Penetrate next to the point of maximum tenderness of the trigger point (TrP)/tender spots (TSs) into normal tissue where 0.1 to 0.5 mL of 1% lidocaine is infiltrated at one stop. Then withdraw the needle to subcutaneous level, redirect to the next stop, and repeat multiple stops as per black circles in the diagram. Spread the anesthetic in this way along the normal tissue side of the taut band (TB), which will be needled and infiltrated post-PIB. This blocks pain nociceptor afferents from reaching the dorsal horn and allows pain-free, more extensive needling of the TrP/TS/TB without amplifying central sensitization. (Adapted from Fischer AA. New injection techniques for treatment of musculoskeletal pain. In Rachlin E, Rachlin I, eds. *Myofascial Pain and Fibromyalgia*. 2nd ed. St. Louis: Mosby; 2002:403–419.)

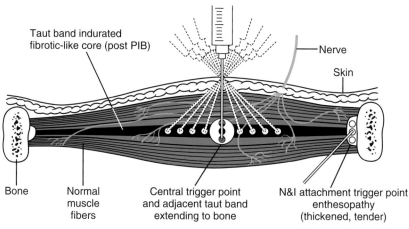

Fig. 70.2 The effect of a preinjection block (PIB) and technique of needling and infiltration (N&I) of the trigger point (TrP)/taut band (TB) are shown. PIB relieves neurogenic muscle fiber contraction and shrinks the TB to about 20% of its original thickness (width). The remaining fibers (solid black) demonstrate very hard linear, fibrotic-like resistance on palpation and needling penetration. N&I consist of repetitive N&I of the central TrP with 1% lidocaine, fanning out along both sides of the TB with N&I (fast in and fast out) at multiple stops (white circles in diagram). Needling of the TB elicits local twitch response. Attachment TrPs (enthesopathy) should also have N&I where the TB attaches to the bone. N&I aims primarily to disrupt the central TrP contraction knots/sensitized nociceptor mechanism and mechanically break up the indurated fibrotic-like core of the TB. (Adapted from Fischer AA. New injection techniques for treatment of musculoskeletal pain. In Rachlin E, Rachlin I, eds. *Myofascial Pain and Fibromyalgia*. 2nd ed. St. Louis: Mosby; 2002:403–419.)

FIBROMYALGIA

21. What are the origins and manifestations of FM?

Chronic myofascial pain bilaterally and "all over" the body is the hallmark clinical presentation of **fibromyalgia (FM)**. FM is a complex clinical syndrome attributed to central neuromodulatory dysregulation with amplification of sensory impulses due to central sensitization. The clinical manifestations include chronic widespread MSK pain with focal pressure sensitivity at anatomically defined tender points, sleep disturbance, severe fatigue, stiffness,

---

Box 70.1 Postinjection Segmental Physical Therapy

Immediate Therapy
- Moist heat
- Spray and passive stretch or
- Spray and active limbering, relaxation exercises
- Eyes down, exhale, and relaxation by activation of antagonist(s) with stretch specific for muscles of the involved myotome
- Electrical stimulation of treated muscle (tetanizing and sinusoid surging currents)
- Subsequent therapy
- Home program of relaxation and self-stretching exercises
- Postural correction and elimination of perpetuating factors (see question 9)
- Strengthening and aerobic conditioning

---

dysphoric affect, and cognitive dysfunction ("**fibrofog**"). Predictably, FM can have a more significant negative impact on quality of life than osteoarthritis or chronic obstructive pulmonary disease. At work, 36% are absent 2 or more days per month, 31% lose employment; and 26% to 55% receive disability or social security payments.

Price DD, Stoud R. Neurobiology of fibromyalgia syndrome. *J Rheum Suppl.* 2005;75:22–28. Available at: https://www.jrheum.org/content/jrheumsupp/75/22.full.pdf.

22. **How are the diagnostic criteria integrated to make the diagnosis of FM, recognize exacerbations, and gauge response to therapy?**

Recognition of the syndrome begins with widespread distribution of pain for greater than 3 months, extending above and below the waist, to the right and left sides of the body, and axially. Confirming FM requires a discriminating history and physical examination, incorporating a complete assessment of the joints, nervous system, muscle palpation, and strength testing. As a prelude, the Fibromyalgia Rapid Screening Tool (FiRST), with six yes or no questions, gives an 89.7% initial screening identification rate of FM patients, with 90.5% sensitivity and 85.7% specificity. Past diagnostic scores have emphasized the total number of tender points at defined sites. More recent diagnostic paradigms incorporate many non-painful FM symptoms into the criteria, including disturbances of affect and cognition, fatigue, stiffness, and non-restorative sleep, along with the tender point exam and widespread pain for greater than 3 months as described in the previous criteria.

The current widely accepted criteria come from the American College of Rheumatology (ACR). For a diagnosis of FM, as specified by ACR in 2010, the following three conditions need to be met:
1. WPI ≥7 and SS Score ≥5 or WPI 4–6 and SS Score ≥9
2. Generalized pain—in at least 4 of 5 regions
3. Symptoms present at a similar level for at least 3 months

The **Widespread Pain Index (WPI)** consists of 19 body areas where patients may be experiencing pain, with a score range of 0 to 19. These zones include the neck, chest, abdomen, upper and lower back, bilateral shoulder girdle, upper and lower arm, hip, upper and lower leg, and jaw.

The **Symptom Severity (SS) Scale** includes two sections. The first quantifies fatigue, unrefreshed waking, and cognitive symptoms, each on a Likert scale of 0 to 3 (from 0 representing "no problems" to 3 representing "severe"). The second presents 41 different symptoms that can be associated with FM. Patients with no symptoms receive a score of 0, 1 to 10 symptoms receive a score of 1, 11 to 24 symptoms receive a score of 2, while 25 or greater symptoms receive a score of 3. The completed SS scale distributes in a range of 0 to 12.

In 2016, an alternative set of criteria for the diagnosis of FM was developed, modifying the 2010/2011 criteria. These alternative criteria lessen the misclassification of FM as regional pain syndrome. The modification adds widespread pain criteria to the older criteria. With 92% to 96% accuracy, this new set of criteria allows a clinician to diagnose FM without excluding other clinically relevant diagnoses. Additionally, the new criteria simplify the diagnosis of FM by eliminating confusing diagnostic exclusions. The 2016 criteria introduce one set of criteria. Instead of having a separate physician and patient criteria, it replaces the physician's estimate of somatic symptoms with the ascertainment of the presence of headaches, pain or cramps in the lower abdomen, and depression in the previous 6 months. The new 2016 criteria permit quantitative measurement of the severity of FM symptoms without measuring the pain threshold with a dolorimeter.

The new 2016 criteria for FM serve as an effective screening tool. They introduce a **Fibromyalgia Severity (FS) score** polysymptomatic distress scale, which is equal to the sum of the WPI and a symptom severity scale SSS (FS = WPI+SSS >12 to 13). For patients whose scores exceed the cutoff FS score of 12 for the diagnosis of FM, increasing scores up to 31 may indicate an increasing level of severity of FM. As with the earlier criteria, all undiagnosed patients should receive a detailed interview, a physical examination, and laboratory tests for alternative diagnoses before screening for FM.

In 2018, yet another proposal for FM diagnostic criteria was designed as part of the concept of a consistent diagnosis for all types of chronic pain disorders. This was devised by the Analgesic, Anesthetic, and Addiction Clinical Trial Translations Innovations Opportunities and Networks (ACTTION) in conjunction with the American Pain Society (APS). Their collaborative pain taxonomy, or AAPT, bases diagnosis on five "dimensions:" (1) core diagnostic criteria; (2) common features; (3) common medical comorbidities; (4) neurobiological, psychosocial, and functional consequences; and (5) putative neurobiological and psychosocial mechanisms, risk factors, and protective factors. The framework remains theoretical and has not yet been validated clinically.

Galvez-Sánchez CM, Reyes Del Paso GA. Diagnostic criteria for fibromyalgia: critical review and future perspectives. *J Clin Med.* 2020;9(4):1219. doi:10.3390/jcm9041219Available at: https://www.ncbi.nlm.nih.gov/pmc/articles/PMC7230253/pdf/jcm-09-01219.pdf.

2016 Fibromyalgia Diagnostic Criteria Form. Available at: https://people.clarkson.edu/~lrussek/2016FMS.pdf.

1990 Fibro Files: 1990 ACR classification pdf and Tender Points image for diagnosing Fibromyalgia - FibroFlutters Patient Advocacy Organisation | Chronic Illness & Rare Disease Network. Available at https://fibroflutters.com/2016/04/08/fibro-files-1990-acr-classification-pdf-and-tender-points-image-for-diagnosing-fibromyalgia/.

23. What comorbid, concomitant, and other disorders may be associated with FM? Why is it important to identify them?

The physician should search for comorbid, concomitant, and associated disorders (Box 70.2) because treatment strategies are specific and different from those required for FM alone. The presence of another clinical disorder does not exclude FM as a comorbidity.

Bennett R. Fibromyalgia: present to future. *Curr Pain Headache Rep.* 2004;8(5):379–384. doi: 10.1007/s11916-996-0011-5.

Yunus MB. Central sensitivity syndromes: a new paradigm and group nosology for fibromyalgia and overlapping conditions, and the related issue of disease versus illness. *Semin Arthritis Rheum.* 2008;37(6):339–352. doi: 10.1016/j.semarthrit. 2007.09.003.

24. Can epidemiology and precipitation ("triggers") contribute to the understanding and management of "triggering" factors?

A female-to-male ratio of 6:1 to 9:1 has been shown in some studies, but more recent studies have shown a 2:1 ratio. Initial diagnosis is made between 20 and 55 years of age, with an increasing prevalence that peaks at 70 to 79 years for 7% of women and 1% of men. Genetic susceptibility is suggested by family clustering, serotonin and catecholamine metabolism abnormalities, and associations with autoimmune conditions.

There is increasing evidence that FM is one of many overlapping clinical sensitization syndromes capable of being "triggered." Triggering stressors include physical trauma (e.g., motor vehicle collision), surgical procedures, acute infection, emotionally catastrophic events, autoimmune diseases, or other pain syndromes that may lead to central sensitization.

Stressors such as these have been shown to be temporally associated with the onset of FM, and the symptoms and signs of FM persist well after the "stressor" has abated. Evidence in the medical literature suggests

---

Box 70.2 Comorbid, Concomitant, and Other Disorders Associated With Fibromyalgia

Comorbid Central Sensitivity Syndromes	Systemic Lupus Erythematosus
Chronic fatigue syndrome	Sjögren's syndrome
Migraine/tension headaches	Ankylosing Spondylitis
Irritable bowel syndrome	Other Associated Disorders
Regional soft tissue/Myofascial Pain Syndrome	Lyme disease
Temporomandibular joint and myofascial dysfunction	Human Immunodeficiency Virus
Primary dysmenorrhea	Hepatitis C
Interstitial cystitis	Hypothyroidism
Restless legs syndrome	Hypoestrogenism
Concomitant Rheumatic Disorders	Hypermobility
Rheumatoid Arthritis	Multiple region myofascial trigger points
Osteoarthritis	Arnold Chiari syndrome

that motor vehicle collision (MVC) trauma or other stressors in concert with genetic factors may lead to the development of FM.

McLean SA, Williams DA, Clauw DJ. Fibromyalgia after motor vehicle collision: evidence and implications. *Traff Inj Prevent.* 2005;6(2): 97–104. doi: 10.1080/15389580580590931545.

25. **How do imaging, laboratory, and electrodiagnostic tests contribute to the diagnosis of FM and MPS?**
    Testing helps diagnose or excludes other conditions that might be associated with or perpetuating both syndromes. Detection of other pathologies on imaging tests does not exclude the presence of FM, MPS, or both. There are no diagnostic gold standard tests.

26. **What common peripheral pain generators should you look for in FM?**
    A skilled search for nociceptive pain generators is essential. Focal treatment can reduce total pain by eliminating regional sources, thereby decreasing the perpetuation and amplification of central sensitization. Common peripheral pain generators include MTrPs, enthesopathies, bursitis, tendonitis, degenerative and inflammatory joint disease, radiculopathies, and visceral pain and dysfunction.

Borg-Stein J. Management of peripheral pain generators in fibromyalgia. *Rheum Dis Clin North Am.* 2002;28(2):305–317. doi: 10.1016/s0889-857x(02)00004-2.

27. **What are the main differences between MPS and FM?**
    See Table 70.2.

Table 70.2 Differentiation Between Myofascial Pain Syndrome and Fibromyalgia

	MYOFASCIAL PAIN SYNDROME	FIBROMYALGIA
Pain	Pain caused by trigger points in taut bands of muscle that can be identified by palpation. Activation by compression reproduces the patient's local and/or referred pain complaint	Pain diffuse and not limited to a taut band. Pain on compression of tender points. Pain complaint not reproducible by activation of a tender point and no referral pattern
Gender	Equal	Mostly female (8:1 ratio)
Critical level of tenderness	2 kg/cm^2 lower than normosensitive opposite side or surrounding area	4 kg pressure or less (thumbnail blanch) algometer more reliable
Symmetry	Asymmetric	Symmetric
Pain distribution	Usually limited to 1 region, but may involve multiple regions	Widespread sites: right and left sides, above and below waist and axial
Tissues involved	MTrPs limited to muscle tissue only. MTrPs initiate sensitized spinal segment with resultant allodynia/hyperalgesia of dermatome, sclerotome, and MTrPs within muscles of the involved myotome	Muscular tender points in upper trapezius, supraspinatus, and gluteus; tender points in other tissue sites such as medial knee fat pad, humeral epicondyles, insertion of muscles in occiput, costochondral junction, greater trochanter
Pathophysiologic basis	Local dysfunction in part of involved muscle with MTrP formation and peripheral nociceptive sensitization (see question 10)	Diffuse CNS sensitization and dysfunction related to sensory *processing* and autonomic and neuroendocrine regulation
Mode of onset	Frequently, acute muscle strain or overuse of a specific group of muscles	Usually insidious, leading to chronic generalized pain and fatigue; cause unknown, but one-third result in onset following a triggering event (see question 13)
Response to treatment	Immediate relief of pain by needling of TrPs and/or infiltration with local anesthetic. Manual TrP release techniques may be effective (see question 18)	Local injection of anesthetic does not relieve diffuse tenderness and pain. MTrPs present in FM/MPS complex can be treated by TrP therapy, but needling is more painful, post-needling soreness is increased, and shorter duration of relief

FM, Fibromyalgia; *MPS,* myofascial pain syndrome; *MTrPs,* myofascial trigger points.

28. What is the FM/MPS complex?

FM and MPS can coexist in the same patient and may interact with one another. MTrPs can be found in over 70% of patients with FM if revealed by skilled palpation. Therefore, patients with widespread pain and tender points at classic sites for FM may have FM exclusively, an FM/MPS complex, or multiple intermingled MPS segmental origins.

29. How would you treat a patient with FM?

The treatment goals for FM are to improve function, reduce symptoms, and develop patient participation in self-care through effective patient education. FM requires pharmacologic, movement, and psychological therapies in an integrated approach. A targeted pharmacologic intervention aimed at central and peripheral pain mechanisms dampens CNS sensitization and enhances analgesia. FM is a dynamic matrix of symptoms with interrelated mechanisms requiring a flexible multimodal treatment. Various strategies are required to manage dysfunctional sleep, fatigue, emotional stress, mood disorders, cognitive dysfunction, and comorbid/associated disorders.

Education programs should explain that the illness is real and treatable, regardless of unrevealing laboratory and imaging tests. Simultaneous instruction in **relaxation techniques** and **self-efficacy** commands a comprehensive perspective. Transcutaneous electrical nerve stimulation (TENS) and acupuncture provide a brief, targeted therapy. Treatment of concomitant MTrPs as well as other peripheral pain generators can improve the overall symptoms of FM.

Exercise has been shown to improve not only patient fitness but also reduce many FM symptoms. Individualized **aerobic fitness programs** have been shown to improve cardiovascular fitness and deconditioning. There is low-quality evidence from Cochrane reviews that **resistance training** is better than **flexibility exercises** for improving pain and multidisciplinary function. Still, aerobic exercise is superior to both for pain in women with FM. Creative, socially connected, person-centered options that address multiple symptoms can be particularly effective. A Tai Chi program has been shown to be equal or greater benefit than a standard care aerobic exercise program alone.

Cognitive-behavioral therapy (CBT) is helpful for FM patients to develop confidence in their coping abilities, which improves self-management and corrects maladaptive thoughts and expectations. Individuals with less social support, fewer coping skills, or greater emotional distress seem most likely to respond to CBT.

Hydrotherapy has been shown to have short-term beneficial effects on pain and health-related quality of life. There is limited evidence for the use of spinal manipulation and supplements. Still, a 2013 Cochrane review showed low-to-moderate evidence for the use of acupuncture to relieve pain and stiffness, and electro-acupuncture may also improve overall well-being, fatigue, and sleep.

Goldenberg DJ, Burkhardt C, Crofford L. Management of fibromyalgia syndrome. *JAMA*. 2004;292(19):2388–2395. doi: 10.1001/jama.292.19.2388. Available at: https://jamanetwork.com/journals/jama/fullarticle/199786.

Lemstra M, Olszynski WP. The effectiveness of multidisciplinary rehabilitation in the treatment of fibromyalgia: a randomized controlled trial. *Clin J Pain*. 2005;21(2):166–174. doi: 10.1097/00002508-200503000-00008.

Morris CR, Bowen L, Morris AJ. Integrative therapy for fibromyalgia: possible strategies for an individualized treatment program. *South Med J*. 2005;98(2):177–184. doi: 10.1097/01.SMJ.0000153573.32066.E7.

30. Is there one word that summarizes FM treatment that helps visualize patient outcomes?

ExPRESS summarizes interventions that help patients "express their true selves" by maximally participating in life.

Ex: Exercise

P: Psychiatric comorbidities

R: Regain function

E: Education

S: Sleep hygiene

S: Stress management

31. What medications have proven to be efficacious in treating FM?

Antidepressants—exert a direct effect on FM symptoms, not due to any effects on depression.

TCAs are more effective than SSRIs or SNRIs, and the most popular TCA is **amitriptyline**.

Serotonin/norepinephrine-reuptake inhibitors (SNRIs) approved by FDA are **duloxetine** and **milnacipran**. Once-daily dosing of duloxetine has been shown to significantly improve function and quality of life without interfering with sleep. It is superior to milnacipran for the mentioned issues and for reducing pain. Milnacipran is superior to duloxetine for reducing fatigue.

The anticonvulsant drugs **pregabalin** and **gabapentin** have been shown to improve pain, patient global assessment, function, fatigue (pregabalin), and sleep.

Other medications can be used as an adjunct to help with specific symptoms, e.g., the short-acting nonbenzodiazepine sedative zolpidem to help with sleep or cyclobenzaprine as a muscle relaxant.

NSAIDs and glucocorticoids may also help treat comorbidities but are not recommended as a primary option for FM treatment.

Benzodiazepines are not recommended for FM treatment.

Simple analgesics and anti-inflammatory drugs are of limited benefit, addressing peripheral pain mechanisms only. **Tramadol**, acting centrally, has been shown to decrease pain in FM. Opioids also act centrally but should be avoided because of the risk of tolerance, addiction, and other adverse effects. They can be used judiciously as in any other chronic pain state but not as a first-line medication. Potent opioids do not have a role in the treatment of FM.

Other medications directed at central mechanisms are listed in Table 70.3.

In conclusion, treatments need to be sequenced, alternated, and linked to achieving the most consistent patient participation in the entire program with the overall aim of meeting personal and life goals unburdened by chronic pain conditions. Procedures and medications help reduce pain so that FM patients can progress to tolerate and maintain the most important treatment—exercise.

Table 70.3 Medications for Treating Fibromyalgia

Antidepressants	
Tricyclics (low dose) Amitriptyline—improves sleep architecture Doxepin—improves pain and depression	Most commonly used; significant improvement in pain, sleep, mood, and fatigue in multiple randomized controlled trials (RCTs) versus placebo.
Selective serotonin reuptake inhibitors (SSRIs) Fluoxetine enhanced with Amitriptyline or Cyclobenzaprine Citalopram Paroxetine	More effective than placebo; SSRIs may improve mood and fatigue but have little effect on pain when given alone.
Serotonin/norepinephrine-reuptake inhibitors (SNRA) Duloxetine (FDA approved) Venlafaxine Milnacipran (FDA approved)	Action like tricyclics but fewer side effects. Significant decrease in pain, depression, and anxiety versus placebo in RCTs.
Anti-epileptic drugs. Gabapentinoids Gabapentin New studies show that long term pain improvement is insignificant. (FDA approved) Pregabalin some pts experienced 50% pain reduction after 12 or 13 weeks	Improved pain, sleep, fatigue, and quality of life in multicenter RCT versus placebo.
Muscle Relaxants: Cyclobenzaprine (similar to tricyclics in chemical structure.)	Improved sleep, pain, mood.
Cannabinoids Dronabinol reduced pain and depression Nabilone reduced pain and anxiety, improved quality of life	
Serotonin (5-HT3) receptor antagonists Tropisetron	Reduces pain and sensory gating, enhances GABA.
Selective hypnotics (use for resistant adjunctive symptoms only) Zopiclone Zolpidem NMDA receptor antagonists	Improve sleep and fatigue but not pain versus placebo.
Ketamine	Effective for pain relief but cognitive side effects limit use.

Medications commonly utilized individually as part of treatment designs for fibromyalgia are categorized by receptor activity and drug categories. Resistant prominent symptoms are targeted to enable full exercise and life participation. Patients need to be followed closely for symptom improvement and side effects. Sufficient trial of any medication should extend at least three weeks or more with dosing adjustments to recognize improvements.

Data from Tzadok R, Ablin JN. Current and emerging pharmacotherapy for fibromyalgia. *Pain Res Manag.* 2020;Article ID 6541798
Available at:
Current and Emerging Pharmacotherapy for Fibromyalgia (hindawi.com)
https://www.cochrane.org/CD012188/SYMPT_gabapentin-pain-adults-fibromyalgia
https://www.cochranelibrary.com/cdsr/doi/10.1002/14651858.CD011790.pub2/full?highlightAbstract=fibromyalgi%7Cfibromyalgia

WEBSITES

1. Physical Medicine and Rehabilitation for Myofascial Pain. Medscape. Available at www.emedicine.com/pmr/topic84.htm.
2. NIH US National Library of Medicine. Medline Plus. Fibromyalgia. Available at www.nlm.nih.gov/medlineplus/fibromyalgia.html.

BOOKS

Baldry PE, ed. *Acupuncture, Trigger Points and Musculoskeletal Pain.* 2nd ed. New York, NY: Churchill Livingstone; 1998.
Donnelly J, ed. *Travell, Simons, & Simons' Myofascial Pain and Dysfunction, The Trigger Point Manual.* 3rd ed. Philadelphia, PA: Walters Kluwer; 2019.
Fischer AA, ed. *Muscle Pain Syndrome and Fibromyalgia.* New York, NY: Haworth Medical; 1998:158.
Gunn CC. *The Gunn Approach to the Treatment of Chronic Pain: Intramuscular Stimulation for Myofascial Pain of Radiculopathic Origin*, 2nd ed. New York, NY: Churchill Livingstone; 1996.
Maigne R, Nieves WL, eds. *Diagnosis and Treatment of Pain of Vertebral Origin: A Manual Medicine Approach.* 2nd ed. Florence, KY: Taylor & Francis; 2006:103–112.
Rachlin E, Rachlin I, eds. *Myofascial Pain and Fibromyalgia.* 2nd ed. St. Louis: Mosby; 2002:624.
Simons D, Travell J, Simons L, eds. *Myofascial Pain and Dysfunction: The Trigger Point Manual, vol. 1: Upper Half of Body.* 2nd ed. Baltimore, MD: Williams & Wilkins; 1999:626.

BIBLIOGRAPHY

Dommerholt J, Hooks T, Finnegan M, et al. A critical overview of the current myofascial pain literature—February 2019. *Myofascial Pain Treat Edit.* 2019;23(2):295–305. doi: 10.1016/j.jbmt.2019.02.017. Available at: https://www.bodyworkmovementtherapies.com/article/S1360-8592(19)30088-9/fulltext.
Ueda H, Neyama H. LPA1 receptor involvement in fibromyalgia-like pain induced by intermittent psychological stress, empathy. *Neurobiol Pain.* 2017;1:16–25. doi: 10.1016/j.ynpai.2017.04.002. Available at: https://www.ncbi.nlm.nih.gov/pmc/articles/PMC6550118/.

COURSE

Israeli Society of Musculoskeletal Medicine: Theory of Myofascial Pain Course. Available at: (ismm.org.il) Introduction—Theory of Myofascial Pain Lecture 1 (Dr. Negev Bar)—YouTube.

CHAPTER 71

PERIPHERAL NEUROPATHIC PAIN: CLASSIFICATIONS, MECHANISMS, AND TREATMENTS

Michael Flamm, DO, Miroslav "Misha" Backonja, MD, and Steven A. Stiens, MD, MS

When one considers the body in relation to dance, it is then that one truly realizes what suffering is: it is a part of our lives. No matter how much we search for it from the outside, there is no way we can find it without delving into ourselves.
— Tatsumi Hijikata (Founder and Original Choreographer of Butoh Dance 3/9/1928–1/21/1986)

KEY POINTS

1. Peripheral neuropathic pain generally starts a with a peripheral nerve lesion
2. Peripheral neuropathic pain usually presents with positive and negative neuropathic symptoms and signs
3. Diagnostic specificity is essential for classification and selection of a treatment regime
4. Treatments of peripheral neuropathic pain address the underlying pathophysiology, and symptoms with vitamins, medications, therapeutic modalities, neuromodulation, and surgery

1. What is peripheral neuropathic pain?

When a patient experiences an injury or disease that affects the somatosensory nervous system, there is a chance they may experience **neuropathic pain**. Not every injury to the peripheral nerves will result in this type of pain, and only a subset of patients will develop persistent symptoms. When the injury or disease affects the peripheral nervous system, then associated pain is called **peripheral neuropathic pain**. In contrast, an injury to the central nervous system or disease affecting central nervous system sensory pathways in some patients results in **central neuropathic pain**.

2. What clinically distinguishes peripheral neuropathic pain from other types of pain, and how is it characterized?

Peripheral neuropathic pain arises as a direct consequence of a lesion or disease affecting the peripheral nerve itself. It is characterized by negative sensory phenomena such as loss of sensory perception, often reported as numbness, and positive sensory findings such as pain, allodynia, and hyperalgesia. This translates to the physical examination findings of a deficit in at least one modality, for example, light touch, and concurrent positive sensory phenomena to another sensory modality, such as dysesthesia to cold.

3. How prevalent is peripheral neuropathic pain?

Peripheral pain with distinct neuropathic characteristics is found in 6.9% to 10% of the general population. **Painful Diabetic Peripheral Neuropathy** occurs in one-third of patients with **Diabetic Peripheral Neuropathy (DPN)**, including up to 5.7 million patients in the United States alone.

Abbott CA, Malik RA, van Ross ER, et al. Prevalence and characteristics of painful diabetic neuropathy in a large community-based diabetic population in the U.K. *Diabetes Care*. 2011 Oct;34(10):2220–2224. doi: 10.2337/dc11-1108. Available at: https://pubmed.ncbi.nlm.nih.gov/21852677/#:~:text=Results%3A%20Prevalence%20of%20painful%20symptoms,neuropathy%20(NDS%20%3E8).

4. How is neuropathic pain diagnosed, defined, and subclassified?

Possible Neuropathic Pain requires a history of a relevant neurological lesion or disease and a neuroanatomically plausible sensory and pain symptom distribution (dermatome, nerve, brachial, or lumbosacral plexus)

Probable Neuropathic Pain is associated with demonstrable sensory signs in the same neuroanatomical distribution **on neurological** examination. Examples of peripheral neuropathic pain that do not match peripheral neuroanatomical distribution include pain in the entire limb, found in complex regional pain syndrome, and the stocking and glove patterns found in diabetic peripheral painful neuropathy.

Definite Neuropathic Pain requires diagnostic testing confirming a lesion or disease of the somatosensory nervous system to suggest a mechanism for the experienced pain symptoms.

5. Does diagnostic testing confirm the causality of pain?

No, diagnostic testing, such as **nerve conduction study (NCS)** and **electromyography (EMG),** is generally more specific in detecting and quantifying impairment or injury than in determining etiology. For example, **NCS/EMG** could detect median neuropathy in a patient with hand pain, but the pain may be caused by (or contributed to from) a C6 radiculopathy.

6. Can negative sensory signs to one sensory modality, such as loss of perception of light brush, coexist with positive sensory signs to another sensory modality, such as pinprick hyperalgesia?

Yes, demonstrating these dichotomous sensory findings in the same area is the defining characteristic of neuropathic pain.

7. How is peripheral neuropathic pain clinically defined and subclassified?

Symmetric (neuropathologically) and asymmetric (neuroanatomically) patterns lead to diagnosis.

Symmetrical conditions include peripheral neuropathy (diabetic, HIV, chemotherapy-induced, idiopathic, genetic). **Asymmetric conditions** include radiculopathy, trigeminal neuralgia, chronic regional pain syndromes, and painful post-herpetic neuralgia. However, asymmetric peripheral neuropathy occasionally presents bilaterally—e.g., a multiple sclerosis patient with bilateral trigeminal neuropathy— although this is not through a process that is likely to cause a symmetrical condition such as metabolic or chemical irritation of peripheral nerves.

Freeman R, Edwards R, Baron R, et al. AAPT diagnostic criteria for peripheral neuropathic pain: focal and segmental disorders. *J Pain.* 2019;20(4):369–393. doi:10.1016/j.jpain.2018.10.002.

8. What are specific positive and negative sensory signs? Which signs are most strongly associated with peripheral neuropathic pain?

Positive sensory signs can be elicited and described as:

 i. **Allodynia** is pain due to an innocuous stimulus (brush or touch) that does not usually provoke pain
   • Subtypes have been established based on stimulus: **Mechanical** (Dynamic: Stroke, Static: touch), **thermal** and **passive movement**
 ii. **Dysesthesia** is an unpleasant abnormal sensation, whether spontaneous or evoked.
   • Vibration can provoke an allodynia/dysesthesia type response commonly in neuropathic pain syndromes
 iii. **Hyperalgesia** is an increased experience of pain from a noxious stimulus that normally provokes pain.
 iv. **Hyperesthesia** is increased sensitivity to stimulation, excluding special senses.
 v. **Hyperpathia** is a painful syndrome characterized by an abnormally painful reaction to stimulus, especially a repetitive stimulus and an increased threshold.
   • For example, light brush begins as tolerable but soon becomes painful after several repetitions.
 vi. **Paresthesia is** an abnormal sensation, whether spontaneous or evoked.

Negative sensory signs are indicative of diagnosis particularly when they follow a specific neuroanatomic pathway. Reduced light touch, pinprick, vibration, or temperature all suggest various nerve conduits and pathways. Sensory deficits without pain suggest a painless peripheral neuropathy.

IASP Terminology homepage. Available at: https://www.iasp-pain.org/Education/Content.aspx?ItemNumber51698.

9. Which neuropathic pain condition is preventable by vaccine?

Post-herpetic neuralgia can be prevented by the herpes zoster vaccines designed to prevent shingles eruption.

CDC recommendations: Available at: https://www.cdc.gov/vaccines/vpd/shingles/hcp/index.html.

Oxman MN, Levin MJ, Johnson GR, et al. A vaccine to prevent herpes zoster and post-herpetic neuralgia in older adults. *N Engl J Med.* 2005;352(22):2271–2284. doi:10.1056/NEJMoa05101.

10. What are the focal and segmental peripheral neuropathic pain disorders?

Trigeminal Neuralgia, Postherpetic Neuralgia, Persistent Post-traumatic Neuropathic Pain, and Chronic Regional Pain Syndrome are all classified under Focal and Segmental Peripheral Neuropathic Pain Disorders.

11. What is the differential diagnosis of asymmetrical facial pain?

Trigeminal neuralgia is a focal, segmental, peripheral, neuropathic pain disorder of the fifth cranial nerve. The crux of treating this debilitating condition is an accurate diagnosis and differentiating the pain from a dental process (such as odontalgia, irreversible pulpitis, osteomyelitis of the maxillary bone) or Temporomandibular joint dysfunction and headache.

12. How does trigeminal neuralgia present, and what are some common features?
Pain in the distribution of the **trigeminal nerve** alone is not synonymous with **trigeminal neuralgia (TN)**. **TN** is a pain syndrome with specific clinical features and evidence of nerve injury. **TN** is distinguished from **Trigeminal Neuropathy**, which follows a similar distribution but has different clinical features. They are also known as **TN type I (classical)** and **TN type II (Trigeminal Neuropathic Pain)**. **TN type I** is a paroxysmal disorder limited to only one branch of the **trigeminal nerve** and is characterized by normal sensory exam except for the presence of **trigger zone**, a very small area that triggers onset of trigeminal neuralgia. In contrast, trigeminal neuropathy is a constant pain usually affecting more than one branch of the trigeminal nerve and is characterized by abnormal neurological examination.

Cruccu G, Gronseth G, Alksne J, et al. AAN-EFNS guidelines on trigeminal neuralgia management. *Eur J Neurol.* 2008;15(10): 1013–1028. doi:10.1111/j.1468-1331.2008.02185.x.

Cruccu G, Finnerup NB, Jensen TS, et al. Trigeminal neuralgia: new classification and diagnostic grading for practice and research. *Neurology.* 2016;87(2):220–228. doi:10.1212/WNL.0000000000002840.

13. What are the core diagnostic criteria for trigeminal neuralgia type I:
Pain in the territory of one or more contiguous distributions of the trigeminal nerve without extending to the posterior third of the scalp, the back of the ear, or angle of the mandible. The pain is reported as paroxysmal, and the paroxysms are associated with distribution-specific muscle spasms with tactile stimulation or facial movement. There must be an identifiable etiological basis for the pain, e.g., an identifiable lesion on MRI.

14. What are the demographics and common clinical features of TN type I?
Typical onset occurs between age 60 and 70 years with the right side affected 2:1. There is **no gender preference**. If two distributions are involved, it is most commonly the maxillary and mandibular divisions. Involvement of the ophthalmic branch is rare. Sixty-three percent of patients experience a period of remission. There is not a progression of the disease. There does not appear to be an association with either premorbid or depression resultant of the condition.

Maarbjerg S, Gozalov A, Olesen J, et al. Trigeminal neuralgia—a prospective systematic study of clinical characteristics in 158 patients. *Headache J Head Face Pain.* 2014;54:1574–1582. Available at: https://doi.org/10.1111/head.12441.

15. What is a trigger zone?
A **trigger zone** is an area of skin that sets off pain paroxysms and muscle spasms when lightly stroked with a soft brush or cotton ball.

16. TN type I must have a cause. What are the likely etiologies and mechanisms of this disorder?
The underlying mechanism is demyelination of the trigeminal nerve as a result of damage of the trigeminal root **at its entry course to and within the pons**. The most likely cause is a vessel, likely the **Posterior Inferior Cerebellar Artery**, compressing the trigeminal root. In secondary subtypes, a separate process can result in similar pathology. In Multiple sclerosis, a plaque can form on primary afferents **after** entry to the pons. A cerebellopontine tumor may compress the primary afferents **prior to** entry to the pons. The **looping artery may be compressed** between the pons and the trigeminal root. In healing, peripheral myelin may be **substituted by central myelin extending from the Pons.**

17. In what disease does TN type I develop bilaterally?
Ten percent of MS-related TN cases develop bilateral disease.

18. What two oral medications are most commonly used for TN, and how are they similar? What are their mechanisms of action and adverse effects?
Carbamazepine binds voltage-gated Na ion channels in their inactive conformation. Three major adverse effects of **Carbamazepine** are agranulocytosis, Syndrome of inappropriate antidiuretic hormone secretion (SIADH), and hepatic impairment. **Oxcarbazepine** has a similar mechanism of action (MOA) but is better tolerated because it does not have as much central effect.

19. Is the risk of Syndrome of Inappropriate Antidiuretic Hormone Secretion lower with oxcarbazepine?
No, while both drugs pose a risk and require monitoring for SIADH, the risk is likely higher than with carbamazepine.

20. Does lamotrigine have a role in treating TN? What is its mechanism of action and risk profile? How do TN patients respond to it?
Lamotrigine is a Na channel blocker, which blocks Glu and Asp neurotransmitter release. Its major adverse effect is a serious rash, which affects children (0.8%) and adults (0.3%) respectively. The risk of rash can be reduced with slow titration. Clinically, fewer patients respond to lamotrigine but those who do have a more profound response than with carbamazepine or oxcarbazepine; they also have fewer side effects.

21. What surgical options are available for TN? What are its major risk factors?
Microvascular decompression (MVD) is a dissection of the **PICA** from the **Trigeminal Nerve**. It is often offered to patients who do not improve with medication therapy. It can result in persistent pain and ipsilateral hearing loss.

22. What treatment options are available for TN exacerbation?
Lidocaine infusion can be used for acute increase in pain.

23. What is the mechanism of action of lidocaine?
Lidocaine is a Na channel blocker that blocks the initiation and propagation of a neuronal impulse.

24. What oral medication is similar to lidocaine, and what class of antiarrhythmic are both drugs?
Mexiletine, they are both class 1B antiarrhythmics. Oral mexiletine can provide relief for some patients, particularly if they respond to lidocaine infusion.

25. What is an absolute contraindication in an otherwise healthy patient for the use of mexiletine and lidocaine infusion? What tests could be considered prior to initiating therapy?
Structural heart disease. Class 1B antiarrhythmics have a deleterious effect on structural heart patients. An ECG should always be considered, and further consideration would be for a transthoracic echocardiogram.

Pratt CM, Moyé LA. The cardiac arrhythmia suppression trial. Casting suppression in a different light. *Circulation*. 1995;91:245–247. Available at: https://doi.org/10.1161/01.CIR.91.1.245.

26. What are the diagnostic criteria for post-herpetic neuralgia?
Herpes zoster is a unilateral, dermatomal rash with grouped vesicles on an erythematous base that never crosses the midline. The Core diagnostic criteria for post-herpetic neuralgia (PHN) include a history of herpes zoster; pain persisting for 4 or more months following the rash; one or more positive or negative sensory signs on physical exam limited to the affected dermatomes with no better explanation for the pain's etiology. Varicella is a disease of the same virus that affects children and remains dormant in the spinal cord dorsal root ganglia until re-expression of the disease as herpes zoster. Both diseases are resultant of the varicella-zoster virus.

27. What is the incidence and course of the herpes zoster disease (also known as shingles)?
Herpes zoster's lifetime incidence is 20% to 30% of the general population, with ~50% of patients older than 85 years old developing the disease. Zoster rash follows dermatomes and with the thoracic dermatomes most commonly affected. The rash typically takes 2 to 3 weeks to heal.

28. How is Postherpetic Neuralgia differentiated from zoster-related pain, and what are risk factors for the progression of the disease?
Factors predictive for PHN development are older age, increased pain severity, greater severity of the rash, and presence of painful prodrome. Pain within 30 days of rash onset is considered "acute zoster" and is related to the eruption inflammation. Pain experienced for more than 30 days but less than 4 months is considered "subacute herpetic neuralgia." Pain experienced for more than 4 months is **PHN**. **PHN** pain is typically associated with dynamic mechanical allodynia.

Arani R, Soong S, Weiss H, et al. Phase specific analysis of herpes zoster associated pain data: a new statistical approach. *Stat Med*. 2001:20(16):2429–2439.

29. What is persistent posttraumatic neuropathic pain?
Persistent posttraumatic neuropathic pain (PPTNP) is neuropathic pain resulting from a lesion of a peripheral nerve. It contrasts with Chronic Regional Pain Syndrome type II (CRPS II) by sharing signs and symptoms of ongoing pain, sensory deficits, allodynia, and hyperalgesia with the main distinction being that CRPS II includes centrally modulated autonomic symptoms such as thermoregulatory instability, swelling, and regional perspiration while PTTNP does not.

30. What are the core diagnostic criteria for PPTNP?
- History of trauma or surgery associated with nerve injury
- Pain for more than 3 months, with the onset temporal to injury (days to weeks)
- Positive with or without negative signs of sensory disturbance following distribution of the injured nerve with one or greater of the following:
  - Mixed areas of hypo-and/or hypersensitivity to sensory modalities
  - Hyposensitivity to nonpainful warmth
  - Hypersensitivity to brush or pinprick
- No other condition better explains the symptoms/signs
The **prevalence** of PPTNP is 10% to 20% of the general population

31. What is the mechanism for PPTNP?

Maladaptive changes in primary afferent neurons, known as **peripheral sensitization**, result in inappropriate signaling that is amplified in the central nervous system, resulting in the phenomenon known as **central sensitization**.[ii]

32. What are the most common types of postsurgical PPTNP?

Post-thoracotomy and post-mastectomy pain syndrome and affecting the **intercostal nerve(s)**; post-hernia repair and abdominal surgeries affecting the **ilioinguinal**, **iliohypogastric**, and **genitofemoral** nerves.

THIS SUBTYPE DOES NOT ENCOMPASS ENTRAPMENT NEUROPATHIES.

SYMMETRICAL PAINFUL NEUROPATHIC PAIN DISORDERS

33. What are the MOAs of painful polyneuropathy?

Damaged C-and A-delta pain fibers, central sensitization, and impaired descending inhibition (**windup phenomenon**).

Gewandter JS, Gibbons CH, Campagnolo M, et al. Clinician-rated measures for distal symmetrical axonal polyneuropathy: ACTTION systematic review. *Neurology.* 2019;93(8):346–360.

Gylfadottir SS, Christensen DH, Nicolaisen SK, et al. Diabetic polyneuropathy and pain, prevalence, and patient characteristics: a cross-sectional questionnaire study of 5,514 patients with recently diagnosed type 2 diabetes. *Pain.* 2020;161(3):574–583.

Scott W, Garcia Calderon Mendoza Del Solar M, Kemp H, et al. A qualitative study of the experience and impact of neuropathic pain in people living with HIV. *Pain.* 2020;161(5):970–978.

Van Hecke O, Kamerman PR, Attal N, et al. Neuropathic pain phenotyping by international consensus (NeuroPPIC) for genetic studies: a NeuPSIG systematic review, Delphi survey, and expert panel recommendations. *Pain.* 2015;156(11):2337–2353.

34. What is a small fiber neuropathy?

Small fiber neuropathy (SFN) is a length-dependent neuropathy affecting the A-delta fibers and/or C-fibers while sparing large A-beta fibers. A-delta and c-fibers register and transmit signals about the detection of temperature, pain, and itch. They also participate in functions of the autonomic nervous system (sudomotor, thermoregulatory, cardiovascular, gastrointestinal, urogenital).

Terkelsen AJ, Karlsson P, Lauria G, et al. The diagnostic challenge of small fibre neuropathy: clinical presentations, evaluations, and causes [published correction appears in Lancet Neurol. 2017 Dec;16(12):954]. *Lancet Neurol.* 2017;16(11):934–944. doi:10.1016/S1474-4422(17)30329-0.

35. What are the most common symptoms of small fiber neuropathy?

Painful burning of the feet is most common followed by numbness and tingling of the feet.

36. What are the current diagnostic etiologies of SFN? What portion is deemed idiopathic?

Etiologies include autoimmune diseases, genetic disease, diabetes mellitus, vitamin B12 deficiency, alcohol abuse, chemotherapy, monoclonal gammopathy of undetermined significance haemochromatosis. Fifty percent are idiopathic.

37. Which genetic channelopathies are associated with SFN, where are they found, and what is their MOA?

Voltage-gated Na channelopathies SCN9A, SCN10A, SCN11A found on peripheral nerves. Their proposed MOA is hyperexcitable DRG neuron or spontaneously active DRG.

38. Which genetic disease is associated with SFN, and what is its defective enzyme?

Fabry disease with defective alpha-galactosidase.

39. Which vitamin deficiency is most likely linked to SFN?

Vitamin B12 is most likely, and its deficiency has a prevalence of less than 3% among 20-to 39-year-olds and ~10% among adults 70 years and older.

de Greef BTA, Hoeijmakers JGJ, Gorissen-Brouwers CML, et al. Associated conditions in small fiber neuropathy—a large cohort study and review of the literature. *Eur J Neurol.* 2018;25(2):348–355. doi:10.1111/ene.13508.

40. What is the gold standard for diagnosis in painful polyneuropathy?

Immunohistochemistry staining demonstrating reduced intraepidermal nerve fiber density is the gold standard for diagnosis in painful polyneuropathy. For patients with suspected SFN, an in-office biopsy is obtained. Obtaining it from a site known to be painful generally yields better results.

41. How useful are historical screening tools in painful polyneuropathy?
    The Michigan Neuropathy Screening Instrument questionnaire (MNSIq) has a sensitivity of forty percent and specificity of ninety two percent regarding Diabetic Painful Neuropathy.

Karlsson P, Hincker A, Jensen T, et al. Structural, functional, and symptom relations in painful distal symmetric polyneuropathies: a systematic review. *Pain*. 2019;160(2):286–297.

42. What is the role of Duloxetine in the treatment of painful neuropathies?
    Duloxetine is FDA approved for diabetic peripheral neuropathic pain (Major depressive disorder, Generalized anxiety disorder, fibromyalgia, and chronic musculoskeletal pain). In practical terms, duloxetine is useful in treating all other painful neuropathies, and it is part of most national and international guidelines for the treatment of painful neuropathies. Duloxetine is a selective serotonin, norepinephrine reuptake inhibitor, which more significantly amplifies norepinephrine.

BIBLIOGRAPHY

Bates D, Schultheis BC, Hanes MC, et al. A comprehensive algorithm for management of neuropathic pain. *Pain Med*. 2019;20(Suppl 1):S2–S12. doi:10.1093/pm/pnz075.
Endrizzi SA, Rathmell JP, Hurley RW. *Chapter 32—Painful Peripheral Neuropathies*. In Benzon HT, Raja SN, Liu SS, Fishman SM, Cohen SP, eds. *Essentials of Pain Medicine*. 4th edn. Philadelphia: Elsevier. 2018:273–282.e2. ISBN 9780323401968.

COMPLEX REGIONAL PAIN SYNDROME: DIAGNOSIS AND MANAGEMENT

Nathan J. Rudin, MD, MA, Bryan J. O'Young, MD, CAc, FAAPMR, Cynthia D. Ang-Muñoz, MD, MSc, and Ninghua Wang, MD, PhD

Pain ... seems to me an insufficient reason not to embrace life. Being dead is quite painless. Pain, like time, is going to come on regardless. Question is, what glorious moments can you win from life in addition to the pain?
— Barrayar, Lois McMaster Bujold (1949–)

KEY POINTS: MANAGEMENT OF CRPS

1. Initiate treatment quickly.
2. The best treatment for complex regional pain syndrome (CRPS) is a combination of pain control (with medications, modalities and interventional procedures), rehabilitation, and behavioral treatment.

1. What are common descriptive terms for neuropathic pain?
   - Allodynia: Pain from a normally nonpainful stimulus.
   - Hyperalgesia: Increased pain from a stimulus that is normally less painful.
   - Hyperesthesia: Stronger than normal sensation elicited by a stimulus.
   - Summation: Increasing sensation of pain with repetitive stimulation (e.g., tapping).
   - Hyperpathia or Aftersensation: Prolonged sensation of pain that persists after repetitive stimulation.

CLINICAL PRESENTATION AND DIAGNOSIS

2. What is complex regional pain syndrome (CRPS)?
   CRPS is a syndrome characterized by continuous and severe pain in a region of the body, usually a limb. The affected area is hypersensitive to contact, and patients may have trouble tolerating clothing, water contact, even wind. Edema, temperature change, weakness, and limited motion are common. More severe cases may progress to contracture, thinning of the skin, and nail abnormalities. Pain and weakness often cause significant disability.

3. What is reflex sympathetic dystrophy (RSD)?
   RSD is an old term for CRPS. It is still in popular use but is considered outdated.

4. What are the clinical features of CRPS?
   The initial and primary complaint in one or more extremities is described as severe, constant, burning, and/or deep aching pain generally worse than that expected from the initial injury. Any contact with the skin may be perceived as painful (allodynia). Summation and aftersensation may be present. At first, the pain may be localized to the site of injury, but it may become more diffuse with time, generally spreading proximal to the injury site.
   Besides pain, CRPS may include:
   - vasomotor abnormalities (temperature and skin changes)
   - sweating changes (usually increased, sometimes decreased)
   - edema
   - weakness, tremor, limited motion, contracture
   - trophic changes (thinning of skin, brittle nails, changes in nail growth, decreased or increased hair, contracture)
   - juxta-articular osteoporosis
   CRPS may have an early phase with local swelling, erythema, and increased skin warmth. Patients then develop a chronic phase characterized by coolness, mottling, edema, and increased sweating.

5. How is CRPS diagnosed?
   CRPS is diagnosed by history and physical examination. The current ("Budapest") clinical diagnostic criteria are reproduced here.

DIAGNOSTIC CRITERIA FOR COMPLEX REGIONAL PAIN SYNDROME

1. Continuing pain that is disproportionate to any inciting event
2. At least one *symptom* reported in at least three of the following categories:
   a. Sensory: Hyperesthesia or allodynia
   b. Vasomotor: Temperature asymmetry, skin color changes, skin color asymmetry
   c. Sudomotor/edema: Edema, sweating changes, or sweating asymmetry
   d. Motor/trophic: Decreased range of motion, motor dysfunction (e.g., weakness, tremor, dystonia), or trophic changes (e.g., hair, nail, skin)
3. At least one *sign at time of evaluation* in at least two of the following categories:
   a. Sensory: Evidence of hyperalgesia (to pinprick), allodynia (to light touch, temperature sensation, deep somatic pressure, or joint movement)
   b. Vasomotor: Evidence of temperature asymmetry ($>1°C$), skin color changes or asymmetry
   c. Sudomotor/edema: Evidence of edema, sweating changes, or sweating asymmetry
   d. Motor/trophic: Evidence of decreased range of motion, motor dysfunction (e.g., weakness, tremor, dystonia), or trophic changes (e.g., hair, nail, skin)
4. No other diagnosis better explaining the signs and symptoms
   All four criteria must be met to make the diagnosis of CRPS. Criteria for use in CRPS research are modified to require symptoms in all four categories and signs in at least two categories.

Harden RN, Oaklander AL, Burton AW, et al. Complex regional pain syndrome: practical diagnostic and treatment guidelines, 4th edition. *Pain Med.* 2013;14(2):180–229.

6. How does CRPS type I differ from CRPS type II?
   CRPS type I is initiated by a noxious event (e.g., crush, soft tissue injury) or immobilization (e.g., casting, frozen shoulder). In type II, there is a known injury to a specific nerve. The two CRPS types may appear clinically identical.

7. Can diagnostic tests help identify CRPS?
   No. CRPS is diagnosed by history and physical examination only. X-rays, triple-phase bone scan, and infrared thermography may be helpful but cannot confirm or rule out the diagnosis.
   Electromyography/nerve conduction studies can help confirm CRPS type II but may be too painful to tolerate. Musculoskeletal ultrasound can confirm nerve injury underlying CRPS II. Vascular ultrasound can exclude peripheral vascular disease.
   Sympathetic block is used to diagnose sympathetically maintained pain (SMP) (see #16 below).

Birklein F. Complex regional pain syndrome. *J Neurol.* 2005;252:131–138.

van Eijs F, Stanton-Hicks M, Van Zundert J, et al. Evidence-based interventional pain medicine according to clinical diagnoses. 16. Complex regional pain syndrome. *Pain Pract.* 2011;11(1):70–87.

8. What are typical imaging findings in CRPS patients?
   - **X-rays** of the affected limb may be normal. Periarticular osteoporosis may develop later.
   - **Triple-phase bone scan:** Blood flow and blood pool phases may show asymmetric uptake between limbs whereas the static phase (most sensitive) shows increased periarticular uptake in the affected limb. Sensitivity and specificity for CRPS are low, limiting the study's usefulness.
   - **MRI** may demonstrate edema and bony changes but lacks sensitivity and specificity. MRI may help identify focal nerve injury in individuals with CRPS type II.

9. Are there specific abnormal laboratory findings in CRPS?
   No. Complete blood count and inflammatory markers are normal but may help exclude infectious or rheumatologic disease.

10. Are there gender differences in the experience of CRPS?
    CRPS is two to four times more common in women than in men; however, gender differences mostly concern psychological functioning. Men with CRPS are more likely to experience depression and kinesiophobia (fear of movement) and may more often use extreme words to describe the emotional dimension of pain. Women with CRPS cope more adaptively, often acting more proactively about their disease, and are more likely to seek early intervention.

van Velzen GAJ, Huygen FJPM, van Kleef M, et al. Sex matters in complex regional pain syndrome. *Eur J Pain.* 2019;23(6): 1108–1116.

11. What is the prognosis for adults with CRPS?

Guarded. Early diagnosis and treatment can improve the prognosis, but in many cases CRPS does not remit.

Lee J, Nandi P. Early aggressive treatment improves prognosis in complex regional pain syndrome. *Practitioner.* 2011;255(1736):23–26.

12. How do the clinical presentation and course of CRPS differ in children?

The biggest difference is that with appropriate treatment, the prognosis in children is generally favorable. Children often have complete or near-complete recovery. This suggests that pediatric and adult CRPS may be quite different disorders. Preceding neurologic or traumatic events may be very mild or entirely absent, and the lower extremity is affected more often. Regional nerve blocks, often with temporary indwelling catheters, are increasingly employed along with rehabilitation to promote rapid return of motion and functional restoration.

Individual and family psychological issues can be key contributors to pediatric CRPS. Careful attention to these issues is necessary and may be essential to treatment success.

Berde CB, Lebel A. Complex regional pain syndromes in children and adolescents. *Anesthesiology.* 2005;102:252–255.

Logan DE, Guite JW, Sherry DD, et al. Adolescent-parent relationships in the context of adolescent chronic pain conditions. *Clin J Pain.* 2006;22(6):576–583.

13. What is shoulder-hand syndrome?

Shoulder-hand syndrome is a variant of CRPS found in the weakened upper limb in patients with hemiplegic or hemiparetic stroke. Edema, pain, and limited motion are present in the affected shoulder, wrist, and hand. Shoulder-hand syndrome may respond to early treatment with moderate doses of oral cortico steroid combined with aggressive range of motion and edema control.

14. What other disorders should be considered in the differential diagnosis of CRPS?

- Neuropathic pain syndromes: nerve entrapment, radiculopathy, plexopathy, stroke, central post-stroke pain, and postherpetic neuralgia.
- Vascular disorders: Raynaud disease, erythromelalgia, peripheral arterial disease, venous stasis disease, and deep venous thrombosis.
- Lymphatic obstruction (cancer, hematoma, other).
- Inflammatory diseases: rheumatoid arthritis, cellulitis, septic arthritis, systemic lupus erythematosus, and scleroderma.
- Musculoskeletal disorders: overuse injuries, myofascial pain syndrome, fracture, edema and contracture of disuse, sprain, and muscle or tendon tear.
- Paraneoplastic syndromes.
- Factitious disorder (limb ligation, injection, others).
- Somatic symptom disorder.

PATHOPHYSIOLOGY

15. What causes CRPS?

The exact mechanisms underlying CRPS are not clear, but it appears to be caused and maintained by a combination of processes.

- **Tissue trauma** is the trigger for most CRPS. Soft tissue injury, fracture, nerve injury, and burns are common initial injuries. Surgery, especially fracture repairs and arthroscopic procedures, is a known risk factor. Immobilization (e.g., casts or splints), hypoxemia, and inflammation can increase the odds of developing CRPS. Stroke and traumatic brain injury can also precipitate CRPS.
- **Abnormal pain processing:** The nervous system adapts protectively to injury by increasing its response to pain. This protective response normally resolves as healing proceeds. In CRPS, the response is enhanced and fails to resolve.
  - Injury-induced inflammation causes peripheral nociceptive afferents to become more responsive to stimuli and fire spontaneously (*peripheral sensitization*).
  - The ongoing "nociceptive barrage" from hypersensitized pain afferents causes chemical and structural changes in the dorsal horn of the spinal cord (*central sensitization*). Wide-dynamic-range neurons in the dorsal horn develop a lower firing threshold and respond to a broader range of stimuli ("*wind-up*" response, mediated by glutamate via NMDA receptors).
  - The painful area becomes larger and still more sensitive, leading to hyperalgesia and allodynia.
  - Neurogenic inflammation can also be seen in the basal ganglia with alterations in its outputs to thalamus, subthalamic nuclei, spinal cord motor centers, and frontal cortex.
  - Cortical alterations also occur, including shrinkage and distortion of the somatosensory cortex representing the affected limb.

- **Autonomic dysregulation:** Although the sympathetic nervous system was originally thought to be overactive in CRPS, this is no longer considered to be the case. However, there is dysfunction of the sympathetic and parasympathetic systems. At the site of tissue injury, nociceptive afferent fibers may become abnormally responsive to circulating catecholamines, causing abnormal nociceptive firing ("sympatho-afferent coupling"). Vagal activity, which opposes and balances sympathetic activity, may be decreased.
- **Immune dysfunction:** The cerebrospinal fluid and circulatory systems of CRPS patients show increased concentrations of cytokines and other compounds which promote inflammation, edema, and changes in vascular tone. Autoimmune processes may also be involved.
- **Other mechanisms:** Genetics, psychological factors, levels of circulating catecholamines, medications, smoking, and other factors may contribute to the development and/or perpetuation of CRPS.

Azqueta-Gavaldon M, Schulte-Gocking H, Storz C, et al. Basal ganglia dysfunction in complex regional pain syndrome—a valid hypothesis? *Eur J Pain.* 2017;21:415–24.

Bruehl S. Complex regional pain syndrome. *BMJ.* 2015;350:h2730.

Harden RN, Rudin NJ, Bruehl S, et al. Elevated systemic catecholamines in complex regional pain syndrome and relationship to psychological factors: a pilot study. *Anesth Analg.* 2004;99:1478–1485.

Russo M, Georgius P, Santarelli DM. A new hypothesis for the pathophysiology of complex regional pain syndrome. *Med Hypotheses.* 2018;119:41–53.

16. What is SMP?

    SMP is pain maintained by sympathetic efferent innervation or by circulating catecholamines. Some CRPS is sympathetically mediated. SMP is diagnosed by performing a sympathetic block, that is, anesthetizing the sympathetic ganglion supplying the painful region. If sympathetic block produces significant pain relief, the condition is categorized as SMP; however, if there is no relief, the condition is classified as sympathetically independent pain (SIP). CRPS patients with SMP may respond to sympathetic blocks and noradrenergic blocking agents as part of treatment.

17. What is the difference between CRPS and SMP?

    CRPS is a clinical diagnosis whereas SMP refers to a pain mechanism. A patient with CRPS may have SMP or SIP and CRPS patients with SMP or SIP may appear clinically identical. SMP may contribute to other pain syndromes including peripheral neuropathies, postherpetic neuralgia, and phantom limb pain.

MANAGEMENT

18. What are the basic principles for treating CRPS?
    - Early diagnosis and treatment lead to better outcome.
    - Immediate and aggressive pain control is essential to improve comfort, reduce suffering, permit rehabilitation, and help reestablish normal limb use.
    - Rehabilitation (physical and/or occupational therapy) is necessary to encourage normal use of the limb, address contracture, control edema, and restore strength and motion.
    - Psychological treatment enhances coping and pain management skills while addressing comorbid depression and anxiety. Techniques include cognitive-behavioral therapy, acceptance and commitment therapy, and relaxation training.
    - Psychiatric treatment is essential for patients with comorbid depression, who have significant risk factors for suicidal ideation.

Lee D-H, Noh EC, Kim YC, et al. Risk factors for suicidal ideation among patients with complex regional pain syndrome. *Psychiatry Investig.* 2014;11:32–38.

19. What medications are used to treat CRPS?

    Medications commonly used to treat CRPS are chosen based on the type and characteristics of the patient's pain (see Table 72.1). Medications from different classes may be combined for synergistic effect, taking care to avoid potentially dangerous drug-drug interactions. No medication currently has a specific US Food and Drug Administration (FDA) indication for use in CRPS. A bisphosphonate (neridronic acid) has received FDA approval for CRPS clinical trials. There are no data on the efficacy of marijuana or its compounds in CRPS.

20. Which rehabilitative modalities are used to treat CRPS?
    - **Desensitization techniques** may increase the patient's tolerance of normal sensory input, reducing allodynia and hyperalgesia. Graduated sensory stimuli are commonly used (very light touch, progressing slowly to greater pressure and larger surface area).
    - **Elevation, massage, gentle range of motion, isometric strengthening exercises, and stress loading** can improve the motor functioning of the affected limb.

Table 72.1 Medications Used to Treat Complex Regional Pain Syndrome

SYMPTOMS	MEDICATIONS
New-onset CRPS	$\alpha2\delta$ ligands (gabapentin, pregabalin), corticosteroid "pulse" (prednisone, methylprednisolone), NSAIDs and/or short-acting opioids as needed to promote increased mobility
Continuous dysesthetic and/or burning pain	Tricyclic antidepressants (amitriptyline, nortriptyline, doxepin, *et al.*), SNRI antidepressants (e.g., duloxetine), gabapentin, pregabalin, mexiletine, intravenous lidocaine, topical lidocaine, clonidine
Lancinating or paroxysmal pain	Carbamazepine, baclofen, mexiletine, intravenous lidocaine, clonidine, other anticonvulsants (gabapentin, pregabalin, topiramate, zonisamide, valproate, others), topical agents
Inflammatory pain	NSAIDs (both standard and COX-2 selective), acetaminophen, topical NSAIDs, topical capsaicin (where tolerated), low-dose naltrexone
Myofascial pain	NSAIDs, antispasticity agents (baclofen, tizanidine), "muscle relaxants" (cyclobenzaprine)
Sympathetically maintained pain	Clonidine (oral or transdermal), nifedipine, tizanidine, local anesthetic (sympathetic ganglion block)
Bone pain	Intravenous bisphosphonates, nasal calcitonin
Pain with sleep disturbance	Tricyclic antidepressants, trazodone, mirtazapine, nighttime baclofen, nighttime gabapentin or pregabalin
Dystonia	Botulinum toxin injection, baclofen, tizanidine
Refractory, severe pain	Opioid analgesics, intrathecal ziconotide, intravenous ketamine

CRPS, Complex regional pain syndrome; *COX-2*, cyclooxygenase-2 enzyme; *NSAIDs*, nonsteroidal anti-inflammatory drugs; *SNRI*, serotonin-norepinephrine reuptake inhibitors.

- **Graded motor imagery,** including **mirror therapy,** left-right limb judgment tasks, and imagining movement of the affected limb may be beneficial.
- **Contrast baths** (alternating cool and warm water) for the affected limb help reduce vasomotor instability.
- **Transcutaneous electrical nerve stimulation (TENS)** may be used proximal to the affected area to modulate afferent input to the dorsal horn, reducing pain severity.
- **Ultrasound** may be used proximal to the affected area to address secondary myofascial pain and contracture, increasing motion, and reducing pain.
- **Specialized garments or wrappings** may be used to reduce edema and sensory overload of the affected limb.

Goh EL, Chidambaram S, Ma D. Complex regional pain syndrome: a recent update. *Burns Trauma.* 2017;5:2.

21. Does amputation relieve the pain of CRPS?
    Sometimes. For some patients, amputation of the painful limb results in pain relief, improved mobility, and ability to use a prosthesis. However, there is a risk (24% in one series) of phantom pain and/or recurrence of CRPS. Meticulous patient screening and informed consent are advised if contemplating amputation.

Krans-Schreuder HK, Bodde MI, Schrier E, et al. Amputation for long-standing, therapy-resistant type-I complex regional pain syndrome. *J Bone Joint Surg Am.* 2012;94(24):2263–2268.

22. What regional anesthetic procedures are helpful in CRPS?
    - Paravertebral sympathetic block: Stellate ganglion block (for upper limb CRPS), lumbar sympathetic block (for lower limb CRPS).
    - Bier block with sympatholytic agent (guanethidine, reserpine).
    - Regional catheter (epidural, plexus, peripheral nerve) for anesthetic infusion.
    - Epidural injection.
    - Brachial or lumbosacral plexus block.
    - Trigger point injection (for myofascial pain proximal to region affected by CRPS).

23. How is a stellate ganglion block performed?

The stellate ganglion lies medial to the vertebral artery at the level of the C6 vertebra, near the recurrent laryngeal nerve. Given the risk of intravascular, intrathecal, or intrapleural injection, fluoroscopic guidance is recommended. Recurrent laryngeal nerve block is a potential complication.

With the patient in the supine position and the neck extended, the needle is directed toward the tubercle of the C6 vertebral body (Chassaignac's tubercle). Once the needle comes into contact with bone, it is withdrawn a few millimeters. After aspiration to rule out intravascular or intradural position, a test dose of anesthetic plus contrast is administered. If the patient tolerates the test dose without difficulty and the pattern of contrast spread is appropriate, the remainder of the anesthetic is slowly administered with periodic syringe aspirations.

Lennard TA (Ed.). *Pain Procedures in Clinical Practice.* 2nd ed. Philadelphia, PA: Hanley & Belfus; 2000.

24. What signs and symptoms suggest an effective stellate ganglion block?

Pain relief, Horner's syndrome (miosis, ptosis, nasal congestion, and anhidrosis), and an increase in skin temperature of the limb. Patients must be instructed that pain relief from the injection may be short-lived (24 to 48 hours), though longer periods of efficacy are common. Greater and longer-lasting relief may justify repeat injections.

25. What is a bier block?

In this technique, sympatholytic agents (e.g., guanethidine, reserpine) are infused intravenously into the affected limb. Circulation in the limb is restricted by a tourniquet, creating a high concentration of drug in the limb. The infused drug is then allowed to circulate in a high concentration in the affected limb, producing local chemical sympatholysis.

26. What is the role of intravenous infusion therapies in managing CRPS?

Bisphosphonates may be effective in reducing bone pain, though the quality of available evidence is low. Complications may include osteonecrosis.

Intravenous **lidocaine** (local anesthetic) is safe and well tolerated. In one study, infusion of lidocaine at 5 mg/kg/h improved spontaneous pain better than placebo. However, further studies are needed.

Ketamine (NMDA receptor antagonist, general anesthetic) holds some promise but must be used cautiously due to hallucinogenic, dissociative, and tranquilizing effects. No standard protocol exists for its use in CRPS and randomized controlled trials and multicenter studies are needed.

Intravenous immunoglobulin (IVIG) was reported to have beneficial effect on patients with CRPS, suggesting CRPS has an autoimmune component. Similarly, plasma exchange therapy has been shown to be helpful in some CRPS patients.

Xu J, Yang J, Lin P, et al. Intravenous therapies for complex regional pain syndrome: a systematic review. *Anesth Analg.* 2016;122(3): 843–856.

Aradillas E, Schwartzman RJ, Grothusen JR, et al. Plasma exchange therapy in patients with complex regional pain syndrome. *Pain Physician.* 2015;18(4):383–394.

27. What is the role of implantable neurostimulation in managing CRPS?

Dorsal column (spinal cord) stimulation is an effective and FDA-approved modality for treating refractory CRPS. There is high-level evidence for improvements in pain and quality of life. Effects on functional status, sleep, mood, and analgesic use are not well defined.

Complication rates are relatively high (34.6% in one series), with hardware problems being the most common issue. Moreover, the therapeutic effect may be lost within a few years of implantation, sometimes prompting explant.

Newer techniques currently under study include high-frequency dorsal column stimulation (10 kHz; does not produce paresthesia) and dorsal root ganglion stimulation.

Hayek SM, Veizi E, Hanes M. Treatment-limiting complications of percutaneous spinal cord stimulator implants: a review of eight years of experience from an academic center database. *Neuromodulation.* 2015;18(7):603–608; discussion 608.

Visnjevac O, Costandi S, Patel BA, et al. A comprehensive outcome-specific review of the use of spinal cord stimulation for complex regional pain syndrome. *Pain Pract.* 2017;17(4):533–545.

28. What complementary and alternative modalities are employed in CRPS?

Scant evidence exists to support the use of complementary therapies in CRPS; however, many have been employed including acupuncture, massage, and mindfulness techniques—all of which are safe, well tolerated, and unlikely to cause harm.

29. Does CRPS spread to other limbs?

Occasionally. Spread usually follows a contralateral or ipsilateral pattern. Spread is associated with younger age and more severe disease. Trauma may precede onset in the second limb, but spontaneous spread also occurs and may result from both spinal and supraspinal processes.

van Rijn, MA, Marinus J, Putter H, et al. Spreading of complex regional pain syndrome: not a random process. *J Neural Transm (Vienna).* 2011;118(9): 1301–1309.

30. Can CRPS be prevented?

CRPS is a known complication after distal radius fracture, with incidence of 10.5% to 37.0%. Daily supplementation of 500 mg of vitamin C per day for 50 days has demonstrated a decrease the 1-year risk of CRPS type I after wrist fracture and surgery.

Aïm F, Klouche S, Frison A, et al. Efficacy of vitamin C in preventing complex regional pain syndrome after wrist fracture: a systematic review and meta-analysis. *Orthop Traumatol Surg Res.* 2017;103(3):465–470.

BIBLIOGRAPHY

Ballantyne J, Fishman S, Rathmell J (Eds.). *Bonica's Management of Pain.* 5th ed. Alphen aan den Rijn: Wolters Kluwer; 2018.
McMahon S, Koltzenburg M, Tracey I, et al. (Eds.). *Wall and Melzack Textbook of Pain.* 6th ed. Philadelphia, PA: Elsevier; 2013.

CHAPTER 73

PEDIATRIC REHABILITATION: MAXIMIZING POTENTIALS ONE STEP AT A TIME

Rochelle Dy, MD, Melissa K. Trovato, MD, and Sarah Korth, MD

We do not remember days, we remember moments.

— Cesare Pavese (1908–1950)

KEY POINTS

1. Birth trauma to the brachial plexus results in Erb palsy and typically not Klumpke palsy.
2. Child abuse is physical, sexual, or emotional maltreatment, or neglect of a child.
3. Ability to utilize power mobility is not necessarily based on age but on cognitive and perceptual skills.

1. **What is the difference between habilitation versus rehabilitation?**
   Habilitation helps the children achieve developmentally appropriate functional skills that will be newly developed. An example is therapy provided for a child with developmental delay.
   Rehabilitation helps the child achieve developmentally appropriate functional skills that existed previously. An example is a teenager receiving services following a traumatic brain injury (TBI). Both work to promote function, prevent compensation patterns, decrease the effects of impairments on children's activities, participation and provide adaptive strategies.[1]

2. **Why do more infants have flattened skulls? What can be done about it?**
   One of the surprising effects of the Back to Sleep campaign, which has reduced the incidence of sudden infant death syndrome by more than 50% since 1992, has been the increase in the incidence of babies with positional plagiocephaly, which is the term used to describe an asymmetrically shaped head. Positional brachycephaly is the term used to describe a symmetrically flat head across the occiput and parietal areas associated with biparietal width and increased posterior head height. These are both deformational and not related to premature closure of the cranial sutures. Recent prevalence is documented at 1:5 infants. When identified early, repositioning and supervised tummy time is an appropriate intervention. More severe flattening or asymmetry may be treated with a cranial orthosis or helmet. Both repositioning and the orthosis have been shown to provide improvement. The orthosis requires an average wearing time of 3 to 6 months for 23 hours per day. They are FDA-approved for use up to 18 months of life. In-depth education on repositioning and tummy time may be provided by the physician or a physical therapist.[2]

3. **Does congenital torticollis resolve on its own?**
   Congenital muscular torticollis is a postural deformity of the neck that may be noted at birth or within the first few months of life. It typically presents as a head tilt to one side with rotation to the opposite side due to tightness of the sternocleidomastoid muscle. Other muscles such as scalenes and trapezius may also be involved. These babies will have a higher incidence of hip dysplasia and plagiocephaly. Range of motion testing will reveal passive and active range of motion limitations, and a SCM mass or fibrosis coli may be noted. Early intervention results in the best outcomes. If it does not resolve, the patient should be evaluated for non-muscular problems such as benign paroxysmal torticollis, Klippel-Feil syndrome, hemivertebrae, or congenital absence of one of the cervical muscles. An appropriate evaluation for non-resolving torticollis would include x-rays of the cervical spine. A head tilt may reoccur, and episodes are generally brief and are associated with fatigue, illness, and growth spurts.[3]

4. **Should you be concerned if a newborn presents with an isolated Klumpke's palsy?**
   Yes. Birth trauma to the brachial plexus results in Erb palsy, not Klumpke palsy. In Erb palsy, there is a downward lateral traction of the brachial plexus away from the roots anchored to the cervical spinal cord, putting the greatest stretch on the upper roots as a result of the increased angle between the head and the shoulder during shoulder delivery (see Table 73.1).[4]

5. **What is the management of neonatal brachial plexus palsy (NBPP)?**
   Management of NBPP is controversial. Consistent recommendations include a period of physical therapy (PT), observation for evidence of recovery, and if functional recovery is not observed in 3 to 9 months, then referral to a surgical center with expertise in the management of NBPP is suggested.

Table 73.1 Brachial Plexus Injuries

NEONATAL PALSIES	NERVES AFFECTED	MUSCLES AFFECTED	POSITION	POTENTIAL CAUSES
Erb Palsy	Upper roots of brachial plexus (C5-C6, sometimes C7) NOTE: *If there is any lower plexus involvement related to birth trauma, it is seen in addition to upper plexus involvement, but not in isolation*	PROXIMAL INVOLVE-MENT (damage may extend to include some distally inner-vated muscles, but *always* includes prox-imal involvement) SHOULDER Deltoid Supraspinatus Infraspinatus ELBOW Brachioradialis Biceps Supinator *May also include:* FOREARM/HAND • Wrist extensors • Long finger extensors	Upper arm ad-ducted, internally rotated, and fore-arm pronated. Hand spared if it involves upper roots only, but if damage extends to include low roots as well, may also see distal involve-ment of wrist, hand, and fingers.	Most common: (1) Obstetrical factors including fetal position and forces of labor* Force of la-bor = Endogenous (maternal expulsion forces with impacted shoulder), and/or ex-ogenous (2) Large fetal size
Klumpke Palsy	Lower roots of brachial plexus only (C8-T1) *extremely rare in neo-nate*	**DISTAL INVOLVEMENT** FOREARM/HAND • Flexor carpi ulnaris • Flexor digitorum profundus, ulnar half • Hand intrinsics (interossei, thenar and hypothenar muscles)	Forearm supinated, wrist extended, and fingers in claw position	*If seen in a neonate, must rule out other causes than birth trauma, such as spinal cord injury, outlet tumors (rare), and anomalous brachial plexus (very rare). Most common in an older child due to traction on abducted arm.

Contractures are a primary cause of functional disability. PT should be involved early for contracture prevention with early passive range of motion, splinting, and strengthening.

In select cases with severe nerve injury or if functional recovery does not ensue in 3 to 9 months, surgery may be warranted. Surgical options depend on the findings but may include nerve transfers, muscle transfers, and/or soft tissue reconstruction for contracture release. Improvement in function has been reported in infants who un-derwent surgical repairs, but there is no consensus on the timing of surgery.[5]

6. **How do you spot signs of child abuse or neglect?**
Child abuse is the physical, sexual, or emotional maltreatment or neglect of a child. A high index of suspicion (in-consistent or questionable history, delay in seeking care), backed up by appropriate physical and medical findings, is the key to identifying non-accidental childhood trauma. Fractures suggestive of abuse include multiple fractures in various stages of healing, such as growth plate fracture; transverse metaphyseal fracture (bucket-handle frac-ture) near the growth plate of the femur, tibia, and humerus; spiral fractures of long bones; and unusual locations of fracture, such as the posterior rib, vertebrae, sternum, and scapula. Any injury to a young, pre-ambulant child or non-ambulant individual, or injury to non-bony or unusual locations such as the torso, ears, face, neck, or upper arms should raise suspicion. Abusive head trauma (aka Shaken Baby Syndrome) findings include retinal hemor-rhages and subdural hemorrhages, especially when multiple and appearing at different ages. Reporting suspected child abuse and/or neglect is required by law. If you're wrong, the result of the investigation is inconvenience and ruffled feathers. If you're right, the result may well save a life.[6]

7. **Do children suffer from stroke too?**
Yes, they do. Although arterial ischemic stroke (AIS) is relatively rare (1 to 8/1000/year) compared to adults, it can result in significant sensorimotor and cognitive deficits with lasting and lifelong morbidity. An International Pediatric Stroke study reported cardiac disorders accounting for 30% of the cases, with half due to congenital heart disease. They tended to occur in younger children, with stroke developing within 72 hours of cardiac surgery

or catheterization in about 20% of the time. Other causes of stroke include vasculopathy (dissection, moyamoya), sickle cell disease, immune disorders, coagulation disorders, and head or neck trauma. Very young premature babies (<28 weeks age of gestation) are also at a greater risk, with hemorrhagic etiology being more common.

Presenting symptoms may be non-specific, such as headache and seizure. Focal motor deficits are present at a later time, especially in younger children. An index of suspicion for those at risk can help hasten diagnosis and treatment and hopefully lessen the degree of morbidity and impairment.[7]

8. What is the WeeFIM and pediatric evaluation of disability inventory (PEDI)?

The WeeFIM (Functional Independent Measure for Children) is similar to the FIM. It is used to measure functional abilities and the need for assistance associated with disability in children ages 6 to 7 years. It was developed in 1987. The data is centrally collected at the Uniform Data System for Medical Rehabilitation in the USA. The PEDI assess functional skills, level of independence, and the extent of modifications required to perform functional activities in young children. PEDI could be used in children up to 8 years of age. There are floor and ceiling effects for both, with the lowest or highest score unable to assess a patient's ability. Limitations of the PEDI is that it does not adequately assess cognitive skills. The WeeFIM does not capture small changes in function and lower-level changes in ease of care, arousal, and response.[8]

9. What is the earliest age at which a child can operate power mobility safely?

The ability to utilize power mobility is not necessarily based on age but on cognitive and perceptual skills. Motivation, understanding and cause of effect, attention and the ability to access the control method are necessary. Use of power mobility does not limit or decrease gross motor function or ability. The Pediatric Powered Wheelchair screening test may be utilized as a screening tool. Studies show that children as young as 18 to 20 months can learn to drive a powered wheelchair safely with training. Supervision may be required based on the age of the child.[9,10]

10. What is distraction osteogenesis and what diagnosis may be appropriate for this procedure?

In 1951, Professor Ilizarov developed a surgical procedure for lengthening limbs utilizing distraction osteogenesis. An osteotomy of the bone, is done followed by the application of an external fixator to apply controlled osseous distraction. The gap caused by the slow separation of the ends of the bone is filled with new bone tissue. The rate of lengthening is approximately 1 mm/day. Post procedure, intensive therapy for stretching of the soft tissues and muscles to accommodate the lengthening bone is essential. The procedure is still utilized today for congenital limb deficiencies, limb length discrepancy from a variety of causes, and skeletal dysplasias. Distraction osteogenesis may be combined with other procedures such as pelvic osteotomy for tibial/fibular hemimelia, uniplanar external fixation for diaphyseal fractures, and epiphysiodesis for treatment of limb length discrepancy. Limb lengthening with an intramedullary motorized nail is a newer method.[11–13]

11. What are the earliest signs of Duchenne muscular dystrophy (DMD)?

The early developmental history of children with DMD is normal with age-appropriate achievement of milestones, such as raising their head from prone and sitting independently. In retrospect, there is often a history of difficulty arising from the floor, frequent falls, or an abnormally loud noise when walking. Neck flexor muscles are involved early, and these children have a characteristic difficulty in raising their heads when supine. At approximately 3 to 6 years of age, the lag in motor development becomes inescapable. The child shows difficulty with climbing stairs, develops a waddling gait to compensate for proximal weakness with lordosis, and develops toe-walking to maintain the center of gravity over the feet and prevent collapse at the knees. Placing them on daytime AFO's would render them unable to walk without the risk of falling.

12. What is the COAT?

COAT stands for Children's Orientation and Amnesia Test. It is a 16-item test of orientation and memory designed for children recovering from TBI. It assesses general orientation, temporal orientation, and memory. On the COAT, a score within 2 standard deviations (SD) of the mean for age defines the end of post-traumatic amnesia (PTA), the period after injury during which the brain is unable to store and recall new events or information. The duration of PTA is important to define, especially in someone assumed to have a mild to moderate TBI, because it correlates strongly with long-term cognitive and memory outcomes. In pediatrics, many clinicians use 7 days of PTA as a marker for severe TBI. More than 50% of children who meet this criterion have persistent behavioral and/or psychiatric problems.[14]

13. What injury prevention strategies are most effective?

The main principles of brain injury prevention include decreasing the amount and rate of energy transfer; using passive or automatic strategies rather than strategies based solely on behavioral change, and using focused and specific recommendations. Don't say, "be careful," instead say, "use a car seat, a bike helmet, and throw out the baby walker"! Prevention needs to be approached from multiple simultaneous angles, including passive strategies, education, financial incentives (e.g., bicycle helmet coupons/subsidies), and mandatory legislation. The first step is for all professionals working with children to remember the need for and importance of prevention. The Centers for Disease Control and Prevention (CDC) has put out guidelines and educational materials for care providers, patients, and families on the prevention and management of mild brain injury.[15,16]

14. **Does outcome after TBI follow the general pediatric brain injury rule that outcome is better with earlier insults (due to brain plasticity)?**

Unfortunately, for younger children, this is not the case. Although some studies using narrower age ranges have shown no significant differences with age, others have shown that older children and adolescents do better than younger children. Plasticity, which is so important in recovery from focal brain injuries such as infantile strokes, may be at a disadvantage because of the diffuse nature of the injuries. The physical and neurochemical properties of the younger brain may make it more susceptible to injury. Also, because *new* learning is affected after TBI, the development of the younger child is much more compromised. Toddlers and infants with severe TBI tended to have a negative developmental trajectory, especially in the realm of communication, gross motor, problem-solving, and social-emotional domains.

15. **What is executive function?**

The executive system describes those mental processes necessary for formulating goals, planning how to achieve them, and carrying out the plans effectively. Executive function can also be thought of as those processes that allow mental flexibility—the ability to mentally initiate and sustain thoughts and plans appropriately, inhibit unwanted thoughts and actions, and yet mentally shift gears when appropriate.

16. **How may executive dysfunction manifest in children after closed head trauma?**

Executive dysfunction in children after closed head trauma is related in part to the frontal lobe injuries. Failure to develop higher-level executive functions in these children may be misinterpreted as the development of new deficits. This often manifests itself when students are expected, based on normal development, to have reached a stage of increased independence. A common example of this is when children go from elementary to middle school. Elementary school is a highly structured environment that does not expect students to independently organize their day, whereas middle school expects students to independently organize many diverse activities and responsibilities (multiple classrooms, multiple teachers, increased homework, lockers, etc.).

17. **Will children return to their pre-trauma abilities after sustaining a moderate TBI?**

Although children with moderate TBI can be expected to score within the normal range on neuropsychological and behavioral tests, their performance will be less than their predicted pre-trauma abilities level, based on very closely matched controls. These persisting deficits impact on real-life functioning, as evidenced by school achievement tests and grades after both moderate and severe TBI. There is a strong correlation between severity and neurobehavioral outcome within the moderate and severe range.

REFERENCES

1. Houtrow A, Murphy N; Council on Children with Disabilities. Prescribing physical, occupational, and speech therapy services for children with disabilities. *Pediatrics*. 2019;143(4):1–14.
2. Dörhage KWW, Wiltfang J, von Grabe V, et al. Effect of head orthoses on skull deformities in positional plagiocephaly: evaluation of a 3-dimensional approach. *J Craniomaxillofac Surg*. 2018;46(6):953–957.
3. Kaplan SL, Coutler C, Fetters L. Physical therapy management of congenital muscular torticollis: an evidence-based clinical practice guideline: from the Section on Pediatrics of the American Physical Therapy Association. *Pediatr Phys Ther*. 2013;25(4):348–394.
4. Darras BT, Jones HR, Ryan MM, et al., eds. *Neuromuscular Disorders of Infancy, Childhood, and Adolescence*. 2nd ed. London, UK: Elsevier; 2015.
5. Smith BW, Daunter AK, Yang LJ, et al. An update on the management of neonatal brachial plexus palsy-replacing old paradigms: a review. *JAMA Pediatr*. 2018;172(6):585–591.
6. Christian C. Committee on Child Abuse and Neglect. The evaluation of suspected child physical abuse. *Pediatrics*. 2015;135(5): e1337–e1354. https://pediatrics.aappublications.org/content/pediatrics/135/5/e1337.full.pdf. Accessed on June 23, 2020.
7. Dowling MM, Hynan LS, Lo W, et al. International paediatric stroke study: stroke associated with cardiac disorders. *Int J Stroke*. 2013;8 Suppl A100:39–44.
8. Williams KS, Young DK, Burke GAA, et al. Comparing the WeeFIM and PEDI in neurorehabilitation for children with acquired brain injury: a systematic review. *Dev Neurorehabil*. 2017;20(7):443–451.
9. Kenyon LK, Jones M, Livingstone R, et al. Power mobility for children: a survey study of American and Canadian therapists' perspectives and practices. *Dev Med Child Neurol*. 2018;60:1018–1025.
10. Rosen L, Arva J, Furumasu J, et al. RESNA position on the application of power wheelchairs for pediatric users. *Assist Technol*. 2009;21:218–226.
11. Paley D, Kovelman HF, Herzenberg JE. Ilizarov technology. *Adv Oper Orthop*. 1993;1:243–287.
12. Hamdy RC, Bernstein M, Fragomen AT, et al. What's new in limb lengthening and deformity correction. *J Bone Joint Surg Am*. 2017; 99:1408–1414.
13. Horn J, Hvid I, Huhnstock S, et al. Limb lengthening and deformity correction with externally controlled motorized intramedullary nails: evaluation of 50 consecutive lengthenings. *Acta Orthop*. 2019;90(1):81–87.
14. Brown G, Chadwick O, Shaffer D, et al. A prospective study of children with head injuries: III. Psychiatric sequelae. *Psychol Med*. 1981;11:63–78.
15. Lumba-Brown A, Yeates KO, Sarmiento K, et al. Centers for Disease Control and Prevention Guideline on the diagnosis and management of mild traumatic brain injury among children. *JAMA Pediatr*. 2018;172(11):e182853.
16. *Centers for Disease Control and Prevention*. Available at: https://www.cdc.gov/headsup/index.html. Accessed June 23, 2020.

CHAPTER 74

DEVELOPMENT: THE HEAD-TO-TOE CONTINUUM AND LIFE COURSE

Scott E. Benjamin, MD, Melissa K. Trovato, MD, Elizabeth A. Stiens, MEd, and Edward A. Hurvitz, MD

The aim of life is self-development. To realize one's nature perfectly—that is what each of us is here for.
— Oscar Wilde (1854–1900)

KEY POINTS: MOST USEFUL DEVELOPMENTAL MILESTONES

1. Gross motor: Cruising/walking (12 months)
2. Fine motor: Pincer grasp (10 to 12 months)
3. Speech: 10 words/body parts (18 months)
4. Social: Social interaction (4 years)

1. **What is normal development?**
   Simply formulated, development is the continuous process of personal adaptive change, driven by nature and nurture. Genetic determinants, available substrate, a permissive environment, sufficient stimulus, and social and family guidance are essential for the fullest self-actualization and participation throughout the life course.

2. **Name and explain three theories of childhood development**
   - **Neuromaturational theory:** Motor development takes place in a cephalocaudal direction, from proximal to distal.
   - **Dynamic systems theory:** Motor development occurs as the end product of multiple internal and external components or subsystems.
   - **Neuronal group selection theory:** The interaction of genetics and environment (nature–nurture leads to a dynamic regulation of neural networks by cell migration and neuronal growth.

   Helders PJM, Engelbert RHH, Custers JWH, et al. Creating and being created: the changing panorama of paediatric rehabilitation. *Pediatr Rehabil.* 2003;6(1):5–12.

3. **Are there other theories of development? How can the process be conceptualized?**
   There are three general categories for theories of human development: endogenous, exogenous, and constructivist. **Endogenous** perspectives focus on causes that "come from within," like genetics or the developmental milestone stages described by Erik Erickson that all persons are expected to experience regardless of environmental influences. **Exogenous** perspectives stress the influence of the environment on the person to determine developmental outcomes, such as theories of Behaviorism from BF Skinner. Although **constructivist** perspectives view development as a synthesis of progressive organization and reorganization that is constructed in the process of adapting. Each clinician must develop a **paradigm** as a collection of understandings of the processes and methods to positively intervene. Educational experience and interdisciplinary patient and family collaborations provide for problem definition. Rehabilitative care is designed to enable the patient to be the best they can be in the best places they should be as they participate in life each day.

   Fox G, Katz DA, Eddins-Folensbee FF, et al. Teaching development in undergraduate and graduate medical education. *Child Adolesc Psychiatr Clin N Am.* 2007;16(1):67–94.

4. **How can one understand developmental milestones instead of just memorizing the events and ages at which they take place?**
   Think of development in a logical progression as a continuum with one function building on top of another. Development proceeds in a head-to-toe direction as follows: head control, then trunk control, followed by rolling (which includes head, trunk, and some limb control), then sitting, crawling, pulling to stand, cruising with handheld assistance or along furniture, then independent walking, running, etc.
   In addition, think of mass activity being replaced by individual, specific actions. Infants react to a stimulating toy with their whole body, whereas an older child will reach, crawl, or walk toward the toy.

5. **What are handy mobility milestones to remember?**
   - Rolling (first prone to supine, then reversed, starts lifting head): 4 to 5 months.
   - Sitting independently (trunk stability): 6 to 7 months.
   - Walking (Standing balance): 1 year.
   - Running: 2 years.
   - Stairs (adult style): 4 years.
   - Skipping: 5 years (boys later than girls).

6. **How does muscle tone differ between premature and term infants? What is the sequence and pattern of tone development?**
   The muscle tone of an infant born at 28 weeks' gestation is completely **hypotonic**. Muscle tone first increases caudally, beginning with flexion of the thigh at the hip at approximately 30 weeks' gestation and progresses cephalad. Flexion of the four limbs appears at 36 weeks. In the full-term newborn, flexor tone predominates.

7. **What is the parachute response?**
   The infant is held in prone vertical suspension and then suddenly thrust downward by the examiner. The infant's upper and lower extremities extend and reach for support to protect him from falling. These postural responses appear at 6 to 7 months. They are not suppressed and persist for life. The postural responses, if delayed or absent, may indicate central nervous system CNS dysfunction, immaturity, or motor neuron disease.

8. **How is the hip examination important in the evaluation of children in a physiatry practice? What is Galeazzi's or Allis sign?**
   The hip examination is essential in the assessment of newborns, infants, and children who are either non-ambulatory or have abnormal muscle tone. As a physiatrist, one may encounter children with hip problems caused by diagnoses such as cerebral palsy, spinal cord injury, or spina bifida. These conditions may carry an increased risk of hip subluxation or dislocation. In older infants and children with conditions such as these, hip range of motion (ROM) and knee height difference should be evaluated. **Galeazzi's** or **Allis sign** refers to the comparison of knee height, making note of a discrepancy between the height of both knees. A discrepancy may be a positive sign of hip subluxation.

9. **At what age do 50% of children walk independently?**
   Most children can walk with one hand held at 12 months. If a child has not passed this milestone by 13 months of age, there may be a need for closer monitoring of the child's progress in attaining other milestones.

10. **How do you approach the child with persistent toe-walking that lasts more than 3 to 6 months beyond the initiation of independent walking?**
    Persistent toe-walking may not be associated with any orthopedic or neurologic problems in 7% to 24% of the normal childhood population. This is generally referred to as **idiopathic or idiosyncratic toe-walking.** The differential diagnoses should include mild cerebral palsy, spastic diplegia, transient focal dystonia of infancy, hereditary spastic paraparesis, and congenital short tendocalcaneus. Toe-walking has also been associated with mental retardation, autism, and childhood schizophrenia. Evaluation should consist of a thorough birth history (e.g., prematurity, complications at birth), family history of toe-walkers or other neurologic problems (e.g., hereditary spastic paraparesis), developmental history, physical exam for gait, spasticity/dystonic findings, and ROM. Electromyography has been used to rule out spasticity during gait. Close monitoring over several months to years will either demonstrate spontaneous resolution of the toe-walking over time or more apparent persistence of increased tone or mild to moderate developmental issues. Treatment of idiopathic toe-walking includes monitoring, ROM, and gait training. If not treated, planter-flexion, contracture can develop, requiring bracing, serial casting, and, potentially, soft tissue release.

Caselli MA, Rzonca EC, Lue BY. Habitual toe-walking: evaluation and approach to treatment. *Clin Podiatr Med Surg.* 1988;5(3):547–549.

Sobel E, Caselli MA, Velez Z. Effect of persistent toe walking on ankle equinus. Analysis of 60 idiopathic toe walkers. *J Am Podiatr Assoc.* 1997;87(1):17–22.

11. **At what ages do children typically begin to go up and down stairs, alternating their feet?**
    Children typically begin going *up* stairs with alternating feet at 3 years of age; they typically begin going *down* stairs with alternating feet at 4 years of age.

12. **What are handy fine motor milestones to remember?**
    - Grasping items: 4 to 5 months
    - Hand-to-hand transfers: 6 months
    - Pincer: 10 to 11 months
    - Feeding with spoon: 18 months
    - Scribbling: 18 months
    - Copying circle: 3 years
    - Copying cross: 4 years

- Copying triangle: 5 years
- Babbling: 7 to 8 months
- Single words: 1 year
- Body parts: 18 months
- Short sentences: 2 years
- Full sentences: 3 years
- Paragraphs: 4 years
- Knowing colors: 5 years

13. What do the words squeeze, palmar, scissor, chuck, and pincer have in common?
They are different types of grasp through which an infant progresses, beginning at approximately 4 months of age. The **squeeze grasp** is first achieved, with progression through the other grasp types until a **fine pincer grasp** is achieved at approximately 10 to 11 months of age.

14. At what age is hand dominance usually established?
Usually by 2 years of age. Early hand dominance may be a sign of a neurologic deficit, such as weakness caused by hemiplegic cerebral palsy, with a resultant decreased use of the affected side.

15. Why have you not mentioned toilet training?
Toilet training varies by culture and by family. It generally starts at approximately 18 months and is usually completed by 3 years. There is a wide variance, especially with overnight continence. Suffice it to say that children should be dry all day by age 3. Children with disabilities will often toilet train later because of cognitive, mobility, sensory, or other problems relating to their diagnoses.

16. What are handy social skill milestones to remember?
- Interactive games (pat-a-cake): 9 months
- Taking off clothes (shoes): 15 months
- Copying housekeeping: 18 months
- Parallel play: 3 years
- Social interaction: 4 years

17. When does stranger anxiety appear?
Beginning at 5 months, the infant starts the process of **operation** and **individuation,** differentiating between the mother and self. Eventually, the infant develops a sense of belonging to a central person, and by 7 to 8 months, behavior toward strangers differs from that with familiar people. This behavior, termed **stranger anxiety**, is manifested by crying or a look of wariness when handled by strangers.

18. What do I do if language development is delayed?
Order an **audiology evaluation** to check for hearing and make sure that the child is in an environment that stimulates language. It is important to start speech and language intervention as early as possible.

19. How can the life course health development framework be utilized in contemporary practice?
Life Course Theory integrates the expertise of many disciplines by looking at individuals as they develop personal life trajectories in time and place considering genetics, nutrition, social, environmental, economic, educational, and vocational resources throughout the life span.

Bates RA, Blair LM, Schlegel EC, et al. Nursing across the lifespan: implications of lifecourse theory for nursing research. *J Pediatric Heath Care.* 2018;32(1):93–97.

20. Can clinicians integrate theories and provide a shared paradigm for continual redesign of interventions to anticipate patient needs throughout all the transitions in each patient's life trajectory?
Principles of the applied **Life Course Developmental Framework** include roles of: location, time in history, opportunities, barriers, constraints and continued life choices that are self-determining. Health development, therefore, is responsive to the synchronization of micro- to macro-level ecological pathways from molecular to social and cultural functions. Interdisciplinary understanding of the patient, early recognition of deficits, and a creative anticipatory design for the achievement of life aspirations are the essential ingredients for contemporary program design.

Gautreau S, Gould ON, Forsythe ME. Aging and orthopedics: how a lifespan development model can inform practice and research. *Can J Surg.* 2016;59(4):281–286. DOI: 10.1503/cjs.008215.

21. How can spina bifida be used a good model for life long development understanding.
Life with spina bifida/myelomeningocele provides a good model for discussing development and rehabilitation concepts as it is a complicated diagnoses that affects multiple systems, including neurological, bowel, bladder,

cognition, and musculoskeletal. All have separate consequences. The impact on parents, siblings, and other family members is complex. Early dependency with care and continued intimate care beyond what is typical for age challenges the family. Medical, motor, and cognitive issue related to spina bifida impact teenagers and adults from being self-managers/directive, socially integrated and financially productive. The Life Course Model provides a framework for understanding and arranging services, treatment, and research to continue development and success to the greatest extent possible.

Grayson NH, Alriksson-Schmidt AI, Bellin MH, et al. A family perspective: how this product can inform and empower families of youth with spina bifida. *Pediatr Clin N Am.* 2010;57:919–934.

See Fig. 74.1.

22. **What are some critical milestones to remember by age?**
Table 74.1 is a guideline. Use it for a rough estimate, not for diagnostic purposes (*see* question 16). These are 50th percentiles.

www.aap.org/healthtopics/stages.cfm

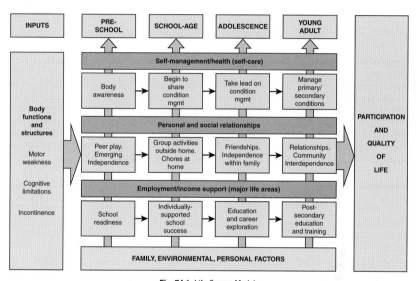

Fig. 74.1 Life Course Model.

Table 74.1 Critical Milestones by Age

AGE	GROSS MOTOR	FINE MOTOR	LANGUAGE	SOCIAL
6 months	Sitting	Hand to hand, palmar grasp	Makes sounds	
1 year	Cruising (walks by holding on), early walking	Pincer grasp	Mama, Dada; one or two other words	Interactive game
18 months	Walks upstairs with help	Scribbling	10 words, body parts	Takes off clothes, feeds self, copies housekeeping
2 years	Running	Circular scribbling	Short sentences	
3 years	Stands on one foot, rides tricycle	Copies circle	Full sentences	Parallel play
4 years	Upstairs adult style	Copies cross	Speaks in paragraphs	Social interaction
5 years	Skips (boys later)	Copies triangle	Knows colors	

23. **How do I use developmental milestones in practice?**
One has to approach the child with a disability with an understanding of normal development in order to use adaptive equipment to assist the child in gaining increased interaction with the environment. For example, for a child with spina bifida, one might consider the following:
   - **3 to 8 months:** Use **tumble form chair** to allow the child to visually inspect the environment.
   - **8 to 14 months:** Place child in a 90-degree seat to allow bimanual interaction with the environment, sitting experience, and exploration. Also, use a sitting cart to allow exploration.
   - **14 to 25 months:** Place child in a **standing frame** to provide standing experience and weight-bearing for developing bones and muscles.

24. **How can development be assessed more formally?**
Some of the more popular assessments are described in Table 74.2.

25. **What if a child has poor motor development in the absence of any neuromuscular pathology?**
Developmental coordination disorder (DCD) has been defined as an impairment of both functional performance and quality of movement that is not explicable by age, intellect, or other diagnosable conditions. This syndrome has many names, including developmental dyspraxia and the clumsy child. Idiopathic toe-walking (*see* Question 9) and the sensory integration syndrome may be a part of this same clinical picture. DCD is a diagnosis of exclusion and is treated through a variety of therapy approaches.

---

www.canchild.ca

---

26. **Are there developmental phases later in life and how are they associated with end of life fulfillment?**
Erikson discussed **generativity** as the seventh developmental task in his first publication of the stages and defined it as "the concern with establishing and guiding the next generation." He put this responsibility into middle adulthood and included the concepts of productivity, creativity, leadership, and mentorship. Participation requires "belief in the species" and "a trust in the welcoming of the community." In early life, patients need to be exposed to and develop the largest variety of interests, passions, and capabilities during the **industry phase**. Later in generativity opportunities to contribute need to be creatively identified and utilized to support life roles and retain fidelity to principles understood and supported by the strengths of the individual.

Schoklitsch A, Baumann U. Generativity and aging: a promising future research topic? *J. Aging Stud.* 2012;26:262–272.

BOOKS

Illingworth RS. *The Development of the Infant and Young Child.* 10th ed. India: Harcourt; 2013:408.

Molnar GE, Alexander MA, eds. *Pediatric Rehabilitation.* 5th ed. New York: Demos Medical Publishing, LLC.; 2015:636.

Learner RM. *Concepts and Theories of Human Development.* 4th ed. Oxfordshire, England, UK: Routledge; 2018:606.

Erickson EH, Erickson JM. *Life Cycle Completed.* New York: W.W. Norton & Company;1998:134.

Maslow AH. *Future Visions: The Unpublished Papers of Abraham Maslow.* In: Hoffman E, ed. Thousand Oaks, CA: Sage Publications;1996:210.

Table 74.2 Assessments of Developmental Milestones

TOOL	ASSESSMENT
DDST—Denver Development Screening Test	Screening tools that can be administered in the office. Administration requires anywhere from 2 to 15 min.
PEDS—Pediatric Evaluation of Development	Some are just questions, some (e.g., DDST) involve small items to test specific tasks.
ASQ—Ages and Stages Questionnaire	
CDI—Child Development Inventory	
Bayley Infant Neurodevelopmental Screen	Full developmental test to assess risk for infants aged 3–24 months.
Peabody Developmental Test of Motor Proficiency	An assessment of gross and fine motor skills from birth to 83 months.
B & O—Bruininks-Oseretsky	A scale of motor proficiency for children aged 4.5–14.5 years.

BIBLIOGRAPHY

Carpenter DL, Batley RJ, Johnson EW. Developmental evaluation of infants and children. *Phys Med Rehabil Clin North Am.* 1996;7:561–582.

Hafton N, LarsonM, Lu M, et al. Lifecourse health development: past, present and future. *Matern Child Health J.* 2014;18(2):344–365.

CHAPTER 75

NEURAL TUBE DEFECTS: PATHOLOGY, COMPLICATIONS, AND REHABILITATION

Sam S. H. Wu, MD, MA, MPH, MBA, Sarah A. Korth, MD, and Steven A. Stiens, MD, MS

The farther back you can look, the farther forward you are likely to see.
— Winston Churchill (1874–1965)

KEY POINTS: NEURAL TUBE DEFECTS

1. Neurogenic bowel and bladder are present in most people with myelomeningocele.
2. The higher the lesion, the greater the likelihood of cognitive impairment.
3. Children born today with a neural tube defect have a near normal life span.
4. Mobility is dependent on the motor level, orthotics, wheelchairs, and power.
5. Folic acid supplementation greatly reduces the risk for neural tube defects.
6. Renal failure is an important preventable cause of death in adults with spina bifida.

1. How are neural tube defects (NTDs) categorized?

NTDs **(myelodysplasia)** result from disruption in neural tube closure (neurulation). The neural tube closes in a zipper-like fashion between the 23rd and 28th days after conception. There are three major types of NTDs:

- **Anencephaly**: A failure of closure of the anterior neuropore, resulting in variable loss of cranial structures and is almost universally lethal.
- **Encephalocele**: A cystic structure that forms at the craniocervical junction, resulting in mild to severe impairment, depending on cyst contents.
- **Spina bifida (SB)**: A general term used to describe a group of NTDs with failure of the vertebrae to fuse posteriorly.

Greene NDE, Copp AJ. Neural tube defects. *Annu Rev Neurosci.* 2014;37:221–242. doi: 10.1146/annurev-neuro-062012-170354.

2. What are the subtypes of SB?

- **Spina bifida occulta:** Posterior vertebral defect with no herniation of the spinal cord or the meninges, and no neurologic symptom. This is the most common type and is present in up to 10% of the population. The bony defect can usually be seen on plain radiographs. There may be cutaneous manifestations overlying the defect, such as a hairy tuft, dimples, or hemangioma.
- **Meningocele:** Herniation of meninges through a vertebral defect with no involvement of the underlying nervous system. This defect is usually repaired at birth.
- **Myelomeningocele (MMC):** Herniation of the spinal cord and meninges through a vertebral defect. The lumbosacral junction is the most common site. Associated conditions may include neurogenic bowel and bladder, motor and sensory impairments, hydrocephalus, Chiari malformations, spinal cord tethering, and syringomyelia. Motor and sensory deficits depend largely on the level of the herniation.

3. What are the etiology and prevalence of NTDs?

The etiology of NTDs is multifactorial, involving genetic, environmental, and/or geographical factors. Maternal risk factors include personal or family history of NTD, prior pregnancy with NTD, use of certain anticonvulsant medications, diabetes, obesity, and mutations in folate-related enzymes. Other associations include maternal hyperthermia, parental exposure to Agent Orange, and low socioeconomic status.

The wide-ranging estimates for the prevalence of NTDs worldwide (0.3 to 199.4 NTDs per 10,000 births) are likely due to a combination of variation in data collection methodology, inconsistent documentation, and differences resulting from nutritional factors, genetics, and routine folic acid supplementation. The majority of NTD cases could be prevented with sufficient maternal consumption of folic acid prior to conception and during early pregnancy. In 1998, the US mandated fortification of flour and cereal grain products with folic acid as a primary prevention measure, which led to a significant decrease in the prevalence of NTDs.

Prevalence of NTDs in the US is estimated to be 5.1 to 5.4 cases per 10,000 births (95% confidence interval).

Zaganjor I, Sekkarie A, Tsang BL, et al. Describing the prevalence of neural tube defects worldwide: a systematic literature review. *PLoS One.* 2016;11(4):e0151586. Available at: https://doi.org/10.1371/journal.pone.0151586.

4. What are the recommendations for folic acid supplementation?
   The CDC and US Preventive Services Task Force recommends that women of reproductive age take daily folic acid supplements of 0.4 mg. For women with a history of NTD-affected pregnancy, 4 mg of folic acid daily beginning at least 1 month prior to the pregnancy and through the first trimester reduces the risk of NTD in the active pregnancy by about 70%.

5. What prenatal testing is available for detecting NTDs?
   Elevated serum alpha fetoprotein (AFP) levels are associated with NTD and are routinely screened for during pregnancies. In addition, consensus by the American College of Obstetricians and Gynecologists indicates that high-resolution, second-trimester fetal anatomy ultrasonography is an appropriate screening test for NTDs between 18 and 22 weeks of gestation. However, routine screening with amniotic fluid AFP is not considered a cost-effective approach. Invasive tests such as amniocentesis or chorionic villus sampling are reserved for high-risk pregnancies or when noninvasive screening test results are inconclusive.

Flick A, Krakow D, Martirosian A, et al. Routine measurement of amniotic fluid alpha-fetoprotein and acetylcholinesterase: the need for a reevaluation. *Am J Obstet Gynecol.* 2014;211(2):139.e1-6.

6. What are the determinants for morbidity and mortality in MMC?
   See Table 75.1.

7. What other common central nervous system (CNS) complications ARE associated with NTDs?
   A Chiari II malformation (herniation of the cerebellar tonsil through the foramen magnum) is the most common complication, followed by hydrocephalus, tethered cord syndrome, and syringomyelia.

8. How are cognitive functions affected in MMC?
   - **General intelligence:** Lower IQ scores are associated with higher-level lesions, CNS infections, and shunt malfunctions.

Table 75.1 Factors Affecting Morbidity and Mortality in Meningomyelocele

LEADING FACTORS	MORBIDITY AND MORTALITY
Hydrocephalus	May occur in 95% of all children with meningomyelocele (MMC) and requires shunt placement in up to 85%.
Renal failure	A preventable complication that may lead to death. Reflux, hydronephrosis, and recurrent infection are the primary causes of renal failure.
Pressure ulcers	A major cause of morbidity in adolescents and adults.
Tethered cord	A defect caused by the abnormal attachment of the spinal cord at its distal end (filum terminale), which prevents the normal ascension of the conus medullaris with growth from its earlier distal position to the adult L1–L2 vertebral level. This defect can occur in 11%–15% of children after MMC repair. The average age at diagnosis is 6 years. Signs and symptoms can include recent changes in lower-extremity motor strength or sensation; recent changes in functional mobility; and the new onset of spasticity, back pain, scoliosis, or new bowel or bladder incontinence.
Hydromyelia	A cavitation in the spinal canal, which can present as neck rigidity, pain, weakness, or spasticity in the upper or lower extremities, rapidly progressive scoliosis, or worsening in bowel or bladder function.
Obesity	A frequent problem in individuals with MMC. Their reduced daily energy expenditure is caused by paralysis, lack of muscle mass, and decreased physical activity.
Latex hypersensitivity	Develops over time and can occur in up to 80% of patients with spina bifida. A negative diagnostic test does not rule out future sensitization. Therefore, these patients should avoid all exposure to latex-containing material, including catheters and other medical and nonmedical equipment.

- **Higher-order cognitive functions:** Regardless of IQ, many with SB have impairments in problem-solving, conceptualization, efficiency of processing, and mental flexibility. Neuropsychological testing is particularly valuable for the quantification and remediation of these deficits.

Brown TM, Ris MD, Beebe D, et al. Factors of biological risk and reserve associated with executive behaviors in children and adolescents with spina bifida myelomeningocele. *Child Neuropsychol.* 2008;14(2): 118–134. Available at: https://doi: 10.1080/0929704060 1147605.

9. What bowel and urologic deficits are associated with MMC?
   Neurogenic bowel dysfunction can involve dyssynergy of intestinal peristalsis, a total or partial absence of rectal fullness sensation, and/or a lack of anorectal sphincter control. More than 80% of children with MMC have neurogenic bowel dysfunction.
       Neurogenic bladder dysfunction affects greater than 80% of those with MMC. They may have partial or complete denervation of the bladder with poor compliance and poor contractility. In the vast majority (86%), the internal sphincter is incompetent. In a third, there is detrusor–sphincter dyssynergy resulting from a partially functional external sphincter.

10. What are the determinants for ambulation potential in MMC?
    The ambulatory status is dependent on multiple factors, including motor level (with higher levels less likely to ambulate than lower levels), musculoskeletal complications, history of shunted hydrocephalus, cognitive function, obesity, motivation, and age (see Table 75.2).

11. How are orthopedic deficits associated with MMC?
    See Table 75.3.

12. What orthotics improve ambulation in MMC?
    See Table 75.4.

Ivanyi B, Schoenmakers M, van Veen N, et al. The effects of orthoses, footwear, and walking aids on the walking ability of children and adolescents with spina bifida: a systematic review using International Classification of Functioning, Disability and Health for Children and Youth (ICF-CY) as a reference framework. *Prosthet Orthot Int.* 2015;39(6):437–443. Available at: https://doi.org/10.1177/0309364614543550.

13. What are the risks and benefits of prenatal surgery for MMC closure?
    The **Management of Myelomeningocele Study (MOMS)** trial demonstrated that open fetal surgery (OFS) to repair SB aperta improves hindbrain herniation, reduces ventriculoperitoneal shunting, and improves motor function in comparison to postnatal surgery. The maternal and fetal risks include uterine wall thinning, peripartum bleeding, and premature birth. Perinatal mortality of OFS is comparable to that of postnatal surgery. The MOMS trial demonstrated Level 1 efficacy for prenatal closure and should be offered for all fetuses diagnosed with MMC.

Table 75.2 Motor Strengths Determining Ambulation Potential in Meningomyelocele

AMBULATION POTENTIAL	ASSOCIATED MOTOR STRENGTH
Community ambulation without assistive devices	Grade 4–5 gluteal and tibialis anterior function
No complete reliance on wheelchair use; majority are community ambulators	Grade 4–5 iliopsoas and quadriceps function
Partial or complete reliance on wheelchair use	Grade 0–3 iliopsoas function

Table 75.3 Orthopedic Deficits Associated With Meningomyelocele

LEVEL OF SPINAL INVOLVEMENT	MUSCULOSKELETAL DEFICITS AND COMPLICATIONS
T6–T12	Kyphosis, scoliosis, hip and knee flexion contractures, and equinus foot
L1–L3	Scoliosis, hip flexion and adduction contractures, hip dislocation, knee flexion contractures, and equinus foot
L4–L5	Scoliosis, lordosis, hip and knee flexion contractures, hip dislocation, knee extension contractures, and calcaneovarus or calcaneus foot
S1–S4	Cavus foot

Table 75.4 Orthoses to Improve Ambulation in Meningomyelocele

LEVEL OF INJURY	AMBULATION POTENTIAL	ORTHOTICS	GAIT AND ASSISTIVE DEVICE
Mid-thoracic	Therapeutic ambulation in early age, but later requiring wheelchair.	Parapodium	• Provides structural support from the mid-thoracic level to the feet and allows for both standing and sitting. Children can ambulate therapeutically with a swing-through gait using a walker or crutches. However, as the child grows, the base plate of the parapodium needs to be enlarged to maintain stability; ambulation thus becomes more difficult in older children.
		Swivel walker	• A modification of the parapodium with a footplate attachment that translates lateral trunk movement to forward propulsion. It has increased ambulation efficiency over the parapodium.
Low thoracic/ high lumbar	Household-level ambulation	Reciprocal gait orthosis	• Composed of bilateral hip-knee-ankle-foot orthoses with a cross-connecting cable system that translates hip flexion into contralateral hip extension. • Energy expenditure for ambulation with this orthosis approaches that of wheelchair locomotion.
Mid lumbar	Limited community ambulation	Hip-knee-ankle-foot orthosis	• Assistive device may be needed for ambulation in presence of hip instability.
		Knee-ankle-foot orthosis	• Correct or prevent knee deformity.
		Ankle-foot orthosis	• May be adequate when knee extension strength is >3/5. • Stabilizes knee in extension, assists in push-off in late stance phase and prevents foot drop in swing phase.
Low lumbar/ sacral	Community ambulation	Floor reaction orthosis	• For non-fixed calcaneal foot deformity, to increase knee extension moment.
		Ankle orthosis	• For ankle stabilization. • Improves gait pattern including reduced stance-phase knee flexion and increased walking velocity.
		Shoe modifications	• For foot deformities. • Arch support.

WEBSITES

1. Spina Bifida Association. Available at: https://www.spinabifidaassociation.org.
2. *Guidelines for the Care of People with Spina Bifida.* 4th ed. 2018. Available at: https://www.spinabifidaassociation.org/resource/guidelines.
3. National Center on Birth Defects and Developmental Disabilities. Available at: www.cdc.gov/ncbddd.
4. Medline Plus. Available at: www.nlm.nih.gov/medlineplus/neuraltubedefects.html.

BIBLIOGRAPHY

Dicianno BE, Karmarkar A, Houtrow A, et al. Factors associated with mobility outcomes in a National Spina Bifida Patient Registry. *Am J Phys Med Rehabil.* 2015;94(12):1015–1025.
Joyeux L, Danzer E, Flake AW, et al. Fetal surgery for spina bifida aperta. *Arch Dis Child Fetal Neonatal Ed.* 2018;103:F589–F595.

CHAPTER 76

CEREBRAL PALSY

Jessica Pruente, MD, Edward A. Hurvitz, MD, Rita Ayyangar, MD, and Mindy Aisen, MD

There are only two lasting bequests we can hope to give our children. One is roots; the other, wings.
— Hodding Carter

KEY POINTS: TREATMENT OF HYPERTONIA

1. Focal Tone: Stretching, therapy, serial casting, splinting and orthotics, botulinum toxin injections, phenol neurolysis
2. Regional Tone: Selective dorsal rhizotomy, SEMLS (single event multilevel surgery), therapy
3. Generalized Tone: Oral medications, therapy, specialized seating system, baclofen pump

1. What is cerebral palsy (CP)?

In 2005, the following definition of CP was published by an international working group on the topic:

> CP describes a group of permanent disorders of the development of movement and posture, causing activity limitation that are attributed to non-progressive disturbances in the fetal or infant brain. The motor disorders of cerebral palsy are often accompanied by disturbances of sensation, perception, cognition, communication, and behavior, by a seizure disorder and by secondary musculoskeletal problems.

The fetal or infant range allows some latitude as to the upper limit of age of diagnosis. It is generally accepted that the onset occurs before the age of 2 or 3 years and, practically speaking, the disturbance has occurred before the affected function has developed (for example, walking or talking). It is also important to note that the lesion resulting in CP is static. Some children with progressive neurological disorders may be misdiagnosed as having CP before evidence of progressive neurological impairment is evident. As children grow, their muscles may become tighter, and as they age, they may have increasing functional deficits generally related to secondary effects of spasticity and other primary problems.

Bax M, Goldstein M, Rosenbaum P, et al. Proposed definition and classification of cerebral palsy, April 2005. *Dev Med Child Neurol.* 2005;47:571.

2. What causes CP?

CP has a heterogeneous etiology. The principal distinction of CP from other phenotypically similar disorders is time of onset of the damage to the nervous system. The damage or malformation occurs before the affected function has developed. Preterm birth is the most important risk factor for CP; risk of CP increases steadily with declining gestational age at birth. In very low-birth-weight premature infants, electrophysiological studies have suggested that brain damage happens in the first 24 hours after birth. The neuronal damage is thought to have an inflammatory mechanism (e.g., from chorioamnioitis), and the resulting pattern of brain injury is periventricular leukomalacia. Other common findings in this population are intraventricular hemorrhage, often resulting in hydrocephalus. In full-term infants, risk factors include hypoxic ischemic encephalopathy, neonatal stroke, poor fetal growth, heavy metal exposures (e.g., lead, mercury), kernicterus, chorioamnioitis, head trauma (shaken baby syndrome), encephalitis, and meningitis. Genetic causes of CP-type syndromes are gaining more attention, and their place in CP etiology is being defined.

Wu YW, Colford JM Jr. Chorioamnionitis as a risk factor for cerebral palsy: a meta-analysis. *JAMA.* 2000;284(11):1417–1424.

3. How is CP diagnosed?

Clinical diagnosis based on the definition mentioned in Question 1 is the most common way. In less severe cases, developmental delays and manifestations of spasticity may not be present for up to a year. However, early diagnosis at around 6 months is possible in infants presenting with perinatal risk factors using the Generalized Movement Assessment and neuroimaging. The common presenting complaints are developmental delay (e.g., not sitting by 9 months), hand preference prior to 1 year, trouble feeding, drooling, and arms and/or legs feeling stiff with the legs often crossing over each other (scissoring). The most important thing to determine is that there is *no loss of milestones*, which would indicate a neuro-degenerative disorder, hydrocephalus, or even a tumor. Metabolic testing to rule out other diagnoses is often indicated. An MRI or brain CT may demonstrate the findings noted above.

Part of the diagnosis is a description of the clinical manifestations; individuals with *spastic diplegia* have more leg involvement than arms. Those with *spastic quadriplegia* have total body involvement, while *spastic hemiplegia* involves only one side, with an arm usually affected more than the leg. Some children may often have dystonia, chorea, athetosis, or ataxia, in addition to spasticity. Pure ataxia is rare and is usually associated with a problem in the posterior fossa.

Novak I, Morgan C, Adde L, et al. Early, accurate diagnosis and early intervention in cerebral palsy: advances in diagnosis and treatment. *JAMA Pediatr.* 2017;171(9):897.

4. What is the gross motor function classification system (GMFCS)?

The GMFCS is used to classify the mobility of people with CP and allows for more universal descriptions when discussing function of people with CP. Interrater reliability is highest when used to classify the gross motor function of children 2 to 12 years old. This is a *five-level classification* with best function at I and least capability at V:

I. Ambulatory with no assistive device in the home and outdoors.
II. Ambulatory in most settings but may have difficulty on uneven terrain.
III. Walk using a handheld mobility device; requires wheelchair in the community.
IV. Requires wheelchair for household mobility.
V. Very limited movement even with the use of an adaptively controlled power wheelchair.

There are similar classifications for upper extremity function (Manual Ability Classification System, or MACS), language (Communicative Function and Classification System or CFCS), and feeding.

Palisano R, Rosenbaum P, Walter S, et al. Development and reliability of a system to classify gross motor function in children with cerebral palsy. *Dev Med Child Neurol.* 1997;39:214.

5. Will the child walk?

The best gauge of how a child will do is how they are doing currently. *Head control* by 9 months and *sitting balance* at age 2 are positive indicators of future walking. Bleck listed seven *primitive reflexes* and found that a child whose response was abnormal for two of these reflexes by age 12 months had a poor prognosis for walking. These are:

Should Be Absent	*Should Be Present*
Asymmetric tonic neck reflex	Parachute reaction
Symmetric tonic neck reflex	Foot placement
Moro response	
Neck righting reflex	
Extensor thrust	

Walking in these studies includes use of a walker or crutches. Absence of certain comorbidities associated with CP are also positive predictors for ambulation. These include an absence of visual impairment, intellectual disability, and epilepsy.

Bleck EE. *Orthopedic Management of Cerebral Palsy.* London: Mac Keith; 1987.

Keeratisirog O, Thawinchai N, Siritaratiwat W, et al. Prognostic predictors for ambulation in children with cerebral palsy: a systematic review and meta-analysis of observational studies. *Disabil Rehabil.* 2018;40(2):135.

6. How does CP gait look?

Children with hemiplegia will *toe walk* with plantar flexion and excess knee flexion on the involved side and their involved arm held in flexion synergy. Diplegic children often have bilateral *equinovarus* deformity, *knees that are flexed and in valgus*, and *"scissoring"* (feet crossing in front of each other with each step). With time, the gait may transition to a crouched pattern with the feet in excessive dorsiflexion and knees and hips flexed. Rotational problems, including *femoral anteversion* and *tibial torsion*, will often cause internal rotation of the feet.

7. Is CP associated with intellectual and behavioral impairments?

Not necessarily. CP covers a wide spectrum of clinical presentations. Many children have normal to above normal cognition, while others are severely impaired. Cognitive impairments include language delays, perceptual-motor deficits, and attentional deficits, and are reported in approximately 30% to 75% of children with CP. Learning disorders, psychosocial behavioral issues, and psychiatric impairments (including autism spectrum symptoms) are more common in children with CP and must be addressed to promote academic success and emotional/behavioral development.

8. How can schools help?

Parents should obtain early intervention services for the child. The law requires that every state provide education for every child, with appropriate services for children with special needs. Parents should contact their school district, inform them that they have a child with special needs, and have their child evaluated. The family will have an Individual Family Service Plan (IFSP) if the child is less than 3. These children generally receive physical or occupational therapy weekly through early intervention services. If the child is older than 3, an IEPC (Individual Education Planning Committee) with the school staff is created and determines the child's service eligibility.

9. Should you be concerned about seizures?

Many children with CP have seizures. Children with spastic quadriplegia are most prone, followed by those with spastic hemiplegia. There is no need for a baseline electroencephalogram (EEG); evaluation and management can wait until there are symptoms.

10. What about sleep?

Sleep disturbances are common in children with CP. Compared to age-matched controls; children with severe CP had more apneas and hypopneas per hour of sleep, resulting from fewer body position changes, macroglossia, glossoptosis, and aspiration from gastroesophageal reflux. There may also be a primary disturbance in sleep organization due to brainstem dysfunction. Sleep logs and actigraphy may be helpful to those with sleep onset insomnia and circadian rhythm abnormalities. Melatonin, given 30 to 60 minutes before bed, may be very useful in conjunction with an established calming bedtime routine. Nocturnal polysomnography is critical to evaluating sleep maintenance difficulties. The EEG segment can help distinguish epileptic and non-epileptic arousals.

Kotagal S, Gibbons VP, Stith JA. Sleep abnormalities in patients with severe cerebral palsy. *Dev Med Child Neurol.* 1994;36:304.

Stores, G., & Wiggs, L. (2001). Sleep Disturbance in Children and Adolescents with Disorders of Development. Cambridge University Press.

11. What kinds of visual problems occur?

Strabismus is a common problem in CP due to an imbalance in eye musculature. It is often treated with ophthalmologic surgery. *Hemianopsia* may be present with dense hemiplegia, with a middle cerebral artery lesion.

12. What problems does hypertonicity cause?

Spasticity is defined as a velocity-dependent resistance to stretch. It is a common manifestation of the upper-motor-neuron syndrome (decreased dexterity, hyperreflexia, spasticity, paralysis). *Dystonia* is a movement disorder in which involuntary sustained or intermittent muscle contractions cause twisting and repetitive movement, abnormal postures, or both. The most prominent findings in both are hypertonicity of the musculature and impaired motor control. Reducing spasticity improves motor control but does not normalize it; factors such as weakness, impaired coordination, and impaired sensation also play a role.

Spasticity can cause *contractures* secondary to muscle tightness, especially in the gastrocnemius-soleus group, hamstrings, adductors, hip flexors, biceps, wrist flexors, and opponens pollicus. *Hip dislocation* can occur due to tightness in hip flexors and adductors (see Question 13). *Scoliosis* or *lordosis* from spasticity and weakness is another frequently noted problem that may worsen rapidly as the child goes through a growth spurt (see Question 13). Spasticity can also cause difficulty with seating and interfere with caretakers' ability to perform transfers and other aspects of care.

Sanger TD, Delgado MR, Gaebler-Spira D, et al. Classification and definition of disorders causing hypertonia in childhood. Task Force on Childhood Motor Disorders. *Pediatrics.* 2003;111:e89.

13. What should be done about the hips?

Hip dislocation affects a third of children with CP but almost 90% of those with very high tone or CP with GMFCS Level V. In children with tight hip musculature, especially the adductors and hip flexors, the hips should be followed with plain x-rays on a schedule based upon GMFCS level. This includes yearly radiographs in Levels IV–V but less frequent at Levels I–III. Orthopedic procedures such as *adductor tenotomies* or *derotational osteotomies* help prevent dislocation. Surgical reduction of a dislocated hip is indicated for ambulatory children or for non-ambulatory children with pain or seating difficulties. In younger children, hip dislocation can lead to improper development of the hip joint and painful arthritis in young adulthood.

14. What should be done about the spine?

Occurrence of scoliosis increases with greater neurologic involvement, with an incidence of 60% in children with spastic quadriplegia. Scoliosis in CP progresses more rapidly and produces different curve patterns than idiopathic scoliosis. Hip dislocation and pelvic obliquity can contribute to worsening curves. Seating problems, pressure sores, and cardiopulmonary compromise are potential complications. Ambulatory children are managed with bracing and surgery (fusion, rod placement). Non-ambulatory children are often best managed with molded seating but may need other interventions as well.

15. **What should be done for other limbs and joints?**
Spasticity often leads to contracture, especially in muscles that cross two joints. Contractures worsen with growth, as bones grow faster than muscles. The main joints at risk are the ankles (plantarflexion) and flexion contractures at the knees, hips, elbows, and wrists. First-line treatment is repeated, gradual, sustained *stretching*. *Serial casting* and *orthoses* are used, especially for the ankles, knees, and elbows. Casting can be combined with nerve/motor point blocks (see Question 17). If these methods fail, *orthopedic surgery* is indicated for muscle and tendon lengthening. Muscles that are lengthened will lose about a grade of strength. As children grow, these interventions (including surgery) will need to be repeated.

16. **When should anti-spasticity medications be used?**
Oral anti-spasticity medications (**diazepam**, **baclofen**, **dantrolene**, **tizanidine**, etc.) are indicated for the treatment of *generalized spasticity*. They are useful in severely involved children to aid with hygiene and prevent mass extensor spasm. They are less commonly used in more functional children due to adverse effects. They may be used; see if the child might be a candidate for a rhizotomy or other more extensive interventions. Each drug has its own complications; diazepam, tizanidine, and baclofen are sedating; baclofen and dantrolene sodium cause hepatic problems (liver functions must be monitored); and baclofen can lower the seizure threshold.

17. **What are nerve/motor point blocks?**
Motor point/nerve blocks are indicated for *spasticity affecting specific muscle groups*. They are commonly done to decrease scissoring due to adductor spasticity, equinovarus foot deformity during gait, and hamstring, elbow flexor, or wrist/finger flexor tightness.

    Botulinum toxin injections lead to presynaptic inhibition of motor nerve function. Tone reduction peaks at 2 to 4 weeks after injection, and effects can persist 3 to 6 months. A variety of injection techniques are used, with some practitioners using EMG guidance, nerve stimulation, ultrasound or visually/anatomically locating motor points. The child's skin is commonly treated with **EMLA cream** (a mixture of lidocaine 2.5% and prilocaine 2.5%) or **ethyl chloride** spray for local anesthesia. **Sedation or general anesthesia** are used for younger children or more involved blocks. **Phenol** and, less commonly, **alcohol** are neurolytic, and effective for 3 to 6 months. The injection needle is used as a cathode for nerve stimulation, and amperage is reduced for precise localization. An aggressive stretching and motor reeducation program is indicated after block procedures.

18. **When is a rhizotomy indicated? What can it do?**
The selective dorsal rootlet rhizotomy is a neurosurgical procedure designed to decrease the excitatory input to the motor neuron, thereby decreasing spasticity. The procedure consists of a laminectomy and exposure of the cauda equina. The dorsal roots are electrically stimulated, and various criteria are used for determining which parts of the root contain more fibers involved with abnormal reflexes. The involved rootlets are then severed. This technique allows for decreased tone without sacrificing significant sensation.

    The ideal patient is a *young child (ages 3 to 8) with spastic diplegia, who is ambulatory with a spastic gait.* Generally, any child who could make significant functional gains if his or her spasticity were reduced could benefit as well as children with significant seating problems. Children with poor head and trunk control, and children who use spasticity for functional purposes (e.g., extensor spasms to stand) are less-classic candidates for the procedure. Many centers are performing rhizotomies for these children for spasticity reduction and improved care and comfort rather than other functional goals. After surgery, the children require extensive physical and occupational therapy programs to recover from postoperative weakness and to maximize functional gains. When discussing the surgery, parents should be given a good understanding of potential complications and realistic goals.

Dudley RWR, Parolin M, Gagnon, B, et al. Long-term functional benefits of selective dorsal rhizotomy for spastic cerebral palsy. *J Neurosurg Pediatrics.* 2013;12(2):142.

19. **When is the intrathecal baclofen (ITB) pump best used in patients with CP?**
The ITB pump is an electronic, programmable pump device that is implanted under the skin and connected to a catheter with its tip usually at T12 or higher so that it releases baclofen directly into the cerebrospinal fluid. ITB therapy is indicated in children with CP who have moderate to severe generalized spasticity and/or dystonia. It may be used in non-ambulatory or ambulatory children weighing more than 28 lb who have enough torso room for the pump and can maintain and refill it. In general, acceptance has been high by patients despite relatively high maintenance required for refilling and reprogramming the pump and managing complications. Common problems include CSF leaks, catheter kinks or breaks, infections (such as pump pocket infections and meningitis), pump programming errors leading to drug over- or under-dosage, and pump malfunction.

    Another unanticipated concern is that as the child grows, catheters may need to be replaced. Also, though insurance may cover the costs of ongoing maintenance of the ITB in children, as they age into adulthood they may encounter difficulty finding appropriate medical care, so a comprehensive approach does require that care through the life span be considered.

Winter G, Beni-Adani L, Ben-Pazi H. Intrathecal baclofen therapy–practical approach: clinical benefits and complication management. *J Child Neurol.* 2018;33(11):734.

20. When should I consult orthopedics? Neurosurgery?

The rhizotomy and baclofen pumps *decrease spasticity* but have no effect on shortened, contracted muscles. Orthopedic surgery can *lengthen muscles* and change the biomechanics of gait through tendon transfers but does not change the basic neurology. A combination of techniques is often required to gain greatest improvement in gait. Motion analysis laboratories for three-dimensional gait analysis are useful in determining appropriate interventions.

21. What's new in CP therapy?

In the past, strength training was considered bad for spastic musculature. However, there is now evidence that strengthening and resistive exercises result in improved gait patterns. Several new programs and treatment philosophies have emerged based on increased intensity of therapy. Some, like *conductive education*, require a short-term, but very intensive commitment by the family. The effectiveness of these programs is being investigated. *Hippotherapy* uses a horse as a tool in physical therapy; several beneficial effects have been suggested, and the programs are fun and motivate children. Newer technologies such as robotics are also gaining popularity for treating children, including using Lokomat technology for gait training.

Recently there has been a greater focus on therapy for the upper extremity. *Constraint-Induced Therapy (CIT)* techniques improve upper extremity function in children with hemiplegia. CIT, first used in adult stroke patients, involves restraining the less-involved extremity with a cast or splint and *mass practice* for the more involved side through an intensive therapy/activity program. *Bimanual Therapy* involves planned repeated practice of two-handed games and activities to improve use of a hemiplegic arm.

GAME (Goals–Activity–Motor Enrichment) is a motor-learning, environmental enrichment intervention done at home. This program is still being studied for infants 3 to 6 months old.

Novak I, McIntyre S, Morgan C, et al. A systematic review of interventions for children with cerebral palsy: state of the evidence. *Dev Med Child Neurol.* 2013;55:885.

22. What are ankle foot-orthoses (AFOS)?

AFOs aid in gait by controlling an equinus or equinovarus deformity. Articulated AFOs have an ankle joint and are capable of dorsiflexion. Some braces, called *ground reaction AFOs*, are designed to prevent crouching by producing a knee extension moment with anterior shin pressure during stance phase. They are effective only in the absence of significant knee or hip flexion contractures. For children with spasticity, AFOs are designed with features to decrease abnormal reflexes, including a foot plate that extends past the toe to discourage toe flexion and a metatarsal support to discourage stimulation to a particularly reflexogenic area of the foot. Non-ambulatory children wear AFOs prevent contracture and during supported standing.

23. What are some seating issues in CP?

The goals of seating are *proper postural alignment, comfort, and mobility.* Positioning should protect the joints and skin, support the trunk and pelvis to prevent deformity, and discourage abnormal reflexes. Extensor reflexes can be inhibited by keeping the hips, knees, and ankles at *a minimum of 90°.* Head support can discourage the asymmetric tonic neck reflex. Power chairs are important mobility devices for many children.

24. What oropharyngeal/swallowing problems accompany CP?

Children with CP may have difficulty with swallowing, speech, and drooling due to oral motor control problems. *Dysphagia* can lead to difficulty with adequate nutrition or aspiration. *Fiberoptic endoscopic evaluation of swallowing* (FEES) is a direct visualization technique that gives a better view of the sequence and timing of swallowing as well as the amount of residual food left with each swallow. Interventions include positioning, such as chin tuck, using the wheelchair head rest to control the head position, and dietary changes, usually involving soft foods over liquids and full solids. Swallowing evaluations are helpful in resolving conflicts between families and the school about safety and appropriateness of oral feeding. With severe aspiration or caloric need problems, a gastrostomy tube is indicated. If the aspiration is asymptomatic, placing a G-tube is somewhat controversial and less of an absolute indication.

Significant drooling problems are managed with **glycopyrrolate**, **scopolamine patches**, and **surgery** (realignment of the salivary ducts) in the most severe cases. **Botulinum toxin** injections into the salivary glands utilizing ultrasound guidance are also used as a safe alternative to manage severe drooling. The effect can last up to 24 weeks.

Jongerius PH, Rotteveel JJ, van Limbeek J, et al. Botulinum toxin effect on salivary flow rate in children with cerebral palsy. *Neurology.* 2004;63(8):1371–1375.

25. What are some of the growth and physical development problems that children with CP face?

Children with spastic quadriplegic CP are at high risk for poor growth and undernutrition. However, ambulatory children with CP face problems with obesity. Children with CP are at higher risk for osteopenia due to decreased weight bearing, poor oral intake, limited exposure to sunlight, and the concurrent use of anti-seizure medications (which interferes with absorption and metabolism of calcium and vitamin D).

26. How do I help kids who have communication problems?

Speech problems are often accompanied by spasticity, dystonia, decreased coordination, and choreoathetosis. Augmentative communication devices must compensate for lack of speed and accuracy. Special switches have been developed to improve access to technology, as well as software that allows for greater options with fewer demands for accurate keyboard use.

27. What other equipment should I consider?

Various ADLs may require specialized seating. There are *feeder seats, car seats, corner seats*, and *bath seats. Prone or supine standers* are used to encourage weight bearing and standing activities. If children have difficulty sleeping at night, a *supine lying orthotic* can position them more comfortably. Computers are important for school and recreation, and voice-activated devices open up new possibilities. An assisted technology assessment can aid with access problems. Specialty equipment may be commercially available or custom-modified. Adaptive bicycles are also available to accommodate children with CP.

28. Describe some adapted recreational options.

Most recreational activities can be adapted depending on the resources and willingness of the community. *Special Olympics* offers the child a way to participate in peer-level athletic competition. There are many adapted *horseback-riding programs*. Horseback riding can be recreational as well as therapeutic. Many communities offer adaptive recreation activities in a variety of sports, including basketball, hockey, soccer, rock climbing, archery, etc. *Computers* can open up many recreation opportunities. In today's world, a child who is severely impaired can interact on an even plane with others through the Internet.

29. What are some critical psychosocial issues to address?

Children with CP are at high risk for developing psychological and behavioral problems. Like other children with disabilities, they often have difficulties with peer interaction and other issues of social competence. Higher-functioning kids will have more awareness of disability with resultant adjustment issues. Vocational issues, long-term care concerns, advocacy training, and access to proper resources are all factors to be considered when managing a family with a child who has CP.

30. What issues do those with CP face as they become adults?

Life span with CP has improved. However, adults with CP have an increased risk of chronic diseases such as cardiovascular disease, musculoskeletal syndromes, and mental health conditions. Pain, fatigue, and early functional loss (sometimes called "early aging") are common. Teens and adults with CP have more health needs than their typically developing peers but have difficulty with access to specialists who are trained to address their needs. Employment, intimate relationships, and living independently are all less prevalent than in the general population. Greater support structure and better access to health care are important goals for improving the lives of adults with CP. Robotic technology, such as autonomous vehicles, offer new opportunities for independence.

Ryan JM, Allen E, Gormley J, et al. The risk, burden, and management of non-communicable diseases in cerebral palsy: a scoping review. *Dev Med Child Neur.* 2018;60(8):753.

31. What is the best thing I can say to the family?

A family needs to hear that there will be support for them down the road from their doctor and from their community. The physician should demonstrate this by listening to the family's concerns, providing medical information, and providing access to resources. They also need to know that CP has a wide spectrum of clinical presentations and functional prognoses, and that the effort they put in can make a difference in the final outcome.

BIBLIOGRAPHY

1. *American Academy for Cerebral Palsy and Developmental Medicine.* Available at: www.aacpdm.org (go to Resources, then Library).
2. Murphy, K. P., McMahon, M. A., & Houtrow, A. J. (2020). Cerebral Palsy. In Pediatric Rehabilitation: Principles and Practice (6th ed., pp. 319–347). Demos Medical.

CHAPTER 77

SPINAL DEFORMITY: RECOGNITION AND INTERVENTION

J. Christian Barrett, BSEng, Theresa J. C. Pazionis, MD, and Steven A. Stiens, MD, MS

Never confuse motion with action.

— Benjamin Franklin (1705–1790)

KEY POINTS

1. Large curves with limited pain typify **adolescent idiopathic scoliosis** (AIS), while significant pain and reduced function define **adult spinal deformity** (ASD).
2. **Spinal bracing** reduces spinal pain intensity and disability in spinal deformity.
3. Degenerative spinal stenosis is a **synchronous process**. Any lumbar presentation (e.g., neurogenic claudication) requires cervical surveillance for latent pathology.
4. **Spinal tumors metastasis** from breast, prostate, and lung (80%) instigates pathologic fractures, kyphotic deformity, and neural impingement.
5. Bowel/bladder dysfunction and peroneal numbness are hallmarks for **cauda equina syndrome** (CES). Surgical decompression within hours is required to prevent permanent "saddle anesthesia" and paralysis.
6. **Vitamin B$_{12}$** deficiency surveillance complements MRI imaging and electrodiagnostic evaluation of spinal impingement.
7. **X-ray** imaging: Static (standing) and dynamic (frontal and lateral bending) films of the entire spine (cervical through sacral) should be captured in both the coronal and sagittal planes.

1. What is spinal deformity?

The dynamic three-dimensional configuration of the spinal column is the foundation for the structural support, flexible motion, and safeguarding of the neural elements which network the entire human body.

Each vertebral element serves as a **structural anchor** tethered by skeletal muscles which maintain an upright posture to support the movements of the upper and lower extremities. **Flexible motion** is directed by the orientation plane of **zygapophyseal (facet) joints** which constrain dynamic forces of bending, rotation, and axial loading while simultaneously protecting the spinal cord and exiting nerve roots.

Facet alignment and segmental motion:

- **Cervical**: flexion, extension, lateral bending, and rotation
  - 45-degree coronal plane orientation
- **Thoracic**: lateral bending and rotation
  - 60-degree coronal plane orientation
- **Lumbar**: flexion and extension
  - 90-degree coronal plane orientation

Disruptions in functional performance of these structural, kinetic, and neural elements manifest across a broad spectrum of clinical presentations (clinically silent to severe disability and paralysis). These abnormalities of spinal alignment and structural configuration are collectively referred to as **spinal deformity**.

DEGENERATIVE SCOLIOSIS: CAUSES, SYMPTOMS, DIAGNOSIS, TREATMENT

Available at: https://www.hss.edu/conditions_degenerative-scoliosis-causes-symptoms-diagnosis-treatment.asp.

2. What spinal abnormalities can cause deformity?

Spinal structural alignment and curvature can be disrupted by many pathologic processes. Causes can be categorized as birth defects, traumatic injury, aging, prior surgery, or adolescent growth. Understanding these acquired, congenital, neuromuscular, or idiopathic mechanisms as **etiology** of the deformity is critical to maximizing treatment outcomes for each patient.

Idiopathic—80% of spinal abnormalities (adolescent and degenerative scoliosis) derive from yet unknown origins, often with insidious onset.

Congenital—embryological malformations of the vertebral spine. These geometric abnormalities can affect any region of the spine altering linear growth and local configuration:

- Incomplete formation—Hemivertebra (wedge/sharp angle in the spine).
- Failure of separation—Boney connectivity bridging adjacent segments prevents growth/elongation of spine.
- Compensatory curves—**Secondary curves** (opposite direction) balance body mass over the center of gravity.

Neuromuscular—mechanical deformation due to central discoordination of the muscle contraction or hypertonia. Weakness, spasticity, axonal, and muscular pathology interfere with postural stability and ambulation. Neuromuscular scoliosis is frequently more rapidly progressive.

- Cerebral palsy, spinal cord trauma, muscular dystrophy, spinal muscular atrophy, and **spina bifida** (congenital and neuromuscular).

Acquired—from a known causative agent, process, or event. Resulting in focal or segmental sequelae.

- High energy trauma
- Repetitive overuse activities
- Inflammatory or infections processes (osteoarthritis, inflammatory arthritis, or thyroid disease)
- Endocrine mineralization disorders (osteoporosis, Paget disease, diabetes)
- Metastasis of malignant neoplasms

Ailon T, Smith JS, Shaffrey CI, et al. Degenerative spinal deformity. *Neurosurgery*. 2015;77(suppl 4):S75–S91. doi:10.1227/NEU.0000000000000938. Available at: https://academic.oup.com/neurosurgery/article-abstract/77/suppl_1/S75/2453587?redirectedFrom=fulltext.

3. What are the strategies to use in ordering and reviewing plane x-ray studies?

Determining the true static imbalance of spinal deformity requires evaluation of **standing** and **lateral bending** X-ray imaging of the entire spine (cervical through sacral). Always utilize upright, full-spine X-ray radiographs in both the coronal and sagittal planes. Standing films demonstrate the effects of gravity and postural reaction to compensate for instability.

Comparative review of each set of films determines the specific contributions **coronal (scoliosis)** and **sagittal (kyphotic)** abnormalities have on the global spinal imbalances unique to each patient.

Takahashi T, Polly D, Martin CT. Full-spine radiographs: what others are reporting—a survey of Society of Skeletal Radiology members. *Skeletal Radiol*. 2019;48(11):1759–1763. doi:10.1007/s00256-019-03194-0. Available at: https://link.springer.com/article/10.1007/s00256-019-03194-0.

4. What is the significance of Cobb angle when assessing spinal deformity?

The most common measure of spinal deformity is **Cobb angle**. This geometric gage of **spinal curvature** is used to assess disease severity, classification, and risk progression, and to predict intervention outcome.

Originally developed to evaluate coronal deformities of **scoliosis** (lateral curves), it has been adapted to characterize sagittal plane deformities of **kyphosis** (forward curves), **lordosis**, (backward curves), and **pelvic tilt** (pelvic angulation).

To measure the Cobb angle:

- Identify the **most tilted** vertebra at the superior and inferior ends of the curve
- Trace one line **parallel** to the top edge of the superior vertebral body
- Trace a second line **parallel** to the bottom edge of the inferior vertebral body
- Two **perpendicular** lines are then drawn (at 90-degree angles to the first lines) so they intersect
- The angle formed above these **intersecting perpendicular lines** represents the **Cobb angle.**

COBB ANGLE MEASUREMENT

Available at: https://youtu.be/SXJvzQ0sxgI.

GNU Free Documentation License 1.2 it appears that Fig 77.1 should be on this line as it's current position does not appear contiguous with the section title s0065: "Cobb Angle Measurement"

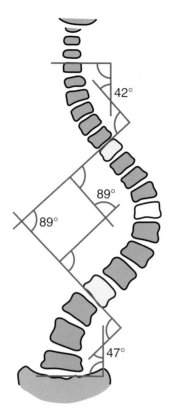

Fig. 77.1 Cobb angle measurement in scoliosis. Copyright © 2005 Skoliose-Info-Forum.de, Skoliose-Info-Forum.de. https://commons.wikimedia.org/wiki/File:ScoliosisF_cobb.svg.

5. What principles guide the use and evaluation of spinal imaging?

Selection of diagnostic imaging is determined by the pathology of interest, as each modality and technique uniquely depict bone, muscle, soft tissue, or continuous fluid spaces. Imaging is required for accurate and positive diagnosis of spinal deformity.

X-ray: Low-resolution radiological evaluation of bony structures (vertebra and joints). Full spine standing, flexion, and extensions views are captured to assess malalignments and curve progression, arthritic changes (bone spurs, joint space narrowing, sub-cortical cysts) fractures, or slippage between vertebrae.

Computed tomography scan (CT or CAT scan): High-resolution X-ray evaluation of the spinal canal (size, shape, contents) and focal change of adjacent boney structures due to infections, fractures, and tumors of the spine.

Magnetic resonance imaging (MRI): Extremely detailed imaging of soft tissue structures of the spine using powerful magnets to generate radio waves. Unlike with X-ray and CT, the spinal cord, nerves, ligaments, and intervertebral discs of the spine are clearly visible on a grey scale determined by water content. Subsequent computer processing "weights" characteristics unique to bone, muscle, and other water-rich tissues to selectively reveal pathologic processes or anatomical disturbances.

- **T1-weighted** images show the best anatomy, suppressing fluid-rich tissues (black) and enhancing muscle/fat (white).
- **T2-weighted** images are most sensitive to pathology, enhancing fluid (white) and suppressing muscle/fat (black).

In general, T1- and T2-weighted images can be easily differentiated by looking at the **CSF**. CSF is dark on T1-weighted imaging and bright on T2-weighted imaging.

Mnemonic: H_2O = **T2** imaging shows **WATER** brightness

Tilson ER, Strickland GD, Gibson SD. An overview of radiography, computed tomography, and magnetic resonance imaging in the diagnosis of lumbar spine pathology. *Orthopaedic Nurs.* 2006;25(6):415–420. Available at: https://www.researchgate.net/publication/ 6667312_An_Overview_of_Radiography_Computed_Tomography_and_Magnetic_Resonance_Imaging_in_the_Diagnosis_of_Lumbar_ Spine_Pathology.

6. Would you notice if your patients were hiding their deformities?

Clues for the "Spinal Sleuth":

- Hip/knee flexion (one or both)
- Unequal foot position
- Tilt or rotation of pelvis
- Neck hyperextension ("craning" increases lordosis)
- Sacral retroversion (sagittal plane X-ray) is prognostic for anterior kyphotic imbalance.

SCOLIOSIS IN ADULTS: SYMPTOMS, DIAGNOSIS, AND TREATMENTS

Available at: https://www.hss.edu/conditions_scoliosis-adults.asp.

7. What hints give you a "hunch" that scoliosis or kyphosis might be part of the problem?

Scoliosis is abnormal lateral deviation of the spine greater than 10 degrees from its natural alignment. These **"S"-shaped curves** most often "show up" with one shoulder higher than the other, or as compensatory pelvic shift to maintain postural balance while standing. Smaller curves are often unnoticed as they are disguised in dynamic posture.

- Pediatric patients respond best to bracing if diagnosed before puberty when the rapid growth spurt can significantly accelerate curve progression. Surgical intervention may be necessary once curves have progressed to **45 to 50 degrees**.
- Adult patients often seek treatment due to pain in their back, pelvis, or lower extremities. Postural imbalance or focal "bulges" of their back may accompany weakness and muscle spasms. Pain management and stabilization of deforming curves are the primary goals of intervention. Curves over 30 degrees may require surgical correction.

Kyphosis is a disproportionate forward curvature of the spine that measures greater than **50 degrees**. This excessive posterior convexity creates a "hunchback" appearance in the thoracic or lumbar spine and can significantly destabilize postural balance and gait.

- Postural and structural abnormalities of the spinal vertebra most often present in pediatric populations, whereas traumatic injury, **osteoporotic compression fractures,** and **junctional kyphosis** following previous spinal surgery are more often present in adult patients.

Scoliosis—"S"-shaped, coronal plane deformity greater than 10 degrees → most common in children/ adolescents.

Kyphosis—"C"-shaped, sagittal plane deformity less than 50 degrees → most common in adults (>65).

OSMOSIS: LORDOSIS, KYPHOSIS, AND SCOLIOSIS

Available at: https://youtu.be/DOi24AH5yiE.

8. How to recognize stenosis in degenerative spinal deformity?

Spinal stenosis is the narrowing of one or more spaces within the spinal column and can result in compression of the spinal cord or nerve roots. Symptomatic recognition can come with use provoking pain, or insidious loss of sensation, muscle mass, or pelvic floor function.

This narrowing most often occurs in the lumbar spine due to osteoarthritis and presents with **Neurogenic claudication**: intermittent pain or weakness of the lower extremities, hips, and lower back. These symptoms are most significant when walking or standing and are relieved when leaning forward or sitting.

While the lumbar spine is most often affected, degenerative spondylosis is a synchronous process which simultaneously affects the cervical spine. Any patient which presents with symptoms of lumbar stenosis should also be evaluated for cervical stenosis and associated neuromotor deficits/symptoms in the upper extremities.

- **Cervical stenosis** is insidious and may be signaled by bilateral intrinsic hand and muscle wasting, particularly the first dorsal interosseous muscle which may exhibit fasciculations.
- **Lumbosacral stenosis** encroaches in a "trifoil" pattern as bone spicules intrude on the spinal canal constructing the cauda equina.

Buckland AJ, Vira S, Oren JH, et al. When is compensation for lumbar spinal stenosis a clinical sagittal plane deformity? *Spine J.* 2016; 16(8):971–981. doi:10.1016/j.spinee.2016.03.047. Available at: https://www.thespinejournalonline.com/article/S1529-9430(16) 30017-1/fulltext.

Available at: https://pubmed.ncbi.nlm.nih.gov/27063925/.

9. How can spinal deformities put patients at risk for radiculopathy and myelopathy?

   Radiculopathy is irritation of a spinal nerve root associated with segmental radiation of pain, dermatomal sensory disturbance, isolated muscle weakness, and hyporeflexia. Impingement is usually at the intervertebral foramen. Compression resulting from disc herniation, spondylotic bone spurs and neoplastic disease (tumors) is generally isolated to a singular nerve root. However, polyradiculopathies can arise with multifocal pathology.

   Myelopathy is pathology of the spinal cord itself resulting in bilateral sensory and upper motor neuron syndrome. The subsequent numbness, decreases in dexterity, and weakness may progress to gait abnormalities and loss of bowel/bladder function. This can present acutely or with insidious progression. Sudden symptoms arise from extremes of range with spondylosis or rapid expansion of a spinal abscess, hemorrhage, or tumor. Progressive difficulty with tasks that require **fine motor skills** (difficulty with buttons or writing) are hallmarks of this disorder.

   Spinal alignment and surgical decompression of the neural elements is most effective to address these focal impingements and limit further progression and permanent injury. Diagnostic MRI imaging and vitamin B_{12} deficiency surveillance are essential to identify myelopathy, focus intervention, and support recovery by optimizing nutrient availability.

MYELOPATHY VERSUS RADICULOPATHY—

Available at: https://youtu.be/3Q-c107NEdY.

10. What is the role of electrodiagnosis when evaluating patients with spinal abnormalities?

    Electrodiagnoses is a set of physiologic assessments of nerve and muscle that can locate nerve impingement, detect the presence and location of muscular denervation, and establish chronicity of processes.

    Nerve conduction velocities compare speed of conductions through nerve segments to locate focal impingement and detect generalized neuropathy.

    Electromyography (EMG) records muscle potentials that reveal spontaneous depolarization after denervation, motor unit size to gauge chronic reinnervation, and recruitment as a measure of voluntary activation

    Somatosensory evoked potentials (SSEPs) are generated by repetitive stimulation of nerves or various dermatomes. Nerve depolarization waves from along the spine and the somatosensory centers of the brain are detected through the skin and averaged to measure latencies.

    Electrophysiological information complements history, examination, and imaging to characterize pathology and provide surveillance for complications, recovery, and progression.

Dr. Grant Performs EMG on 'The Doctors'. Available at: https://www.youtube.com/watch?v=WVsw4v6Ojng&t=98s.

11. How is Cauda Equina syndrome (CES) related to structural changes of the spine?

    CES is a rare, but serious, compromise of the spinal cord motor and sensory nerve roots as they descend from the conus medullaris (~L1–L2) to exit intervertebral and sacral foramina. Dysfunction of the **cauda equina** (Latin for "horse tail") resulting from significant compression or traumatic injury to the lumbar spine requires emergent surgical decompression to prevent permanent paralysis of the lower extremities and genitourinary organs.

    While early stages of CES may present with low back pain, motor weakness, and sensory deficits common to many disorders of the lumbar spine, peroneal numbness and bowel/bladder dysfunction (acute and chronic onset) serve as hallmark "red flags" in diagnosing CES.

Any patient who demonstrates these "red flag" symptoms should be immediately imaged and simultaneously referred for treatment as decompression within hours of symptom onset has demonstrated improved outcomes in continence, strength, and sensation.

Chau AM, Xu LL, Pelzer NR, et al. Timing of surgical intervention in Cauda Equina syndrome: a systematic critical review. *World Neurosurg.* 2014;81(3–4):640–650. doi:10.1016/j.wneu.2013.11.007. Available at: https://pubmed.ncbi.nlm.nih.gov/24240024/.

12. Which tumors metastasize to the spine? How can I remember them?

In the United States, around 350,000 people die each year with bone metastasis. As these neoplastic growths displace healthy bone, they weaken the structural integrity of the vertebral bodies and increase the risk for **pathologic fractures** and **neural impingement**.

Kyphotic deformity most often results due to vertebral collapse, producing debilitating pain and neurologic deficits. While minimally invasive surgical interventions are available to expand vertebral bodies, multiple modality palliative pain management is often the primary goal of therapeutic management for these patients.

Metastatic tumors are the most frequent tumors that involve the spine with 80% of tumors originating from the breast, prostate, and lung.

The memory mnemonic "**Lead Kettle**" (PB-KTL) can be used to remember tumors that metastasize to bone: **Mnemonic**
- **P:** prostate
- **B:** breast
- **K:** kidney
- **T:** thyroid
- **L:** lung

Primary benign spine tumors (osteoid osteoma, osteoblastoma, osteochondroma, giant cell tumor of the bone, aneurysmal bone cyst, eosinophilic granuloma, and neurofibroma) are more common than **primary malignant** ones (osteosarcoma, Ewing sarcoma, and chondrosarcoma).

Memorial Sloan Kettering Cancer Pain: *Introduction to Spinal Tumor Diagnosis and Classification and Review of Intradural Tumors.* Available at: https://www.mskcc.org/videos/introduction-spinal-tumor-diagnosis-and-classification-and-review-intradural-tumors.

13. How are spondylolysis and spondylolisthesis related?

Spondylolysis is a crack or stress-induced fracture affecting the **pars interarticularis** of the vertebra. Subsequent instability at this segment may result in a "slip" forward of the affected vertebral body, known as **spondylolisthesis.**

These injuries most frequently occur in adolescent athletes due to repetitive lumbar hyperextension in gymnastics, weightlifting, and contact sports. Microtears in muscle fibers and ligaments, stress to the tendon, and bruising of the bones of the posterior spine produce the adjacent segment translation seen in these overuse injuries. In adults, spondylolysis results from acute traumatic injuries and affects women (>50 years) most commonly.

Spondylolysis of the Lumbar Spine: Symptoms, Causes & Treatments (braceability.com). Available at: https://www.braceability.com/blogs/info/spondylolysis.

14. What are options for spondylolysis treatment?

Non-steroidal anti-inflammatory drugs (NSAIDs), physical therapy, bracing, and rest accelerate return to sport/daily activities by:
- Reducing pain
- Facilitating bone healing
- Decreasing pars interarticularis stress

When indicated, surgical management focuses on realigning the "slipped" vertebra and a fusion of the adjacent spinal segments via surgical instrument (screws/rods) and bone grafting.

Physical therapy exercise "dos and don'ts":

Highly effective: Core stability and stretching
- Pelvic tilt
- Partial curl
- Gluteal stretch
- Double knee to chest
- Quadruped arm/leg raise

Critical to avoid: Forceful, repetitive, or sustained hyperextension
- Heavy weightlifting
- Twisting or bending (golf, tennis)
- High impact activities (CrossFit, circuit training, running, basketball, etc.)

---

6 Best Spondylolisthesis Exercises, and 3 to Avoid. Available at: https://www.braceability.com/blogs/articles/spondylolisthesis-exercises.

Video Series: Exercises for Spondylolisthesis. Available at: https://www.spineuniverse.com/conditions/spondylolisthesis/video-series-exercises-spondylolisthesis.

15. When is bracing indicated for treatment of spinal deformity?

Pain reduction, deformity/alignment correction, and structural instability are clear indications for bracing, especially in acute traumatic spinal injury and whenever instability is suspected that may cause neurologic damage.

Pain:

Sagittal plane stabilization is correlated with pain reduction from ASD.
- **Hydraulic support** and **ROM reduction** (flexion, extension, rotation) compensate for muscle weakness, reduce stiffness, and facilitate healing. Bracing reduces progression and chance of further injury in degenerative spinal pathologies

Correction:

Large magnitude curves, as well as those presenting before the adolescent growth spurt, are associated with better outcomes when treated with pattern-specific scoliosis braces.
- Most often applied to coronal plane deformities common in adolescent idiopathic scoliosis (AIS).
- Adult patients with severe segmental **listhesis**, hypermobility, or rapidly progressive deformities benefit from both structural realignment and reduction in static muscular tone.
- Aggressive bracing may provide **perioperative traction** in preparation for the major surgical reconstructions often necessary to restore proper alignment.

Instability:

Ridged "three-point stabilization" to relieve anterior (sagittal plane) loading, encourage extension while limiting flexion, lateral bending, and rotation. This rigid support is preferential when treating severe pathologies:
- Kyphotic deformities (osteoporotic compression fractures, tumors, and osteomyelitis)
- High-energy trauma (MVA, high falls, gunshot)
- Post-surgical stabilization (bone healing and limit nerve irritation)

Limitations:
- Muscle atrophy in the setting of inactivity
- Failure to adopt corrective stabilizing muscle strength
- Epidermal irritation and breakdown
- Psychological addiction (use dependence)
- Patient compliance can drive outcomes

Weiss H-R, Turnbull D. In Bettany-Saltikov J, Kandasamy G, eds. *Brace Treatment for Adults With Spinal Deformities, Spinal Deformities in Adolescents, Adults and Older Adults.* IntechOpen; 2020. doi:10.5772/intechopen.92321. Available at: https://www.intechopen.com/books/spinal-deformities-in-adolescents-adults-and-older-adults/brace-treatment-for-adults-with-spinal-deformities.

16. How should clinicians assess symptoms in relation to the severity of spinal pathology?

Physical discomfort, **postural imbalance,** and **chronic pain** are often the main factors which drive ASD patients to seek treatment. They are often unaware of the relationship between their symptoms and structural deformities.

Pediatric and adolescent spine patients generally are **pain free** and remain **highly active** despite significant physical manifestations of their disease. However, traumatic or repetitive-use injuries can present with significant pain and structure instability in both patient populations.

Terran J, Schwab F, Shaffrey CI, et al. The SRS-Schwab adult spinal deformity classification: assessment and clinical correlations based on a prospective operative and nonoperative cohort. *Neurosurgery.* 2013;73(4):559–568. doi:10.1227/NEU.0000000000000012. Available at: https://academic.oup.com/neurosurgery/article/73/4/559/2417509.

17. How is the clinical database categorized and sorted for considerations of treatment design and prognosis?
- **Pain** characteristics as related to **structural deformities** and function
  - Is pain control sufficient to restore function?
  - Can multimodal rehabilitation maintain function and prevent secondary symptoms (short and long term)?

- Is minimally invasive surgery available after failed conservative management?
- Will spinal reconstruction surgery meet the primary goals of the patient?
- Spinal maturity as related to Cobb angle and curve location
  - Is the patient's spine still growing and changing?
  - How severe is the curve (Cobb angle)?
  - Are multiple curves present?
  - Is the primary deformity coronal or sagittal?
  - **Etiology** as risk for **progression**
  - Large curves present before adolescent growth spurt
  - Thoracic curves (scoliosis and kyphosis)
  - Post-operative junctional kyphosis
  - Failure of boney fusion and subsequent instrumentation breakdown

18. How do you "align" treatment with patient expectations of prognosis?
    - Provide an explanation of the problem using terminology familiar to the patient
    - Consider providing pictures or views of X-rays
    - Reassure patients by clarifying/explaining malignant causes less likely
    - Link the symptoms and pathophysiology to proposed treatment and expected outcomes
    - Advanced treatments as compliance and adaptive habits are generated

---

Kim HJ, Yang JH, Chang DG, et al. Adult spinal deformity: current concepts and decision-making strategies for management. *Asian Spine J.* 2020;14(6):886–897. doi:10.31616/asj.2020.0568. Available at: https://www.asianspinejournal.org/journal/view.php?doi= 10.31616/asj.2020.0568.

BIBLIOGRAPHY

Acaroglu E, European Spine Study Group. Decision-making in the treatment of adult spinal deformity. *EFORT Open Rev.* 2017;1(5):167–176. doi:10.1302/2058-5241.1.000013. Available at: https://pubmed.ncbi.nlm.nih.gov/28461944/. https://online.boneandjoint.org.uk/doi/full/10.1302/2058-5241.1.000013.

Buckland AJ, Vira S, Oren JH, et al. When is compensation for lumbar spinal stenosis a clinical sagittal plane deformity? *Spine J.* 2016; 16(8):971–981. doi:10.1016/j.spinee.2016.03.047. Available at: https://www.thespinejournalonline.com/article/S1529-9430(16) 30017-1/fulltext. https://pubmed.ncbi.nlm.nih.gov/27063925/.

Özyemişci Taşkıran Ö. Rehabilitation in adult spinal deformity. *Turk J Phys Med Rehabil.* 2020;66(3):231–243. doi:10.5606/tftrd.2020.6225. Available at: https://www.ncbi.nlm.nih.gov/pmc/articles/PMC7557622/.

WEBSITES

1. *Society on Scoliosis Orthopaedic and Rehabilitation Treatment (SOSORT): Orthopaedic and Rehabilitation Treatment of Idiopathic Scoliosis During Growth.* Available at: https://scoliosisjournal.biomedcentral.com/articles/10.1186/s13013-017-0145-8.
2. North American Spine Society—Clinical Guidelines. Available at: https://www.spine.org/Research-Clinical-Care/Quality-Improvement/Clinical-Guidelines.
3. Scoliosis Research Society. Available at: https://www.srs.org/.
4. American Association of Neurological Surgeons. Available at: https://www.aans.org/.
5. Pediatric Orthopaedic society of North America. Available at: https://posna.org/.
6. Setting Scoliosis Straight: Available at: https://www.settingscoliosisstraight.org/.

CHAPTER 78

JUVENILE IDIOPATHIC ARTHRITIS: CHILDREN CAN GET ARTHRITIS TOO

Roger Rossi, DO, Stephanie Chan, MD, Aakash Thakral, MD, and Sara J. Cuccurullo, MD

It always seems impossible until it's done

— Nelson Mandela (1918–2013)

KEY POINTS

1. Juvenile idiopathic arthritis (JIA) is multifactorial, classified into six subtypes, and characterized by onset less than the age of 16 and the presence of arthritis for more than 6 weeks.
2. Comprehensive treatment requires pharmacologic options including nonsteroidal anti-inflammatory drugs (NSAIDs), corticosteroids, methotrexate, and biologics; rehabilitation emphasizing range of motion (ROM), strength, flexibility, balance, and adaptive equipment; nutrition, calcium/vitamin D supplementation; and integrative medicine such as massage.

1. **What is juvenile idiopathic arthritis (JIA)?**
   JIA encompasses a collection of chronic pediatric arthropathies with onset before the age of 16 years and more than one joint for at least 6 weeks. Joint arthritis presents as swelling/effusion, warm, and limited movement with/without tenderness. Pain is the most common symptom. It is the most common chronic rheumatic disease in children, with prevalence of 1 in 1000.

2. **What are key features of the JIA subtypes?**
   International League of Associations for Rheumatology (ILAR) classification of JIA includes six subtypes: systemic arthritis, oligoarthritis, polyarthritis (RF [−]) and RF [+], enthesitis-related arthritis, psoriatic arthritis, and undifferentiated arthritis. The hallmark of all JIA subtypes is joint inflammation (Fig. 78.1).

3. **How many joints are involved in polyarticular JIA?**
   Polyarticular JIA involves more than five joints. Oligoarticular JIA involves less than four joints.

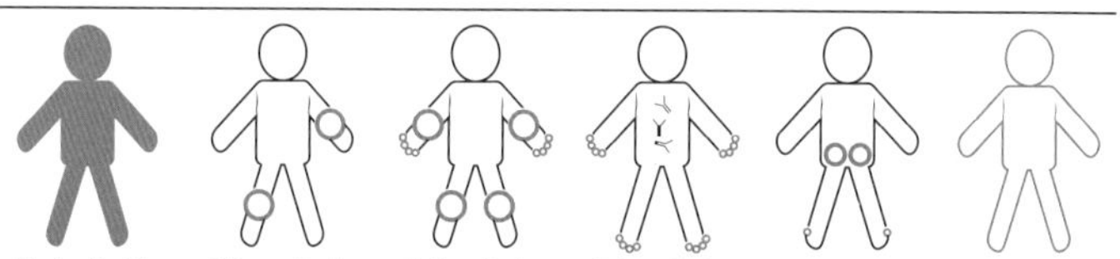

Subtype	Systemic JIA	Oligo articular JIA	Poly articular JIA RF⁻	Poly articular JIA RF⁺	Enthesitis related JIA	Psoriatic JIA
Characteristics	Spiking fever Rash Organomegaly Serositis MAS	≤4 joints affected Mainly large joints Asymmetric	≥5 joints affected Both large and small joints	≥5 joints affected Mainly small joints Erosive	Sacroiliac joints Enthesitis Positive family	Psoriasis Nail pits Dactylitis Positive family
Sex		Female pre-dominance	Female pre-dominance	Female pre-dominance	Male predominance	
Classifying biomarkers	MRP8/14 S100A12 IL-18	ANA⁺ (50%)	ANA⁺ (25%) RF (0%)	RF⁺ (100%) Anti-CCP (48%)	HLA-B27⁺ (85%)	ANA (50%)
Biomarkers for (subclinical) disease activity	MRP8/14 S100A12 IL-18	CRP ESR MRP8/14	CRP ESR MRP8/14	CRP ESR MRP8/14	CRP ESR	CRP ESR
Biomarkers for treatment response		MRP8/14 S100A12	MRP8/14 S100A12	MRP8/14 S100A12		

Fig. 78.1 Characteristics and biomarkers for juvenile idiopathic arthritis (*JIA*) subtypes. (Adapted from Swart J, de Roock S, Prakken B. Understanding inflammation in juvenile idiopathic arthritis: how immune biomarkers guide clinical strategies in the systemic onset subtype. *Eur J Immunol*. 2016;46:2068–2077, Table 1, p. 2070.)

4. How is JIA different from adult rheumatoid arthritis?
   Affected children have more systemic involvement, tenosynovitis, later erosive disease, more ulnar deviation at the wrist with loss of extension, more cervical spine involvement, and more likelihood of being ANA (+) and RF (−).

5. What joint complications occur in JIA? How do you protect these joints?
   See Table 78.1.

6. What laboratory results support the diagnosis of systemic JIA?
   Systemic JIA has lab evidence of systemic inflammation, including leukocytosis, thrombocytosis, anemia due to chronic inflammation, elevated CRP, and potentially elevated D-dimer or ferritin.

Table 78.1 Common Joints Involved in Juvenile Idiopathic Arthritis, Complications, and Protection Mechanisms

JOINT	COMPLICATIONS	PROTECTION MECHANISMS
Cervical Spine	• Atlantoaxial joint subluxation • Painful cervical flexion	• Avoid prolonged cervical flexed positions • Cervical collars can relax posterior cervical musculature • Adjusting chair/table heights for proper ergonomics • Active range of motion (AROM) exercises promoting extension and rotation • Prone lying to prevent flexion contractures • Spinal extension exercises
Temporomandibular Joint (TMJ)	Micrognathia (undersized jaw)	• Holding mouth slightly open and biting big morsels to increase jaw strength
Shoulder	Loss of abduction and internal rotation	• Keep in neutral position • Avoid sitting in soft armchairs, which promotes a flexed, internally rotated shoulder
Elbow	Decreased functional ROM (≥90% flexion needed for most activities of daily living (ADLs))	• AROM exercises • Resting night splints • Hold arms in full extension when sitting/standing • Extensor muscle strengthening • Check for ulnar entrapment neuropathy caused by synovitis and rheumatoid nodules
Wrist	Radiocarpal joint extension and ulnar deviation	• Night/daytime splints
Hand	• Swan-neck deformity (flexion of metacarpophalangeal (MCP), hyperextension proximal interphalangeal (PIP) joint, flexion distal interphalangeal (DIP) joint) • Boutonniere deformity (hyperextension MCP, flexion PIP, hyperextension DIP) • Decreased grip strength and ability to maintain handwriting	• Resting hand and ring splints
Hip	Flexion contractures with internal rotation and adduction	• Sleeping prone • Stretch and strengthen extensor muscles • Traction when hip flexion contracture is reduced to 10–15 degrees
Knee	Pain, weakness, flexion contracture	• Straight leg raises with foot in external rotation helps maintain medial quadriceps strength • Resting night splints • Activities including swimming, going up and down stairs, and kicking a ball
Ankle/Foot	Flat foot gait due to metatarsophalangeal joint pain	• Ankle stretching and casting can improve ROM • Picking up items on the floor with intrinsic foot muscles • Shoes with arch support and slightly raised heels

7. **What are common imaging findings for inflammatory joint disease? What features are specific to children?**
Findings common in adults and children include soft tissue swelling, joint effusion, periarticular osteopenia, erosions, synovitis, and bone edema. Features specific to children include epiphyseal growth disturbances, premature physeal fusion, limb length inequality, and abnormal periosteal reaction (Table 78.2).

8. **What is a common extra-articular manifestation of JIA?**
The most common extra-articular in JIA is chronic anterior uveitis. Although usually asymptomatic, early referral to ophthalmology and follow-up are recommended for all newly diagnosed JIA patients.

9. **How is temporomandibular joint (TMJ) arthritis managed in JIA?**
TMJ arthritis complicates 40% to 96% of cases. MRI with/without contrast is the preferred imaging modality. Intraarticular (IA) corticosteroids have short-term effectiveness, however, long-term safety remains uncertain. Other options to prevent long-term effects include arthrocentesis, splints, biologic therapies, and surgery.

10. **What pharmacologic agents are used for JIA?**
NSAIDs used in children include ibuprofen, naproxen, and tolmetin. Corticosteroids and IA steroid injections are helpful, especially for oligoarticular JIA. Methotrexate (MTX) is first-line treatment in oligoarticular disease and polyarticular disease that persists despite NSAIDs and steroid therapy. Baseline CBC, serum Cr, LFTs, and urinalysis are monitored. Tumor necrosis factor (TNF) inhibitors require yearly tuberculosis screening. If at risk for hepatitis B and C, individuals should be screened prior to MTX and TNF inhibitor administration.

11. **Why is folic acid recommended for those who take MTX?**
MTX can decrease folate levels, which can lead to RBC abnormalities and anemia.

12. **What is the prognosis and mortality rate for JIA?**
At least 50% of children with JIA have risk of arthritis as adults. Children with systemic JIA unresponsive to therapy have worse prognosis compared to those who achieve symptom and disease control; however, prognosis has greatly improved due to advances in biologics. Overall mortality rate is low in children with systemic JIA, but in children with more severe disease and in adults, the mortality risk is higher.

13. **How does JIA affect gait?**
Limitations of lower limb function in JIA can cause a crouch-like gait pattern, reduced walking speed, and restricted push-off phase, especially with bilateral symmetrical lower limb arthritis.

14. **What assistive devices are utilized in JIA?**
Lightweight wheelchairs, angled cups for children with cervical stiffness, clothes with Velcro closures, padded spoons, extended comb handles, and shoehorns are utilized to assist with ADLs.

15. **What should a therapeutic exercise program include for JIA?**
It should include positioning, aquatic exercises, and isometric exercises. Swimming and tai chi are recommended over sporting activities since overuse of ankles may promote injury. Aerobic exercises should be moderate in intensity and last less than 30 minutes per day. Intensive aerobic exercises followed by stretching (10-second hold, 20-second relax) improve ROM. In acute disease with severely inflamed joints, splinting is used to produce immobilization with twice daily full and slow passive range of motion to prevent soft tissue contracture.

16. **How is splinting utilized in JIA?**
Resting splints position and rest the joint in extension. Customized splints are more effective than ready-made splints. Dynamic splints are used for limited time to achieve a therapeutic target. Functional splints are protective

Table 78.2 Imaging for Juvenile Idiopathic Arthritis With Benefits/Limitations

	PROS	CONS
X-ray	• Helpful to evaluate changes in symptoms/management	• Limited role in assessment
Ultrasound	• Can demonstrate subclinical synovitis and enthesitis • Portability	• Anatomic knowledge of sonographic changes over time, immunopathophysiology, standardization, and validation under investigation
CT	• Can evaluate cervical facet joints • Cone-beam CT helpful in temporomandibular joint	• High dose radiation
MRI	• Most complete imaging analysis • Assesses extent of synovitis • Reliably depicts early erosive disease	• Cost • May be difficult to perform

during activity. Ankle-foot orthoses (AFOs) improve load distribution in the foot. Serial casting is recommended for contractures. Casts should remain on for at least 23 hours, be removed at 24- to 48-hour intervals, followed by aggressive 20-minute stretching.

17. How does therapeutic heat and cold affect joints and muscles in JIA?
Heat can decrease joint rigidity, increase joint capsule and tendon flexibility, and decrease muscle spasm and pain. Optimum temperature is 40°C to 45.5°C. Hot showers can alleviate morning stiffness and evening baths may control pain. Ultrasound-generated deep heat may be useful, but there is concern that it can affect the growth plate in children. Cold treatment may be beneficial for analgesia and vasoconstriction in inflamed joints.

18. What is the role of diet in JIA?
Foods such as tea, coffee, gluten, fructose, diet soda, roasted peanuts, and soybean products produce advanced glycation end-products and glycated lipids which form free radicals that may worsen intestinal permeability via inflammation. Elimination diets for autoimmune diseases show occasional symptom improvement. There is some value to a trial of 6-food elimination diet (cow's milk, soy, wheat, egg, peanut/tree nuts, and seafood) with nutrient supplementation.

19. What vitamins should be supplemented in JIA?
Patients with JIA are at a high risk for osteoporosis due to decreased physical activity and systemic steroids. Calcium intake ≥1000 mg/day through food and supplementation is recommended. If deficient in 25-hydroxy vitamin D, children should be supplemented via food, vitamin D2/D3, and sunlight exposure.

20. What are the uses of natural health products in JIA?
The yellow pigment curcumin—found in the spice turmeric—has antioxidant, anti-inflammatory, and antiproliferative effects, which may reduce inflammation and intestinal permeability. Glutamine also has similar beneficial effects. Certain bacterial strains can positively affect intestinal mucosa and gut immunity.

21. What recommendations are there for modalities such as massage, exercise, and acupuncture?
Massages decrease pain, serum cortisol levels, anxiety, and morning stiffness in JIA compared to progressive muscle relaxation. Exercising three times per week for 12 weeks with core exercises, jumping rope, and free weights increases leg strength, bone health, and mental health in JIA. Benefits of acupuncture remain inconclusive in JIA.

RECOMMENDED READINGS

1. Beukelman T, Patkar NM, Saag KG, et al. 2011 American College of Rheumatology recommendations for the treatment of juvenile idiopathic arthritis: initiation and safety monitoring of therapeutic agents for the treatment of arthritis and systemic features. *Arthritis Care Res (Hoboken)*. 2011;63:465–482.
2. Cakmak A, Bolukbas N. Juvenile rheumatoid arthritis: physical therapy and rehabilitation. *South Med J*. 2005;98:212–216.
3. Cavallo S, Brosseau L, Toupin-April K, et al. Ottawa panel evidence-based clinical practice guidelines for structured physical activity in the management of juvenile idiopathic arthritis. *Arch Phys Med Rehabil*. 2017;98:1018–1041.
4. Dimitriou C, Boitsios G, Badot V, et al. Imaging of juvenile idiopathic arthritis. *Radiol Clin North Am*. 2017;55:1071–1083.
5. Farr S, Girsch W. The hand and wrist in juvenile rheumatoid arthritis. *J Hand Surg Am*. 2015;40:2289–2292.
6. Guillaume S, Prieur AM, Coste J, et al. Long-term outcome and prognosis in oligoarticular-onset juvenile idiopathic arthritis. *Arthritis Rheum*. 2000;43:1858–1865.
7. Kuntze G, Nesbitt C, Whittaker JL, et al. Exercise therapy in juvenile idiopathic arthritis: a systematic review and meta-analysis. *Arch Phys Med Rehabil*. 2018;99(1):178–193.
8. Merker J, Hartmann M, Haas JP, et al. Analysis of impaired gait dynamics in children with juvenile idiopathic arthritis and symmetrical lower limb joint involvement requires combined three-dimensional gait analysis and pedobarography. *Gait Posture*. 2016;49:185.
9. Ringold S, Weiss PF, Beukelman T, et al. 2013 update of the 2011 American College of Rheumatology recommendations for the treatment of juvenile idiopathic arthritis: recommendations for the medical therapy of children with systemic juvenile idiopathic arthritis and tuberculosis screening among children receiving biologic medications. *Arthritis Rheum*. 2013;65:2499–2512.
10. Rodríguez-García A. The importance of an ophthalmologic examination in patients with juvenile idiopathic arthritis. *Reumatol Clin*. 2015;11:133–138.
11. Rossi R, Alexander M, Eckert K, et al. Pediatric rehabilitation. In Cuccurullo SJ, eds. *Physical Medicine and Rehabilitation Board Review*. 3rd ed. Philadelphia, PA: Demos Medical; 2015:733–829.
12. Stoll ML, Kau CH, Waite PD, et al. Temporomandibular joint arthritis in juvenile idiopathic arthritis, now what? *Pediatr Rheumatol*. 2018;16:1–14.
13. Swart J, de Roock S, Prakken B. Understanding inflammation in juvenile idiopathic arthritis: how immune biomarkers guide clinical strategies in the systemic onset subtype. *Eur J Immunol*. 2016;46:2068–2077.

CHAPTER 79

GERIATRIC REHABILITATION: MAINTAINING RESILIENCE, SUSTAINING PASSIONS, AND CULTIVATING VIBRANCY

Steven A. Stiens, MD, MS, Naheed Asad-Van de Walle, MD, Jeffrey Lehman, MD, Levi Atanelov, MD, MS, James P. Richardson, M.D., M.P.H., and Mark A. Young, MD, MBA, FACP, FAAPMR, DABPMR

The longer I live, the more beautiful life becomes.

— Frank Lloyd Wright (1867–1959)

KEY POINTS

1. Physical aging is a genetically driven process that is ameliorated by maintaining sustained exercise demands with regular activity and a nutrition-rich diet for ideal weight, primary prevention of disease, minimizing complications, and adaptive functional enablement despite impairments.
2. The aging process can be divided into primary (endogenous; intrinsic phenotypic programming), secondary (exogenous) diseases, and tertiary organ system decline.
3. Medical interventions are focused at minimizing aging gene expression, prevention, and pathophysiology interruption of disease processes and maximizing organ system function to sustain resilience.
4. Rehabilitation aligns with aged patients' needs and includes comprehensive geriatric assessment to address all problems with a comprehensive care plan with referrals as indicated to maximize health span.
5. Interdisciplinary rehabilitation elicits patient life passions, facilitates family and community contributory roles, and encourages depth of relationships and sensitivity.

1. **What are the current trends in the growth of the world's aged population?**
   By 2050, 1 in 6 people will be older than 65 years, up from 1 in 11 in 2019. From 2019 to 2050, the percentage of elderly will increase from 9% to 16% of the world's population. Most growth is expected among the "oldest-old" (i.e., >85).

United Nations. *Population Division.* 2019. Available at: https://www.un.org/development/desa/pd/.

2. **What challenges face the physician treating chronic diseases in the elderly?**
   Chronic conditions are usually preceded by a ***prolonged latent*** or ***preclinical phase*** and develop over several years (Alzheimer disease, osteoarthritis, cardiovascular disease). Given the heterogeneity of the aging population, screening is problematic. Data suggest that preclinical changes in function are the strongest predictors of functional decline. Underlying risk factors, pathophysiologic mechanisms, and maximal performance must all be addressed. Table 79.1 gives three broadly used definitions of healthy aging.
   An ***interdisciplinary team for geriatric assessment*** is the recommended approach because of the often-complex needs encountered among older people. The goal of such teams is to intensively assess older adults who require the skills and experience of several disciplines working together. Teams have the capacity to assess patients in much greater depth, and patients are able to share different kinds of information with different providers. The makeup of the team can vary according to the needs of the patient populations.
   This approach also benefits the physiatrist by involving other specialties that use physical performance measures. For example, the concept of frailty can involve the fields of cardiology, oncology, and surgery because all use gait speed as a means of assessing risk and making decisions regarding care. A team can therefore enhance the physical medicine and rehabilitation (PM&R) physician's outlook and vision about care based on input received from other medical specialties and subspecialties.

Bean JF, Orkaby AR, Driver JA. Geriatric rehabilitation should not be an oxymoron: a path forward. *Arch Phys Med Rehabil.* 2019; 100(5):995–1000. Available at: https://www.sciencedirect.com/science/article/pii/S000399931930084X?via%3Dihubdoi:10.1016/j.apmr.2018.12. 038.

Table 79.1 Results of Aging[a] Beyond Oneself

DECADE	CONCEPTS	OBJECTIVES	OUTCOME
?	Generosity	Family, Charitable giving	Reexpress values
?	"Giving back"	Community enrichment	Focused volunteerism
?	Legacy	Memoir, Digital social networks	Physical/visual/aural records
?	Sharing	Planned giving	Directed gifts
2020s	Digital presence	Databases to augment intelligence	Interactive presence after death

[a]Aging is a process of human development that needs to be creatively addressed with rehabilitation principles to overcome limitations of disability time, and space. This table uses terms from the literature, media, and clinical practice pertinent to care design.

3. What differentiates strategies for primary, secondary, and tertiary aging prevention, disease prevention, and impairment compensation?

Primary prevention aims at stopping the disease before it starts by reducing or eliminating risk factors using *vaccinations* and *chemoprophylaxis*, such as anticoagulation. Health promotion aims to identify health problems for which preventive measures can result in the more appropriate utilization of health services and improvements in health status. This approach emphasizes *behavioral* and *lifestyle changes* to maintain an optimum state of physical health and mental well-being.

Secondary prevention aims to detect and treat disease and its complications in early stages. *Tertiary prevention* aims to decrease the severity and duration of a disease and its potentially disabling sequelae, *reduce complications* from the disease to *minimize suffering*, and help the individual *adjust* to permanent impairments.

Fried LP. Epidemiology of aging. *Epidemiol Rev.* 2000;221:95–106. Available at: https://academic.oup.com/epirev/article/22/1/95/437017/. doi:10.1093/oxfordjournals. epirev.a018031.

National Research Council Panel on Statistics for an Aging Population, Gilford DM, ed. *The Aging Population in the Twenty-First Century: Statistics for Health Policy.* Washington, DC: National Academies Press; 1988. Available at: https://www.ncbi.nlm.nih.gov/books/NBK217737/.

Table 79.2 Evolution of Conceptual Definitions of Healthy Aging

CONCEPT	DECADE	OBJECTIVE	EXAMPLE OF OUTCOME
Longevity	1980s	Avoid disease	Fewer diagnoses
Safety/independence	1980s	Maintain physique	Home maintenance
"Use it or lose it"	1980s	Cognitive sharpness	Social performance
Downsizing	1990s	Emphasize essentials	Vital needs met
Strategic planning	1990s	Prioritize goals	Personal preferences set
Reinforcing	1990s	Practicing skills	Specific abilities retained
Enriching	1990s	Acquiring new skills	Practical aspirations met
Adaptive techniques	1990s	Compensating behaviors	Accomplish in new ways
Adaptive equipment	1990s	Utilize assistive devices	Safety, endurance
Whole system optimization	2000s	Maximize situation	Synergize methods
Building resilience	2000s	Active, healthy aging	Strength/mindset for living
"Aging in place"	2000s	Home accessibility	Extended full use
Optimizing opportunities	2010s	Selective planning	Focused participation
Enhance quality of life	2010s	Enhance experiences	Enjoyment, satisfaction
Health span	2010s	Sustained participation	Longer use of abilities
Generativity	2010s	Sharing philosophy	Self-translating to others

Adapted from Michel JP, Sadana R. "Healthy Aging" Concepts and Measures. *J Am Med Dir Assoc.* 2017;18(6):460-464. doi:10.1016/j. jamda.2017.03.008.

Table 79.3 Interventions to Foster Healthy Aging[a]

AREA	Level		
	1° PREVENTION	2° PREVENTION	3° PREVENTION
Promote health, prevent injury, and manage chronic conditions	Practice healthful, balanced nutrition. No tobacco. No recreational drugs or excess alcohol. Use good sleep hygiene. Keep ideal body weight. Use good oral hygiene. Control stress.	Control hypertension. Monitor lipid level. Treat diabetes. Treat ischemic heart disease.	Use rehabilitation services. Use adaptive equipment. Palliative care, when needed. Avoid effects of polypharmacy.
Maximize cognitive health	Lifelong learning and intellectual activities.	Detect sensory impairment early. Provide caregiver education.	Change community and/or modify environment.
Maximize physical performance	Appropriate calcium and vitamin D intake Routine physical activity (aerobic, resistance, balance).	Fall prevention programs. Osteoporosis screening and treatment, if needed. Dental exams. Osteoarthritis monitoring.	Rehabilitation technologies. Adaptive equipment/ mobility aids. Environmental safety, accessibility.
Maximize mental health	Get enough sleep. Avoid substance abuse. Do meaningful work. Have enriching social activities Seek life's purposes.	Accessible mental health services. Effectively manage mental health disorders. Reduce stigma over mental health.	Screen for elder abuse. Readily available family and social supports. Safety services for seniors.
Pursue social engagement	Create meaningful relation- ships with those who share interests. Pursue civic and spiritual involvement. Able to meet safety, financial, and housing needs.	Education and planning for social networking. Support variety and depth of relationships.	Access to adaptive equipment. Appropriate and safe environment. Personally empowering community outreach.

Adapted from Friedman SM, Mulhausen P, Cleveland ML, et al. Healthy aging: American Geriatrics Society white paper executive summary. *J Am Geriatr Soc.* 2019;67(1):17–20. doi: 10.1111 /jgs.15644.

4. What is the relationship between primary and secondary aging?

Primary (endogenous) aging is a gradual intrinsic process of deterioration that takes place throughout life primarily due to phenotypic programmed biological factors. This leads to age-related changes in vision, graying hair, loss of melatonin, and loss of skin elasticity and wrinkles. However, lifestyle choices such as prolonged exposure to the sun, sedentary habits, and unhealthy dietary choices can accelerate this process and associated morbidities.

Secondary (exogenous) aging occurs as a result of illness and disease. This type of aging is influenced by environmental factors or extrinsic factors such as dietary choices, exercise, smoking, and sanitation.

Tertiary aging processes represent aspects of terminal organ system decline. Mortality-related processes take over and influence changes occurring during the last years of life.

There is an interaction between primary and secondary aging. Although our DNA remains unchanged, gene expression can change. Environmental and lifestyle changes can impact biologic aspects of how we age and the three **lifespan stages: time lived, time disabled,** and **time left.**

Ram N, Gerstorf D, Fauth E, et al. Aging, disablement, and dying: using time-as-process and time-as-resources metrics to chart late-life change. *Res Hum Dev.* 2010;7(1):27–44. Available at: https://www.ncbi.nlm.nih.gov/pmc/articles/PMC3482431.

5. What role does multimorbidity play in various domains of disability (disablement)?

Multimorbidity is defined by the presence of two or more incurable long-term conditions (LTCs), managed with treatment. Multimorbidity is a significant predictor of functional capabilities and outcomes. Functioning and disability of an individual occur in a context, including environmental factors.

The *International Classification of Functioning, Disability, and Health* (ICF) relates to diagnoses, disease, and disability from new perspectives. ICF thus mainstreams the experience of disability, recognizing it as a universal human experience. **Shifting the focus from cause to impact** places all health conditions on an equal functional footing, allowing them to be compared using common metrics (i.e., the standards of health and disability).

Multimorbidity burden rather than specific patterns of multimorbidity is associated with poor performance in all three disability domains, body structure and function, activities, and participation among older adults at risk for disability. Multimorbidity counts may be an excellent tool for risk stratification and identification of those in need of rehabilitation.

Jacob ME, Ni P, Driver J, et al. Burden and patterns of multimorbidity: impact on disablement in older adults. *Am J Phys Med Rehabil.* 2020;99(5):359–365. doi:10.1097/PHM.0000000000001388.

Jette AM. Toward a common language for function, disability, and health. *Phys Ther.* 2006;86(5):726–734. Available at: https://academic.oup.com/ptj/article/86/5/726/2857468.

Yarnall AJ, Sayer AA, Clegg A, et al. New horizons in multimorbidity in older adults. *Age Ageing.* 2017;46:882–888. Available at: https://www.ncbi.nlm.nih.gov/pmc/articles/PMC5860018/.

6. How can differences in the aging process with disability offer opportunities for transformative intervention?

The history of recent care of people with disabilities has included new certified medical subspecialties and consensus on clinical practice guidelines guided by diagnostic and functional epidemiology. Immunization, infection prevention and early management, ventilatory support, reduction in chronic systemic inflammation, joint protection, and prevention of renal failure have all increased the lifespans and healthspans of people aging with disabilities.

Patterns of pathology for diagnostic groups and individual patients are complex and require clinical exploration of their full context and environment. Annual evaluations and screening tests are justified by the increased incidence of many conditions, including infection, hypertension, obesity, diabetes, skin breakdown, and osteoporosis. Although impairments are apparently static, their interactions between systems generate threats that must be addressed.

Aiello A, Farzaneh F, Candore G, et al. Immunosenescence and its hallmarks: how to oppose aging strategically? A review of potential options for therapeutic intervention. *Front Immunol.* 2019;10:2247. Available at: https://www.ncbi.nlm.nih.gov/pmc/articles/PMC6773825/. doi:10.3389/ fimmu.2019.02247.

7. What are the implications of aging for people with disabilities?
- *Vision*: Combined negative effect of cortical visual impairment in people with neurologic problems and age-related cataracts cause worsening of visual deficits.
- *Hearing*: Age-related sensorineural hearing loss combined with underlying conductive hearing deficits such as the propensity of conductive hearing loss in Down syndrome.
- *Taste and smell*: Age-related decline may lead to nutritional deficiencies in cognitively impaired individuals.
- *Somatosensory*: Loss of somatosensory function used in compensation threatens safety.
- *Immunity*: Immunosenescence increases infection and cancer risk, requiring early immunization and bioactive nutrition.
- *Neuromusculoskeletal system*: Changes in collagen associated with aging threaten flexibility leading to changes compounding disability.
- *Muscle strength*: Strength in antigravity muscles is affected most with normal aging, which can cause further functional limitations in patients with disabilities.
- *Posture*: worsening of existing scoliosis with aging further compromises ventilation capacity.
- *Cardiopulmonary*: Changes begin as early as age 24 in normal aging, with decreased lung compliance. Greater incidence of nonischemic heart disease was noted in persons with disabilities compared with age- and gender-matched peers in the general population.
- *Cognitive function*: Normal age-related changes in the brain include volume loss attributed to a decrease in the size of neurons. Changes also include loss of synapses and changes in neuronal structure. In persons with a history of traumatic brain injury (TBI) and cognitive deficits, even slow progression of cognitive decline may become clinically evident at an earlier age.

Jensen MP, Molton IR. Preface: aging with a physical disability. *Phys Med Rehabil Clin N Am.* 2010;21(2):253–450.

Klingbeil H, Baer HR, Wilson PE. Aging with a disability. *Arch Phys Med Rehabil.* 2004;85(7 Suppl 3):S68–S73. doi:10.1016/j.apmr.2004.03.014.

Strax TE, Luciano L, Dunn AM, et al. Aging and developmental disability. *Phys Med Rehabil Clin N Am.* 2010;21(2):419–427.

8. What factors lead to successful aging despite disability?
   - *Resilience*: Reserve capacity to adapt to new circumstances.
   - *Autonomy*: Ability to maintain self-efficacy and choice.
   - *Social connectedness*: Degree to which an individual meaningfully connects with friends, family, social environment, and others with similar disabilities.
   - *Physical health*: Reflected by a sense of wellness and access to health care services to improve or maintain health.

Cook KF, Molton IR, Jensen MP. Fatigue and aging with a disability. *Arch Phys Med Rehabil.* 2011;92(7):1126–1133. Available at: https://www.archives-pmr.org/action/showPdf?pii= S0003-9993%2811%2900130-4. doi:10.1016/j.apmr.2011.02.017.

Molton IR, Yorkston KM. Growing older with a physical disability: a special application of the successful aging paradigm. *J Gerontol B Psychol Sci Soc Sci.* 2017;72(2):290–299. Available at: https://academic.oup.com/psychsocgerontology/article/72/2/290/2632079. doi:10.1093/geronb/gbw122.

9. How is frailty treated?
   Many believe that frailty cannot be reversed and that the best approach is to *utilize a comprehensive geriatric approach*. However, a recent review article showed that *exercise* and *nutritional supplementation* are the most effective methods to delay or reverse frailty. Hormone supplementation and counseling were shown to be ineffective compared with exercise, nutritional supplementation, health education, *comprehensive geriatric assessment* (social supports, financial stability, living environment, medical conditions, mobility, balance, activities of daily living [ADLs], cognition, mood, nutrition), and home visits.

   Strength exercise and nutritional supplements were shown to be the most effective and easiest to implement. A simple intervention would include designing 20 to 25 minutes of activity, 4 days each week at home with exercises to strengthen arms and legs, improve balance and coordination that are repeated 10 times per minute and progressing to 15 times per minute over 2 to 3 months with a 30-second rest between each set, *and increase in protein consumption* (milk, eggs, tuna, and chicken).

Travers J, Romero-Ortuno R, Bailey J, et al. Delaying and reversing frailty: a systematic review of primary care interventions. *Br J Gen Pract.* 2019;69(678):e61–e69.Available at: https://bjgp.org/content/69/678/e61.long. doi:10.3399/bjgp18X700241.

10. What are effective treatments for dementia? Can rehabilitation be designed to meet patients' needs despite cognitive decline?
    There is support for using *acetylcholinesterase inhibitors* (memantine) in cases of moderate dementia and interventions given by *support caregivers*, including those that help to *coordinate care* for patients and caregivers. These may result in small improvements in the short term. Unfortunately, the average effects of these benefits are relatively small and likely not of clinical significance. Any benefits are reduced by the commonly experienced side effects of medications and the limited availability of complex caregiver interventions. *Cognitive stimulation* and training, *exercise* interventions, and other medications and supplements showed some favorable effects on patients' cognitive and physical function, but the trial evidence lacked consistency and the estimates of benefit were imprecise. However, despite the lack of treatments that result in a cure or significant improvement, it is essential to *make the diagnosis,* so that family members understand the patients' behavior, keep them safe (e.g., prevent them from wandering or driving), and plan for the future as patients continue to decline (e.g., appoint a *health care surrogate* and do financial planning).

Littbrand H, Rosendahl E, Lindelöf N, et al. A high-intensity functional weight-bearing exercise program for older people dependent in activities of daily living and living in residential care facilities: evaluation of the applicability with focus on cognitive function. *Phys Ther.* 2006;86(4):489–498. Available at: https://academic.oup.com/ptj/article/86/4/489/2805059. doi:10/1093/ptj/ 86.4.489.

Patnode CD, Perdue LA, Rossom RC, et al. *Screening for Cognitive Impairment in Older Adults: An Evidence Update for the U.S. Preventive Services Task Force.* Rockville, MD: Agency for Healthcare Research and Quality; 2020. doi.org/10.1016/j.apmr. 2011.02.017.

Oh ES, Fong TG, Hshieh TT, et al. Delirium in older persons: advances in diagnosis and treatment. *JAMA.* 2017;318(12):1161–1174. Available at: https://www.ncbi.nlm.nih.gov/ pmc/articles/PMC5717753/. doi:10.1001/jama.2017.12067.

11. What types of interventions help to counter social isolation and loneliness?
    Increasing one's social networks can have positive effect on health. Maintain social connections via phone and social media when in-person contact is not possible. Socially isolated people with contact once or twice a week showed the least amount of depression.
    Features common to successful interventions include adaptability, community participation, and activities involving productive engagement. Relevant systemic reviews of interventions for people at risk for social isolation

and loneliness have also been studied by National Institute for Health Research (UK)-funded research (available at: https://www.nihr.ac.uk/).

Social Networking Using the Internet. Available at: https://www.pewresearch.org/internet/2010/08/27/older-adults-and-social-media/.

Chopik WJ. The benefits of social technology use among older adults are mediated by reduced loneliness. *Cyberpsychol Behav Soc Netw.* 2016;19(9):551–556. Available at: https://www.ncbi.nlm.nih.gov/pmc/articles/PMC5312603/. doi:10.1089/cyber.2016.0151.

Alcarez KI, Eddens KS, Blase JL, et al. Social isolation and mortality in US Black and White men and women. *Am J Epidemiol.* 2019;188(1):102–109. doi.org/10.1016/j.apmr.2011.02.017. doi:10.1093/aje/kwy231.

Gardiner C, Geldenhuys G, Gott M. Interventions to reduce social isolation and loneliness among older people: an integrative review. *Health Soc Care Community.* 2018;26(2):147–157. Available at: https://onlinelibrary.wiley.com/doi/pdf/10.1111/hsc.12367i: 10.1111/hsc.12367.

FURTHER READING

Fillit HM, Rockwood K, Young JB. *Brocklehurst's Textbook of Geriatric Medicine and Gerontology.* 8th ed. Philadelphia, PA: Elsevier; 2016.
Ornish D. *Love and Survival: 8 Pathways to Intimacy and Health.* New York, NY: William Morrow Paperbacks; 1999.

Bonus questions and answers available online.

CHAPTER 80

PHYSIATRIC SPORTS MEDICINE: FUNCTIONAL DIAGNOSIS, FOCAL INTERVENTIONS, AND REHABILITATION FOR PREVENTION

Omar M. Bhatti, MD and Joel M. Press, MD

What lies behind us and what lies before us are tiny matters compared to what lies within us.
— Ralph Waldo Emerson (1803–1882)

KEY POINTS

1. Physiatric sports medicine addresses the patient as an athlete to achieve exceptional personal and athletic actualization with sustained play.
2. Success is attained with sport-specific knowledge of injury mechanisms, prevention planning, relative rest after injury, successive performance approximation, and rehabilitation beyond the resolution of symptoms.
3. A classic sign of plantar fasciitis is worse pain upon awakening with the first few steps in the morning.
4. Iliotibial band syndrome is lateral knee pain caused by overuse from repetitive knee flexion activities and occurs commonly in running and cycling.

1. What is the philosophy of sports medicine?

Sports medicine is a patient-centered approach to the athlete that emphasizes injury prevention, play performance, and mechanism-directed diagnosis. A comprehensive, problem-oriented plan utilizes a full spectrum of evidence-based outcomes for focused, directed interventions. The therapeutic "team" includes family, coaches, therapists, athletic trainers, sports organizations, and equipment providers. Like other clinicians from various backgrounds, physiatrists integrate rehabilitation methods, modalities, bracing, and interdisciplinary collaboration to achieve exceptional athlete actualization.

Fredericson M. The evolution of physical medicine and rehabilitation in sports medicine. *PM R.* 2016;8(3 suppl):S1–S7. doi:10.1016/j.pmrj.2015.09.020.

2. What are the key questions to ask when discussing an injury with an athlete?
   - What was the **mechanism** of injury?
   - When was the onset of injury? Is this a **recurrent injury, repetitive overload**, or an **acute traumatic** event? Previous injury to the same area may imply inadequate rehabilitation or the progression of chronic microtraumatic injury.
   - Where else has the patient been injured? A **kinetic chain analysis** of injuries often reveals deficits proximal or distal to the site of acute injury, which has rendered the symptomatic site vulnerable to overload.
   - What **treatment** has the patient received? Ask which specific exercises were performed in physical therapy. An alarming number of musculoskeletal injuries do not receive adequate prevention and proper rehabilitation.
   - What **other medical conditions** does the patient have? Do not assume that the patient is healthy just because he or she is an athlete. Many individuals with asthma, cardiac conditions, and metabolic and hormonal disorders are active participants in sports. Treatment regimens need to take this information into account.
   - **An athlete-centered history** builds on understanding the **context of injury**. Perceptive attention to athlete performance goals, general health, psychological processes, fitness when injured, training methods, and impact of injury guides problem definitions.

3. What are the primary goals of the preparticipation history and physical evaluation (PPE)?
   - Provide an access point for medical care by promoting the physician–athlete relationship
   - Screening for potentially life-threatening conditions and sports-specific risk factors
   - Determine general health, flexibility, strength, coordination, and endurance
   - Review injury history to plan prevention, psychological responses, and adaptation

- Identify current systemic illnesses (cardiovascular, respiratory, or endocrine disorders) or focal conditions that may worsen with activity
- Detect conditions that may restrict participation or performance
- Review current medications and educate in the use
- Guide individuals with chronic conditions toward safe participation
- Provide sports-specific education for safe technique and equipment use
- Fulfill medical–legal requirements
- Provide medical clearance to participate in sport

Available at: https://www.tandfonline.com/doi/abs/10.3810/psm.1999.08.941.

Available at: https://www.aafp.org/afp/2015/0901/p371.html.

4. What is a musculoskeletal examination?

In a complete musculoskeletal examination, the examiner quantifies **biomechanical deficits** such as inflexibilities and motion restrictions at the level of the joints, connective tissue, muscle, and fascia. **Static and dynamic strength and proprioception** assess performance. These findings, along with the **neurologic exam**, can reveal diagnosis with functional implications. Biomechanical deficits and imbalances can be determined that may be important in prescribing a comprehensive rehabilitation program. **Key components of the physiatric examination** include inspection, range of motion, palpation, ligament testing, strength testing, biomechanics and functional evaluation, sensation, and reflexes. For example, evaluation of the functional range of motion may include assessing for scapular dyskinesis or glenohumeral internal rotation deficit (GIRD) in an overhead athlete. An example of functional strength testing may include assessing for weak hip abduction in the patellofemoral pain syndrome (PFPS).

5. What is the fourth leading risk factor for death worldwide?

Physical inactivity is a significant health problem and is now the **fourth leading risk factor for mortality**. The medical literature demonstrates numerous beneficial effects of physical activity and exercise. It is essential to counsel and educate patients on the significance of maintaining a physically active lifestyle.

PODCAST. Available at: https://soundcloud.com/bmjpodcasts/physical-inactivity-a-global-public-health-problem-episode-368.

Available at: https://www.who.int/news-room/fact-sheets/detail/physical-activity.

6. What are common sports-specific injuries?

Specific movement in various sports can result in injury patterns unique to athletes (Table 80.1). Athletes involved in high-impact sports that require jumping and landing on hard surfaces (e.g., basketball, volleyball) are at risk for injuries in the knee and ankle, such as anterior cruciate ligament (ACL) tears, meniscal tears, and ankle sprains. Activities involving more upper-extremity movement (e.g., tennis, baseball, racquetball) may cause injury to the

Table 80.1 Common Sports-Specific Injuries

SPORT	INJURIES
BASEBALL	Rotator cuff tendinosis, glenoid labral tear, UCL injury, medial epicondylitis, OCD of the capitellum
BASKETBALL	Ankle sprain, ACL tear, patellar and quad tendinopathy, mallet finger, finger dislocations
BOXING	Facial and ocular injuries, fifth metacarpal fracture, concussion
DANCE AND FIGURE SKATING	Spondylolysis, Achilles tendinopathy, ankle sprain, foot stress fractures, flexor hallucis tendinosis
AMERICAN FOOTBALL	Stinger, concussion, spine injuries, shoulder dislocation, Acromioclavicular (AC) joint sprain, Medial collateral ligament (MCL) sprain tear, Anterior cruciate ligament (ACL) tear, ankle sprain, leg fractures
SOCCER	Athletic pubalgia, adductor strain, hamstring strain, ACL tear, meniscus tear, Jones fracture
GYMNASTICS	Spondylolysis, disc herniation, wrist fractures, ACL tear, shoulder dislocation, Achilles rupture, ankle sprain, stress fractures

ACL, Anterior cruciate ligament; *OCD,* osteochondritis dissecans; *UCL,* ulnar collateral ligament.

rotator cuff and elbow. Sports such as cheerleading, volleyball, track, gymnastics, and weight lifting may predispose to back injuries resulting from repetitive hyperextension.

Hootman JM, Dick R, Agel J. Epidemiology of collegiate injuries for 15 sports: summary and recommendations for injury prevention initiatives. *J Athl Train.* 2007;42(2):311–319.

7. What is a stinger?

Stingers result from an impact to the head/neck/shoulder region, commonly seen in contact sports such as football. This creates sudden traction or compression of the brachial plexus (most commonly the upper trunk) or cervical nerve roots (most commonly C5 and C6). There are **two primary mechanisms**: (1) shoulder depression while the neck is forced laterally in the opposite direction, resulting in a **stretch injury to the brachial plexus**, or (2) **nerve root compression** by ipsilateral cervical rotation with flexion or hyperextension (Fig. 80.1). **Sharp, burning pain radiates down one upper extremity** and generally lasts from seconds to minutes. Return to play requires complete resolution of symptoms and a normal neurologic exam. When there are transient neurologic symptoms in more than one extremity, cervical spinal cord neuropraxia must be ruled out while the spine is stabilized.

Stingers and Burners. Available at: https://now.aapmr.org/stingers-and-burners/.

Available at: https://www.wheelessonline.com/bones/transient-brachial-plexopathy-stinger-burner/.

8. What is cervical cord neuropraxia?

Cervical cord neuropraxia (transient quadriparesis) is an injury to the spinal cord during contact sports. It can result from a hyperextension, hyperflexion, or axial force to the neck. This results in transient neurologic symptoms in two or more limbs (most commonly bilateral upper extremities). Symptoms typically resolve quickly (seconds to minutes); however, they rarely can last up to 36 hours. Spinal precautions and advanced imaging must be obtained. Return to play is controversial, given the unknown consequence of reinjury and the possibility of sustaining permanent neurologic deficits.

Cantu RV, Cantu RC. Current thinking: return to play and transient quadriplegia. *Curr Sports Med Rep.* 2005;4(1):27–32.

Allen CR, Kang JD. Transient quadriparesis in the athlete. *Clin Sports Med.* 2002;21(1):15–27.

Qureshi SA, Hecht AC. Burner syndrome and cervical cord neuropraxia. *Semin Spine Surg.* 2010;22(4):193–197.

9. What injuries are associated with running?

Most running-related injuries occur in the lower extremities. Forces up to three times the body's weight is translated through the lower limb joints during running. Injuries include plantar fasciitis, medial tibial stress syndrome (MTSS), Achilles tendinopathy, stress fractures, PFPS, and iliotibial band (ITB) friction syndrome. Stress fractures commonly occur in the tibia, metatarsals, and fibula, and less commonly in the femur and pelvis. The most common site for a stress fracture is the **posteromedial aspect of the mid-distal tibia**.

Available at: https://www.aafp.org/afp/2018/0415/p510.html.

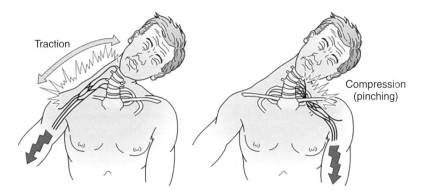

Traction

Compression (pinching)

Fig. 80.1 Stinger mechanism of injury. (From Magee DJ. Chapter 3: Cervical spine. In *Orthopedic Physical Assessment.* Elsevier; 2014:148–223 (Fig. 3.10).

10. What is plantar fasciitis?

Plantar fasciitis is a common cause of heel pain in adults. It is caused by the overload of the plantar fascia and foot muscles. It is commonly found in runners as a result of overuse. Biomechanical abnormalities include decreased dorsiflexion, overpronation, and weakness of plantar flexors. A classic sign is worse pain with the first few steps in the morning. Treatment includes relative rest, correction of biomechanics, stretching and strengthening, night splints, orthotics, and injections in refractory cases. It is usually self-limiting, and time until resolution is often 6 to 12 months.

Available at: https://www.aafp.org/afp/2011/0915/p676.htm.

11. When patients complain of diffuse shin pain, what could be a cause?

Medial tibial stress syndrome (MTSS), "**shin splints,**" is caused by an overload of structures that originate at the posteromedial calf. MTSS is a continuum of pathology that may include posterior tibial tendinosis, medial soleus enthesitis, tibial periostitis, tibial stress responses, and tibial stress fracture. A common mechanism of injury occurs when excessive pronation of the subtalar joint stretches the soleus, causing increased stress and traction at the fascial origin over the medial tibia. Management includes reduction of inflammation, stretching, arch support, and applying sports-specific techniques (e.g., running, jumping, and landing).

Available at: www.wheelessonline.com/ortho/shin_splints_medial_tibial_stress_syndrome.

12. What are other common causes of calf pain in the athlete?

Chronic exertional compartment syndrome manifests as gradually increasing calf pain during physical exertion. There are four fascial compartments in the calf (anterior, lateral, superficial posterior, and deep posterior). The anterior compartment is most frequently affected. Symptoms include tightness, aching, cramping, pressure, and sometimes weakness and paresthesias in the calf and foot. Symptoms typically subside at rest. These symptoms result from **increased intramuscular pressure within the affected compartment**. Diagnosis is made by measuring intercompartmental pressures before and after exercise. Treatment involves modifying the training regimen (reduce volume), addressing deficiencies in strength and flexibility, using insoles, and correcting running technique. If symptoms persist despite conservative treatment, then fasciotomy can increase compartment volume.

Paik RS, Pepple DA, Hutchinson MR. Chronic exertional compartment syndrome. *BMJ.* 2013;346:f33.

Meehan WP, O'Brien MJ. Chronic exertional compartment syndrome. In Fields KB, ed. *UpToDate*; 2018. Available at: https://www.uptodate.com/contents/chronic-exertional-compartment-syndrome.

13. What is the most common type of ankle sprain in athletics?

Ankle sprains are some of the most common injuries in many sports (e.g., basketball, football, gymnastics, soccer, and ballet). A lateral ankle sprain is the most common and results from an inversion injury. This type of sprain results in damage to the lateral ligament complex, which includes the **anterior talofibular ligament** (most common ankle ligament injured). Disruption of the syndesmosis is called a **high ankle sprain** (usually during eversion).

Kirschner J, Geer R. *Ankle Sprain.* Available at: https://now.aapmr.org/ankle-sprain/.

14. What is a common cause of low back pain in young athletes?

Spondylolysis, which is a defect in the pars interarticularis, is a common injury found in many athletes (e.g., gymnasts, dancers, football, track, and wrestlers) who are subject to twisting and hyperextension loading of the lumbar spine. The defect most commonly occurs at L5 and is best seen on single positron emission computed tomography (SPECT) scan, because radiographs and MRI may be negative. Treatment remains controversial, with some authors recommending rigid bracing (to prevent excessive spine extension) for varying durations. However, the vast majority of patients seem to do well with conservative care (physical therapy with core strengthening, rest, and NSAIDs) and can return to play with few or no symptoms.

Standaert CJ, Herring SA. Expert opinion and controversies in sports and musculoskeletal medicine: the diagnosis and treatment of spondylolysis in adolescent athletes. *Arch Phys Med Rehabil.* 2007;88(94):537–540.

Gagnet P, Kern K, Andrews K, et al. Spondylolysis and spondylolisthesis: a review of the literature. *J Orthop.* 2018;15(2):404–407.

Berger RG, Doyle SM. Spondylolysis 2019 update. *Curr Opin Pediatr.* 2019;31(1):61–68.

15. What is the female athlete triad?

The female athlete triad is a metabolic injury that results from three interrelated medical conditions among female athletes (**low energy availability, menstrual dysfunction, low bone mineral density**). This disorder often goes unrecognized and is the result of maladaptive patterns of diet and exercise adopted to improve body image or performance. The consequences of this disorder impair functioning of metabolic rate, menstruation, bone health (including fractures), immunity, and cardiovascular health. Early recognition of the female athlete triad can be accomplished through risk factor assessment and screening questionnaires. Treatment involves a multidisciplinary approach, and preventive measures start with educating parents, coaches, and athletes in the health risks of the disorder.

Chamberlain R. The female athlete triad: recommendations for management. *Am Fam Physician*. 2018;97(8):499–502. Available at: https://www.aafp.org/afp/2018/0415/p499.html.

Daily JP, Stumbo JR. Female athlete triad. *Prim Care Clin Office Pract*. 2018;45:615–624.

Statuta S. The female athlete triad, relative energy deficiency in sport, and the male athlete triad: the exploration of low-energy syndromes in athletes. *Curr Sports Med Rep*. 2020;19(2):43–44.

16. What are two common sports-related injuries to the wrist and hand?

Skier's thumb is the instability of the metacarpophalangeal (MCP) joint of the thumb caused by the tearing of the **ulnar collateral ligament (UCL)** (Fig. 80.2). The injury occurs when the thumb is pulled into a valgus position (commonly seen in skiers). Partial tears of the thumb UCL may be treated conservatively with a molded spica splint or cast. A **Stener lesion** occurs when the aponeurosis of the adductor pollicis interpositions between the ruptured UCL. When this occurs, the ligament cannot heal, and surgery is indicated because of chronic instability at the MCP joint.

Scaphoid fractures are another common upper extremity injury in athletes. These most commonly occur after a **fall onto an outstretched hand (FOOSH)**. Pain is localized to the anatomic snuff box. The scaphoid has a tenuous blood supply, especially at the middle and proximal poles. Thus, fractures can sometimes lead to nonunion. Conservative treatment includes a spica splint or cast. If there is evidence of displacement or nonunion, then surgery is warranted.

Kundu N, Asfaw S, Polster J, et al. The Stener Lesión. *Eplasty*. 2012;12:ic11. Available at: https://www.ncbi.nlm.nih.gov/pmc/articles/PMC3406613/.

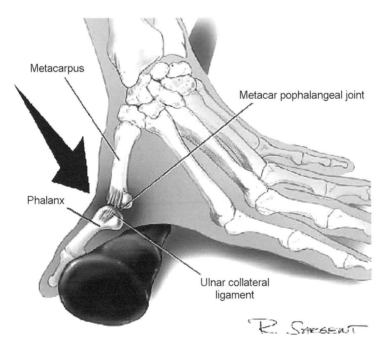

Metacarpus

Metacar pophalangeal joint

Phalanx

Ulnar collateral ligament

R. SARGENT

Fig. 80.2 Skier's thumb (carried over from the previous edition).

17. Is surgery necessary for a meniscal tear of the knee?

Not always. Meniscal injuries associated with mechanical locking, painful catching, loss of full range of motion, and persistent pain that limits daily activity may require surgical intervention. The **outer one-third** of the meniscus has the potential for healing secondary to adequate vascular supply. The **inner two-thirds** are not well vascularized. Many meniscal injuries that minimally affect daily activities during the first few weeks after injury respond to rehabilitation. Exercise, in conjunction with symptomatic surveillance, may allow the return to baseline. In patients with non-mechanical symptoms, it has been demonstrated that **physical therapy**, exercise (i.e., quad sets, hamstring curls, hip abductor strengthening, knee mobilization), and training have outcomes comparable to surgery. However, if symptoms persist after 4 to 8 weeks (depending on the demands of the athlete), surgical consultation may be indicated.

Van de Graaf VA, Noorduyn JCA, Willigenburg NW, et al. Effect of early surgery vs physical therapy on knee function among patients with nonobstructive meniscal tears: the ESCAPE randomized clinical trial. *JAMA.* 2018;320(13):1328–1337, 2018.

Valdez G, Haque A, Chang RG. *Meniscus Injuries of the Knee.* Available at: https://now.aapmr.org/meniscus-injuries-of-the-knee/.

18. What is athletic pubalgia?

Athletic pubalgia (**core muscle injury**) is groin pain in an athlete without a demonstrable hernia. The specific location of the injury can vary depending on what structures are injured. Commonly injured structures include the rectus abdominus, external oblique aponeurosis, internal oblique, adductors, and pectineus. Athletes report acute or insidious onset unilateral pain at the **groin or pubic symphysis**. Physical examination may reveal tenderness in the groin, pubic symphysis, or lower abdominal musculature. Provocative tests such as Valsalva, resisted sit-ups, or resisted hip adduction may reproduce symptoms. Diagnostic injections may be useful to differentiate from intraarticular hip pathology. Ultrasound and MRI are preferred imaging modalities to reveal the location of the injury. Occurrence is more common in men and athletes that participate in **twisting and explosive sports** that require sudden changes in direction. Treatment includes physical therapy (strengthening core, abductors, and adductors), NSAIDs, rest, icing, improvement in sports-specific movement patterns and biomechanics, and possibly platelet-rich plasma (PRP) injection or surgery.

King E, Ward J, Small L, et al. Athletic groin pain: a systematic review and meta-analysis of surgical versus physical therapy rehabilitation outcomes. *Br J Sports Med.* 2015;49(22):1447–1451.

19. Is it possible to participate in sports without surgical reconstruction of a torn ACL?

ACL injuries can be managed operatively or nonoperatively. The ACL prevents **anterior translation of the tibia relative to the femur** and provides rotatory stability at the knee. In ACL-deficient knees, stability during deceleration, lateral, and twisting movements is lost. Most high-level athletes and young recreational athletes who wish to return to the same level of sports competition typically undergo surgical reconstruction. Reconstructive surgery reestablishes the restraint to rotatory and anterior instability. Some patients will do well without surgery and can return to sports activities, particularly "straight-ahead" sports such as cycling. Both nonoperative and postoperative treatment require aggressive rehabilitation (regaining range of motion, gait retraining, core, quad and hamstring strengthening), neuromuscular, and proprioceptive training.

Micheo WF, Rosas OR, Rivera A, et al. *ACL Injury and Rehabilitation.* Available at: https://now.aapmr.org/acl-injury-and-rehabilitation/.

Anterior Cruciate Ligament Injuries. Available at: https://www.aaos.org/anteriorcruciateligamentinjuries/?ssopc=1.

20. What important considerations are involved in the rehabilitation of patellofemoral pain syndrome?

PFPS is one of the most common diagnoses seen in young athletes. The evaluation of anterior knee pain is guided by the age of the competitor and sports activities. PFPS results from **maltracking of the patella** in the **trochlear groove** with knee flexion and extension. Emphasis needs to be placed on dynamic realignment by stretching posterior, lateral, and kinetic chain structures that may be tight (i.e., the ITB, hamstrings, gastrocsoleus), strengthening (e.g., vastus medialis, gluteus medius, and minimus), proprioceptive retraining of patellofemoral motion (e.g., taping versus bracing), and exercises that do not excessively increase patellofemoral joint reaction forces.

Gaitonde DY, Ericksen A, Robbins RC. Patellofemoral pain syndrome. *Am Fam Physician.* 2019;99(2):88–94. Available at: https://www.aafp.org/afp/2019/0115/p88.html.

21. What sports exacerbate ITB friction syndrome?

ITB syndrome is lateral knee pain caused by overuse from repetitive knee flexion activities. Pain is produced as the ITB rubs **over the lateral femoral condyle**, typically between 20 degrees and 30 degrees of flexion. This commonly occurs in **running and cycling**. Causes include running on uneven surfaces, sudden mileage increase, poor flexibility, poor seat height and pedal positioning in cycling, and incorrect footwear causing biomechanical alterations.

Dinescu L, Mukherjee V, Guerzon A, et al. *Iliotibial Band Syndrome.* Available at: https://now.aapmr.org/iliotibial-band-syndrome/.

22. What is the difference between turf toe and a Jones fracture?

A fracture of the proximal fifth metatarsal is called a **Jones fracture**. These can result from an inversion-plantarflexion injury or with sudden force to the lateral foot. Stress fractures in this area may also occur. Initial treatment may include non-weight bearing in a casting or boot; however, many athletes undergo screw fixation as this area is prone to nonunion. **Turf toe** is another common injury to the foot. This is an injury to the plantar plate and capsule of the great toe metatarsophalangeal joint caused by excessive forces during push-off. Splinting for 7 to 10 days and/or taping to limit dorsiflexion may prevent further injury.

23. Describe the important aspects of the rehabilitation of rotator cuff injuries.

Rehabilitation should include assessment of the entire kinetic chain (e.g., cervical, thoracic, lumbar, and upper and lower extremities). This is especially important in the overhead athlete. Muscles should be strengthened both concentrically and eccentrically, individually, and in group motor patterns. Progression should lead to sports-specific exercises that approximate play. Rotator cuff rehabilitation must address the following:

- **Flexibility deficits,** particularly in the external rotators and posterior capsule.
- **Joint motion restriction** within the sternoclavicular, acromioclavicular, scapulothoracic, and glenohumeral articulations.
- **Strength deficits,** particularly in the scapular stabilizers (rhomboids, lower and middle trapezius, and serratus anterior) as well as the cuff muscles (supraspinatus, infraspinatus, subscapularis, and teres minor).

Martinez-Silvestrini JA, Micheo W, Zaremski JL. *Shoulder Pain in the Throwing Athlete.* Available at: https://now.aapmr.org/shoulder-pain-in-the-throwing-athlete/.

24. How is tennis elbow treated?

Lateral epicondylitis, "tennis elbow," is the result of a repetitive overload of the extensors and supinators of the wrist, most commonly at the origin of the extensor carpi radialis brevis (ECRB). Rehabilitation focuses on stretching tight wrist extensors, eccentric strengthening, and avoiding aggravating factors. Limitations of motion at the shoulder, poor cervicothoracic posture, and kinetic chain mechanics must be corrected. Ice, massage, wrist splinting, counterforce brace, and PRP injections are options.

Tennis Elbow—Lateral Epicondylitis. Available at: http://www.wheelessonline.com/ortho/tennis_elbow_lateral_epicondylitis.

25. What is "Little League elbow"?

Little League elbow is the consequence of repeated **valgus overload** of the skeletally immature elbow. During late cocking and acceleration, medial structures are stretched while lateral structures are compressed. The distraction forces on the medial side may cause avulsion of the medial epicondyle and UCL injuries, while the lateral compressive forces may induce radial head and capitellum growth disturbances, osteochondritis dissecans (OCD) of the capitellum, fractures, and articular cartilage breakdown.

Abbasi D, Ahmad CS. *Little League Elbow.* Available at: https://www.orthobullets.com/shoulder-and-elbow/3086/little-league-elbow.

Throwing Injuries in the Elbow in Children. Available at: https://orthoinfo.aaos.org/en/diseases—conditions/throwing-injuries-in-the-elbow-in-children/.

26. What is biker's palsy?

Biker's palsy refers to an entrapment or pressure neuropathy of the ulnar nerve at the wrist within **Guyon canal**. It may occur in distance cyclists because of direct pressure on the ulnar side of the hand, especially in the drop-down handlebar position. Sensory and motor symptoms are confined to the ulnar-innervated structures distal to this area, with sparing of the flexor carpi ulnaris muscle and the dorsal ulnar cutaneous sensory patch. Methods of prevention include wearing padded cycling gloves, changing hand position frequently, and the use of "aero-bars," which allow weight bearing through the forearm. Carpal tunnel syndrome is also common in long-distance cyclists.

Cyclist's Palsy. Available at: https://www.physio-pedia.com/Cyclist%27s_palsy.

27. **What is "functional" musculoskeletal rehabilitation?**

Functional rehabilitation is designed to provide comprehensive injury treatment with the goal of return to play for a specific sport. It implies that the exercises performed by the patient for a specific musculoskeletal disorder can be sequentially approximated in the planes of motion for their sport, incorporating flexibility, strengthening, agility, and proprioceptive training. A coordinated sports-specific, functional rehabilitation program should "look like" the activities an athlete performs in play. Straight-leg raises, for example, would be a means of strengthening lower-extremity musculature, including the quadriceps and hip flexors of a swimmer. However, there are very few "functional" activities that a person would do during the day that would simulate this motion. A more appropriate functional activity might be a partial squat or a step-up or step-down exercise to activate the quadriceps and hip flexors.

Lee H, Plastaras C. *Functional Rehabilitation.* Available at: https://now.aapmr.org/functional-rehabilitation/.

28. **What are open and closed chain exercises, and why are they used?**

A **closed kinetic chain (CKC)** is operational when the distal segment of the motion chain is fixed in space, and movement at one segment will move the other segments in a predictable pattern. An **open kinetic chain (OKC)** is operational when the distal segment moves freely. An example of a CKC movement is a simple squat, whereas an example of an OKC movement is throwing a baseball. Both types of exercises are used in sports injury rehabilitation, depending on the type of motion that is being functionally addressed. Most running injuries involving the lower extremities will emphasize CKC activities, whereas rehabilitation of shoulder and elbow injuries in tennis and throwing sports may emphasize OKC exercises.

Chu SK, Jayabalan P, Kibler WB, et al. The kinetic chain revisited: new concepts on throwing mechanics and injury. *PM R.* 2016;8 (3 suppl):S69–S77.

29. **What does "rehabilitation beyond the resolution of symptoms" mean?**

Many musculoskeletal injuries appear to resolve despite the treatment patients are given. After treatment of the acute inflammation, symptoms from many ailments disappear, and athletes mistakenly assume it is safe to return to sport. However, the absence of pain does not always imply the absence of pathology, and stopping rehabilitation at this point is inadequate. Most musculoskeletal injuries in sports are the result of chronic overload, in which biomechanical alterations and microtraumatic tissue injury have occurred. These biomechanical changes, consisting of muscle imbalances, inflexibilities, and weaknesses, need to be addressed to prevent recurrence of injury.

BIBLIOGRAPHY

Bruckner P, Khan K. *Clinical Sports Medicine.* Sydney: McGraw-Hill; 2017.
Eiff MP, Hatch RL. *Fracture Management for Primary Care Updated Edition.* 3rd ed. Philadelphia, PA: Saunders; 2018.
Fredericson M. The evolution of physical medicine and rehabilitation in sports medicine. *PM R.* 2016;8(3 suppl):S1–S7. doi:10.1016/j.pmrj.2015.09.020.
Krabak BJ. *Sports Medicine. Physical Medicine and Rehabilitation Clinics of North America.* Vol. 25(4). Philadelphia, PA: W.B. Saunders; 2014.

CHAPTER 81

VOCATIONAL REHABILITATION AND PERSONHOOD: A PHYSIATRIST'S VITAL CALLING

Mark A. Young, MD, MBA, FACP, FAAPMR, DABPMR, Steven A. Stiens, MD, MS, and Benjamin S. Carson Sr., MD

Every disability conceals a vocation. If only we can find it, we shall turn "necessity" to a "glorious gain."
— C. S. Lewis (1898–1963)

KEY POINTS: ACHIEVING VOCATIONAL REHABILITATION OUTCOMES

1. Set the expectation, even from the initial rehabilitation stages, that resuming or pursuing a career is a viable and desirable rehabilitation goal.
2. Optimize physical, emotional, and cognitive functioning.
3. Utilize professional vocational rehabilitation services and return-to-work incentive programs.
4. Facilitate work adaptation through retraining, assistive technology, accommodations, housing support, and communication.

1. **How are employment and vocational satisfaction fundamental to wellbeing of a person (despite "disability")?**
   Work is an essential force in defining one's life and destiny. Employment fulfills an identity and provides structure, income, housing possibilities, and social networks. Often, disability interferes with one's vocational role. This can impact self-worth, social status, and housing and living conditions, and diminish quality of life (QOL).

2. **What is the philosophy and ideology of the vocational rehabilitation (VR) process?**
   Motivated by Sigmund Freud's now legendary proclamation—**"The cornerstone of humanness is Love and Work**,"—the rehabilitation clinician often plays a critically important role in promoting the independence of persons with disability through VR. The physiatrist, in concert with the VR team, is well-positioned to steward the vocational recovery process. PM&R's specialty-specific emphasis on measuring functional ability, recognizing motivation, uncovering strengths, and creatively promoting inclusion and productivity stands at the center of the VR process.

3. **Is VR essential to the rehabilitation continuum of care (COC)?**
   VR is a critical and indispensable component of the rehabilitation COC, as it offers a coordinated and systematic process of professional services that allow people with disabilities to obtain and sustain employment. The heart of the VR mission is the altruistic goal to promote economic self-sufficiency, dignity, and independence. In attaining this powerful "functional outcome," the VR team successfully completes the concluding step in the COC.

4. **How is the VR process initiated during the acute rehabilitation phase?**
   Recognizing current or potential disability-related employment vulnerabilities among rehabilitation patients is an important early duty of the clinician. Vocational information must be collected in the initial clinical encounter to determine past roles, passions, skills, and anticipated community contributions. Early referral to the physiatry-directed VR team is mission-critical as it will allow for early planning.

5. **Is VR relevant to the "musculoskeletal physiatrist" and/or the interventional pain physiatrist?**
   No matter what a physiatrist's work concentration is (MSK/interventional versus classic rehabilitation, e.g., CVA, SCI), VR can play a critically important role in the COC. An illustrative example:
   A 37-year-old male presents with discogenic lumbar pain after sustaining a workplace injury. You perform a series of epidural injections and are asked by the workers' compensation RN to complete a "functional capacity evaluation" form in order to determine the feasibility of a VR program helping to return the patient to gainful employment.

6. **Describe the value of VR to governmental, legislative, and public policy makers.**
   Although the primary benefit of VR to clinicians is the restoration of self-esteem and dignity through employment of persons with disability, there are other practical advantages accruing from VR including economic and societal

gains. As Eleanor Roosevelt once bluntly said, "**It is not more vacation we need—it is more vocation**." By compassionately empowering a citizen with a disability to return to work, the VR process is helpful to the government, policy makers, and society by enhancing employment, improving the economy, cultivating affordable housing standards, and optimizing the tax base. More importantly and humanely, VR restores the pride and self-worth of persons with disabilities

7. How does the VR process help? Which patients benefit?

VR can help those with disabilities retain or maintain current employment by changing work schedules, providing accommodations, and using accessible/assistive technology (AT). Those who have lost employment or need to change careers may also benefit from transferable skills analysis, career development, or retraining. Those not previously employed, or who have not developed career skills because of childhood disability or extended chronic illness can also receive VR services (e.g., career exploration through job shadowing and/or work skill development). Often the VR team includes a PT, OT, SLP, RN, audiologist, and addictions counselor—all led, ideally, by a PM&R physician.

8. Describe the clinician's role in establishing an interdisciplinary blueprint for employment outcomes.

As a medical specialist trained in assessing physical, functional, and behavioral aspects of illness and disease, and gauging its important impact on disability, the PM&R physician often plays a preeminent role in the VR process. From the initial phase of the medical care continuum, when the physiatrist performs a "Medical Functional Evaluation" (MFE), through the later stages of job assessment and placement, physiatrist input is critical in formulating a vision and coordinating and directing the multidisciplinary team. When medical and behavioral complications arise during the assessment process, the physiatrist is often helpful in assessing and directing an effective response from the selected disciplines. The physiatrist, with their knowledge of medicine and mastery of the neurological and MSK systems, serves as an indispensable "quarterback" in the VR work process. Important members of the VR team, including PT, OT, SLP, et al., often look to the physiatrist for guidance and direction.

9. How does the VR process often begin?

With the active recommendation of the physiatrist and the endorsement of the multidisciplinary rehabilitation team, VR services can be most effective when initiated during inpatient rehabilitation by an onsite VR counselor. Upon discharge, a referral to a VR counselor is often made. In many jurisdictions, there is a local "**Division of Vocational Rehabilitation (DVR)**," a state and federal partnership. Funded by the Rehabilitation Services Administration (RSA) and state governments, DVR offices are in every state.

Individuals may also be able to access other VR counseling services (depending on eligibility requirements) through the following sources: a workers' compensation or personal injury insurance carrier, transition-to-work programs in high schools, disabled student services centers at postsecondary institutions, or other community rehabilitation agencies (e.g., county social services, veterans' agencies, mental health centers, religious and spiritual community resources).

Rehabilitation Services Administration. Available at: https://rsa.ed.gov/ and https://www2.ed.gov/about/offices/list/osers/rsa/index.html.

10. Who is eligible for VR services?

Potential VR candidates must meet several qualifications: have a physical or mental impairment posing a substantial impediment to employment, be capable of benefitting from VR employment services, and require VR services to prepare for, enter, engage in, and retain employment. More information is available from the RSA (available at: https://www2.ed.gov/about/offices/list/osers/rsa/index.html).

11. How are VR services compensated?

Virtually all states in the US have VR programs through a DVR. These entities fund services, education, and equipment for eligible persons through a partnership of state and federal (RSA) funds. Other VR services are sometimes provided through: funding from workers' compensation, Social Security Disability, private health, motor vehicle payments, disability insurance, county or local social service, legal settlements, or nonprofit agencies serving persons with disabilities through donations and grant funding (e.g., Easter Seals, Goodwill Industries).

Large employers having disability management or employee assistance programs may provide VR services, as well as schools, colleges, and universities (e.g., high school work transition services, university offices for students with disabilities). As VR services are viewed as an "empowerment" program rather than an "entitlement" initiative, careful matching of the patient with eligible VR services and continual case management surveillance is required.

12. Who are the key members of the VR team?

Key collaborators in the VR team include the rehabilitation physician, PT, OT, SLP, RN, addictions counselor, psychologist, and AT specialist. As leader of the VR team, the physiatrist catalyzes the VR process by linking work and independent living goals through a well-considered and carefully coordinated team effort focused on health care, psychosocial, educational, occupational, technological, and vocational objectives.

Specific members of the VR action team include: rehabilitation counselors (RC), vocational evaluators, work adjustment specialists, job developers, job-placement specialists, job coaches, and disability-management case managers. VR clients with sensory disabilities may require additional services such as low-vision specialists, rehabilitation teachers for vision impairment, and sign-language interpreters.

13. **Describe the role of the RC.**

   With the assistance of the VR team, RCs procure services that meet specific rehabilitation needs, identify programs and resources, and provide skill development and counseling for independent living and vocational functioning. Examples are:

   - Gather vocational, educational, psychological, and **medical background information** to understand the VR client's current physical and **functional status**, capabilities, and interests.
   - Arrange for relevant **analyses and diagnostics** (e.g., career interests, educational aptitude, physical demands, reasonable accommodations) so the person can make an informed choice about career options.
   - Identify **knowledge, skills, and added training** needed to nurture a career aligned with the person's abilities and interests.
   - **Assist in designing a plan** (blueprint) for independent living and vocational success.
   - **Develop an individualized plan (IEP)** for achieving employment that lists the steps needed to reach the person's job goal.
   - Assess and **review labor market data** and other resources to obtain job leads.
   - Follow the **person's work progress** to help maintain the job and foster adherence.

14. **How does case management play a role in the VR arena?**

   VR counselors serve as case managers who facilitate reintegration into school, work, recreation, and independent living. VR counselors often interact with health care providers, employers, third-party payers, community agencies, and schools. The goal is to promote patient involvement with work and/or school, minimize costs, and secure benefits and resources that improve outpatient rehabilitation outcomes.

15. **Do environmental influences affect VR planning and services?**

   An individual's characteristics and functional capacities are not the only determinants of independent living and employment outcomes. Discriminatory policies and practices, as well as environmental barriers such as poor access to transportation, limited entrance into or movement within buildings, and lack of modified tools and equipment are also major handicapping factors. VR services must address modifications in both the physical and interpersonal aspects of the worksite, including physical structures.

   Physical elements (e.g., equipment and/or architecture):
   - Modify the physical environment of the workplace.
   - Restructure job duties or processes so that essential functions are possible.
   - Provide augmentative or AT equipment, qualified readers, or interpreters.
   - Coordinate accessible transportation.

   Interpersonal elements (e.g., co-workers and supervisors)
   - Teach direct supervisors to facilitate accommodation needs involving production and performance requirements.
   - Solicit supportive co-workers (natural supports) to provide accommodations or assistance.

   Interventions will be most effective when the client, VR counselor, and individuals from the targeted environment closely collaborate.

16. **How can a state VR program successfully achieve these objectives?**

   While many state VR programs exist, one author (Young) is more familiar with the program in Maryland. In 1973, the Maryland Rehabilitation Center was established and was later renamed the Workforce and Technology Center (WTC; Available at: https://dors.maryland.gov/Pages/default.aspx) to more accurately reflect its vision.

   The Center was a landmark event for PM&R in the Chesapeake Bay region, as it was envisioned as a wellspring of empowerment rather than entitlement. Its mission is to comprehensively assess those with disabilities, provide needed services, and compassionately have them re-enter the workplace. The WTC is the only facility of its kind in Maryland to maintain continuous Commission on Accreditation of Rehabilitation Facilities certification under physiatric and medical leadership

---

WTC. Available at: https://dors.maryland.gov/Pages/default.aspx

Young MA, Siebens HC, Wainapel SF. A tale of two cities: evolution of academic physiatry in Boston and Baltimore. Part 2: from flower shop to full bloom in Baltimore. *PM R*. 2020;12(2):202–210. Available at: https://pubmed.ncbi.nlm.nih.gov/32198832/

17. **Describe historical examples of VR program interaction with academic medicine that positively affected medical residency education and research objectives?**

   VR programs in Baltimore aligned with PM&R residency and fellowship training programs in 1998, fulfilling a critical ACGME PM&R training requirement. In addition to training residents on the fundamentals of VR, it also gave them exposure to novel vocational initiatives for diabetics with blindness seeking to return to work who required AT, such as talking and implanted transmitting glucometers.

Cross-collaboration between major funding and grant organizations, including the National Science Foundation and NIH, and local universities, have facilitated research and discovery relating to VR and AT. During the COVID era, a portion of these programs has transitioned to an online format, leveraging social media technology such as Zoom and Google Hangouts (see Young et al.).

18. **What VR programs exist for employees with cancer who wish to return to work and stay at work?**
Work Stride: Managing Cancer at Work, an innovative program at Johns Hopkins Hospital, is designed to meet the needs of employees and their families who want to be proactive in preventing and mitigating cancer's impact in the workplace, as well as for those who are dealing with a cancer diagnosis, or caring for someone with cancer. It also provides information specifically for supervisors on how best to support employees through a cancer journey. Pioneered and nurtured by Professor of Surgery Lillie Shockney and the late administrator of the hospital, Terry Langbaum, the program has helped countless cancer survivors.

Work Stride: Managing Cancer at Work. Available at: https://www.workstride.org/about/

19. **Do alternatives exist for persons with work tolerance restrictions?**
    - *Work-hardening programs* (i.e., conditioning programs that focus on increasing work-specific physical activities such as sitting, standing, and lifting).
    - *Modified return-to-work plans* involving reduced work hours and gradually increasing work tasks and hours.

20. **What solutions are available for those with very limited work capacities?**
    - Supportive employment that provides a job coach in a competitive work environment, places and trains the individual directly in the workplace, builds work supports and accommodations with the employer and coworkers, and gradually reduces the job coach's involvement.
    - Day programs (e.g., day centers with flexible hours).
    - Working from home.
    - Sheltered or enclave work (i.e., a group of workers with disabilities with their own supervisor in competitive settings).

21. **What is a "determination of severity" of disability for VR services? What does "order of selection" disability mean?**
Determination of severity is a phrase used by the state/federal DVR system to clarify the level of physical and mental limitations and functional capacities that may influence employment outcomes (e.g., mobility, communication, self-care, self-direction, interpersonal skills, work tolerance, work behavior skills). *Order of selection* refers to the system that state/federal agencies use to prioritize individuals eligible for service. When funding is limited, waitlists may be used, with individuals having the most severe disabilities being served first, based on the order of selection system.

22. **Describe a possible VR plan for an individual with chronic low back pain who is returning to a pre-injury job.**
Vocational intervention at the *personal level*:
    - Effective pain management, regular physician management and follow-up, and support groups.
    - Analysis of the person's functional capacities compared to demands of former work.
    - Counseling regarding the impact of the injury on the individual's career.
    - Coordinating rehabilitation efforts to maximize the individual's confidence, strength, endurance, and flexibility to perform the demands of the job.
    Vocational intervention at the *environmental level*:
    - Detailed analysis of the work environment (physical and interpersonal) and job demands.
    - Modifications to accommodate current functioning and reduce possible further aggravation of the condition; ergonomic adaptations.
    Vocational plan: Developing and negotiating gradual return to work or temporary modified duty, with all parties assisting the individual in an early transition back to work.

23. **Describe a plan for an individual with traumatic brain injury who was unemployed at the time of injury.**
    - Vocational intervention at the *personal level*—Assess residual skills, attention span, self-monitoring, and learning styles; determine interests and aptitudes; develop a career plan.
    - Vocational intervention at the *environmental level*—Consider requirements of suitable occupations, work environments, and potential accommodation strategies (i.e., maximize residual functions, reorganize tasks into discrete, observable, and monitorable steps).
    - **Vocational Plan:**

- Provide social skills training focused work.
- Provide occupational retraining through continuing education or on-the-job training.
- Use volunteer placement to develop general work behaviors or supported employment with a job coach to teach work skills at the job site.
- Provide placement assistance or continue supported employment services depending on severity and capacities.
- Provide adaptive technology for improving work performance.

Trexler LE, Parrott DR. Models of brain injury vocational rehabilitation: the evidence for resource facilitation from efficacy to effectiveness. *J Vocat Rehabil*. 2018;49(2):195–203. Available at: https://www.ncbi.nlm.nih.gov/pmc/articles/PMC6218150/

24. An individual with spinal cord injury wishes to return to a former job, but has substantial limitations performing essential job duties—even with accommodations. What are the options?
There are VR options other than returning to the same job with the same employer. Employment options may exist with the same employer by using existing transferable skills in a different position. However, it may be more beneficial to return to a similar job, but with a new employer. Volunteering, self-employment, telecommuting, and/or retraining for new job skills may be other options that lead to a paid position.

25. How can physiatry and other medical specialties facilitate VR for people with disabilities?
Physicians can facilitate the VR process by approaching patients with the expectation that each will reach his or her full potential and by communicating an expectation of return to work with patients and their families. Other steps that can facilitate the VR process are:
- Promote and build endurance for daily schedules that would accommodate work.
- Communicate with VR counselors and employers to determine appropriate job duties and work modifications for a safe and timely return to work.
- Assist in developing trial work situations or volunteer positions at medical facilities or in the community for patients who require job tryouts.
- Include return to work as a goal at medical follow-up visits.

26. Can VR optimize housing opportunities for those with disabilities?
The process of VR, which skillfully facilitates employment and compassionately enhances QOL, often can play an instrumental role in fostering financial independence, economic stability, and improved housing possibilities for persons with a disability. Workfare, in contrast to welfare, is a potent therapeutic remedy and can result in profound improvement in housing and living conditions. The home is an essential environment in which those with disabilities can carry out ADLs and attain functional independence.

Being able to live independently in one's own home can help sustain independence, self-esteem and individuality for persons with neurological, musculoskeletal, and age-related impairments. At least one study demonstrated the critical relationship between environmental factors such as housing and vocation. QOL is a compelling and potent outcome measure frequently shaped by a person's housing and living conditions. Another seminal study demonstrated that the International Classification of Function Model (ICF), which considers critical environmental factors such as housing, is a far better indicator of QOL and carries a higher predictive value than traditional QOL measures.

Recently, federal agencies such as the Department of Housing and Urban Development, under the capable direction of neurosurgeon Ben Carson, have incorporated time-honored concepts of self-empowerment and self-sufficiency into their important work. Truly, vocational rehab is a critical step in the process of promoting well-being and independent housing.

Private enterprise and corporate enterprise have the powerful capacity to help in the self-sufficiency journey. A notable example of a regional housing and vocational partnership success was begun by Orlando, FL hotelier Harris Rosen, President and CEO of Rosen Hotels & Resorts. His Tangelo Park Program, launched in 1995, has greatly empowered disadvantaged people to attain educational and vocational success. Best of all, this model promotes free market partnerships/philanthropy between private industry and government.

While the Veterans Administration has been acutely aware of the relationship between VR and housing for veterans, novel private sector ventures, though fewer, have also achieved positive outcomes. Harris Rosen, has—through his generous support of the Tangelo Park community—helped facilitate employment in the hospitality industry for many within the disabled and disadvantaged community around Orlando. Attaining safe and affordable housing has thereby become a welcome reality for them.

Alvarez L. One man's millions turn a community in Florida around. *New York Times 2015 May 15*. Available at: https://nyti.ms/1LyHtkf

BBA. *Tangelo Park Program (Orlando, Florida): A Broader, Bolder Approach to Education*. Available at: https://www.boldapproach.org/index.html@p=548.html

Fleming AR, Fairweather JS, Leahy MJ. Quality of life as a potential rehabilitation service outcome: the relationship between employment, quality of life, and other life areas. *Rehabil Coun Bull*. 2013;57(1):9–22 2013. Research.summary at: http://research2vrpractice.com/wp-content/uploads/2014/10/QualityofLife.pdf

27. Can housing contribute to health, function, self-actualization, and wellbeing?
As a center of the present-day family, home is a major factor in risk reduction, conditioning, productive interde-pendence, and success to the community. Models of housing related to health have addressed cost, conditions, consistency, and context. With the occurrence of new disabilities, all these pillars of support are invitations for creative adaptation and generate patient outcomes. Proactive policy to address family interdependence and cost of home requires a rehabilitation perspective in order to integrate income and functional capacities. Conditions must be safe, healthy, accessible, and adapted for interdependent function and connected for full participation.

Swope CB, Hernandez D. Housing as a determinant of health equity: a conceptual model. *Soc Sci Med.* 2019;243:112571. Available at: https://www.ncbi.nlm.nih.gov/pmc/articles/PMC7146083/. doi: 10.1016/j.socscimed.2019.112571

The critical nexus between housing and health was the subject of another landmark public health study which demonstrated the importance of housing stability, affordability, quality, safety, and neighborhood opportunity as key determinants of health:

Hernández D, Swope CB. Housing as a platform for health and equity: evidence and future directions. *Am J Public Health.* 2019;109(10):1363–1366. Available at: https://www.ncbi.nlm.nih.gov/pmc/articles/PMC6727307/ doi:10.2105/AJPH.2019.305210

FURTHER READING

Article
Andersson J, Ahgren B, Axelsson SB, et al. Organizational approaches to collaboration in vocational rehabilitation—an international literature review. 2011;11(4):e137. Available at: https://www.ijic.org/articles/abstract/10.5334/ijic.670/. doi:10.5334/ijic.670

TEXTS
Harsløf I. *New Dynamics of Disability and Rehabilitation: Interdisciplinary Perspectives.* New York, NY: Springer; 2019.
Koch LC, Rumrill PD Jr. *Rehabilitation Counseling and Emerging Disabilities: Medical, Psychosocial, and Vocational Aspects.* New York, NY: Springer; 2017.
Moroz A, Flanagan S, Zaretsky H, eds. *Medical Aspects of Disability for the Rehabilitation Professional.* 5th ed. New York, NY: Springer; 2017.
Strauser DR. *Career Development, Employment, and Disability in Rehabilitation: From Theory to Practice.* 2nd ed. New York, NY: Springer; 2020.
Tarvydas V, Hartley MT, eds. *The Professional Practice of Rehabilitation Counseling.* 2nd ed. New York, NY: Springer; 2017.
Wilson KB, Acklin CL, Chao S-Y, eds. *Case Management for the Health, Human, and Vocational Rehabilitation Services.* Linn Creek: Aspen; 2018.

WEBSITES
Multidisciplinary Association of Spinal Cord Injury Professionals. *Vocational Rehabilitation Guidelines.* 2017. Available at: https://www.mascip.co.uk/wp-content/uploads/2017/11/Mascip-vocational-rehab-guidelines-Sept-2017.pdf
National Institute for Health and Care Excellence. *Workplace Health: Long-Term Sickness Absence and Capability to Work.* 2019. Available at: https://www.nice.org.uk/guidance/ng146

CHAPTER 82

IMPAIRMENT AND DISABILITY RATING: ESTIMATION OF WORK CAPACITY

Richard T. Katz, MD and Robert D. Rondinelli, MD, PhD

Although the world is full of suffering, it is also full of the overcoming of it.

— Helen Keller

KEY POINTS: IMPAIRMENT AND DISABILITY RATING

1. The occupational definition of disability varies among institutions.
2. The Social Security Administration defines disability as the "inability to engage in any substantial gainful activity by reason of any medically determinable physical or mental impairment(s)."
3. The operational definition of disability in the workplace is inability to carry out the activities of the occupation.
4. Definitions of disabled by insurance companies typically imply that a person can no longer perform the substantial and material duties of an occupation.

1. What are the differences among impairment, disablement, and being disabled for an occupation?[a]
   - **Disablement** is the summation of impairment, disability, and handicap as defined by the World Health Organization (1980).
   - **Impairment** is an abnormality of structure, appearance, and/or function at the end-organ level. For example, herniated discs, ligament inflammation, and weak muscles with trigger points are all examples of impairment.
   - **Disability** is the inability of a person to perform an activity. The inability to carry a bag of groceries to the car or walk up a flight of stairs is a disability.
   - **Handicap** is an environmentally defined abnormality reflecting societal bias experienced by the individual trying to fulfill a role. The absence of braille signage in a building would be considered a handicap to a blind person, while the blindness would be considered an impairment.

2. What constitutes disability in the workplace?
   Disability as understood in relation to employment means inability to carry out the activities of an occupation. When a mover with his co-workers can no longer lift several 300-pound refrigerators in a day, the patient is *disabled* for performing that particular job. When a nurse can no longer bend over and stoop on a frequent basis—which most job analyses require for a ward nurse—he or she can no longer work *full duty* and must be placed temporarily or permanently on *light duty*.

3. How is disability officially defined?
   In 2001, the World Health Organization revised terminology for impairment, handicap, and disability and promoted a new model describing body "functions and structures." Under this new model, impairment is defined as the loss of organs or deviations in organ function. Disability is renamed as activity limitation, and barriers to *life opportunities* are termed barriers to *participation*. The new model provides a theoretical framework for the impact of an injury on a person. Current definitions of disability vary between various institutions that provide compensation.
   Unfortunately, this leads to confusion due to the differing definitions government and insurance have for disability. Insurance companies typically use "disabled" to imply that the person can no longer perform the "substantial and material duties of an occupation."[1] In contrast, to be disabled in the context of the Social Security Administration means that a person must be disabled for all "substantial gainful activity"[2] in order to receive benefits.

4. How are levels of disability determined?
   When a patient with low back pain (LBP) has an acute musculoskeletal back injury, we may place the patient on *temporary disability,* but it is unlikely there will be any *permanent disability*. When treatment for LBP has continued

---

[a]These terms of disablement are ubiquitous in their use and applications across the various U.S. and Canadian disability systems and hence are defined here. They have since been updated by the World Health Organization (WHO 2001) in the International Classification of Functioning, Disability and Health (ICF) in which the terms "*disability*" and "*handicap*" have been replaced by "*activity limitations*" and "*participation restrictions*," respectively. Although the ICF model is contemporary, integrated, and interactive, and conceptually robust, we have continued using the traditional terms defined above to minimize confusion in the context of workers' compensation and personal claims management and litigation.

without improvement for more than 12 months, many would consider that the patient's *temporary disability* has become a *permanent disability*. A disability rating is then required by many workers' compensation jurisdictions and will determine whether the patient's disability affects 100% of the whole person *(total disability)*, or some fraction thereof *(partial disability)*.

The terms *impairment* and *disability* are used somewhat interchangeably and incorrectly. For example, physicians may be asked in certain jurisdictions to use the *American Medical Association Guides to the Evaluation of Permanent Impairment* to provide a disability rating, although the title and introduction to the book clearly state it was intended to rate *impairment* and not *disability*. The reason is simple: different jurisdictions rate and provide compensation for physical impairments differently. There is no way the *Guides* can satisfy the rules of disability ratings in all of these different settings.

5. **How prevalent is occupational disability in Western countries?**
One must distinguish between persons with disability and people disabled from work. About 56.7 million people (19% of the population) had a disability in 2010.[3,4] The number of disabled workers grew steadily until 1978, declined slightly until 1983, started to increase again in 1984, and began to increase more rapidly beginning in 1990. The growth in the 1980s and 1990s was the result of demographic changes, a recession, and legislative changes.

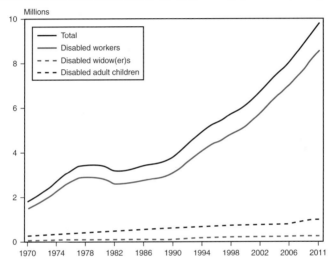

6. **What are the costs of occupational disability?**
Costs include medical expenditures, lost wages and production, consumer cost increases, employee retraining, and litigation. Alaska leads the nation in workers' compensation employer costs ($2.58 per $100 of covered wages). New York and California have seen the most dramatic increases. Extensive information about workers' compensation benefits can be found at

---

Worker's Compensation. Available at: https://www.nasi.org/wp-content/uploads/2021/10/2021-Workers-Compensation-Report-2019-Data.pdf.

7. **What is workers' compensation?**
The critical language of workers' compensation statutes is that employees must suffer "accidental... personal injury... arising out of and in the scope of employment." Using LBP as an example, this language is troublesome for the clinician. LBP is an essentially ubiquitous condition, and yet statutes indicate that LBP must arise clearly through the course of employment. A key concept in the workers' compensation statues is that of "no-fault" or "tort immunity." In exchange for the employer caring for the injured worker, the worker offers the employer tort immunity from legal suit in response to being injured. Workers' compensation usually offers the worker between 50% and 70% of preinjury wages as an incentive to return to work.[5-7]

Compensation varies greatly among states. Some states provide scheduled awards based on the physician-determined disability rating or the permanent partial loss of function of the body part or person as a whole. Others compensate in a nonscheduled fashion, as a function of the loss of the ability to be gainfully employed in a part of the workplace.

8. **How does the Social Security Administration define disability?**
Social Security is the second major system for providing a social safety net for persons with disability. For a worker to become eligible for Social Security disability benefits, the patient must have a disability defined as "the

inability to engage in any substantial gainful activity by reason of any medically determinable physical or mental impairment(s) which can be expected to result in death or which has lasted or can be expected to last for a continuous period of not less than 12 months."

9. What other groups of American workers have coverage for disability?
Although most physicians are aware of the workers' compensation statutes and Social Security disability programs, they may not be aware that there are special programs for other specific populations. Various workers, including veterans and government employees, may be protected under the *Federal Employees' Compensation Act, Longshore and Harbor Workers' Compensation Act, Veterans Administration, and Federal Employers' Liability Act.*

10. How does the physician determine if and when a patient is ready to return to work?
The physician can decide based on clinical judgment, or he or she may rely on a **functional capacity evaluation** (FCE). An FCE is simply a quantified physical ability test in which various parameters are measured over time. These parameters include how long and how much a given patient can perform in a given day in regard to strength, flexibility, endurance, lifting, carrying, pushing, pulling, bending, crawling, sitting, standing, walking, and ascending steps/ladders. These parameters are quantified in terms of weight and frequency. Terms used to modify frequency include *occasional* (typically ≤33% of the time), *frequent* (34% to 66% of the time), and *constant* (≥67% of the time). Although there is an intuitive attractiveness to FCE, there is debate over the reproducibility of these tests, as well as the degree to which they are limited by patient motivation.[8,9] An FCE in a highly cooperative patient may be of value, while a FCE in a patient with poor motivation may be expensive and often invalid. Utilizing FCEs, the physician may designate permanent restrictions for an employee and may indicate that they can return to work within certain strength requirements, ranging from sedentary work through very heavy work. These classifications are discussed in detail at: www.occupationalinfo.org/appendxc_1.html.

11. How does the *Americans with Disabilities Act* define disability?
The *Americans with Disabilities Act* (ADA) defines disability as a "physical or mental impairment that substantially limits one or more of the major life activities of the individual, or a record of such an impairment, or being regarded as having such an impairment." The ADA is intended to protect persons who can perform the essential functions of a job with reasonable accommodation. The employer may not inquire about a potential employee's impairment or medical history when the potential employee applies for a job. Upon offering the potential employee a job, a medical examination may be performed. The position may be withdrawn if the medical officer, based on receiving more information about the worker's abilities, impairments, or past medical history, feels that the particular position offered would be a direct threat to the health of the worker or those around him or her. If the worker cannot perform all aspects of a job, the employer is obligated to make a reasonable accommodation by modifying the job description, providing adaptive equipment, or offering physical assistance. Further, an accommodation which might otherwise be considered "reasonable" may be legally denied if it can be shown to pose an "undue hardship" to the employer or a "direct threat" to the health and safety of the injured worker and/or their co-workers.[10]

12. If an employee is injured on the job, how are coverage and disability determined?
If the patient is injured in a workers' compensation setting, the first task at hand is understanding the laws of the state. These can be obtained on a search of the state's website, by contacting a human resources department, or by speaking to an attorney who handles workers' compensation claims. All workers' compensation jurisdictions have "specified time limits" from date of onset to filing a claim and notifying the employer. Typically, the employer must be notified within 30 days of the illness or injury, and a claim must be filed within 1 year for disability and 2 years for death.

For most jurisdictions injuries are excluded from coverage for wage-loss benefits if they do not produce disability beyond a minimum "waiting period" which is intended to minimize administrative overhead and excessive costs for minor or "inconsequential" injuries.

Impairment and disability under workers' compensation. In Novick A, Rondinelli R, eds. *Impairment Rating and Disability Evaluation*, Philadelphia, PA: W.B. Saunders Co.; 2000:146.

State law varies on whether the employer or employee selects the clinician who will care for the "injured worker" covered under worker's compensation. Certain states, such as Florida, Minnesota, and California, have their own schedules for rating disability, and the physician should consult those statues before proceeding. Veterans are rated according to their own schedule, which can be found at: https://www.va.gov/disability/compensation-rates/veteran-rates/.

13. Is there a standard method for evaluation and documentation of physical disability?
In many jurisdictions, the physician will be asked to provide a disability rating, and the best available document to do so (and one that will often be mandated by that state's workers' compensation statute) is the *AMA Guides to the Evaluation of Permanent Impairment*.

14. **What are the AMA Guides?**

    The *Guides* began to take form in the 1950s and have evolved into a widely recognized impairment-rating document, used in 40 of 53 jurisdictions.[11] The fifth edition was published in 2001, and the sixth edition in 2009.

    The AMA Guides are not scientific documents based on demographic or epidemiologic data. It was developed with a "Delphi" panel to produce a consensus among informed experts. Although some complain of its inadequacies, it can be argued that no superior document is available. The *Guides* rate impairments (not disabilities, not schedule for compensation, not employability) for each organ system in the body.

15. **According to the *Guides*, what constitutes permanent disability?**

    A suitable period must elapse before an impairment is considered to be permanent. This is generally 12 months, according to the present *Guides*. Raters need to determine within their jurisdiction how long a patient needs to remain at his or her "therapeutic plateau" before being considered at maximal medical improvement, also called permanent and stationary.

16. **What are long-term disability insurance and Social Security?**

    At least 51 million working adults in the United States are without disability insurance other than the basic coverage available through Social Security.[12] The leading causes of long-term disability are musculoskeletal disorders, cancer, pregnancy, and mental health. An important differentiating feature among long-term disability policies is the distinction between "own occupation" versus "any occupation" coverage.
    - **Own occupation coverage** provides the insured with disability benefits (typically in the range of 60% of normal salary reimbursement to provide incentive to return to work) if they are not able to provide the essential elements of their particular job.
    - **Any occupation coverage** means, within limits, the employee would be reimbursed only if he or she could no longer perform meaningful work in any related occupation.

    Less expensive *group* long-term disability plans tend to have own occupation coverage for approximately 2 years; then the worker must be disabled from any occupation to receive further benefits. More expensive *individual* long-term disability plans tend to have more restrictive own occupation provisions.

    Social Security is the second major system for providing a social safety net for persons with a disability. In order for a worker to become eligible for social security disability benefits, the patient's disability must be defined as "the inability to engage in substantial gainful activity by reason of any medically determinable physical or mental impairments(s) that can be expected to result in death or that has lasted or can be expected to last for a continuous period of not less than 12 months." (Code of Federal Regulations §404.1505. See https://www.ssa.gov/OP_Home/cfr20/404/404-1505.htm)

17. **What are the challenges of maintaining objectivity that the independent medical examiner faces?**

    The independent medical examiner faces the significant challenge of remaining objective. If the person to be evaluated is a patient, the physician must honestly offer a disability rating in an objective fashion without being biased in the patient's interest. If a physician sees a patient at the behest of a workers' compensation carrier, insurer, or attorney who regularly refers business to the practice, the examiner must be mindful of this potential bias.

18. **When a physician is performing an independent medical exam (IME), who assumes patient care?**

    When performing an IME, the physician does not assume care of the patient. Make it clear that the evaluation is for IME purposes and that there is to be no ongoing physician–patient relationship. It is advised that the patient sign a disclosure indicating that he or she understands that the evaluation is only for the purpose of an IME and you will not be assuming care.

19. **What is the legal definition of medical probability?**

    The IME physician is asked to comment on causality. For example, "Within a reasonable degree of medical certainty, doctor, can you state that A caused B?" The real question that the attorney is asking is whether it is more likely than not ($>$50% probability) that A caused B. If the answer is yes, you are satisfying the legal requirement that it is "probably true." This is the level of certainty that the attorney is requesting. It is not the standard of "beyond a reasonable doubt" that holds in criminal cases. If the answer is that A possibly caused B, the real meaning of the statement is that it is less than likely ($<$50% probability) that A caused B. This statement suggests evidence against causality.

20. **How are benefits apportioned?**

    While impairment rating certainly presents an ethical dilemma, the concept of apportionment is additionally precarious. IME physicians may be asked, "Doctor, you felt the patient's back condition is worthy of a 20% whole person impairment. But the patient had back injuries in 1986, 1992, 1994, and 1996! How much of that 20% do you apportion to each injury?" It is safe to say that there is no scientific way to answer this question.

21. **What are the two basic types of depositions?**

    Finally, IME physicians may be asked to participate in depositions and trial appearances in their roles as expert evaluators. Depositions come in two varieties—discovery and evidentiary.

- **Discovery depositions** offer the plaintiff and defense attorneys a chance to hear what the other's experts have to say, with the intention of laying out the weight of truth for each side. The rules of evidence do not apply in discovery deposition, and the physician's testimony can be introduced into the courtroom only if it conflicts with testimony that the physician offers at the time of trial.
- In distinction, **evidentiary depositions** represent legal testimony according to the formal rules of evidence and may be videotaped in lieu of the physician appearing at trial. The physician's testimony may be read verbatim at the trial (or the videotape played) as part of the trial record.

BIBLIOGRAPHY

1. *American Medical Association: Guides to the Evaluation of Permanent Impairment.* 6th ed. Chicago, IL: American Medical Association; 2009.
2. Demeter SL, Andersson GBJ, eds. *Disability Evaluation.* St. Louis: Mosby; 2003.
3. Rondinelli R, Katz RT, eds. *Impairment Rating and Disability Evaluation.* Philadelphia, PA: W.B. Saunders; 1999.
4. *Social Security Administration Office of Disability Programs: Disability Evaluation Under Social Security.* SSA Publication Number 64–039, ICN 468600, January 2005.
5. *Fact Sheet: Social Security.* Available at: https://www.ssa.gov/news/press/factsheets/basicfact-alt.pdf

REFERENCES

1. What is own-occupation disability insurance? Available at: https://www.policygenius.com/disability-insurance/own-occupation-disability-insurance/#what-is-a-definition-of-disability
2. *Disability Benefits. How You Qualify.* Available at: https://www.ssa.gov/planners/disability/qualify.html#anchor3
3. *Nearly 1 in 5 People Have a Disability in the U.S., Census Bureau Reports. Report Released to Coincide with 22nd Anniversary of the ADA.* Available at: https://www.census.gov/newsroom/releases/archives/miscellaneous/cb12-134.html
4. *Annual Statistical Report on the Social Security Disability Insurance Program.* 2011. Available at: https://www.ssa.gov/policy/docs/statcomps/di_asr/2011/sect01.html
5. *Temporary Disability Benefits.* Available at: https://www.dir.ca.gov/dwc/TemporaryDisability.htm
6. *Workers' Compensation Commission.* Available at: http://www.wcc.state.md.us/gen_info/wcc_benefits.html
7. *Alabama Department of Labor.* Available at: https://labor.alabama.gov/wc/faq.aspx
8. Reneman MF, Roelofs M, Schiphorst Preuper HR. Reliability and agreement of neck functional capacity evaluation tests in patients with chronic multifactorial neck pain. *Arch Phys Med Rehabil.* 2017;98(7):1476–1479.
9. De Baets S, Calders P, Schalley N, et al. Updating the evidence on functional capacity evaluation methods: a systematic review. *J Occup Rehabil.* 2018;28:418. Available at: https://doi.org/10.1007/s10926-017-9734-x
10. *Reasonable Accommodations in the Workplace.* Available at: https://adata.org/factsheet/reasonable-accommodations-workplace
11. *AMA Guides.* Available at: https://www.amaguides.com/
12. *Disability Statistics.* Available at: http://disabilitycanhappen.org/disability-statistic/
13. Impairment and disability under workers' compensation. In Novick A, Rondinelli RD, eds. *Impairment Rating and Disability Evaluation.* W.B. Saunders Co.; 2000:146.

CHAPTER 83

PERFORMING ARTS REHABILITATION: HARMONIC PERFORMER ORCHESTRATIONS

Scott E. Brown, MD, and Steven A. Stiens, MD, MS

Great art is as irrational as great music. It is made with its own loveliness.
— George Jean Nathan (1882–1958)

KEY POINTS: REHABILITATION OF THE PERFORMING ARTIST

1. Performer-centered methods include specific anatomical and functional diagnostic assessment.
2. Environmental ergonomic considerations are critical.
3. Severity is measured as well as methods modified.
4. Strength and endurance for performance is developed with specific exercises.
5. The greatest number of injuries among university-level student musicians are seen with piano, guitar, and harp players.
6. The female athlete triad includes disordered eating, amenorrhea, and osteoporosis.

1. **What is arts medicine and how can rehabilitation principles be applied?**
   Performing arts medicine dates back to the 1713 treatise of Bernardino Ramazzini titled "Diseases of Tradesmen" summarizing the occupational diseases of musicians. Contemporary interdisciplinary practice includes occupa-tional, rehabilitation, orthopedic, sports, podiatric, and otolaryngology medical methods. They collaborate with specialized therapists, trainers, and educators achieving performer-centered holistic care. This requires a preven-tive, primary, and rehabilitative practice that is informed with contemporary interventions customized to enhance artists' performance and minimize complications.

   Dawson WJ, Charness M, Goode DJ, et al. What's in a name?-terminologic issues in performing arts medicine. *Med Probl Perform Art.* 1998;13:45–50.

2. **Are performing artists really injured in the line of duty? How many artists are injured by performing their art? What is the rate of injury for performing artists in music and in dance?**
   In a survey of the members of the International Conference of Symphony and Opera Musicians, 76% reported having had at least one medical problem severe enough to interfere with performance, and 36% reported four severe prob-lems. A recent review of the literature concludes that the lifetime prevalence of injuries that impair performance of professional musicians is between 62% and 93%. The annual incidence of injury in student musicians is 5.7% for men and 11.5% for women at conservatories. In some studies, injuries have affected as many as 90% of dancers.

   Brandfonbrener AG. Special issues in the medical assessment of musicians. *Phys Med Rehab Clin No Amer.* 2006;17(4);147–753.

3. **What are the special considerations in the diagnosis and treatment of a musician?**
   Injured musicians often expect a greater level of expertise from their doctors in specificity of diagnosis and treat-ment. A music medicine history should include a detailed performance history including age began playing, what instruments and genres played, average usual time spent playing, recent change in playing time and/or technique, and upcoming performance demands.

   If possible, musicians should be **examined while playing their instrument**. Although most patients will be able to bring their instruments to the examination, a piano is needed in the office for pianists. Problems with **embouchure (**the position of the lips and mouth in playing a wind or brass instrument), focal dystonia, and ergonomic and other technical problems will be missed if the musician is not examined while playing. **Videotaping** in the office as well as during rehearsal and performance can be a helpful adjunct. A thorough but directed musculoskeletal and neurologic exam should be undertaken. Underlying medical problems may present earlier in musicians, who are more sensitive to the functional effects of minor impairment early in the course of disease. A careful search for contractures and tendon anomalies should be done, especially in string and wind instrument players. A common problem that can cause difficulties in the left hand of violin players and the right hand of clarinet players is the **conjoined flexor sublimis tendons** of the small and ring fingers. Other specific problems for which to examine include **hypermobility**, hand span, **dyscoordination** and uneven playing**, muscle tension**, and excessive gripping or pressure on the instrument.

Teacher involvement in student musician's care is essential, especially in non-operative management, which can include a modified playing schedule and instrument and technique modifications. A working knowledge of musical terminology as well as biomechanical demands of different instruments is helpful to communicate effectively with the musician and their teacher to ensure the modifications are feasible and increase compliance with treatment.

Dommerholt J. Performing arts medicine—instrumentalist musicians part I—general considerations. *J Bodyw Mov Ther*. 2009;13(4): 311–319. DOI: 10.1016/j.jbmt.2009.02.003

4. What areas should be included in the biomechanical evaluation of dancers?
   - Upper **body alignment** and center of gravity position **(plumb line)**
   - Lumbar range of motion (ROM)
   - Pelvic tilt and lumbar lordosis
   - Hip joint internal and external rotation with the hip in neutral (0 degrees flexion or extension)
   - Femoral anteversion or retroversion
   - Hamstring flexibility
   - Q angle
   - Tibial torsion
   - Toe out
   - Ankle ROM
   - Foot pronation
   - First metatarsophalangeal (MTP) joint ROM

     As with musicians, it is often necessary to see the dancer demonstrating basic movements such as the five basic foot positions, **plie, pointe,** and leg **"extension"** (actually forward flexion in turned out position). The **pointe position** permits analysis of **toe shoe and insert fit and function.**

5. What are the common nerve entrapments seen in musicians?
   Carpal tunnel syndrome, **ulnar neuropathy at the elbow**, and **thoracic outlet syndrome** present most often. A few retrospective studies suggest that **left arm entrapment syndromes**, specifically ulnar neuropathy at the elbow is predominant in string players most likely due to playing position that involves sustained elbow flexion and repetitive loading of the flexor carpi ulnaris muscle. Studies suggest that electrodiagnostic studies can be normal in symptomatic compressive peripheral neuropathies in musicians, especially in ulnar neuropathy early in the disease course.

   No commonly agreed upon diagnostic criteria exist for **thoracic outlet syndrome.** The most common pattern of involvement is entrapment of the lower most nerves of the brachial plexus, resulting in the symptom complex of numbness and tingling in the medial forearm and the small and ring fingers. Most instruments are held or played in front of the body, which potentially tightens the anterior chest and neck muscles. The resulting symptoms, suggestive of **medial cord entrapment,** may involve some nonaxonotmetic process or may only be a referred symptom. The neurologic examination and electro-diagnostic studies usually appear normal. If a **focal dystonia** is recognized, a thorough search for an associated **entrapment neuropathy** should be undertaken as pain and partial denervation of muscles can be contributory.

Dommerholt J. Performing arts medicine—instrumentalist musicians, part II—examination. *J Bodyw Mov Ther*. 2010 January;14(1): 65–72. doi: 10.1016/j.jbmt.2009.02.004.

Wilson RJ, Watson JT, Lee DH. Nerve entrapment syndromes in musicians. *Clin Anat*. 2014;27(6):861–865.

6. What are the most and least dangerous instruments? Can music rehabilitation medicine detect dissonance and harmonize interventions?
   Highest injury rates in university-level student musicians seem to be with piano, guitar, and harp. Intermediate risk includes the bowed strings, percussion, clarinet, saxophone, flute, and organ. Lower risk appears to include all brass instruments, the oboe, and the bassoon.

Cayea D, Manchester RA. Instrument-specific rates of upper-extremity injuries in music students. *Med Probl Perform Art*. 1998;13: 19–25.

Dommerholt J. Performing arts medicine—instrumentalist musicians: part III—case histories. *J Bodyw Mov Ther*. 2010;14(2): 127–138. DOI: 10.1016/j.jbmt.2009.02.005.

7. What is meant by "overuse" in performing artists?

Overuse practice is an activity in which anatomically normal structures have been used in a so-called normal manner, but to a degree that has exceeded their biologic limits. **Overuse syndromes** are the pathologic changes that may result from overuse practices and symptomatology depends on the tissues affected and the degree and type of damage (i.e., inflammation, fatigue, structural change). Many of the commonly used synonyms for overuse (i.e., repetitive stress injury) combine cause and effect into a single entity rather than considering them as separate events, which in turn reduces diagnostic precision.

Kok LM, Huisstede BM, Voorn VM, et al. The occurrence of musculoskeletal complaints among professional musicians: a systematic review. *Int Arch Occup Environ Health.* 2016;89(3):373–396.

8. A professional opera singer reports a history of hoarseness (a sense of something stuck in upper throat), vocal fatigue, dysphoria, and coughing up thin mucus after a night in the bar followed by a midnight meal of hot chili. What is the differential diagnosis leading into your acute, rehabilitation, and preventive management?

The history suggests **laryngopharyngeal reflux (LPR)** due to recumbent position after eating. Visualization of the vocal folds reveal mild edema and redness. Treatment includes antacids before bedtime and a short course of proton pump inhibitors, with voice rest, and education in **vocal hygiene** (maintaining hydration and moistness of vocal folds). History of sudden voice change with extreme volume of overuse and evidence of vocal fold ecchymoses suggests the emergency of **vocal fold hemorrhage** requiring voice rest and ENT consultation. **Singer's voice quality** can be followed with **Handicap Index** (VHI, **Singing VHI**) and **Reflux Symptom Index (RSI)**.

Franco RA, Andrus JG. Common diagnoses and treatments in professional voice users. *Otolaryngol Clinic N Amer.* 2007;40:1025–1061.

9. Is there consensus opinion regarding assessing readiness to dance en pointe?

There is no universally agreed on protocol for assessing readiness to start pointe work. For serious dancers, this transition likely occurs in early adolescence. The **Relevé Endurance Test** and **Airplane Test** have shown statistical differences between pointe and pre-pointe students, indicating calf muscle endurance rather than absolute strength as well as balance may be predictive of pointe readiness.

DeWolf A, McPherson A, Besong K, et al. Quantitative measures utilized in determining pointe readiness in young ballet dancers. *J Dance Med Sci.* 2018;22(4):209–217.

10. What is turnout?

Turnout refers to the total amount of external rotation of both lower extremities. Ideally, most of a dancer's turnout should come from true external rotation at the hip joint. The ideal classical ballet aesthetic stresses 180 degrees of turnout, which would require the dancer to have 90 degrees at each hip. This rarely occurs, and in order to meet expectations of teachers and company directors in attaining the 180 degrees, the dancer has to cheat biomechanically. The **biomechanical evaluation** (Question 3) helps break down the components of turnout. Turnout may be improved using isolated joint stretch and myofascial release techniques.

Lohr C, Schmidt T. Turnout in classical dance: is it possible to enhance the external rotation of the lower limb by a myofascial manipulation? A pilot study. *J Dance Med Sci.* 2017;21(4):168–178.

Air ME, Grierson MJ, Davenport KL, et al. Dissecting the doctor–dancer relationship: health care decision making among American Collegiate dancers. *PM R.* 2014;6(3):241–249.

11. How is the female athlete triad relevant to dancers?

In June 2017, The American College of Obstetrics and Gynecology committee on Adolescent Health Care updated their recommendations for assessment and treatment of the **triad**: (1) **low energy availability** with or without disordered eating, (2) **menstrual dysfunction**, and (3) **low bone density**. They noted dancers are at the highest risk with a prevalence of secondary amenorrhea of up to 69%, and low bone density up to 50%. Disordered eating is a common response to the pressures of meeting an aesthetic ideal of thinness. Exercise and anorexia produce a state of **hypothalamic hypogonadism**. Decreased ovarian hormone production and **hypoestrogenemia** result from hypothalamic amenorrhea, which ultimately produces osteoporosis. If even one component of the triad is detected, a high index of suspicion for osteoporosis and other less obvious medical sequelae, such as arrhythmias, depression, and stress fractures, must be considered. Strategic management includes synergistic multimodal interdisciplinary rehabilitation designs with focus on the pathophysiology, impairments, performance, and health outcomes.

American College of Obstetricians and Gynecologists, Committee on Adolescent health Care. *Female Athletic Triad*. Available at: https://www.acog.org/Clinical-Guidance-and-Publications/Committee-Opinions/Committee-on-Adolescent-Health-Care/Female-Athlete-Triad?IsMobileSet=false

12. Who is Pilates?

Joseph Pilates (1883–1967) was a German athlete who initially developed a philosophy of physical conditioning as he rehabilitated German soldiers after World War I. His approach incorporated physical exercise and stressed the mind–body interaction. After coming to the United States in the 1920s, he opened an innovative studio that quickly became popular with dancers. His program allowed jumping and other analogous dance activities to be performed supine (gravity eliminated). This program continues to be popular in the dance world for cross-training and injury rehabilitation. His example is an aspiration for rehabilitation teams designing custom treatment programs for each performer.

13. What is the differential diagnosis of groin pain in a dancer?

A clunk or pop, often described as a feeling of the hip joint coming out of place, occurs when the **iliopsoas** snaps across the **iliopectineal** eminence, especially when the flexed, abducted, externally rotated hip returns to the neutral position. Other causes of hip/groin pain include a torn acetabular labrum, femoral neck stress fracture, adductor strain (as can occur during momentum transfers in pirouette), rectus femoris tendinitis, and myofascial pain, especially in a poorly trained dancer who incorrectly uses the rectus femoris to raise the leg forward.

14. Can dancers return to dance after platelet-rich plasma (PRP) injections?

Numerous conditions of the lower extremities have been treated with PRP including various tendinopathies, plantar fascia problems, and first MTP joint capsule. In a small study of elite dancers, following ultrasound-guided injection and strict adherence to post-injection protocols, most were able to return to asymptomatic and unrestricted dance in 6 months or less. Foot and ankle conditions most often required a protracted recovery with rehabilitation, and in some, a second injection.

Jain N, Bauman PA, Hamilton WG, et al. Can Elite dancers return to dance after ultrasound-guided platelet-rich plasma (PRP) injections? *J Dance Med Sci.* 2018;22(4):225–232.

WEBSITES

1. Performing Arts Medicine Association (PAMA). www.artsmed.org
2. International Association for Dance Medicine and Science. Available at: www.iadms.org

BOOKS

Sataloff RT, Brandfonbrener AG, Lederman RJ, eds. *Performing Arts Medicine.* 3rd ed. Narberth, PA: Science & Medicine; 2010.
Ryan AJ, Stephens RE. *Dance Medicine: A Comprehensive Guide.* Chicago, IL: Pluribus Press; 1987.
Rose CF. *Neurology of the Arts.* London, UK: Imperial College Press; 2004:433.

BIBLIOGRAPHY

Dawson WJ. Performing arts medicine-a bibliographic retrospective of the early literature: an historical examination of bibliographic references pre-1975. *Med Probl Perform Art.* 2013;28(1):47–53.
Manchester RA. Globalization of performing arts medicine. *Med Probl Perform Art.* 2007;22(4):133–135.

HEALTH POLICY, LEGISLATION, AND REIMBURSEMENT: IMPORTANT FACETS OF PHYSIATRIC PRACTICE

Sam S. H. Wu, MD, MA, MPH, MBA, Peter Thomas, JD, Sergey Filatov, MD, Leela Baggett, JD, and Leighton Chan, MD

CHAPTER 84

For he who has health has hope; and he who has hope, has everything.
— Owen Arthur (1949–2020)

KEY POINTS

1. There are more than 1 billion persons with disability worldwide, and nearly 200 million of them experience significant functional deficits.
2. The Americans with Disabilities Act of 1990 prohibits discrimination based on disability in employment, state and local governments, places of public accommodation, transportation, and telecommunications.
3. The Individuals with Disabilities Education Act provides free appropriate public education to eligible children with disabilities and ensures special education and related services to those children.
4. Medicare provides payments to help cover the costs of approved residency programs.

1. **What is the difference between impairment, disability, and participation?**
   Impairment is a diminished or loss of a body structure or function.
   Disability is a diminished or loss of ability to engage in the performance of major life activities due to *mental or physical* impairment.
   Participation is the ability to fulfill roles such as employment and it is impacted by impairment and disability.

2. **What is the World Report on Disability and why is it important?**
   Published in 2011 by World Health Organization (WHO), the World Report on Disability emphasized that "More than one billion people in the world live with some form of disability, of whom nearly 200 million experience considerable difficulties in functioning."
   According to Professor Stephen W. Hawking in the Foreword, "This report makes a major contribution to our understanding of disability and its impact on individuals and society. It highlights the different barriers that people with disabilities face—attitudinal, physical, and financial... In fact, we have a moral duty to remove the barriers to participation, and to invest sufficient funding and expertise to unlock the vast potential of people with disabilities."
   The report also contains concrete recommendations for policy and practice to improve the lives of persons with disability.

3. **Why should physiatrists get involved in advocacy?**
   Physiatrists offer a unique perspective in advancing public policies that improve access to quality rehabilitation services. As leaders of the rehabilitation team, physiatrists can speak to the clinical implications of such policy proposals that will either harm or advance patient care from a physician's perspective. Physiatrists are well positioned to discuss the clinical literature as well as the real-world patient implications of these policies being considered by decision makers.

4. **What is the Americans with Disabilities Act of 1990 (ADA) and why is it important?**
   The ADA is a landmark civil rights law that prohibits discrimination based on disability in employment, state and local governments, places of public accommodation, transportation, and telecommunications. The precursor of the ADA is the Rehabilitation Act of 1973 which prohibits discrimination based on disability in the federal government as well as federal grantees and contractors. Together, these laws provide comprehensive federal protection against disability discrimination and have become model laws replicated by countries around the world. Along with changing legal standards, these laws have had the effect of changing attitudes about persons with disabilities. The ADA and other key disabilities laws are based on fundamental principles of fairness including equality of opportunity, full participation, independent living, and economic self-sufficiency.
   One issue with the ADA is its omission of comprehensive disability protections applicable to private health insurance. However, Title V of the ADA does lay the foundation for equal access to health benefits in employment.

Employers must provide equal access to health benefits to all employees, with or without disabilities, who are similarly situated (e.g., full-time versus part-time employment). Employers may make certain distinctions among employees for risk classification purposes if those distinctions do not act as a "subterfuge" to evade the purposes of the ADA. Disability-based distinctions that single out a particular disability or disability overall are prohibited. Comprehensive disability discrimination protections in private health insurance would not become federal law until 2010 with enactment of the Patient Protection and Affordable Care Act (ACA).

5. How does the ACA affect persons with disabilities?

The precursor to the ACA was enactment in 1996 of the Health Insurance Portability and Accountability Act (HIPAA), which prohibited discrimination based on health status in large group and employer-provided health plans. However, the small group and individual insurance market continued to permit discrimination based on health status, which was responsible for some of the most egregious practices of health insurers to reduce risk and avoid covering individuals with a wide variety of health conditions.

ACA created a set of federal standards for private small group and individual market health insurance which prohibits discrimination based on health status, medical condition, or history, claims experience, genetic information, disability, or evidence of insurability. ACA guarantees issue and renewability of health insurance, prohibits rescission of health insurance policies, bans pre-existing condition exclusions as well as lifetime and annual caps in insurance benefits, limits factors that can impact premium rating, and creates an essential health benefits package that includes coverage of rehabilitative and habilitative services and durable medical equipment (DME) as well as physician, hospital, and related health care services.

These improvements in health insurance practices greatly benefit all individuals particularly those with disabilities, chronic conditions, and other diagnoses where insurance plans routinely denied coverage in the past. Under the ACA, even individuals with the most disabling conditions are guaranteed access to coverage of essential benefits, including rehabilitation services, with premiums that are community-rated with no arbitrary caps in benefits. In addition, individuals who cannot afford premiums under ACA exchanges can obtain federal subsidies to purchase insurance or join Medicaid programs in states that have chosen to expand coverage of the uninsured.

6. What is the difference between Medicare and Medicaid?

Medicare is a federal public health insurance program that provides benefits to individuals who are age 65 or older, have end-stage renal disease, or qualify on the basis of disability. In 2019, the Medicare program covered 61.5 million people, with Medicare expenditures totaling approximately $799.4 billion.

Medicare is divided into four distinct parts: Part A, B, C, and D. Medicare Part A covers inpatient hospital services, home health services, skilled nursing facility services, and hospice care. Inpatient rehabilitation services provided to Medicare fee-for-service beneficiaries are paid under Medicare Part A. Most Medicare beneficiaries are automatically enrolled in Part A and do not pay premiums. Medicare Part B is a voluntary program that covers the services of physicians, outpatient clinic visits, and ancillary items and services, such as x-rays, laboratory tests, DME, prostheses, orthoses and certain drugs. Beneficiaries are responsible for paying monthly premiums and co-payments for Medicare Part B items and services. Medicare Part C, also known as "Medicare Advantage," is an optional managed care program. Under Medicare Part C, the Centers for Medicare and Medicaid Services (CMS) contracts with qualifying private organizations to administer benefits that would otherwise be covered under Medicare Parts A and B and usually Part D. In 2018, approximately 36% of Medicare beneficiaries were enrolled in Medicare Part C plans. Medicare Part D is voluntary and requires premium payments and cost sharing for coverage of medically necessary outpatient prescription drugs. In addition, private insurance companies offer "Medigap" or supplemental health insurance policies to help pay the costs of care not covered by fee-for-service Medicare.

In contrast, **Medicaid** is a medical assistance program that is funded jointly by the federal government and the states and is designed for individuals with low incomes. According to February 2019 Medicaid data, Medicaid covers approximately 65.6 million individuals. Federal law requires Medicaid to provide health coverage to low-income families, children, pregnant women, seniors, and persons with disabilities. The ACA permits states to expand Medicaid to individuals under age 65 solely based on low-income status. According to the Henry J. Kaiser Family Foundation, as of May 2019, 36 states and the District of Columbia have adopted Medicaid expansion under the ACA. States also have the option to cover additional groups of individuals. Federal law requires state Medicaid programs to cover the cost of certain "mandatory services" and offers states flexibility to cover additional services designated as "optional services." All states may also apply for waivers of certain Federal Medicaid requirements in order to cover specific subgroups of individuals. Accordingly, Medicaid coverage varies widely from state to state.

Low-income seniors and individuals with disabilities may qualify for both Medicare and Medicaid and are referred to as "dual eligibles."

7. What US federal legislation mandates education for children with disabilities?

In 1975, Congress passed the Education for All Handicapped Children Act, now known as the Individuals with Disabilities Education Act (IDEA) which "makes available a free appropriate public education to eligible children with disabilities throughout the nation and ensures special education and related services to those children."

The intent of IDEA is to promote the "mainstreaming" of children with disabilities into regular classrooms, which improves the education of both disabled and nondisabled students. However, "mainstreaming" is not appropriate for all children with disabilities, and for some individuals a more controlled setting may represent the "least restrictive environment." Although not directly involved in creating the Individual Education Plan (IEP) produced by the school district for the educational goals of each student with disabilities, the physiatrist can be very helpful in (1) identifying children who might be candidates for educational assistance; (2) providing written guidance to the school concerning the educational impact of the disability; and (3) outlining a child's health maintenance activities, such as medication prescriptions, urinary catheterization, and g-tube feedings, as well as writing therapy orders.

8. **What is workers compensation?**
Workers compensation is a type of insurance purchased by employers to provide replacement of wages and medical benefits to employees injured in the course of employment. By using workers compensation benefits, employees surrender the right to sue their employer for negligence and tort. Benefits vary among insurances and may include wage replacement, compensation for the past and future losses, and reimbursement for medical expenses.

Patients with workers compensation typically arrive with their case workers to health care appointments. Case workers are liaisons between the patient and the insurance company. The patient can choose to have or not to have their case manager in the exam room during an appointment. However, the workers compensation insurance company will have access to that patient's medical records.

The goal of rehabilitation within workers compensation is to return the injured workers to the functional level which would allow them to return to their previous duties. If a patient is not able to resume the previous duties, the workers compensation will either be required to provide alternative training or pay out compensation. Usually, workers compensation has comprehensive coverage for treatment options.

9. **What is supplemental security income (SSI) and social security disability insurance (SSDI)?**
There are two major federal programs to provide income assistance to individuals with disabilities: SSI and SSDI.

SSI is linked to the Medicaid system and provides financial assistance to low-income individuals who are elderly, blind, or disabled. To qualify on the basis of disability, a person must be "unable to engage in any substantial gainful activity by reason of a medically determined physical or mental impairment expected to result in death or that has lasted or can be expected to last for a continuous period of at least 12 months." SSI determination for children is different and based on a categorical definition of disability.

SSDI is similar to SSI, but the benefits are more generous. In addition, it is linked to the Medicare program. To be eligible for SSDI benefits, the person must have worked and paid into the Social Security system. Applicants for SSDI must meet a definition of disability similar to that for SSI. Physician assessment is required when a person cannot work or is ready to return to work. Eligibility is reevaluated approximately every 3 years.

10. **How are post-acute care services reimbursed?**
Post-acute care consists of rehabilitation or palliative services that are rendered after, or in certain cases instead of, an acute care hospital stay. The providers of these services generally include long-term acute care hospitals (LTACHs), inpatient rehabilitation facilities (IRFs), skilled nursing facilities (SNFs), and home health agencies (HHAs). Medicare pays for post-acute care services under separate prospective payment systems specific to each setting of care. The Medicare rates differ under each prospective payment system to reflect the level of resources necessary to serve each patient in these various settings. Under the IRF and LTACH prospective payment systems, Medicare pays a predetermined amount per discharge for services provided to Medicare Part A beneficiaries. Under the SNF prospective payment system, Medicare provides "a per diem payment of a predetermined rate for inpatient services furnished to Medicare beneficiaries." Under the home health prospective payment system, HHAs receive "a unit of payment equal to a national, standardized prospective 60-day episode payment amount" for episodes beginning on or before December 31, 2019. For periods beginning on or after January 1, 2020, Medicare pays HHAs "a unit of payment equal to a national, standardized prospective 30-day payment amount."

According to the Medicare Payment Advisory Commission ("MedPAC"), an independent legislative branch agency that advises Congress on the Medicare program, the Medicare fee-for-service program spent nearly $60 billion on post-acute care services in 2017. MedPAC has been working on post-acute care payment reform for more than a decade. MedPAC believes that the fee-for-service Medicare program overpays for post-acute care services and that there should be equity in payment across all post-acute care settings. MedPAC continues to explore the design of a unified post-acute care prospective payment system that would be based on the patient's characteristics rather than the setting of care. Such a system, proponents argue, would remove the silos of post-acute care, enable providers to be more efficient in providing services to patients as they move through the post-acute care continuum, and enable stakeholders to compare quality, costs, and patient outcomes across the four main settings of post-acute care.

11. **What governmental programs fund physician residency programs in the US?**
Medicare is the largest payer of resident education in the United States. The type of Medicare payment, however, depends on the type of health care provider furnishing resident education. Certain health care providers, such as SNFs, do not receive any residency education-related payments from Medicare. For inpatient prospective payment system hospitals, Medicare provides two types of payments to help cover the costs of approved residency programs: (1) direct graduate medical education (DGME) payments and (2) indirect medical education (IME) payments.

Approved residency programs are those that are approved by Accreditation Council on Graduate Medical Education, American Osteopathic Association, American Dental Association, or American Podiatric Medical Association.

Medicare provides DGME payments to compensate hospitals for costs directly related to running an approved residency program. These costs include the salaries and fringe benefits of residents and teaching physicians, overhead costs associated with the residency program, and other direct costs. DGME payments are separate pass-through payments. Medicare calculates DGME payments, in part, by multiplying the hospital's "approved amount" times the hospital's Medicare "patient load" which is the "fraction of the total number of inpatient-bed-days... during the period which are attributable to patients with respect to whom payment may be made under" Medicare part A. The "approved amount" is calculated by multiplying the hospital's approved full-time equivalent (FTE) resident amount for the cost reporting period by the weighted average number of FTE residents (as determined according to the DGME statute). For cost reporting periods beginning on or after October 1, 1997, Medicare statute imposes a cap on the number of allopathic and osteopathic FTE residents that may be counted for purposes of determining DGME payments. For more information on the DGME payment methodology, please refer to 42 U.S.C. § 1395ww(h) and 42 C.F.R. §§ 413.75-413.83.

Medicare also provides IME payment to compensate hospitals for higher operating costs incurred due to supporting an approved residency program. Unlike DGME payments, IME payments are percentage add-on payments to the Medicare severity diagnosis related groups (MS-DRG) payment. Medicare calculates IME payments through a formula that reflects the number of FTE interns and residents, the number of a hospital's beds, a measurement factor for teaching activity, and a statutory IME multiplier. Similar to DGME payments, for discharges occurring on or after October 1, 1997, Medicare imposes a cap on the number of allopathic and osteopathic FTE interns and residents that may be counted for purposes of IME payments. For more information on the IME payment methodology, please refer to 42 U.S.C. § 1395ww(d)(5)(B) and 42 C.F.R. § 412.105.

IRF that are teaching institutions or units of teaching institutions receive a "teaching status adjustment" for discharges on or after October 1, 2005, in addition to DGME payments. The teaching status adjustment modifies the IRF prospective payment by a factor specified by CMS. The teaching status adjustment accounts for the higher indirect operating costs experienced by facilities that participate in graduate medical education programs.

Other federal and state programs provide graduate medical education funding, including the Department of Defense, the Department of Veterans Affairs, Medicaid, and the Health Resources and Services Administration.

BIBLIOGRAPHY

About IDEA. Available at: https://sites.ed.gov/idea/about-idea/#IDEA-History; Accessed on April 16, 2021.

Benefits for People with Disabilities. Available at: https://www.ssa.gov/disability/; Accessed on April 16, 2021.

MDCR ENROLL AB 1 Total Medicare Enrollment: Total, Original Medicare, and Medicare Advantage and Other Health Plan Enrollment, Calendar Years 2014–2019 (cms.gov). Available at: https://www.cms.gov/files/document/2019cpsmdcrenrollab1.pdf; Accessed on April 18, 2021.

Medicare Program; Inpatient Rehabilitation Facility Prospective Payment System for FY 2006, 70 Fed. Reg. 47,880, 47,928 (August 15, 2005).

MedPAC. *March 2019 Report to the Congress: Medicare Payment Policy.* Available at: https://www.medpac.gov/document/march-2019-report-to-the-congress-medicare-payment-policy/; Accessed August 14, 2022.

MedPAC. *Post-Acute Care,* Available at: http://www.medpac.gov/-research-areas-/post-acute-care#; Accessed April 16, 2021.

NHE Fact Sheet. Available at: https://www.cms.gov/Research-Statistics-Data-and-Systems/Statistics-Trends-and-Reports/NationalHealthExpendData/NHE-Fact-Sheet#:~:text=Historical%20NHE%2C%202019%3A%201%20NHE%20grew%204.6%25%20to,16%20percent%20of%20total%20NHE.%20More%20items...%20; Accessed on April 18, 2021.

The Board of Trustees, Federal Hospital Insurance and Federal Supplementary Medical Insurance Trust Funds. *2019 Annual Report of the Board of Trustees of the Federal Hospital Insurance and Federal Supplementary Medical Insurance Trust Funds,* 6 (April 22, 2019). Available at: https://www.cms.gov/Research-Statistics-Data-and-Systems/Statistics-Trends-and-Reports/ReportsTrustFunds/Downloads/TR2019.pdf; Accessed April 16, 2021.

World Report on Disability. Available at: https://www.who.int/teams/noncommunicable-diseases/sensory-functions-disability-and-rehabilitation/world-report-on-disability; Accessed on April 16, 2021.

INTERNATIONAL PHYSICAL MEDICINE AND REHABILITATION: GLOBAL SYNERGY AND COLLABORATION TO MAXIMIZE REHABILITATION POTENTIAL

Bryan J. O'Young, MD, CAc, FAAPMR, Sam S. H. Wu, MD, MA, MPH, MBA, Jorge Lains, MD, Carlotte Kiekens, MD, Fary Khan, MD, MBBS, FAFRM (RACP), Rochelle Coleen Tan Dy, MD, Dongfeng Huang, MD, Mark A. Young, MD, MBA, FACP, FAAPMR, DABPMR, Filipinas G. Ganchoon, MD, DPBRM, FPARM, and Akiko Ito, LLM, LLB, MA

Physiatrists can make the world a better place and create a better tomorrow.

Haim Ring (1944–2008)

(Ring H. International rehabilitation medicine: Closing the gaps and globalization of the profession. *Am J Phys Med Rehabil.* 2004; 83(9):667–669 [invited editorial]).

KEY POINTS

1. International rehabilitation medicine allows the synergistic exchange of ideas and resources among nations and cultures, strengthens scientific knowledge, and increases and disseminates research in rehabilitation.
2. Rehabilitation is not only for people with long-term or physical impairments. Instead, it is a *core health service* for anyone with an acute or chronic health condition that limits functioning and should be available for anyone who needs it.
3. "Historic" health indicators, ***morbidity*** and ***mortality***, no longer adequately respond to health needs. Hence, ***functioning*** became a crucial health indicator and was introduced in WHO's *International Classification of Functioning, Disability, and Health* (ICF) to identify the dimensions of the functional impact of health conditions on an individual's experience in the context of their life.
4. The collaboration of international societies of rehabilitation professionals with the United Nations and the World Health Organization is essential to strengthening rehabilitation worldwide.
5. You and all PM&R practitioners should be involved in international PM&R.

1. **What is international physical medicine and rehabilitation (PM&R)?**
   It is a term to broadly describe the specialty of Physical Medicine and Rehabilitation (PM&R) as practiced in each nation and ***collaborating*** with other nations on a global scale. The specialty of PM&R has steadily gained international recognition because of its unique and essential role in assisting people with disabilities or disabling health conditions gain greater functional independence in the face of aging and disease. International physical medicine and rehabilitation involves a synergistic exchange of ideas and resources among different nations and cultures. It focuses on strengthening scientific knowledge, increasing and disseminating research in PM&R, providing humanitarian rehabilitation assistance, and optimizing the quality of life for persons with disabilities.

   Participation in international rehabilitation medicine organizations leads to a broader and more enlightened view of the world. Traveling physiatrists acquire a keen understanding of the world and develop a transcendent sense of caring by experiencing, learning, teaching, and sharing. Rehabilitation medicine is internationally recognized because of its unique and vital role in helping those with disabilities. International rehabilitation medicine allows the synergistic exchange of ideas and resources among nations and cultures, strengthens scientific knowledge, and increases and disseminates research in rehabilitation.

Ring H. International rehabilitation medicine: Closing the gaps and globalization of the profession. *Am J Phys Med Rehabil.* 2004; 83(9):667–669. doi: 10.1097/00002060-200409000-00001

2. Why is this issue important?

PM&R is a unique and vitally important medical specialization that helps facilitate care for people with disabilities. Disability is a "universal feature of the human condition, and everyone will experience or is at risk of experiencing limitations of capacity and performance problems in one or several domains of functioning." Health is complete physical, mental, and social well-being and not merely the absence of disease or infirmity.

Rehabilitation Medicine is the answer for those experiencing some form of limitation in functioning. Internationalization and international cooperation are essential to achieve the United Nations' Sustainable Development Goal 3: Ensure healthy lives and promote well-being for all ages.

The health of the world's population is steadily improving. Global life expectancy at birth is dramatically increasing. Communicable, maternal, neonatal, and nutritional (CMNN) diseases are decreasing, and non-communicable diseases are increasing. As a result, global life expectancy at birth and chronic diseases are increasing rapidly. Currently, in high-level SDI (Socio-Demographic Index) countries, the main concern is not premature mortality but functional health loss.

The Universal Health Coverage Collaborators demonstrated lagging performance on effective coverage indicators for non-communicable diseases and that many health systems are not keeping pace with the rising non-communicable disease burden and associated population health needs.

The "historic" health indicators **morbidity** and **mortality** no longer adequately respond to health needs. Hence**, functioning** became a crucial health indicator and was introduced in the World Health Organization (WHO)'s *International Classification of Functioning, Disability, and Health* (ICF) to identify the dimensions of the functional impact of health conditions on an individual's experience in the context of their life. Rehabilitation Medicine is the answer for those experiencing some form of limitation in functioning. Internationalization and International Cooperation are essential to achieve the UN's Sustainable Development Goal 3: Ensure healthy lives and promote well-being for all at all ages.

3. What resources are needed?

About 2.4 billion people are currently living with a health condition that would benefit from rehabilitation. Therefore, rehabilitation is an essential part of universal health coverage, along with promoting good health.

Rehabilitation is an integral component of health services; it must be effectively integrated into the health system, and the ministry of health is the appropriate agency for governing rehabilitation. Efforts must be made to increase the quality, accessibility, and affordability of services. In addition, access to appropriately trained rehabilitation providers is needed. In many parts of the world, however, the capacity to provide rehabilitation is limited or nonexistent and fails to address the population's needs adequately.

Rehabilitation services are required at all levels of health systems (primary, secondary, and tertiary) and in the continuum of care throughout a person's recovery. It is also necessary to ensure that hospitals include specialized rehabilitation units for inpatients with complex needs, providing intensive, comprehensive, and highly specialized interventions for restoring functioning to patients with complex rehabilitation needs. A multi-disciplinary workforce in health systems ensures that the range of rehabilitation needs exists. Therefore, investment in the education, development, and maintenance of a multi-disciplinary rehabilitation workforce should be factored in health sector planning and budgets.

In 2017, WHO hosted the meeting, "Rehabilitation 2030: A Call for Action." The participants, worldwide rehabilitation professionals, highlighted the ever-increasing unmet need for rehabilitation trans-nationally and the importance of considering rehabilitation as a health strategy relevant to all people across the lifetime and the continuum of care.

4. What are the barriers?

Health systems must be structured to respond to the population's needs. In the past, the primary concerns were mortality and morbidity. Epidemiological trends, demographic shifts, an aging population, the predominance of non-communicable and chronic diseases, and expanded access to health care make disability a significant health issue and concern. Rehabilitation services are imperative for health systems in the 21st century. Rehabilitation is the solution, but health systems are not keeping pace with the rising non-communicable disease burden and associated population health needs.

Nonetheless, there are some misconceptions about rehabilitation. Rehabilitation is not only for people with long-term or physical impairments. Instead, it is a *core health service* for anyone with an acute or chronic health condition that limits functioning and should be available for anyone who needs it.

Rehabilitation is not an optional service to try only when other interventions designed to prevent or cure a health condition fail. Rehabilitation is not a luxury health service that is available only for those who can afford it. Like education, rehabilitation is not an expense but an *investment*. Rehabilitation can reduce care costs and enable participation in education and gainful employment.

Global rehabilitation needs continue to be unmet due to multiple factors, including:

- Lack of prioritization, funding, policies, and plans for rehabilitation at a national level.
- Lack of available rehabilitation services outside urban areas and long waiting times.
- High out-of-pocket expenses and nonexistent or inadequate means of funding.
- Lack of trained rehabilitation professionals.
- Lack of resources, including assistive technology, equipment, and consumables.
- The need for more research and data on rehabilitation.
- Ineffective and under-utilized referral pathways to rehabilitation.

5. What organizations are involved?

PM&R has different names in different regions of the world. For example, in many parts of the world, PM&R is known as Physical and Rehabilitation Medicine (PRM), which some believe enhances the specialty's cohesiveness. In other areas, it may just be known as rehabilitation medicine. The International Society of Physical and Rehabilitation Medicine (ISPRM) comprises 72 national PRM societies from 70 countries. Please see Table 85.1.

Table 85.1 ISPRM National Societies

COUNTRY[a]	NATIONAL SOCIETY
Algeria, People's Democratic Republic of	Algerian Society of Physical Medicine and Rehabilitation
Argentina, Republic of	Argentine Society of Physical Medicine and Rehabilitation Sociedad Argentina de Medicina Física y Rehabilitación
Australia, Commonwealth of	Rehabilitation Medicine Society of Australia and New Zealand
Austria, Republic of	Austrian Society for Physical Medicine and Rehabilitation Österreichische Gesellschaft für Physikalische Medizin und Rehabilitation
Bangladesh, People's Republic of	Bangladesh Association of PM&R
Belgium, Kingdom of	Royal Belgian Society of Physical Medicine and Rehabilitation
Bolivia, Plurinational State of	Bolivian Society of Physical Medicine and Rehabilitation Sociedad Boliviana de Medicina Fisica y Rehabilitacion
Brazil, Federative Republic of	Brazilian Association of Physical Medicine and Rehabilitation Associação Brasileira de Medicina Fisica e Reabilitação
Bulgaria, Republic of	Bulgarian Association of Physical Medicine and Rehabilitation
Canada	Canadian Association of Physical Medicine & Rehabilitation
Chile, Republic of	Chilean Society of Physical Medicine and Rehabilitation Sociedad Chilena de Medicina Física y Rehabilitación
China, People's Republic of	Chinese Association of Rehabilitation Medicine
China, People's Republic of	Chinese Society of Physical Medicine and Rehabilitation
Colombia, Republic of	Colombian Association of Physical Medicine and Rehabilitation Asociación Colombiana de Medicina Física y Rehabilitación
Congo, Democratic Republic of	National Council of Physicians and Rehabilitation of the Democratic Republic of Congo Conseil National de Medecins Physiques et de Readaptation
Costa Rica, Republic of	Asociación de Fisiatría de Costa Rica
Cuba, Republic of	Cuban Society of Physical Medicine and Rehabilitation Sociedad Cubana de Medicina Física y Rehabilitación
Cyprus	Cyprus Society of Physical Medicine and Rehabilitation
Czech Republic	Czech Society of Rehabilitation and Physical Medicine
Dominican Republic	Dominican Society of Physiatry Sociedad Dominicana de Fisiatria
Ecuador, Republic of	Ecuadorian Society of Physical Medicine and Rehabilitation Sociedad Ecuatoriana de Medicina Física y Rehabilitación
Egypt, Arab Republic of	Egyptian Society of Rheumatology and Rehabilitation
Finland	Finnish Society of Physical Medicine and Rehabilitation

Continued

Table 85.1 ISPRM National Societies—cont'd

COUNTRY[a]	NATIONAL SOCIETY
France, Republic of	French Society of Physical Medicine and Rehabilitation Société Française de Médecine Physique et de Réadaptation
Georgia	National Association of Medical Rehabilitation and Sports Medicine of Georgia
Germany, Federal Republic of	German Society of Physical Medicine and Rehabilitation Deutsche Gesellschaft für Physikalische Medizin und Rehabilitation
Greece (Hellenic Republic)	Greek Society of Physical Medicine and Rehabilitation
Guatemala, Republic of	Guatemalan Association of Physical Medicine and Rehabilitation Asociacion Guatemalteca de Medicina Física y Rehabilitación
Honduras, Republic of	Honduran Association of Physical Medicine and Rehabilitation Asociación Hondureña de Medicina Física y Rehabilitación
Hong Kong, Special Administrative Region of China	Hong Kong Association of Rehabilitation Medicine
India, Republic of	Indian Association of Physical Medicine & Rehabilitation
Indonesia, Republic of	Indonesian Society of Physical Medicine and Rehabilitation
Iran, Islamic Republic of	Iranian Society of Physical Medicine and Rehabilitation
Israel, State of	Israeli Association of Physical and Rehabilitation Medicine
Italy, Republic of	Italian Society of Physical Medicine and Rehabilitation Società Italiana di Medicina Fisica e Riabilitativa
Japan	Japanese Association of Rehabilitation Medicine
Jordan, Hashemite Kingdom of	Jordanian Society of Physical Medicine and Rehabilitation
Korea, Democratic People's Republic of	Medical Rehabilitation Committee of Hospitals Association of Korea
Korea, Republic of	Korean Academy of Rehabilitation Medicine
Kuwait, State of	Kuwait Society of Physical Medicine and Rehabilitation
Madagascar, Republic of	Association of Physical and Rehabilitation Medicine of Madagascar Association de Médecine Physique et de Réadaptation de Madagascar
Malaysia	Malaysian Association of Rehabilitation Physicians
Mexico (United Mexican States)	Sociedad Mexicana de Medicina Física y Rehabilitación
Mongolia	Mongolian Society of Physical and Rehabilitation Medicine
Morocco, Kingdom of	Morocco Society of PMR
Myanmar, Republic of the Union of	Myanmar Society of Rehabilitation Medicine
New Zealand	Australasian Faculty of Rehabilitation Medicine
Nicaragua	Asociación Nicaragüense de Medicina Física y Rehabilitación
Pakistan, Islamic Republic of	Pakistan Society of Physical and Rehabilitation Medicine
Panama, Republic of	Panamanian Society of Physical Medicine and Rehabilitation Sociedad Panameña de Medicina Física y Rehabilitación

Table 85.1 ISPRM National Societies—cont'd

COUNTRY[a]	NATIONAL SOCIETY
Paraguay	Paraguayan Society of Physical Medicine and Rehabilitation Sociedad Paraguaya de Medicina Física y Rehabilitación
Peru	Society of Rehabilitation Medicine of Peru Sociedad de Medicina de Rehabilitación del Perú
Philippines, Republic of the	Philippine Academy of Rehabilitation Medicine
Poland	Polish Rehabilitation Society Polskie Towarzystwo Rehabilitacji
Portugal, Republic of	Portuguese Society of Rehabilitation Medicine Sociedade Portuguesa de Medicina Física e de Reabilitação
Puerto Rico, Commonwealth of	Puerto Rico Society of Physical Medicine and Rehabilitation
Qatar, State of	Physical & Rehabilitation Medicine Physicians Club of Qatar
Romania	Romanian Society of Rehabilitation Medicine Societatea Romana de Reabilitare Medicala
Romania	Romanian Society of Physical and Rehabilitation Medicine & Balneoclimatology
Russian Federation	Russian Association of Regenerative Medicine and Medical Rehabilitation Specialists
Saudi Arabia	Saudi Arabian Society for Physical & Rehabilitation Medicine
Serbia, Republic of	Serbian Association for Physical Medical and Rehabilitation Udruženje za fizikalnu medicinu i rehabilitaciju Srbije
Singapore, Republic of	Society of Rehabilitation Medicine—Singapore
Slovenia	Slovenian Society of Physical & Rehabilitation Medicine
South Africa, Republic of	The South African Society of Physical and Rehabilitation Medicine
Spain	Spanish Society of Physical Medicine and Rehabilitation Sociedad Española de Rehabilitación y Medicina Física
Sudan, Republic of the	Sudanese Society for Physical and Rehabilitation Medicine
Sweden	Swedish Society of Rehabilitation Medicine
Swiss Confederation	Swiss Society of Physical Medicine and Rehabilitation Schweizerische Gesellschaft für Physikalische Medizin und Rehabilitation/ Société Suisse de Médecine Physique et Réadaptation
Syria	Syrian Society Association for Physical Medicine and Rehabilitation
Taiwan, Province of China	Taiwan Academy of Physical Medicine & Rehabilitation
Thailand, Kingdom of	Royal College of Physiatrists of Thailand
The Netherlands	Dutch Association of Rehabilitation Doctors Nederlandse Vereniging van Revalidatieartsen
Tunisia	Tunisian Society of Physical Medicine, Rehabilitation and Functional Rehabilitation Société Tunisienne de Médecine Physique, de Rééducation et de Réadaptation Fonctionelles

Continued

Table 85.1 ISPRM National Societies—cont'd	
COUNTRY[a]	**NATIONAL SOCIETY**
Turkey, Republic of	Turkish Society of Physical Medicine and Rehabilitation Türkiye Fiziksel Tıp ve Rehabilitasyon Derneği
UK, The Kingdom of Great Britain and Northern Ireland	British Society of Rehabilitation Medicine
Ukraine	Ukrainian Society of Physical and Rehabilitation Medicine
Uruguay, Oriental Republic of	Uruguayan Society of Physiatrists Sociedad Uruguaya de Medicos Fisiatras
USA, United States of America	Association of Academic Physiatrists
Venezuela	Venezuelan Society of Physical Medicine and Rehabilitation Sociedad Venezolana de Medicina Física y Rehabilitación
Vietnam, Socialist Republic of	The Vietnam Rehabilitation Association

[a]Country names are aligned to United Nations terminology.
ISPRM National Societies. Available at https://www.isprm.org/natsoc/. Accessed May 19, 2022.

6. Who should be involved?

The simple answer is that *you* should be involved! You can then help get others involved, because all of us in the PRM community should be engaged at some level with international PM&R.

As we have seen throughout history, a single person can make a world of difference. Unfortunately, with busy lives and professional obligations, we all have come across roadblocks to being involved with issues. Lack of knowledge about the issues, lack of time, lack of focus, and lack of comfort with the international healthcare advocacy process discourage many. The essential step is to decide to be involved.

Consider that a series of small successes at the national level can make the process of getting involved in international healthcare issues manageable and less overwhelming. One way is to connect with your national society. You can participate in activities on the national level, which is where many global healthcare issues stem from. Getting involved with national societies provides many opportunities to build alliances with other national societies. Building strong national societies is crucial to give the specialty a powerful and unified global voice on key health policy issues. When you are comfortable, consider joining an international society such as ISPRM.

7. What are ISPRM'S activities and goals?

ISPRM serves as the global agency for PRM and comprises over 70 national PRM societies. As a non-governmental organization (NGO) in relation to WHO and the UN, it is an international umbrella organization for PRM physicians and a catalyst for international PRM research. In addition, ISPRM has humanitarian or civil/societal, professional, and scientific mandates.

ISPRM. *Mission and goals.* Available at: https://www.isprm.org/discover/mission-goals.

8. What has been done so far?

Since its founding in 1999, ISPRM has been increasingly successful in achieving its mission, both within PRM and through its collaboration with WHO and the UN. With its emergence as the preeminent international scientific and educational society for practitioners in PRM and its evolving policy role, ISPRM has supported various WHO and UN initiatives. For example, ISPRM has contributed to WHO's *International Classification of Functioning, Disability, and Health* (2001), *World Report on Disability* (2011), *WHO Disability Action Plan* (2014 to 2021), and *Rehabilitation 2030–A Call for Action*, to name a few. In addition, ISPRM has supported the UN's *Sustainable Development Goals* (SDGs).

9. What is the UN? What are the 17 sustainable development goals? What is ISPRM'S involvement?

The United Nations is an international organization that seeks to maintain international peace and security, protect human rights, deliver humanitarian aid, and promote sustainable development. It was established in 1945, just after World War II, to prevent future wars and "promote social progress and better standards of life." It currently consists of 193 member states.

The SDGs are the blueprint for achieving a better and more sustainable future for everyone, everywhere, leaving no one behind. They address global issues that everyone faces, including poverty, inequality, environmental degradation, climate change, peace, and justice. The 17 goals are interconnected and were unanimously adopted by the UN General Assembly in 2015 with the goal of achieving them by 2030.

To support the implementation of the SDGs, ISPRM—through the UN Liaison Committee—has collaborated with the UN Secretariat for the Convention on the Rights of Persons with Disabilities as an NGO in support of the goals and the objectives of the UN Convention on the Rights of Persons with Disabilities (CRPD): the full and equal participation of persons with disabilities in all aspects of society and development. The mission is to support the UN on the SDG goals, particularly those related to disabilities, including *Good Health and Well-Being* (SDG3), *Quality Education* (SDG 4), *Decent Work and Economic Growth* (SDG 8), *Sustainable Cities and Communities* (SDG 11), and *Partnerships* (SDG 17) to optimize the abilities of persons with disabilities and ensure that no one is left behind toward an inclusive, accessible, and sustainable world.

In recognition of ISPRM's support of persons with disabilities and collaboration with the UN as partners in maximizing person's with disabilities potential, ISPRM was granted NGO with special consultation status with the UNCRPD in 2017 and United Nations Economic and Social Affairs in 2021.

UN. *Sustainable Development Goals.* Available at: https://www.un.org/sustainabledevelopment/sustainable-development-goals/

10. What is the World Health Organization (WHO), and how is international rehabilitation involved?

WHO is the lead agency for international health within the UN. Its goal is to achieve better health for all and expand universal health coverage. ISPRM is a non-State actor in official relations with WHO, can participate in WHO meetings, and make statements on agenda topics. WHO and ISPRM signed a collaboration agreement to strengthen rehabilitation worldwide and achieve the goals of "Rehabilitation 2030" and WHO's World Health Assembly resolution on improving access to assistive technology.

ISPRM-WHO-Liaison Committee. Available at: https://www.isprm.org/collaborate/who-isprm/

BIBLIOGRAPHY

Bickenbach J, Rubinelli S, Stucki G. Being a person with disabilities or experiencing disability: Two perspectives on the social response to disability. *J Rehabil Med.* 2017;49(7):543–549. doi:10.2340/16501977-2251

Bradley SM, Rumsfeld JS, Ho PM. Incorporating health status in routine care to improve health care value: The VA patient-reported health status assessment (PROST) system. *JAMA.* 2016;316(5):487–488. doi: 10.1001/jama.2016.6495

Cieza A, Causey K, Kamenov K, Hanson SW, Chatterji S, Vos T. Global estimates of the need for rehabilitation based on the Global Burden of Disease study 2019: a systematic analysis for the Global Burden of Disease Study 2019. Lancet. 2021 Dec 19;396(10267):2006-2017. doi: 10.1016/S0140-6736(20)32340-0. Epub 2020 Dec 1. Erratum in: Lancet. 2020 Dec 4;: PMID: 33275908; PMCID: PMC7811204.

DeLisa JA. What is the American physiatrist's role in the international physical medicine and rehabilitation organization? *Am J Phys Med Rehabil.* 2006;85(11):935–937. doi: 10.1097/01.phm.0000242743.02969.eb.

Florent V. Global health: Time for radical change? *Lancet.* 2020;396(10258):1129. doi: 10.1016/S0140-6736(20)32131-0

GBD 2019 Universal Health Coverage Collaborators. Measuring universal health coverage based on an index of effective coverage of health services in 204 countries and territories, 1990–2019: A systematic analysis for the Global Burden of Disease Study 2019.

ISPRM. Available at: www.isprm.org

Jimenez J, Peek W, Grabis M. *The International Society of Physical Medicine and Rehabilitation-Society History.* Available at https://www.isprm.org/discover/society-history/

Lancet. 2020;396(10258):1250–1284. Available at: https://www.thelancet.com/action/showPdf?pii=S0140-6736%2820%2930750-9

Melvin JL. How does globalization of the specialty of PM&R impact US physiatrists. *PM R.* 2009;1(3):205–207. doi:10.1016/j.pmrj.2008.11.009.

O'Young B, Young M, Stiens S, et al. International rehabilitation medicine: maximizing ability through global synergy and collaboration. In O'Young B, Young M, Stiens S, eds. *Physical Medicine and Rehabilitation Secrets.* 3rd ed. Philadelphia: Elsevier; 2008:699–703.

Stucki G, Bickenbach J, Melvin J. Strengthening rehabilitation in health systems worldwide by integrating information on functioning in national health information systems. *Am J Phys Med Rehabil.* 2017;96(9):677–681. doi: 10.1097/PHM.0000000000000688

United Nations Development Programme. *Sustainable development goals;* 2016. Available at: http://www.undp.org/content/undp/en/home/sustainable-development-goals.html

World Health Organization. *The Constitution of the World Health Organization.* Available at: https://www.who.int/about/governance/constitution

World Health Organization. *International Classification of Functioning, Disability, and Health. Geneva:* World Health Organization; 2001.

World Health Organization. *Decade of Healthy Ageing: The global strategy and action plan on ageing and health 2016–2020.* Available at: https://apps.who.int/gb/ebwha/pdf_files/WHA73/A73_INF2-en.pdf.

World Health Organization. *Rehabilitation: Key facts.* Available at: https://www.who.int/news-room/fact-sheets/detail/rehabilitation

World Health Organization & World Bank. *World report on disability.* Geneva: WHO; 2011.

World Health Organization. *Rehabilitation 2030: A call for action.* Available at: https://www.who.int/initiatives/rehabilitation-2030

WHO. *Rehabilitation 2030: A call for Action. Concept note.* Available at: https://cdn.who.int/media/docs/default-source/documents/health-topics/rehabilitation/call-for-action/conceptnoteen.pdf?sfvrsn=9c87be26_5

WHO. *Rehabilitation 2030: A call for action. The need to scale up rehabilitation.* Available at: https://www.who.int/initiatives/rehabilitation-2030

Bonus questions and answers are available online.

CHAPTER 86

EPILOGUE: THE PAST, PRESENT, AND FUTURE OF PHYSICAL MEDICINE AND REHABILITATION

Leonard S.W. Li, MBBS, FRCP FAFRM(RACP) FHKAM(Medicine) and
Sam S. H. Wu, MD, MA, MPH, MBA

The important thing is not to stop questioning. Curiosity has its own reason for existing. One cannot help but be in awe when one contemplates the mysteries of eternity, of life, of the marvelous structure of reality. It is enough if one tries merely to comprehend a little of this mystery every day.

— Albert Einstein (1879–1955)

This textbook that you are now holding in your hands represents the collective wisdom of physiatry practitioners worldwide. The essential physical medicine and rehabilitation (PM&R) topics preciously presented in this volume range from the anatomy of individuals, the diseases that affect them, the environment they live in, and the hopes and dreams they hold dear. To be true to the hallowed roots and traditions of our specialty, this book also covers important moments in the history of PM&R. From this solid foundation of the past and the present, this book aims to carry the reader to the future of the specialty.

THE PAST

The specialty of PM&R, also known as rehabilitation medicine or physical and rehabilitation medicine (PRM) in many parts of the world, has its origins in antiquity. Historians have indicated that in ancient civilizations such as Egypt, Greece, and China venerated practitioners of medicine such as Hesy-Ra, Hippocrates, and Hua Tuo have used various physical medicine modalities such as procedures (e.g., tooth extraction), heat, and exercises in the treatment of their infirmed patients. In the Middle Ages, Maimonides emphasized exercise along with a healthy diet as preventive medicine. During the Renaissance, Girolamo Mercuriale published "De Arte Gymnastica," which encouraged gymnastics to maintain and improve health.

Physiatry's modern beginnings reside in European facilities decades before the First World War. In 1897, a facility was established in Saint Petersburg to train men with physical disabilities to manufacture orthopedic devices. A decade later in 1908, a school was founded in Charleroi, Belgium, where those men maimed in industrial accidents were taught crafting skills to earn a living. The first school for injured veterans was created in Lyon, France, in December 1914, four months after the outbreak of the Great War. This school was thought to be the inspiration for other similar schools that followed.

In the aftermath of this Great War, the field of rehabilitation boomed due to the sense of urgency accompanying the 20 million wounded veterans returning home and the youthfulness of the field. A proliferation of orthopedic and career development facilities took place to return veterans to the active workforce. The Red Cross Institute for the Crippled and Disabled Men was founded in 1917 in New York City based on this concept. This institution currently exists as the Institute for Career Development (ICD). It has remained in New York City to help "people with barriers to employment to gain skills, enter the workforce and live happy, productive lives."

The development of PM&R was also hastened by the ravages of the poliomyelitis epidemics in the early 1900s. These frequent epidemics spread to developed countries and were rampant in cities. Franklin Delano Roosevelt (FDR), who contracted polio in 1921, was an avid proponent for rehabilitation and turned his property in Warm Spring, Georgia, into what most historians believed to be the first comprehensive rehabilitation facility.

In 1928, Dr. Frank H. Krusen founded the first department of PM&R at Temple University School of Medicine which is now the Lewis Katz School of Medicine. His research focused on helping his patients recover from illnesses such as back pain and postsurgical musculoskeletal complications using physical modalities (e.g., short wave diathermy, electrical stimulation, and ultraviolet radiation). He is also credited with coining the term "physiatrist." In 1941, Dr. Krusen published *Physical Medicine,* the first comprehensive physiatry textbook.

After this publication, the US government established the Army Air Forces Convalescent Training Program in 1942 and appointed Dr. Howard A. Rusk to direct comprehensive rehabilitative services, including physical, neuropsychological, and occupational therapies. After spending some time with the Red Cross Institute for the Crippled and Disabled Men in New York City, Dr. Rusk founded the world's first university-affiliated comprehensive rehabilitation center at New York University in 1951. This center was renamed the Howard A. Rusk Institute of Rehabilitation Medicine and continues to serve persons with disabilities to this day.

The tremendous growth of PM&R in the 1940s to 1960s was lifted by a combination of the peaking of the polio epidemics and the surge of World War II veterans with disabilities. Opportunities for successful vocational rehabilitation emerged. During this growth period, the American Board of Physical Medicine Rehabilitation (ABPMR) was established in 1947. The ABPMR is the world's first organization to certify physiatrists.

Over time, postgraduate medical education PM&R residency training opportunities continued to proliferate to meet the flourishing demand for physicians dedicated to serving the needs of persons with disability. The emergence and prodigious growth of academic training programs in major medical centers was soon to become a reality.

THE PRESENT

PM&R focuses on caring for persons with disabilities to help optimize their function and reduce their suffering both mentally and physically. This means that physiatrists practice physical medicine to diagnose and treat patients' musculoskeletal ailments, including pain, and practice rehabilitation for patients with permanent impairments from various organs to restore and optimize their functional abilities.

With advancement of medicine and technologies, current tools used in the process or collaborating with rehabilitation include ultrasound, electromyography, antispastic medications, implantable devices, fluoroscopic guided axial skeletal injections, team-based treatment algorithms, pharmacological agents, computer-aided gait analysis, gene therapy, and deep brain stimulation for Parkinson disease, and cognitive-behavioral treatments. Moreover, a team approach in collaborations with physical therapists, occupational therapists, and speech/language pathologists is the current frontline conservative treatment.

Exoskeletons, carbon fiber orthotics, microchip-embedded prosthetics, and infrared imaging diagnostic devices are making their way out of the research settings to the clinical settings.

Evidence-based practice in rehabilitation is further strengthened with the establishment of a division of Cochrane Rehabilitation within the Cochrane Library.

THE FUTURE

The future of PM&R depends on our ability to imagine a better world where everyone, meaning persons with and without disabilities, can live fulfilling and productive lives. However, like all those who came before us who not only imagine new ways to care for their patients but worked hard to discover those pathways, we must similarly also work hard to extrapolate from our current tools and find the new "killer apps" to create the infrastructure for that better world.

These so-called killer apps may be minimally invasive brain-computer interfaces, gene therapy for Parkinson disease and musculoskeletal ailments, nanobots for targeted drug delivery to ameliorate low back pain or tissue repair of rotator cuff tears, or portable nerve regeneration devices for polio survivors. What appears to be science fiction today could be the gold standard treatments for tomorrow. Your efforts may be that needed ingredient to transform these and other fantasies into reality.

The *PM&R Secrets,* 4th edition, showcases much of the current tools and practices that physiatrists around the world are using. Let this textbook help you to make the leap to land our specialty onto that higher future platform. The world is depending on you!

REFERENCES

Atanelov L, Stiens SA, Young MA. History of physical medicine and rehabilitation and its ethical dimensions. *AMA J Ethics.* 2015;17(6): 568–574. doi: 10.1001/journalofethics.2015.17.6.mhst1-1506.
Cochrane Rehabilitation at: https://rehabilitation.cochrane.org/
Girolamo Mercuriale. Available at: https://en.wikipedia.org/wiki/Girolamo_Mercuriale. Accessed on August 8, 2021.
Hesy-Ra. Available at: http://en.wikipedia.org/wiki/ Hesy-Ra. Accessed on August 8, 2021.
Hippocrates. Available at: http://en.wikipedia.org/wiki/Hippocrates. Accessed on August 8, 2021.
History of Polio. https://en.wikipedia.org/wiki/History_of_polio. Accessed on August 8, 2021.
Hua Tuo. Available at: http://en.wikipedia.org/wiki/Hua_Tuo. Accessed on August 8, 2021
ICD-Institute for Career Development. https://www.icdnyc.org/history. Accessed on August 8, 2021.
Krusen, Frank H. Available at: https://en.wikipedia.org/wiki/Frank_H._Krusen. Accessed on August 9, 2021.
Maimonides. Available at: https://en.wikipedia.org/wiki/Maimonides. Accessed on August 8, 2021.
The Red Cross Institute for Crippled and Disabled Men and the "Gospel of Rehabilitation". Available at: https://nyamcenterforhistory. org/2018/08/27/gospel-of-rehabilitation/. Accessed on August 8, 2021.
Wu SSH, Welch DG, Hoppe KM, Weinstein SM. Pathways to certifications in physical medicine and rehabilitation in the United States: past, present, and future. *Eur J Phys Rehabil Med.* 2013 Jun;49(3):385–393. PMID: 23276900.
Young MA, Siebens HC, Wainapel SF. A Tale of Two Cities: Evolution of Academic Physiatry in Boston and Baltimore. Part 2: From Flower Shop to Full Bloom in Baltimore. *PM&R.* 2020 Feb;12(2):202–210. doi: 10.1002/pmrj.12252. Epub 2019 Nov 25. PMID: 31593359.

Page numbers followed by *f* indicate figures, *t* indicate tables, and *b* indicate boxes.

A

Abdomen, acute, 411.e4
Abdominal binder, 411.e2
Abdominal blunt trauma, 296
Abdominal cramps, 411.e4
Abdominal CT, 239
Abdominal reflex, 75.e2
Abdominal x-ray, 239
Abducens nerve palsy, 438.e7t
Ableism, 44
Abnormal Involuntary Movement Scale (AIMS), 425
Abnormal pain processing, 543
Access-friendly kitchens, 58
Accreditation Council for Graduate Medical Education
    (ACGME) Program, 40
Acetaminophen
    as analgesics, 500
    for low back pain treatment, 372–373
Acetylcholine (Ach), 109, 109–111
Acetylcholinesterase inhibitors, 584
Acetylcysteine, 167
Achilles pain, 194
Achilles tendinitis, 194
Achilles tendinosis, 356
Ach receptor (AChR), 109
ACL. *See* Anterior cruciate ligament (ACL)
Acoustic measurements, 221
Acquired language disorder, 217–218
Acquired myopathies, 300, 300t
Acromioclavicular (AC) joint, 19, 327f, 327–329
    osteophytes, 330f, 330
    separation, 333, 333t
    shear test, 332f, 330
Acromioclavicular ligament, 329
Action observation therapy (AOT), 425
Action potential, 32
Action tremor, 420, 420t
Active compression test, 332f, 333f, 330
Active control systems, 121
Active listening, 46
Active range of motion (AROM), 72
Active trigger point, 522
Activities of daily living (ADLs), 47
Activity-based restorative therapy (ABRT), 144
Activity limitations, 116
Acupressure, 131
Acupuncture, 185, 472.e1–472.e2
    biological effects of, 188
    brain stimulated by, 188
    for chronic pain, 503.e2
    common problems, 187
    contraindications for, 186
    fascia and, 622.e31–622.e32
    as myofascial pain syndrome treatment, 527

Acupuncture *(Continued)*
    for pain management, 187
    placebo, 187
    points, 186
    practice of physiatrist, 189
    safe and risks, 186
    therapeutic effect of, 186
    treatment, 187
Acupuncturist, 188–189
Acute cell-mediated rejection, 493
Acute flaccid myelitis (AFM), 388
Acute flaccid paralysis, 90
Acute hypertension, 166
Acute illness, 585.e3
Acute inflammatory demyelinating polyradiculoneuropathy
    (AIDP), 103
Acute pain, 497
Acute quadriplegic myopathy (AQM), 108.e1
Acute rehabilitation phase, 594
Acute transient radiation myelopathy (ATRM), 471
Acute treatment, 8–9
Adaptive equipment, for Parkinson's disease patients,
    422–423
Adhesive capsulitis, 332, 332t
Adipose-derived stromal/stem cell (ADSC), 298
Adjuvant pain medications, 500
Adolescent idiopathic scoliosis, 568
Adult botulism, 114
Adult spinal deformity, 568
Adult stem cells, 181
Advanced glycosylation end products, 585.e2
Aerobic capacity, maximum, 448
Aerobic endurance exercise, 135f
Aerobic exercise
    diabetics and, 142
    for JIA, 578
    for spinal cord injury patients, 451
    for stroke patients, 450
Aerobic fitness, 140
Afferent sensory systems, 34
AFO. *See* Ankle foot orthosis (AFO)
Age
    critical milestones by, 555, 555t
    with disability, 585.e2
Aged population, current trends in, 580
Agent Orange, as neural tube defect cause, 558
Aging, 142
    definitions of healthy, 581t
    dementia treatment and, 584
    with disabilities, 585.e2, 585.e3
        cardiovascular disease, 585.e2
        diabetes, 585.e2
        factors to, 585.e2–585.e3
        implications of, 583